Biomechanics of Impact Injuries and Injury Tolerances of the Abdomen, Lumbar Spine, and Pelvis Complex

PT-47

Edited by
Stanley Backaitis

Published by:
Society of Automotive Engineers, Inc.
400 Commonwealth Drive
Warrendale, PA 15096-0001
U.S.A.
Phone: (412) 776-4841
Fax: (412) 776-5760

Copyright © 1995 Society of Automotive Engineers, Inc.

ISBN 1-56091-592-7

Library of Congress Catalog Card Number: 94-074713
All rights reserved. Printed in the United States of America.

Permission to photocopy for internal or personal use, or the internal or personal use of specific clients, is granted by SAE for libraries and other users registered with the Copyright Clearance Center (CCC), provided that the base fee of $5.00 per article is paid directly to CCC, 222 Rosewood Dr., Danvers, MA 01923. Special requests should be addressed to the SAE Publications Group.
ISBN 1-56091-592-7/95 $5.00

SAE Order No. PT-47

PREFACE

This publication, <u>Biomechanics of Impact Injury and Injury Tolerances of the Abdomen, Lumbar Spine, and Pelvis Complex</u> (PT-47) is the third of four books in the Progress in Technology series published by the SAE as a means of presenting to the reader the best selection of papers published on the subject. Available information on the subject is so vast and so varied in quality that a learned panel of experts in this field of knowledge from throughout the world was invited to review the papers and render judgement on their suitability for inclusion in this publication.

The content of this book was derived from a three stage evaluation process. The selection process was initiated by the SAE publications office by a search for relevant data in the SAE Global Mobility Database. The database includes papers published by the SAE, ESV (Experimental Safety Vehicles) and the European based IRCOBI conference proceedings. It was also recognized at the outset that there are many other outstanding technical papers of non-SAE origin, but their full text inclusion in this publication could not be realized because of proprietary rights or other restrictions. At best they could be cited in the book as suitable references. Upon receipt from the SAE of over 500 candidate papers, the editor made the first stage of selections by removing from the compiled list all of the marginal and/or irrelevant publications. This reduced the listing to over 180 papers for further consideration. The set was then transmitted to the panel of experts for the second review cycle. Several lists of relevant non-SAE publications were also included in this package. The reviewers were asked to determine their suitability for inclusion in this book as recommended references to relevant and important information. The panel was asked to observe the following guidelines when reviewing and scoring the papers during the selection process:

1. Long term reference value of the paper,
2. Contribution of the paper towards the development of scientific basis,
3. Soundness of experimental data,
4. Uniqueness of data reduction and interpretive techniques to explain injury mechanisms and/or to derive injury tolerances,
5. Uniqueness of experiments and/or technical procedures,
6. Experimental or analytical novelty towards explaining the injury,
7. Citation of the paper in subsequent publications by other authors.

They were asked to rate the papers by placing each of them into one of three categories:

1. Essential,
2. Desirable,
3. Marginal or irrelevant.

The reviewers were further instructed to focus their selections primarily on research work that could be related to the biomechanics of injury in automotive accidents. Paper selections were to include not only those based on direct biomechanical experiments, but also those based on accident simulations and reconstructions. The panelists were reminded that while the primary interest was in biomechanics and injuries resulting from occupant impacts in vehicle interiors, they have also to consider research related to pedestrians, motorcyclists, sports, and injuries resulting from falls, diving and semi-static or static loading exposures.

Upon receipt of the second round of selections from the panel, the editor compiled the ratings and based on the merits each paper received, established a list of 96 papers that were worthy for further consideration. The panel members were provided this list and asked to review and rate them again. The third review cycle was based on the same selection criteria as the second cycle, except that the reviewers were also asked to select those papers that would avoid duplication of the topic, assure that paper would fit in specific topic areas, and that they were indeed of superior quality and usefulness to the reader needing this information. The last review yielded a selection of 59 papers that were judged to be worthy of full text reprint and 33 papers for placement in the recommended reading list. The scoring process for the final selection of papers were established as follows: 2 points for essential, 1 point for desirable and 0 points for marginal. Inasmuch as the panel included 18 reviewers, the maximum number of points any paper could receive is 36. An arbitrary cut of 18 points was selected to admit a paper for full reprint, those that received 9 to 18 points were entered into the reprint of abstract only (recommended reading) category, and all others were placed into the recommended reading category. In addition, any paper scheduled for full reprint had to have at least 6 or more points in the essential category. The nominated entries were further reviewed to avoid repeating the same data in a parallel but different or later publication.

The contents of this book is divided for the reader's convenience into topical chapters covering 1) the anatomy and principles of biomechanics of abdomen, lumbar spine and pelvis; 2) biomechanics, impact response and trauma in frontal impacts; 3) biomechanics, impact response and trauma in lateral impacts; 4) biomechanical response of cadaveric spine in tension and compression; 5) biomechanical data and response of children; and 6) modeling, simulation and instrumentation. In quite a few instances, the subjects covered in various chapters are intertwined and therefore, some overlap between them is unavoidable.

The expert review panel was made up of the following individuals:

L. M. Patrick, Professor Emeritus
Wayne State Univ.
Hendersonville, NC

Professor Allan Nahum, M.D.
University of California San Diego
La Jolla, CA

Dr. Dominique Cesari
INRETS
Bron Cedex, Lyon, France

Annette L. Irwin, Ph.D.
General Motors Corp.
Warren, MI

Harold J. Mertz, Ph.D.
General Motors Corp.
Warren, MI

Professor Donald F. Huelke
University of Michigan
Ann Arbor, MI

Dr. J. M. Cavanaugh
Wayne State University
Detroit, MI

Dr. rer. nat. Dimitrios Kallieris
University of Heidelberg
Heidelberg, Germany

Frank A. Pintar, Ph.D.
University of Wisconsin
Milwaukee, WI

Professor Walter B. Pilkey
University of Virginia
Charlottesville, VA

Mr. Roger Saul, Ph.D. cand.
Vehicle Research Test Center, NHTSA
East Liberty, OH

Pria Prasad, Ph.D.
Ford Motor Co.
Dearborn, MI

Lawrence Schneider, Ph.D.
The University of Michigan
Ann Arbor, MI

Professor Raymond Neathery
Oklahoma State University
Stillwater, OK

Stephen W. Rouhana, Ph.D.
General Motors Corp.
Warren, MI

Anna-Lisa Osvalder, Ph.D.
Chalmers University of Technology
Goteburg, Sweden

Prof. Dr. Jac Wismans
TNO Crash-Safety Research Center
Delft, The Netherlands

Professor Barry Meyers
Duke University
Durham, NC

Professor Patrick J. Bishop
University of Waterloo
Waterloo, Ontario, Canada

Professor Murray McKay (first review only)
University of Birmingham
Birmingham, UK

The editor is grateful to all panel members for their cooperation, timely responses and constructive participation in the extremely time consuming review process. Their contribution is even more remarkable because all of the expert review work was performed on a voluntary basis and no one received any compensation. It attests dedication to their profession and also their deep commitment in the health and safety of the motoring public.

The final selection of papers for this publication reflects the consensus of the review panel. While the selection of any particular paper is by no means unanimous, it nevertheless reflects the best judgement of the majority. The editor is confident that these selections are the very best in the field and perhaps the most complete resource ever garnered on the subject matter. It is hoped that this publication will become the premiere source of the best and most reliable information for those in the need of this knowledge.

The editor is grateful to Mr. Barry Felrice, Associate Administrator, Rulemaking and Dr. Patricia Breslin, Director, Office of Vehicle Safety Standards, National Highway Safety Administration, for their support in carrying out this work. Sincere thanks for cooperation and assistance are due to a number of people who helped bring this publication to reality, particularly the SAE Publications staff in Warrendale, PA for their patience, enthusiastic assistance and support in collecting the fragmented materials into such an outstanding book.

Stanley H. Backaitis
Chairman, SAE Occupant Protection Committee

Table of Contents

Section 1: The Human Abdomen, Lumbar Spine, and Pelvis Complex

Synopsis of Anatomy and Medical Terminology (700195) 3
    D. Huelke

Thoracic and Abdominal Anatomy (700195) 15
    A. Burdi

Joint Range of Motion and Mobility of the Human Torso (710848) 33
    R. Snyder, D. Chaffin, R. Schutz

Biomechanics of the Spine and Pelvis (730413) 55
    A. King

Secton 2: Biomechanics, Impact Response and Trauma Assessed with Volunteers, Cadavers, Animal, and Mechanical Surrogates in Frontal Impacts

Impact Tolerance and Resulting Injury Patterns in the Baboon: Air Force Shoulder Harness—Lap Belt Restraint (720974) 71
    T. Clarke, D. Smedley, W. Muzzy, C. Gragg, R. Schmidt, E. Trout

Spinal Loads Resulting from $-G_x$ Acceleration (730977) 97
    P. Begeman, A. King, P. Prasad

Results of 49 Cadaver Tests Simulating Frontal Collision of Front Seat Passengers (741182) 115
    G. Schmidt, D. Kallieris, J. Barz, R. Mattern

Injury to Unembalmed Belted Cadavers in Simulated Collisions (751144) 125
    L. Patrick, R. Levine

Static Bending Response of the Human Lower Torso (751158) 163
    G. Nyquist, C. Murton

Lumbar and Pelvic Orientations of the Vehicle Seated Volunteer (760821) 193
    G. Nyquist, L. Patrick

Biomechanical Experiments with Animals on Abdominal Tolerance Levels (770931) 223
    E. Gögler, A. Best, H. Braess, H. Burst, G. Laschet

Dynamic Characteristics of the Human Spine During -G_x Acceleration (780889) 263
    N. Mital, R. Cheng, R. Levine, A. King

Biodynamics of the Living Human Spine During -G_x Impact Acceleration (791027) 289
    R. Cheng, N. Mital, R. Levine, A. King

Biodynamic Response of the Musculoskeletal System to Impact Acceleration (801312) 309
    P. Begeman, A. King, R. Levine, D. Viano

Submarining Injuries of 3 Pt. Belted Occupants in Frontal Collisions—Description, Mechanisms and Protection (821158) 325
    Y. Leung, C. Tarrière, D. Lestrelin, C. Got, F. Guillon, A. Patel, J. Hureau

Impact Response and Injury of the Pelvis (821160) 359
    G. Nusholtz, N. Alem, J. Melvin

Study of "Knee-Thigh-Hip" Protection Criterion (831629) 401
    Y. Leung, B. Hue, A. Fayon, C. Tarrière, H. Hamon, C. Got, A. Patel, J. Hureau

Mechanism of Abdominal Injury by Steering Wheel Loading (851724) 415
    J. Horsch, I. Lau, D. Viano, D. Andrzejak

Thoraco-Abdominal Response to Steering Wheel Impacts (851737) 425
    G. Nusholtz, P. Kaiker, D. Huelke, B. Suggitt

Interaction of Human Cadaver and Hybrid III Subjects with a Steering Assembly (872202) 473
    D. Schneider, A. Nahum, D. Dainty, J. Awad, S. Forrest, R. Morgan, R. Eppinger, J. Marcus

Assessing Submarining and Abdominal Injury Risk in the Hybrid III Family of Dummies (892440) 489
    S. Rouhana, D. Viano, E. Jedrzejczak, J. McCleary

Experimental Investigation of Rear Seat Submarining (896032) 513
    T. MacLaughlin, L. Sullivan, C. O'Connor

Steering Assembly Impacts Using Cadavers and Dummies (902316) 525
    P. Begeman, J. Kopacz, A. King

Intraabdominal Injuries Associated with Lap-Shoulder Belt Usage (930639) 547
    D. Huelke, G. Mackay, A. Morris

Visocelastic Shear Responses of the Cadaver and Hybrid III Lumbar Spine (942205) 557
    P. Begeman, H. Visarius, L. Nolte, P. Prasad

High Chest Accelerations in the Hybrid III Dummy Due to Interference in the Hip Joint (942224) 571
    E. Abramoski, K. Warmann, J. Feustel, S. Nilkar, N. Nagrant

Section 3: Biomechanics, Impact Response and Trauma Assessed with Volunteers, Cadavers, Animal, and Mechanical Surrogates in Lateral Impacts

The Pathology and Pathogenesis of Injuries Caused by Lateral Impact Accidents (680773) 585
    J. States, D. States

Side Impact Response and Injury (766064) 605
    J. Melvin, D. Robbins, R. Stalnaker

Synthesis of Human Tolerances Obtained from Lateral Impact Simulations (796033) 615
    C. Tarrière, G. Walfisch, A. Fayon, J. Rosey, C. Got, A. Patel, A. Delmas

Thoraco-Abdominal Response and Injury (801305) 631
    G. Nusholtz, J. Melvin, G. Mueller, J. MacKenzie, R. Burney

Evaluation of Pelvic Fracture Tolerance in Side Impact (801306) 657
    D. Césari, M. Ramet, P. Clair

Development of a Dummy Abdomen Capable of Injury Detection in Side Impacts (811019) 669
    J. Maltha, R. Stalnaker

Pelvic Tolerance and Protection Criteria in Side Impact (821159) 701
    D. Césari, M. Ramet

Tolerance of Human Pelvis to Fracture and Proposed Pelvic Protection Criterion to be Measured on Side Impact Dummies (826036) 711
    D. Césari, M. Ramet, R. Bouquet

Human Response to and Injury from Lateral Impact (831634) 721
    J. Marcus, R. Morgan, R. Eppinger, D. Kallieris, R. Mattern, G. Scmidt

Abdominal Trauma—Review, Response, and Criteria (851720) 735
    R. Stalnaker, M. Ulman

Synthesis of Pelvic Fracture Criteria for Lateral Impact Loading (856028) 751
    M. Haffner

Lower Abdominal Tolerance and Response (861878) 773
    J. Cavanaugh, G. Nyquist, S. Goldberg, A. King

The Effect of Limiting Impact Force on Abdominal Injury: A Preliminary Study (861879) 797
  S. Rouhana, S. Ridella, D. Viano

How and When Blunt Injury Occurs—Implications to Frontal and Side Impact Protection (881714) 813
  I. Lau, D. Viano

The Effect of Door Topography on Abdominal Injury in Lateral Impact (892433) 833
  S. Rouhana, C. Kroell

Comparison of EUROSID and Cadaver Responses in Side Impacts (896084) 843
  E. Janssen, J. Wismans, P. de Coo

Biomechanics of the Human Chest, Abdomen, and Pelvis in Lateral Impact (896113) 861
  D. Viano, I. Lau, C. Asbury, A. King, P. Begeman

Biomechanical Response and Injury Tolerance of the Pelvis in Twelve Sled Side Impacts (902305) 869
  J. Cavanaugh, T. Walilko, A. Malhotra, Y. Zhu, A. King

Regional Tolerance of the Shoulder, Thorax, Abdomen and Pelvis to Padding in Side Impact (930435) 881
  J. Cavanaugh, Y. Huang, Y. Zhu, A. King

Pelvic Biomechanical Response and Padding Benefits in Side Impact Based on a Cadaveric Test Series (933128) 889
  J. Zhu, J. Cavanaugh, A. King

Section 4: Biomechanical Response of Cadaveric Spine in Tension and Compression

Static and Dynamic Articular Facet Loads (760819) 903
  N. Hakim, A. King

Biomechanical Investigations of the Human Thoracolumbar Spine (881331) 935
  N. Yoganandan, F. Pintar, A. Sances, Jr., D. Maiman, J. Myklebust, G. Harris, G. Ray

Section 5: Biomechanical Data and Response of Children in Automotive Impact Environment

Airbag Effects on the Out-of-Position Child (720442) 947
  L. Patrick, G. Nyquist

Comparison Between Child Cadavers and Child Dummy by Using Child Restraint Systems in Simulated Collisions (760815) 957
    D. Kallieris, J. Barz, G. Schmidt, G. Heess, R. Mattern

Biomechanical Data of Children (801313) 987
    G. Stürtz

Responses of Animals Exposed to Deployment of Various Passenger Inflatable Restraint System Concepts for a Variety of Collision Severities and Animal Positions (826047) 1011
    H. Mertz, G. Driscoll, J. Lenox, G. Nyquist, D. Weber

Interpretations of the Impact Responses of a Three-Year-Old Child Dummy Relative to Child Injury Potential (826048) 1029
    H. Mertz, D. Weber

Section 6: Modeling, Simulation, and Instrumentation

A Biodynamic Model of the Human Spinal Column (760771) 1039
    S. Tennyson, A. King

Finite Element Simulation of the Occupant/Belt Interaction: Chest and Pelvis Deformation, Belt Sliding and Submarining (933108) 1053
    D. Song, P. Mack, C. Tarriere, F. Brun-Cassan, J. LeCoz, F. Levaste

Finite Element Modeling of Gross Motion of Human Cadavers in Side Impact (942207) 1075
    Y. Huang, A. King, J. Cavanaugh

Development of an Abdominal Deformation Measuring System for Hybrid III Dummy (942223) 1095
    S. Ishiyama, K. Tsukada, H. Nishigaki, Y. Ikeda, S. Sakuma, F. Matsuoka, Y. Kanno, S. Hayashi

Mathematical Modelling of the BioSID Dummy (942226) 1111
    M. Fountain, P. Altamore, J. Skarakis, O. Spiess

Simulation of the Hybrid III Dummy Response to Impact by Nonlinear Finite Element Analysis (942227) 1127
    T. Khalil, T. Lin

Recommended Reading 1147

Related Reading 1159

Section 1:
The Human Abdomen, Lumbar Spine, and Pelvis Complex

Synopsis of Anatomy and Medical Terminology

Donald F. Huelke
University of Michigan

THIS PAPER by no means represents a complete presentation of gross anatomy as would be given to medical students. It is merely intended to present some very elementary anatomical principles in a simplified form for the beginner or semiprofessional interested in automobile collision research and the production of occupant injury. Anatomical details and injuries in various body areas will be described in the other chapters. This paper includes, in Appendix A, reference books to which the reader may go for further information and more detailed study. Also listed in the appendix is a series of anatomical and medical related terms, many of which must become a part of the engineers' terminology so that communication with physicians and nurses will be enhanced, and medical records more understandable.

Anatomy is the study of human body structure. The field of anatomy is conveniently subdivided into gross anatomy and microscopic anatomy. A special area of study of the nervous system is called neuroanatomy. The study of the development of the human body before birth is called embryology. In each area are subdivisions which, for our purposes, need not be detailed.

In order for us to understand various body parts, a standardized orientation of the body—the anatomical position—is used. This is a standing individual facing forward with the palms of the hands outward (Fig. 1). From this orientation then, various directions can be more clearly related (Table 1). That portion of the body which is closer to the head or above another part is said to be cranial (or superior). Conversely that which is closer to the feet would be caudal (or inferior). The front of the body is referred to as the anterior or ventral side, and the back of the body then is the posterior or dorsal side. Especially in the limbs there are two other terms used to reference the relative position of one structure to another. A structure or part that is closer to the attachment of the limb to the torso, would be proximal; any part farther away from the root of the limb than some other structure is distal. For example, the shoulder joint is proximal to the elbow joint, and conversely the wrist is distal to the elbow. Thus, in hospital descriptions you may see, for example, that the distal end of the radius is fractured. The radius, one of the bones of the forearm, has a fracture that is closer to the wrist than to the upper end of the bone which is at the elbow joint. Similarly in the lower limb, the knee joint is proximal to the foot.

Table 1 - Positional and Descriptive Terminology

Anterior - or ventral - Toward the front of the body.
Posterior - or dorsal - Toward the back of the body.
Medial - Nearer the median plane than some other part.
Lateral - Toward the side, or farther from the median plane.
Internal - Deeper to some other part.
External - More superficial than some other part.
Superior - or Cranial - Toward the head, or closer to the head than some other structure.
Inferior - or caudal - Toward the tail, or farther from the head than some other structure.
Central - In the center of the body, or nearer the center than some other part.
Peripheral - The surface of the body, or farther from the center than some other part.
Proximal - Nearer the root of the limb than some other part.
Distal - Farther from the root of the limb than some other part.

ANATOMICAL TERMINOLOGY

The terms used in anatomy and medicine in general all have specific meanings and have been derived from Latin and Greek

Planes Of Direction

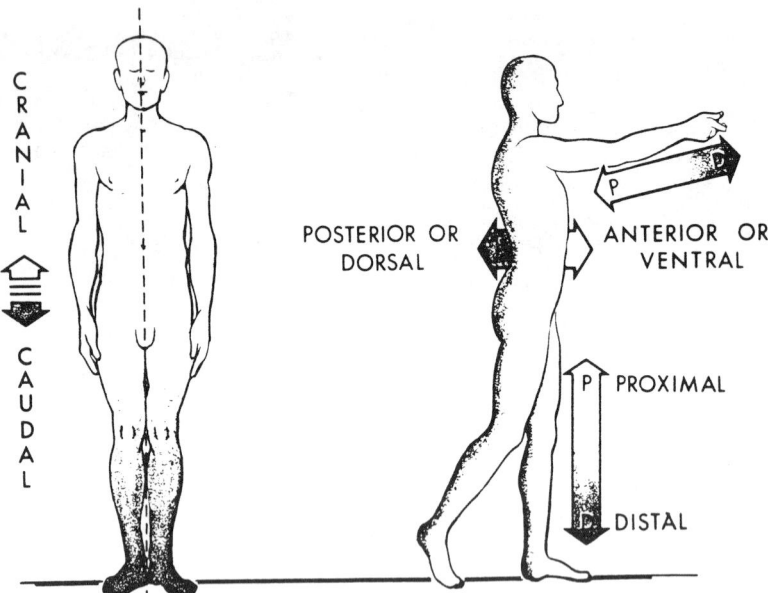

Fig. 1 - Planes of direction

origins. It is highly recommended that a medical dictionary be within arms reach of anyone learning this new terminology —the language of the healing arts. In addition, the dictionary will aid in the proper pronounciation of the word. Nothing is more annoying to a physician or health scientist than to hear medical or anatomical terms mispronounced! In Tables 1 and 2 are presented the beginnings of this new medical language.

Anatomical and medical terms are frequently formed from several subterms. The familiar "biceps brachii" muscle is in the arm—between the shoulder and elbow. Actually, its name tells one where it is located—brachii (the arm); the word biceps indicates a two (bi-) headed (-ceps) muscle. Thus, triceps brachii is the three-headed muscle in the arm. Arteries, for example, frequently take the name of the area in which they are located (brachial artery, facial artery, etc.) or their area of supply (coronary artery, gastric, splenic, femoral, etc.) Frequently, structures have even more descriptive names; the external abdominal oblique is that muscle of the abdominal wall which has fibers running obliquely and is the outermost muscle in the area. Its name also indicates that there must be an internal abdominal oblique muscle, for if there would be only one abdominal oblique muscle, that would be its name, for anatomists do not use more words than are necessary in naming body parts. One last example: the longest named muscle in the body is the levator labii superioris dilator alaequae nasi. This small muscle is found on the side of the nose. Its name tells one that it lifts (levator) the upper lip (labii superioris) and dilates the nose (dilator alaequae nasi). Thus anatomical terminology has a rational basis; but to understand and to use such terms, one must know the body regions and related structures which often form the basis for the name of a specific structure.

REGIONS OF THE BODY

The body is divisible into many parts and regions, but for ease in classification seven areas will be recognized: head, neck, thorax, abdomen, pelvis, upper and lower extremities. Specific subregions must also be studied for many of the structures in a specific area take on the name of the region in which they are found (Table 2).

The head is that area above the chin including the skull and surrounding soft tissue. Most importantly, the skull encloses the brain, and two separate subdivisions of the head are recognized—the face and cranium (Fig. 2). Many of the external environmental stimuli are received in the facial area; food and water are taken in through the mouth and air through the mouth or nose. The special sense organs for taste, smell, and vision are also found in the facial area. The cranium encloses the brain and the organs of hearing and equilibrium.

The neck region consists of the throat structures in front and the cervical portion of the vertebral column and associated muscle mass behind. On each side of the neck, covered by muscles, are the large vessels that traverse the neck to supply structures of the head and the brain. The lower extent of the neck is approximately at the level of the clavicles (collar bones).

The thorax can be considered as the area outlined by the ribs. Posteriorly, the ribs articulate with the vertebral column and, anteriorly, with the sternum (breast bone). Below, the thorax is closed by respiratory diaphragm, which forms the roof of the abdominal cavity. The thorax houses the lungs, heart, and great vessels, and the lower portion of the trachea (windpipe).

Extending from the diaphragm above, the abdominopelvic cavity is limited by the vertebral column posteriorly, the soft

Table 2 - Anatomical Terminology of Body Regions

Region	The Region of the:
Antibrachial	forearm
Axilla	armpit
Brachial	shoulder to elbow (arm)
Cervical	neck
Cubital	elbow
Epigastric	above the stomach
Femoral	thigh
Hypochondriac	under the rib cartilages
Hypogastric	below the stomach
Iliac (inguinal)	over the hips
Lumbar	small of back
Pectoral	anterior chest
Popliteal	back of knee
Thoracic	chest
Umbilical	navel

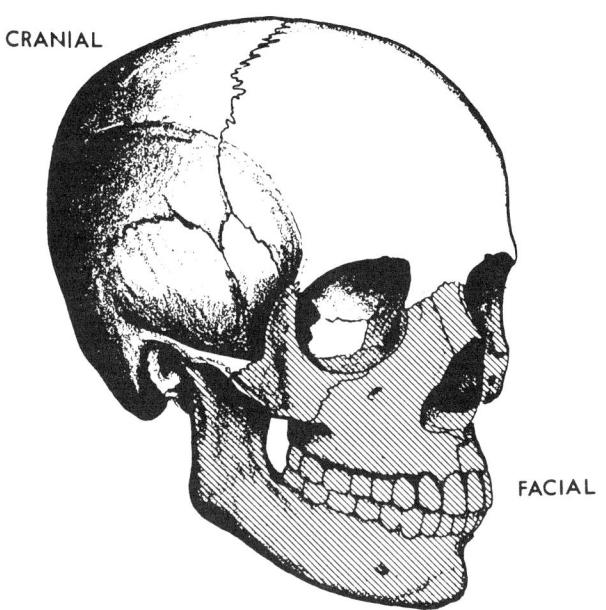

Fig. 2 - Units of the skull

flat abdominal muscles in front and to the sides, and below by the bony pelvis. A clear-cut division of abdomen and pelvis is not possible. However, the pelvic area can be considered that portion which contains the internal reproductive organs, and the lower portions of the gastrointestinal tract and the urinary system. Within the abdomen is the greater portion of the digestive tract—stomach, small intestines, colon—and its associated organs—liver, pancreas, gallbladder, etc.

The upper extremity includes the shoulder girdle, consisting of the scapula (shoulder blade) and clavicle (collar bone). Extending from these structures are the subregions of the upper extremity: the arm, forearm, wrist, and hand. Each area is interconnected by freely movable articulations (joints). Similarly, the lower extremity is attached to the pelvic girdle and is divided into the thigh, leg, ankle, and foot.

It is very important that correct terminology be used for these various named regions. Thus, the thigh is that area between the hip and knee joints; it is not the upper leg. The upper leg is that area just below the knee. Likewise, in the upper extremity the terms are "arm and forearm," not the "upper arm" and "lower arm."

THE SKELETON

The skeleton is the structural framework of the body. It consists of an internal set of bones which in the complete adult skeleton number 206. For convenience, the skeleton is divided into the axial and the appendicular skeletons. The axial skeleton consists of the skull, the hyoid (a small bone underneath the chin), the vertebral column, the ribs, and the sternum (breast bone) (Fig. 3). The appendicular skeleton is composed of the upper and lower limbs. Many of the bones of the skeleton—especially those of the upper and lower limbs—have a length greater than their breadth. These are the long bones of the body. Even though some of these bones may be quite short, such as those in the fingers and toes, they are still considered long bones for their length is greater than their breadth. On the other hand, short bones are those which are small cuboidal or rectangular in character; they are typified by the bones in the wrist and ankle. Flat bones are those of the skull which enclose the brain. In addition, the sternum (breast bone), the ribs, and the scapulae (shoulder blades) are also flat bones. Flat bones are characterized by having thin plates of compact bone separated by thin sponge-like bony spaces.

Long bones consist of three parts, a shaft, or diaphysis, and two ends, the epiphyses. Quite a few of the long bones have a smooth and more or less spherical end which is called the "head," beneath which there is generally a constriction called the "neck." The other end of some of the bones, as the humerus and femur, have smooth and rounded eminences called "condyles," while others, as the metacarpals (hand bones) and metatarsals (foot bones) have squarish rough ends called "bases."

Long bones are not solid, but have a cavity in the shaft which is called the "marrow cavity." The epiphyses are not hollow but are porous and spongy, and also contain marrow.

The shaft of long bones is hard and dense, and is called "compact bone," while the porous epiphyses of long bones, the bodies of vertebrae, and the inside of flat bones are made up of spongy bone.

In Table 3 is presented the distribution of the various bones in the body. It is strongly recommended that the parts of the major bones of the body be well learned.

The skull, in particular, is a unit of the body which is made up of 29 bones. Almost all of these bones are well joined together through immovable joints called "sutures." The only movable bone of the skull is the mandible (lower jaw). That

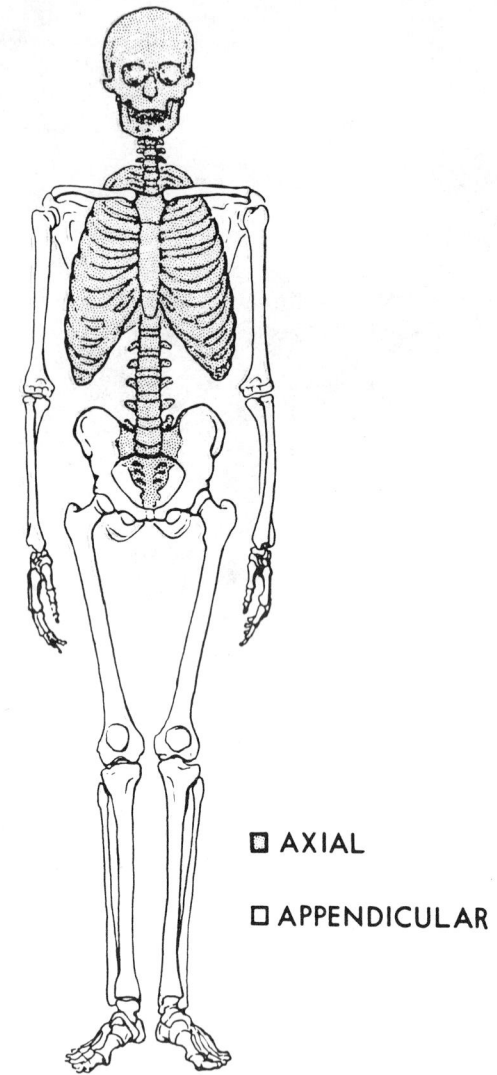

Fig. 3 - Axial and appendicular skeleton

Table 3 - The Number of Skeletal Elements

Skull		22
Cranium	8	
Face	14	
Ear bones		6
Hyoid		1
Thorax		25
Ribs	24	
Sternum	1	
Vertebral column		26 (in adult)
Upper extremities		64
Lower extremities		62
Total		206

part of the skull which encloses the brain is called the "cranium" and consists of eight individual flat bones. The face consists of 14 bones (Fig. 2). The jaw bones are those portions of the skull which support the teeth. The lower jaw is named the mandible and the upper jaw, the maxilla.

The names of the various portions of the extremities are important for knowledgeable conversation with those in the medical sciences. The shoulder girdle is that portion of the upper extremity which includes the scapula (shoulder blade) and clavicle (collar bone), (Fig. 3). These two interconnect at the shoulder joint with the bone of the arm, the humerus. The elbow joint is made up of the distal end of the humerus and the proximal ends of the radius and ulna. The area of the body between the elbow joint and wrist is the forearm. The wrist is a group of articulations (joints) between the forearm and the hand.

In the lower extremity the pelvic girdle articulates with the femur at the hip joint. The femur is the bone of the thigh; it joins with the leg at the knee joint. Within the leg are two bones—the larger one, the tibia, and the small thin bone on the outside called the fibula. These articulate with the foot bones through the ankle joint.

THE JOINTS

Wherever one bone joins with another, there always is a joint between the two; not always are these joints movable. Typically, movable joints are surrounded by ligaments which are strong and tough, but yet pliable; as a group they have very little elasticity to them. At the ends of the bones in a movable joint there is a covering of cartilage and within the enclosed joint space a bit of lubricant called synovial fluid. This allows for the smooth movement at the joint area. The joints are generally classified according to their degree of movement.

JOINT CLASSIFICATION BASED ON THE DEGREE OF MOVEMENT

I. NONMOVABLE (Synarthroses) - joints where no movement is possible—the sutures of the skull.

II. MODERATELY MOVABLE (Amphiarthroses) - joints where only slight movement is possible.

    A - Symphysis—symphysis pubis, sacroiliac joint, and the intervertebral joints.

    B - Syndesmosis—the distal tibiofibular joint, articulation between the shafts of the ulna and radius, coracoclavicular joint, etc.

III. FREELY MOVABLE (Diarthroses) - joints permitting free movement in various directions.

    A - Hinge—elbow (humerus-ulna), knee (femur-tibia), and the interphalangeal joints.

    B - Pivot—atlanto-axial and proximal radioulnar joints.

    C - Ball and socket—the shoulder and hip joints and the humeroradial articulation.

    D - Gliding—the joints of the vertebral column, intercarpal joints of the wrist, intertarsal joints of the ankle, sternoclavicular joint.

    E - Saddle—the joint between the greater multiangular and the first metacarpal bones.

F - Condyloid—metacarpophalangeal, metatarsophalangeal joints, etc.

G - Ellipsoidal—Temporamandibular and wrist joints.

A synarthrosis joint is one in which there is no movement possible typified by the sutures of the skull. An amphiarthrosis joint is one in which there is slight movement whereas a diarthrosis is a joint that has free movement.

The strength of a joint is determined by several factors: its bony structure, the ligaments that span the joint, the muscles and tendons that also cross over the joint, the tightness of fit between the articulating surfaces of the bones as well as the skin and connective tissue (fascia), muscles, and other soft-tissue structures.

All the joints of the body do not have the same degree of strength or stability. Some, as the hip joint, sacroiliac, and intervertebral joints, are fairly stable, while the shoulder, knee, and ankle joints are less stable and, as a result, are more easily injured. The strength and degree of movement of joints varies. In the shoulder joint, stability is sacrificed for movement, while in the hip joint or intervertebral joints, movement is sacrificed for stability.

THE MUSCLES

Myology is a study of muscles and their properties. Muscles form almost half of the body weight and, although they appear bulky and solid, they are approximately 75% water.

It is almost impossible to make a definite statement as to the exact number of muscles in any one human body. The reasons for this are: (1) Some individuals have extra muscles that do not usually occur. (2) Some muscles can be considered either as a separate muscle, or as a part of a larger muscle. (3) Some muscles may be absent on one or both sides of the body. It is safe to say, however, that there are over 600 main muscles in the average human body, 240 of which have different names. The difference in the two figures is due to the fact that many of the muscles occur in two or more pairs (Fig. 4).

Muscles vary in size, shape, weight, structure, and manner of attachment. Some muscles, as the latissimus dorsi, are large, while others, as the rotatores, are very small. Muscles in the forearm or the back of the thigh are long and narrow, while others between the ribs, the intercostal muscles, are short and wide; the gluteus maximus of the buttock is thick and heavy, the eyelid muscles are thin and delicate. There are muscles, such as the quadratus femoris, that are square in shape, others, as the pronator teres, are round, while still others are triangular, rhomboid, or trapezoid in shape. Muscles also vary in the direction they run; the rectus femoris runs vertically on the front of the thigh, the external abdominal oblique extends obliquely across the abdomen, and the transverse abdominus and muscles run horizontally.

The names of muscles are quite descriptive and are derived as follows:

1. *Action Produced* - Adduction (bringing toward the median plane), extension (decreasing the dorsal angle), supination (turning the palm upward, etc.

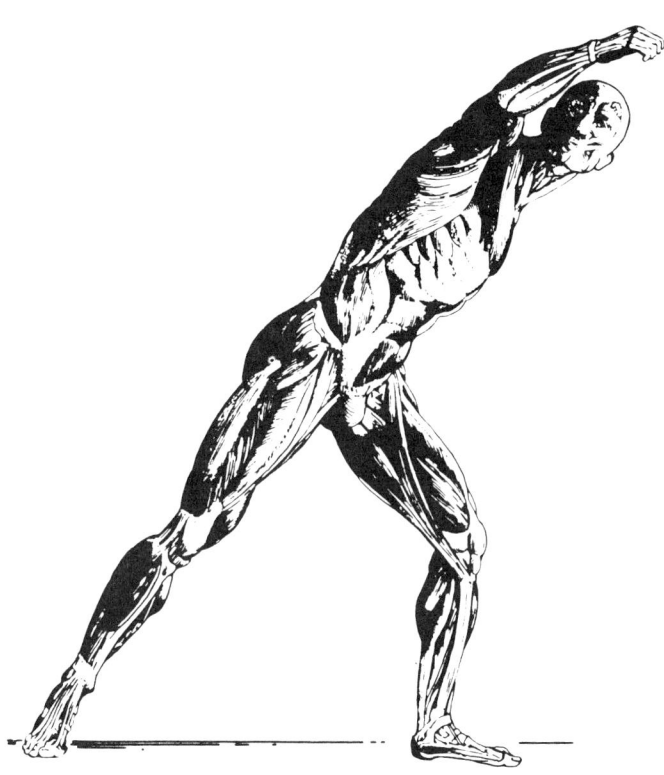

Fig. 4 - Superficial muscles of the body

2. *Attachment* - Omohyoid (shoulder to hyoid bone), Sternocleidomastoid (sternum-clavicle-mastoid process).

3. *Direction* - Oblique (at an angle), rectus (straight), transversus (horizontal).

4. *Location* - Brachii (arm), pectoralis (chest), spinatus (spine), tibialis (tibia).

5. *Relative Size* - Major (large), medius (intermediate), minor (small), minimus (smallest).

6. *Shape* - Serratus (saw-toothed), teres (round), trapezius (trapezoid).

7. *Structure* - Biceps (two heads), diagastric (two bellies), quadriceps (four heads), triceps (three heads).

8. *Combinations of the Above* - It is usually by the combination of two or more of the above terms that muscles are named: biceps brachii, gluteus maximus, pectoralis major, flexor carpi ulnaris.

Muscles may produce one or several of the following actions:

Abductors pull skeletal elements away from the median line, as in spreading the legs apart.

Adductors pull skeletal elements toward the median plane, as holding the arm against the body.

Extensors decrease the dorsal angle between skeletal elements, as in straightening the elbow when pointing. Extension of the arm is represented by the backward movement of the arm in bowling or pitching a softball.

Flexors increase the dorsal angle between skeletal elements (except knee) as pulling the forearm toward the arm (bending the elbow).

Rotators revolve a skeletal element around a long axis, as

Table 4 - The Nervous System

Central Nervous System	Peripheral Nervous System
Brain	Cranial nerves - 12 pairs
Cerebrum	Spinal nerves - 31 pairs
Brain stem	Autonomic nervous system
Spinal cord	Parasympathetic
	Cranial part
	Sacral part
	Sympathetic
	Thoracic part
	Lumbar part

turning the arm around an axis running the length of the humerus with the forearm extended.

Lateral rotation of the arm or thigh occurs when the thumb or great toe is turned away from the median line.

Medial rotation of the arm or thigh occurs when the thumb or great toe is turned toward the median plane.

Circumduction is the movement of the arm or thigh in the shape of a cone, as in throwing the arm around in a circle. Sometimes a pitcher's windup approaches circumduction. It is a sequential combination of the above actions.

Pronators turn the palm of the hand downward when the arm is flexed.

Supinators turn the palm of the hand upward when the arm is flexed.

THE NERVOUS SYSTEM

The muscles are powerless to produce movement without some mechanism to stimulate them into action. This control mechanism is supported by the nervous system which supplies individual fibers to all muscles, as well as to the skin, viscera, and joints.

The general function of the nervous system is to bring about an integration of the body (Fig. 5). Not only does the nervous system provide the means by which muscles are controlled and made to respond either at will or automatically, but it controls the action of all organs of the body, thus causing them to act in a coordinated manner. It is by means of nervous connections between our eyes, ears, nose, and skin and our muscles that we are aware of our surroundings and are able to respond in an intelligent manner to external stimuli. All motor nerves going to skeletal muscle are connected directly or indirectly with the motor area of the cerebral cortex, and as a result, are under its control (Table 4).

The nervous system is analogous to our lighting or telephone systems in which a predominating control system exists. The cerebrum represents the main exchange, whereas the large cables leading away from the central exchange are represented by the spinal cord. The wires going to the various parts of the city are represented by the spinal nerves, and the wires to the factories or homes or office buildings are represented by individual nerve fibers going to various muscles, organs, and other tissues.

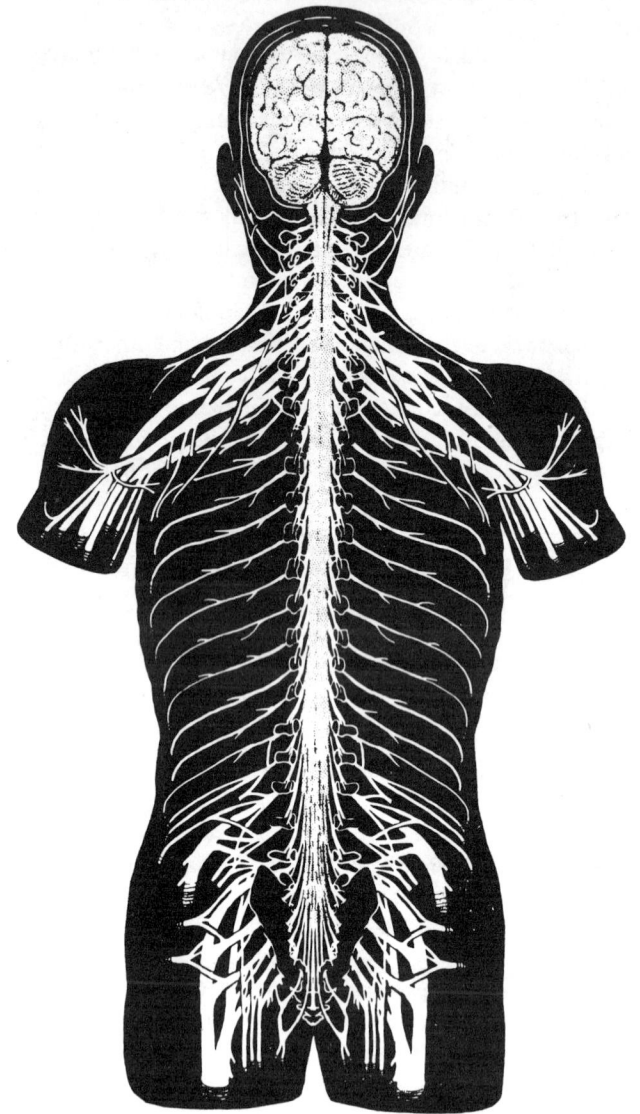

Fig. 5 - General plan of the nervous system

In the telephone system there are subexchanges that make connections independently of the main exchange, so in the nervous system there are subexchanges that make connections with other nerves without the impulse going to the cortex. These subexchanges, or connecting places, are distributed throughout the brain stem, cord, and in the body ganglia between the spinal cord and viscera, and in the walls of the viscera themselves. A connection place in the central nervous system (CNS) is called a nucleus and is defined as a group of nerve cell bodies and connections inside the central nervous system. A ganglion is defined as a group of nerve cell bodies and its connections outside the central nervous system. Impulses making connections in subexchanges without going to the cortex bring about reflex action, that is, an action produced without cerebral involvement.

There are three kinds of nerves—afferent, efferent, and

mixed. The afferent or sensory nerves are those which conduct nerve impulses from the periphery (for example, the skin, the eyes, the nose, etc.) to the central nervous system (the spinal cord or brain). Efferent nerves are those which conduct impulses from the central nervous system to the periphery (glands and muscles). The efferent nerves that conduct nerve impulses to the voluntary muscles are motor nerves. Those nerves which conduct nerve impulses to the visceral muscles, glands, and the heart belong to the autonomic nervous system. The mixed nerves are composed of both afferent and efferent fibers and hence conduct nerve impulses either to or from the central nervous system. Of the 12 pairs of cranial nerves, some are afferent, some are efferent, and some are mixed. The 31 pairs of spinal nerves are all mixed (motor and sensory) nerves.

In certain regions of the body—neck, shoulder, pelvic—the spinal nerves join together after they leave the vertebral canal to form nerve plexuses. A nerve plexus is defined as an intermingling and redistribution of nerve fibers.

THE CIRCULATORY SYSTEM

This closed transportation system consists of a pump (the heart), an aeration unit (the lungs), arteries to transport blood to all parts of the body, and veins for the return of the blood with the metabolic waste products to the heart. Interconnecting the arteries and veins are meshworks of very small vessels called capillaries. It is through the capillary walls that food and other substances pass into the tissue spaces.

The heart is a four-chambered reservoir pump; it can also be thought of as being two individual pumps joined together. Blood from all parts of the body enters the right reservoir (the right atrium; passing through valves blood enters the pump chamber (right ventricle) which upon contraction forces the blood into the artery (pulmonary artery) leading to the lungs. Returning to the left side of the heart via the pulmonary vein the blood enters the left atrium, passes into the left ventricle, and then is pumped out through the aorta (Fig. 6).

The aorta is the largest artery of the body; from it arteries branch to all structures except the lungs. Each artery of the body is named, usually according to the area that it supplies. The splenic, uterine, ovarian, and femoral arteries are typical examples.

Veins return blood to the heart. Receiving blood from the capillaries, small veins (venules) join together to form larger veins. Always at least one or two veins accompany each artery.

THE SKIN

The skin is the largest organ of the body. It has many functions, most of which are protective. It not only protects the deeper structures against mechanical injury and bacterial invasion but prevents loss of body fluids, protects the body from harmful sun rays via skin pigments, and acts as an excretory organ via perspiration.

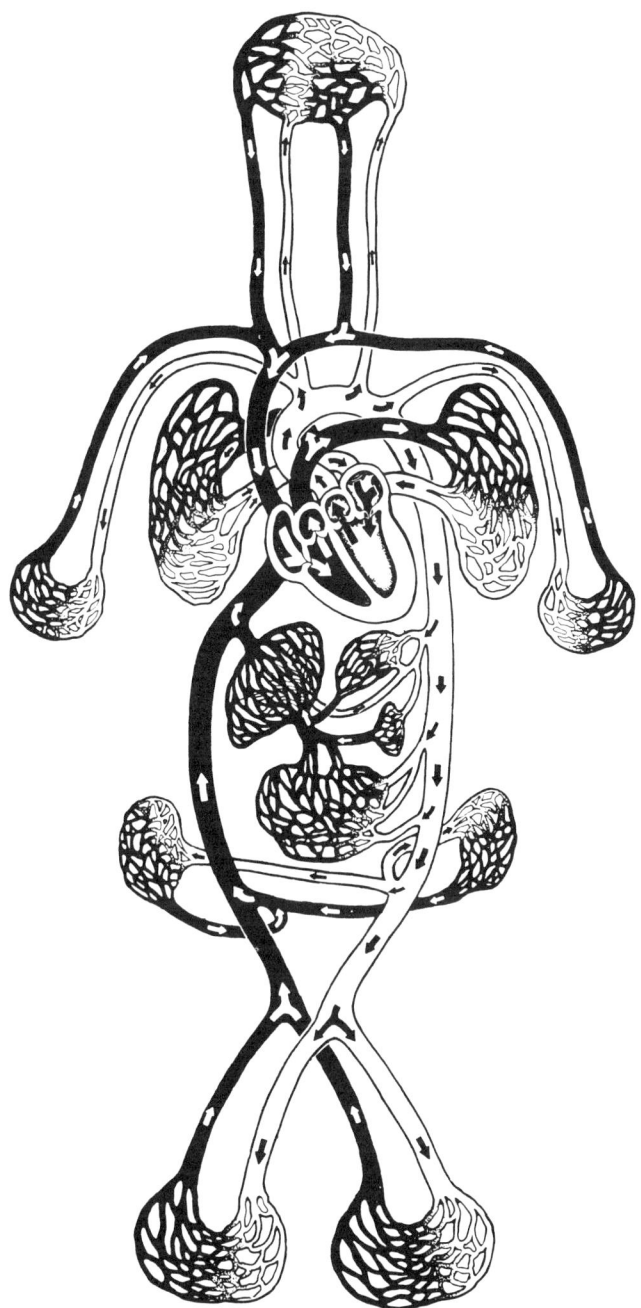

Fig. 6 - Generalized plan of the circulatory system

The skin is the most frequently injured organ of the body; however, fortunately, almost all mechanical injuries to the skin typically found in motor vehicle crashes are not life-threatening.

Some of the more common skin injuries are:

1. Abrasion - a scrape
2. Amputation - cutting off of a limb or other part
3. Avulsion - tearing away of a part or structure
4. Contusion - a bruise; produced without laceration
5. Laceration - a cut
6. Rupture - forceful tearing or breaking of a part

9

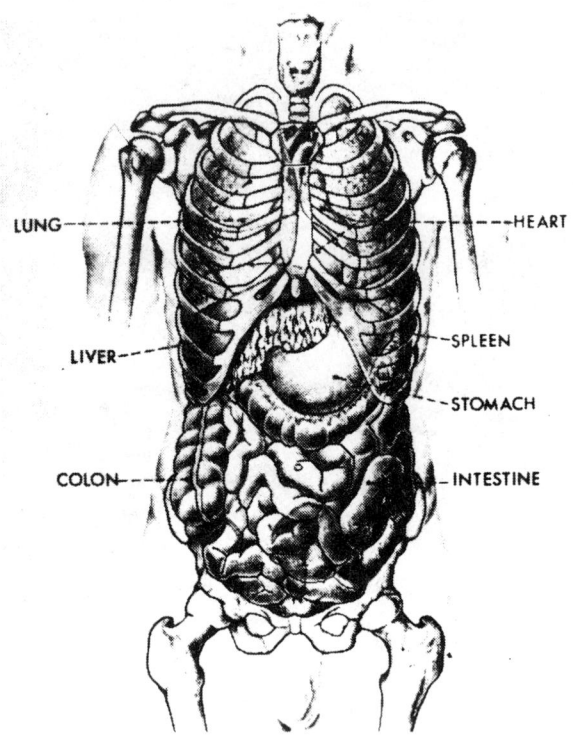

Fig. 7 - Thoracic and abdominal viscera

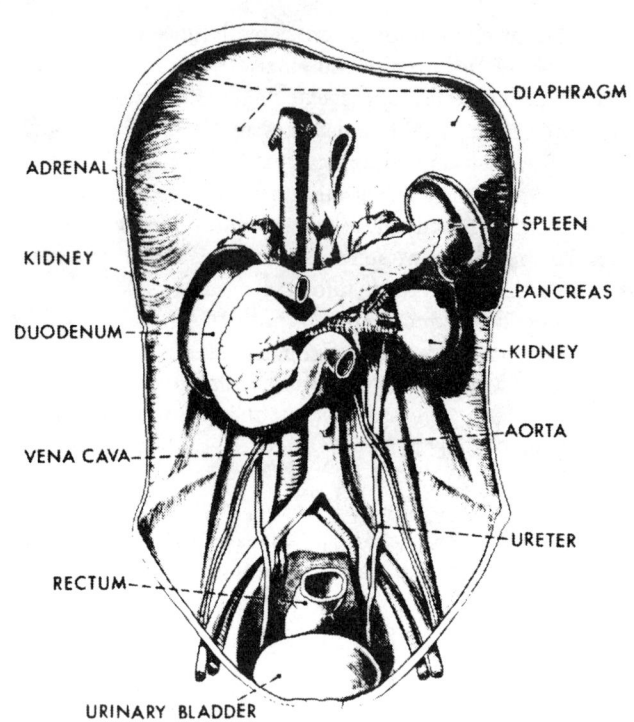

Fig. 8 - Deep abdominal viscera

THE THORAX

The thorax or chest is bounded by the thoracic portion of vertebral column posteriorly, the ribs, and in front of the sternum. Below, the respiratory diaphragm separates the thorax from the abdominal cavity. The diaphragm is dome-shaped, with its margins attached to the lower ribs. The dome of the diaphragm varies in position during respiration extending as high as the level of the nipples in forced expiration. Between the ribs are muscles and blood vessels. These intercostal arteries and veins course along with the ribs.

The thorax can be divided into three compartments—the right and left pleural (chest) cavities and the mediastinum. The mediastinum is a partition; it is a group of structures—the trachea, heart, aorta, large veins, esophagus—that together form a central partition separating the right from the left chest cavity (Fig. 7).

THE ABDOMEN AND PELVIS

For our discussion the abdomen and pelvis will be considered together. Bounded above by the diaphragm, the lumbar portion of the vertebral column posteriorly and the flat abdominal muscles on the sides and in front, and the bony pelvis below, the abdomen and pelvis contain the digestive, urinary, and reproductive systems.

The viscera found in the abdominal cavity are:

Stomach	Small intestine	Spleen
Liver	Large intestine	Adrenals
Gallbladder	Sigmoid colon	Kidneys
Pancreas	Rectum	Ureters

Urinary bladder	Vas deferens	Inferior vena cava
In the Male:	Seminal vesicles	Portal vein
Uterus	Prostate gland	Nerves
Vagina	In the Female:	Nerve plexuses
Abdominal aorta and	Ovaries	
its branches	Uterine tubes	

Because of the lack of adequate protection by bones, the abdominal contents are highly susceptible to blunt trauma. Abdominal organs are either thin-walled (stomach, intestines, etc.) or are spongelike and blood-filled (liver, spleen, kidney). In addition, numerous blood vessels are found in the abdomen for the supply of these organs (Fig. 8).

Thus, blunt impact to the abdomen can cause rupture of the stomach or intestines which release their contents into the abdominal cavity. Bacterial contamination thus can occur (peritonitis). Also, massive bleeding can occur if the blood-filled liver or spleen is ruptured, or if major arteries are damaged. Surgical repair of blunt abdominal injuries is almost always indicated.

The liver is one of the most frequently injured organs of the abdomen. It is about one-fortieth of the total body weight and occupies the upper right area of the abdomen. It is attached to the undersurface of the right side of the diaphragm and usually does not extend below the rib margins. Thus, although the liver is an abdominal organ, it is under the cover of the lower ribs on the right side. Hence, it is not unusual to have a blunt impact to the thorax which produces a liver injury.

Abdominal injuries can be produced by the unrestrained occupants of the car impacting the steering wheel, instrument panel, door panel, or the front seat back. Also, seat belts, when worn improperly, can cause injuries to viscera by direct pressure on the soft abdominal wall.

Within the bony pelvis are located the lower end of the gastrointestinal tract, the urinary bladder, and the uterus in the female. Also, numerous blood vessels and nerves, not only for the supply of pelvic structures but also for the lower extremities, are found here. The urinary bladder and uterus (especially the pregnant uterus) can be sheared off from its attachments by blunt, low abdominal impacts. Fractures of the bony pelvis can injure the organs or blood vessels within. The forces of walking are transmitted through the bony pelvis; thus, a pelvic fracture will be incapacitating and debilitating.

ANATOMICAL PROBLEMS ASSOCIATED WITH AGE

The infant and small child have specific anatomical characteristics which are unique to them. The skulls of these children are relatively thin bones not affording the impact protection as found in the adult. The sutures only incompletely join the skull bones together. Deciduous teeth (baby teeth) may not yet have erupted and the permanent teeth are yet forming in the jaws. Thus, jaw fractures can have a marked effect upon future tooth eruption and proper tooth alignment.

The soft tissue and bones of children heal rapidly, for they are in the growing stages. Not infrequently scars of soft tissue can hardly be found some years later because of tissue repair and growth.

Infants and children live in an adult world of automobile design. Thus, the child requires special and unique considerations for impact protection. Because they are smaller, they frequently will not contact areas in the car that have been designed for adult impact-force amelioration.

The bones of children and early teenagers are not completely formed. In infants the bones are small with cartilage separating the epiphysis from the diaphysis. This is the growth center of the bones and if disrupted can produce growth disturbances in terms of bone length, normal joint arrangements, and possibly in limiting the range of motion at a joint.

The bones of children are highly elastic and the greenstick fracture just above the wrist is a characteristic fracture of children. The bony thorax is no exception. Infants have highly elastic ribs. The space for the mediastinal structures is very small. Thus, chest impacts could easily deform the chest wall, and the heart and great vessels, producing fatal injuries with minimal forces.

In children the liver is massive in relation to the size of the other abdominal organs. Therefore, it is very susceptible to blunt impacts. The potbelly abdomen and the narrow space between the abdominal wall and the front of the thigh in the sitting position makes restraining children with a lap belt very difficult.

In children the head is large and sits on a thin neck which has muscles of minimal strength. Thus, neck injuries from violent head movements can be expected.

The elderly have similar and also different problems from those of children. Whereas bones of children are elastic and incompletely formed, older people have fully formed brittle bones. Thus, rib and long bone fractures are not uncommon in the elderly as well as the potential internal organ injuries associated with blunt impact. The elderly, as a group, heal much more slowly; bones take longer to unite, joints longer to repair, and soft tissue more time to heal. Also, long-term immobilization can cause problems of blood clots, pneumonia, and other complications. Many of the elderly have medical problems which when associated with impact trauma can unite to produce a serious if not fatal outcome. Problems in blood clotting, the body reflexes to prevent or minimize shock, etc., may play a significant role in the final outcome.

APPENDIX A

Selected References

Listed below are suggested references in ascending order of difficulty. Those marked with an asterisk (*) are strongly recommended for those unacquainted with anatomy and medical terminology.

1. Beginning Texts:

   *"The Question and Answer Book About the Human Body," Ann McGovern, New York; Random House, 1965.

   *"The How and Why Wonderbook of the Human Body," Martin Keen, New York; Wonderbooks, 1961.

   *"The Wonders of the Human Body," Martin Keen, New York; Grosset and Dunlap, 1966.

   "Textbook of Anatomy and Physiology," C. P. Anthony, C. V. Mosby Co., Seventh edition, 1967.

   Data-Guides, Human Anatomy Reference Charts, Data-Guide, Inc., Flushing, New York.

   Elementary Human Anatomy - Andrew J. Berger, John Wiley & Sons, Inc., 1964.

   Introduction to Human Anatomy - Carl C. Francis, C. V. Mosby Co., Fourth edition, 1964.

   Human Anatomy and Physiology - B. G. King and M. J. Showers, W. B. Saunders Co., Fifth edition, 1966.

2. Advanced Texts:

   Essentials of Human Anatomy - R. T. Woodburne, Oxford University Press, Fourth edition, 1969.

   Anatomy of the Human Body - H. Gray, Lea & Febiger, edited by C. M. Goss, Twenty-seventh edition, 1959.

   Anatomy of the Human Body - R. D. Lockhart, et al, J. B. Lippincott Co., 1959.

   Outline of Human Anatomy - Saul Wischinitzer, McGraw-Hill Book Co., Blakiston Division, 1963.

3. Gross Anatomy Atlases:

   Illustrations of Regional Anatomy - E. B. Jamieson, The Williams & Wilkins Co., Eighth edition, 1959.

   An Atlas of Anatomy - J. C. B. Grant, The Williams & Wilkins Co., Fifth edition, 1962.

4. Medical Dictionaries:

   Dorland's Medical Dictionary - W. B. Saunders Co., Twenty-fourth edition, 1965.

   Blakiston's New Gould Medical Dictionary - The Blakiston Co., First edition, 1949.

   Stedman's Medical Dictionary - The Williams & Wilkins Co., Twenty-first edition, 1966.

APPENDIX B

A SELECTED GLOSSARY OF ANATOMICAL TERMINOLOGY

A- (G prefix, without).

Ab- (L prefix, away from).

Acetabulum (L, a vinegar cup). A large cup-shaped cavity in which the head of the femur fits.

Acromion (G, *akros*, top; *omos*, shoulder). A projection on the scapula forming the point of the shoulder.

Ad- (L prefix, toward, upon).

Afferent (L, *ad*, to; *fero*, bear or bring). To bring to—a sensory nerve that carries impulses to the central nervous system.

Alveolar (L, a little cavity).

Ankylosis (G, *ankylos*, bent). To make a joint immobile.

Aorta (G, *aorte*, to lift). Large blood vessel leading from the left ventricle of the heart.

Atlas (G, *tlao*, to bear). First cervical vertebra.

Atrium (L, a court). One of the chambers of the heart; an expanded place.

Atrophy (L, not; to nourish). A deficiency or reduction in the size of a structure.

Auricle (L, *auricula*, a little ear). An earlike projection of the atrium of the heart.

Axilla, axillary (L, *axilla*, a little axis). Refers to the armpit.

Biceps (L, *bi*, two; *caput*, head). A two-headed muscle.

Brachial (L, *brachium*, arm). Refers to the arm, or any arm-like process.

Bronchus (G, *bronchos*, windpipe). A division of the trachea.

Carpal (L, *carpalis*, wrist). Refers to the wrist, as the carpal bones.

Caudal (L, *cauda*, tail). Refers to the tail.

Cephalic (G, *kepnale*, head). Refers to the head.

Cerebellum (L, a little brain). A division of the brain, lying inferior to the cerebrum, and posterior to the brain stem.

Cervical (L, *cervix*, neck). Refers to the neck region.

Circulation (L, *circulo*, to form a circle). To flow in a circle. The flow of blood through its blood vessels through the body.

Clavicle (L, clavis, key). The key-like bone of the shoulder girdle.

Colon (G, *kolon*, member). The portion of the large intestine between the cecum and the rectum.

Costal (L, *costa*, rib). Refers to the ribs.

Cutaneous (L, *cutis*, skin). Refers to the skin.

Deltoid (L, *deltoides,* triangular). A triangular-shaped muscle of the shoulder.

Diaphragm (G, *dia*, between; *phragnymi*, to enclose). A membrane that closes a cavity, or separates two cavities, as the respiratory diaphragm.

Dura mater (L, hard mother). The thick outermost meningeal layer around the brain and cord.

Efferent (L, effero, to bear away from). Carrying a fluid or nerve impulse away from a certain part; as efferent nerves which carry impulses away from the cord.

Eip- (G prefix, upon).

Epidermis (G, *epi*, upon; *derma*, skin). Outermost layer of the skin.

Epiphysis (G, an outgrowth). The terminal ends of long bones.

Esophagus (G, to carry; to eat). The upper part of the alimentary tract, extending from the pharynx to the stomach.

Ex- (L prefix, out, outside).

Fibula (L, *fibula*, clasp, buckle). Lateral and smaller of the two bones of the leg.

Gastric (L, *gaster*, stomach). Refers to the stomach.

Gluteus (G, *gloutos*, rump). Refers to the buttocks.

Ileum (G, *eilo*, twist). Refers to the distal two-thirds of the small intestine.

Infra (L prefix, below).

Inguinal (L, *inguen*, groin). Refers to region of the groin.

Intestine (L, *intestinus*, inside or internal). The part of the digestive tract extending from the stomach to the anus.

Jejunum (L, dry or empty). That portion of the digestive tract extending between the duodenum and the ileum.

Jugular (L, *jugulum*, the collar bone or throat). Refers to veins in the neck, draining the head.

Manubrium (L, handle). Superior part of the sternum.

Maxilla (L, *maxilla*, jaw bone). The upper jaw bone.

Membrane (L, *membrum*, member). A thin layer of tissue which covers or lines an organ or surface, or divides a space or organ.

Mesentery (G, *mesos*, middle; *enteron*, gut). Fold of peritoneum which attaches the intestine to the posterior abdominnal wall.

Met-, meta- (L or G prefix, between, after, reversely).

Metacarpal (G, *meta*, after; *karpos*, wrist). Refers to bones between the wrist and fingers.

Metatarsal (G, *meta*, after; *tarsos*, a flat surface of the foot). Refers to bones of the foot between the tarsal bones and the toes.

Occipital (L, *occiput*, back of the head). Pertaining to the back of the head, as the occipital bone.

Omo- (G prefix, *omos*, shoulder). Shows some relation to the shoulder.

Oral (L, *os*, mouth). Refers to the mouth as the oral cavity.

Orbital (L, *orbita*, orbit). Pertains to the orbit or eye socket.

Ossification (L, os, ossis, bone; facio, to manufacture). The conversion of any substance into bone.

Pectoral (L, *pectoralis*, chest). Refers to the breast or chest.

Pericardium (L, around; heart). Membranous sac around the heart.

Peritoneum (G, *peri*, around; teino, stretch). A serous membrane that lines the abdominal walls and invests the organs contained therein.

Peritonitis (G, *peri*, around; *teino*, stretch, inflammation). Inflammation of the peritoneum.

Pharynx (G, *pharynx*, throat). Proximal end of the digestive tract into which the oral and nasal cavities empty.

Pia mater (L, tender mother). Innermost layer of the meninges around the brain.

Pleura (G, *pleura*, rib, side). The serous membrane that lines the thoracic cavity and invests the lungs.

Plexus (L, braid or interweaving). Refers to a network or interweaving of nerves and veins.

Portal (L, *porta*, gate). A hilum through which vessels and nerves enter a gland or organ. In the circulatory system refers to a vein entering the porta of the liver.

Pre- (L prefix, before).

Pro- (L or G prefix, before).

Pulmonary (L, *pulmon*, lung). Refers to the lungs.

Renal (L, *renes,* kidneys). Pertains to the kidneys.

Retro- (L prefix, back, backward).

Serratus (L, *serra*, saw). A saw-toothed muscle of the shoulder girdle.

Sternum (G, *sternon*, breast bone). The bone of the axial skeleton to which the costal cartilages of the true ribs attach.

Sub- (L prefix, under).

Supine (L, *supino*, to put on the back). The position a person is in when lying on the back.

Supra- (L prefix, above).

Tendon (L, *tendo*, to stretch). A fibrous cord coming from muscles.

Tissue (L, *texo*, to weave). An aggregation of similar cells united in the performance of a particular function. Examples: muscle tissue, lung tissue, etc.

Trachea (G, *trachys*, rough). The part of the air passage leading from the larynx to the bronchii.

Triceps,(L, *tri*, three; *caput*, head). A three-headed muscle.

Umbilical (L, *umbilicus,* navel). Refers to the umbilicus or navel.

Ventricle (L, *venter*, belly). A cavity, especially in the heart and brain.

700195

Thoracic and Abdominal Anatomy

Alphonse R. Burdi
University of Michigan

IN GENERAL, THE WALLS of the body cavities are constructed to meet the demands of the contained organs. For example, the brain, not varying in size, is housed in and protected by a rigid bony box (the skull). The heart and lungs expand and contract in their functions and are housed in a cage (the thorax). The thoracic wall is composed of bone, cartilage, and muscle. Still more flexibility is required by the abdominal organs; they are housed in a rather flexible cavity whose walls are chiefly muscular.

The bony cage of the thorax (Fig. 1) consists of 12 thoracic vertebrae behind, the 12 pairs of ribs at the sides, and the breast bone (the sternum) in front. All ribs are connected to the vertebrae via joints, but some ribs do not have anterior connections. The upper seven ribs (true ribs) terminate as cartilage bars that attach to the sternum. "False ribs" (ribs 8-10) also have cartilaginous ends; they attach to the cartilage of the rib above each of them, thus forming the lower margin of the thorax. The eleventh and twelfth ribs remain unattached at their anterior ends, although they are in a matrix of soft tissue. These latter two ribs are "floating ribs." Rib size increases in length from the first to the seventh ribs, thereby increasing the girth of the chest. The ribs move relatively freely at their vertebral attachments in order to allow the chest to expand and contract in size during respiration.

Although chest girth fluctuates with activity, girth changes with age—an observation that has bioengineering significance. At birth the chest is circular in cross section. As the infant grows, the transverse dimension becomes larger than the anteroposterior dimension, giving the cross-sectional shape of the chest an elliptical appearance. At birth, the chest circumference is about 1/2 in. smaller than the head. At 1 year, the chest is equal to or exceeds head circumference slightly; after 1 year, the chest becomes progressively larger than the head. Thus, with the fairly marked change in shape of the infant's chest from that of a circular one to an elliptical one, a problem arises in adequate restraint of the upper torso of the child by the use of restraint belts (straps) which would not fit tightly to the chest wall.

Muscles of the thorax are concerned with forming a protective cage for the thoracic organs. These muscles actually fill in the spaces between successive ribs, thus making the cage a completely enclosed one. However, this is not a rigid cage for it must be alternately expanded and contracted to draw air into the lungs and to force it out again. Thus, muscles of the thoracic wall are also muscles of respiration. They include three muscular sheaths (or layers) arranged in such a way that fibers of each layer run perpendicular to the others. The two outer layers consist of the external intercostal (intercostal = between ribs) and the internal intercostal muscles. Blood vessels also run between the intercostal muscles, near the lower borders of each rib. They are an important source of bleeding if ribs are fractured. Because of its compressibility, the thoracic wall provides varying protection for the vital thoracic organs. The degree of protection, however, varies with age. Thoracic injuries in young children submitted to blunt impacts usually occur to the chest organs due to the smaller size of the child's thorax and the plasticity of the cage. Thoracic walls are thinner and the ribs more elastic in infants and children than in the adult. Therefore, impact to the thorax of an infant or small child will produce larger amounts of chest wall deflection (compression) onto vital thoracic organs, (for example), the heart, lungs, and blood vessels. The highly elastic nature of the young chest wall does have advantages however. As clinicians well know, closed cardiac massage in infants can be performed by using only one or two fingers. The resistance of the chest wall increases with age; the ribs become more bony and thus less elastic and their soft-tissue matrix thickens. However, in the elderly the ribs become more brittle and less resistant to blunt trauma.

LUNGS AND LOWER RESPIRATORY PASSAGES - With each breath, the human body takes in oxygen and discharges carbon dioxide by means of breathing or external respiration. This process consists of inspiration (to take air into the lungs) and expiration (to expel air from the lungs). Inspired air passes through the nasal chambers, pharynx, larynx, trachea, the right and left bronchi, and, finally, the air sacs of the lungs. The red blood cells, coursing through the lungs, take in, by diffusion, oxygen from the air and discharge carbon dioxide into it. Expired carbon dioxide returns to the outside via the same passageways.

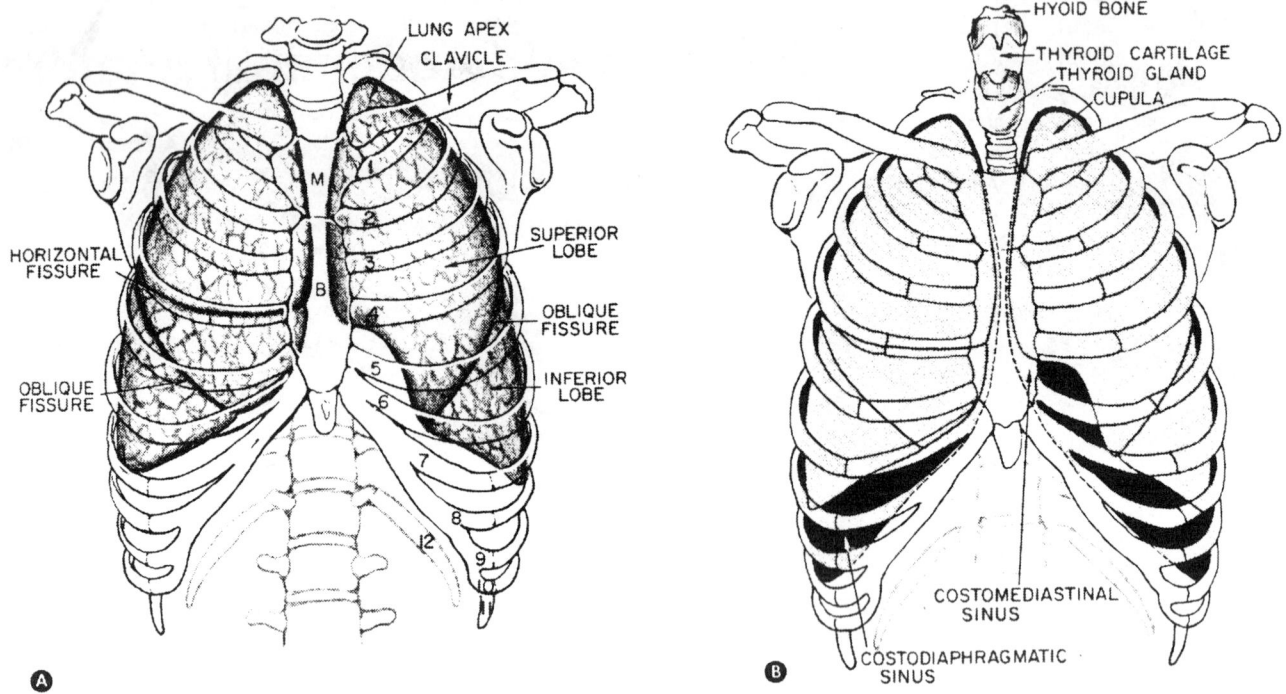

Fig. 1 - Surface projection of the thoracic cage, lungs (A) pleural and pleural sacs (B)

Air is not drawn into the lungs by the mere force of inspiration alone; instead, the diaphragm (which is actually a great, dome-shaped muscle separating the chest from the abdominal cavity) and the chest muscles contract (Fig.2). When the diaphragm contracts, it moves downward (flattens); the ribs move upward and outward, through muscular contractions, increasing the size of the chest cavity. In this manner a partial vacuum is created in which the air pressure in the lungs is also increased. Air flows to areas in which the pressure is below atmospheric level; consequently, this pressure gradient causes an influx of outside air into the lungs. In expiration, the diaphragm and chest muscles relax so that the chest wall returns to its original position prior to inspiration, the intrathoracic pressure increases, and air is expelled from the thorax. Expiration can be, and usually is, modified by a number of muscles which act on the rib cage. Since the air passes over the vocal cords, the cords act as a valve to protect the deep air passages from foreign objects and, secondly, the cords vibrate and produce functional speech sounds.

The consumption of oxygen within individual cells constitutes internal respiration. In the cells of the body, circulatory blood rich in oxygen gives off oxygen (O_2) and replaces it with carbon dioxide (CO_2). Oxygen in the cells combines with other substances which are repeatedly broken down so that only CO_2 and water remain. This chemical exchange (oxidation) releases energy to the cells for use in bodily activities. Some tissues, such as muscles and glands, which use a great deal of energy, especially in strenuous exercise, discharge more carbon dioxide and require large amounts of oxygen. (Oxygen itself cannot be stored in the body but must constantly be replenished through the mechanism of blood circulation.)

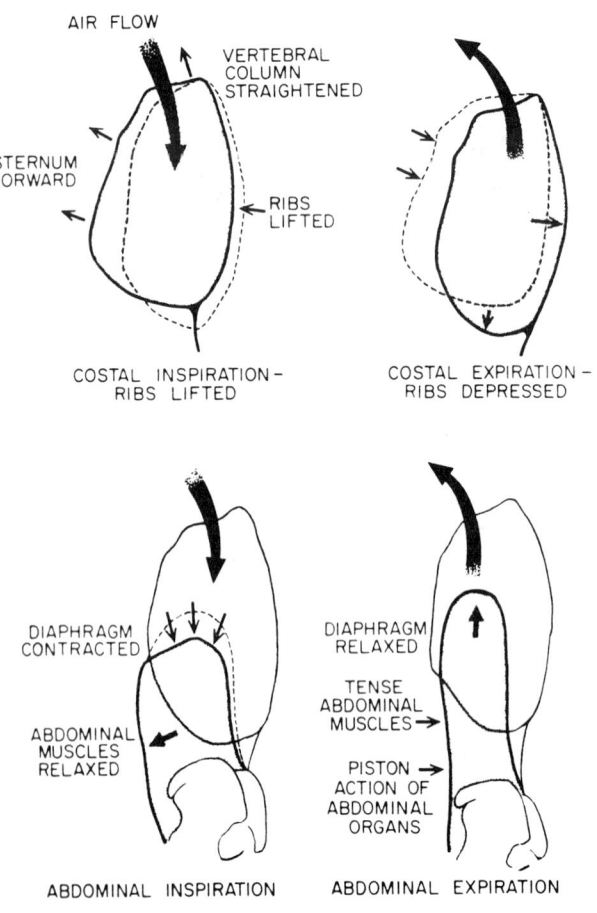

Fig. 2 - Pattern of trunk muscle actions and pressures during costal (above) and abdominal (below) respiration

In this discussion of respiration, as it is a part of thoracic anatomy, it is important to review the larynx and follow its continuity with the respiratory passages of the lungs. The nose and throat have been considered elsewhere.

The "voice box," or larynx, is the tubular channel connecting the throat (pharynx) with the trachea. It consists of nine cartilage plates embedded in a sheet of elastic membrane. The triangular thyroid cartilage or "Adam's apple" consists of two prominent, broad plates on the anterior surface of the throat. The epiglottis, another of the nine cartilages, forms a lid over the opening of the larynx to prevent the entrance of food or water into the respiratory passages. Within the walls of the larynx are found a pair of true vocal folds (vocal cords) which are involved in sound production.

The trachea, or windpipe, is a tubular structure which extends from the larynx (at the level of the sixth cervical vertebra) into the chest cavity, where it divides into two main tubular branches (the primary bronchi). The division of the trachea occurs at the fifth thoracic vertebra. The trachea is lined by a mucous membrane and is supported by 16-20 C-shaped cartilage rings. The open part of each C-shaped ring is directed posteriorly; it is closed off by membranous tissue and is immediately in front of the esophagus.

Functionally the trachea constitutes the main passageway through which air from the nasal chambers, throat, and larynx flows on its route to the bronchi and lungs. Obstructions often lodge in the trachea and may impede the normal flow of air, sometimes to such an extent that a tracheotomy (an operation to open the trachea) becomes necessary to prevent asphyxiation.

The branches into which the trachea divides are the two primary bronchi (singular = bronchus). The right bronchus, about 1 in. long, is wider than the left and lies almost in a straight line with the trachea. The left bronchus is longer, narrower, and is more horizontally oriented. Consequently, foreign objects are more prone to lodge in the right bronchus. Bronchi have walls supported by numerous cartilage rings and are lined by mucous membranes with microscopic hairlike endings which beat rhythmically to lend direction to the air.

Immediately after entering the lungs, each primary bronchus divides into smaller (secondary) bronchi, with two in the left lung and three in the right. These secondary bronchi continue to subdivide into smaller and smaller bronchi within the lung tissue. With decreasing diameter of each subdivision, cartilage support of the tubes disappears, leaving only the membranous air tubes or bronchioles. Again, the bronchioles repeatedly divide until their branches reach into the microscopic ducts (alveolar ducts) leading into the air sacs (alveolar sacs) whose walls have numerous rounded projections, that is, the alveoli. It has been estimated that the lungs contain 600 million alveoli which have a surface area of 600 sq ft. The lining of the bronchioles provides an easy exchange of gases between the air and numerous surrounding blood capillaries.

In respiratory diseases, such as pneumonia, the air spaces of the respiratory tree may close because of inflamed alveoli which then produce mucous secretions that further occlude the spaces. Infection or inflammation of the bronchi may cause bronchitis (-itis = inflammation) or other diseases marked by inflammation, chronic coughing, and congestion.

The two lungs are cone-shaped, spongy, elastic, and are the chief organs of respiration. Each lung fills a substantial portion of the chest cavity. The portion of the chest cavity between the right and left lungs is the mediastinum, or a partition formed by organs, for example, heart, great vessels, and connected tissues.

The left lung is narrow, longer, and smaller than the right. It is divided into two lobes (upper and lower), thereas the right lung is divided into three lobes (upper, middle, and lower). After arising from the trachea, the two primary bronchi enter each lung through a regional passageway (the hilum), on the medial lung surface. Also passing through this hilum are the pulmonary blood vessels. At this point, each lung appears to be suspended in the chest cavity by bronchi, blood vessels, lymph vessels, and nerves.

The pointed top (apex) of the lung rises to a level just above the first rib and sternum. Its lower surface (base) rests on the diaphragm. Within each lung are millions of air sacs (alveoli), along with alveolar ducts, bronchioles, and bronchi. The lungs lie in a double-layered, mucous membrane-lined sac (the pleura). The clearest way to describe the lung coverings is to recall the situation when a clenched fist is pushed into an inflated balloon (Fig. 3). One wall of the balloon intimately adheres to the fist and it is separated from the other wall by a space. Similarly, the embryonic lung invades a sac, and one sac layer covers the lung (visceral pleura) while the other lines the inner chest cavity (parietal pleura). A mucus-like fluid lubricates the two pleural layers and fills the interspace so that the lungs may move without friction during respiration. Pathologically, when there is no mucous interface, the lung may adhere to the chest wall (adhesions) and can be partially immobilized. Other serious disorders may affect the pleura. If air enters the pleural cavity as a result of penetrating injury or disease, the lungs will collapse since they no longer can be inflated. In some cases of lung disease, treatment may include the actual injection of air into the pleural cavity in order to collapse the lung for the purpose of resting it temporarily. Based on the concept that the lung is composed of functionally and structurally independent units (bronchopulmonary segments), improved surgical methods have made it possible to remove only the diseased or damaged portions of the lung.

MEDIASTINUM - The mediastinum is, strictly speaking, the septum between the two lungs, but the name is in general use for the space or compartment between the two pleural sacs. It extends from the sternum in front to the thoracic vertebrae behind, and from the thoracic opening above to the diaphragm below. It is divided, for descriptive purposes, into superior and inferior compartments, and the latter is further divided into anterior, middle, and posterior compartments. Specifically, the superior mediastinum contains such structures as the trachea (lower end), esophagus, aorta, and some of its major branches, the superior vena cava and its tributaries, nerves, and lymphatic vessels. The anterior mediastinum is the compartment between the two pleural sacs just behind the sternum. Its contents are chiefly fat and the remnants of the thymus

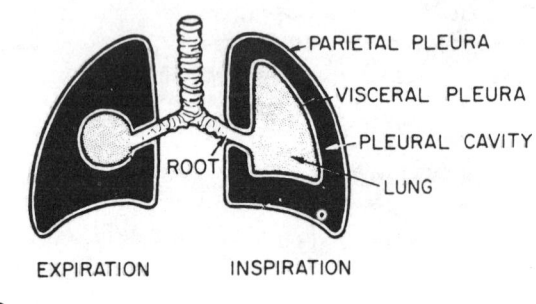

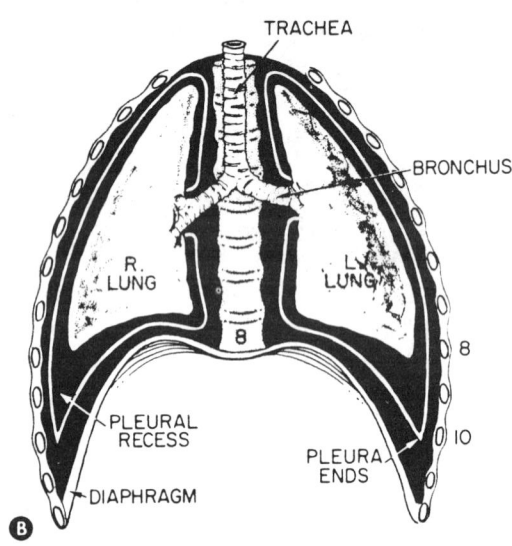

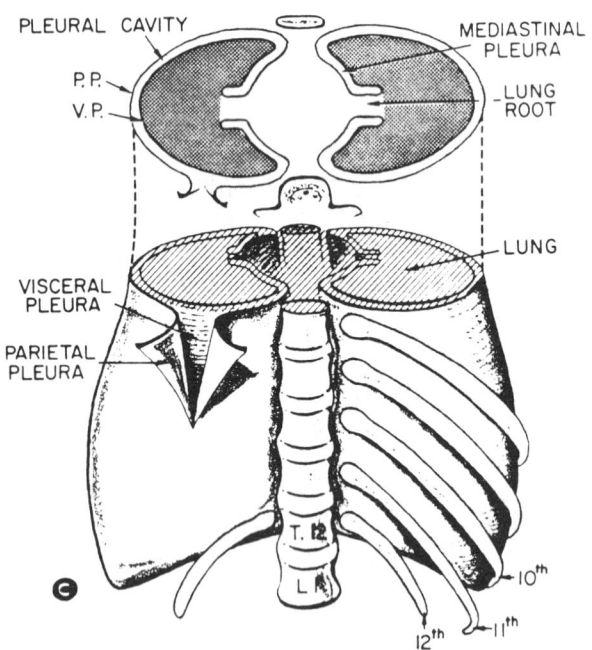

Fig. 3 - The development (A) and adult arrangements (B & C) of the lungs and pleura

gland. The middle mediastinum contains the heart sac (pericardium) with its contents, the bronchi, and blood vessels. The posterior mediastinum contains most of the longitudinally arranged structures passing from the trunk to the neck, for example, the aorta, esophagus, veins.

HEART AND PERICARDIUM - The heart is a muscular pump with two functions to perform: (1) it must pump venous blood (rich in CO_2 to the lungs, so that the red blood cells may exchange their CO_2 for oxygen; (2) it must pump this oxygenated blood, received from the lungs, to all parts of the body. Thus the heart is a double pump whose two parts work together. The right pump (side) receives venous blood and pumps it to the lungs; the left pump propels oxygenated blood to the body at large.

The heart is a hollow organ located between the lungs (in the middle mediastinum) with about two-thirds of its area to the left of the midline of the body (Fig. 4). This organ is about 5 in. long and 3-1/2 in. wide or about the size of an adult human fist. On a weight basis, it is about 10 oz in man and slightly less in the female. Its upper portion, or base, lies at the level of the second rib while its lower portion, or apex, points downward and to the left, resting on the diaphragm at the level of the fifth rib.

The position of the heart changes with age. At birth the infant heart lies midway between the top of the head and the buttocks. The long axis of the heart is directed horizontally in the fourth intercostal space with its apex lateral to a line passing perpendicular from the floor through the nipple (midclavicular line). These relations are maintained until the fourth year, and, later, the heart gradually shifts downward, due to the elongation of the thorax, until it comes to lie at the fifth intercostal space with its apex inside the midclavicular line. Until the first year, the width (or length) of the heart is no more than 55% of the chest width taken at the bottom of the chest plate. After the first year, heart width is slightly less than 50% of the chest width.

The heart and roots of the great arteries and veins are enclosed by a white fibrous sac, the pericardium (Fig. 5). This conically shaped sac lies in the middle mediastinum and is attached both to the great vessels of the heart and to the diaphragm. The sac has two layers between which is a lubricating (serous) fluid which facilitates movement of the heart as it contracts (systole) and expands (diastole). The inner layer of the sac forms the outer lining of the heart and is called the epicardium or visceral pericardium. It becomes continuous with the outer or parietal layer of the pericardium at the roots of the great vessels. The outer surface of the slippery parietal pericardium is covered by a dense fibrous covering.

In general, besides the epicardium, the heart wall has a middle layer, the myocardium, consisting of thick bands of muscular tissue. This heart muscle is of a very special kind. It is an involuntary muscle. Among the special features of heart muscle is that it cannot "cramp." Cramping of a muscle is caused by a failure to relax after contracting, or by a second contraction before a relaxation from the previous contraction. The heart muscle cannot begin a new contraction until it has

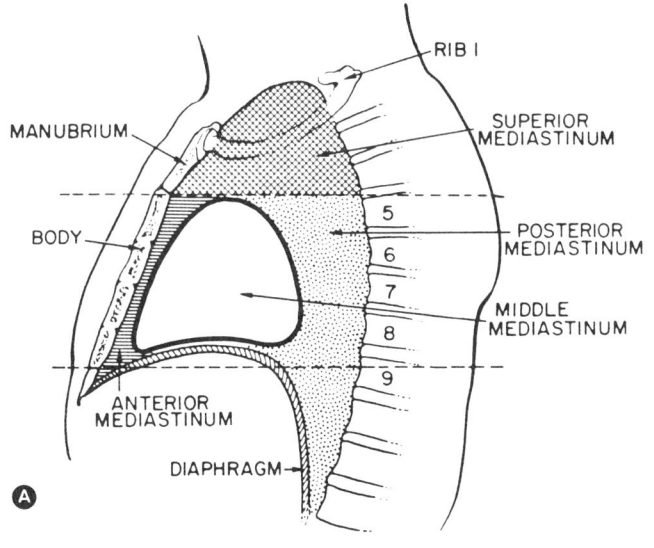
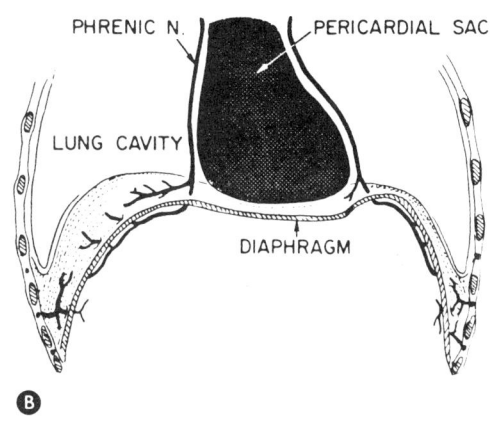
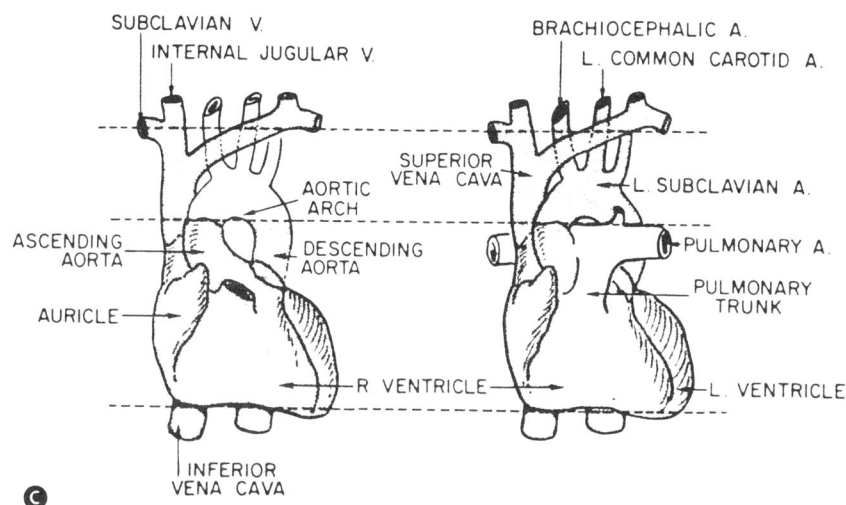

Fig. 4 - Compartments of the thoracic cavity (A) as related to the position (B) and anatomy of the heart (C)

rested from the previous one. The heart also has a third layer, the endocardium, which is a thin layer lining the inner surface of the heart cavities and heart valves.

The heart has two upper chambers (the left and right atria) and two lower chambers (the left and right ventricles). The auricles are earlike outpocketings from the walls of the atria; there are two auricles, right and left. On the outside of the heart can be seen a groove on each side, separating the atria from the ventricles. On the inside a septum (partition) separates the two atria and another septum (the interventricular septum) separates the two ventricles.

In general, the ventricles are larger than the atria in size and capacity and have thicker walls needed for pumping the blood against the pressure in the arteries. This feature is especially noticeable in the left ventricle, which pumps blood to the entire body excepting the lungs. The lungs receive blood pumped by the right ventricle.

The heart has four valves. These allow blood to flow in one direction only. The right atrioventricular channel is guarded by the right artioventricular valve which is also called the tricuspid valve because it has three flaps or cusps. The bicuspid or left atrioventricular valve has two cusps. The cusp tips are free to move into the ventricular chambers allowing blood ejected by the atria to flow freely into the relaxed or expanded ventricles. As the ventricles contract, the pressure of blood flow against the flaps (cusps) closes them to prevent backflow and directs the bloodstream instead into the aorta and pulmonary artery. The latter carries blood rich in carbon dioxide to the lungs to be oxygenated. The atrioventricular valves are kept in place by attached fibrous cords which are connected, at the other end, to muscular elevations of the inner ventricular walls. Similarly, the valves guarding the openings into the outflow vessels from the right and left ventricles, respectively, the pulmonary artery, and aorta, close to prevent a backflow of blood into the heart when the ventricles relax after completing their contraction. These semilunar valves, however, do not have attached fibrous cords but are pushed closed by the gravitational drop of the columns of blood in

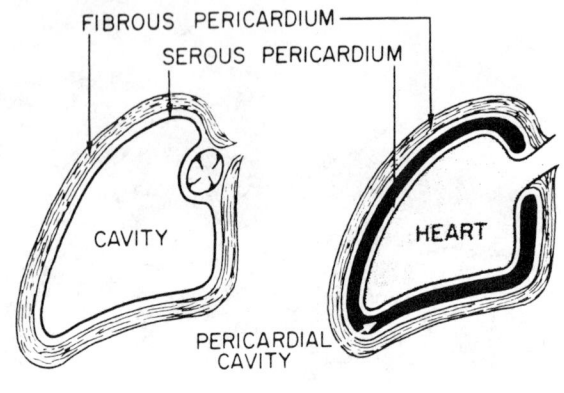
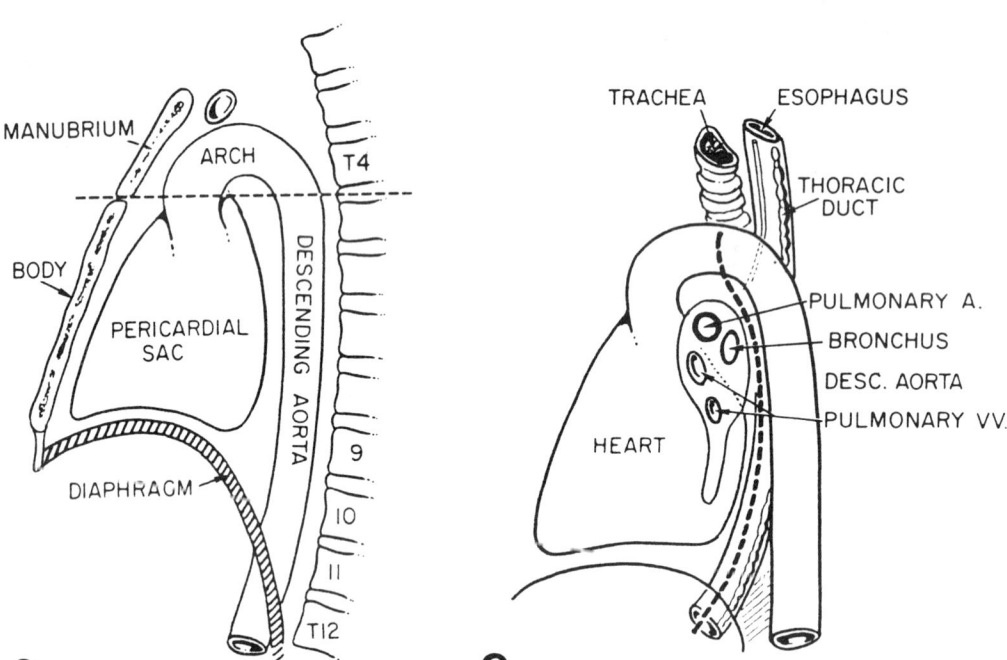

Fig. 5 - The human adult heart: its coverings (A), location (B), and main relations (C)

the pulmonary artery and aorta (the largest artery in the body).

If heart valves become deformed by inflammation and scarring, as in some cases of rheumatic fever, the ventricular outflow may leak back through them in the wrong direction. In the opposite condition, mitral stenosis, the bicuspid valve grows smaller and blood flow into the left ventricle is obstructed. The heart attempts to compensate for such interference by pumping blood more forcibly and faster, causing heart walls (muscle) to grow larger and the heart chambers to expand or dilate. In such a condition, strenuous activity may be ill-advised because the heart muscle cannot overcome the added heavy load imposed by the abnormal valve function. This condition can lead to "heart failure," as evidenced by shortness of breath (dyspnea) and by the accumulation of excessive fluids (edema) in the lungs, liver, and lower limbs.

The normal heart beat consists of the alternate contractions and relaxations of the atria and ventricles. As heard through a stethoscope, the beat has two sounds—lub-dupp—the first longer and lower sound arises from closure of the bicuspid and tricuspid valves and contraction of the ventricles. The shorter and snapping "dupp" sound results from closure of the semilunar valves.

The pumping action of the heart is one of contraction (systole) and relaxation (diastole), followed by a brief period of rest. The normal adult heart beats about 70 times per minute and is highly sensitive or dependent on a balanced supply of calcium, sodium, and potassium in the heart muscle. Each contraction and relaxation of the heart muscle is a heart beat. The rate of the heart beat depends somewhat on the body size the heart is serving. In general, female hearts beat six to eight times a minute faster than the hearts of men. The heart beat of a newborn may be as high as 130 per minute. Heart beat rate also fluctuates with activity. For example, a hedgehog's heart beats 250 times per minute, but in winter, the rate drops to 3 per minute. The heart actually beats more than 100,000 times a day; yet, it is resting more time than it is working. Each beat pumps about 2 oz of blood which results in about 13,000 qt of blood being pumped each day.

In the child before birth, that is, the fetus, the lungs and digestive tract do not function as in the adult. Fetal blood flows through arteries in the umbilical cord to the placenta, which provides nutrition and oxygen from the mother's system. Within the placenta blood passes through capillaries, is oxygenated, and returns to the fetus via the umbilical vein. After reaching the fetal heart, blood in the right atrium of the fetus passes through an opening in the interatrial wall (foramen ovale) and passes directly into the left atrium (by passing the right ventricle, then either through the left ventricle and aorta or through a small duct connecting the pulmonary arteries to the aorta. At birth, this small duct, the foramen ovale, and the umbilical vein close. If the duct of the newborn fails to close sufficiently unoxygenated blood gets through directly to the left atrium instead of passing to the lungs to be aerated—the result being the "blue baby."

Blood pumped from the heart circulates in a double circuit, one called pulmonary (supply only the lungs), and the other systemic supplying the rest of the body, (Fig. 6). The round trip of a drop of blood from the heart to distant parts of the body and back normally takes less than 1 minute. As the right ventricle contracts, in the pulmonary circuit, blood is forced into the pulmonary artery through which it is sent to the lungs where carbon dioxide in the blood is replaced by oxygen. This oxygen-rich blood is then carried back to the left atrium via the pulmonary veins. (Note that vessels carrying blood to the heart are veins whereas arteries carry blood away from the heart. However, not all arteries carry blood rich in oxygen, namely, the pulmonary arteries. Vessels which connect arteries and veins are capillaries.)

In the systemic circuit, the left atrium contracts sending blood past the left atrioventricular valve into the left ventricle which pumps it into the aorta, then into branching arteries and arterioles to capillaries of body tissue and organs. Blood spurts into the aorta at a speed of about 1 mph. As blood flows into smaller and smaller vessels, its pace slows down. In the smallest vessels (the capillaries), its speed is about 1/800 mph. Also when blood is propelled into the aorta, a pressure is exerted against the sides of the aorta and, in turn, all arteries. This pressure is called blood pressure, and a normal blood pressure is some degree of indication of the person's health. Pressure also varies with age. It is low in the baby and, as the body grows older and the elasticity of the vessel wall declines, the blood pressure increases. Blood returns from these body structures via capillaries to veins of increasing size which lead to the superior and inferior vena cavae. The vena cavae empty into the right atrium. This blood in the right atrium begins its pulmonary circuit again with the contraction of the right atrium and, then, right ventricle.

Because of the current interest in heart transplants to replace diseased hearts, it is appropriate to review the circulatory needs of the heart itself, especially since it is the master cog of the blood vascular system. As a functioning muscular pump the heart requires a constant blood supply for its own

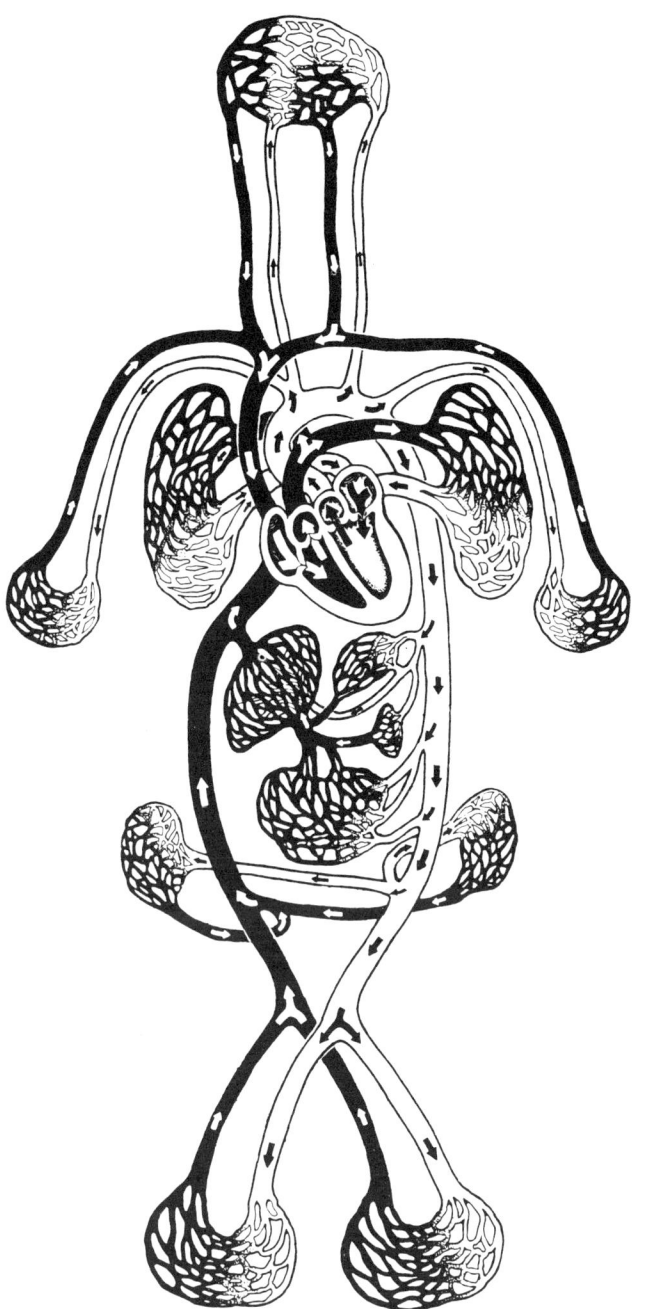

Fig. 6 - Generalized plan of the circulatory system

nutrition and oxygen needs. This supply is furnished by the right and left coronary arteries which originate at the base of the aorta. These two coronary arteries send branches to all parts of the heart. These branches, however, are highly regional and there are few connections between neighboring arteries. Blood from the heart tissue returns to the right atrium via the large cardiac veins.

Insufficient blood supply to the heart gives rise to chest pains (angina pectoris). Since heart muscle is highly dependent on a rich oxygen supply for its longevity, prolonged coronary insufficiency can lead to progressive tissue deterioration and a "heart attack." Such coronary inadequacy can be

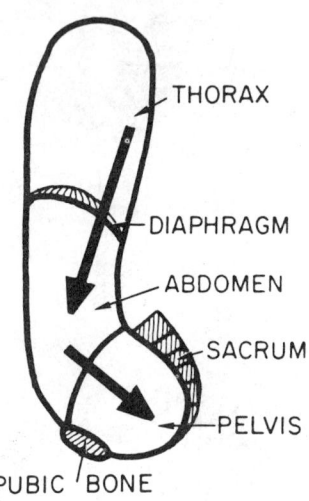

Fig. 7 - The topography of the thoracic, abdominal, and pelvic cavities

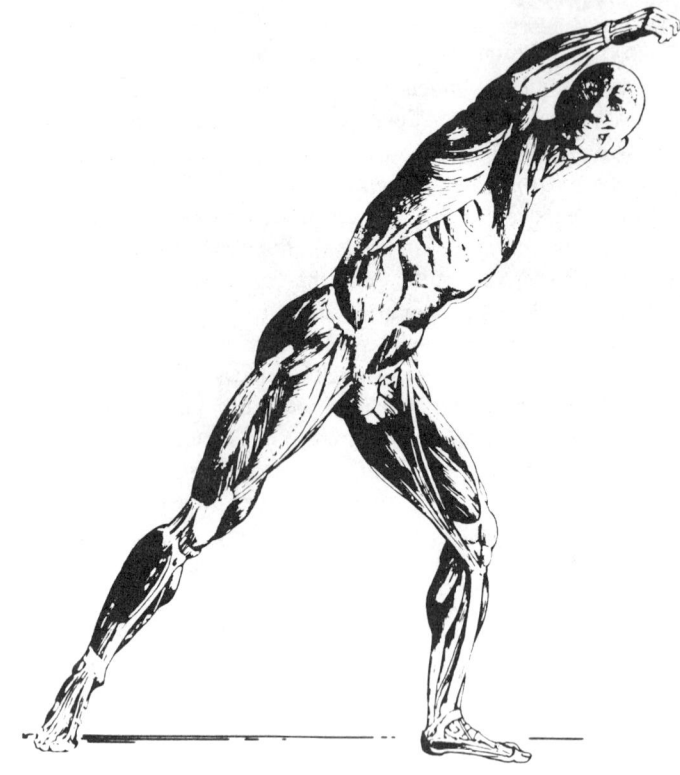

Fig. 8 - Superficial muscles of the body

caused by a blood clot occluding the channel (coronary occlusion or thrombosis) or a thickening of the wall of the vessels with a decrease in its lumen.

The activity of the heart is controlled by nerve impulses from the brain. These impulses, acting via nerve bundles coursing throughout the heart, may either accelerate or decelerate the heart rate. If impulses are blocked as a consequence of disease in this conduction system, the ventricle may contract at a very slow rate independently ("heart block"). The heart is affected also by sensory impulses received in other parts of the body. However, not all body stimuli have the same reactions on the heart. For example, a sudden emotional reaction may accelerate heart rate, while other stimuli, such as a blow to the abdominal region, may reduce it. Chemicals also affect heart rate either in a decelerating (pilocarpine, digitalis) or accelerating (atropine, thyroxin) manner. A rise in body temperature associated with fever or physical exertion also accelerates the heart rate.

Disturbances in normal heart function and rate can also be detected electronically via the electrocardiograph (EKG). This analysis is based on the fact that the cardiac contraction produces electrical charges which reach the body surface and can be detected, recorded, and analyzed.

ABDOMEN AND PELVIS

ABDOMINAL AND PELVIC WALLS - The abdominal and pelvic cavities form the lower portion of the body's trunk. These two areas are continuous with each other at the region of the pelvic bones (Fig. 7). The abdomen is separated from the thorax by the muscular respiratory diaphragm. Also, the abdomen and pelvis contain many organs (viscera) which will be described later.

Similar to the thoracic wall, the anterior abdominal wall is built on a simple plan consisting chiefly of laminated muscular walls lined by a sac (peritoneal sac). Abdominal muscles fall into two groups (Fig. 8). Group 7 muscles are composed of three sheetlike masses of interlacing muscles which enrich the abdominal region at its front and sides (anterolateral). These muscles arise from extensive attachments between the lower ribs above, the vertebral column, and associated tissues posteriorly, and the pelvic girdle below. Muscles of the first group are the external and internal abdominal oblique muscles and the transverse abdominus muscle. These muscles consist of fibers that do not run in the same plane. The external and internal muscles surround the abdomen in such a way that the direction of muscle fibers of the external oblique on one side is continued by the fibers of the internal oblique of the opposite side. Since the thoracic and abdominal muscles are regional components of the same spiraling sheets of muscle, it should be noted that a given abdominal muscle is a direct continuation lower down of a similar muscle in the thorax. The transverse abdominus muscle runs horizontally around the abdomen.

Each of the three flat abdominal muscles fall short of the anterior midline of the abdomen for they form broad flat tendons (aponeuroses) that surround the longitudinally arranged rectus abdominus muscle. This rectus (L., = straight) muscle is formed embryonically by several midline muscle masses; the marks of fusion of these muscles are shown in the adult by horizontal tendinous lines on the surface of a lean, well-developed body.

Acting like dynamic corsets, these four pair of abdominal muscles perform many functions which can be summarized as follows:

1. Protection of the abdominal viscera by tensing the abdominal wall
2. Maintenance of the cylindrical form of the trunk by compression of the abdominal wall
3. Increasing interabdominal pressure as needed in coughing, vomiting, and straining
4. Indirectly aiding visceral functions by assisting, through compression and increased intraabdominal pressure, in the evacuation of the digestive tract.

The base of the trunk, or more specifically, the base or bottom of the bony pelvis is closed off by a funnel-shaped muscular floor which serves to support the contents of the pelvis, for example, bladder, uterus, vagina. Besides acting as a support for the pelvic organs, many fibers of this muscular floor contribute to the voluntary control of the lower digestive tube or rectum.

Within this large muscular envelope that forms the walls of the abdominal and pelvic cavities are the viscera and their related coverings and blood supply. On a systemic basis, these viscera are components of the digestive, excretory, and reproductive systems.

ABDOMINAL VISCERA - Since the abdomen and its organs are closely related to the digestive process, a review of some basic facts about digestion will be helpful. Digestion is the process of breaking down complex foods, as sugars, fats, proteins, into soluble, absorbable materials, then absorbing or storing them and, finally, eliminating the waste products. The digestive system includes all the organs which act on ingested food, both mechanically and chemically. Mechanical processes include the action of the teeth or the muscular movements of the walls of the various parts of the alimentary tract. Changes in food form induced by enzymes produced by accessory digestive glands comprise the chemical processes. The two general divisions of the system are the alimentary canal and the accessory digestive glands. The alimentary canal consists of all the passages and spaces from the oral cavity to the anus (Fig. 9). By comparison, the gastrointestinal tract extends from the stomach to the anus. Organs of this division include, above the diaphragm, the mouth and associated structures, pharynx, and esophagus. Below the diaphragm, the division includes the stomach, small intestine, and large intestine. The accessory digestive glands include the salivary glands, the liver, and pancreas (Fig. 10).

In general, the alimentary canal is a tube that extends throughout the length of the body. In the embryo, the tube runs along the anterior surface of the developing spinal cord; it is, therefore, at first relatively straight and uncomplicated, that is, uncoiled. As development proceeds, this simple tube becomes markedly coiled in the abdominal region as a result of rapid increase in its length, and it becomes of varying caliber as a result of differing rates of growth of its walls. Abdominal anatomy and the continuity of digestive passages can be discussed by picking up a quantity of food in the esophagus, after it has passed through the mouth and pharynx.

The esophagus is a highly muscular tube about 10 in. in length extending from the pharynx to the stomach. Its upper

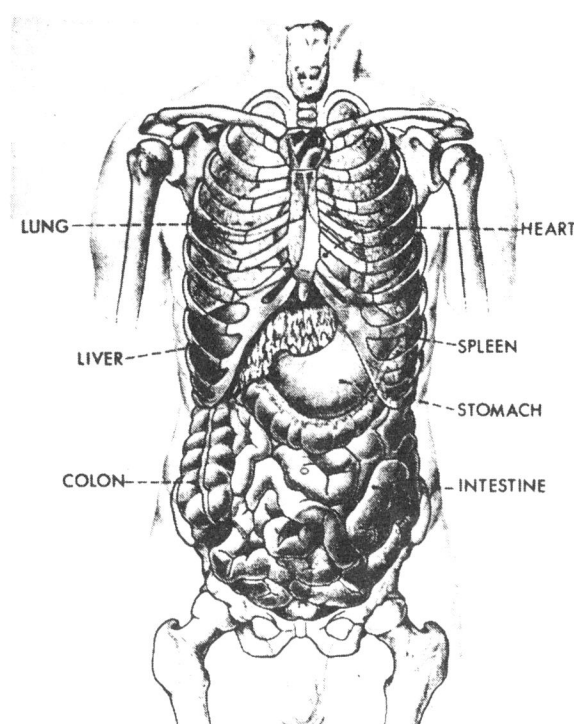

Fig. 9 - Thoracic and abdominal viscera

2 in. lie in the neck, anterior to the bodies of the cervical vertebrae and behind the trachea (windpipe). Its lower 8 in. pass downward into the thoracic cavity continuing through the posterior mediastinal space to the diaphragm through which it passes, and, turning to the left, enters the stomach.

With the beginning of the esophagus, the muscular wall of the digestive tube assumes the characteristic arrangement of an outer longitudinal coat and inner circular one. The longitudinal muscle begins in the laryngeal region at which point a gradual transition occurs from a voluntary (striated type) muscle complex to an involuntary (nonstriated) muscular tube. Muscles of the esophagus propel the food through it downward into the stomach by means of successive contractions (peristalsis). Automatic peristaltic contractions thus begin in the esophagus so that food does not fall downward by gravity alone. That is why, for example, it is possible to drink a glass of water while standing on one's head. It may be noted that all muscle actions in the swallowing process are reflex acts (except for those of the tongue). Semisolid foods usually require about 6 sec or longer.

The stomach is continuous with the esophagus and is the first part of the alimentary tract within the abdomen. It is the most dilated portion of the tract and has a normal average capacity of about 1 qt. It is subject to considerable variation in shape and size, but an average stomach is J-shaped in general outline and has a maximum length of about 10 in. and a maximum width of about 4-1/2 in. As for location, apart from being in the abdomen, the stomach is located in the upper left portion of the abdominal cavity with its concave inside border (the lesser curvature) facing upward and to the right toward the bulging liver; its convex outside border (the greater curvature) faces to the left and downward. About

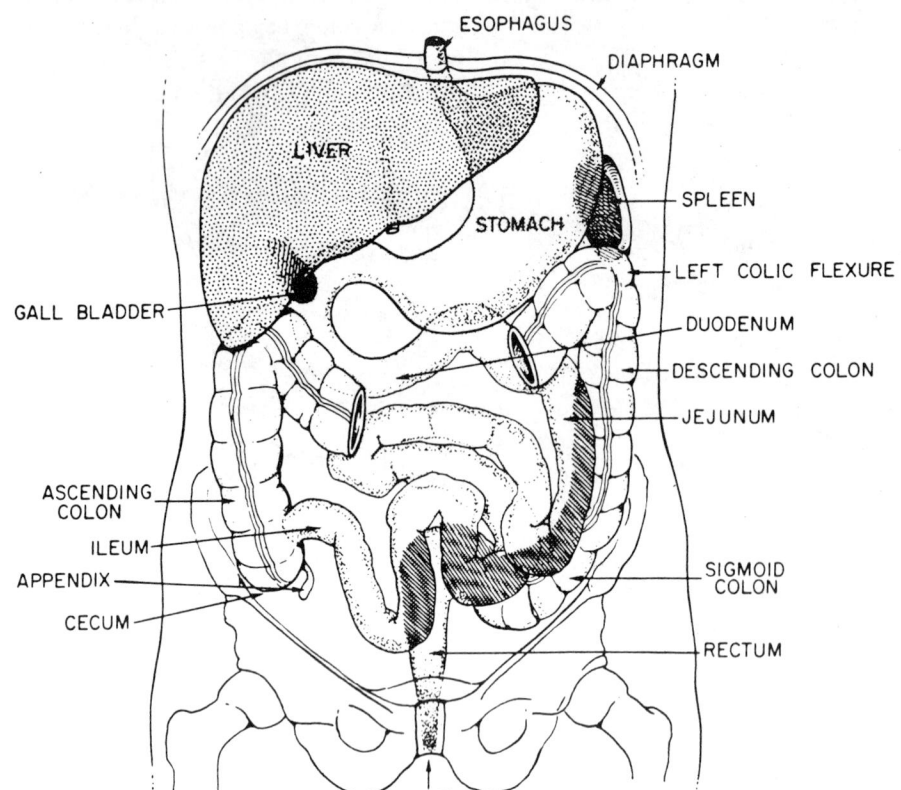

Fig. 10 - The locations and names of key organs of the digestive tract

85% of the stomach mass lies to the left of the body midline. Its four major parts are (Fig. 11):

1. The portion with the opening (cardiac orifice) from the esophagus
2. The fundus, an upward-ballooned recess lying above the level of the cardiac orifice which usually contains small amounts of swallowed air
3. The body (main portion) of the stomach
4. The pyloric portion, with an expanded part (the pyloric antrum), a narrow canal (the pyloric canal), and an opening (pyloric orifice) into the duodenum. The pyloric portion varies in position, depending upon the individual's stature and body position, the amount of food distending the stomach, and the pressure of the adjacent organs.

There are two functional valves in the stomach. The cardiac orifice at the stomach's entrance has no true anatomic valve though the passage of the esophagus through the diaphragm may enable the muscle of the diaphragm to offer some valve-like action. The opening from the lower end of the stomach (the duodenum) is protected by a true anatomical valve, the pyloric sphincter. This pyloric sphincter is quite powerful due to a marked increase in the normal circular muscle of the gut tube; the orifice, slightly open most of the time, permits food to be squirted out, but prevents escape of solids.

Similar to the walls of the entire gut tube, the stomach wall has four layers:

1. An innermost coat of a secreting and absorbing mucous membrane (or mucosa)
2. A backing layer of loose connective tissue

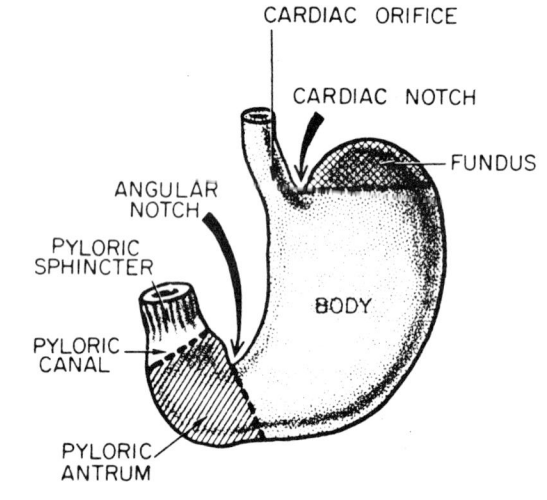

Fig. 11 - The regions of the stomach

3. A muscular layer
4. A thin outer coat of serous membrane.

When the stomach is empty, the innermost lining curves into many folds which vanish when food distends the organ. In this inner lining, there are also many glands of which some secrete pepsin and others hydrochloric acid. Gastric juices secreted by other glands also contain mucin and inorganic salts. Pepsin catalyzes proteins but only in the acidic environment provided by the hydrochloric acid. Muscular movements and enzyme actions convert the food to a semiliquid substance (chyme), an acid material which causes the pyloric sphincter to open so that food can be propelled into the small intestine. In general, it takes 3 to 4 hr for a meal to be digested.

The small intestine is a highly coiled tube approximately 22 ft long that extends from the stomach exit (the pylorus) to the large intestine. It has three continuous tubular sections which are in constant action. The first section, the duodenum, is about 10 in. in length and receives secretions from the bile and pancreatic ducts; the jejunum, about 9.5 ft long, is continuous with the duodenum. The third segment of the small intestine, the ileum, is about 12 ft long and extends from the jejunum to the large intestine. It is important to note that the foregoing measurements apply only to adult cadavers, since contractions of the muscular walls of the gut reduce the length of the small intestine to about 5 or 6 ft in living subjects.

The main digestive juices of the small intestine are bile, pancreatic juice, and intestinal wall secretions. The liver secretes about 500 cc of bile daily which is stored and concentrated in the gallbladder until it passes to the duodenum. Of its many functions, bile makes fatty acids more soluble, conveys waste products, and helps in the full utilization of proteins and carbohydrates. Pancreatic juice contains various enzymes which digest proteins, starches, and fats. Intestinal juice contains secreations from glands in the lining of the small intestine.

The large intestine, about 5 ft in length, begins at the end of the ileum, that is, the ileocecal valve, and continues as a widened tube to the rectum. It begins as an arch to the right of the ileum, extends upward as the ascending colon, then crosses the entire abdomen horizontally to the left (transverse colon), and, finally, extends downward again as the descending colon on the left side of the abdomen. At the lower end, the large intestine curves to the right or midline (the sigmoid colon) to flow into the rectum. Thus, as an analog, the ascending, transverse descending, and terminal portions of the large intestine form the sides of a "picture frame" which is deficient in its right lower corner. Lying within this framework is the small intestine.

Observe that the first and lowest part of the large intestine is the cecum. Next to the stomach, the cecum, about 3 in. long, is the widest channel of the alimentary tract. It is a large blind pouch lying in the right iliac fossa which has attached to it a wormlike tube called the vermiform (= wormlike) appendix. The appendix, varying in length from 1 to 8 in. is the narrowest part of the gut tract. This slender appendage is a cul-de-sac which opens into the cecum near the ileocecal junction. The appendix possesses a large amount of lymphoid material which causes it to resemble the tonsils. Like the tonsils, the appendix is frequently infected and requires removal.

The upper end of the cecum is continuous with the second portion (the ascending colon) of the large intestine. The cecum receives the contents of the terminal part of the small intestine (the ileum) via the ileocecal valve. This valve regulates the flow of digested food from the ileum into the cecum and prevents food from flowing back into the ileum from the large intestine.

In review, the ascending colon makes a sharp left turn near the underside of the liver and becomes the transverse colon.

The latter is highly mobile and extends across the abdomen to the left side. This transverse colon, being twice as long as the abdominal width, hangs down at its middle—sometimes into the pelvis when the person is standing. This horizontal gut segment lies below the stomach and in front of coils of the small intestine. As it reaches the left side, near the spleen and kidney, it turns downward to become the descending colon. This descending colon, at its lower end, turns toward the midline where it becomes the sigmoid colon which continues into the depths of the pelvic cavity as the rectum.

The rectum (= straight), about 5 in. long, lies in the midline in front of the sacrum and connects distally with the anal canal. In the anal canal are two sphincter muscles which compress the rectal wall and, working with muscles of the pelvic floor, control the closure of the canal. Of the two sphincters, the upper (internal) one is a mere thickening of the gut wall and is not controllable (involuntary). The lower or external sphincter is voluntary and relaxes only during defecation.

The main functions of the large intestine are to absorb water (so that the feces are excreted as semisolid) and to excrete waste products as calcium, iron, magnesium, and phosphates. In addition, bacteria in the large intestine cause food fermentation, decomposing the carbohydrates into alcohol and acids. Acting on proteins, normal bacteria inhabitants produce amines, acids, and the gases that impart a typical odor to feces.

Accessory digestive glands include the salivary glands of the oral region, the liver, and the pancreas. Below the diaphragm in the upper right region of the abdomen is the liver, the largest gland of the body. It is about 10 in. wide and weighs about 3 or 4 lb (or about 1/40 of the normal adult body weight.) This solid, blood-packed organ has four lobes separated by fissures (or cracks). Through one of these interlobar fissures runs the common bile duct. The common bile duct carries bile produced in the liver to a point on the small intestine wall near the stomach. The gallbladder is a pear-shaped sac and lies in a depression in the inferior surface of the right lobe of the liver. It is in contact with the anterior abdominal wall at the point where the border of the right rectus abdominus muscle crosses the ninth costal cartilage. This sac is about 3 or 4 in. long, has a capacity of about 50 cc, and is not vital to life. Some mammals possess a gallbladder; others do not. A duct from the liver joins with the duct draining the gallbladder to form the common bile duct which leads to the small intestine. During a meal the gallbladder contracts and bile is squirted into the duodenum.

One of the main functions of the liver is to secrete bile. (Other liver functions include blood formation and manufacture of anticlotting heparin, and storage of proteins and sugars.) The gallbladder concentrates and stores bile. Crystallized fat particles (particularly cholesterol) may accumulate in this sac or in the bile ducts and gradually form gallstones. Passage of these stones through the ducts may be painful. If there is a complete obstruction, bile is absorbed into the bloodstream, causing jaundice which is characterized by a yellowish coloring of the skin by bile pigments. The main functions of bile include the emulsification of fats, the ability to increase fat solubility, the vehicle for excretion of waste sub-

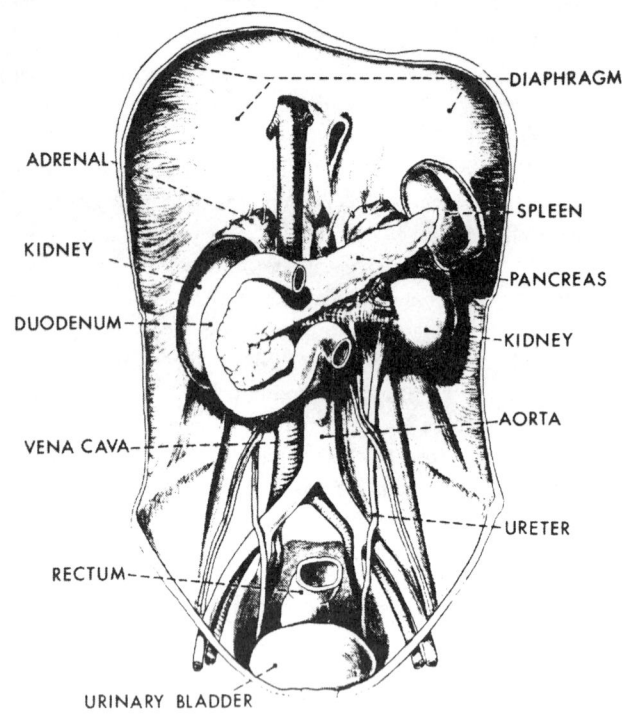

Fig. 12 - Deep abdominal viscera

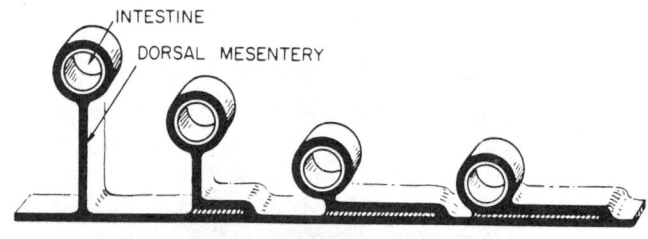

Fig. 13 - Varying lengths of supporting mesentery

stances, such as those resulting from the destruction of blood pigments in the liver.

Below the liver and stomach lies the pancreas, which is a soft, pliable, solid, and fragile organ (Fig. 12). This rather long organ is flattened from front to back and is about 6 or 7 in. long; on the average, the adult pancreas weighs about 3-1/2 oz. The gland has two main parts: its head occupies and overflows the concavity of the curved duodenum and lies in front of the bodies of the first and second lumbar vertebrae where it is firmly fixed to the posterior abdominal wall; its elongated body, about 1 in. wide and 6 in. long, is continuous with the bend and crosses almost horizontally to the left in front of the left kidney toward the spleen.

The pancreas produces a potent digestive juice which its duct conveys to the duodenum. Besides producing a digestive juice, special cells of the pancreas manufacture insulin. Insulin, as a hormone, is carried by the bloodstream rather than in a duct system. It is necessary for the proper utilization of blood sugar. Reduced insulin production results in sugar diabetes (diabetes mellitus).

As mentioned earlier, the abdominal viscera are highly mobile; this is made possible by a slippery membrane that covers most abdominal organs as well as lines the inner surface of the abdominal wall. This slippery membrane is the peritoneum.

Inside this fibrous sac, however, the viscera and related structures do not float or hang free. They also have a covering or investing membrane and this, too, forms a saclike structure called the peritoneal sac. The region of the peritoneal sac lining the abdominal wall is continuous with and reflected over the organs occupying the abdominal cavity. Throughout the abdomen, the peritoneal sac has a fibrous underlying base.

The interior of the sac is called the peritoneal cavity; actually, it is only a potential cavity and contains nothing more than a lubricating fluid which reduces friction between adjacent organs and between the linings and organs.

Organs and vessels normally found in the abdominal cavity develop and grow in the posterior part of the abdominal cavity, along the vertebral column, and, therefore, outside the peritoneal sac. As these organs, for example, stomach, intestines, liver, increase in size they attain more room by pushing the peritoneal sac ahead of them into the peritoneal cavity—"the fist-in-the-balloon" concept. Some organs do not push forward and always remain outside (retroperitoneal) the peritoneal sac; for example, urinary bladder, kidneys, pancreas, parts of the duodenum, and the great blood vessels. Peritoneal linings, however, almost completely surround and cover the stomach, parts of the small intestine, and transverse colon. Only partial peritoneal covering is offered to the liver, cecum, ascending colon, descending colon, rectum, and uterus. In all cases except those organs lying completely behind the peritoneum, there is a double fold of peritoneum which sweeps off the body wall and is pushed ahead of the specific organ into the center of the abdomen away from the posterior body wall—almost as though the peritonealized organs are suspended from the body wall by this double fold of peritoneum. This suspensory peritoneum (mesentery) provides the main passageway of nerves and blood vessels to and from the organs which have grown inward away from the posterior body wall. Since the aorta and inferior vena cava lie in front of the vertebral column at the point from which the mesentery hangs, branches of these major vessels conveniently pass, in the mesentery, to the gut (Fig. 13).

Although not a part of the digestive system, the spleen is an abdominal organ which belongs to the lymphatic system. The lymphatic system, by definition, is a type of circulatory system that is concerned with removing waste products from the tissue fluids closely surrounding body cells. This system consists of tiny ducts, filtering centers (nodes), and lymphoid organs. The spleen is a lymphoid organ as are the tonsils. In fact, the spleen is the chief lymphoid organ of the body. A person's spleen is about the size of a fist and weighs about 200 gm. This solid, pulpy organ lies in the upper left part of the abdominal cavity in contact with the diaphragm. The diaphragm separates it from the left pleural sac. The spleen, in the adult, is offered some protection by ribs 9-11 (Fig. 14). This organ is covered by the peritoneum by which it hangs

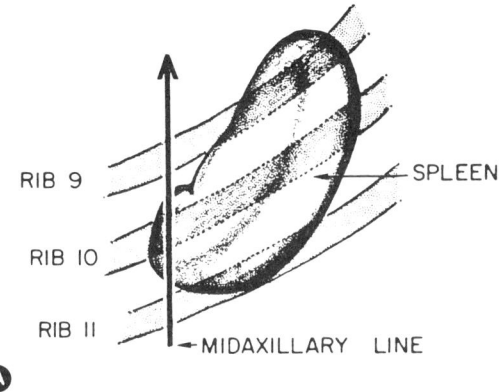

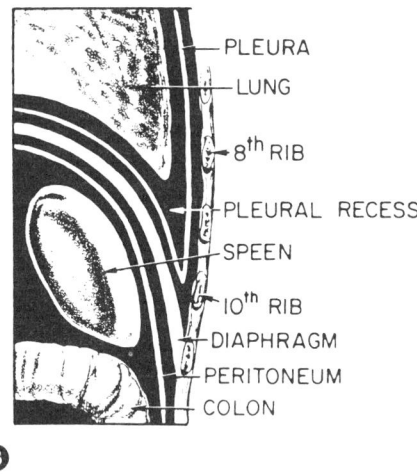

Fig. 14 - The protection of the spleen as provided by the ribs (A) and surrounding soft tissues (B)

from the posterior body wall; it can move freely with movements of the surrounding viscera. The spleen performs several functions, all of them concerned with blood and the body's protective system against foreign matter. In prenatal life and for a short time after birth, the spleen produces all types of blood cells. In the adult, it produces one kind of white blood cell (lymphocyte), and the organ is the chief residence of all the scavenger cells of the body. It removes debris of red blood cells that have broken in circulation, destroys worn out blood cells, and filters bacteria from the body. This protective function of the spleen against foreign matter is especially important in organ transplants, for example, heart transplants, in which the spleen is rendered incapacitated to prevent any rejection of the transplanted organ by the recipient's system. The presence of contractile tissues in the spleen allows it to undergo marked and rapid changes in volume. Contractions of the organ expel red blood cells to increase the number of them circulating. Size of the spleen is much reduced during exercise and after hemorrhage or oxygen lack.

Closely related to the digestive system are the organs of the urinary system. This system, lying behind the peritoneal sac, consists of two kidneys, two ureters (excretory tubes), one urinary bladder (a "bag" for storage and expulsion of urine),

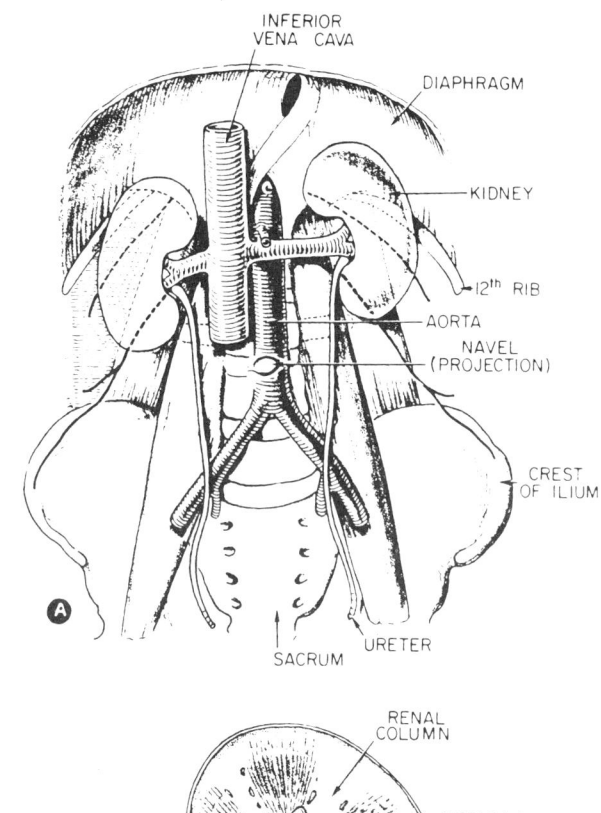

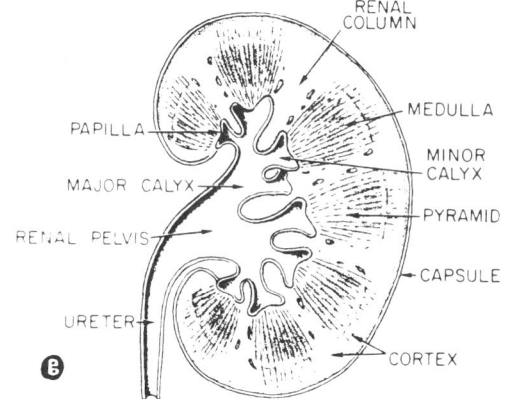

Fig. 15 - The location (A) and internal structure (B) of the kidneys

and a single urethra (a duct from the bladder to the outside of the body). Functionally, this vital system is concerned with maintaining constant alkalinity and chemical compositon of the body's blood while maintaining the proper amounts of water and salts in circulation.

The kidneys, in the adult, are paired bean-shaped organs measuring about 4 in. long, 2 in. wide, and a little over 1 in. thick (Fig. 15). They are buried in a mass of fat on each side of the vertebral column, just behind the peritoneum of the upper abdominal wall. (Their fatty envelope actually helps to cushion them from mechanical trauma.) Kidneys are placed higher on the abdominal wall than popularly supposed. They extend vertically from a level above the waistline upward to the level of the twelfth rib. The right kidney is covered in front by the large right lobe of the liver so that it is somewhat lower than the left kidney. The left kidney is usually placed a little higher and in contact with the spleen and tail of the pancreas. Since the kidneys lie high in the abdomen and touch the diaphragm, they necessarily move with the diaphragm as air is drawn into the lungs.

The lateral border of each kidney is full and rounded. In the middle of each kidney medial surface is a concavity (the hilum) through which blood vessels, lymph vessels, and nerves pass and from which the ureter emerges.

The longitudinal cut through the kidney discloses its internal structure which is not of uniform color. The outer, pale, granular area, about 3/4 in. thick is the cortex. The inner striated zone, the medulla, consists of about half a dozen isolated cone-shaped pyramids whose bases abut the cortex and whose apices are directed to the hilum. Each pair of pyramids is separated by columns (renal columns) extending from the cortex into the medulla as far as the concave hilum. The apex of each pyramid is cupped in the hilum region by a branch of the ureter.

Microscopic study shows each kidney to consist of more than a million (possibly more than four million) units called nephrons. Each nephron consists of a filter unit (renal corpuscle) and a tubule. The corpuscle consists of a cluster of looped capillaries (glomeruli) which rest in a cup-like depression (glomerular capsule) formed by an invagination of the dilated, blind end of the nephron tubule. The parts of the nephron tubule are the first (proximal) and second (distal) convoluted tubules between which is a loop (of Henle). The distal tubule drains into a straight collecting duct. The many straight collecting ducts give the medulla of the kidney its striated appearance; parts of the nephron, other than the straight ducts have about 45 miles of tubing.

Kidneys produce urine by filtering the water and minerals brought to each nephron by the glomerular capillaries while leaving blood cells in the capillaries. The fluid and materials thus taken out of the blood by passing through the glomerular capsule passes toward the ureter via the collecting tubules of the nephron. Additional materials are absorbed from the tubule contents by other capillaries that completely entwine the nephron tubule system. During this process of tubular absorption, 99% of the fluid originally passing into the tubule system is reclaimed by the blood as glucose (sugar) and other elements. Urinalysis may disclose the presence of substances which are not normally found in the urine, for example, sugar in the urine may indicate sugar diabetes (diabetes mellitus). Since waste products such as urea, uric acid, and phosphates are not readily passable through the walls of the tubule system, they remain in the urine and are eliminated with it.

About 1500 cc of urine are excreted daily, the amount varying with diet, water ingestion, wastes lost via lungs and skin, and the degree of physical activity. Nerve impulses stimulating the kidney vessels can alter the normal production of urine. Specific hormones have similar effects. When diseased, kidneys allow deleterious products to circulate in the blood stream resulting in uremic poisoning. Inflammation of the kidney is nephritis which may be acute or chronic. Kidneys are obviously vital organs; however, one may be removed without serious side-effects, provided the other is healthy. Removal of both kidneys is possible in modern medicine, yet a kidney machine must be substituted to carry out the functions of the removed organs.

Urine excreted by the kidneys passes through ducts (ureters) which descend vertically behind the peritoneum and on the muscles of the posterior abdominal wall. Each of the ureters is about 10-12 in. long and connects the kidney with the urinary bladder. Actually one half of the ureter's length lies in the abdominal region while the remaining portion is in the pelvic basin. The ureter contracts and relaxes to effectively squirt urine downward and into the bladder.

PELVIC VISCERA - The urinary bladder is a hollow, thick-walled muscular organ located in the pelvis immediately behind the pubic bones (Fig. 16). In the male, it lies anterior to the rectum; in the female, it lies in front of the uterus and vagina. Size and shape of the bladder, which is a reservoir for urine, vary with the amount of urine stored in it as well as with age. In the latter stages of pregnancy, size and volume capacity of the bladder are reduced since the enlarged uterus compresses the bladder against the pubic bones.

The bladder receives urine from the ureters, which pass through the posterior bladder wall obliquely and about 1 in. apart. Owing to this oblique course by which ureters enter the bladder and the presence of a fold at each opening, which acts as a lid, urine is prevented from re-entering the ureters as the bladder fills and walls pinch shut the ureters.

The bladder wall consists chiefly of virtually the same layers as found in the ureters. The wall consists of three layers of interlacing muscle fibers lined on the inner surface by a specialized bladder lining capable of stretching.

Leading from the bladder is the urethra which conducts urine to the exterior of the body. The beginning of the urethra in both sexes is advantageously situated at the lower end of the bladder like the mouth of a funnel. However, the remainder of the channel differs with the sexes of the individual. In the male, the urethra is about 8 in. long and carries both urine and semen. Its first portion is surrounded by a large gland (the prostate gland), which in older groups of men may enlarge and compress the lumen of the urethra; if this condition seriously impedes the flow of urine, surgical relief may be warranted. The second part of the male urethra is the shortest and narrowest, extending from the prostate gland to the base of the penis; the third portion extends the entire length of the penis. In the female, the urethra serves only as an excretory duct. It is about 1.5 in. long, extending along the front of the vagina and opening into the genital cleft (vestibule) between the clitoris and vaginal opening.

In review, as urine is excreted by the kidneys, it enters the ureters, through which it is forced into the bladder by the wavelike contractions of the muscles in the ureteral walls. While urine is slowly collecting in the bladder, muscle of the bladder wall relaxes and adjusts its tone to the increased volume. When about 300 cc of urine has collected, in the adult, sensory stretch receptors in the bladder wall are stimulated, and brings about the desire to urinate. At this time, under the control of the will, other impulses cause the bladder to contract. As a consequence, urine is discharged (about 3 pt daily) through the urethra with considerable velocity. This is known as urination or micturition. It is important to note that all steps involved in emptying the bladder are reflex in nature,

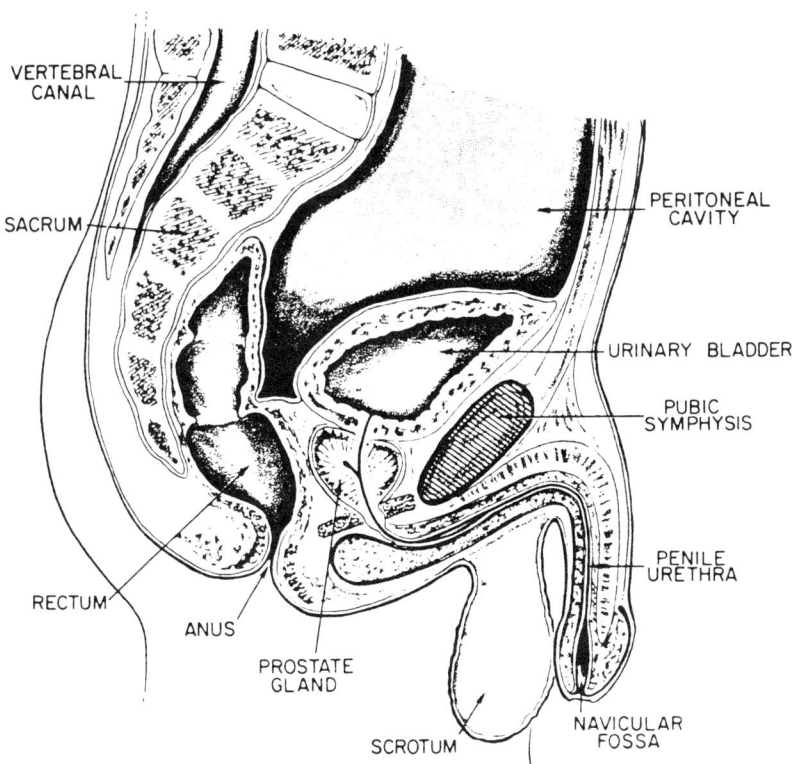

Fig. 16 - Relations of the male pelvic organs within the pelvic girdle

but that they are susceptible to voluntary control or training and, within limits, can be inhibited or initiated at will.

Expulsion of urine also involves contraction of the abdominal walls which increases the intra-abdominal pressure and usually is enough to start micturition. At the same time, muscles of the abdominal floor (pelvic diaphragm) relax in synchrony with contraction of muscles around the urethra which then bring about expulsion of any urine remaining in the urethra.

The reproductive system, closely related to the urinary system, consists of lower abdominal region (pelvic) organs concerned with perpetuation of the species. In addition to these reproductive functions, this system exerts widespread effects on the entire life of the individual through chemical substances produced by the sex glands, that is, hormones. These hormones, carried by the bloodstream, influence bodily development and behavior—in fact, the whole psychosomatic complex of the individual.

Male genital organs, in general, function to manufacture male sex cells (sperm), provide means of copulation, secrete seminal fluid, and transport sperm to the reproductive organs of the female. Reproductive organs of the male include the two testes, a duct system, accessory glands, and the penis.

The testis is oval in shape, about 2 in. long, 1 in. wide, less than 1 in. thick, and with a rounded front border. Its upper posterior portion contains many ducts connecting it with a tube (the epididymis). The two testes are enclosed within a skin like outpocketing of the lower abdominal wall. This pendant sac is the scrotum. It is interesting to note that in the embryo the testes move down from a site high on the posterior abdominal wall (near the kidneys) and pass, in a descending course, through the ventral abdominal wall into the scrotum. In this process ("the descent of the testes"), they travel (along with a cordlike arrangement of ducts, blood vessels, and nerves) through a canal, the inguinal canal. The canal has an internal or deep entrance and a rather superficial or external exit, that is, inguinal rings. (Since the external ring or opening is larger in the male than in the female, abdominal fat or even an intestinal loop can pass through it more easily, either indirectly, along with the spermatic cord, or directly through the external ring through the lower front abdominal wall which is normally weak in structure. For this reason, this outward push of abdominal fat or intestine (rupture, or inguinal hernia, is more common in men than in women). The scrotal position of the testes in man and other warm-blooded animals is an evolutionary adaption favoring the production of sperm cells. Sperm cells are temperature-sensitive, and the production of viable cells is favored by temperatures lower than the body normally maintains. The temperature within the pendant scrotum is several degrees lower than the abdominal temperature.

Within the tough capsule of the testis itself, the organ is subdivided by partitions into about 250 compartments. Each compartment contains 1-3 coiled tubules which join to form a straight tubule which leads sperm cells, produced in that compartment, to a center where straight ducts from many compartments join to form a highly coiled tubule system capping each testis. This coiled system, the epididymis, leads into the major sperm duct, the ductus deferens. It is this latter duct which extends upward inside the spermatic cord and through the inguinal canal, then crosses the pelvis, and subsequently descends over the top and posterior border of the urinary bladder toward the ureter. As it passes the ureter, it turns sharply downward and is joined by a duct from an accessory sex gland (the seminal vesicle). Together these two ducts form a single common duct, the ejaculatory duct, which extends through the prostate gland toward the ureter.

Sperm cells and seminal fluids are produced by cells lining the minute ducts within the testis. The number of spermatozoa produced by both testes in the course of an average lifetime has been estimated at 400 billion and about 200 million are discharged in a single ejaculation averaging about 3 cc. They may maintain their free-swimming motility for several days, but their ability to fertilize is limited to about 24 hr. Only one sperm cell is needed to fertilize a single egg.

Accessory reproductive glands of the male are the seminal vesicles, the prostate gland, and smaller glands at the base of the penis. The two seminal vesicles, located above the prostate gland and behind the neck of the bladder, produce a thick, viscous fluid which is added to sperm cells coming, via the ductus deferens, from the testes. The prostate gland is the largest male accessory sex gland forming a cuff around the bladder neck. As mentioned earlier, enlargement of the prostate causes a compression of the urethra so that urine cannot pass readily to the outside of the body. In severe cases, surgical removal of the prostate is required. The gland pours its secretion into the urethra; the secretion is thin, slightly alkaline, and functions to activate the motility of the sperm cells by raising the pH of the urethra. The small glands, at the base of the urethra, also drain into the urethra. Fluids from the accessory glands contribute to the seminal fluid, or semen, which also has in it sperm cells. Seminal fluid thus serves to nourish sperm cells as well as provide a medium for their transport through the male urethra toward the female genital tract. Seminal fluid may also serve as an often needed lubricant and as a neutralizer of acid normally found in the male urethra and in the vagina.

The male copulatory organ is the penis. Copulation (L., = copula, a bond), coitus (L., = a coming together) or sexual intercourse entails the insertion of the erect penis into the vagina of the female. The penis consists of a root, shaft, and glans. The root attaches the penis to the trunk; whereas the glans is the cone-shaped terminal end of the penis. The body of the penis consists of masses of spongy tissue which contain large blood spaces that, under sexual excitement, become engorged with blood, bringing about erection of the penis. Erection is maintained when blood is prevented from leaving the penis. Erection is normally involuntary, originating in higher brain centers, though it can be voluntarily triggered by the stimulation of various structures, in particular the sex organs. It may occur even while asleep or as a result of pressure on the prostate gland created by a full bladder. Pyschic stimuli (erotic thoughts) are prime factors in voluntary sexual arousal. On the other hand, these arousal mechanisms are easily overridden or superceded by negative stimuli, for example, fright, which prevent erection, a situation referred to as impotence. Temporary impotence may be caused by a variety of factors.

Principal organs of the female reproductive tract are the ovaries which produce eggs (ova), the uterine tubes, by which ova are carried from the ovaries to the site of fertilization, the uterus, in which the fetus develops, the vagina, which serves both as a copulatory organ and as a birth canal for delivery of the child, and the external genitalia, which include the structures of the genital cleft.

The ovaries are two almond-shaped bodies, about one-half the size of a testis, which develop near the kidney. Similar to the testis, the ovary is found outside the peritoneal sac at the posterior body wall. Although early in development it is located high in the abdomen, also like the testis, it migrates downward but no farther than the side wall of the pelvis where it assumes a permanent position. Each ovary lies almost free, hanging only by a sheet-like connection to the body wall. The surface of each ovary is covered by a layer of its own specialized cells (the germinal layer) which produces eggs or ova (ovum = singular) numbering about 200,000 in the life cycle of the adult.

The two uterine tubes (fallopian tubes, oviducts) convey the ova that are discharged by the ovary, usually one per month, to the uterus. Each tube lies under cover in the upper part of the pelvic cavity and averages about 4 in. long. One end of the tube empties into the uterus whereas its opposite or lateral end remains as a wide, unattached, expanded opening whose mouth is guarded by many finger-like projections. Although the uterine tube is not connected to the ovary, many of the tube's finger-like processes move in wave-like fashion near the ovary.

When an egg (or ovum) matures it is freed from the ovary and allowed to float free in the abdominal cavity. Fortunately, it usually rolls, falls, or is attracted into the uterine tube whose broad mouth is in the immediate vicinity of the ovary. After the ovum enters the tube, further movement is accomplished primarily by muscular contractions of the uterine tube. Fertilization usually occurs in about one-half the length of the tube. Should fertilzation occur before the ovum enters the tube, the fertilized egg (or zygote) may continue to develop as an extrauterine or ectopic pregnancy; if the zygote remains in the tube, a tubal pregnancy may develop.

The uterus or womb is a thick-walled, hollow, muscular organ about the size of a 3-in. long pear and with the stalk down. Functions of the uterus are to house and nourish the developing embryo. This organ lies in the pelvic cavity between the bladder and the rectum; however, during successive months of pregnancy, it increases in size considerably as well as changes its position upward and forward. The fact that it overrides the bladder means that, in the later days of pregnancy, the bladder can hold very little urine (Fig. 17). The uterus is anchored in its normal position by various ligaments which attach to the body walls.

The uterus has three distinct regions in its inverted "pear-like" shape. Most familiar is the lower constricted portion called the neck or cervix of the vaginal canal where it is cupped by the vaginal walls.

The cavity of the uterus is very small in the nonpregnant woman. Its walls are about 1/2 in. thick and formed chiefly by voluntary muscle. In pregnancy the cavity expands enor-

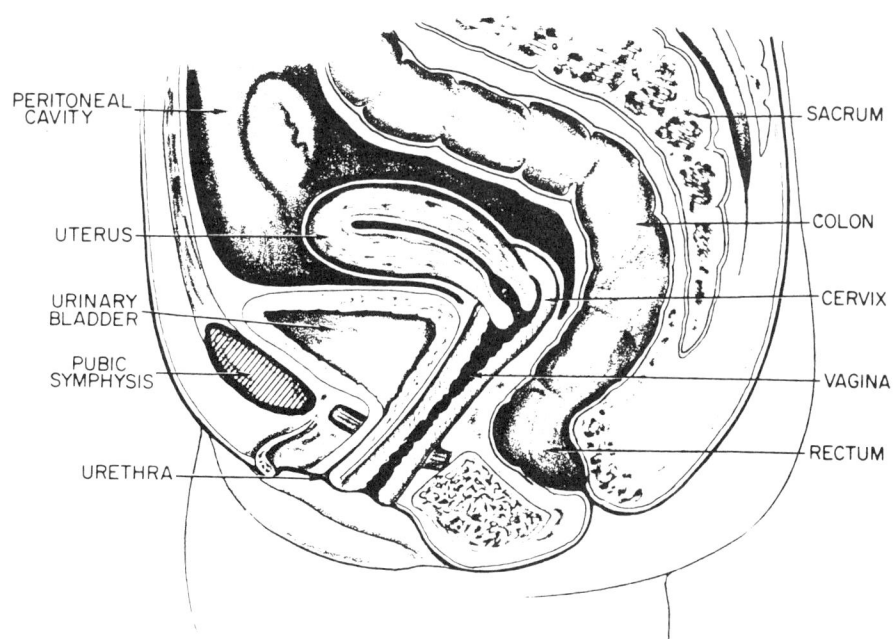

Fig. 17 - Relations of the female pelvic organs within the pelvic girdle

mously, and there is considerable increase in its walls. The nonpregnant uterus weighs about 50 gm and has a capacity of about 2-5 cc. The pregnant uterus at full term increases to about 20 in. in length, weighs about 1000 gm, and has a capacity of 5000-7000 cc. When a fertilized egg reaches the cavity of the uterus for attachment (implantation), the inner, vascular ining of the organ has thickened in advance to receive the zygote. On the other hand, if the egg is not fertilized, the thickened lining of the uterus sloughs off—in a process of menstruation. In other words, release of an egg occurs approximately half way between successive menstrual periods. Sloughing off of the uterine lining lasts several days after which the lining repairs itself only to undergo the same destructive processes if fertilization does not occur after the next egg is released.

The vagina is the tubular canal (about 4 in. long) which leads downward from the uterus to the exterior of the body, where its opening is surrounded by the external genitalia. Normally the highly muscular walls of the vagina are collapsed but they are capable of enormous stretching at various times, especially during the delivery of a child. Lying at about a 40 deg angle to the long axis of the uterus, the vagina lies between the rectum and the urinary bladder. In the virgin female, the external opening of the vagina is partially closed by a thin membrane (the hymen), which is usually ruptured at the first intercourse. Main functions of the vagina are to receive seminal fluid from the male during copulation, to discharge the menstrual flow, and to provide a canal for the passage of the child during birth.

The lower end of the vagina and the hymen are covered by paired longitudinal folds, the labia minora (labium, singular, L. = lip). The labia minora exhibit considerable variation in size and development, especially after menopause and in women who have given birth to many children. Lateral to these small lips are two rather prominent folds of skin (labia majora) bearing pubic hair which unite anteriorly near a rounded prominence covering the pubic bones, known as the mons pubis. Hidden by the labia majora, the front ends of the labia minora meet to form a small finger-like projection called the clitoris. Although the clitoris is developmentally similar to the erectile bodies of the penis, it does not house the female urethra. The area between these female external genitalia and the anal opening is known as the obstetrical perineum where an incision (episiotomy) is sometimes made to minimize tissue tearing during childbirth.

710848

Joint Range of Motion and Mobility of the Human Torso

Richard G. Snyder, Don B. Chaffin and Rodney K. Schutz
University of Michigan

ABSTRACT

The objective of this study has been to develop a quantitative description of the mobility of the human torso, including the shoulder girdle, neck, thoracic and lumbar vertebral column, and pelvis. This has been accomplished by a systematic multidisciplinary investigation involving techniques of cadaver dissection and measurement, utilizing cineradiofluoroscopy for joint center of rotation location, anthropometry, radiography and photogrammetry for selected positions and motions of living subjects, and computer analysis. Positional and dimensional data were obtained for 72 anthropometric dimensions on 28 living male subjects statistically representative of the 1967 USAF anthropometric survey of 3542 rated officers, including bone lengths of the extremities and vertebral landmarks. Normal excursion of these limbs were measured in the living, utilizing the landmarks established in initial cadaver dissection. Centers of joint rotation (link and positions) for the torso and limbs, lengths of functional torso links, and link excursions were correlated with linear body dimensions and landmarks obtained in traditional anthropometry. Some thirty-five positions for each subject were analyzed utilizing an off-line data coder system to determine how arm position affects the three-space surface coordinates. Three simultaneous regression equations were used to develop predictive models for torso positions referenced to a sitting or standing position or task.

The major results of the study are, 1) prediction equations and graphs describing how the base of the spine reference point (fifth lumbar spinal surface marker) moves in relation to defined seated and standing reference points for given reaches, and 3) the development of techniques by which the lengths and excursions of torso and limb links may be estimated and located. It was found that the surface landmarks selected could predict precise location of the underlying anatomical landmarks. The results of this study provide initial basic data regarding human torso motion, joint center of motion and link relationships.

ALTHOUGH STUDIES OF THE EXTREMITIES have identified the structure, range, and type of motions of the limbs, and examined geometric, kinematic and mechanical aspects of space requirements for the seated operator, no previous study has attempted to define similar relationships for the human torso itself. Traditionally, anthropometry has been limited to stereotyped dimensions describing the body surface and reproducible through palpable (and precisely defined) landmarks. While such studies have contributed greatly to many areas of application, such measurements are often inadequate when applied dynamic or functional descriptions are necessary. Design of automotive vehicle occupant seating or control placement, as well as aircraft cockpit or aerospace crew capsules, for example, require both kinematic and geometric (ergospheric) information. The ability of the operator to reach controls with maximum efficiency and minimum fatigue, as well as his ability to move them, perform tasks, apply pressure torques, and make required motions are determined by his range of motion at joints of the body. For any population a range of individual capabilities will be found. For an individual, range of joint motion is determined by the skeletal configuration, by the muscle, tendon and ligamental attachments, the amount of tissue, and the articulation. Some data are presently known for kinematic characteristics of the extremities, however, no knowledge of the link systems of the torso are available. Such basic information of the human body is of major importance to design engineers, and can form a basis for a major advance in the construction of anthropomorphic dummies.

During movements, dimensional changes occur linearly over body joints, causing linear distance increase over the convex surface of a joint when it is bent, and a linear decrease on the concave surface of the joint as tissue is bunched-up. This has been an important consideration in the design of pressure suits (1).* Factors influencing the range of motion have been reviewed by Damon, et al. (2). Mobility of the joint has been found to decrease only slightly between ages 20 and 60, declining about 10% by age 70 (3). No significant differences in mobility have been described between young and middle-aged subjects (4,5). Beyond age 45 arthritis increases markedly resulting in a decreased joint mobility in an older population (6). While no studies have compared racial differences, Sinelnikoff and Grigorowitsch (1931) found that females may exceed males in range of motion of all joints except the knee, and female wrist motion may exceed that of the male by as much as 14 degrees (7). Similarly, thin individuals appear to have greater range of motion than more obese individuals, with average and muscular body builds being intermediate (8). Sinelnikoff and Grigorowitsch (1931) found such variations could exceed 10 degrees. Physical exercise may also contribute to increasing joint range of motion if not excessive (9). There appears to be little more than 4 degrees bilateral difference between left and right limb motion (4,10). Body position or movement in one body part influences range of motion of another part, resulting in greater wrist flexion with the hand pronated than supinated, or in greater hand rotation if shoulder girdle movements are added to those at the elbow. For flight crews, flight clothing may restrict unimpeded motions (11,12), decreasing them by as much as 20 degrees (13).

In a now classic study conducted at The University of Michigan for the Aerospace Medical Research Laboratory and published in 1955, Dempster (17) studied the structure of limb joints and the range and type of motions utilizing materials from eight cadavers ranging from 52 to 83 years of age (averaging nearly 69 years). Previous work by Harless in 1860 (15) and Braune and Fischer in 1889 (16) had provided only limited information from cadaver studies. Thirty-nine living subjects representative of the 1950 Air Force population were studied, resulting in maximum dimensions of workspace for the seated individual, and kinematic motions (17, 18,19). In later work supported by Public Health Service, Dempster developed a means of estimating limb bone and link dimensions from over-body measurements (20).

Range of motion of the neck is still poorly defined. In our review of 203 clinical papers concerning cervical

---
*Number in parentheses designate References at end of paper.

hyper-extension/hyper-flexion injury none of the authors claimed to have measured the actual degree of dorsal or ventral flexion of the neck; thus the limits of motion beyond which trauma occurs is not known. In animal subjects anesthesia produces an artifact and has been shown to impair the stretch reflex (21). Cervical joint motion has been studied by multiple-exposure films (18), and cyclograms (22). Other photographic techniques were devised by Taylor and Blaschke (23), and Eberhart and Inman (24). The normal range of neck flexion has been the subject of several studies, but reproducibility, range of variation in individuals, and lack of adequate landmark standards have been difficulties encountered in voluntary human tests. Glanville and Kreezer (25) demonstrated range of normal voluntary motion of males (ages 20 - 40) to be 59.8 degrees (S.D. 11.7 degrees) ventral flexion, and 61.2 degrees dorsal flexion. Defebaugh (26) found a mean flexion of 57.9 degrees (S.D. 7.9 degrees) and 79.2 degrees extension. The lower limit for both studies was found to be 41 degrees.

Sensors attached to the skin have been found to inaccurately reflect motion of vertebrae in relation to each other during movements of the torso. Experimental work at Berkeley has involved insertion of 3/32-inch diameter threaded steel pins through the skin and anchoring them to the spinous processes at various levels of the thoracolumbar spine under local anesthetic, and using sensing devices to analyze the motion (27).

Other studies have involved range of motion of the wrist on 79 male subjects (28). While numerous investigators have treated the mechanics of joint motion, generally of the extremities, a comprehensive coverage is found in Steindler (29). Kinematic characteristics of the limbs are known to a limited extent, however, similar information concerning joint range of motion of the torso has been previously unavailable.

This study represents a first major attempt to obtain torso mobility data using a systems approach. The human torso is not a few long solid links with simple articulations but is rather a complex group of short links that move as a functional group. Thus only through a systems approach can the total functional mobility of the torso be described. It is believed that this study contributes major insights into torso mobility modeling.

ANTHROPOMETRY

CADAVER DISSECTION - It was necessary to initially define and establish the relationship of surface anthropometry and landmarks to anatomical landmarks and spatial points related to joint centers of rotation. Cadaver dissection was believed to be essential to define and establish the anatomical reference system, not only as related to the surface anthropometry, but also to make precise measurements as a check on radiographic methods. The cadaver also proved to be of particular value in establishing the radiographic techniques since it could be subjected to multiple radiation exposures and provided necessary baseline information prior to use of living human subjects.

The cadaver utilized was a Caucasoid male, approximately 55 years old, weighing 197 pounds, and 171.2 cm stature. To assist in more realistic positioning and joint motion of the cadaver, it was prepared by manually exercising the primary joints of the cervical (neck), shoulder girdle (gleno-humeral joint), pelvic girdle (acetabular joint), elbows and knees. Radiographs were taken of the entire torso and adjacent structures to determine that there were no anomalies, and to provide a complete set of x-ray films for use as a basic measurement tool.

Several experimental techniques for precise spatial measurement during cadaver dissection were utilized in order to measure the cadaver center of joint rotation in space and precisely orient surface and anatomical landmarks dissected and exposed. Figure 1 illustrates the apparatus finally used, consisting of a 6 X 3 foot box fitted with a plexiglass top and leveled with the autopsy table upon which it was positioned. The specimen was placed upon this device in the supine position. A metal framework was leveled with the surface of the autopsy table auxiliary table top. Moveable scales, with plumb bobs attached, allowed 3 coordinate X, Y, Z axis measurements relative to the zero point, which was arbitrarily selected at the vertex. A plumb bob was used to obtain a precise measurement in the X (vertical) axis. While this technique is slow, it proved to be simple and accurate.

The subject was measured in accordance with the selected criteria and conventional anatomical landmarks were located and marked. Marking of landmarks was accomplished in several different ways. Round lead pellet markers were affixed with Kadon to various selected surface landmarks. The lead markers were located on the cadaver specimen at the following landmarks: vertex, right and left tragion, nasal root depression, opisthocranion, cervicale, right and left sterno-clavicular joints, right and left acromion, right and left lateral epicondyles, right and left medial epicondyles, right and left anterior superior iliac spines, right and left trochanterion, and upon the dissected spinous processes of each vertebra. These showed up clearly on x-ray film and provided accurate reference points.

Landmarks were also located in depth through use of long pins. These were positioned at the surface landmark and dissection of underlying soft tissues proceeded until the anatomical landmark of the hard tissue was located. In each case the surface landmark was found to have been located almost identically (within 1 - 3 millimeters) with the underlying anatomical landmark.

In these initial measurements the surface sites were jointly cross-checked by three investigators. Surface anthropometry, however, could not be taken accurately on the cadaver specimen because of tissue differences and compressibility in comparison to the living, and landmarks were thus selected based upon critical relationship to the major torso hinge points and ability to obtain them. Since definitions of landmarks are at variance in the literature, and many may be inprecise in practice, an initial problem concerned agreement on anatomical surface landmark definitions, and subsequently precise definition of the internal skeletal landmarks as identified and measured on the radiographic film of the living subjects.

Dissection of major joints was meticulously performed leaving the surface pins in place to determine precision with which the surface landmark would coincide with anatomical landmark. Results were surprisingly accurate, as previously noted. Once the joint (sterno-clavicular, head of the humerus, trochanter, and all dorsal vertebral spines) were exposed and overlying muscle removed additional markers were implanted. Centers of movement in the X, Y, Z axis for the head of the right humerus and trochanter of the femur were determined and marked by insertion of 3/4 inch steel nails (Figures 2 and 3). Nails were also inserted for x-ray reference planes at the sterno-clavicular, acromial, lateral articular aspect of the clavicle, and lateral and medial epicondyles. Subsequent x-ray evaluation of the location of these reference points demonstrated the difficulty in precisely orienting the axis (angle) of the nail, although the skeletal surface entrance point as marked by the nail was found to be quite accurate for calculation of intersecting planes upon the x-ray. It is not felt that the nails could be placed any more accurately by this technique.

The cadaver was next moved to an x-ray table and the left shoulder (gleno-humeral) and hip (acetabular) joints were then pinned as above while under constant fluoroscopic observation. In addition, a 16 mm cinefluoroscopic motion picture film was taken and reviewed to ensure pins were accurately centered while the joint was moved in all three axes.

Despite the accuracy obtained in the above techniques, it soon became apparent that use of further cadavers, as originally planned, would not provide sufficient additional useful data to be worthwhile. Our experience with the initial cadaver indicated that it was not nearly as critical for reference purposes to the living subject study as had been believed. Secondly, although considerable efforts were made to obtain the clearest possible x-rays of the cadaver, it was found that poor definition of tissue contrast rendered many measurements anticipated to be useful and necessary to this study impossible to obtain. These factors, coupled with problems in obtaining usable x-rays of living subjects in certain arm positions led to an early decision to change the initial experimental design to place greater reliance upon the living study and to add photogrammetry as a necessary adjunct technique.

LIVING SUBJECT SELECTION AND MEASUREMENT - Selection of the experimental subjects were based upon the Air Force population as surveyed in 1967* and the statistical basis for selection, matching on the single variable of stature, is after Churchill, "Selection of Experimental Sample Subjects," (30) for a total of 28 subjects comprized of male University of Michigan students. The statistics for matching the subjects to the USAF population are shown in Table I.

Mean stature was found to be 178.45 cm for the University of Michigan sample, compared to 177.34 cm. Our sample also compares very closely with the 1967 USAF population in measures of weight and sitting height. The mean weight for the 28 subjects was 174.61 pounds, comparing closely to the USAF mean weight of 173.60 pounds. The University of Michigan sample had a mean sitting height of 93.11 cm, almost identical to the USAF mean sitting height of 93.18 cm. Our sample, as predicted, thus is representative of the larger USAF population in these critical measurements.

Prior to commencement of subject anthropometry it was necessary to agree on specific definition of landmarks, decision of required sites, and ensuring that the measurements were actually taken in precisely the same way as was done in the 1967 survey. All measurements were taken by the same investigator to eliminate inter-measurer variability. A number of non-standard anthropometric measures were included, such as extremity bone lengths, to increase compatibility of our results with previous work by Dempster (17-20) relative to skeletal linkages of the appendages.

To facilitate measurement 35 landmarks were initially palpated and marked. A total of 72 measurements were recorded, including several required for determining physique assessments. Following measurements, lead markers were placed at predetermined landmarks to be utilized as surface reference points in the subsequent photogrammetric and radiographic analysis. Several measurements were rechecked directly from the radiographic films, and one measurement, clavicular length, was obtained solely from subject x-ray

---

*Unpublished data, 1967 survey of 2,385 USAF flying population. Anthropology Branch, Aerospace Medical Research Laboratory, Wright-Patterson Air Force Base, Ohio.

films. Although many measurements, particularly the bone lengths, could be most accurately measured from x-ray films, the restrictions on radiation dosage of our subjects severely limited the number and exposure allowable and prevented obtaining films of the extremities for this purpose.

SOMATOTYPES - To provide another measure of the body physique somatotype ratings were plotted for the 28 subjects. The system utilized was the Heath-Carter technique (31). It is expressed as a three-number rating, each number representing evaluation of one of the three primary components of physique which describe individual variations in human body form and composition. This system differs from the classical technique of photographing the nude subject in three views and then subjectively assigning ratings (31), in that it is claimed to be entirely objective and based solely on objectively obtained measurements. A computer program designed by Dr. C. C. Snow at the Civil Aeromedical Research Institute, Oklahoma City, was utilized to reduce these somatoype data. We have previously utilized this technique in a study of Air Force test sled volunteers at Holloman Air Force Base (32,33).

Ten measurements are required to compute the Heath-Carter somatotype and include weight, stature, humeral biepicondylar diameter, femoral biepicondylar diameter, flexed biceps, circumference, calf circumference, and skinfold measures at the triceps, subscapular, suprailiac, and calf sites. Dimensions are uniformly taken on the right side of the body. The skinfolds were obtained with the Lange caliper, which is adjusted to exert a constant pressure of 10 gm/mm^2 over an area of 20 to 40 mm^2. Skinfold sites selected were the right subscapular, right suprailiac, right posterior mid-calf, and right triceps. A triaxial plot of the somatotype ratings indicated that in general the scatter of subject positions appears to fall into the general mesomorphic-endomorphic area normal for young U.S. males in better than average physical condition. These somatotypes are listed in Table II.

PHOTOGRAMMETRY PROCEDURE AND RESULTS

Early in this investigation it became apparent that the cadaver data were of more limited value than previous studies had led us to believe, and as a result emphasis was placed upon radiographic techniques in the living. Radiographic data from the initial cadaver revealed poor contrast between tissues which made many contemplated measurements impossible. Similarly, initial radiographic data from preliminary test subjects revealed density problems impossible to technically overcome when the subject's arm was rotated in certain position (longitudinal to axis of the humerus), which necessitated omitting certain planned arm movements. In addition, restrictions in the safe x-ray exposures for the living subjects limited the amount of available data from each subject. These preliminary findings suggested the addition of photogrammetry to the experimental design.

The basis for the use of photogrammetry was to allow a single person to be studied in a greater number of body positions than was possible with the x-ray procedure. In addition, the larger "viewing area" of a photograph provided the means to study whole torso configurations rather than simply the torso sectors permitted by the x-ray exposure limits.

During the initial anthropometry of each subject surface markers, consisting of 1/2 inch tubular black markers (Figures 4-7), were attached at 16 body landmarks.* Each subject

---
*Nasal root depression, left and right tragion, left and right acromion, suprasternale, cervicale (7th cervical), 4th, 8th, and 12th thoracic vertebral spines, 2nd and 5th lumbar vertebral spines, right anterior superior iliac spine, right lateral and medial femoral epicondyles, center of rotation of the head of the right humerus and surface location.

was brought to the photogrammetry laboratory after being x-rayed, thus the precise location of the surface markers was known for each subject from the radiographic film measurements. The photogrammetry apparatus consisted of four orthogonal cameras placed so as to obtain simultaneous views of the subject from above, behind, in front, and to the side. Front and rear view Praktina SLR cameras, with 135 mm Solidor pre-set lens, were positioned 35 feet from the origin. Side and top view Praktina SLR cameras, having Solidor automatic lens, were stationed 15 feet from the origin, and 75 watt spotlights were positioned at each camera sighting point. All four cameras were simultaneously triggered by electronic shutter release, and the motor driven films automatically indexed while the subject is positioned for the succeeding photograph. The frame identification numbers are changed by the photographer. The subject photometric station provides exact alignment markers so that all subjects can be positioned in the same relative positions for each body motion.

The design of the photogrammetric study required only 20 of the 28 subjects, taking into consideration subject size and position effects to prevent bias. Because all of the surface markers on the body had to be clearly visualized by at least two cameras for each of the 35 torso positions, there was a high probability of losing data, however, 15 of the 20 subjects selected provided adequate data for analysis.

Each subject was asked to make movements chosen to require various levels of torso strain. In both standing and seated positions, the subject was asked to reach out (forearm vertical) and touch a dull stylus target with the medial/posterior aspect of his elbow. To assure intersubject consistency an inked dot was placed on each subject's elbow for reference. Target positions were selected for 70 different body configurations, with 48 seated positions and 22 standing positions. The total series of 70 tests were divided into 10 sets of 7 positions each, and each subject was required to perform 35 tests; one replication on each of three sets and two replications on a fourth set.

The capability of determining both the inter-subject and intra-subject variance was provided by the repetitions. Each subject was required to perform seven tests twice. The sets were orthogonal (balanced), thus, there was no risk of having the angles or distances confounded by the subject's height and weight. Any given subject never performed more than two tests at one particular shoulder angle or at one particular reach distance.

The subjects were assigned to the test sequences according to their height and weight measurements. Although a one-dimensional ranking was not very precise, it was possible to contrast subjects at the top and bottom of the ranking scale, thus further reducing the chance of intra-subject variance changing general inferences about the torso mobility.

PHOTOGRAPH DATA REDUCTION - The location of each of the surface markers in each photograph is obtained by rear projecting each photograph onto a Datacoder,* moving a cursor over the point of interest and activating the system, a punched-paper tape of the coordinates is prepared.

The punched-paper tapes from the Datacoder were then

---

*Manufactured by the BBN Company of Los Angelos, California.

analyzed by a special computer algorithm.** This algorithm solves for the three space coordinates of each point by simultaneously considering the two dimensional locations of each point viewed from two orthogonal directions. The mean repeatability of the procedure has been found to be 0.4 inches.

PREDICTION MODEL DEVELOPMENT - The photogrammetric data of the surface markers previously listed for the trunk and shoulders was analyzed by developing linear and non-linear least squared error regressions for the coordinates of each jth surface marker (X_j, Y_j, Z_j) on each of the elbow coordinates (X_e, Y_e, Z_e). This modeling does not include anthropometric variables, and hence it is referred to as a General Model. Since at least 400 data points were available for each surface point good estimates were obtained of how each surface point moves in three-space as a function of the elbow positions. A second predictive model was developed which included anthropometric variables. Both the 5% and 95% percentile values were chosen from the 1967 survey of USAF rated officers for the anthropometric variables that were included in this model. In general, it was found that the primary anthropometric variables in torso mobility modeling are the sitting and/or standing heights, which have a directly proportional effect on the vertical height of the surface markers, and a secondary but significant effect on the horizontal movements of the surface markers.

The torso prediction models developed in this study appear to give good representations of torso mobility over a large number of elbow positions, though a great deal of variability between subjects still exists which is not explained by the models. Variation in subject physical dimensions does not account for the noted differences in skeletal mobility. The skin movements and resulting marker movements are not believed to be major contributors to the residual errors of the prediction models.

Two important practical aspects of the torso geometry prediction models should be noted. The models contain ten surface markers which describe the geometry of the torso, as opposed to the often used two or three internal links. With a computer graphics capability, these prediction models could be used to depict a more human-like form on a CRT for design reference than the commonly used stick figures. To be capable of doing this, however, computer speed (i.e., program simplicity) is needed. The prediction model approach used in this project provides the fastest possible means to torso mobility determination. This technique could provide complete torso geometry predictions in 30 to 40 milliseconds, and with a minimum of computer memory. Thus a designer of a man-machine system could easily work "on-line" for the evaluation of various work place layouts and other manual task design variables.

PHYSICAL ENVIRONMENT REFERENCE POINT DETERMINATIONS - The preceding torso surface marker coordinates have all been developed in reference to the location of the L5 spine surface marker, since the major orientation of this study was to model human torso geometry. In an attempt to assist the designer a prediction model has been developed which describes how the L5 surface marker moved in relation to the seat reference point (SRP) for the seated operator, and the floor reference point (FRP), the intersection of the mid-sagittal plane with the floor directly between the posterior

---

**The basis for this algorithm is described in a PhD dissertation by Kerry Kilpatrick, entitled "A Model for the Design of Manual Work Station," University Microfilms, August, 1970.

aspects of the heels, for the standing operator.

It is obvious that any relationship between a body point and a reference point in the physical environment will be greatly dependent upon how the body is supported and restrained. For example, a softly padded seat will cause variations in the body to SRP distances due to body weight, while a hard bench can cause subjects to shift their pelvic positions to alleviate pressure points. Thus the following relationships must be understood to be dependent upon the specific physical environment used in the study.

For the seated operator studies, a hard seat was utilized, similar to that used by Kennedy (34). It had a seat pan angle of 6° from the horizontal, and the seat pan was 15 inches deep by 16 inches wide. A low back support was utilized at 13° from the vertical. It rose only six inches above the seat pan, thus serving as a pelvis support only. No seat belt was used, but the subjects were instructed to keep their thighs in contact with the seat pan. The SRP was considered to be at the center of the intersection of the seat pan and seat back. When the subjects sat down in the chair they were positioned so the visualized mid-sagittal plane of the torso passed through the SRP. Direct measures of the SRP to L_5 surface marker distances of persons seated with their hands in their laps (i.e., a normal seated rest position) resulted in a value of 5.7 inches in the vertical axis being assumed as representative of the subject/seat condition. For the standing operator studies, the subjects were instructed to keep both heels on the floor. The average FRP to L_5 surface marker distance was 41.4 inches in the vertical axis with the subjects in a relaxed standing position, arms at their sides. These values were added to the prediction equations developed to depict the L_5 surface marker movements for the seated and standing individuals as a function of right elbow positions.

RADIOGRAPHIC STUDIES

A primary problem in the construction of human linkage representations, (e.g., computerized biokinematic models or anthropographic dummies) is the lack of data regarding how the joints move during the various volitional tasks. The objective of utilizing x-rays was to precisely determine vector distances between various bone articulations and surface markers for subjects maintaining specified body positions, and to develop graphs and prediction equations.

Radiographic data were obtained on 22 of the 28 total subjects according to an experimental design which was constructed to assure that all of the desired body configurations were included by allocating different configurations to different subjects. To maintain as low an x-ray exposure as possible, only nine 14" X 17" radiographic plates were obtained from each subject, resulting in a potential for a 108 total. Since the shoulder x-rays had to be taken in pairs, as well as some of the lumbar and thoracic exposures, a total of 84 body configurations could be studied. This allowed some repetition of certain positions such as the effect of trunk rotation and lateral flexion. However, because of inter-subject tissue density variations, some x-rays were not clear enough to provide good bone definitions, even though extreme care was taken in the taking and processing of the x-rays. This resulted in the loss of data from 3 subjects. Other limitations were that x-rays of a subject could not be repeated due to the exposure limit, established by the University's Committee on Human Use as a maximum of 1.1 roentgens, although 5 roentgens is considered permissible total body irradiation for occupational exposure.

Hence, even when it was known that a loss of several

points occurred, it could not be corrected. In addition, to establish a vector distance, a pair of bone and surface points must be visualized. Many vectors were lost due to one point being covered by similar density tissue, or by the limited film size forcing its sacrifice to gain a few other points on the opposite side of the film. On an average, 18 clear bone readings were obtained for each vector, representing about 50% loss rate. Nevertheless, the results are believed to be adequate to infer skeletal motion relative to the selected surface markers when a male subject is executing various specific arm and torso movements.

RADIOGRAPHIC PROCEDURE - The HSRI Radiology Laboratory was modified for this study by rotating the x-ray table vertically, and building an adjacent platform with seat and fixtures. The x-ray unit consisted of a Piker KM200 Centurian II 300 M.A. @ 125 KVP x-ray generator, a motor driven x-ray table with bucky and grid ancillary capability including a manual spot device, twin tube stand with magnetic locks, and radiographic collimator. The vertical position of the x-ray table allowed full travel of the x-ray tube about the seated subject for positioning at different angles and elevations. As illustrated in Figure 8, a fixture was designed to locate the right elbow in a set of predetermined positions for the seated subject. Cervical spine motion was determined for sagittal plane flexion and extension, with lateral x-rays taken in the "normal" seated, extended, flexed forward, and hyper-flexed forward positions. Some lateral flexion and cervical rotation data were obtained but were insufficient for inclusion.

Since the arm blocked the visualization of skeletal reference points due to density variations in several positions, the positions used included 4 positions in an upper plane, 3 positions in a normal plane, 4 positions in a lower plane, and 1 each with the arm extended vertically upward and the arm relaxed at the side. For each of these arm positions, a pair of oblique x-rays were taken (anode offset from the mid-sagittal plane by $\pm 30°$).

To determine how the torso bone-to-surface distances could change with different trunk configurations, a set of five lumbar and three thoracic configurations were obtained. These are (1) lumbar extension (in sagittal plane), (2) lumbar normal seated rest, (3) lumbar flexion, (4) lumbar hyperflexion, (5) lumbar lateral flexion, (6) thoracic hyper-extension, (7) thoracic normal seated rest, (8) thoracic flexion.

These positions were duplicated with an instruction for the person to rotate to the right "as far as possible," thus allowing the evaluation of trunk rotation, per se. For each of these positions either lateral (sagittal plane), or A/P (frontal plane), or both views were x-rayed, depending upon which would produce the clearest depiction of the bone positions. For example, if obtained, the rotated trunk positions required both views.

It was belived that the configuration of the cervical neck would also effect the surface-to-bone distances as low as the C_7/T_1 level. To study the cervical spinal column, five positions of the neck were sought: (1) cervical hyper-flexion, (2) cervical normal seated, (3) cervical flexion, (4) cervical hyperflexion, and (5) cervical lateral flexion. As with the thoracic and lumbar studies, both lateral and A/P x-rays were obtained.

RADIOGRAPHIC DATA REDUCTION - To develop the procedure a cadaver was positioned in each of the body positions described above, and radiographics taken. Previous partial dissection had allowed the placement of small lead shot markers to be positioned accurately on the palpable bony landmarks, and in reference to general anatomical bone geometry data, the cadaver radiographs were marked with a felt tip ink pen.

To provide both a consistent alignment of different x-rays and to scale the x-rays to the actual dimensions of the body, (i.e., parallax causes distortion magnification) a fixture was built which would display a set of reference points into each radiograph. By having the x-ray anode, film plane and reference points known distances from a reference point on the body (i.e., the right anterior superior iliac spine), it was possible to compute the actual bone distances of the subjects. In actual practice, the measurements were established by "calibrating" the radiology room. This was accomplished by placing markers on the walls and floor from which dowel pins could be projected to precisely position the x-ray anode in reference to the film, and subject. Once these measurements were established for the different viewing angles, they were entered into a computer program which was written to compute the bone locations, as shown in the flow chart, Figure 9.

After the radiographs were marked, the X-Y coordinates were punched into computer cards. The x-ray data for each bone and surface point was reduced to a listing of 3-space coordinates relative to the right anterior superior iliac spine for each subject and position by the computer program marker distances, in terms of vector distances and directions between points were also imputted to a second program. These vectors represent the "links," and show how the surface markers move relative to the skeletal points.

RESULTS OF RADIOGRAPHIC STUDIES - Presentation of the detailed results of the radiographic studies in terms of both prediction equation and graphical form may be found in reference 35. In general, study of the movement of the cervical spine in the sagittal plane showed that above the C_5/C_6 level the spine consistently moved with the degree of head inclination, with greatest mobility achieved at the C_2/C_3 and C_3/C_4 levels (average 0.6 degrees per degree of head tilt). In addition, although the C_7 surface-to-bone distance changes significantly with head inclination, this was not found to occur at either C_5 or C_2 markers. The greatest change in direction was found to be at the C_2 level with the least change at C_5. An overlay of average cervical disc center locations for the normal resting (Fig. 10), extension (Fig. 11), and hyperflexed positions (Fig. 12) are shown.

The radiographic study of the thoracic vertebral movement indicated that the thoracic spinal column can be considered to be a single link whose magnitude and direction can be determined from surface measurements, provided a correction is given for the orientation of the column when the measurements are taken. The distances between both assumed large links of the thoracic column, and surface-to-column links, remain constant with various degrees of flexion and extension; however, the distances of the surface-to-surface vectors vary with the degree of flexion and extension, thus demonstrating that there is a separate movement of the skin. The region slopes for the direction of the vectors between the surface markers and vertebral interspaces indicate that there is more movement relative to the column at the T_8 level than at the T_{12} or T_4 levels. Thus, the T_{12} and T_4 markers would be better for determining the direction of the thoracic spine movement.

The shoulder x-ray data demonstrated the complex mobility of the shoulder. In this study the individuals right elbow was systematically positioned in widely varying angular deviations (humeral reference angle) ranging from -45° (left of the sagittal plane) to +135° (right and back of the frontal plane). Distances for all of bone-to-bone vectors were found to remain constant, regardless of the arm angle. The lack of consistent directional movement of the three long links from the spine to the distal shoulder during arm horizontal movement leads to the conclusion that the subjects executed the movements without rotating their upper trunks. The one bone-to-surface vector distance that changed consistently with the arm angle was the vector from the projected humeral head to the humeral surface marker. Consistent skin movement occurs at the spine at C_7/T_1 level, acromion, and at the humeral marker, thus projections of bone positions in respect to these three surface points must consider arm position.

In regard to the lumbar spine, the vector distances (both from the surface to the spinal interspaces and from vertebral interspace to the interspace) did **not** significantly vary with the general inclination of the lumbar spine from the vertical. It was also found that the vertebral column and the surface markers move consistently with the general lumbar spine. To be specific, the regression slopes show that approximately 20% more mobility is contributed by the lower segments (L_5/S_1 to L_3/L_4 levels) than by the upper segments (L_3/L_4 to L_1/L_2 levels). The surface markers remained statistically constant in direction from the vertebral interspaces. This is particularly true for the L_5 surface marker. Apparently skin movement over the spines during lumbar flexion compensates for the angular changes of the vertebrae. The consistency of the vector distances with the angle of the lumbar spine suggests that in bio-kinematic models a single vector representing the lumbar spinal column is appropriate, and that its length and position is well predicted by the locations of L_2 and L_5 surface markers.

The effect of subject anthropometric dimensions on surface-to-bone distances was analyzed in some detail. The best predictive relationship was found to be dependent on the subject stature.

DESIGN USE OF COMBINED PHOTOGRAMMETRY AND RADIOGRAPHIC DATA - The x-ray and photogrammetric data presented can be combined for engineering design as illustrated in Figure 13. The general procedure for determining torso configuration from graphical data involves three steps.

1. Given the right elbow coordinates relative to the L_5 surface marker location, consult graphical data to estimate the position of the seat or floor reference marks. (It should be noted that the seat conversion data is highly dependent on the type of seat configuration and general restraint, and that the included data is for only one particular seat).

2. Determine the surface marker locations at L_2, T_{12}, T_8, T_4, C_7, acromion, and suprasternale from given prediction equations (for "average" seated male, or for "average" standing male, or from "tall" or "short" male).

3. Project adjacent bone reference points from surface reference points defined in step 2, by referring to prediction equations from x-rays.

Because the dimensions depicted in all of the graphs are empirically defined, as opposed to assuming a set of "hard" links which have specific known degrees of freedom, the undefined variability in the data will cause some misallignment of the bone reference points when they are projected from two or more adjacent points. Thus a single, unique linkage describing the torso mobility is not possible from this study but rather alternative internal linkages can be defined by the designer. The complexity and accuracy of each linkage assumed by the designer will necessarily depend on the range and type of reach simulation.

Because there are so many interactive factors that

affect the movements of both the internal and surface reference points, it is expected that the greatest benefit from this study will be in the improvement of computerized man-geometry simulations. These models will be based on the mobility prediction equation coefficients combined with internal links generated from the bone movement data.

SUMMARY AND CONCLUSIONS

A cadaver study was initially performed to define precise bone and surface landmarks, and to determine orthogonal radiographic procedures. Reference points on the radiographs of the cadaver in various torso configurations were marked to provide a standard reference system for later interpretation of living subject radiographs. A special radiographic facility was constructed for obtaining dimensionally accurate radiographs from widely varying angles. A four-camera photogrammetric facility was also constructed. Special computer programs were written to reduce the radiographic and photographic data to the three-space coordinates of each reference point.

Seventy-two anthropometric dimensions were measured on a sample of 28 male subjects statistically representative of the 1967 USAF anthropometric survey of 3,542 rated officers, including bone lengths of the extremities and vertebral landmarks. Nineteen subjects provided the final radiographic data, and 15 provided the final photographic data. These data consisted of bone and surface marker coordinates obtained while each subject positioned his body in various different torso configurations. To obtain different torso configurations, the subjects reached with their right elbow to various target locations while in either a seated or standing position.

Statistical analysis of the radiographic data provided prediction equations depicting the movements of the ten surface markers relative to adjacent bone structures. In addition, normal torso skeletal dimensions and excursions were determined. Correlations of these dimensions with specific anthropometry were developed for a set of torso configurations. A statistical analysis of the sagittal plane mobility of the cervical neck was determined from the radiographic data. This provided a quantification of the degree of mobility at the various cervical levels for various head orientations, as well as developing the surface-to-bone vectors.

The photogrammetric data depicted the surface marker coordinates for a wide range of torso configurations. In addition, it provided a means of determining the whole torso mobility. This was considered necessary since the torso is a group of relatively small bone links that function as a geometric unit. Statistical analysis of the photogrammetric data (over 4500 marker coordinates were included) resulted in prediction equations that depict the coordinates of each surface marker as a function of the elbow position. These prediction equations were developed for the "general" male population (averaged over all the subjects anthropometric variability), and for specific anthropometric variables. Graphs of the movement of each surface marker as a function of elbow positions were constructed for both general and selected anthropometric conditions. From inspection of these graphs a designer can readily determine with known dimensional accuracy the torso configuration of a seated or standing person whose right arm is required to be in various positions. The inspection of the anthropometric prediction model graphs also clearly describe the affects of major anthropometric variables on torso mobility.

It is generally concluded that this study has provided the means for developing new techniques for the study of human torso mobility, and may be of particular value to the design of anthropomorphic dummies. These techniques have been applied to the quantification of torso mobility during one-arm reaches without a back support. The resulting data analysis has provided many specific concepts regarding torso geometry, and the effects of specific anthropometric variables. The use of prediction equations to describe torso mobility appears to be justified. The accuracy seems to be comparable to other "hard link" biokinematic models of the seated operation, while the speed of predicting a specific configuration could possibly reduce computer modeling time to less than 1/10 th of its present value. It now remains to develop the torso mobility prediction models such that they will reflect such practical considerations as, (1) varying seat configurations, (2) different restraint systems, (3) tasks involving two hands, (4) various hand force requirements, and (5) different forearm and hand orientations.

ACKNOWLEDGEMENTS

The study presented in this paper was conducted under Contract F-33615-70-0-1777 for the Anthropology Branch, 6570th Aerospace Medical Research Laboratories, Wright-Patterson Air Force Base, United States Air Force, under joint Army-Navy (JANAIR) program support, to obtain basic data critical to cockpit geometry evaluation. We wish to gratefully acknowledge the guidance of Kenneth W. Kennedy of the Anthropology Branch during the course of this work. Invaluable support was also provided by Professor F. Gaynor Evans of the Department of Anatomy, The University of Michigan Medical School, and by Joseph W. Young, Chief, Anatomy Laboratory, Civil Aeromedical Research Institute, Federal Aviation Administration, Oklahoma City, who were instrumental in the development of the concepts and anatomical dissections. Dr. Walter M. Whitehouse, Professor of Radiology and Chairman of the Department of Radiology provided advice and expert assistance in establishing the radiographic protocols. William Price, HSRI Supervisory Radiologic Technician, gave unstintingly of his time and experience in the initial portion of the experimental radiographic studies, and Wayne L. Harris, conducted much of the radiographic analysis. Dr. Kerry Kilpatrick, now of the University of Florida, was instrumental in setting up the experimental modeling, and throughout the study James Foulke, also of the Deparment of Industrial Engineering, provided knowledgeable assistance. Peter M. Fuller, presently at the Department of Physiology, University of Virginia, assisted with the initial cadaver work. Pamela Bradley of the Kresge Research Institute, assisted with cineradiographic fluoroscopy and fluoroscopic study of the specimen. Doctoral candidate Frederick Schanne assisted with the photogrammetry. Doctoral candidate Kenneth Park, assisted by Terry Cavanaugh, was responsible for much of the computer programming. Graduate students James Sinnamon, Michael Becker, and Mark Bolton executed much of the final data analysis. Stephen Vanek analyzed the radiographic measurements, managed the subject pool, and assisted with the data reduction. Peter Van Eck contributed immensely to the subject data reduction, analysis of the final data, and final report preparation.

REFERENCES

1. I. Emanuel and J. Barter, "Linear Distance Changes

over Body Joints." WADC Tech. Rept. 56-364, Wright Air Development Center, Wright-Patterson Air Force Base, Ohio. February 1957.

2. A. Damon, H.W. Stoudt, and R.A. McFarland, "The Human Body in Equipment Design." Harvard University Press, Cambridge, Mass., 1966.

3. C.C. West, "Measurement of Joint Motion." Archives of Physical Medicine 26:414-425, 1945.

4. N. Salter and H.D. Darcus, "The Amplitude of Forearm and of Humeral Rotation." J. Anatomy 87:407-418, 1953.

5. D. Hewitt, "Range of Active Motion at the Wrist of Women." J. Bone & Joint Surgery 10:775-787, 1928.

6. C.J. Smyth, "Rheumatism and Arthritis." Annals of Internal Medicine 50:366-801, 1959.

7. E. Sinelnikoff and M. Grigorowitsch, "Die Beweglichkeit der Gelenke als sekündares geschlechtliches und konstitutionelles Merkmal." Zeitschrift fur Konstitutionslehre 15:679-693, 1931.

8. J.T. Barter, I. Emanuel and B. Truett, "Statistical Evaluation of Joint Range Data." WADC Tech. Note 57-311, Aeromedical Research Laboratory, Wright Air Development Center, Wright-Patterson Air Force Base, Ohio. (AD-131-028), 1957.

9. J.J. Keegan, "Evaluation and Improvement of Seats." Industrial Medicine and Surgery 31:137-148, 1962.

10. A.R. Gilliland, "Norms for Amplitude of Voluntary Joint Movement." J. American Medical Assoc. 77:1357, 1921.

11. E.V. Saul and J. Jaffe, "Effects of Clothing on Gross Motor Performance." Tech. Rept. EP-12, U.S. Army Quartermaster Research and Engineering Command, Natick, Mass., 1955.

12. C. Nicoloff, "Effects of Clothing on Range of Motion in the Arm and Shoulder Girdle." Tech. Rept. EP-49, U.S. Army Quartermaster Research and Engineering Center, Natick, Mass., 1957.

13. E.R. Dusek, "Encumberance of Artic Clothing." Tech. Rept. EP-85-USAREC, Natick, Mass., 1958.

14. E. Dzendolet and J.F. Rievley, "Man's Ability to Apply Certain Torques While Weightless." WADC Tech. Rept. 59-94, Aeromedical Research Laboratory, Wright Air Development Center, Wright-Patterson Air Force Base, Ohio. 1959.

15. E. Harless, "Die Statischen Momente der menschlichen Gliedmassen." Abh. d. math.-phys. Cl. d. königl. Bayer Akad. d. Wiss. 8:69-96, 257-294, 1860.

16. W. Braune and O. Fischer, "The Center of Gravity of the Human Body as Related to the Equipment of the German Infantry Man." Leipzig, USAAF, AMC Translation No. 379, Dayton, Ohio. (ATI-138-452, available from Defense Documentation Center), 1889.

17. W.T. Dempster, "Space Requirements of the Seated Operator: Geometrical, Kinematic, and Mechanical Aspects of the Body with Special Reference to the Limbs." WADC Tech. Rept. 55-159, Wright Air Development Center, Wright-Patterson Air Force Base, Ohio, 1955.

18. W.T. Dempster, "The Anthropometry of Body Action." Annals of the New York Academy of Sciences 63(4):559-585, 1955.

19. W.T. Dempster, "The Range of Motion of Cadaver Joints: The Lower Limb." The University of Michigan Medical Bulletin, Vol. 22, 1956.

20. W.T. Dempster, L.A. Shen and J.G. Priest, "Conversion Scales for Estimating Humeral and Femoral Lengths and the Lengths of Functional Segments in the Limbs of American Caucasoid Males." Human Biology 36(3), September, 1964.

21. S.M. Reichel, "Moderate Auto Injuries: The Role of Reflexes in Pathogenesis and Symptomatology." American Assoc. Auto. Med., Holloman Air Force Base, New Mexico, November 11, 1966.

22. R.J. Drillis, "The Use of Sliding Cyclograms in the Biomechanical Analysis of Movements." Human Factors 1:1-11, 1959.

23. C.L. Taylor and A.C. Blaschke, "A Method for Kinematic Analysis of Motion of the Shoulder, Arm and Hand Complex." Annals of the New York Academy of Sciences 51: 1251-1265, 1951.

24. H.D. Eberhart and V.T. Inman, "An Evaluation of Experimental Procedures Used in a Fundamental Study of Locomotion." Annals of the New York Academy of Sciences 51: 1213-1228, 1951.

25. A.D. Glanville and G. Kreezer, "The Maximum Amplitude and Velocity of Joint Movements in Normal Male Human Adults." Human Biology 9:197-211, 1937.

26. J.J. Defebaugh, "Measurement of Head Motion." Physical Therapy 44(3):157-163, 1964.

27. M. Sabanas and G. Porter, "Volunteers Get Stuck for Spinal-Motion Research." Machine Design pp. 3-32, October 12, 1967.

28. G.S. Daniels and H.T.E. Hertzberg, "Applied Anthropometry of the Hand." American Journal of Physical Anthropology 10:209-215, 1952.

29. A. Steindler, "Kinesiology of the Human Body." Charles C Thomas, Springifeld, Illinois, (second printing), 1964.

30. E. Churchill, "Selection of Experimental Sample Subjects." Antioch College, Yellow Springs, Ohio. Unpublished manuscript, 1961.

31. B.H. Heath and J.E.L. Carter, "A Modified Somatotype Method." Amer. J. Phys. Anthrop. 27:57-74, 1969.

32. H. Robbins and V. Roberts, "Anthropometrics to Support Program in Integrated Restraint Systems." Task 23. National Highway Safety Bureau, U.S. Department of Transportation, Final Report Contract FH-11-6962, July 1971.

33. D.H. Robbins, J.H. McElhaney, R.G. Snyder and V.L. Roberts, "A Comparison Between Human Kinematics and the Predictions of Mathematical Crash Victim Simulators." Proceedings, 15th Stapp Car Crash Conference, San Diego, California, November 16-18, 1971.

34. K.W. Kennedy, "Reach Capability of the USAF Population - Phase I. The Outer Boundaries of Grasping-Reach Envelopes for Shirt-Sleeved, Seated Operator." Aerospace Medical Research Laboratories, Wright-Patterson Air Force Base, Ohio. Rept. AMRL-TDR-64-59, 1964.

35. R.G. Snyder, D.B. Chaffin and R.K. Schutz, "Link System of the Human Torso." Aerospace Medical Research Laboratory, Wright-Patterson Air Force Base, Ohio, Report No. AMRL-TR-71-88, (in press) 1971.

Table I - Statistical Basis for Subject Selection Based Upon Single Variable of Stature to Match 1967 Air Force Population

Stature (Cm)	USAF (1967)	%	X28	Sample Required	Sample Obtained
162.75 - 165.74	48	2.01	.56	1	1
165.75 - 168.74	132	5.53	1.55	1	1
168.75 - 171.74	237	9.93	2.78	3	2
171.75 - 174.74	401	16.81	4.71	5	4
174.75 - 177.74	443	18.57	5.20	5	5
177.75 - 180.74	459	19.24	5.39	5	5
180.75 - 183.74	309	12.95	3.63	4	4
183.75 - 186.74	198	8.3	2.32	2	4
186.75 - 189.74	117	4.9	1.37	1	1
189.75 - 192.74	41	1.71	.48	1	1
Totals	2385			28	28

Table II - Somatotype Computations for Each Subject in 1/2 Intervals on a Scale From 1/2 to 9

Component

Subject Number	1 Endomorphy	2 Mesomorphy	3 Ectomorphy
1	3.5	6.5	1.0
2	6.0	5.5	1.5
3	6.0	6.0	0.5
4	1.5	7.0	2.5
5	4.0	4.5	2.5
6	2.0	5.0	2.5
7	1.5	6.5	1.5
8	1.5	6.0	2.0
9	2.5	7.0	1.0
10	1.0	7.5	1.5
11	3.0	5.0	2.5
12	3.0	5.0	2.5
13	3.5	5.0	2.0
14	6.0	5.5	1.0
15	1.0	3.5	4.0
16	2.5	6.5	2.0
17	1.5	4.5	3.5
18	2.5	5.0	2.0
19	3.5	7.0	1.0
20	2.5	5.0	3.5
21	1.0	2.5	5.0
22	1.5	4.5	3.0
23	5.0	5.5	1.0
24	6.0	5.5	1.5
25	6.0	6.0	1.5
26	1.0	5.5	1.5
27	4.0	5.5	1.5
28	6.5	5.5	0.5

<u>Somatotype Ratings</u> (Assessment Based upon Measurements Taken at Four Sites on Each Subject and Calculated After Heath-Carter Technique).

1. Endomorphy (relative fatness)
   N = 28
   Mean = 3.2
   Standard Deviation = 1.85
   Range = 1.0 - 6.0

2. Mesomorphy (relative musculo-skeletal development)
   N = 28
   Mean = 5.5
   Standard Deviation = 1.09
   Range = 2.5 - 7.5

3. Ectomorphy (relative linearity)
   N = 28
   Mean = 2.0
   Standard Deviation = 1.07
   Range = 0.5 - 5.0

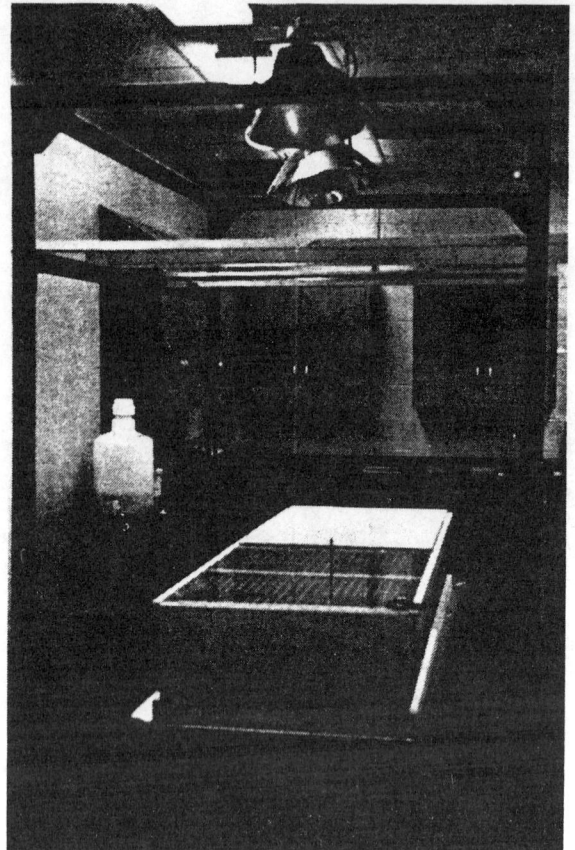

Fig 1 - Dissection measurement apparatus used to determine spatial relationships. Overhead scales allow three axis plots of anatomical landmarks

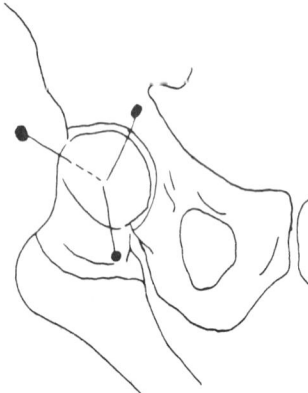

Fig. 2 - Sites of 3-axis pinning of the head of the femur (hip joint) to locate the center of joint rotation

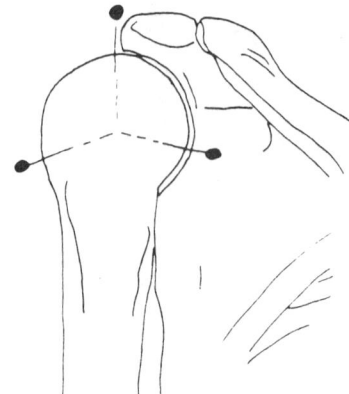

Fig. 3 - Location of steel pins placed in the head of the humerus to locate the center of rotation of the shoulder (gleno-humeral) joint

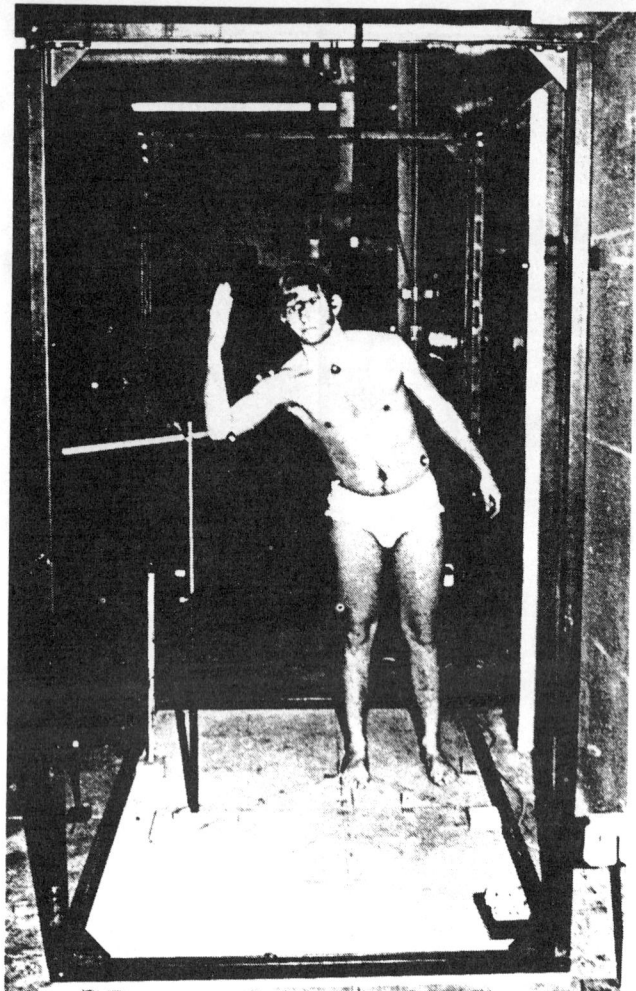

Fig. 4 - Frontal view of subject as seen by camera No. 1

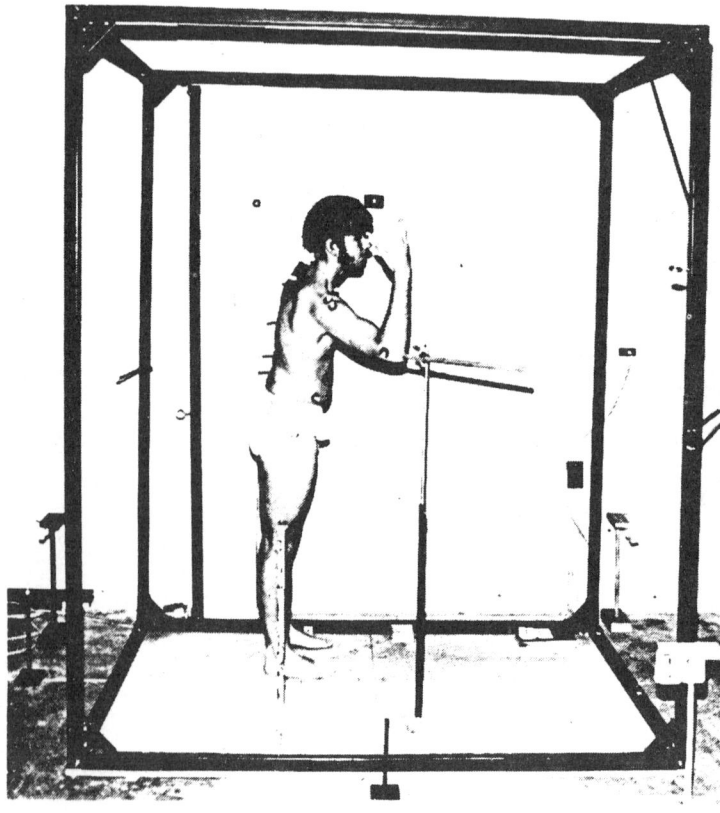

Fig. 5 - Side view of subject as seen by lateral camera No. 2, with subject in same position as in preceding figure

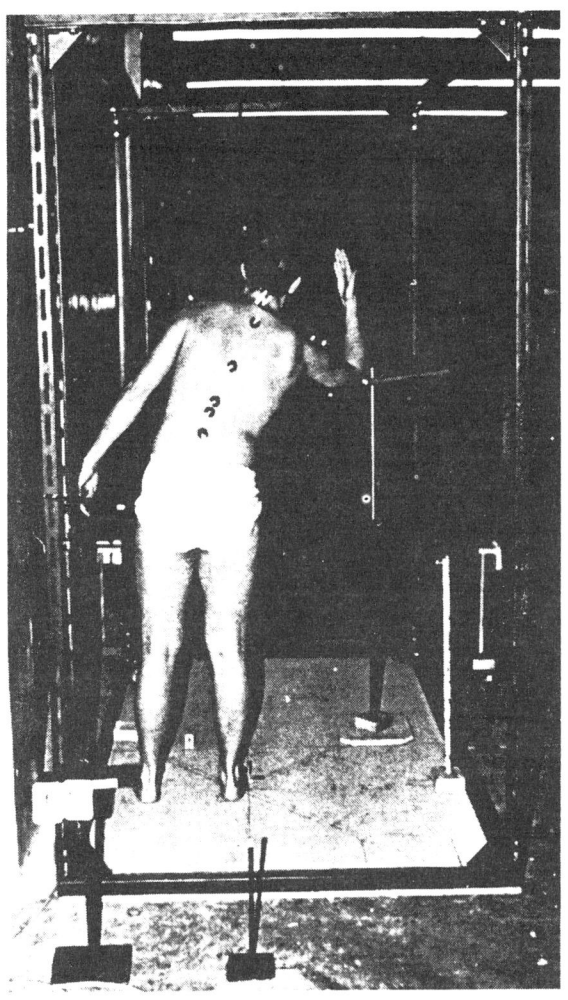

Fig. 6 - Rear view of subject as seen by rear camera No. 3, with subject in same position as in preceding figures

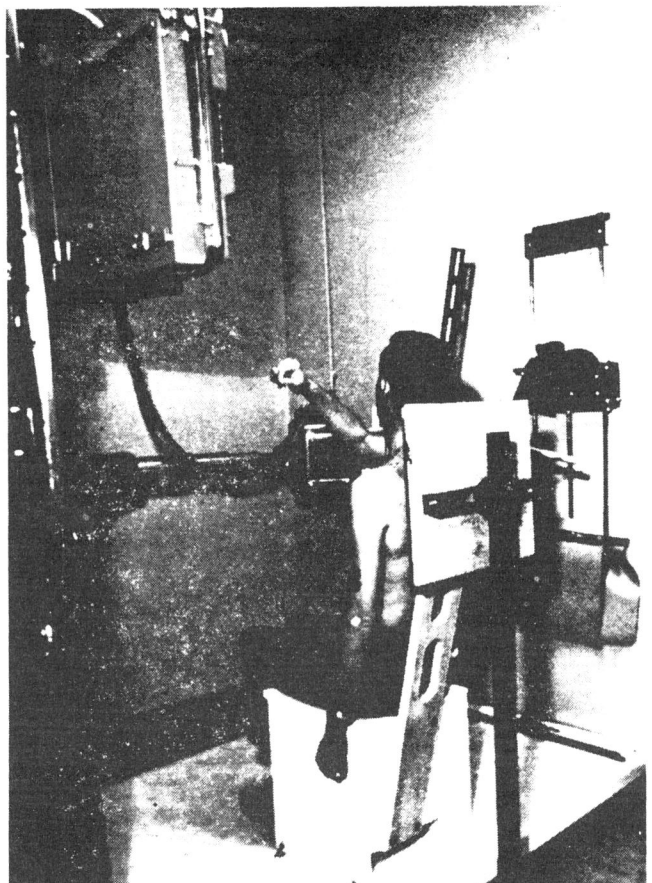

Fig. 8 - View of subject in seated position for 30 deg radiograph

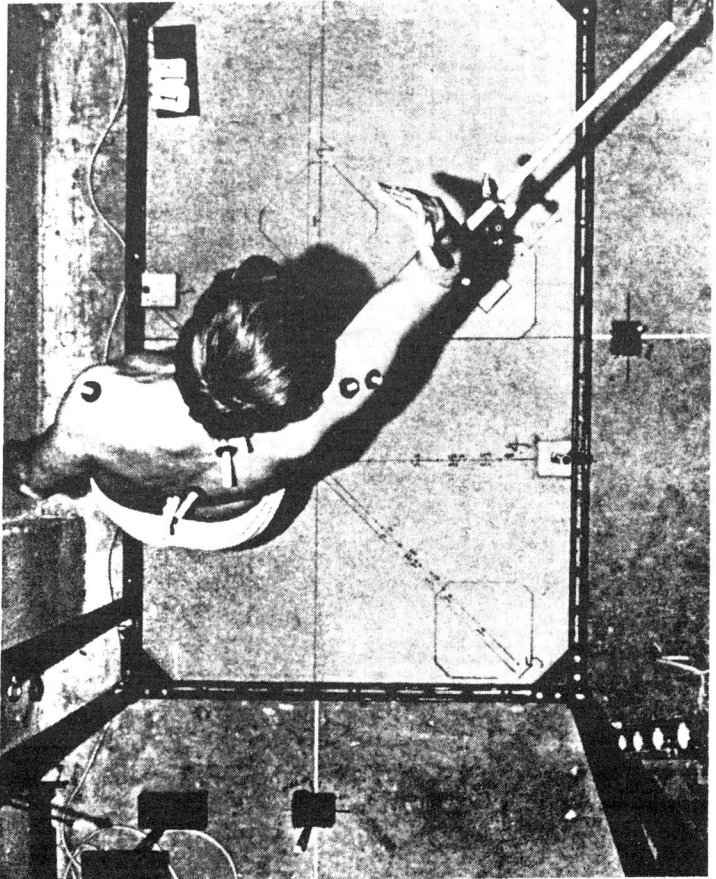

Fig. 7 - View from overhead camera No. 4 of subject in same position as in preceding figures

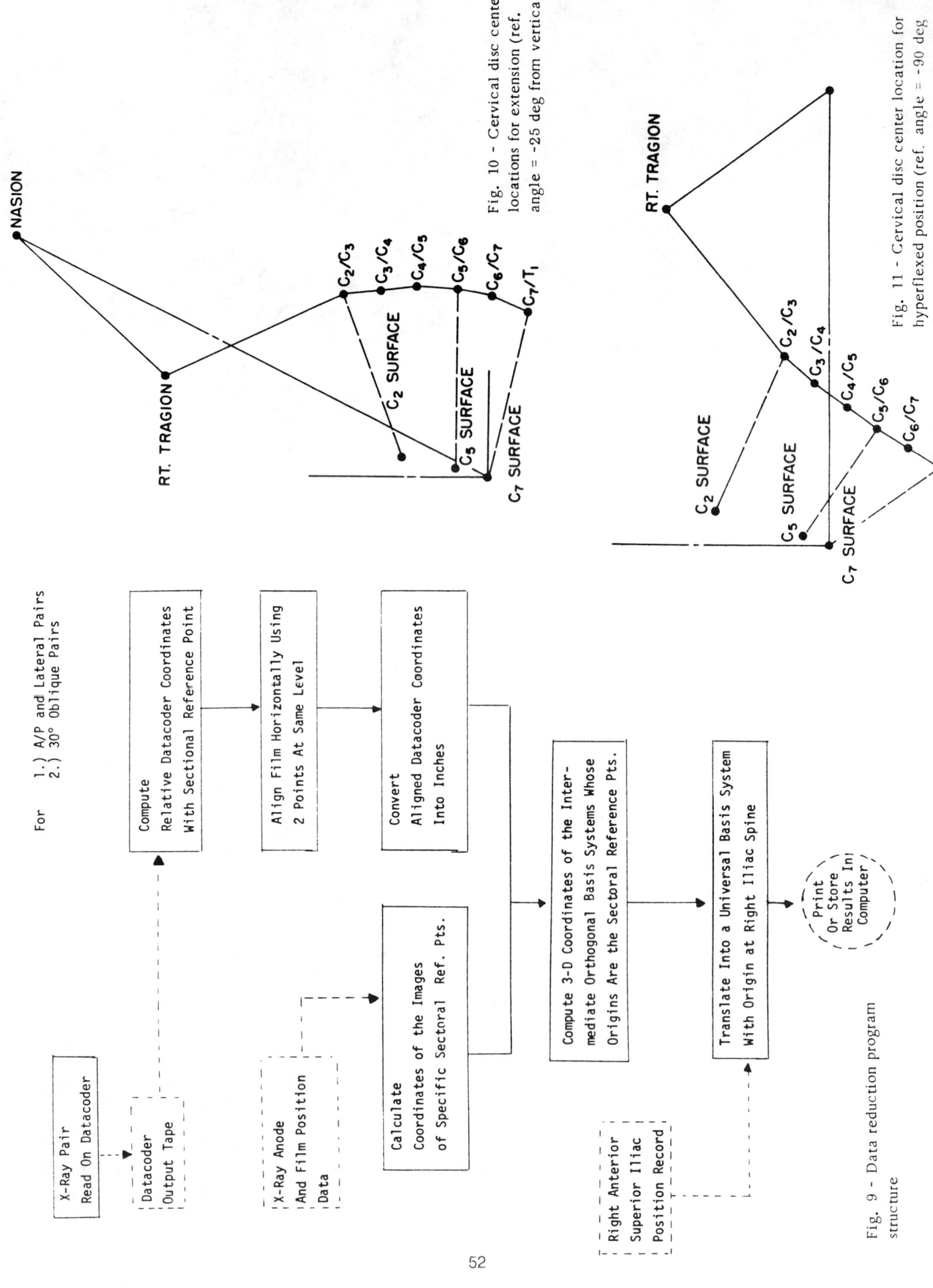

Fig. 10 - Cervical disc center locations for extension (ref. angle = -25 deg from vertical)

Fig. 11 - Cervical disc center location for hyperflexed position (ref. angle = -90 deg from vertical)

Fig. 9 - Data reduction program structure

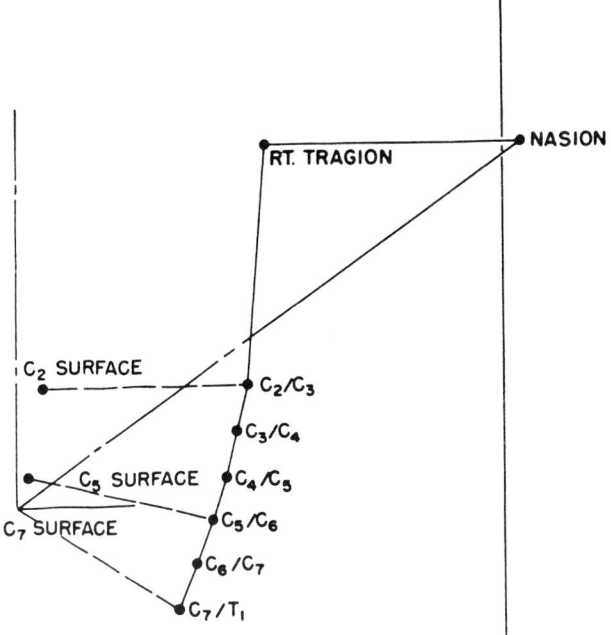

Fig. 12 - Cervical disc center locations for normal resting (ref. angle = -55 deg from vertical)

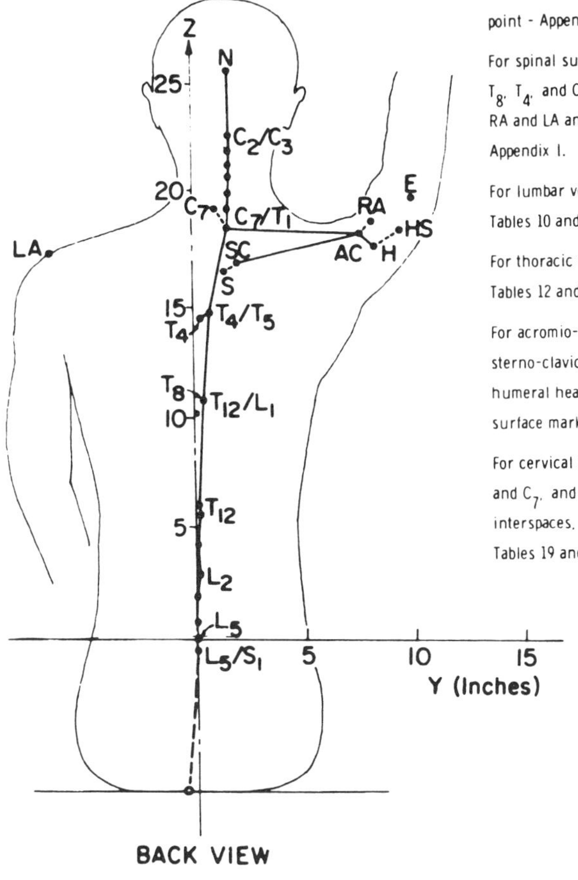

DATA FOR LOCATING REFERENCE POINTS ARE PRESENTED IN THE FOLLOWING:

For seat reference point to L_5 surface point - Appendix L

For spinal surface points L_5, L_2, T_{12}, T_8, T_4, and C_7 and for acromions RA and LA and suprasternales - Appendix I.

For lumbar vertebral interspaces - Tables 10 and 11.

For thoracic vertebral interspaces - Tables 12 and 13.

For acromio-clavicular junction AC, sterno-clavicular junction SC, humeral head center H, and humeral surface marker HS - Tables 14 and 15.

For cervical surface points C_2, C_5 and C_7, and cervical vertebral interspaces, and nasion N - Tables 19 and 20.

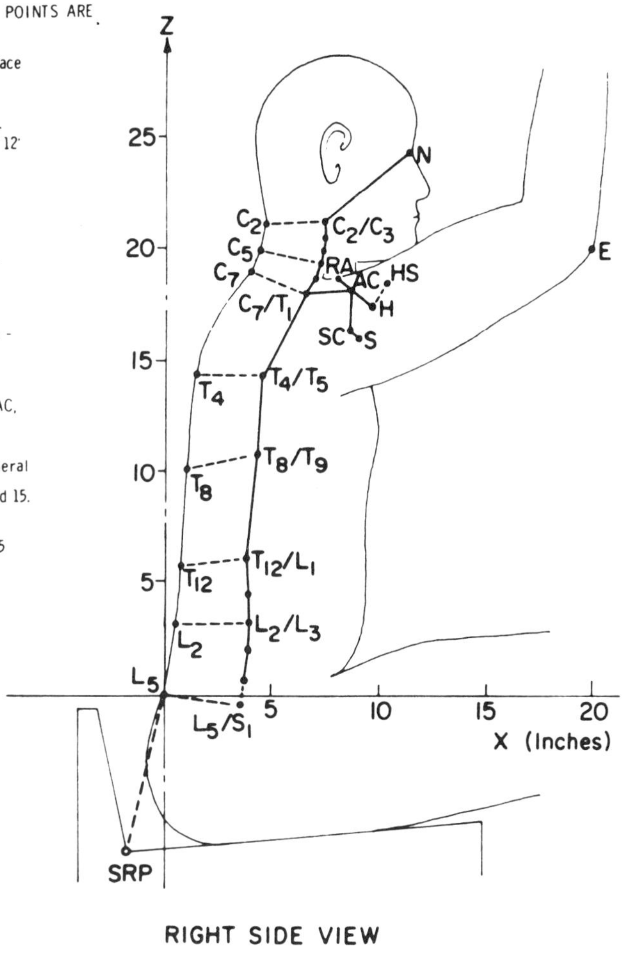

BACK VIEW

RIGHT SIDE VIEW

730413

Biomechanics of the Spine and Pelvis

A. I. King
Wayne State University

THE SPINAL COLUMN and the pelvis act as the major structural member of the human torso. Despite their great strength and ability to serve a variety of purposes, they form an intricately designed and delicate mechanical unit. During normal human activities, the spine is a column which is fixed in the pelvic ring and maintains the torso in an upright position. It carries the thoracic cage and serves as a post of anchorage for many powerful muscles which maintain the balance of the spine and perform all spinal movements. It also provides mechanical protection to the spinal cord which is encased within the vertebral column.

During dynamic function of the body the alternate elements of the spine, the bone and intervertebral discs, constitute a viscoelastic system which efficiently absorbs the innumerable jars and jolts associated with human locomotion. However, in an impact acceleration environment such as in the crash of an automobile or an aircraft, the spinal column and pelvis are called upon to sustain extremely high forces and moments to maintain the integrity of the human torso. In view of the large number of elements involved and the complexity of the anatomical structure, a thorough understanding of their biodynamic response to impact acceleration has not been achieved. Research work is in progress at several laboratories to delineate their functions during impact acceleration and to determine the major mechanisms of injury. Such information is essential to the establishment of tolerance limits of the spinal column and pelvis to impacts in several directions.

The bioengineering emphasis on the osseous and ligamentous structures of the spine and pelvis is not an attempt to ignore the significance of spinal cord injury but is, on the contrary, a recognition of the catastrophic finality of the resulting lesion to the spinal cord when the protective spinal column is traumatized.

ANATOMICAL REVIEW

The anatomical description of the vertebral column can be divided into three broad categories. The vertebral bony column and its attendant ligaments and muscles constitute the first group, which is referred to as the vertebral unit. The second category is composed of the spinal cord and its associated nerve roots and membranes, including the dura. This is the cord unit. The third category is the spinal vascular unit which comprises the vasculature of the spinal cord.

This review will concentrate on the vertebral unit which is the main structural member of the trunk. In addition, it provides protection for the spinal cord, one of the key components of the nervous system. The relationship of the vertebral column to the remainder of the skeleton is shown in Fig. 1.

The weight of the head, upper limbs, and rib cage and its contents are carried by the vertebral column. An examination of the location of these masses indicates that the center of gravity of the upper torso plus head and upper limbs should be anterior (forward) of the centerline of the column. Experimental determination of this center of gravity, as described by Vulcan (1)* confirms this fact.

The vertebrae which comprise the column are usually grouped as follows:

7 cervical (C1 to C7)
12 thoracic (T1 to T12)
5 lumbar (L1 to L5)
5 sacral—fused in the adult to form the sacrum
4 coccygeal—fused in later life to form the coccyx

These are illustrated in Fig. 2. The vertebrae of each group can usually be identified by special characteristics and individual vertebrae have distinguishing characteristics of their own.

The bodies of all vertebrae, except C1 and C2 are separated by a resilient, cartilagenous intervertebral disc. These discs represent approximately 1/4-1/5 of the total height of the vertebral column. They allow relative movement between

---

*Numbers in parentheses designate References at end of paper.

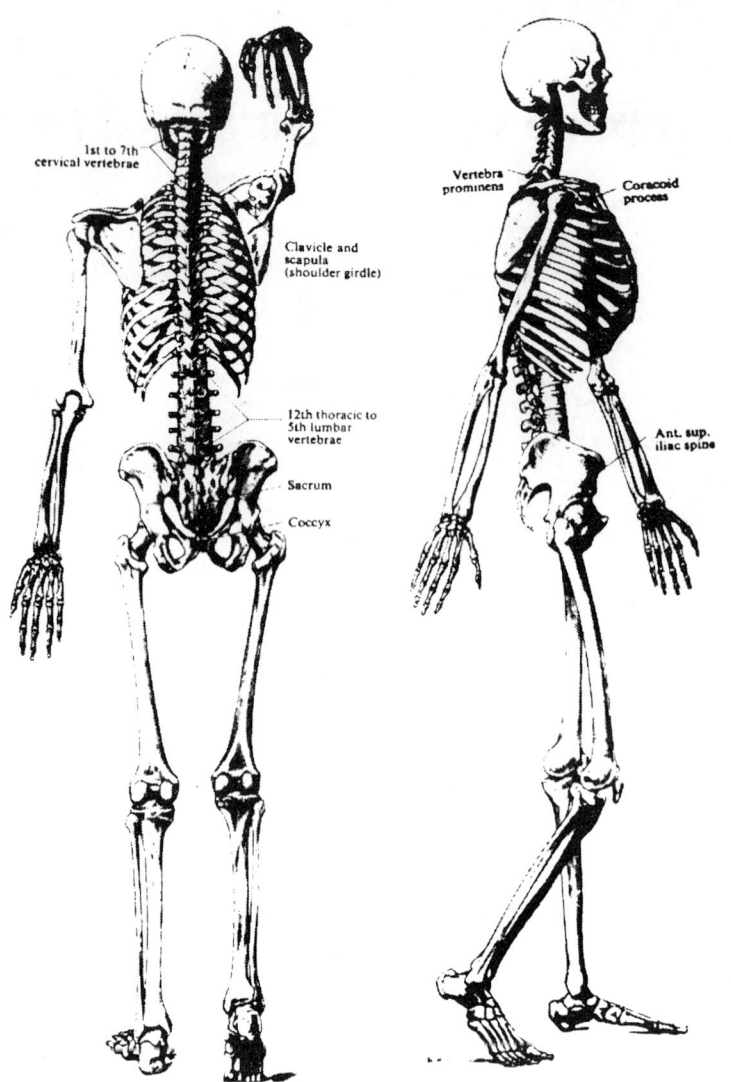

Fig. 1 - The skeleton: (left) posterior aspect (right) lateral aspect. Reproduced from R. D. Lockhart, G. F. Hamilton, and F. W. Fyfe, "Anatomy of the Human Body." Philadelphia: J. B. Lippincott Co., 1959 (with permission)

adjacent vertebrae, resulting in flexion (forward bending), extension (backward bending), and lateral flexion (sideway bending). A small amount of relative rotation (torsion about a vertical axis) is also possible. Under the action of axial forces, small relative movements in the axial direction occur, resulting in shortening or lengthening of the column. In each case, total motion is the summation of up to 23 individual small relative movements. The amount of relative movement varies according to the region. Thus, most flexion takes place in the lumbar and cervical regions, rather than in the thoracic region. Also, as shown in Fig. 2, the intervertebral discs in the lumbar region are considerably thicker than those in the thoracic regions, which should allow more relative axial movement in the lumbar than the thoracic region.

The stability of the column depends mainly upon the ligaments and muscles joining individual vertebrae. Further stability is provided by the shape of the column and its constituent parts.

The adult vertebral column has four curvatures in the midsagittal plane (a vertical plane parallel to the median plane which divides the body into left and right halves), the cervical, thoracic, lumbar, and sacral (Fig. 2). The thoracic and sacral curves are called primary because they are in the same direction (concave forward) as the vertebral column in the fetus. These curves are due to differences in height between the front and back of the vertebral bodies. The secondary curves, cervical and lumbar, are due mainly to differences in thickness between the anterior and posterior parts of the intervertebral discs. The secondary curvatures being concave rearward compensate for the primary curvatures and for a normal human, bring the centerline of C1 approximately over that of L5. Spinal curvature varies considerably between normal persons (Fig. 3) and also, of course, depends upon posture. Brinkley (2) has recorded this variation among different persons seated in two types of aircraft ejection seats.

Curvature of the vertebral column in the direction of primary curvature (concave anteriorly) is termed kyphosis, while that in the direction of secondary curvature (concave posteriorly) is termed lordosis. These terms are usually reserved for exaggerated curvature resulting from pathological conditions which are not considered in this paper.

Lateral curvature of the column (to the left or right) is termed scoliosis. Slight functional scoliosis may occur in the thoracic region and is attributed to inequality of muscle ac-

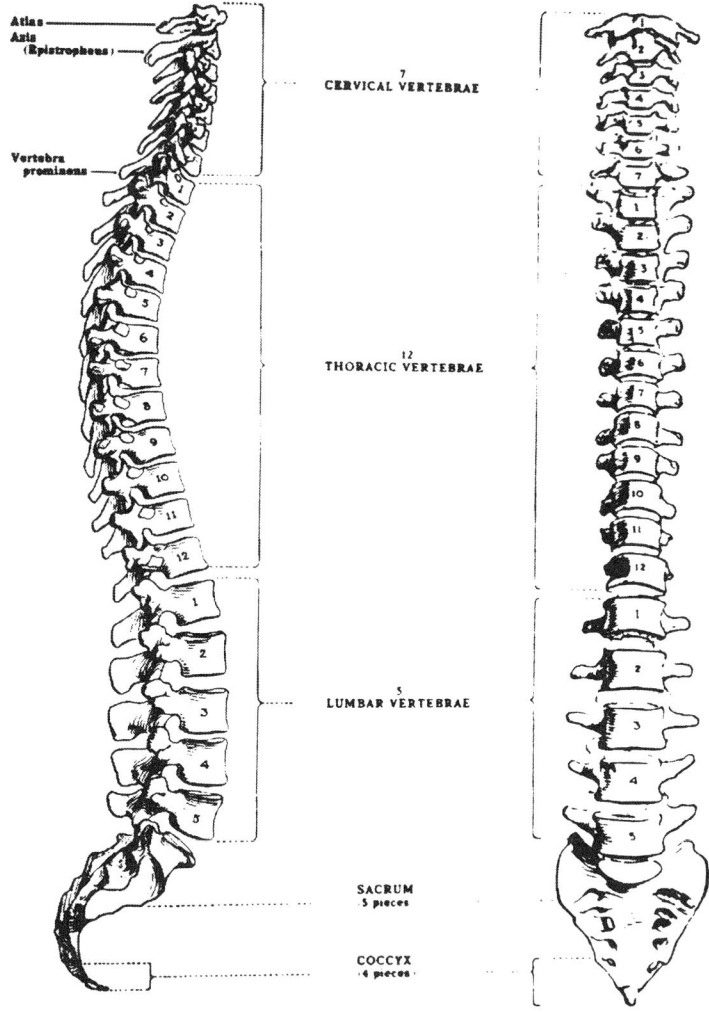

Fig. 2 - The vertebral column: (left) side view, (right) front view. Reproduced from J. C. Boileau Grant, "An Atlas of Anatomy." Baltimore: Williams & Wilkins Co., 1962 (with permission)

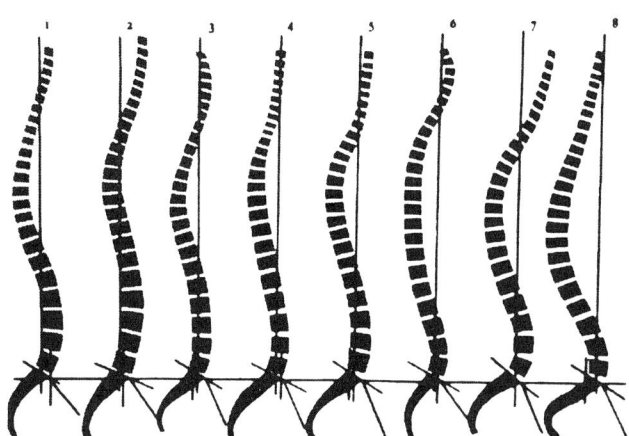

Fig. 3 - Eight normal vertebral columns. Reproduced from W. Spalteholz and R. Spanner, "Atlas of Human Anatomy." Philadelphia. 1967 (with permission)

tions in walking, or perhaps to differences in weight between the two halves of the body. More severe structural scoliosis resulting from pathological conditions will not be considered here.

The weight of the vertebral column and the structures supported by it is transferred to the ilium (the upper portion of the hip bone) at each sacroiliac joint. This is a synovial joint, though there is usually little movement here. When the human is standing, the weight is then transferred at each hip joint to the femur and hence down the lower limb to the ground. When seated the weight is transferred by the hip bone, via the ischial tuberosities, through a comparatively thin layer of gluteal muscle and skin to the seat. During caudocephalad acceleration of the seated human, upward forces are transferred along the same path but in the opposite direction.

Some further details of the structure of the vertebral column, with emphasis on the lumbar and lower thoracic regions, which are the main areas of interest, will now be given. A typical vertebra consists of a body, a vertebral arch, and several processes to which muscles and ligaments are attached. It is considered that the body of the vertebra is the part which gives strength and carries most of the compressive force transmitted by the column. The body consists of spongy bone that contains red marrow and is surrounded by a thin layer of compact bone. The compact bone is very thin on upper and lower surfaces of the body except at the margins, which in the adult are raised by fusion to them of the ring epiphysis. Usually there is

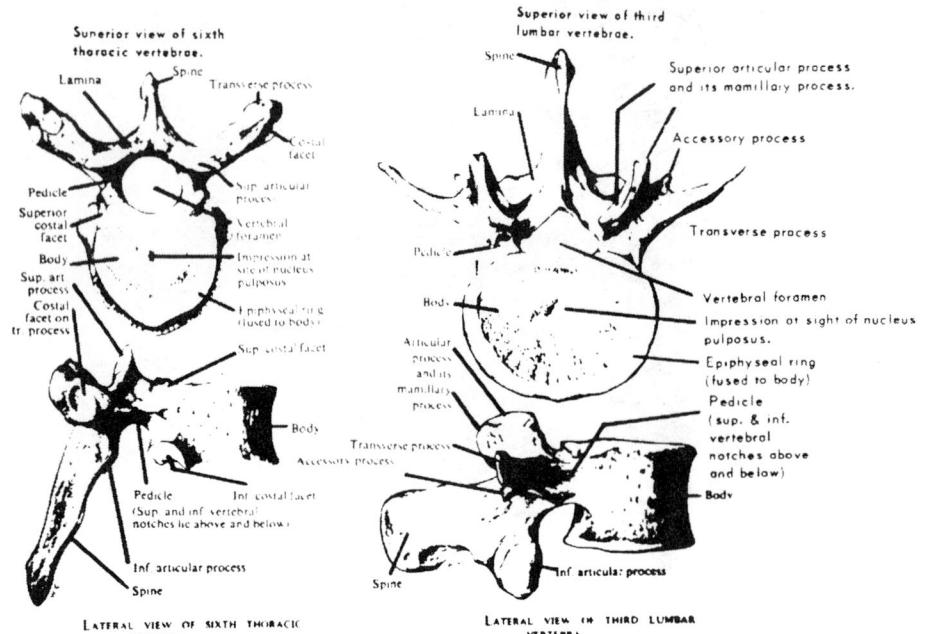

Fig. 4 - Typical thoracic and lumbar vertebra. Reproduced from Lockhart et al., see Fig. 1 (with permission)

a gradual increase in size and a change in shape of each body as one proceeds down the column. This may be seen in Fig. 2. Fig. 4 shows a typical thoracic and a typical lumbar vertebra.

Posterior to the body is the vertebral arch, which, with the posterior surface of the body, forms the walls of the vertebral foramen (foramen—a passage or opening). These walls enclose and protect the spinal cord. The vertebral arch is composed of right and left pedicles and right and left laminae. A spinous process extends backward from each vertebral arch, at the junction of the two laminae. Transverse processes project on either side from the junction of the pedicle and the lamina. A deep notch is present on the lower edge of each pedicle and a shallow notch on its upper edge. Two adjacent notches, together with the intervening body and intervertebral disc form an intervertebral foramen, through which a spinal nerve and its vessels pass. Thus, large deformation of the intervertebral disc would cause a reduction in the size of the intervertebral foramen, possible accompanied by compression of the spinal nerve.

There are also superior and inferior articular processes bearing articular facets on each side of the vertebral arch. The joint between the superior articular process of one vertebra and the inferior articular process of the vertebra immediately above it is the only place, apart from the intervertebral disc where significant compressive forces could be transmitted between vertebrae. This joint is a plane synovial joint that allows gliding between the articular facets. As this joint lies almost in a vertical plane for the lumbar and lower thoracic regions (Fig. 5), it is often assumed that only small vertical compressive forces can be transmitted by it. That is, almost all of the compressive force transmitted by the vertebral column must be carried by the body of each vertebra and be transmitted by the intervertebral disc. As will be discussed later, this assumption is questionable and recent data show that both compressive and tensile forces can be transmitted by the facets.

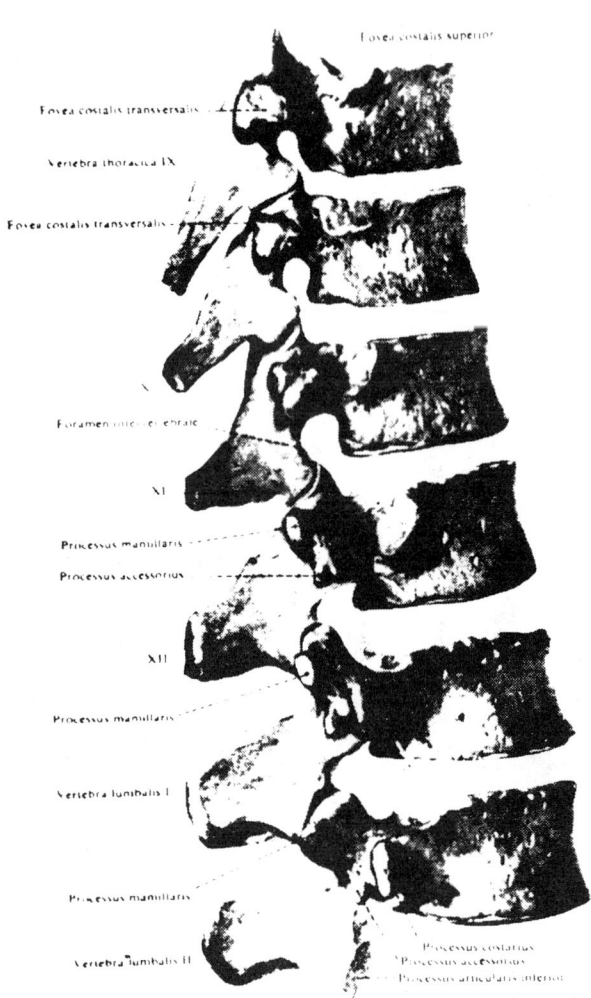

Fig. 5 - Inferior thoracic and lumbar vertebrae. Reproduced form W. Spalteholtz, see Fig. 3 (with permission)

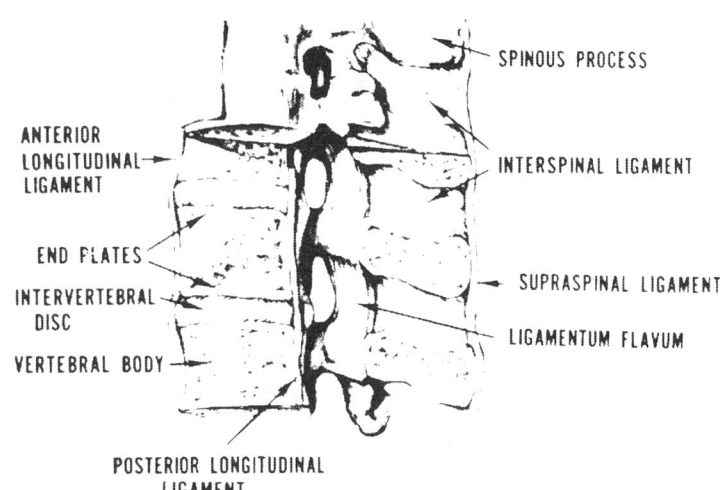

Fig. 6 - Anatomy of intervertebral stabilization. Reproduced from L. E. Kazarin, H. E. von Gierke, G. C. Mohr, 6570th Aerospace Med. Res. Labs., WPAFB Ohio, "Anatomy of Intervertebral Stabilization, Mechanics of Vertebral Body Injury As a Result of G_z Spinal Impact" (with permission)

There are numerous differences between the shape of a typical thoracic and lumbar vertebra, as illustrated in Fig. 4. For example, the lumbar vertebra has thicker pedicles and laminae, the spinous process is more solid and extends horizontally backward, whereas the longer, more slender thoracic spinous process extends downward considerably further. However, the main structural difference is that each of the 12 thoracic vertebrae usually carry a pair of ribs, attached at the costovertebral joint. This joint consists of two synovial joints, one between the tubercle of the rib and the costal facet on the transverse process of the vertebra, the other formed by the head of the rib and the superior costal facet of that vertebra together with the inferior costal facet of the vertebra above plus the intervertebral disc. A number of ligaments strengthen this joint. The weight of the thoracic cage and upper limbs causes both a vertical force and a bending moment (tending to cause flexion) to be exerted on each vertebra from T1 down to T10. This applies to a lesser extent at T11 and T12 because the ribs attached to these vertebrae are "floating," that is, they are not attached to the sternum at the front.

As has already been stated, the intervertebral disc forms a fibrocartilagenous joint between the bodies of adjacent vertebrae, except between C1 and C2. The structure and arrangement of the disc varies with age. In a young adult, it consists of two hyaline cartilage plates, the nucleus pulposus and the annulus fibrosus.

The thin hyaline cartilage plates cover the upper and lower aspects of the vertebral body. The nucleus pulposus, which occupies the center of the disc, contains five bundles of collagenous fibers, connective tissue cells, cartilage cells, and much amorphous cellular material. It behaves like a fluid and is held in shape by the hyaline cartilage plates and the annulus fibrosus. The nucleus pulposus often degenerates with age. The annulus fibrosus consists of a series of lamellae of collagenous bundles, arranged spirally. Above and below, the fibers of the annulus are anchored to the ring epiphysis and to the margins of the hyaline plates. The outermost fibers of the annulus blend with the anterior and posterior longitudinal ligaments.

The bodies and processes of adjacent vertebrae are joined by a number of ligaments which will now be described. The anterior longitudinal ligament runs from the base of the skull along the front of the vertebral bodies to the sacrum, increasing in thickness and width as it descends. If fuses with the anterior margins of each vertebral body and also the annulus fibrosus of the discs, as seen in Figs. 6 and 7.

The posterior longitudinal ligament lies within the vertebral canal, on posterior aspects of the vertebral bodies and the intervertebral discs. Above it is continuous with the membrane tectoria, which is attached to the occipital bone (of the skull). Below it enters the sacral canal. This ligament narrows behind each vertebral body, being only loosely attached to its posterior aspect, but widens at the intervertebral disc and fuses with the posterior aspect of each annulus fibrosus. It may be seen in Figs. 6-8.

At the rear surface of the vertebral canal, the laminae of each vertebra are connected to those of the adjacent vertebra by the left and right ligamenta flava (Fig. 7). The intertransverse ligaments connect adjacent transverse processes, and again are only well developed in the lumbar region. The tips of the spinous processes are connected by the supraspinous ligament which runs the full length of the column. Both of these ligaments may be seen in Fig. 6.

In the living human, the muscles of the back are important in controlling extension and flexion of the vertebral column and in the maintenance of posture in a "1 g environment." However, during impact acceleration, the effectiveness of muscular response is unknown. Although large muscular forces are usually present, it is not known whether they are developed in sufficient time and in the appropriate directions to provide the vertebral column with added stability. Thus, a discussion of the muscles of the back will not be made here.

The pelvis is formed by the sacrum (and coccyx) and the two hip bones, which are attached to the sacrum posteriorly via the sacroiliac joint described previously, and are joined to each other anteriorly at the pubic symphysis, as shown in Fig. 9. Each hip bone has three components, the ilium, the ischium, and the pubis. The ilium is fan-like and splays up-

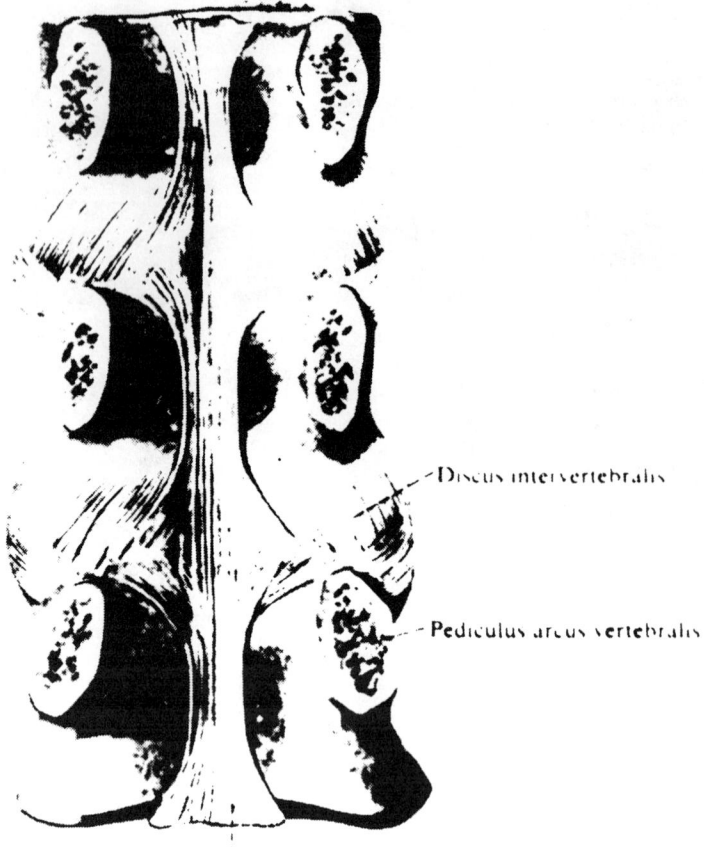

Fig. 7 - Ligamenta flava in lower thoracic region. Reproduced from Lockhart, et al., see Fig. 1 (with permission)

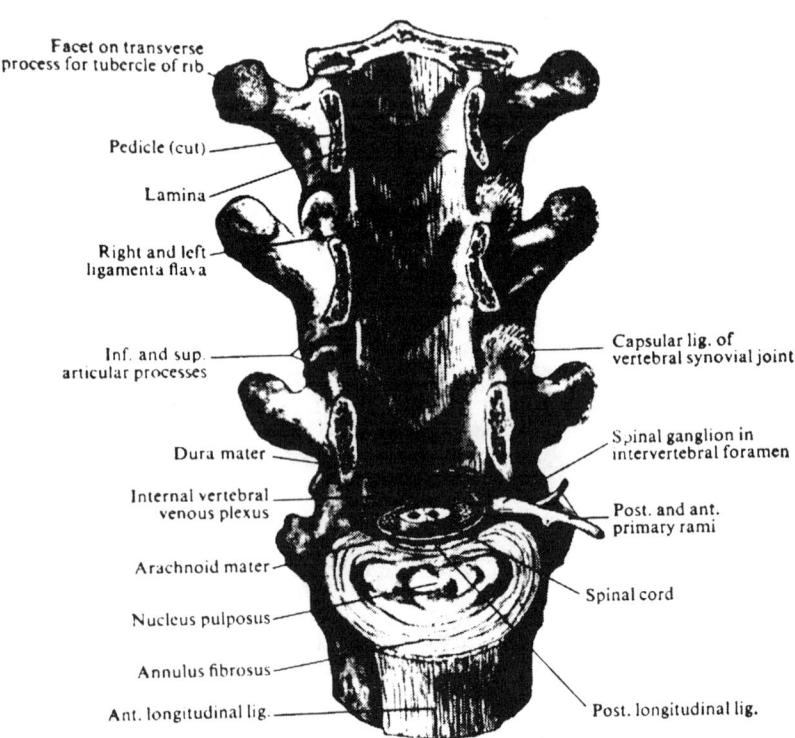

Fig. 8 - Posterior longitundinal ligament of vertebral column, lumbar region, posterior aspect. Reproduced from W. Spalteholtz, see Fig. 3 (with permission)

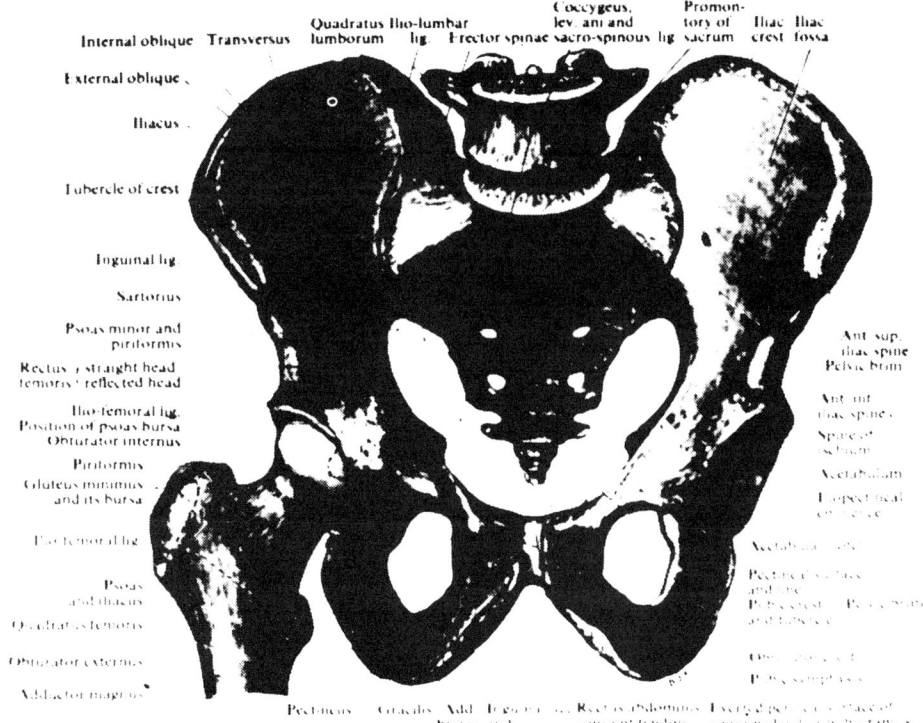

Fig. 9 - Anterior view of pelvis. Reproduced from Lockhart et al., see Fig. 1 (with permission)

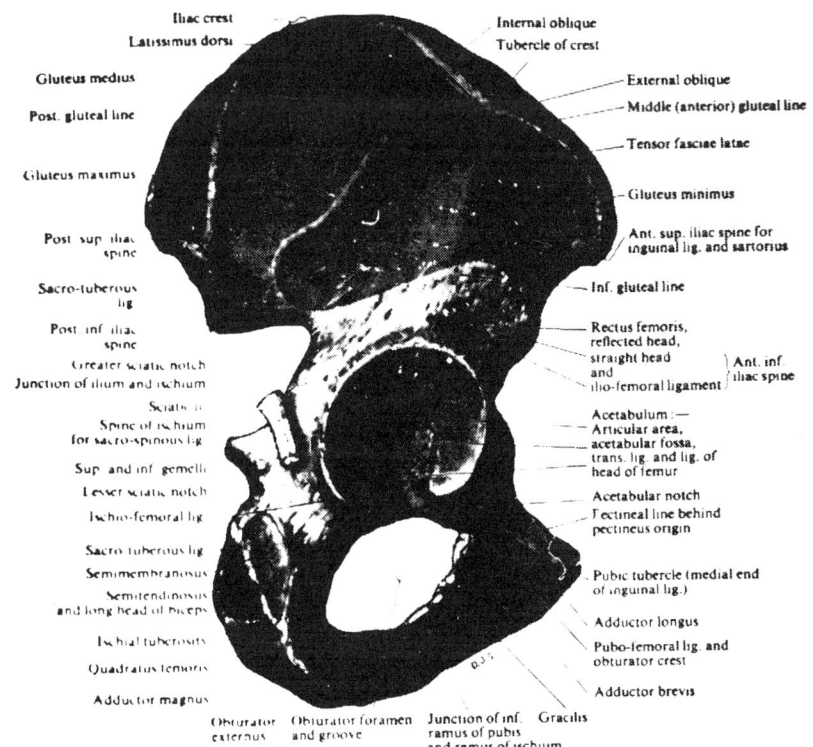

Fig. 10 - Lateral aspect of hip bone. Reproduced from Lockhart et al., see Fig. 1 (with permission)

ward, while the pubis in front and the ischium behind form the lower portion of the pelvic cavity and enclose an oval aperture called the obturator foramen. Fig. 10 is a lateral view of the hip bone showing the three parts, each of which contribute to the formation of the acetabulum through which the body weight of a standing individual is transmitted to the lower limbs via the femoral head. The acetabulum and the head of the femur form a ball-and-socket joint which is surrounded by many ligaments and allows the femur great freedom of motion.

The anterior superior iliac spine shown in Fig. 9 provides the best bearing surface for the lap belt, since it is the strongest structure in the anterior abdominal region. Also, for a seated individual the body weight borne by the chair is transmitted to the latter via the ischial tuberosities which are directly below the obturator foramen. (See Fig. 10.) It can be seen that the bony pelvis is a strong shell-like structure which carries the body weight in either the standing or sitting position. Collapse of the shell is prevented by strong ligaments among the three components of the hip bone, among the hip bones, the sacrum, the coccyx, and the lower lumbar vertebrae.

SUMMARY OF RESEARCH DATA

CAUDOCEPHALAD ACCELERATION ($+G_z$) - A considerable amount of experimental and theoretical work in the area of spinal injury due to impact acceleration has been carried out in the past 30 years. One of the principal reasons for continuing interest is the relatively high incidence of vertebral fracture during emergency egress from disabled aircraft. The results, however, are valid for other impact situations, such as helicopter and light aircraft crashes, and certain types of falls. A major goal in the study of the effects of caudocephalad acceleration on the vertebral column is the understanding of the mechanism of injury, after which it would be possible to establish tolerance limits for humans.

Experimental studies on the strength of the vertebral column can be generally classified under four different headings. They involve research work using human volunteers, animals such as subhuman primates, intact human cadavers, and fresh or embalmed segments of the human spine. It is interesting to note that humans were the first test subjects. Glaister (3) described some of the early tests on ejection seats carried out by the German Luftwaffe during World War II. Incidence of vertebral fracture was high due to the inconsistent use of restraint harnesses. Tests conducted by the British on the Martin-Baker seat were also described by Glaister (3). Painful flexion of the neck was observed and the introduction of a face blind, as a means of firing the seat, proved to be an effective way to restrain forward movement of the head. In the United States, Watts et al. (4) carried out tests on an ejection tower using a number of different catapults. The volunteers were all restrained by a lap belt and shoulder harness. They found the face curtain to be effective in preventing the extreme forward flexion of the head and shoulders which was otherwise encountered. Eiband (5) has reproduced 22 frames of high-speed motion pictures from another report by Watts et al. (6) showing this violent forward rotation of the head.

Tests on human vertebral segments were first carried out by Ruff (7) in 1940. He obtained static breaking strength of fresh vertebrae under uniaxial compression. Numerous investigators have since extended the work to combined axial and bending tests, dynamic studies on vertebrae and discs, measurement of intradiscal pressure, and fatigue of vertebral segments. A complete survey of this area of investigation would be beyond the scope of this paper, but the work of Perey (8), Brown et al. (9), Evans and Lissner (10), Roaf (11), Hirsch (12), Nachemson (13), and Crocker and Higgins (14) are referenced. It is quite apparent from these papers that the effects on nonaxial loading were felt to be important, but there was no quantitative correlation with the bending effects in the intact vertebral column of a seated human.

Experiments using intact cadavers were carried out at Wayne State University by Patrick (15), Evans et al. (16), Hodgson et al. (17), Vulcan and King (18, 19) and Ewing et al. (20).

Recently, animal studies have been performed at Wright-Patterson Air Force Base by Kazarian et al. (21) on soft tissue injury. Subhuman primates were subjected to caudocephalad acceleration, and it was possible to observe and associate spinal injuries with those of the thoracic and abdominal organs, resulting from caudocephalad acceleration. Interpretation of the data is somewhat hampered by the unknown scaling laws between humans and subhuman primates, and by the anatomical differences between the species.

The effects of jerk and seat cushions were studied by Hodgson et al. (17). It was found that the ratio of the peak to the mean strain increased with jerk up to a certain magnitude, beyond which the ratio was independent of jerk. The use of seat cushions produced undesirably high strain peaks, particularly when the cushion bottomed out. This result is consistent with the findings of Bondurant (22).

The effects of bending on the vertebral column during caudocephalad acceleration were first reported by King and Vulcan (18) and subsequently in greater detail by Vulcan et al. (19). Forward rotation of the head was observed during pilot ejection as reported by Eiband (5), who also reproduced a roentgenogram showing an anterior wedge fracture "resulting from flexion of the vertebral column during headward acceleration." Crocker and Higgins (14) showed photographs and radiographs of an ejection fracture of L1 which was also of the anterior wedge compression type. Ewing et al. (20) also report this predominance of anterior wedge fractures in 80 ejection vertebral fracture cases. From anatomical considerations, the weight of the chest wall, the thoracic contents, and part of the arm and shoulder complex exert a bending moment on the spine via the rib cage. The eccentricity of this load is magnified by caudocephalad acceleration as forward flexion of the torso takes place.

In view of these considerations, it was postulated that fracture resulted from the combined action of bending and axial compression. To determine whether bending strains were significant or not, a series of runs were carried out on eight cadavers which were fully restrained and extensively instrumented with strain gages. The head was allowed to rotate forward in most of the runs, but it was restrained in some cases to reproduce earlier results. Strain gages were installed on the anterior and lateral aspects of the lumbar and lower thoracic vertebrae. A complete description of the experimental procedure is given by Vulcan (1). A typical oscillograph tracing of the strain data is shown in Fig. 11. The anterior gages are denoted by the letter A and the lateral gages by the letter D or V.

The vertebral strain show two peaks instead of one, when

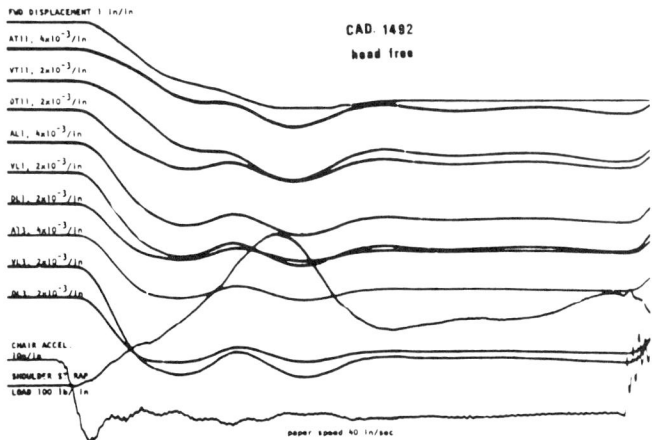

Fig. 11 - Typical oscillograph tracing of vertebral strain data (Vulcan, et al., Ref. 19)

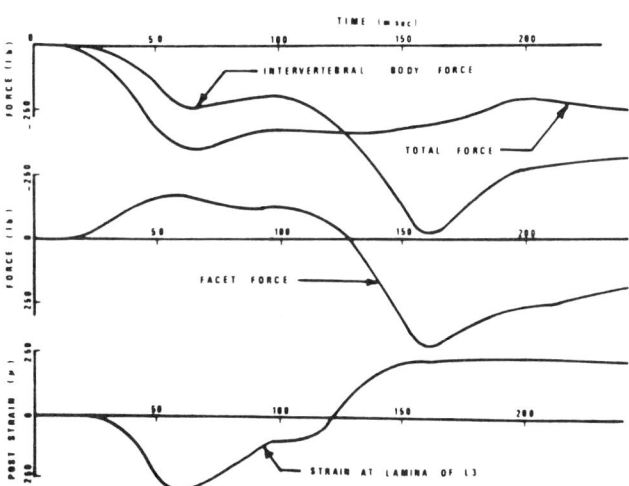

Fig. 12 - Measured Intervertebral forces and strain

the head was unrestrained. In general, the magnitude of the second peak is larger than the first and this difference is more pronounced for the anterior gages than that of the lateral gages. Since anterior gages are more sensitive to bending, while the lateral gages indicate mainly axial compression, it follows that the second peak results from an increase in bending, moment rather than merely an increase in axial force. It should also be noted that the second peak occurs at approximately the same instant as the head and torso reach their maximum forward position. This confirms the postulate that the increase in bending moment is caused by forward rotation of the head and torso.

It was also shown by King and Vulcan (23) that the observed differences in the strain data, such as those between the first and second peaks and those between the head free and head tied back cases, are statistically significant ($p \leq 0.05$).

In a further study by Ewing et al. (20), the restraint system was utilized to raise the acceleration level necessary to cause fracture. The bending hypothesis and the theory that the articular facets can possibly carry axial load were the basis for this study. By moderately hyperextending the lumbar spine, the average fracture level for cadavers was raised from 10.4 ± 3.79 g to 17.75 ± 5.55 g, with a confidence level of better than 95% (20). The age of the cadavers used averaged about 60 years and since the strength of vertebrae in the second decade of life is twice that in the sixth (24), the projected fracture level can be raised from roughly 20 to 36 g.

Thus, tolerance limits for the spine are highly dependent on the restraint system used and Eiband's curve (5) is a simplified representation of a complex problem. The use of a severity index to denote tolerance is also unsatisfactory. Stech (25) proposed such an index in 1963. It is called the Dynamic Response Index (DRI), and is based on Payne's model (26), which was simply the base-excitation problem of a single degree-of-freedom spring-mass system. A linear single degree-of-freedom system can have a dynamic overshoot but ignores the bending phenomenon which plays a dominant role in causing vertebral fracture. Physically, DRI is the ratio of the force in the spine to the body weight. For a simple base-excitation model, this force is proportional to the acceleration of the mass, which can exceed the input acceleration by a factor equal to the dynamic overshoot. Thus, the DRI is an acceleration tolerance value in g's which accounts for the overshoot. The recommended peak DRI for 5% probability of injury is 18. If the overshoot is 50%, the allowable input acceleration is 12 g. For low rates of onset, there is minimal overshoot and the limit becomes 18 g. This is, for a given input g-level, the DRI is solely a function of the rate of onset of the input acceleration pulse. Vulcan's results (27) are not in agreement with this conclusion.

The role of the articular facets in the transmission of load was investigated further in a recent series of experimental runs using cadavers. An intervertebral load cell was fabricated to measure the axial force and its line of action with respect to the center of the load cell. It was inserted in the spine below L3 by removing the inferior part of L3 and the superior part of the L3-L4 disc. Strain gages were installed on both the anterior aspects of the bodies, as well as on the posterior surfaces of the laminae. The runs were carried out with the head free to rotate and the upper torso and pelvis restrained by a shoulder harness, lap belt, and inverted V-belt. Fig. 12 shows the results of a typical run. During $+G_z$ acceleration, the force transmitted by the vertebral bodies has a second peak higher than the first as a result of the unloading of the facets when the torso rotates forward. It is measured by the intervertebral load cell and is initially less than the total axial force. The load carried by the facets is the difference between the two curves. The zero cross-over point for the facet force corresponds with that of the posterior strain gage output.

Controlled experiments studying the dynamic response of the pelvis to $+G_z$ impact acceleration were conducted by Evans and Lissner (28). Two series of tests were conducted.

In the first series of tests, 22 pelves, 16 from embalmed dissecting room cadavers and 6 from fresh unembalmed bodies, were used. The age of the specimens were from individuals between 29 and 85 years of age.

The pelvis and lumbar spine were removed from the body and defleshed. In some specimens, the sacrospinal and the sacrotuberal ligaments were also removed, but in others they were preserved until ready for testing. The pelves from embalmed bodies were kept in embalming fluid and those from unembalmed bodies in a deep freezer.

The pelves were coated with stresscoat, a brittle strain sensitive lacquer. Each specimen was suspended over a 140 lb steel block and a force dynamically applied to the ischial tuberosities by burning the supporting string. The pelvis was dropped so that both ischial tuberosities struck the steel block simultaneously. The specimen was caught by hand on the rebound so that it struck the block just once. Because of the low magnitude of the energy used in the tests (33 to 112.5 in-lb), it was assumed that, for all intents and purposes, all the available kinetic energy of a test was expended in deforming and/or fracturing the pelvis. The amount of energy transferred from the specimen to the steel block and absorbed by it would be neglibible.

A minimum tensile strain pattern was produced in the embalmed pelvis of a white male 64 years of age with 103.4 in-lb of energy. An extensive strain pattern occurred in the embalmed pelvis of a 29-year-old Negro male with 60 in-lb of energy. An equally extensive strain pattern was produced in the unemblamed (fresh) pelvis of a 63-year-old Negro man with 90.2 in-lb of energy. No fractures were produced in the first series of tests.

In the second series of tests, eight almost intact bodies of persons 47-82 years of age were used to determine the effect of the mass of the head, the trunk, and the upper limbs on pelvic deformations and fractures. In these cadavers, all of which were embalmed, the lower limbs, pelvic musculature, and viscera were removed and the pelvis stresscoated.

The body was then suspended over the steel block and dropped as in the first test series. Care was taken so that the ischial tuberosities struck the block simultaneously and that no other part of the body contacted the block. In some specimens, 0.5 in of soft tissue (mainly gluteus maximus muscle and skin) was left under the ischial tuberosities to determine what effect this might have on the strain patterns produced in the pelves. The energy applied to the pelves ranged from a minimum of 200 in-lb to a maximum of 450 in-lb.

In the tests, 240 in-lb of energy produced a fracture of the right ischiopubic ramus near the acetabulum in the embalmed pelvis of a 79-year-old white man. No other fractures were produced with applications of 200-450 in-lb of energy. The latter amount of energy, applied to a specimen with some soft tissue under the ischial tuberosities, produced a minimal tensile strain (stresscoat) pattern, indicating that soft tissue is a very good energy absorbing material.

Fasola et al. (29) also conducted impact tests on human pelves. The unembalmed specimens were subjected to impacts from a weight that was dropped on to L3 or L4. A force of 830 lb was required to produce bilateral disjunction of the sacroiliac joint from failure of the bone at the point of attachment of the ligaments. The ligaments themselves were not ruptured.

In a second, completely intact specimen, a load of 7500 lb was required to produce a unilateral fracture of the superior pubic ramus and a fracture disjunction of the sacroiliac joint.

BODY REGION	INCIDENCE OF INJURY
HEAD AND NECK	104 — skull 33, facial area 32, neck 20, scalp 19
LOWER EXTREMITIES	74
UPPER EXTREMITIES	59
CHEST	39
ABDOMEN	21
PELVIS	20

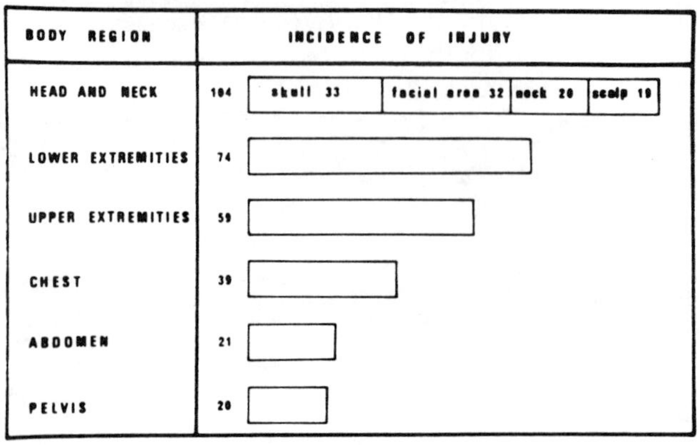

Fig. 13 - Frequency of injury to various regions of body in 1019 business aircraft crashes in 1965 (31)

The incidence of pelvic fractures during $+G_z$ acceleration was found to be low. Braunstein et al. (30) reported that only 3.2% of the 800 survivors of light plane crashes sustained pelvic injuries. In a study of 1019 business aircraft accidents during 1965, the FAA (31) reported that the frequency of pelvic injury was the lowest, as shown in Fig. 13.

FORWARD DECELERATION ($-G_x$) - There is very little research work concerned with the dynamic response of the thoracic and lumbar sping during $-G_x$ acceleration. This is not unusual since the loading on the spine is expected to be rather minimal in most cases involving automobile occupants. With the introduction of lap belts in cars, a vertebral injury commonly referred to as the seat belt syndrome has been reported by several authors. Dehner (32) made an excellent survey of the literature and cites over 20 references of original articles on seat belt trauma. Many of these papers discuss case reports of a variety of spinal injuries, which were generally restricted to the vertebrae L2 and L3. These vertebrae sustained anterior compression fractures, posterior tension fractures, fracture-dislocations, and Chance fractures which were first described by Chance (33) as a horizontal splitting and separation of the posterior vertebral arch, involving the lamina, the pedicles, and the transverse and spinous processes.

The injury is apparently due to extreme hyperflexion of the torso about the lap belt (34) and is thought to be more severe when the belt is improperly worn above the iliac crest (35).

Although recent statistics are not available, the study by Garrett and Braunstein (36) revealed that there were only 12 lumbar spine injuries out of a total of 944 injured occupants who were restrained by a lap belt. Perry and McClellan (37) reported in 1964 4 cases of spinal injury out of 64 automobile occupants who were autopsied.

Injuries attributable to the shoulder harness and lap belt combination were reported by Hamilton (38). The cervical-thoracic junction of the spine appeared to be vulnerable. However, Nelson (39) showed that as a result of the use of the lap-and-shoulder belt, the severity of the injury to the pelvis and the lumbar spine sustained by both the driver and front passenger was reduced when compared with lap belted or unrestrained occupants. That for the neck remained approximately the same for the lap belted and lap-and-shoulder belted occupants. This information was based on 160 cases of United States accidents. An earlier Swedish survey by Bohlin (40) also showed a decrease in injury severity to the spine and pelvis, but the sample size related to these body regions is small despite the large number of accidents investigated.

At present, a research program is underway at Wayne State University to determine the existence and cause of large axial forces generated in the spine during $-G_x$ acceleration. Cadavers, fully restrained by a military-type harness, are being used as test subjects.

Injuries to the pelvis as a result of $-G_x$ acceleration take on many forms as a result of different injury mechanism. Various components of the hip bone can be fractured due to high-velocity impact with hard surfaces. The acetabulum appears to be a common site for fractures and for fracture/dislocations involving the femoral head. For automobile occupants, these injuries can occur from impact of the knee against the instrument panel.

In 1957, Braunstein et al. (36) reported a 2.3% frequency of pelvic injury to 1678 persons involved in automobile accidents. Perry and McClellan (37) reported that there were 27 cases of pelvic and lower extremity injuries out of 64 autopsied patients who were automobile occupants while they sustained a variety of fatal injuries.

The various types of pelvic fractures have been categorized by Conolly et al. (41) based on 200 cases treated at Sydney Hospital in Australia. There were 109 major fractures which involve the line of weight transmission from the spine to the acetabulum or which involve the rami on both sides of the symphysis pubis. Remaining fractures were classified as minor. It was found that the fatality rate for major fractures was 1 in 3, while only 2 out of 91 with minor fractures died. The five major categories are fractures of the acetabulum, bilateral fractures of the pubic rami, fractures of the hemi-pelvis (multiple fractures), separation of the symphysis pubis, and isolated fractures of the sacrum. The associated injuries include retroperitoneal hemorrhage, injury to the abdominal and urinary organs, and to the central nervous system. Injury mechanisms were not described by the authors.

Levine and Crampton (42) reported on the results of a 10-year study of 425 cases of pelvic fractures (1952-1962). The etiology as related to the type of fracture sustained is shown in Table 1. It can be seen that fracture of the acetabulum was most frequent among the automobile occupants, presumably as a result of impact of the knees with the instrument panel. The authors also do not give any explanation of the injury mechanism, but describe the major complications that can arise from this injury.

A controlled experimental study was carried out by Patrick et al. (43). Intact human cadavers were seated on a car crash simulator and subjected to various levels of deceleration. The knees were made to impact against padded targets simulating the instrument panel. Among the 10 cadavers tested, the peak force on the right hip varied 950-3850 lb and that on the left was 1400-2650 lb.

Table 1 - Relationship of Etiology of Pelvic Fracture and Type of Fracture Sustained (42)

Type of Fracture	Automobile Driver	Automobile Passenger	Struck by Vehicle	Crush Injury	Full	Other	Total
One or more pubic rami	15	41	51	8	71	8	194
Acetabulum	36	10	4	2	8	3	63
Ischium	2	1	2	0	4	0	9
Pubic body	4	5	5	1	10	0	25
Ilium	2	0	6	7	0	1	16
Multiple fractures	24	26	44	7	16	1	118
Total	83	83	112	25	109	13	425

Fractures of the right hip were found to occur at 1400, 1900, 2550, and 3850 lb. Severe multiple fractures of the right hip were produced in one cadaver at 1900 lb, in another at 3850 lb, and in the third at 2550 lb. Fractures of the superior and inferior rami of the left pubis were caused by a force of 1600 lb and severe multiple fractures of the left hip with 2650 lb. A possible fracture of the superior ramus of the pubis was produced with a force of 1950 lb.

The authors also obtained voluntary tolerance force levels at the knee. Eight male volunteers, ranging in age 18-45 years, subjected their knees to maximum forces of 400-1050 lb without pain or injury. The authors concluded that a conservative estimate for tolerance of the knee-thigh-hip complex was 1400 lb.

DISCUSSION AND CONCLUSIONS

A brief survey of the existing knowledge on the impact biomechanics of the spine and pelvis has been made. It reveals that there is much to be learned before a complete understanding of all of the injury mechanisms can be achieved and accurate tolerance levels can be established. This paper does not discuss the effects of lateral impact, very little of which is known, nor does it consider the combined effects of $+G_z$ and $-G_x$ acceleration, or of other off-axis directions, of which even less is known. Snyder (44) made an extensive survey of the state-of-the-art on human impact tolerance and found very few references on these subjects.

In going through the clinical literature on spinal and pelvic injuries, it appears that injury to the two regions are equally severe but considerably more information concerning the spine is available. There is a need to do more work on the mechanisms of pelvic fractures, particularly in the protection of pedestrians. The hip bone is complex in terms of its geometry and bony structure. Nevertheless, it is the only load-bearing structure which usually supports all of the weight of the head and torso, whether the individual is seated or standing. A complete analysis of the problem will not only be challenging, but also be an extremely valuable contribution to our meager store of biomechanical knowledge.

A discussion of mathematical modeling of the spine and

pelvis was deliberately left out, not because models do not exist but rather because there are very few which have been validated. Such simulations, if validated, can provide valuable assistance to an analysis of an impact event and point to the areas in which further experimentation is required. Vulcan (1) made a substantive survey of existing spinal models prior to 1969 and more recent models can be found in a 1971 USAF publication (45). It is not known whether models of the pelvis have been proposed.

Based on our present knowledge of the spine, it can be seen that the dual load path through the vertebral bodies and the articular facets increases the difficulty in providing for its protection against $+G_z$ acceleration. At each level, the spinal curvature and eccentricity of the load carried by the vertebra must be carefully adjusted so that no excessive load is transmitted via either path. The use of a hyperextension device increases the acceleration level for fracture by transferring a portion of the inertial load to the posterior structures of the vertebral column. Whether an optimum transfer has been achieved is not known at this time.

Finally, it should be pointed out that in the search for methods of protection against various types of impact acceleration, it is essential that the solution of a specific problem does not create serious difficulties affecting other areas of the body. An awareness of the overall safety of the individual must be kept in mind in the design of restraint systems and protective environments.

REFERENCES

1. A. P. Vulcan, "Response of the Lower Vertebral Column to Caudocephalad Acceleration." Ph. D. dissertation, Wayne State University, 1969.

2. J. Brinkley, personal communication, 6570th Aerospace Medical Research Labs., Wright Patterson AFB, Ohio.

3. D. H. Glaister, "The Effects of Acceleration of Short Duration." A Textbook of Aviation Physiology (Ed., J. A. Fillies), Chap. 26, pp. 746-794. Oxford: Pergamon Press, 1965.

4. D. T. Watts, E. S. Mendelson, H. N. Hunter, A. T. Kornfield, and J. R. Poppen, "Tolerance to Vertical Acceleration Required for Seat Ejection." Aviation Med., Vol. 18 (1947), pp. 554-564, 616, 618.

5. A. M. Eiband, "Human Tolerance to Rapidly Applied Accelerations: A Summary of the Literature." NASA Memo. 5-59-59E, 1959.

6. D. T. Watts, E. S. Mendelson, and H. N. Hunter, "Evaluation of a Fact Curtain and Arm Rests for Use on Ejection Seats." TED No. NAM 256005, Rep. No. 4, Naval Air Material Command, 1947.

7. S. Ruff, "Brief Acceleration: Less than one second." German Aviation Med. World War II, Chap. VI-C, 1950.

8. O. Perey, "Fracture of the Vertebral End Plate in the Lumbar Spine." Acta Ortho. Scand., Suppl. 25, 1957.

9. T. Brown, R. J. Hansen, and A. J. Yorra, "Some Mechanical Tests on the Lumbosacral Spine with Particular Reference to the Intervertebral Discs." J. Bone Jt. Surg., 1957, pp. 1135-1164.

10. F. G. Evans, and H. R. Lissner, "Biomechanical Studies on the Lumbar Spine and Pelvis." J. Bone Jt. Surg., Vol. 41A (1959), pp. 278-290.

11. R. Roaf, "A Study of the Mechanics of Spinal Injuries." J. Bone Jt. Surg., Vol. 42B (1960), pp. 810-823.

12. C. Hirsch, "The Reaction of Intervertebral Discs to Compression Forces." J. Bone Jt. Surg., Vol. 37A (1955), pp. 1188-1196.

13. A. Nachemson, "The Load on Lumbar Discs in Different Positions of the Body." Clin. Orthop., Vol. 45 (1966), pp. 107-122.

14. J. F. Crocker and L. S. Higgins, "Phase IV–Investigation of Strength of Isolated Vertebrae." Final Technical Report, Contract No. NASW-1313, Technol. Inc., San Antonio, Texas, 1966.

15. L. M. Patrick, "Caudo-cephaled Static and Dynamic Injuries." Proc. of Fifth Stapp Automative Crash Conf. Minneapolis: Univ. of Minnesota, 1962.

16. F. G. Evans, H. R. Lissner, and L. M. Patrick, "Acceleration-induced Strains in the Intact Vertebral Column." J. Appl. Physiol., Vol. 17 (1962), pp. 405-409.

17. V. R. Hodgson, H. R. Lissner, and L. M. Patrick, "Response of the seated Human Cadaver to Acceleration and Jerk With and Without Seat Cushions." Hum. Factors, Vol. 6 (1963), pp. 505-523.

18. A. I. King, A. P. Vulcan, and L. K. Cheng, "Effects of Bending on the Vertebral Column of the Seated Human During Cuadocephalad Acceleration." Proc. of 21st Annual Conf. on Engineering in Med. and Biol., 1968.

19. A. P. Vulcan, A. I. King, and G. S. Nakamura, "Effects of Bending on the Vertebral Column During $+G_z$ Acceleration" Aerospace Med., Vol. 41 (1970), pp. 294-300.

20. C. L. Ewing, A. I. King, and P. Prasad, "Structural Considerations of the Human Vertebral Column Under $+G_z$ Impact Acceleration." J. of Trauma, Vol. 9, No. 1 (January 1972), pp. 84-90.

21. L. E. Kazarian, J. W. Hahn, and H. E. von Gierke, "Biomechanics of the Vertebral Column and Internal Organ Response to Seated Spinal Impact in the Rhesus Monkey (Macaca Mulatta)." Proc. of 14th Stapp Car Crash Conf., (p. 33), paper 700898. New York: Society of Automotive Engineers, Inc., 1970.

22. S. Bondurant, "Optimal Elastic Characteristics of Ejection Seat Cushions for Safety and Comfort." WADC Technical Note 58-260, ASTIA Doc. No. AD 203384, 1958.

23. A. I. King, and A. P. Vulcan, "Elastic Deformation Characteristics of the Spine." J. Biomechanics, Vol. 4 (1971) pp. 413-429.

24. J. McElhaney, and V. Roberts, "Mechanical Properties of Cancellous Bone." AIAA Paper 71-111, 1971.

25. E. L. Stech, "The Variability of Human Response to Acceleration in the Spinal Direction." Report No. 122-109, Frost Engineering Dev. Corp., Contract AF 33(657)-9514, 1963.

26. P. R. Payne, "The Dynamics of Human Restraint Systems." Impact Acceleration Stress, Publ. 977, NAS-NRC, 1962, pp. 195-257.

27. A. P. Vulcan, and A. I. King, "Forces and Moments Sustained by the Lower Vertebral Column of a Seated Human During Seat-to-Head Acceleration," "Dynamic Response of Biomechanical Systems," ASME, 1970, pp. 84-100.

28. F. G. Evans, and H. R. Lissner, "Studies on Pelvic Deformations and Fractures," Anat. Rec., Vol. 121 (1955), pp. 141-166.

29. A. F. Fasola, R. C. Baker, and F. A. Hitchcock, "Anatomical and Physiological Effects of Rapid Deceleration," WADC Tech. Report, Wright-Patterson Air Force Base, Ohio, 1955, pp. 54-218.

30. P. W. Braunstein, J. O. Moore, and P. A. Wade, "Preliminary Findings of the Effect of Automotive Safety Design on Injury Patterns," Surg. Gyn. & Obstet., Vol. 105 (1957), pp. 257-263.

31. U. S. Dept. of Transportation, Fed. Aviation Admin., "FAA Statistical Handbook of Aviation," 1968, p. 240.

32. J. R. Dehner, "Seat Belt Injuries of the Spine and Abdomen," Am. J. of Roentgenography, Radium Therapy and Nuclear Med., Vol. 3, No. 4 (April 1971), pp. 833-843.

33. G. Q. Chance, "Note on Type of Flexion Fracture of Spine," Brit. J. of Radiol., Vol. 21 (1948), pp. 452-453.

34. R. G. Snyder, et al., "Seat Belt Injuries in Impact," The Prevention of Highway Injury, Ed. M. L. Slezer, et al. Highway Safety Research Inst., Univ. of Michigan, 1967, pp. 188-210.

35. R. M. Steckler, J. A. Epstein, and B. S. Epstein, "Seat Belt Trauma to the Lumbar Spine: An Unusual Manifestation of the Seat Belt Syndrome," J. of Trauma Vol. 9 (1969), No. 6, pp. 508-513.

36. J. W. Garrett and P. W. Braunstein, "Seat Belt Syndrome," J. of Trauma, Vol. 2 (1962), pp. 220-237.

37. J. F. Perry, and R. J. McClellan, "Autopsy Findings in 127 Patients Following Fatal Traffic Accidents," Surg., Gynecology & Obstet., Vol. 119 (1964), pp. 586-590.

38. J. B. Hamilton, "Seat-belt Injuries," Brit. M. J. 1968, pp. 485-486.

39. W. D. Nelson, "Lap-Shoulder Restraint Effectiveness in the United States," Paper 710077 presented at SAE Automotive Engineering Congress, Detroit, January 1971.

40. N. I. Bohlin, "A Statistical Analysis of 28,000 Accident Cases with Emphasis on Occupant Restraint Value," SAE Transactions, Vol. 76, paper 670925.

41. W. B. Conolly and E. A. Hedberg, "Observations on Fractures of the Pelvis," J. of Trauma, Vol. 9(2) (1969), pp. 104-111.

42. J. I. Levine and R. S. Crampton, "Major Abdominal Associated with Pelvic Fractures," Surg., Gyn. & Obstet., February 1963.

43. L. M. Patrick, C. K. Kroell, and H. J. Mertz, Jr., "Forces on the Human Body in Simulated Crashes," Proc. of 9th Stapp Car Crash Conf., Minneapolis: Univ. of Minn., 1966.

44. R. G. Snyder, "Human Impact Tolerance," SAE Transactions, Vol. 79 (1970), paper 700398.

45. Symposium on Biodynamic Models and Their Applications, AMRL-TR-71-29, Aerospace Med. Res. Lab., Aerospace Med. Div., Air Force Systems Com. WPAFB, Ohio 45433, December 1971.

Section 2:
Biomechanics, Impact Response and Trauma Assessed with Volunteers, Cadavers, Animal, and Mechanical Surrogates in Frontal Impacts

720974

Impact Tolerance and Resulting Injury Patterns in the Baboon: Air Force Shoulder Harness—Lap Belt Restraint

Thomas D. Clarke, David C. Smedley, William H. Muzzy, C. Dee Gragg, Robert E. Schmidt, and Edwin M. Trout
6570th Aerospace Medical Research Laboratory

CRASH SAFETY EXPERTS have long advocated the efficacy of occupant restraints for automobiles and aircraft. Although the lap belt can significantly reduce the incidence of impact fatalities by preventing ejection from the vehicle, this restraint cannot always eliminate lethal head contact with the relatively nonyielding windshield or instrument panel (1).*

Note: The research reported in this paper was conducted by personnel of the Aerospace Medical Research Laboratory, Wright-Patterson Air Force Base, Ohio. This paper has been identified by the Aerospace Medical Research Laboratory as AMRL-TR-72-74. Further reproduction is authorized to satisfy needs of the U.S. Government.

The experiments reported herein were conducted according to the "Guide for Laboratory Animals Facilities and Care," 1965, prepared by the Committee on the Guide for Laboratory Animal Resources, National Academy of Sciences–National Research Council.

*Numbers in parentheses designate References at end of paper.

ABSTRACT

The tolerance to abrupt linear deceleration ($-G_x$) and impact trauma patterns resulting from the use of the Air Force shoulder harness-lap belt restraint were investigated. Eighty-nine deceleration tests were performed with 37 adult male baboons. Peak sled decelerations ranged from 6.5-134 g. The stopping distance varied from 0.5-3.5 ft at 6 in increments.

LD_{50}s were calculated to be 102, 103, and 98 g for the 0.5, 2.0, and 3.5 ft stopping distances, respectively. Since the deceleration pulses were similar, the results imply that for the exposure range of these tests, impact lethality is dependent upon magnitude of peak sled deceleration, irrespective of the pulse duration, sled velocity, or stopping distance.

At all stopping distances, the primary cause of death was lower brainstem or cervical spinal cord trauma. The pelvic, abdominal, and thoracic injury patterns were significantly different at the various stopping distances. Animals impacted at the 0.5 ft stop typically displayed no significant injuries other than head-neck trauma. The predominant injuries at the 2.0 ft stop included pelvic and abdominal myorrhexis, intestinal herniation, urinary bladder rupture, and pelvic fractures in addition to luxation of cervical through thoracic vertebrae. At the 3.5 stop animals received extensive muscular and skeletal injuries of the pelvic, abdominal, and thoracic regions. Brainstem hemorrhage was a significant finding, but there was no evidence of luxation or fractures of cervical vertebrae.

Since World War II, military aviators have used a restraint consisting of a lap belt incorporated with a torso harness. This system not only reduces torso and head contact with the cockpit interior under survivable crash conditions, but also securely restrains the aviator during routine flight or combat maneuvers. The principal function of the harness is the prevention of torso hyperflexion during impact (2); the capability of pilots to tolerate greater decelerative force is secondary.

In 1952, relying upon accident-injury reports of single-engine aircraft crashes, De Haven showed that fatal or nonfatal injuries occurred six times more frequently when shoulder harness restraints were not used (3). This important and pioneering monograph contributed significantly to the adoption of the shoulder harness-lap belt restraint in private and commercial aircraft. Likewise, more recent articles have contributed to the mandatory installation of shoulder belt restraints in all production automobiles (4, 5).

Although many investigators are pursuing the course of dynamic response analysis of safety harnesses (6, 7), the protective effectiveness of the shoulder harness-lap belt restraint remains incompletely documented. Snyder's comprehensive restraint evaluation included only one impact test (34 lb baboon at 20 g) with a full torso harness (8). Numerous dummy and human tests (9-13) have documented the loading characteristics of the harness system by emphasizing its beneficial distribution of force to the torso and pelvis. However, in most tests, the peak vehicle decelerations were far below the maximum capability or potential of the restraint. Limited information can be garnered from aviation pathology reports since many accidents are catastrophic with massive disruption of cockpit integrity. Furthermore, only fragmentary data can be gathered from automobile accident reports because of the dismaying public apathy or, indeed, rejection of shoulder belt usage.

In a recent report, the protective capabilities of the Air Force shoulder harness-lap belt were compared with the lap belt only and the airbag plus lap belt in controlled animal experiments (14). Although the safety potential of the harness at excessive decelerations is less than that of the airbag for a frontal impact (14), the superior cost effectiveness and sensibility of the harness restraint dictate the need for its further evaluation.

Using baboons, the principal objectives of this study were to determine tolerance limits at various stopping distances during exposure to abrupt linear deceleration ($-G_x$) and to investigate impact trauma patterns resulting from the use of the Air Force shoulder harness-lap belt restraint.

MATERIALS AND METHODS

Eighty-nine deceleration tests were performed with 37 adult male baboons *(Papio anubis)* weighing 43-58 lb (20-26 kg). The LC_{50} was the sled deceleration level where impact fatalities were expected in 50% of the animals. The tolerance to impact (LD_{50}) was determined by sequential testing: each successive baboon was impacted at a 10 g increment below or above the peak sled deceleration of the previous test, respectively depending upon whether there was or was not a fatality within 3 h on the previous test. The primary advantage of this method was the concentration of testing near the tolerance level, thus increasing the accuracy of LD_{50} estimation (15, 16):

The experiment was conducted on the Daisy Decelerator (17) utilizing a 1135 lb (515 kg) sled. Peak sled decelerations ranged from 6.5-134 g. The impact pulse was approximately half sine (actually haversine) with the stopping distance varying from 0.5-3.5 ft (0.15-1.07 m) at 6 in (15.2 cm) increments. Table 1 contains the various ranges of peak sled decelerations, velocities, pulse durations, and onsets for the test series. The instant of maximum sled deceleration occurred midway through the brake pattern. The time duration applied to the calculation of sled onset extended from the initiation of the pulse to the instant of peak deceleration.

The animal preparation, instrumentation, photography, data collection, and data reduction methods have been reported previously (14, 18, 19). Although a total of 89 tests were performed, equipment malfunctions and preimpact cancellation of specific data channels resulted in deletions of some recorded information.

Preceding all deceleration tests, the animals were anesthetized with sodium pentobarbital. The baboons were muzzled to mitigate lingual injury; their wrists and ankles were taped to prevent flailing (Fig. 1). Prior to impact, the head was hyperextended approximately 15-20 deg from the neutral anatomi-

Table 1 - Test Parameters

	\multicolumn{7}{c}{Stopping Distance, ft(m)}
	0.5 (0.15)	1.0 (0.31)	1.5 (0.46)	2.0 (0.61)	2.5 (0.76)	3.0 (0.91)	3.5 (1.07)
No. tests	12	7	6	38	6	6	14
Peak sled deceleration, g	21.2-134	11.3-54.7	13.0-61.2	6.5-131	11.4-59.4	8.1-62.2	9.7-112
Peak sled velocity, ft/s (m/s)	20.5-49.1 (6.2-15.0)	21.4-47.4 (6.5-14.4)	26.9-56.2 (8.2-17.1)	21.8-93.2 (6.6-28.4)	33.5-74.2 (10.2-22.6)	31.9-87.0 (9.7-26.5)	37.3-123.5 (11.4-37.6)
Sled pulse duration, s	0.053-0.023	0.077-0.045	0.097-0.049	0.233-0.042	0.154-0.067	0.161-0.071	0.185-0.059
Sled onset, g/s	707-8350	264-2242	239-2155	73-5678	155-1674	92-1673	108-3961

cal position. Masking tape was employed to hold the head in this position against the headrest. The tape did not contribute significantly as a restraint since the inertia of the head easily broke the tape during the initial phase of the impact event.

An extensive series of x-rays was taken immediately postimpact. Gross necropsy was conducted within 1 h postimpact for animals not surviving a deceleration test. Animals that sustained traumatic but nonlethal injuries were euthanized from 6-24 h postimpact. Many animals receiving less than 70 g (particularly at the short deceleration patterns) were not euthanized because of the absence of severe trauma. These baboons were subjected to multiple impacts at low decelerations. An animal was never returned to the cage in a seriously injured condition. Where fatality occurred in excess of 3 h postimpact (two tests), surgical intervention and/or fluid replacement, if used, may have reversed the final outcome.

The proportionately "scaled" Air Force restraint was composed of an inverted Y-yoke shoulder harness and lap belt. All restraint belts consisted of 1 in (2.54 cm) Dacron webbing of 3700 lb (16458 N) tensile test. The two torso straps were attached separately to the lap belt at the midline of the animal. The yoke of the torso harness was formed several inches posterior to the neck and continued horizontally rearward as a single belt to a triaxial load cell (Fig. 2). Each lap belt attach point was similarly instrumented with a triaxial load cell that measured forces in three axes and enabled calculation of resultant force magnitudes and directions. All belts were statically pretensioned at approximately 15 lb (67 N).

Uniaxial accelerometers were affixed to anterior and posterior flanges of a lightweight plastic headmount (Fig. 1). The mount, restraining straps, and accelerometers weighed 6.7 oz (190 g). Head angular accelerations in a spatial reference system were calculated from the two linear acceleration components (20). The design of the angular acceleration system is dependent upon the principle that the tangential acceleration of point A on a rigid body relative to point B on the body, divided by their separation distance, is the angular acceleration of the body within a spatial reference system. Integration of head angular accelerations by computer yielded a listing and plot of angular velocity versus time. Angular displacement of the head was computed by an additional integration. All angular displacements were verified by comparing the twice-integrated accelerometer values with the angular displacements obtained from high-speed movie film. The movie film also served for assessment of torso and extremity kinematics during the impact event.

RESULTS AND DISCUSSION

TOLERANCE - The authors recognize that many physical quantities may be extracted from the exposure conditions for correlation with the limits of tolerance; for example, peak

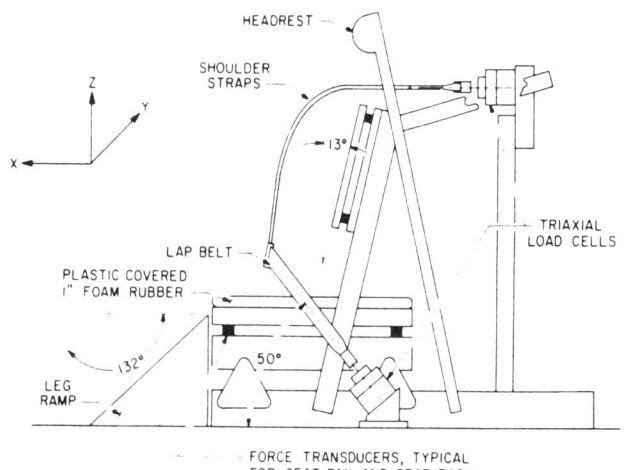

Fig. 2 - Experimental seat layout

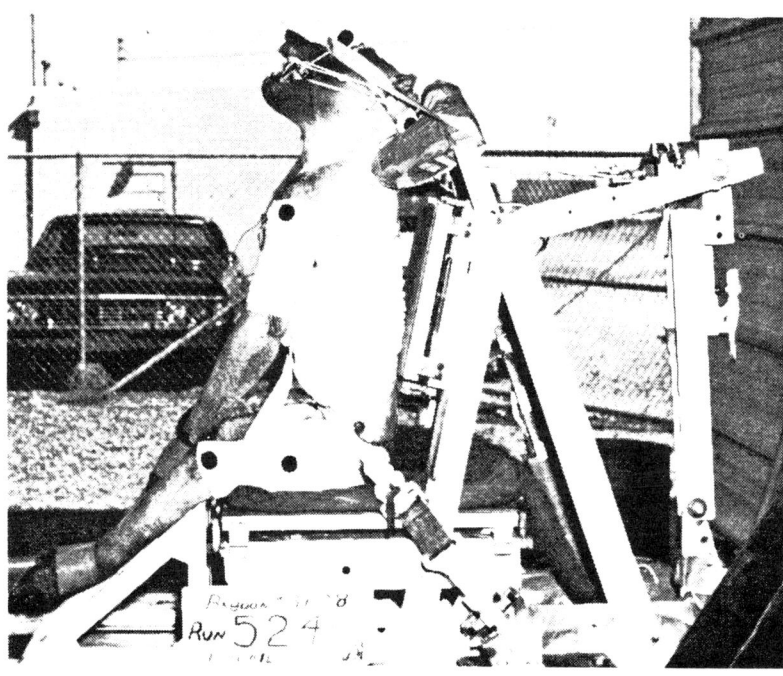

Fig. 1 - Baboon seated on sled before impact (run 5245)

deceleration, duration of exposure, deceleration onset, momentum, etc. In this report, the tolerance to impact was expressed as the percentage of subjects surviving the effects of abrupt linear deceleration ($-G_x$). Employing probit analysis (21), the median lethal sled deceleration (LD_{50}) was calculated to be 102, 103, and 98 g for the 0.5, 2.0, and 3.5 ft (0.15, 0.61, and 1.07 m) stopping distances, respectively (Table 2). Since the deceleration pulses are similar (all half sine with different pulse duration), the results imply that impact lethality is dependent upon the magnitude of peak sled deceleration, irrespective of the pulse duration, sled velocity, onset, energy dissipation, or stopping distance. LD_{50}s were not calculated for the 1.0, 1.5, 2.5, and 3.0 ft (0.31, 0.46, 0.76, and 0.91 m) stopping distances due to limited time and resources. There was no attempt to quantitate fatalities on the basis of injury severity; that is, a fatality was a fatality irrespective of the mode of death.

Fig. 3 is a graphic representation of the tolerance limits to impact. The standard deviations are inconsistent because of the number of tests at each stopping distance (Table 1) and the statistical method of LD_{50} estimation. The dashed line represents the lowest sled deceleration where a fatality occurred; the dotted line indicates the maximum sled deceleration where an animal survived. The parabolic stopping distance curves (Fig. 3) are not equidistant because of the mechanical properties of the decelerator and variations between the anticipated and actual stopping distance of the sled (Table 3).

Superficially, it would appear that these results contradict many of the significant impact manuscripts (22, 23). However, it should be borne in mind that in this report, stopping distance, deceleration, velocity, pulse duration, pulse shape, and onset include only a small range of the conceivable impact parameters. Specifically, fatalities may occur on a centrifuge at less than 20 g. In this case, the duration of the acceleration results in cardiovascular and respiratory distress. Conversely, one can jump from a chair and receive high decelerative force for an extremely short duration, but with no ill effect because of negligible impulse.

PATHOLOGY - Although the reported injuries were produced directly or indirectly by the safety restraint, its disuse would have resulted in comparable or more severe injuries at substantially lower sled decelerations (18).

Table 2 - Tolerance Limits to Impact

	Stopping Distance, ft(m)		
	0.5 (0.15)	2.0 (0.61)	3.5 (1.07)
LD_{50}, sled g	102 ± 5	103 ± 16	98 ± 3
Sled pulse duration, ms	27	46	63
Sled velocity, ft/s (m/s)	44 (13)	83 (25)	117 (36)
Sled onset, g/s	5750	3962	2980
Energy dissipation ft-lb (J)	1507 (2043)	5362 (7271)	10655 (14448)

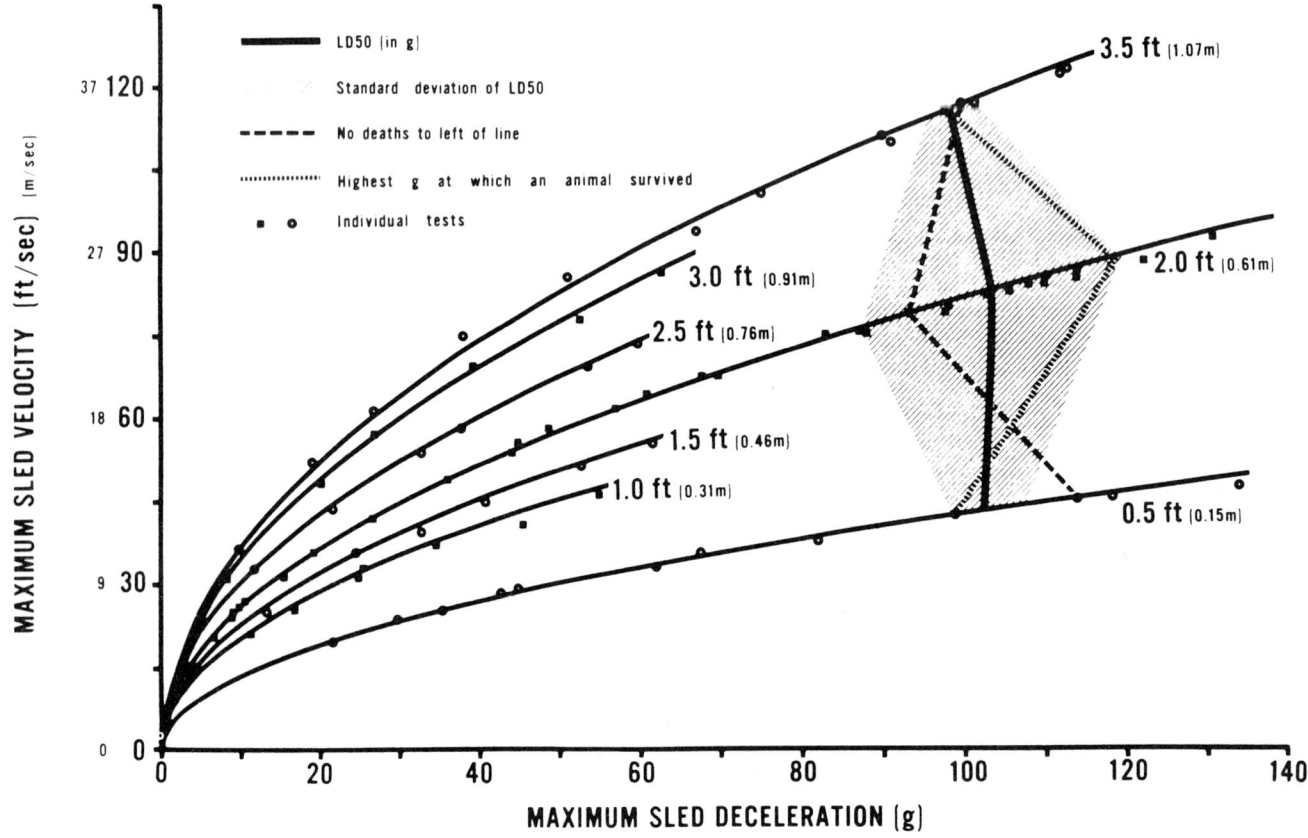

Fig. 3 - Tolerance levels to impact

Predominant Injury Patterns - In the vicinity of 100 g, the injury patterns at the various stopping distances were appreciably dissimilar. At the 0.5 ft (0.15 m) stop, pelvic and abdominal trauma was essentially nonexistent. Most of the significant injuries were indirectly attributable to the torso portion of the restraint. These injuries included hemorrhage of thoracic musculature, myocardial contusion, and transection of the cervical spinal cord resulting from avulsion of the atlanto-occipital articulation (Fig. 4).

The predominant injuries at the 2.0 ft (0.61 m) stop included pelvic and abdominal myorrhexis, intestinal herniation, urinary bladder rupture, and pelvic fractures (Fig. 5). Again, the torso straps of the harness were primarily instrumental in producing the most life-threatening trauma. These injuries included costal, clavicular, and scapular fractures plus luxation of cervical through thoracic vertebrae.

At the 3.5 ft (1.07 m) stop, the pelvic and abdominal injury patterns were similar to those at the 2.0 ft (0.61 m) stop but compounded in severity (Fig. 6). There was a high incidence of transection of the descending colon and musculature or blood vessels in the axillary and cervical regions (Fig. 7). Brainstem hemorrhage was a significant finding, but there was no evidence of luxation or fractures of cervical vertebrae.

A tabulation of impact-related trauma for all animals used in the study can be found in Table 4. Sled deceleration, velocity, onset, and pulse duration can be compared with the radiological and necropsy reports. The authors wish to emphasize equally those injuries that were nonfatal, yet incapacitating.

Several points should be stressed for clarification of Table 4. First, it should be recognized that hemorrhage occurred in all myorrhexic muscle groups, lacerated, ruptured, or transected organs. Therefore, this finding is not specifically delineated within the table. Second, all injuries were bilateral unless indicated otherwise. The severity of injuries was not quantitated due to the complexity of arbitrary scales. Third, the baboons invariably showed evidence of parasitic infestation, particularly

Table 3 - Sled Stopping Distances and Equations of G versus Velocity

Anticipated Sled Stopping Distance, in (cm)	Actual Sled Stopping Distance, in (cm)	Equation of G versus Velocity	Correlation Coefficients
6.0 (15.2)	6.4 (16.26)	$g_{max} = 0.0542V^2$	0.9991
12.0 (30.5)	14.5 (36.83)	$g_{max} = 0.0241V^2$	0.9990
18.0 (45.7)	18.1 (45.97)	$g_{max} = 0.0192V^2$	0.9999
24.0 (61.0)	24.5 (62.23)	$g_{max} = 0.0149V^2$	0.9996
30.0 (76.2)	30.1 (76.45)	$g_{max} = 0.0108V^2$	0.9999
36.0 (91.4)	36.1 (91.69)	$g_{max} = 0.0082V^2$	0.9995
42.0 (106.7)	42.3 (107.44)	$g_{max} = 0.0073V^2$	0.9995

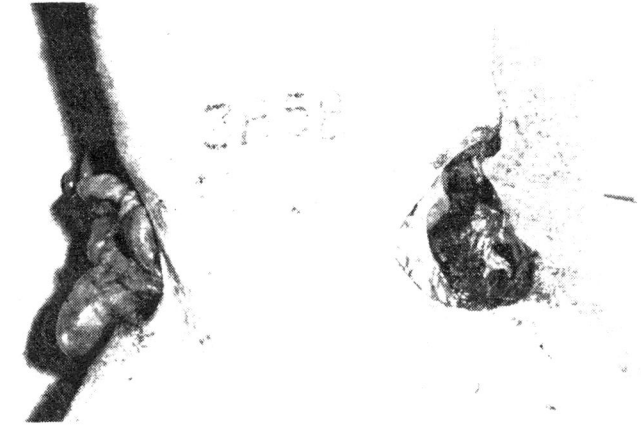

Fig. 5 - Abdominal evisceration. Note apparent lack of injury in midline

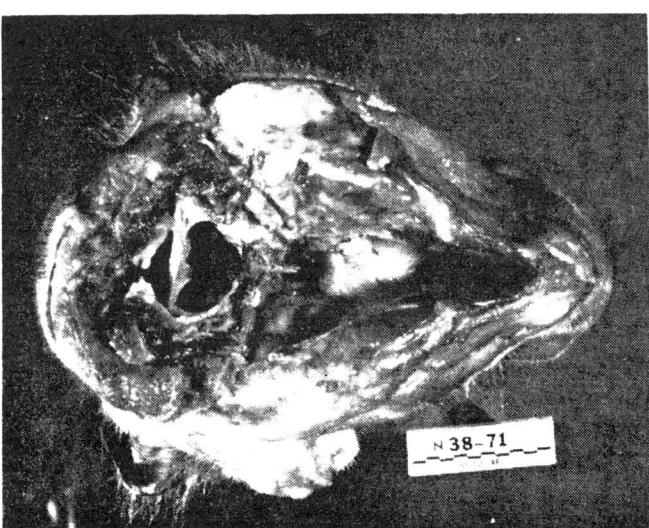

Fig. 4 - Avulsion: basilar portion of occipital bone

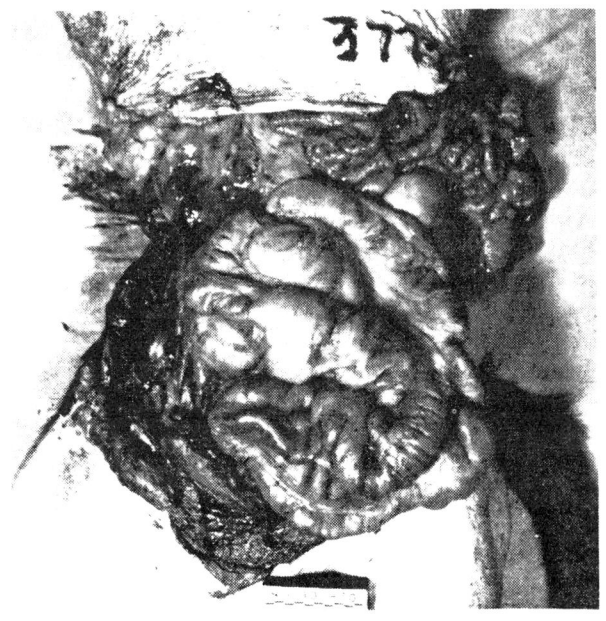

Fig. 6 - Abdominal evisceration and myorrhexis of abdominal and pelvic musculature. Injuries attributable to submarining

Table 4 - Summary of Trauma Attributable to Restraint System

Peak Sled Deceleration, g_{max}	Sled Entrance Velocity, ft/s (m/s)	Sled Onset, g/s	Impact Pulse Duration, ms	Postimpact Survival	Radiographic Report	Comments from Necropsy Report
						0.5 ft Stopping Distance
21.15	20.5 (6.25)	707	53	Indefinite	Normal	No injuries, no necropsy
29.02	24.4 (7.44)	1029	46	Indefinite	Normal	No injuries, no necropsy
35.03	25.9 (7.89)	1352	43	Indefinite	Normal	No injuries, no necropsy
42.14	29.4 (8.96)	1770	39	Indefinite	Normal	No injuries, no necropsy
44.14	30.0 (9.14)	1953	37	Indefinite	Normal	No injuries, no necropsy
61.16	34.3 (10.45)	2829	34	Indefinite	Normal	No injuries, no necropsy
67.27	36.5 (11.13)	3219	33	Indefinite	Normal	Cutaneous lap belt and harness abrasions and contusions, no necropsy
81.99	38.9 (11.86)	4315	31	Indefinite	Normal	Cutaneous lap belt and harness abrasions and contusions, no necropsy
98.88	42.9 (13.08)	5493	28	Euthanized after 24 h	Luxation: sternum	Cutaneous lap belt and harness abrasions and contusions. Laceration: renal cortex (L). Hemorrhage: inguinocrural fascia and musculature, psoas major and minor, kidney, adrenal (L), pancreas, root of mesentery, pectoralis major and minor, intercostals, costal pleura, myocardium adjacent to anterior interventricular artery, cervical spinal cord
113.6	45.6 (14.00)	6682	26	5 min	Avulsion: basilar portion of occipital bone. Luxation: L-3 upon L-4	Cutaneous lap belt and harness abrasions and contusions. Transection: brainstem at pons. Hemorrhage: inguinocrural fascia and musculature, psoas major and minor, root of mesentery, pectoralis major and minor, intercostals, costal pleura, lungs, cervical and thoracic spinal cord, brainstem, temporal cortex. Bone marrow emboli: lung

Fatal injury: brainstem transection resulting from avulsion of basilar portion of occipital bone

| 118.4 | 46.5 (14.17) | 6965 | 25 | 5 min | Avulsion: atlanto-occipital articulation. Fractures: clavicles, ribs 6-8 | Cutaneous lap belt and harness abrasions, contusions, and lacerations. Transection: cervical spinal cord. Hemorrhage: inguinocrural fascia and musculature, psoas major and minor, pectoralis major and minor, intercostals, costal pleura, myocardium adjacent to anterior interventricular artery, cervical spinal cord, brainstem, temporal cortex |

Fatal injury: cervical spinal cord transection resulting from avulsion of atlanto-occipital articulation

| 133.6 | 49.1 (14.97) | 8350 | 23 | 10 min | Avulsion: atlanto-occipital articulation. Luxation: L-3 upon L-4. Fractures: sternum, comminuted iliac crests and fossae | Cutaneous lap belt and harness abrasions, contusions, and lacerations. Myorrhexis: sartorius (L), tensor fascia lata (L), rectus femoris (L), rectus abdominus (R), external and internal obliques (R). Rupture: neck of urinary bladder, descending colon. Transection: cervical and lumbar spinal cord. Hemorrhage: inguinocrural fascia and musculature, sartorius, tensor fascia lata, rectus femoris, rectus abdominus, external and internal obliques, psoas major and minor, root of mesentery, renal capsule, pancreas, retroperitoneal, pectoralis major and minor, costal pleura, intercostals, within mediastinum, pericardium, lungs, cervical and lumbar spinal cord, brainstem |

Fatal injury: cervical spinal cord transection resulting from avulsion of atlanto-occipital articulation.

Table 4 - Continued

Peak Sled Deceleration, g_{max}	Sled Entrance Velocity, ft/s (m/s)	Sled Onset, g/s	Impact Pulse Duration, ms	Postimpact Survival	Radiographic Report	Comments from Necropsy Report
\multicolumn{7}{c}{1.0 ft Stopping Distance}						
11.34	21.4 (6.52)	264	77	Indefinite	Normal	No injuries, no necropsy
16.96	26.0 (7.92)	439	70	Indefinite	Normal	No injuries, no necropsy
24.86	32.4 (9.88)	789	58	Indefinite	Normal	No injuries, no necropsy
25.38	33.5 (10.21)	806	58	Indefinite	Normal	No injuries, no necropsy
34.17	38.7 (10.42)	1335	52	Indefinite	Normal	No injuries, no necropsy
45.74	42.9 (13.08)	1867	51	Indefinite	Normal	No injuries, no necropsy
54.71	47.4 (14.45)	2242	45	20 days	Normal	Cutaneous lap belt and harness abrasions and contusions. Right ventricular hypertrophy. Hemorrhage and necrosis of adrenal cortices, nephritis, hepatitis

Fatal injury: shock resulting from prolonged exposure to freezing temperature. Not impact related

1.5 ft Stopping Distance

12.96	26.9 (8.20)	239	97	Indefinite	Normal	No injuries, no necropsy
24.80	36.1 (11.00)	571	81	Indefinite	Normal	No injuries, no necropsy
32.13	41.2 (12.56)	820	66	Indefinite	Normal	No injuries, no necropsy
40.32	45.9 (13.99)	1146	60	Indefinite	Normal	No injuries, no necropsy
52.20	52.4 (15.97)	1652	53	Indefinite	Normal	Cutaneous lap belt and harness abrasions and contusions, no necropsy
61.20	56.2 (17.13)	2155	49	Indefinite	Normal	Cutaneous lap belt and harness abrasions and contusions, no necropsy

2.0 ft Stopping Distance

6.50 to 26.19	21.8 (6.64) to 43.2 (13.17)	73 to 548	233 to 87	Indefinite	Normal	No injuries, no necropsy (14 tests)
35.89	50.3 (15.33)	897	74	Indefinite	Normal	No injuries, no necropsy
43.87	54.8 (16.70)	1148	69	Indefinite	Normal	Cutaneous lap belt and harness abrasions and contusions, no necropsy
44.47	56.9 (17.34)	1112	66	Euthanized after 6 h	Fractures: clavicle (L). Sternal luxation	Cutaneous lap belt and harness abrasions and contusions. Myorrhexis: rectus abdominus (R). Hemorrhage: inguinocrural fascia and musculature, rectus abdominus, psoas major and minor, urinary bladder, descending colon, omentum, costal pleura, tongue, labial gingiva
48.33	59.2 (18.04)	1343	63	Indefinite	Fractures: clavicle (R)	Cutaneous lap belt and harness abrasions and contusions, no necropsy
56.63	62.8 (19.14)	1821	59	Indefinite	Normal	Cutaneous lap belt and harness abrasions and contusions, no necropsy
60.80	65.4 (19.93)	1842	57	Euthanized after 48 h	Normal	Cutaneous lap belt and harness abrasions and contusions. Hemorrhage: inguinocrural fascia and musculature, urinary bladder
67.52	68.6 (20.91)	2386	54	Indefinite	Normal	Cutaneous lap belt and harness abrasions and contusions, no necropsy
69.36	68.9 (21.00)	2335	53	Euthanized after 6 h	Normal	Cutaneous lap belt and harness abrasions and contusions. Myorrhexis: sartorius, tensor fascia lata, rectus femoris. Hemorrhage: inguinocrural fascia and musculature, root of mesentery, rectus abdominus

Table 4 - Continued

Peak Sled Deceleration, g_{max}	Sled Entrance Velocity, ft/s (m/s)	Sled Onset, g/s	Impact Pulse Duration, ms	Postimpact Survival	Radiographic Report	Comments from Necropsy Report
82.46	76.4 (23.29)	2843	50	Euthanized after 6 h	Fractures: clavicles, scapulae–glenoid fossa to medial border, iliac crest (L)	Cutaneous lap belt and harness abrasions, contusions, and lacerations. Myorrhexis: sartorius, tensor fascia lata, rectus femoris. Rupture: neck of urinary bladder. Bone marrow emboli: lung. Hemorrhage: inguinocrural fascia and musculature, root of mesentery, omentum, pectoralis major and minor, intercostals, costal pleura
87.01	76.3 (23.26)	3108	48	Euthanized after 6 h	Fractures: sternum, clavicles, comminuted iliac crests and fossae	Cutaneous lap belt and harness abrasions, contusions, and lacerations. Myorrhexis: sartorius, tensor fascia lata, rectus femoris, rectus abdominus. Herniation: intestinal. Hemorrhage: inguinocrural fascia and musculature, external and internal obliques, root of mesentery, descending colon, pectoralis major and minor, intercostals, costal pleura, lungs
87.79	76.3 (23.26)	3038	48	Euthanized after 7 h	Luxation: L-3 upon L-4. Fractures: clavicle (R), comminuted acromion process (R), comminuted iliac crests and fossae, transverse through body of sacrum	Cutaneous lap belt and harness abrasions, contusions, and lacerations. Myorrhexis: sartorius, tensor fascia lata, rectus femoris, pectoralis major (L). Hemorrhage: inguinocrural fascia and musculature, rectus abdominus, external and internal obliques, psoas major and minor, lumbar spinal cord, root of mesentery, pectoralis major and minor, intercostals, costal pleura
92.86 Fatal injury: cervical spinal cord and brainstem trauma resulting from avulsion of odontoid process	79.6 (24.26)	3439	48	10 min	Avulsion: odontoid process. Fractures: clavicle (R), comminuted iliac crests and fossae	Cutaneous lap belt and harness abrasions and contusions. Myorrhexis: rectus abdominus, external and internal obliques. Herniation: intestinal. Hemorrhage: inguinocrural fascia and musculature, sartorius, tensor fascia lata, rectus femoris, psoas major and minor, pectoralis major and minor, intercostals, costal pleura, trachea, lungs, cervical spinal cord, medulla, middle cerebellar peduncle (R), occipital cortex (R)
97.14 Fatal injury: cardiorespiratory failure resulting from brainstem hemorrhage	80.0 (24.38)	3507	47	15 min	Fractures: clavicles, sternum, comminuted iliac crests and fossae	Cutaneous lap belt and harness abrasions and contusions. Myorrhexis: sartorius, tensor fascia lata, rectus femoris, rectus abdominus, external and internal obliques. Herniation: intestinal. Hemorrhage: inguinocrural fascia and musculature, psoas major and minor, root of mesentery, pectoralis major and minor, intercostals, costal pleura, within mediastinum, labial gingiva, medulla, cerebellar peduncles
97.42 Fatal injury: thoracic spinal cord transection resulting from luxation of T-4 upon T-5	81.0 (24.69)	3543	47	22 h	Luxation: T-4 upon T-5. Fractures: spinous processes T-4 and T-5, sternum, clavicles	Cutaneous lap belt and harness abrasions and contusions. Myorrhexis: sartorius, tensor fascia lata, rectus femoris. Transection: spinal cord at T-4 and T-5. Hemorrhage: inguinocrural fascia and musculature, rectus abdominus, psoas major and minor, pectoralis major and minor, intercostals, costal pleura, within mediastinum, periaortic, subpleural in thoracic region

Table 4 - Continued

Peak Sled Deceleration, g_{max}	Sled Entrance Velocity, ft/s (m/s)	Sled Onset, g/s	Impact Pulse Duration, ms	Postimpact Survival	Radiographic Report	Comments from Necropsy Report
102.1	82.8 (25.24)	3927	46	Euthanized after 6 h	Fractures: lamina and pedicles of T-12, compression T-12, clavicle (R), scapula (L)–neck of glenoid fossae to medial border, sternum, comminuted iliac crests and fossae, transverse through body of sacrum	Cutaneous lap belt and harness abrasions, contusions and lacerations. Myorrhexis: sartorius, tensor fascia lata, rectus femoris, rectus abdominus, external and internal obliques, psoas major and minor, pectoralis major and minor. Herniation: intestinal. Transection: spinal cord at T-12. Hemorrhage: inguinocrural fascia and musculature, root of mesentery, retroperitoneal, intercostals, costal pleura, within mediastinum, thoracic spinal cord
105.1	83.9 (25.57)	4042	46	1 h	Fractures: clavicles, glenoid neck of scapula (L), comminuted iliac crests and fossae	Cutaneous lap belt and harness abrasions, contusions, and lacerations. Myorrhexis: sartorius, tensor fascia lata, rectus femoris, rectus abdominus, external and internal obliques, psoas major and minor, pectoralis major and minor. Herniation: intestinal. Rupture: neck of urinary bladder. Hemorrhage: inguinocrural fascia and musculature, root of mesentery, stomach mucosa, intercostals, costal pleura, myocardium adjacent to anterior interventricular artery, bronchial lymph nodes, cervical spinal cord, middle cerebellar peduncles, hypophysis, tuber cinereum, posterior perforated substance

Fatal injury: cardiorespiratory failure resulting from brainstem and cervical spinal cord hemorrhage

| 107.3 | 85.4 (26.03) | 4127 | 45 | Euthanized after 6 h | Fractures: compound of humerus (L), clavicles, comminuted of scapular infraspinous fossa (R), iliac crests and fossae adjacent to acetabulum | Cutaneous lap belt and harness abrasions, contusions, and lacerations. Myorrhexis: sartorius, tensor fascia lata, rectus femoris, rectus abdominus, external and internal obliques, pectoralis major (R), psoas major and minor. Herniation: intestinal. Hemorrhage: inguinocrural fascia and musculature, liver, pectoralis major and minor, intercostals, costal pleura, trachea, cervical fascia and musculature |
| 109.9 | 86.3 (26.30) | 4227 | 45 | 5 min | Avulsion: atlanto-occipital articulation. Fractures: clavicles, body of mandible, comminuted iliac crests and fossae | Cutaneous lap belt and harness abrasions, contusions, and lacerations. Myorrhexis: sartorius, tensor fascia lata, rectus femoris, rectus abdominus, psoas major and minor, external and internal obliques, pectoralis major (L). Transection: cervical spinal cord at C-1. Evisceration: abdominal. Laceration: descending colon. Rupture: neck and fundus of urinary bladder. Hemorrhage: inguinocrural fascia and musculature, testes, root of mesentery, pectoralis major and minor, intercostals, costal pleura, cervical fascia and musculature, cervical spinal cord, medulla, midbrain |

Fatal injury: cervical spinal cord transection resulting from avulsion of atlanto-occipital articulation

Table 4 - Continued

Peak Sled Deceleration, g_{max}	Sled Entrance Velocity, ft/s (m/s)	Sled Onset, g/s	Impact Pulse Duration, ms	Postimpact Survival	Radiographic Report	Comments from Necropsy Report
113.4	86.4 (26.33)	~4200	44	5 min	Avulsion: atlanto-occipital articulation. Fractures: clavicles, scapula (R)–neck of glenoid fossa to medial border, comminuted iliac crests and fossae	Cutaneous lap belt and harness abrasions, contusions, and lacerations. Myorrhexis: sartorius, tensor fascia lata, rectus femoris, rectus abdominus, psoas major and minor, external and internal obliques, pectoralis major and minor (L), longus colli and longus capitus. Transection: cervical spinal cord at C-1. Herniation: intestinal. Hemorrhage: inguinocrural fascia and musculature, root of mesentery, descending colon, adrenal (L), pectoralis major and minor, intercostals, costal pleura, tongue, cervical and thoracic spinal cord, medulla, midbrain
Fatal injury: cervical spinal cord transection resulting from avulsion of atlanto-occipital articulation						
113.6	87.0 (26.52)	4287	44	5 min	Avulsion: atlanto-occipital articulation. Fractures: spinous processes of C-7, T-1, and T-2. Subluxation: T-9 upon T-10. Fractures: clavicles, humerus (L), scapulae–neck of glenoid fossae to medial border, rib (R)-8, comminuted iliac crests and fossae, sternum	Cutaneous lap belt and harness abrasions, contusions, and lacerations. Myorrhexis: sartorius, tensor fascia lata, rectus femoris, rectus abdominus, psoas major and minor, external and internal obliques, pectoralis major and minor, longus colli. Herniation: intestinal. Transection: cervical spinal cord at C-1. Hemorrhage: inguinocrural fascia and musculature, root of mesentery, descending colon, kidney (L), liver, intercostals, costal pleura, trapezius, cervical and thoracic spinal cord, cerebral and cerebellar peduncles
Fatal injury: cervical spinal cord transection resulting from avulsion of atlanto-occipital articulation						
118.0	88.7 (27.04)	4370	43	5 min	Fractures: mandible, clavicles, humerus (L), sacrum, comminuted iliac crests and fossae	Cutaneous lap belt and harness abrasions, contusions, and lacerations. Myorrhexis: sartorius, tensor fascia lata, rectus femoris, rectus abdominus, psoas major and minor, external and internal obliques, pectoralis major and minor. Transection: descending colon. Evisceration: abdominal. Bone marrow emboli: lung. Hemorrhage: inguinocrural fascia and musculature, root of mesentery, ilium, urinary bladder, intercostals, costal pleura
Fatal injury: cardiorespiratory failure resulting from hemorrhage and shock						
118.2	89.2 (27.19)	4546	43	12 h	Fractures: sternum, clavicles, scapula (R)–neck of glenoid fossa to medial border, spinous processes T-1 through T-5, arch T-12, sacrum, comminuted iliac crests and fossae	Cutaneous lap belt and harness abrasions, contusions, and lacerations. Myorrhexis: sartorius, tensor fascia lata, rectus femoris, rectus abdominus, psoas major and minor, external and internal obliques, pectoralis major and minor. Transection: spinal cord at T-1. Rupture: neck of urinary bladder. Evisceration: abdominal. Bone marrow emboli: lung. Hemorrhage: inguinocrural fascia and musculature, root of mesentery, descending colon, intercostals, costal pleura, cervical fascia and musculature, cervical and thoracic spinal cord
Fatal injury: cardiorespiratory failure resulting from hemorrhage and thoracic cord transection						

Table 4 - Continued

Peak Sled Deceleration, g_{max}	Sled Entrance Velocity, ft/s (m/s)	Sled Onset, g/s	Impact Pulse Duration, ms	Postimpact Survival	Radiographic Report	Comments from Necropsy Report
121.8	89.6 (27.31)	4511	43	10 min	Luxation: T-1 upon T-2. Fractures: arch and body C-5 and T-12, anterior compression L-3, clavicles, humerus (R), mandible, ribs 3 and 5, comminuted iliac crests and fossae	Cutaneous lap belt and harness abrasions, contusions, and lacerations. Myorrhexis: sartorius, tensor fascia lata, rectus femoris, rectus abdominus, psoas major and minor, external and internal obliques, pectoralis major and minor. Herniation: intestinal. Transection: descending colon, spinal cord at T-1. Rupture: neck of urinary bladder. Hemorrhage: inguinocrural fascia and musculature, intercostals, costal pleura, longus colli, cervical fascia and musculature, root of mesentery, cervical and thoracic spinal cord, brainstem, cerebral cortex
Fatal injury: cardiorespiratory failure resulting from hemorrhage and thoracic cord transection						
130.6	93.2 (28.41)	5678	42	5 min	Fractures: sternum, clavicles, scapula (R) – neck of glenoid fossa to medial border, sacrum, comminuted iliac crests and fossae	Cutaneous lap belt and harness abrasions, contusions, and lacerations. Myorrhexis: sartorius, tensor fascia lata, rectus femoris, rectus abdominus, psoas major and minor, external and internal obliques, pectoralis major and minor, cervical musculature. Transection: brachial arteries. Rupture: neck of urinary bladder. Hemorrhage: inguinocrural fascia and musculature, root of mesentery, intercostals, costal pleura, axillary fascia and musculature, cervical fascia and musculature, cervical and thoracic spinal cord, medulla, cerebellum
Fatal injury: cardiorespiratory failure resulting from hemorrhage and shock						

2.5 ft Stopping Distance

11.43	33.5 (10.21)	155	154	Indefinite	Normal	No injuries, no necropsy
21.34	44.8 (13.66)	389	113	Indefinite	Normal	No injuries, no necropsy
32.19	54.5 (16.61)	712	94	Indefinite	Normal	No injuries, no necropsy
37.43	59.0 (17.98)	847	89	Indefinite	Normal	Cutaneous lap belt and harness abrasions and contusions, no necropsy
53.01	69.7 (21.24)	1421	73	Indefinite	Normal	Cutaneous lap belt and harness abrasions and contusions, no necropsy
59.44	74.2 (22.62)	1674	67	Indefinite	Normal	Cutaneous lap belt and harness abrasions and contusions, no necropsy

3.0 ft Stopping Distance

8.08	31.9 (9.72)	92	161	Indefinite	Normal	No injuries, no necropsy
20.00	49.2 (15.00)	313	118	Indefinite	Normal	No injuries, no necropsy
26.04	57.8 (17.62)	491	101	Indefinite	Normal	No injuries, no necropsy
38.82	70.0 (21.34)	872	88	Indefinite	Normal	Cutaneous lap belt and harness abrasions and contusions, no necropsy
52.07	78.4 (23.90)	1308	78	Indefinite	Normal	Cutaneous lap belt and harness abrasions and contusions, no necropsy
62.22	87.0 (26.52)	1673	71	Indefinite	Fractures: clavicle (L)	Cutaneous lap belt and harness abrasions, contusions, and lacerations, no necropsy

3.5 ft Stopping Distance

9.70	37.3 (11.37)	108	185	Indefinite	Normal	No injuries, no necropsy
18.97	52.7 (16.06)	267	131	Indefinite	Normal	No injuries, no necropsy
26.11	62.1 (18.93)	450	115	Indefinite	Normal	No injuries, no necropsy
37.79	75.6 (23.04)	776	94	Indefinite	Normal	Cutaneous lap belt and harness abrasions and contusions, no necropsy
50.52	86.6 (26.40)	1197	80	Indefinite	Normal	Cutaneous lap belt and harness abrasions and contusions, no necropsy

Table 4 - Continued

Peak Sled Deceleration, g_{max}	Sled Entrance Velocity, ft/s (m/s)	Sled Onset, g/s	Impact Pulse Duration, ms	Postimpact Survival	Radiographic Report	Comments from Necropsy Report
60.63	94.4 (28.77)	1520	74	Indefinite	Normal	Cutaneous lap belt and harness abrasions, contusions, and lacerations, no necropsy
74.61	101.6 (30.97)	2108	69	Euthanized after 24 h	Fractures: clavicles, comminuted iliac crests and fossae	Cutaneous lap belt and harness abrasions, contusions, and lacerations. Myorrhexis: rectus abdominus, external and internal obliques. Herniation: intestinal. Transection: descending colon. Hemorrhage: inguinocrural fascia and musculature, sartorius, tensor fascia lata, rectus femoris, psoas major and minor, urinary bladder, omentum, root of mesentery, small intestine, retroperitoneal, pectoralis major and minor, intercostals, costal pleura, myocardium adjacent to anterior interventricular artery
89.76	111.3 (33.92)	2543	66	5 min	Avulsion: atlanto-occipital articulation. Fractures: sternum, comminuted iliac crests and fossae	Cutaneous lap belt and harness abrasions, contusions, and lacerations. Myorrhexis: sartorius, tensor fascia lata, rectus femoris, psoas major and minor, pectoralis major and minor (R), sternohyoid. Transection: cervical spinal cord. Rupture: neck of urinary bladder. Hemorrhage: inguinocrural fascia and musculature, rectus abdominus, root of mesentery, pectoralis major and minor, intercostals, costal pleura, myocardium adjacent to anterior interventricular artery, cervical fascia and musculature, cervical spinal cord, brainstem
90.36	110.5 (33.68)	2582	67	Euthanized after 24 h	Fractures: comminuted iliac crests and fossae, clavicle (R)	Cutaneous lap belt and harness abrasions, contusions, and lacerations. Myorrhexis: sartorius, tensor fascia lata, rectus femoris, psoas major and minor, rectus abdominus, external and internal obliques, pectoralis major and minor (R). Laceration: descending colon. Herniation: intestinal. Hemorrhage: inguinocrural fascia and musculature, urinary bladder, root of mesentery, pectoralis major and minor, intercostals, costal pleura, cervical fascia and musculature
97.42	116.3 (35.45)	2943	64	Euthanized after 24 h	Fractures: sternum	Cutaneous lap belt and harness abrasions, contusions, and lacerations. Myorrhexis: sartorius, tensor fascia lata, rectus femoris, rectus abdominus, external and internal obliques, psoas major and minor, pectoralis major and minor (L). Rupture: fundus of urinary bladder. Hemorrhage: inguinocrural fascia and musculature, gluteal muscles, root of mesentery, liver, descending colon, pectoralis major and minor, intercostals, costal pleura, lungs, myocardium adjacent to anterior interventricular artery, labial gingiva

Fatal injury: cervical spinal cord transection resulting from avulsion of atlanto-occipital articulation
Lap belt severed during impact. Animal not included in LD_{50} estimate or pathology tabulations

Table 4 - Continued

Peak Sled Deceleration, g_{max}	Sled Entrance Velocity, ft/s (m/s)	Sled Onset, g/s	Impact Pulse Duration, ms	Postimpact Survival	Radiographic Report	Comments from Necropsy Report
99.12 Fatal injury: cardiorespiratory failure resulting from hemorrhage and pneumoperitoneum	117.1 (35.69)	3050	63	10 min	Luxation: L-6 upon L-7. Fractures: comminuted iliac crests and fossae	Cutaneous lap belt and harness abrasions, contusions, and lacerations. Myorrhexis: sartorius, tensor fascia lata, rectus femoris, psoas major and minor, rectus abdominus, external and internal obliques, pectoralis major and minor. Transection: lumbar spinal cord, descending colon colon, iliac arteries, inferior vena cava at L-6. Evisceration: abdominal. Hemorrhage: inguinocrural fascia and musculature, urinary bladder, root of mesentery, retroperitoneal, intercostals, costal pleura, myocardium adjacent to pleura, myocardium adjacent to anterior interventricular artery, cervical fascia and musculature, thoracic and lumbar spinal cord
100.80 Fatal injury: cardiorespiratory failure resulting from brainstem hemorrhage and pneumoperitoneum	117.3 (35.75)	3140	63	10 min	Fractures: body of mandible (L), clavicles, comminuted iliac crests and fossae	Cutaneous lap belt and harness abrasions, contusions, and lacerations. Myorrhexis: sartorius, tensor fascia lata, rectus femoris, psoas major and minor, rectus abdominus, external and internal obliques, pectoralis major and minor (L). Evisceration: abdominal. Rupture: neck of urinary bladder, descending colon. Hemorrhage: inguinocrural fascia and musculature, root of mesentery, pectoralis major and minor, intercostals, costal pleura, cervical fascia and musculature, brainstem, cerebellum, temporal cortex
111.36 Fatal injury: cardiorespiratory failure resulting from brainstem hemorrhage and pneumpoperitoneum	122.9 (37.46)	3867	59	10 min	Luxation: L-6 upon L-7. Fractures: body of mandible (L), clavicles, sternum, comminuted iliac crests and fossae	Cutaneous lap belt and harness abrasions, contusions, and lacerations. Myorrhexis: sartorius, tensor fascia lata, rectus femoris, psoas major and minor, rectus abdominus, external and internal obliques, pectoralis major and minor. Evisceration: abdominal. Transection: lumbar spinal cord, iliac arteries, inferior vena cava, descending colon. Laceration: myocardium (L ventricle). Rupture: neck of urinary bladder. Hemorrhage: inguinocrural fascia and musculature, root of mesentery, retroperitoneal, intercostals, costal pleura, lungs, cervical fascia and musculature, lumbar spinal cord, brainstem
112.10 Fatal injury: cardiorespiratory failure resulting from brainstem hemorrhage and pneumoperitoneum	123.5 (37.64)	3961	59	10 min	Luxation: L-6 upon L-7. Fractures: body of mandible (L), clavicles, sternum, comminuted iliac crests and fossae	Cutaneous lap belt and harness abrasions, contusions, and lacerations. Myorrhexis: sartorius, tensor fascia lata, rectus femoris, psoas major and minor, rectus abdominus, external and internal obliques, pectoralis major and minor. Laceration: endocardium and myocardium. Rupture: neck of urinary bladder. Evisceration: abdominal. Transection: descending colon, lumbar spinal cord. Hemorrhage: inguinocrural fascia and musculature, root of mesentery, intercostals, costal pleura, lungs, cervical fascia and musculature, lumbar spinal cord, medulla, middle cerebral peduncle

of the liver and intestine. The severity of the infestation may have contributed to death in two animals that survived from 12-22 h. Last, it should be noted that the cause of death is a presumption based upon the necropsy findings, radiological examination, and sundry clinical evaluations (blood chemistry, hematology, urinalysis, cerebrospinal fluid, electrocardiogram, etc.).

Fatal Injuries - At all stopping distances, the primary cause of death was lower brainstem or cervical spinal cord trauma. At the 0.5 and 2.0 ft (0.15 and 0.61 m) stops, hemorrhage of the brainstem and spinal cord or transection of the cervical spinal cord typically resulted from avulsion of the atlanto-occipital articulation or luxation of cervical vertebrae. At the 3.5 ft (1.07 m) stop, brainstem hemorrhage concomitant with severe pelvic and abdominal trauma resulted in death. By reviewing Table 5, one notes that avulsion of the atlanto-occipital articulation, dislocation fractures of the vertebral column, or hemorrhage of the brainstem (Fig. 8) occurred at

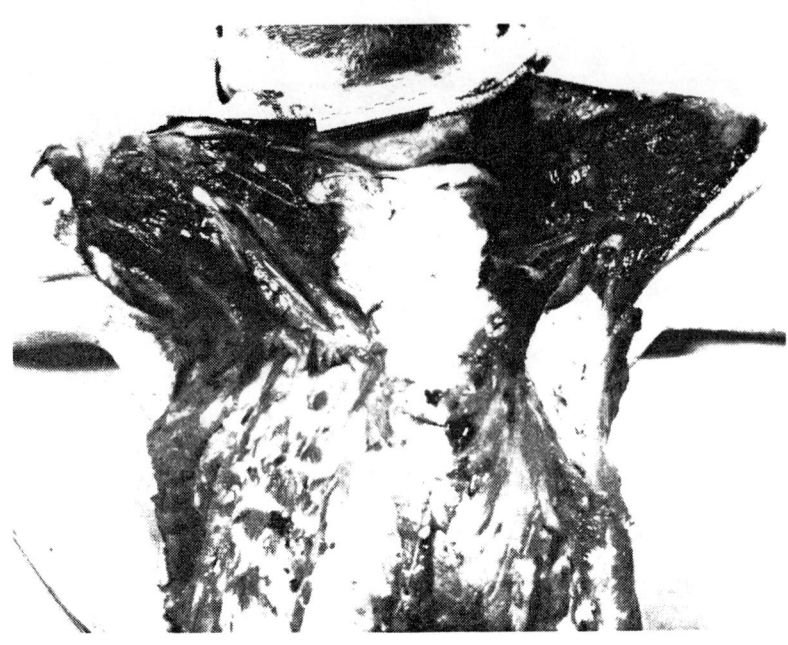

Fig. 7 - Myorrhexis of pectoral musculature. Clavicular and scapular fractures

Table 5 - Sled Deceleration (g_{max}) Required to Produce 50% Incidence of Injuries at Various Stopping Distances, Values Expressed in g_{max}

	Stopping distance, ft (m)				Stopping distance, ft (m)		
	0.5 (0.15)	2.0 (0.61)	3.5 (1.07)		0.5 (0.15)	2.0 (0.61)	3.5 (1.07)
Cutaneous lap belt and harness abrasions and contusions	67 ± 10	35 ± 8	24 ± 11	Hemorrhage: root of mesentery	104 ± 23	85 ± 26	74 ± 8
				Transection: descending colon	>134	125 ± 16	84 ± 14
Cutaneous lap belt and harness lacerations	112 ± 14	91 ± 12	59 ± 8	Hemorrhage: intestine	124 ± 12	100 ± 29	74 ± 8
				Evisceration or herniation	>134	91 ± 8	84 ± 14
Hemorrhage: inguinocrural fascia and musculature	90 ± 11	60 ± 13	69 ± 8	Fracture: pelvis	124 ± 12	85 ± 10	80 ± 14
Myorrhexis: rectus abdominus	124 ± 12	85 ± 22	74 ± 8	Myorrhexis: pectoralis major and minor	>134	96 ± 10	84 ± 8
Hemorrhage: rectus abdominus	124 ± 12	74 ± 19	74 ± 8	Hemorrhage: pectoralis major and minor	90 ± 11	81 ± 8	74 ± 8
Myorrhexis: sartorius, tensor fascia lata and rectus femoris	124 ± 12	74 ± 13	79 ± 8	Hemorrhage: intercostals	90 ± 11	81 ± 8	74 ± 8
Hemorrhage: sartorius, tensor fascia lata and rectus femoris	124 ± 12	69 ± 9	74 ± 8	Hemorrhage: costal pleura	90 ± 11	71 ± 16	74 ± 8
				Myorrhexis: cervical musculature	>134	114 ± 11	>112
Myorrhexis: external and internal obliques	124 ± 12	94 ± 8	74 ± 8	Hemorrhage: cervical musculature	>134	114 ± 11	89 ± 11
Hemorrhage: external and internal obliques	124 ± 12	88 ± 9	74 ± 8	Hemorrhage: myocardium	102 ± 15	155 ± 59	89 ± 18
				Fracture: sternum and ribs	102 ± 15	110 ± 45	99 ± 14
Myorrhexis: psoas major and minor	>134	100 ± 8	84 ± 8	Fracture: clavicle	133 ± 23	65 ± 20	89 ± 18
				Fracture: scapula	>134	108 ± 23	>112
Hemorrhage: psoas major and minor	90 ± 11	81 ± 20	84 ± 8	Fracture: mandible	>134	125 ± 16	102 ± 10
				Fracture or avulsion: vertebrae	101 ± 12	105 ± 26	99 ± 14
Rupture: urinary bladder	124 ± 12	115 ± 23	93 ± 10	Transection: spinal cord	101 ± 12	111 ± 20	99 ± 14
Hemorrhage: urinary bladder	124 ± 12	97 ± 37	74 ± 8	Hemorrhage: spinal cord	90 ± 11	104 ± 14	99 ± 14
				Hemorrhage: brainstem or cortex	101 ± 12	107 ± 19	102 ± 10

approximately the same level of peak sled deceleration as did the LD_{50} at the various stopping distances. For the test series, this observation supports the premise that neurological trauma is related directly to maximum sled deceleration (g_{max}). Furthermore, since the graph of deceleration required to produce a 50% incidence of head-neck trauma (Fig. 9) is a virtual overlay of the tolerance levels to impact (Fig. 3), the cause of death is reasonably substantiated.

Lap Belt-Induced Injuries - The trauma sustained as a result of the impact can generally be attributed to either the lap belt or torso harness portion of the restraint system. Although details of the gross anatomical and microscopic pathology will be reported in a subsequent paper, several of the injuries deserve additional comment.

Cutaneous abrasions, contusions, and lacerations were linear in nature and resulted from impingement of the lap belt portion of the restraint. Hemorrhage of the inguinocrural fascia and musculature is an all-inclusive term for hemorrhage within the superficial and deep fascia of the anterolateral abdominal wall. Likewise, this terminology has been used when hemorrhage existed within the aponeurosis of the external and internal obliques, adjacent to the superior and inferior crura and from the inguinal falx to the femoral ring.

Myorrhexis of the rectus abdominus, sartorius, tensor fascia lata, rectus femoris, and iliopsoas, plus comminuted fractures of the iliac crest and fossa, occurred in an area directly beneath or adjacent to the lap belt (Fig. 10). The injuries of the pelvic and abdominal region did not result strictly as a function of peak sled deceleration (Table 5). These injuries resulted at lower sled decelerations as the stopping distance was increased (Fig. 11).

Torso Harness-Induced Injuries - The trauma resulting di-

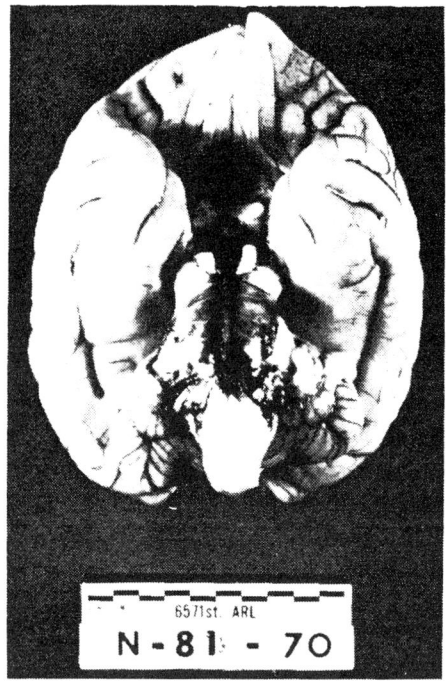

Fig. 8 - Hemorrhage: brainstem and cerebellum

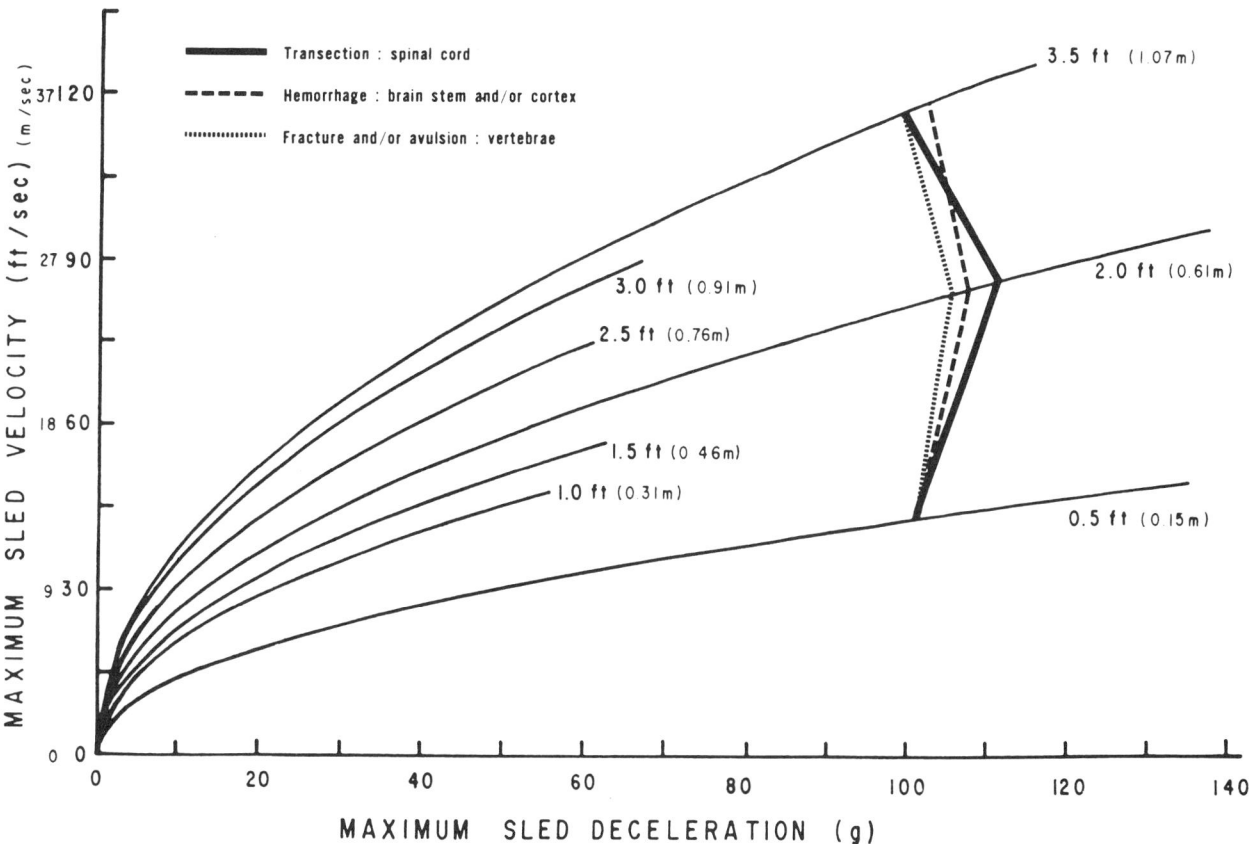

Fig. 9 - Sled deceleration (g_{max}) required to produce 50% incidence of neurological trauma

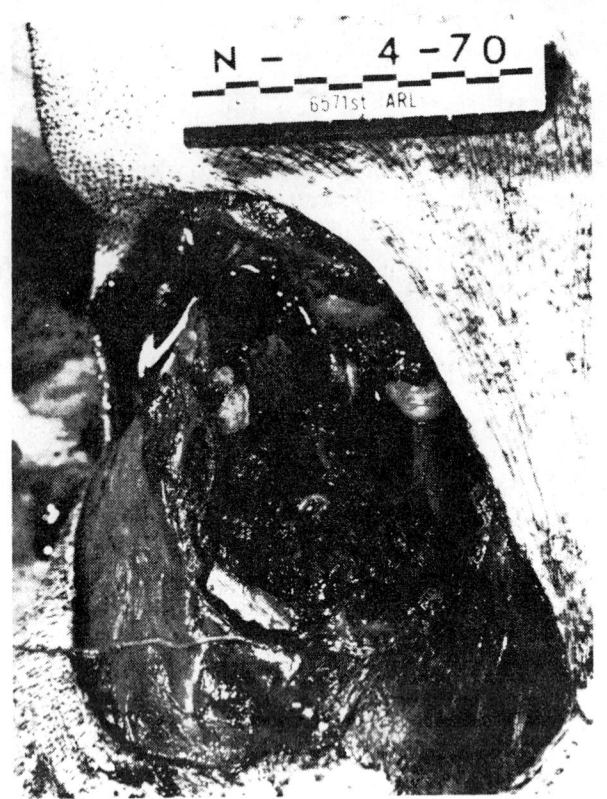

Fig. 10 - Myorrhexis: sartorius, tensor fascia lata, rectus femoris, and iliopsoas. Comminuted fractures of iliac crest and fossa

rectly or indirectly from the torso portion of the restraint was generally more life-threatening than the pelvic or abdominal injuries. The high incidence of sternal, costal, clavicular, or scapular fractures presented the opportunity for pleural perforation and thus pneumothorax. The sternal fractures may have been produced by mandibular contact with the manubrium or body of the sternum. In six cases, the striking force was sufficient to fracture the body of the mandible (Fig. 12). Myocardial hemorrhage was invariable adjacent to the anterior interventricular artery. The injury could actually be described as contusion of the anterior wall of the right and left ventricle. It is presumed that this injury resulted from sternal and costal impingement (compression) coincident with flexion of the thorax or from cardiac displacement relative to the thoracic cage.

Muscular and skeletal trauma of the axillary and cervical regions may be the resultant of an improper restraint for the baboon. Specifically, since the deltoid and trapezoid angles of shoulder slope in humans is an important factor in shoulder harness design (24), one would expect modifications in the existing system to reduce baboon trauma.

Submarining is a phenomenon generally attributed to elongation of the lap belt and torso harness webbing under applied load, causing an unbalanced turning moment on the baboon. Submarining occurred frequently in this study because the lap belt was affixed to the torso portion of the restraint. In es-

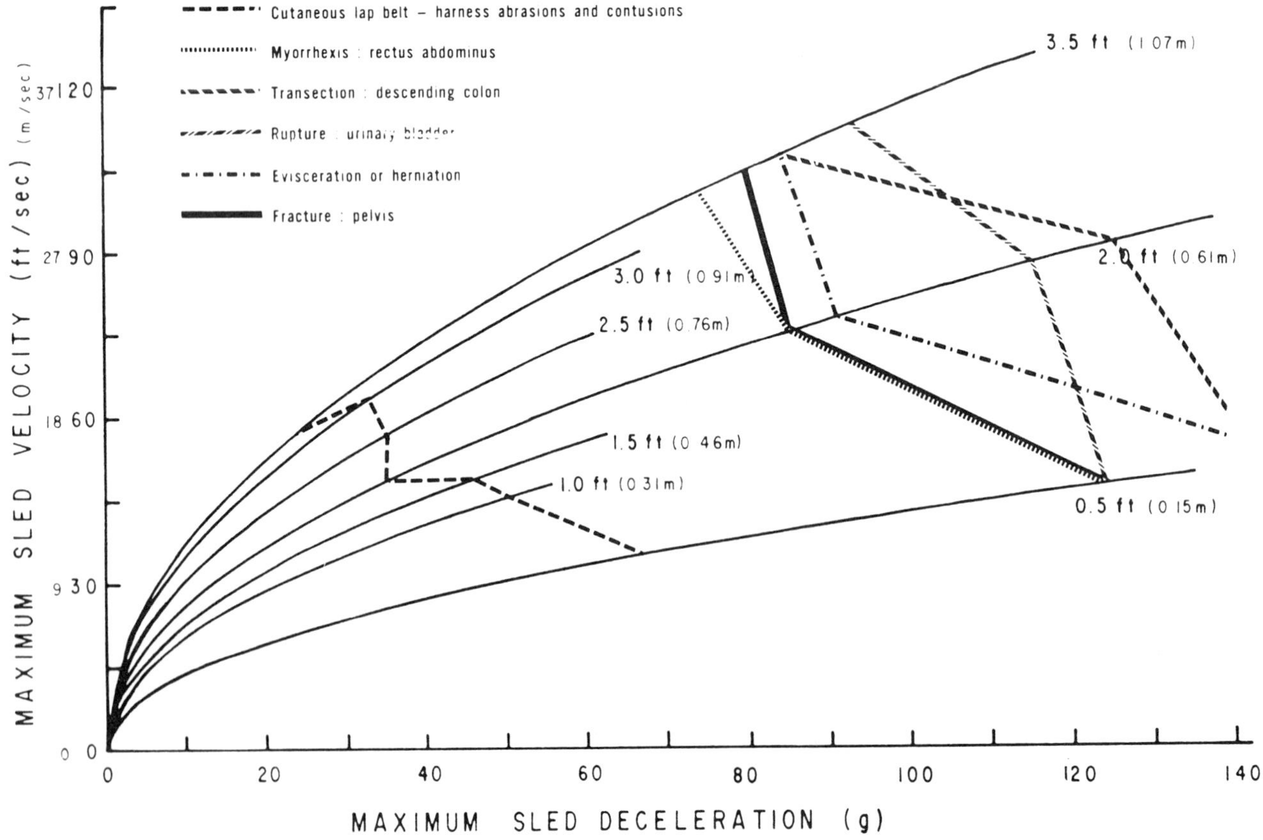

Fig. 11 - Sled deceleration (g_{max}) required to produce 50% incidence of pelvic/abdominal trauma

sence, a vertical displacement of the lap belt was produced as the subject loaded the torso harness.

Submarining was not evident at the 0.5 ft (0.15 m) stop. Moderate to severe submarining was noticed at the 2.0 ft (0.61 m) stop but only in excess of 100 g. The principal resulting injury was intestinal herniation. For the 3.5 ft (1.07 m) stop, the submarining was more severe and occurred first at about 75 g. The injuries directly attributable to submarining included abdominal evisceration and transection of the descending colon.

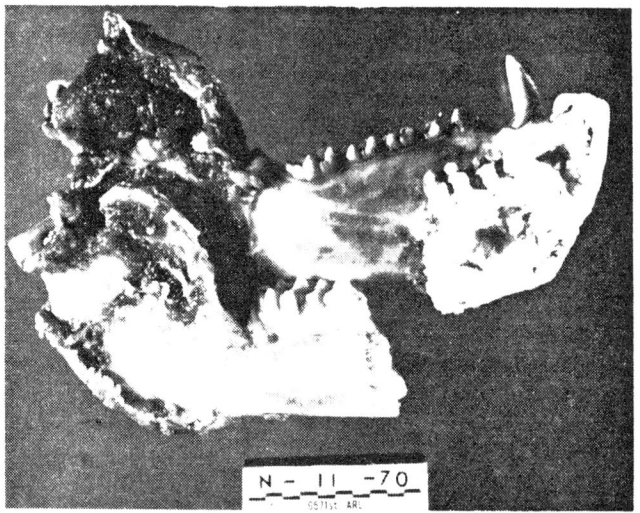

Fig. 12 - Transverse fracture through body of mandible

It is speculated that luxation of lumbar vertebrae also resulted from submarining or from rebound into the seat back. This injury was primarily associated with the 3.5 ft (1.07 m) stop.

FORCE - Many factors relating to decelerative force are significant determinants of injury patterns. Several of these factors include: force magnitude, impulse (time integral of the forces), direction of force application, site of application to the body, area of force distribution, and the mechanism through which the force is applied. In this report, only force magnitude and impulse are emphasized since the other factors remained relatively constant throughout the test series.

The values of x, y, and z refer to a left-handed Cartesian coordinate system where x is parallel to sled movement, y is lateral, and z is vertical. The forces transmitted by the baboon to the lap belt, torso harness, seat pan, and back were recorded and corrected by subtraction of dynamic tare loads—the force/g attributable to the mass of the transducer system acting upon the active portion of the gage. Total lap belt force was calculated from the vector summation of the right and left belt x, y, and z force components.

In Tables 6-12, peak lap belt, torso harness, seat pan, and back forces are presented in relation to maximum sled deceleration. Equations of regression lines and respective correlation coefficients are given for each of the seven stopping distances. The forces and impulses were proportionately adjusted to reflect a standard 50 lb (22.7 kg) animal weight. Impulses were computed by integrating the force-time curves using 1 ms

Table 6 - Equations of Force (lb_f) and Impulse (lb_f - s) Regression Lines
0.5 ft (0.15 m) Stop*

Ordinate	Equation of Regression Line	Linear Correlation Coefficient
Lap belt total	Force = 386.0 + 36.09 (g_{max})	0.9678
	Impulse = 14.0 + 0.47 (g_{max})	0.9402
Lap belt x	Force = 179.7 + 24.57 (g_{max})	0.9729
	Impulse = 8.4 + 0.31 (g_{max})	0.9399
Lap belt y	Force = 160.5 + 18.00 (g_{max})	0.9703
Lap belt z	Force = 326.3 + 19.40 (g_{max})	0.9535
	Impulse = 9.4 + 0.26 (g_{max})	0.9246
Seat pan x (forward)	Force = 21.6 + 7.55 (g_{max})	0.9540
Seat pan z (down)	Force = 265.0 + 10.17 (g_{max})	0.8407
	Impulse = 3.4 + 0.30 (g_{max})	0.9577
Seat back x (rebound)	Force = 6.6 + 9.83 (g_{max})	0.9000
Torso harness total	Force = -0.4 + 26.22 (g_{max})	0.9948
	Impulse = 4.9 + 0.37 (g_{max})	0.9803
Torso harness x	Force = -216.2 + 6.33 (g_{max})	0.8173
Torso harness z	Force = -1.6 + 2.64 (g_{max})	0.7577

*Multiply lb_f by 4.448 for conversion to Newtons and N-s.

intervals from time zero (instant of sled contact with the brake) until the force traces returned to 0 lb. The correlation coefficients indicated a definite linear relationship between force or impulse and peak sled deceleration.

In Table 13, the data from the seven stopping distances were combined to yield equations of force in relation to peak sled deceleration irrespective of the stopping distance. Although many of the correlation coefficients lost minor significance, there was no appreciable difference in the bandwidth of 90% confidence intervals. The lap belt finite forces at 0 g were partially due to pretensioning and to possible nonlinearity of the regression line at low sled decelerations.

Table 7 - Equations of Force (lb_f) and Impulse (lb_f-s) Regression Lines 1.0 ft (0.31 m) Stop

Ordinate	Equation of Regression Line	Linear Correlation Coefficient
Lap belt total	Force = $-39.3 + 52.86 (g_{max})$	0.9920
	Impulse = $6.6 + 1.02 (g_{max})$	0.9730
Lap belt x	Force = $-35.8 + 35.35 (g_{max})$	0.9943
	Impulse = $3.4 + 0.70 (g_{max})$	0.9775
Lap belt y	Force = $-19.7 + 25.02 (g_{max})$	0.9967
Lap belt z	Force = $-9.5 + 30.25 (g_{max})$	0.9942
	Impulse = $4.8 + 0.57 (g_{max})$	0.9578
Seat pan x (forward)	Force = $-4.3 + 10.50 (g_{max})$	0.9945
Seat pan z (down)	Force = $69.1 + 14.55 (g_{max})$	0.8479
	Impulse = $5.3 + 0.38 (g_{max})$	0.8592
Seat back x (rebound)	Force = $-15.3 + 9.34 (g_{max})$	0.9925
Torso harness total	Force = $-33.1 + 33.09 (g_{max})$	0.9949
	Impulse = $3.4 + 0.65 (g_{max})$	0.9575
Torso harness x	Force = $-33.1 + 33.02 (g_{max})$	0.9949
Torso harness z	Force = $-17.6 + 2.45 (g_{max})$	0.9287

Table 8 - Equations of Force (lb_f) and Impulse (lb_f-s) Regression Lines 1.5 ft (0.46 m) Stop

Ordinate	Equation of Regression Line	Linear Correlation Coefficient
Lap belt total	Force = $-132.7 + 49.35 (g_{max})$	0.9880
	Impulse = $4.4 + 1.25 (g_{max})$	0.9839
Lap belt x	Force = $-110.9 + 33.90 (g_{max})$	0.9827
	Impulse = $1.8 + 0.88 (g_{max})$	0.9843
Lap belt y	Force = $-44.9 + 22.91 (g_{max})$	0.9910
Lap belt z	Force = $-65.9 + 27.60 (g_{max})$	0.9914
	Impulse = $3.0 + 0.69 (g_{max})$	0.9827
Seat pan x (forward)	Force = $26.7 + 6.28 (g_{max})$	0.9698
Seat pan z (down)	Force = $47.3 + 18.33 (g_{max})$	0.9759
	Impulse = $2.7 + 0.61 (g_{max})$	0.9786
Seat back x (rebound)	Force = $-63.3 + 8.31 (g_{max})$	0.9169
Torso harness total	Force = $-26.6 + 27.51 (g_{max})$	0.9942
	Impulse = $5.7 + 0.63 (g_{max})$	0.9605
Torso harness x	Force = $-27.3 + 27.49 (g_{max})$	0.9944
Torso harness z	Force = $15.1 + 0.58 (g_{max})$	0.3937

The relationship of lap belt total force to peak sled deceleration (Fig. 13) adheres to Newton's second law of motion. Specifically, 1000 lb (4448 N) was recorded as lap belt force from only 17-22 g, irrespective of the stopping distance (Fig. 13). Indeed, at any force up to 5000 lb (22240 N), there is only a predicted variation of 20 g from the 0.5-3.5 ft (0.15-1.07 m) stop. The same relationship exists with the torso harness total force (Fig. 14), but the variability is slightly less.

It is generally accepted that the ultimate harness restraint should incorporate the features of maximal area and provide equal distribution of force to the torso (25). In this test series, the lap belt received almost 54% of the total restraint load in

Table 9 - Equations of Force (lb_f) and Impulse (lb_f-s) Regression Lines
2.0 ft (0.61 m) Stop

Ordinate	Equation of Regression Line	Linear Correlation Coefficient
Lap belt total	Force = 58.6 + 41.40 (g_{max})	0.9809
	Impulse = 17.7 + 0.87 (g_{max})	0.9783
Lap belt x	Force = −40.9 + 30.77 (g_{max})	0.9904
	Impulse = 8.8 + 0.66 (g_{max})	0.9853
Lap belt y	Force = 62.3 + 17.27 (g_{max})	0.9724
Lap belt z	Force = 100.6 + 21.50 (g_{max})	0.9614
	Impulse = 12.3 + 0.43 (g_{max})	0.9567
Seat pan x (forward)	Force = 38.6 + 4.18 (g_{max})	0.8816
Seat pan z (down)	Force = 179.0 + 6.85 (g_{max})	0.9056
	Impulse = 20.9 + 0.29 (g_{max})	0.8783
Seat back x (rebound)	Force = 21.7 + 4.60 (g_{max})	0.9356
Torso harness total	Force = 99.6 + 24.04 (g_{max})	0.9908
	Impulse = 16.7 + 0.52 (g_{max})	0.9791
Torso harness x	Force = 97.4 + 24.01 (g_{max})	0.9909
Torso harness z	Force = −5.7 + 1.92 (g_{max})	0.8804

Table 10 - Equations of Force (lb_f) and Impulse (lb_f-s) Regression Lines
2.5 ft (0.76 m) Stop

Ordinate	Equation of Regression Line	Linear Correlation Coefficient
Lap belt total	Force = −56.4 + 51.19 (g_{max})	0.9864
	Impulse = 9.8 + 1.53 (g_{max})	0.9672
Lap belt x	Force = −83.2 + 37.57 (g_{max})	0.9770
	Impulse = 4.8 + 1.12 (g_{max})	0.9659
Lap belt y	Force = −4.3 + 23.06 (g_{max})	0.9896
Lap belt z	Force = 7.2 + 26.02 (g_{max})	0.9942
	Impulse = 7.0 + 0.77 (g_{max})	0.9605
Seat pan x (forward)	Force = 50.5 + 4.43 (g_{max})	0.8715
Seat pan z (down)	Force = 160.0 + 13.37 (g_{max})	0.9126
	Impulse = 8.9 + 0.65 (g_{max})	0.9109
Seat back x (rebound)	Force = 0.4 + 2.85 (g_{max})	0.8850
Torso harness total	Force = −53.1 + 29.31 (g_{max})	0.9955
	Impulse = 5.9 + 0.88 (g_{max})	0.9840
Torso harness x	Force = −53.7 + 29.30 (g_{max})	0.9956
Torso harness z	Force = 20.6 + 0.40 (g_{max})	0.2372

the x direction at any of the stopping distances. However, approximately 62% of the restraint total force (vector summation of x, y, and z components) was transmitted to the lap belt portion of the restraint.

Although there is a relatively equal distribution of force with this restraint system, these figures should be used cautiously. The force measurements may be somewhat redundant because the torso portion of the restraint is affixed to the lap belt. Likewise, there exists a force amplification of at least 16% within the restraint system.

IMPULSE - The relationship of peak sled deceleration to lap belt and torso harness impulse (area under the restraint force-time curve) was tabulated for all stopping distances (Tables 6-12). Figs. 15 and 16 show the levels of peak sled deceleration

Table 11 - Equations of Force (lb_f) and Impulse (lb_f-s) Regression Lines
3.0 ft (0.91 m) Stop

Ordinate	Equation of Regression Line	Linear Correlation Coefficient
Lap belt total	Force = $-97.4 + 53.03 (g_{max})$	0.9961
	Impulse = $9.1 + 1.59 (g_{max})$	0.9879
Lap belt x	Force = $-75.0 + 34.31 (g_{max})$	0.9949
	Impulse = $4.3 + 1.06 (g_{max})$	0.9919
Lap belt y	Force = $-48.7 + 25.40 (g_{max})$	0.9961
Lap belt z	Force = $-45.5 + 31.46 (g_{max})$	0.9966
	Impulse = $6.8 + 0.91 (g_{max})$	0.9799
Seat pan x (forward)	Force = $11.8 + 8.08 (g_{max})$	0.9911
Seat pan z (down)	Force = $72.5 + 18.84 (g_{max})$	0.9409
	Impulse = $11.0 + 0.75 (g_{max})$	0.8933
Seat back x (rebound)	Force = $-26.4 + 6.81 (g_{max})$	0.9701
Torso harness total	Force = $46.6 + 32.34 (g_{max})$	0.9837
	Impulse = $11.2 + 1.01 (g_{max})$	0.9532
Torso harness x	Force = $45.7 + 32.33 (g_{max})$	0.9839
Torso harness z	Force = $19.8 + 0.71 (g_{max})$	0.4025

Table 12 - Equations of Force (lb_f) and Impulse (lb_f-s) Regression Lines
3.5 ft (1.07 m) Stop

Ordinate	Equation of Regression Line	Linear Correlation Coefficient
Lap belt total	Force = $129.0 + 45.07 (g_{max})$	0.9910
	Impulse = $30.2 + 1.27 (g_{max})$	0.9606
Lap belt x	Force = $51.8 + 31.80 (g_{max})$	0.9925
	Impulse = $17.4 + 0.95 (g_{max})$	0.9640
Lap belt y	Force = $29.1 + 22.48 (g_{max})$	0.9882
Lap belt z	Force = $145.0 + 22.64 (g_{max})$	0.9841
	Impulse = $22.5 + 0.56 (g_{max})$	0.9196
Seat pan x (forward)	Force = $82.9 + 4.64 (g_{max})$	0.8899
Seat pan z (down)	Force = $448.2 + 6.57 (g_{max})$	0.4042
	Impulse = $30.5 + 0.14 (g_{max})$	0.3114
Seat back x (rebound)	Force = $52.8 + 2.09 (g_{max})$	0.6535
Torso harness total	Force = $39.0 + 27.69 (g_{max})$	0.9913
	Impulse = $17.6 + 0.78 (g_{max})$	0.9696
Torso harness x	Force = $37.2 + 27.70 (g_{max})$	0.9914
Torso harness z	Force = $3.8 + 1.29 (g_{max})$	0.6936

where various impulse values occur at the different stopping distances. The magnitude of impulse is virtually unaffected by the level of peak sled deceleration. That is, the same impulse at the 3.5 ft (1.07 m) stop occurs at the 0.5 ft (0.15 m) stop at considerably higher peak sled deceleration and shorter pulse duration. A significant finding is that the 50% incidence of pelvic and abdominal trauma (Fig. 11) has almost the same relationship (in slope) to sled deceleration and velocity as does impulse (Fig. 15). Therefore, it is not peak restraining force but the level of impulse that appears to be a significant determinant of muscular and skeletal trauma of the pelvic and abdominal region. Also, many of the thoracic injuries may be produced via the same mechanism.

HEAD-NECK RESPONSE - The head reference axes may be depicted using a polar coordinate system where angular displacement of the head was positive with flexion and negative

Table 13 - Equations of Force (lb_f) Regression Lines
Total of All Stopping Distances

Ordinate	Equation of Regression Line	Linear Correlation Coefficient
Lap belt total	Force = 130.2 + 42.44 (g_{max})	0.9793
Lap belt x	Force = −22.4 + 31.38 (g_{max})	0.9897
Lap belt y	Force = 106.1 + 18.27 (g_{max})	0.9637
Lap belt z	Force = 163.0 + 21.71 (g_{max})	0.9636
Seat pan x (forward)	Force = 92.1 + 4.06 (g_{max})	0.8175
Seat pan z (down)	Force = 301.6 + 7.64 (g_{max})	0.7398
Seat back x (rebound)	Force = 34.6 + 4.51 (g_{max})	0.8624
Torso harness total	Force = 88.7 + 25.60 (g_{max})	0.9872
Torso harness x	Force = 86.3 + 25.60 (g_{max})	0.9873
Torso harness z	Force = −6.8 + 1.83 (g_{max})	0.8251

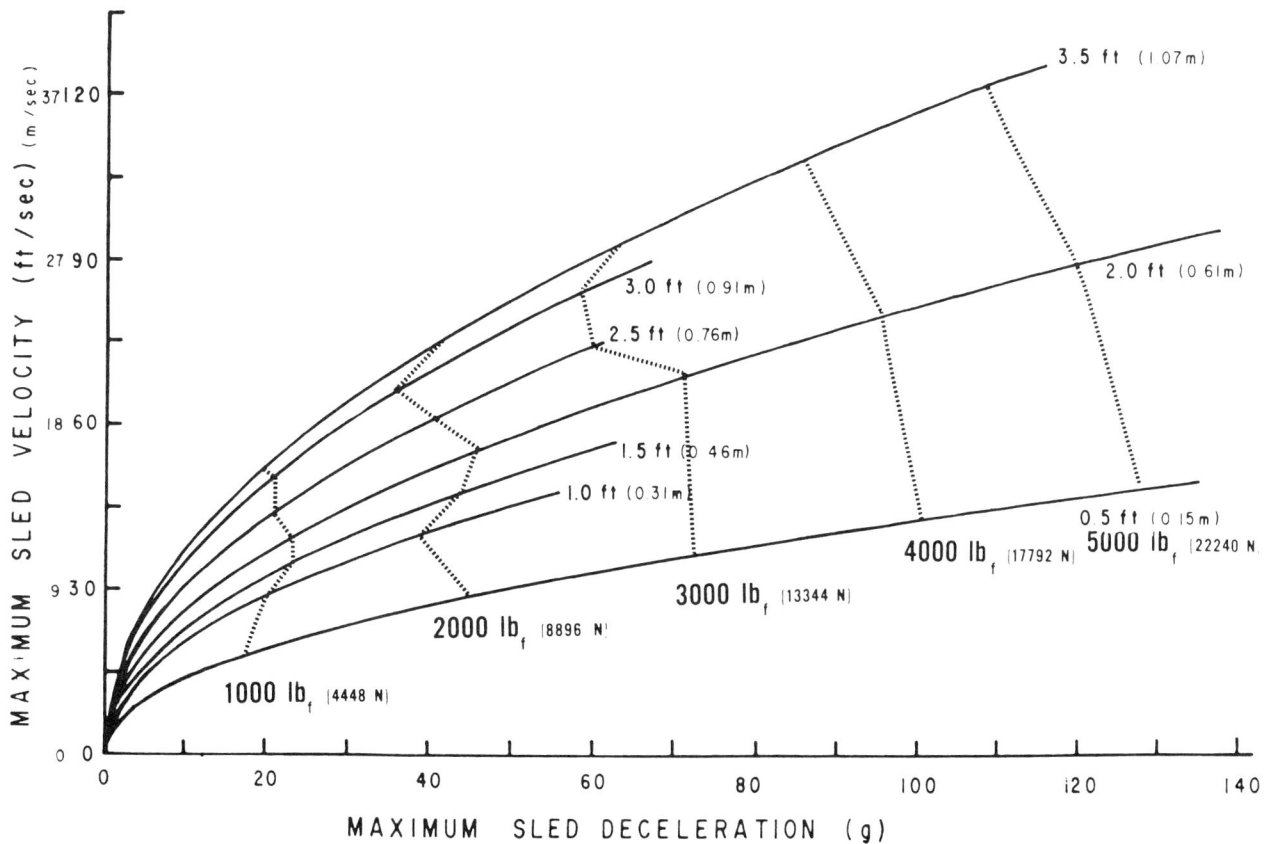

Fig. 13 - Relationship of peak lap belt total force to sled deceleration (g_{max})

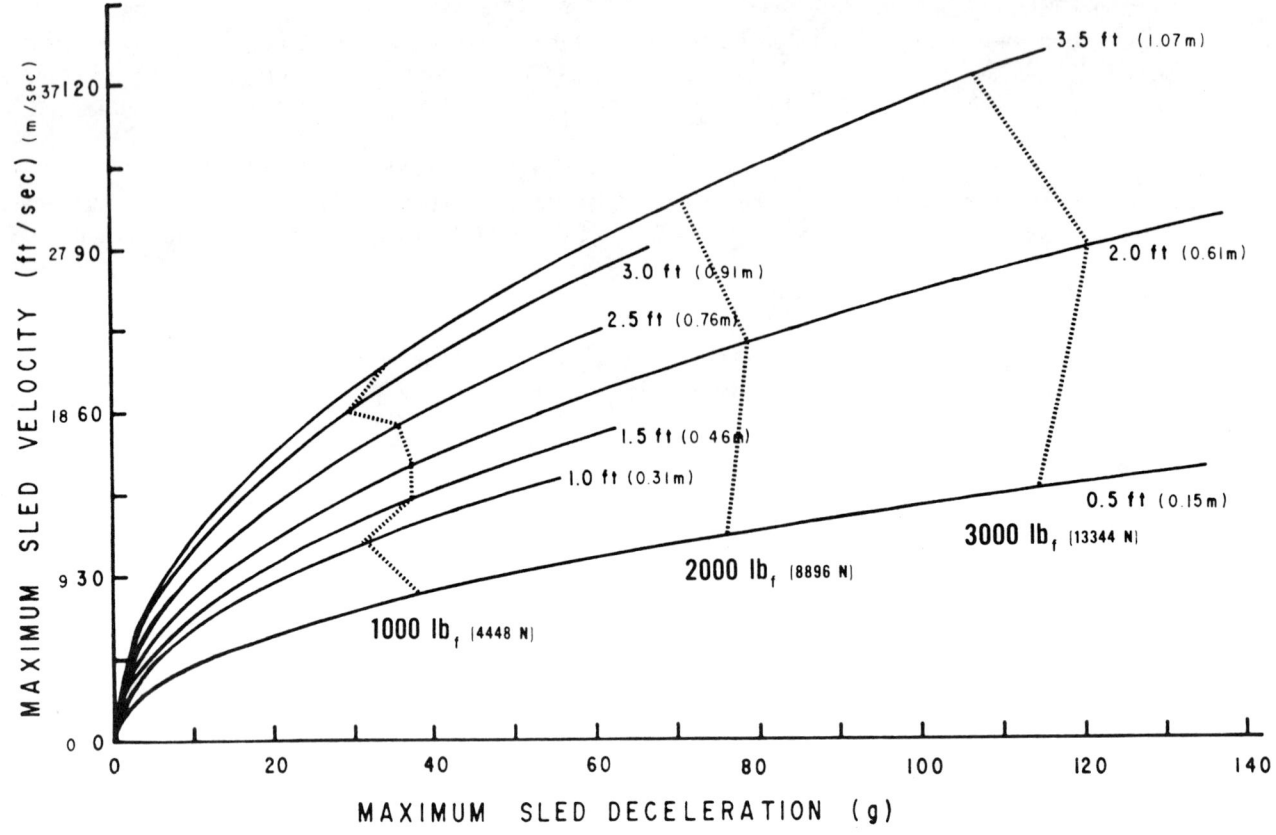

Fig. 14 - Relationship of peak torso harness total force to sled deceleration (g_{max})

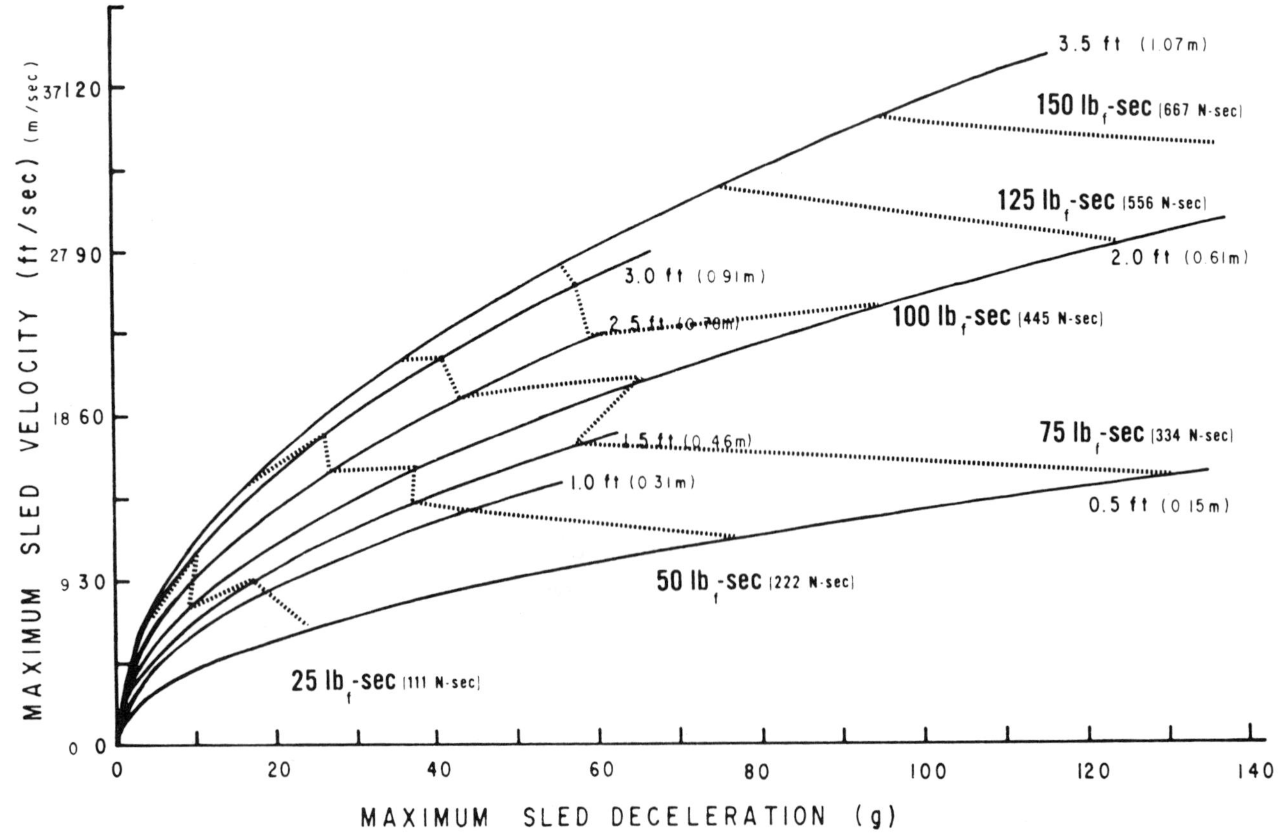

Fig. 15 - Relationship of lap belt total impulse to sled deceleration (g_{max})

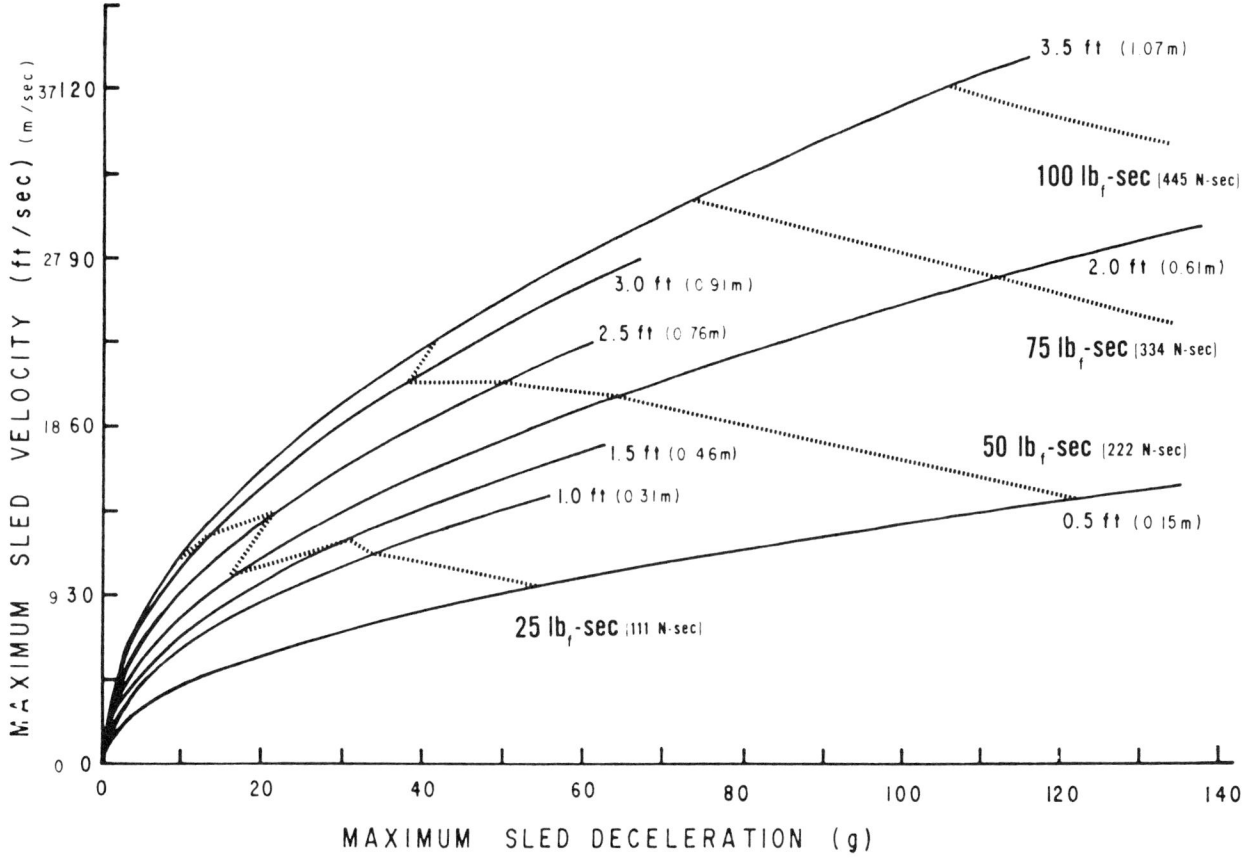

Fig. 16 - Relationship of torso harness total impulse to sled deceleration (g_{max})

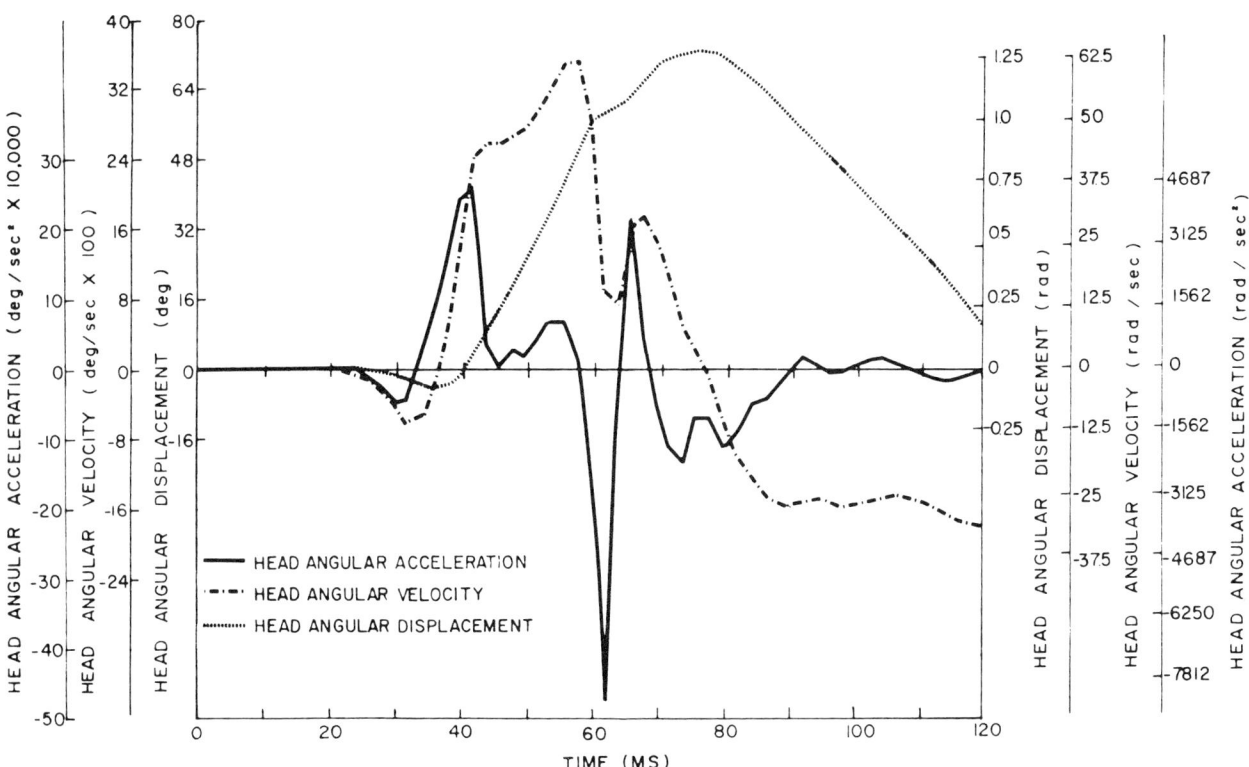

Fig. 17 - Head angular acceleration, head angular velocity and head angular displacement versus time, 0.5 ft (0.15 m) stop, 113.6 g

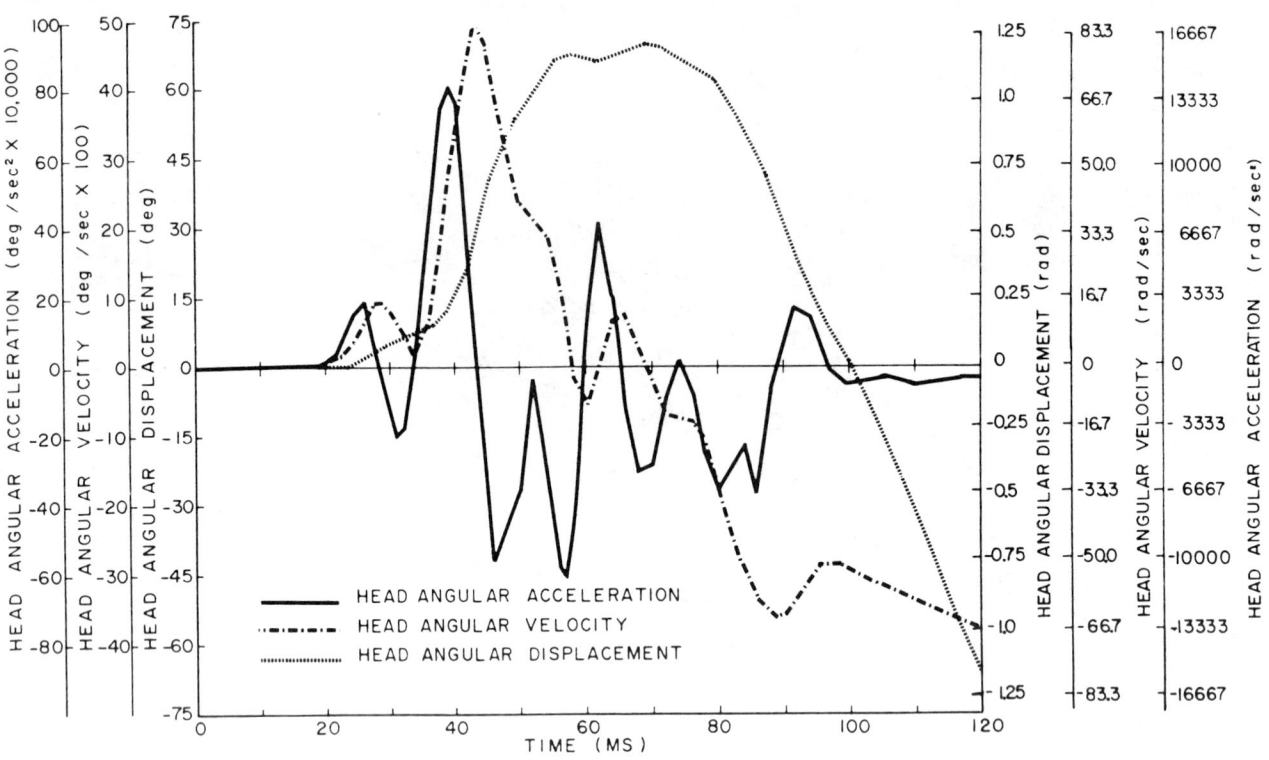

Fig. 18 - Head angular acceleration, head angular velocity and head angular displacement versus time, 2.0 ft (0.51 m) stop, 105.1 g

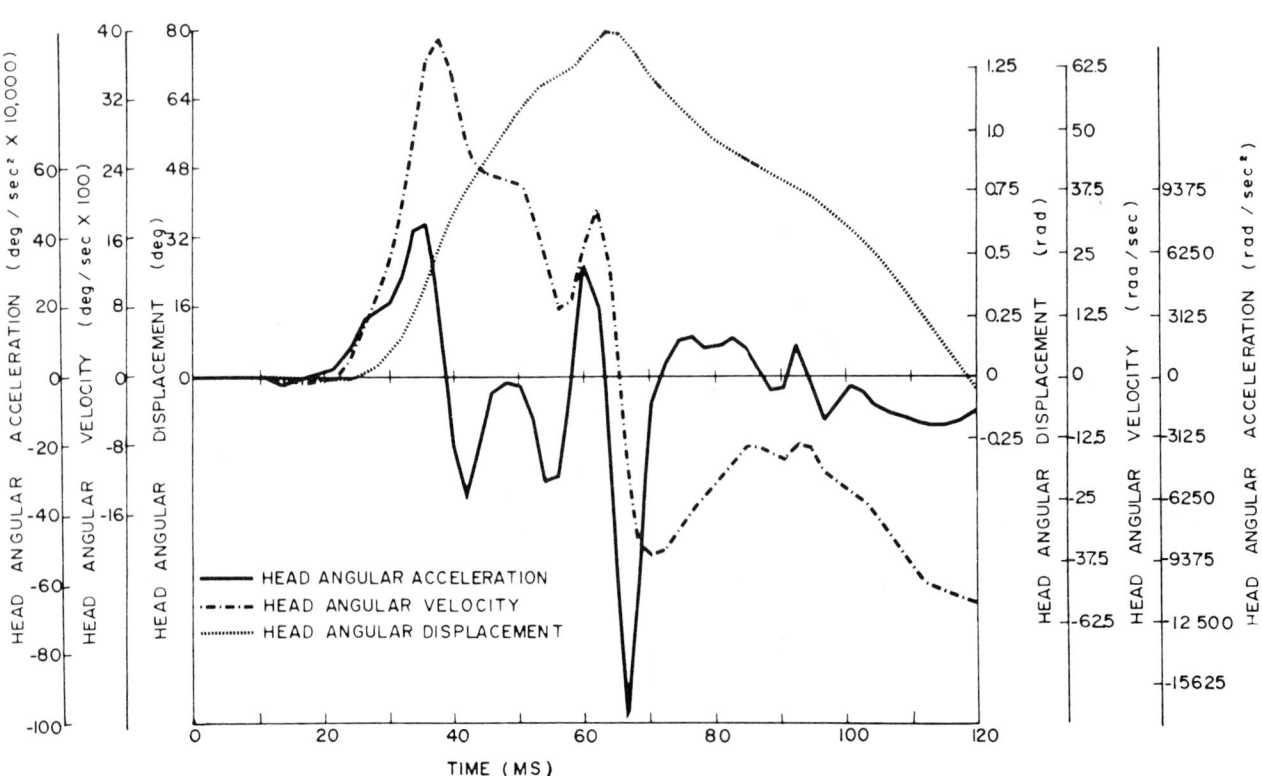

Fig. 19 - Head angular acceleration, head angular velocity and head angular displacement versus time, 3.5 ft (1.07 m) stop, 90.36 g

Table 14 - Comparison of Baboon Head-Neck Responses at Various Stopping Distances

Stopping distance, ft (m)	0.5 (0.15)	2.0 (0.61)	3.5 (1.07)
No. Tests	5	7	8
Max head angular acceleration, deg/s^2 (rad/s^2)	411900* ± 78500** 7188 ± 1370	621400 ± 135000 10843 ± 2356	567300 ± 179100 9899 ± 3125
Max head angular deceleration, deg/s^2 (rad/s^2)	-581300 ± 256700 -10144 ± 4479	-560800 ± 153400 -9786 ± 2677	-540800 ± 268400 -9437 ± 4684
Max positive head angular velocity, deg/s (rad/s)	3260 ± 320 56.9 ± 5.6	4700 ± 820 82.0 ± 14.3	3700 ± 920 64.6 ± 16.1
Max negative head angular velocity, deg/s (rad/s)	-1300 ± 300 -23.2 ± 5.2	-2700 ± 1250 -47.1 ± 21.8	-3000 ± 820 -52.4 ± 14.3
Max head angular displacement—flexion, deg (rad)	85 ± 12 1.5 ± 0.2	84 ± 21 1.5 ± 0.4	64 ± 17 1.1 ± 0.3
Max sled deceleration, g	109 ± 20	116 ± 9	97 ± 12

*Mean of peak values.
**Standard deviation.

with hyperextension. Head angular acceleration, velocity, and displacement of baboons restrained with the Air Force shoulder harness-lap belt are graphically displayed for a 0.5, 2.0, and 3.5 ft (0.15, 0.61, and 1.07 m) stop at 113.6, 105.1, and 90.4 g, respectively (Figs. 17-19).

The primary positive and negative peaks of the head angular acceleration traces occurred at approximately the same time, even though the durations of the impact pulses were quite different. Peak head angular velocities and displacements did occur earlier in time for the tests with the greatest stopping distance and therefore the greatest sled velocity.

The average peak magnitudes for angular accelerations and velocities were approximately equal at the various stopping distances (Table 14). The head angular displacements were considerably less for the 3.5 ft (1.07 m) stop (averaging 64 deg) because of submarining and the forward translation of the thorax preventing full head-neck rotation. Indeed, in all cases at the different stopping distances, the maximum head-neck flexion was determined by mandibular contact with the sternum.

Although in a previous report there was a linear relationship between head angular acceleration and maximum sled deceleration (14), the relatively few tests at the 0.5 and 3.5 ft (0.15 and 1.07 m) stopping distances precluded this type of analysis in this report. It appears that the magnitude of head angular acceleration is related to peak sled deceleration, but the authors did not attempt to correlate lethal head-neck trauma with head angular accelerations. Linear accelerations of the head were not recorded in the x and y directions. Therefore, it is only speculative to assume that lethal trauma may have resulted from translational or angular shear loading at the atlanto-occipital articulation.

SUMMARY

LD$_{50}$s were calculated to be 102, 103, and 98 g for the 0.5, 2.0, and 3.5 ft stopping distances, respectively. Since the deceleration pulses were similar (all half sine with different pulse duration), the results imply that for the pulse range investigated, impact lethality is dependent upon the magnitude of peak sled deceleration irrespective of the pulse duration, sled velocity, onset, energy dissipation, or stopping distance.

At all stopping distances, the primary cause of death was lower brainstem or cervical spinal cord trauma. At the 0.5 and 2.0 ft stops, hemorrhage of the brainstem and spinal cord or transection of the cervical spinal cord typically resulted from avulsion of the atlanto-occipital articulation or luxation of cervical vertebrae. At the 3.5 ft stop, brainstem hemorrhage concomitant with severe pelvic and abdominal trauma resulted in death.

The peak sled deceleration required to produce a 50% incidence of injuries at various stopping distances provided a convenient method of presenting and discussing injury causation. The level of impulse or the time integral of restraint force appeared to be a significant factor contributing to muscular and skeletal trauma of the pelvic, abdominal, and thoracic regions. Additional investigations of injury patterns should improve the understanding of impact trauma causation and provide further guidance for designers of occupant restraint systems.

ACKNOWLEDGMENT

The authors gratefully acknowledge the support by the entire Daisy Decelerator staff of the Land-Air Division, Dynalectron Corp., Holloman Air Force Base, New Mexico. Appreciation is also expressed to Darlene Bach of Systems Research Laboratories, Inc. for assistance in data reduction and analyses.

REFERENCES

1. H. De Haven, "The Site, Frequency and Dangerousness of Injury Sustained by 800 Survivors of Lightplane Accidents." Crash Injury Research, Dept. of Public Health and

Preventive Medicine, Cornell University Medical College, New York, 1952.

2. S. Ruff, "Brief Acceleration: Less Than One Second." German Aviation Medicine, World War II, Vol. 1 (1950), pp. 584-597.

3. H. De Haven and A. H. Hasbrook, "Shoulder Harness: Its Use and Effectiveness." Crash Injury Research, Dept. of Public Health and Preventive Medicine, Cornell University Medical College, New York, 1952.

4. N. I. Bohlin, "Studies of Three-Point Restraint Harness Systems in Full-Scale Barrier Crashes and Sled Runs." Proceedings of Eighth Stapp Car Crash and Field Demonstration Conference, Detroit: Wayne State University Press, 1966, p. 258.

5. N. I. Bohlin, "A Statistical Analysis of 28,000 Accident Cases with Emphasis on Occupant Restraint Value." SAE Transactions, Vol. 76, paper 670925.

6. Y. Hiroshige and L. E. Hackman, "The Dynamics of Crash Restraint Harnesses." AFFTC-TR-55-24, Air Research and Development Command, Air Force Flight Test Center, Edwards AFB, California, 1955.

7. R. R. McHenry, "Analysis of the Dynamics of Automobile Passenger Restraint Systems." The Seventh Stapp Car Crash Conference–Proceedings. Springfield, Ill.: Charles C. Thomas, Publisher, 1965, pp. 207-249.

8. R. G. Snyder, C. C. Snow, J. W. Young, W. M. Crosby, and G. T. Price, "Pathology of Trauma Attributed to Restraint Systems in Crash Impacts." Aerospace Medicine, Vol. 39 (1968), pp. 812-829.

9. B. Aldman, "Biodynamic Studies on Impact Protection." Acta Physiologica Scandinavica, Vol. 192, No. 56 (Suppl.) (1962), pp. 1-80.

10. J. F. Sprouffske, W. H. Muzzy, T. D. Clarke, E. M. Trout, and C. D. Gragg, "The Effect on Data Reproducibility of Dummy Modifications." Paper 710847, Proceedings of Fifteenth Stapp Car Crash Conference, P-29. New York: Society of Automotive Engineers, Inc., 1971.

11. J. F. Sprouffske, T. D. Clarke, C. D. Gragg, E. M. Trout, and W. H. Muzzy, "Evaluation of the Lap Belt, Air Force Shoulder Harness-Lap Belt and Air Bag Plus Lap Belt Restraints During Impact with Anthropomorphic Dummies." AMRL-TR-71-86, Aerospace Medicine, Vol. 43 (1972), pp. 368-371.

12. C. D. Gragg, C. D. Bendixen, T. D. Clarke, H. S. Klopfenstein, and J. F. Sprouffske, "Evaluation of the Lap Belt, Air Bag and Air Force Restraint Systems During Impact with Living Human Sled Subjects." Paper 700904, Proceedings of Fourteenth Stapp Car Crash Conference, P-33. New York: Society of Automotive Engineers, Inc., 1970. Also identified as AMRL-TR-72-42.

13. C. D. Gragg, T. C. Clarke, and J. F. Sprouffske, "Human Weight Distribution During Impact—Lap Belt, Air Bag and Air Force Harness Restraint Systems." Proceedings of Seventeenth Annual Meeting of Institute of Environmental Sciences. Los Angeles, 1971, pp. 365-369.

14. T. D. Clarke, D. C. Smedley, C. D. Gragg, E. M. Trout, and W. H. Muzzy, "Baboon Tolerance to Linear Deceleration ($-G_x$): Air Force Shoulder Harness-Lap Belt Restraint." Aerospace Medicine, 1972. Submitted.

15. W. J. Dixon and A. M. Mood, "A Method for Obtaining and Analyzing Sensitivity Data." Jrl. Amer. Stat. Assn., Vol. 43 (1948), pp. 109-126.

16. A. W. Kimball, W. T. Burnett, Jr., and D. G. Doherty, "Chemical Protection Against Ionizing Radiation. 1. Sampling Methods for Screening Compounds in Radiation Protection Studies with Mice." Radiation Res., Vol. 7 (1957), pp. 1-12.

17. R. F. Chandler, "The Daisy Decelerator." ARL-TDR-67-3, Holloman AFB, New Mexico, 1967.

18. T. D. Clarke, J. F. Sprouffske, E. M. Trout, H. S. Klopfenstein, W. H. Muzzy, C. D. Gragg, and C. D. Bendixen, "Baboon Tolerance to Linear Deceleration ($-G_x$): Lap Belt Restraint." Paper 700906, Proceedings of Fourteenth Stapp Car Crash Conference, P-33. New York: Society of Automotive Engineers, Inc., 1970. Also identified as AMRL-TR-72-44.

19. T. D. Clarke, J. F. Sprouffske, E. M. Trout, C. D. Gragg, W. H. Muzzy, and H. S. Klopfenstein, "Baboon Tolerance to Linear Deceleration ($-G_x$): Air Bag Restraint." Paper 700905, Proceedings of Fourteenth Stapp Car Crash Conference, P-33. New York: Society of Automotive Engineers, Inc., 1970. Also identified as AMRL-TR-72-43.

20. T. D. Clarke, C. D. Gragg, J. F. Sprouffske, E. M. Trout, R. M. Zimmerman, and W. H. Muzzy, "Human Head Linear and Angular Accelerations During Impact." Paper 710857, Proceedings of Fifteenth Stapp Car Crash Conference, P-39. New York: Society of Automotive Engineers, Inc., 1971. Also identified as AMRL-TR-71-95.

21. A. Goldstein, "Biostatistics." New York: The MacMillan Co., 1964, pp. 172-178.

22. J. P. Stapp, J. D. Mosely, C. P. Lombard, and G. A. Nelson, "Analysis and Biodynamics of Selected Rocket-Sled Experiments. Part I. Biodynamics of Maximal Decelerations." Brooks AFB, Texas (SAM), 1964.

23. M. Kornhauser and R. W. Lawton, "Impact Tolerance of Mammals." Proceedings of Fourth AFBMD/STL Symposium, Advances in Ballistic Missile and Space Technology, Vol. 3, Oxford: Pergamon Press, 1961, pp. 386-394.

24. C. C. Snow and H. Hasbrook, "The Angle of Shoulder Slope in Normal Males as a Factor in Shoulder-Harness Design." FAA Tech. Report AM 65-14, 1965, pp. 1-3.

25. H. R. Bierman, and R. M. Wilder, Jr., and H. K. Hellems, "The Principles of Protection of the Human Body as Applied in a Restraining Harness for Aircraft Pilots." Naval Institute, Bethesda, Md., Project X-630, Report 6, 1946.

730977

Spinal Loads Resulting from $-G_x$ Acceleration

P. C. Begeman, A. I. King, and P. Prasad
Wayne State University

Abstract

The biodynamic response of cadaver torsos subjected to $-G_x$ impact acceleration is discussed in this paper, with particular emphasis on the response of the vertebral column. The existence of an axial force along the spine and its manifestation as a load on the seat pan are reported. Spinal curvature appears to be an important factor in the generation of this spine load. In anthropometric dummies, the spine load does not exist. Details of the testing and results are given, and the development of a mathematical model is shown.

THERE IS VERY LITTLE research work concerned with the dynamic response of the thoracic and lumbar spine during $-G_x$ acceleration. This is not unusual, since the loading on the spine is expected to be rather minimal in most cases involving automobile occupants. With the introduction of lap belts in cars, a vertebral injury commonly referred to as the seat belt syndrome has been reported by several authors. Dehner (1)* made an excellent survey of the literature and cites over 20 references of original articles on seat belt trauma. Many of these papers discuss case reports of a variety of spinal injuries, which were generally restricted to the vertebrae L2 and L3. These vertebrae sustained anterior compression fractures, posterior tension fractures, fracture-dislocations and Chance fractures, which were first described by Chance (2) as a horizontal splitting and separation of the posterior vertebral arch, involving the lamina, the pedicles, and the transverse and spinous processes.

The injury is apparently due to extreme hyperflexion of the torso about the lap belt (3) and is thought to be more severe when the belt is improperly worn above the iliac crest (4).

Although recent statistics are not available, the study by Garrett and Braunstein (5) revealed that there were only 12 lumbar spine injuries out of a total of 944 injured occupants who were restrained by a lap belt. In 1964, Perry and McClellan (6) reported four cases of spinal injury out of 64 automobile occupants who were autopsied.

---
*Numbers in parentheses designate References at end of paper.

Injuries attributable to the shoulder harness and lap belt combination were reported by Hamilton (7). The cervical-thoracic junction of the spine appeared to be vulnerable. However, Nelson (8) showed that as a result of the use of the lap and shoulder belt, the severity of the injury to the pelvis and the lumbar spine sustained by both the driver and front passenger was reduced when compared with lap belted or unrestrained occupants. That for the neck remained approximately the same for the lap-belted and lap-and-shoulder-belted occupants. This information was based upon 160 cases of United States accidents. An earlier Swedish survey by Bohlin (9) also showed a decrease in injury severity to the spine and pelvis but the same size related to these body regions is small despite the large number of accidents investigated. Patrick has recent injury data from 148 occupants restrained by a three-point harness. The severest injury was a fractured cervical vertebra (AIS scale of 3).

Although field data indicate an absence of injury to the spine, it was discovered that significant spinal forces can be generated in the spine of an occupant restrained by lap and shoulder belts and subjected to $-G_x$ acceleration. Prasad (11) proposed a mathematical model of the spine that was validated for $+G_z$ acceleration. This model predicted that when the spine was subjected to $-G_x$ acceleration, a compressive force along the vertebral column was generated and revealed itself as a seat-pan load in the seat-to-head direction.

The objective of this research is to determine the validity of the model predictions and to measure the magnitude of this spine load.

Experimental Setup and Procedure

The device used to produce the deceleration is WHAM III (Wayne Horizontal Accelerator Mechanism). This is a flat bed sled approximately 8 × 12 ft to which a chair is bolted. The sled is accelerated slowly, at 0.5 g or less, over a distance of approximately 120 ft to a predetermined velocity and is then decelerated by a hydraulic snubber that can be programmed to give the desired deceleration pulse. Details of WHAM III have been described by Patrick (12).

The chair is of welded steel tubular frame construction with adjustable seat back angle, height, and headrest position. It is equipped with a strain-gage type of load cell under the seat pan to monitor axial seat loads and with load cells at each of the lap belt attachments and at the rear shoulder harness attachment. Accelerometers were mounted on the sled and the chair.

Cadavers were used as test subjects. Their abdominal organs were eviscerated and strain gages applied to the anterior surface of three vertebral bodies, usually T11, L1, and L4, to measure anterior spinal stress.

The cadaver was seated erect in the chair and secured with a lap belt and a double shoulder belt of the military type. The shoulder straps were attached to the lap belt in front and converged to a Y behind the neck. The shoulder belts were horizontal as they passed over the shoulders of the cadaver. The feet were tied to the chair by means of a rope. Fig. 1 shows the cadaver on the sled prior to a test run.

The peak deceleration levels of the sled were between 5-15 g and were either triangular or trapezoidal in shape, with a duration of approximately 170 ms.

Results

The results given in this paper are based on some 40 runs on three cadavers. The spinal gages show high compressive strain levels and all the cadavers sustained spinal fractures. These fractures were of the wedging or the compressive type at L1, T9, or T7. Most gages went into tension during rebound. Typical strain data are shown in Figs. 2 and 3 for runs on two different cadavers at approximately the same input deceleration.

The seat-pan load cell showed an axial load with three distinct peaks: a large peak during the deceleration pulse (50 ms), a second near the end of the pulse (100-150 ms), and a third later on during rebound (270 ms). These data are shown in Figs. 4 and 5 for the same runs as in Figs. 2 and 3, respectively.

The lap belts exerted a vertical force on the seat pan since they were inclined at an angle of 30 deg with respect to the horizontal. The calculated vertical component was subtracted from the seat-pan load and the result is the spine load as shown in Figs. 4 and 5. No vertical component was subtracted for the shoulder belt because it came across the top of the shoulders approximately horizontally and was attached to the lap belt in front. Any downward vertical component on the torso resulting from the shoulder belt had an equal and opposite reaction which could only be taken up by the lap belt, and the lap belt vertical component had already been subtracted.

The spine load also had three peaks, the largest of which varied from 400-800 lb. It is postulated that this spine load is the result of spinal curvature and torso kinematics, giving rise to the first two peaks. The third peak can be due to the body lifting off the seat and then sitting back down. Further evidence of spine load is provided by Figs. 6-9, which show data from four runs made on a third cadaver (No. 2388). Run 328 (Fig. 6) was made at a nominal deceleration of 11.8 g resulting in a peak spine load of 450 lb. The seat pan was not padded. In run 338 (Fig. 7), a 3 in thick foam rubber cushion was added to the seat pan. The nominal g-level was 14 g. Again, a significant spine load of almost 900 lb was generated. The cadaver was decapitated and subjected to a 16.2 g run (No. 340). The results are shown in Fig. 8. The spine load reached a peak of 1250 lb and is obviously not a result of head motion. A final run (No. 341) was made without the shoulder harness. The results of this 4 g run are shown in Fig. 9. The shape of the spine load curve is somewhat different but it still exists.

In an attempt to clarify the cause of the spine load, several runs were made with a 50th percentile anthropometric dummy (Sierra Model 1050). The traces

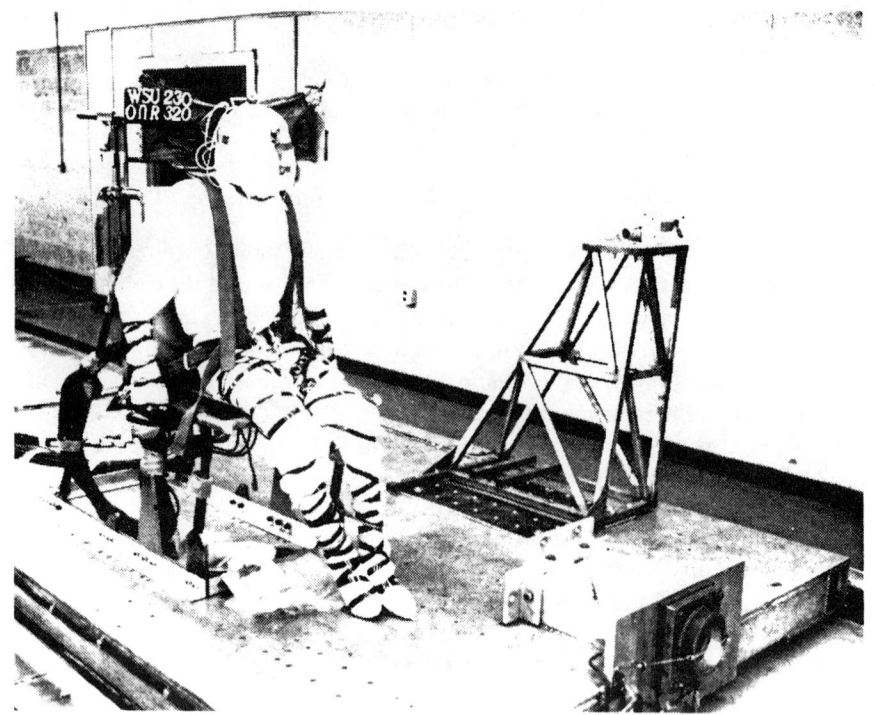

Fig. 1—Seated cadaver on WHAM III

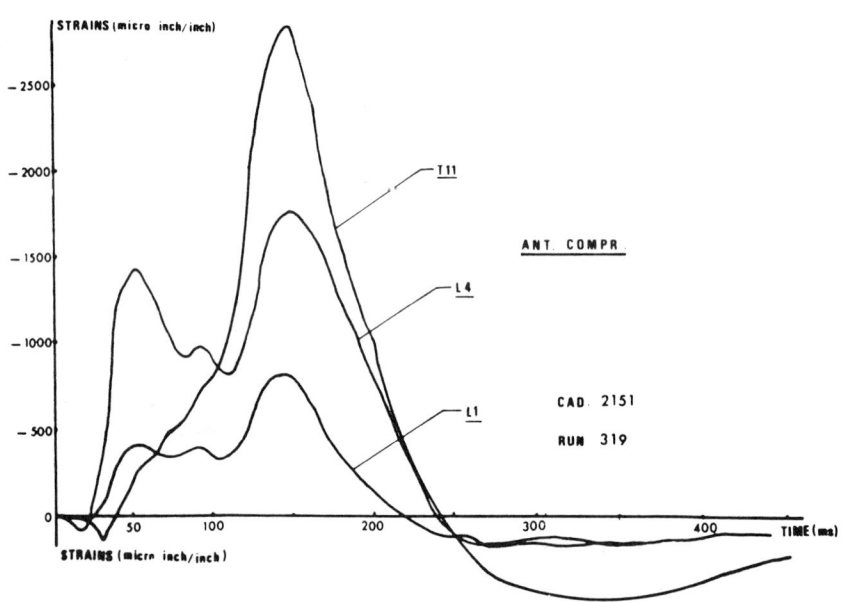

Fig. 2—Strain gage output for run 319

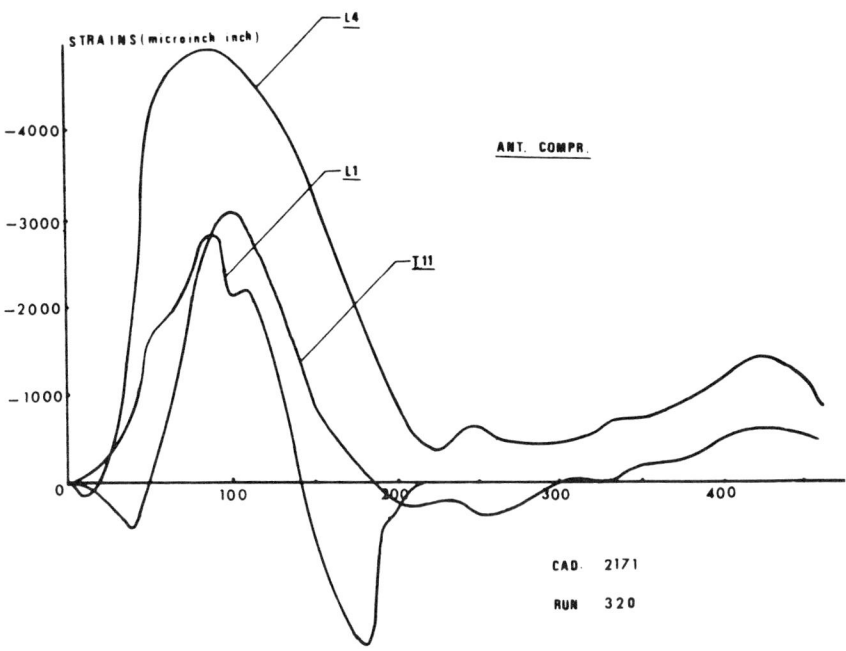

Fig. 3—Strain gage output for run 320

for the seat pan, lap belt, and shoulder belt are shown in Fig. 10. The computed spine load is oscillatory in nature resembling the response of a simple spring-mass system. The patten is quite different from that of the cadaver runs. This difference is attributed to the fact that the dummy does not have a curved articulated spine.

In a further attempt to verify axial load in the spine, a pair of lateral gages was installed on T11 in addition to the anterior gage, since it is impossible to separate out the contribution due to axial load from that due to bending, from the anterior gages. These lateral gages indicate a large axial component. However, they cannot give a quantitative measure of load because they are still subject to bending effects, due to the ability of the articular facets to carry load (11).

Mathematical Model

Several mathematical models have been formulated to study the effect of $\pm G_x$ acceleration to the human body in the mid-sagittal plane. However, all of the existing models concentrate on the prediction of forces and moments in the cervical spine. MacKenzie (13) modified the Orne and Liu (14) mathematical

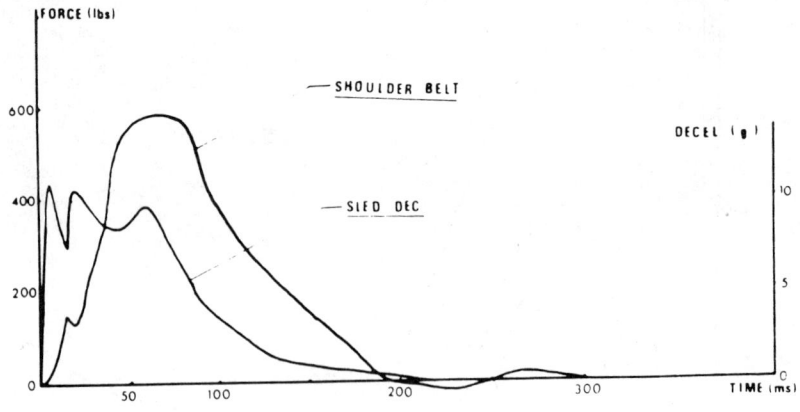

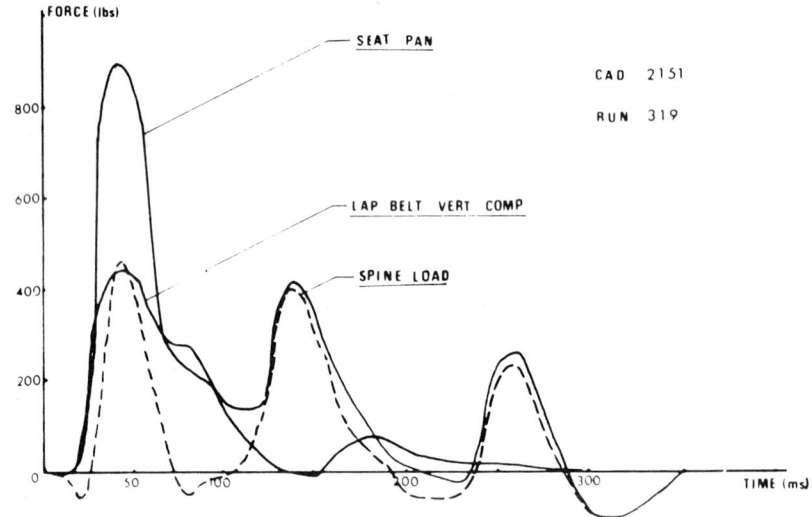

Fig. 4—Spine load and deceleration data from run 319

model of the spine to simulate whiplash situations by considering the head and the seven cervical vertebrae as rigid links having three degrees-of-freedom in the mid-sagittal plane. The cervical discs are modeled as viscoelastic beams. The thoraco-lumbar spine is represented by a rigid link, hence making the study of forces and moments in the thoraco-lumbar spine impossible. Mertz (15) proposed a model for studying the effect of forward deceleration to the human body. Although this model is good for studying neck torques and head dynamics, it is not useful for predicting stresses in the spine. The mathematical model

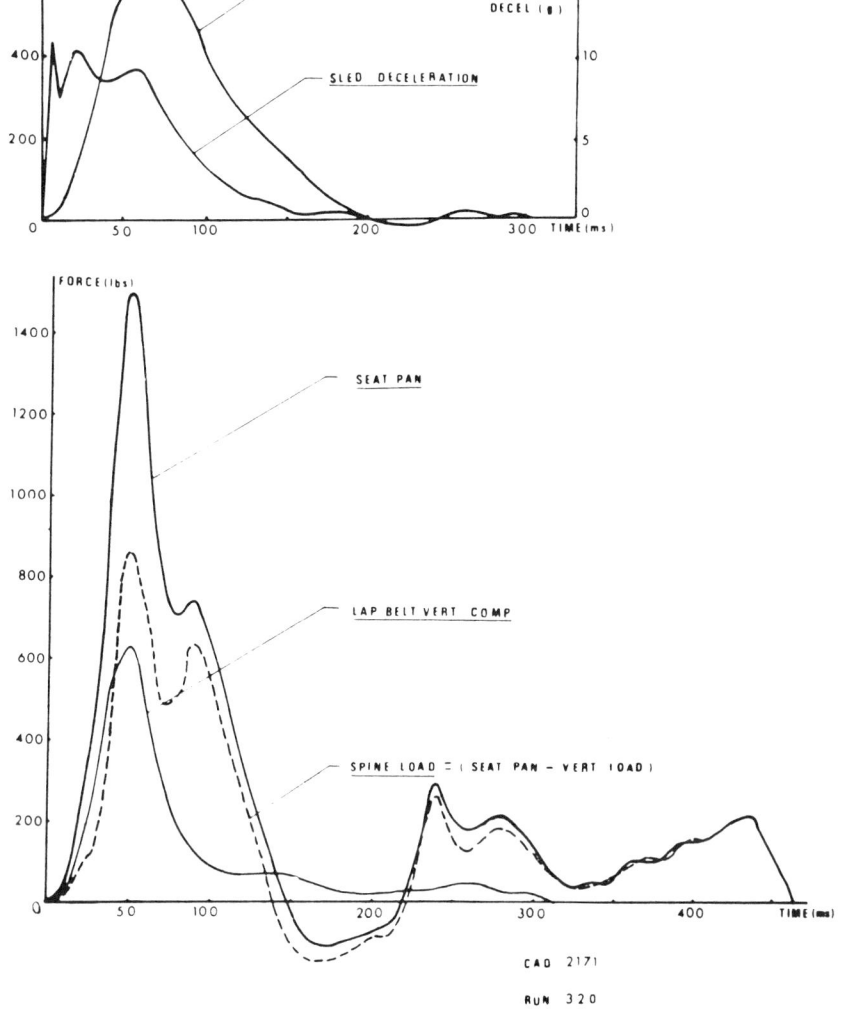

Fig. 5—Spine load and deceleration data from run 320

to be described incorporates the entire upper torso; that is, the head, the cervical, thoracic, and lumbar spine, and the pelvis.

Although the model is restricted to motion in the mid-sagittal plane, it permits the study of the effects of $\pm G_z$, $\pm G_x$ acceleration and a combination of the above on the spine. This resulted in a 78 degree-of-freedom discrete parameter

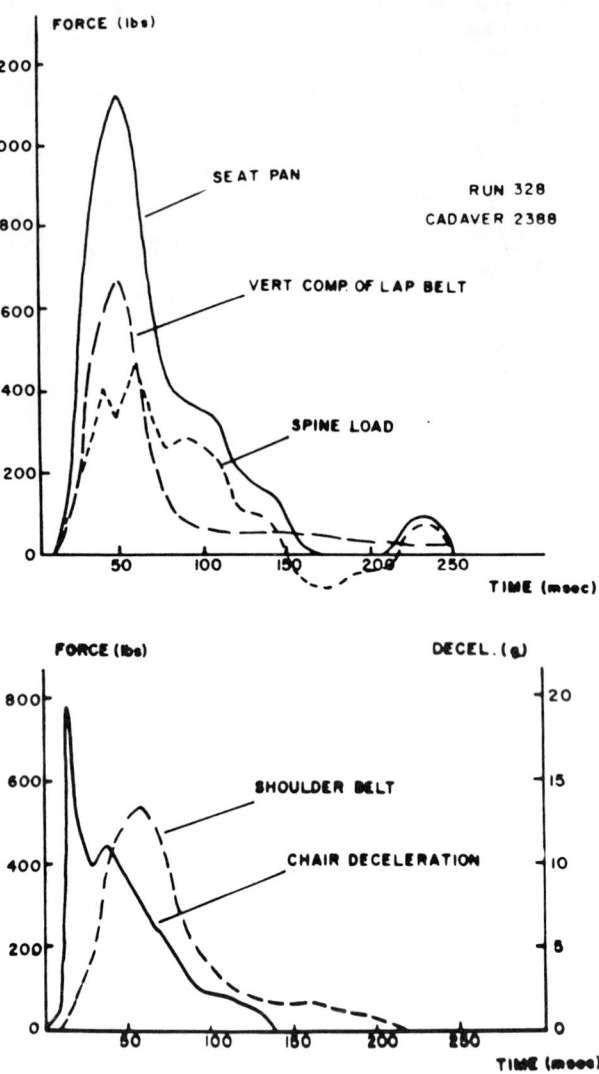

Fig. 6—Spine load and deceleration data from run 328

model incorporating the following features:
1. Flexion and extension of the spine.
2. The natural curvatures of the spine.
3. The eccentric inertial loading of the spine.
4. The head and neck motions.
5. Two load transmission paths—one through the vertebral body and one through the articular facets (11).

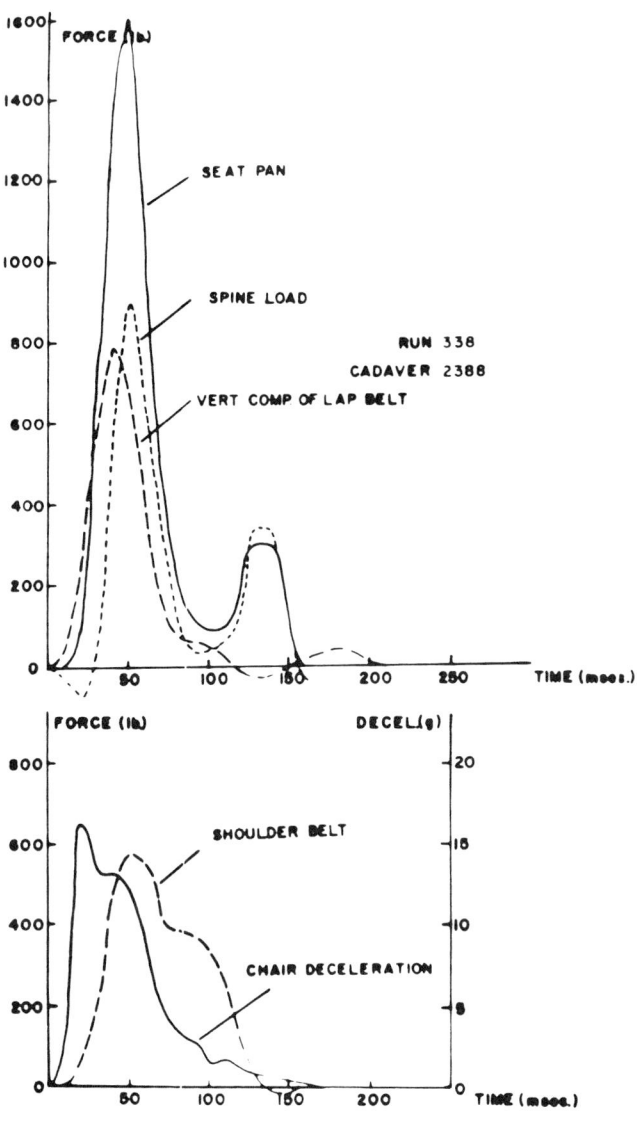

Fig. 7—Spine load and deceleration data from run 338

6. The restraint and support systems.

In the development of the mathematical model, the following assumptions were made:

1. The 24 vertebral bodies, the head, and the pelvis are rigid bodies constrained to move in the mid-sagittal plane.

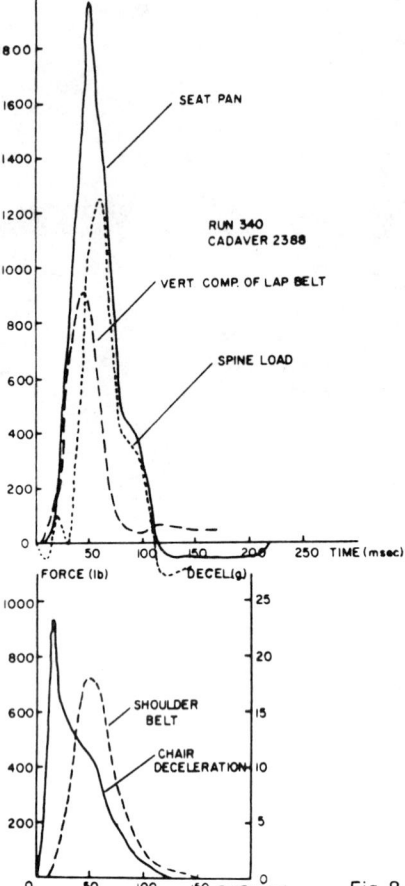

Fig. 8—Spine load and deceleration data from run 340

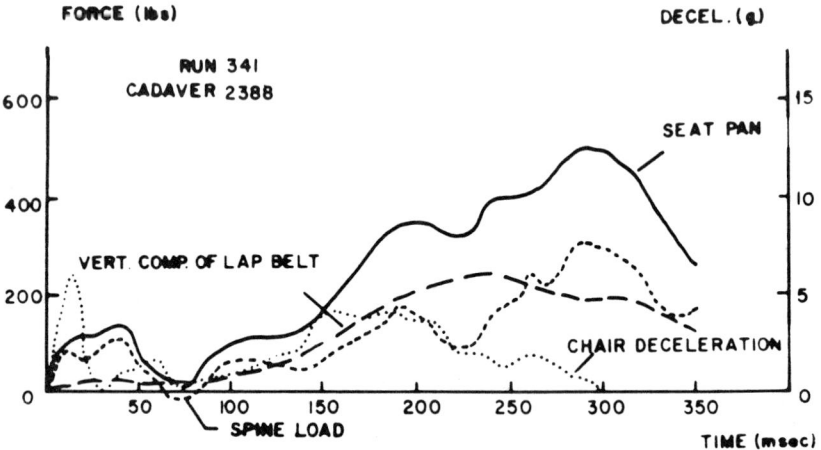

Fig. 9—Spine load and deceleration data from run 341

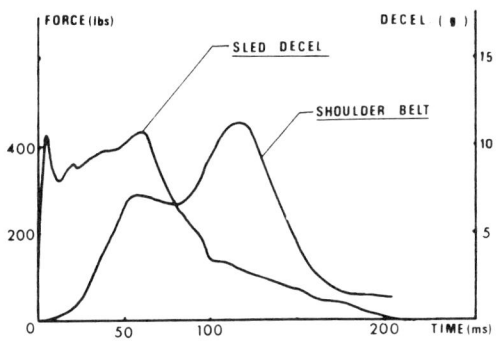

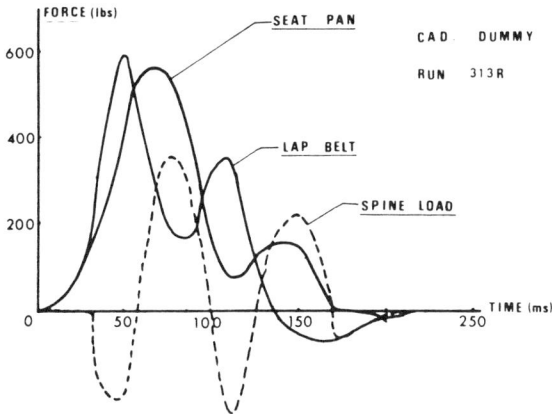

Fig. 10—Load cell output for anthropometric dummy

2. Each rigid body has three degrees-of-freedom in the mid-sagittal plane, two translational and one rotational.

3. The intervertebral discs are massless, and deformation of the spine takes place at the discs.

4. The discs are replaced by a system of springs and dampers—one spring and damper for axial forces, one spring and damper for shear forces, and another spring and damper arrangement for restoring torques due to relative angular motion between adjacent vertebral bodies.

5. The facets and laminae are springs connected to the vertebral body by a massless rigid rod.

6. Each rigid body is assumed to carry a portion of the torso weight which is eccentric with respect to the centerline of the spine.

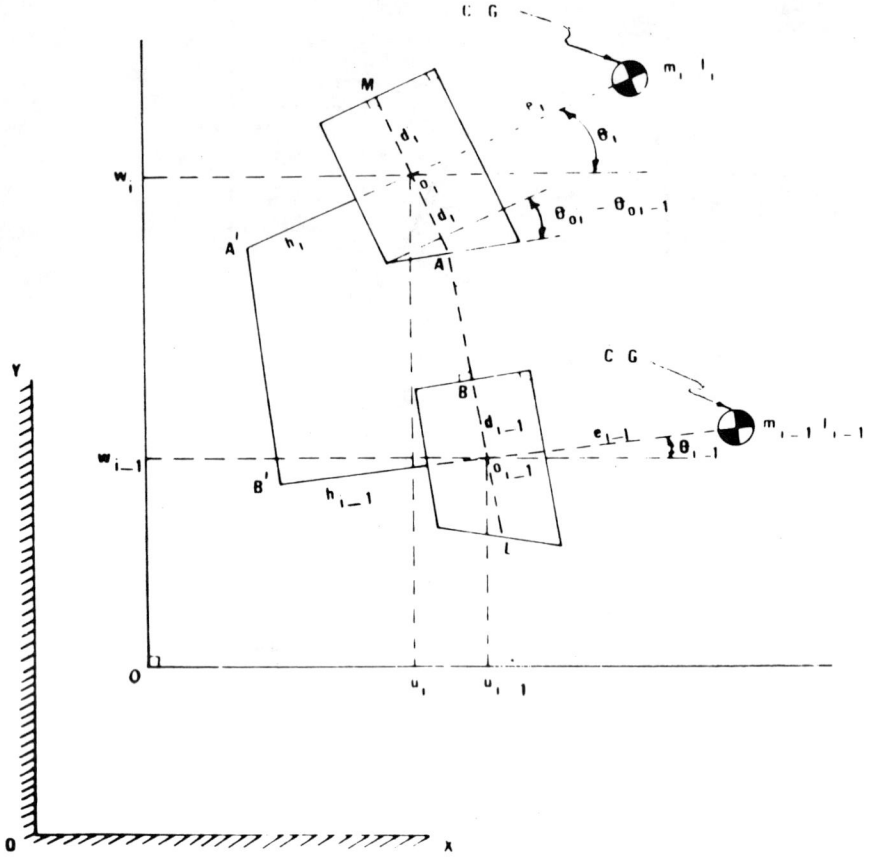

Fig. 11—Initial configuration of two successive vertebrae and intervertebral disc

7. The rigid bodies are arranged to simulate the spinal curvatures as closely as possible.

Fig. 11 shows the initial configuration of two successive links (the vertebrae) and a deformable link (the disc). It has been assumed that the axis of any disc is coincident with the axis of the vertebra immediately below it in the initial configuration of the spine in the normal seated position. Also, it is assumed that the disc is of uniform thickness, which is not necessarily true. The two vertebrae are shown as trapezoids to simulate the change of curvature of the spine. This is a valid assumption because it has been observed that in the lumbar region the vertebral bodies are wedged posteriorly, whereas in the thoracic level they are wedged anteriorly. The position in the mid-sagittal plane of the center of the ith rigid link (vertebral body) is determined by the three generalized coordinates u_i, w_i, and θ_i, as shown in Fig. 11.

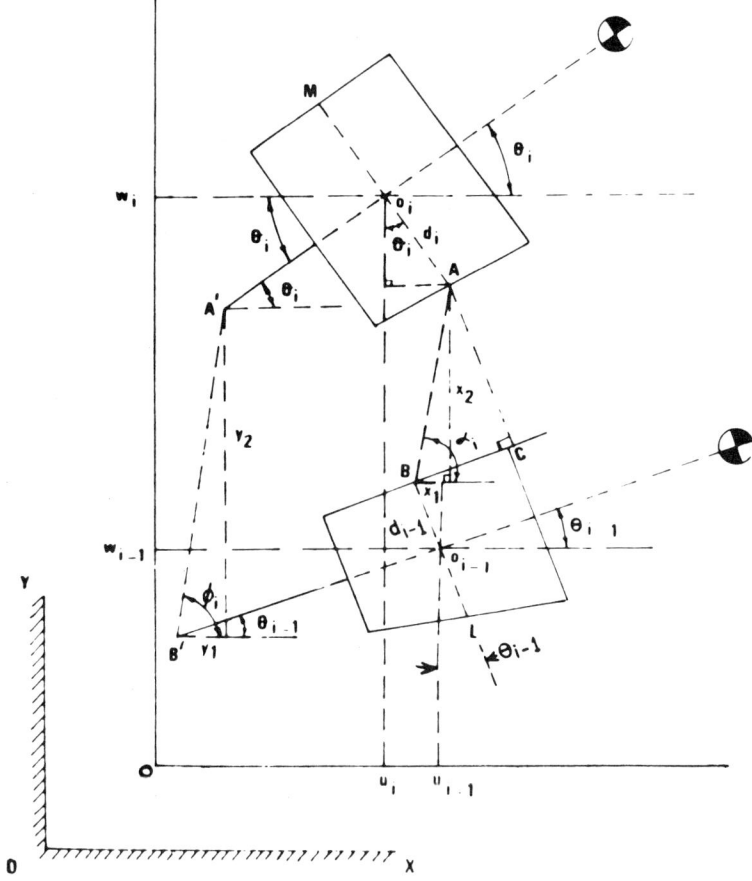

Fig. 12—Configuration of two successive vertebrae after deformation of disc

At time t (t > 0), the configuration of two successive rigid links is shown in Fig. 12. The links have undergone translations and rotations causing axial, shear, and rotational deformations of the discs. The chord length AB_i of the disc is determined by the generalized coordinates u_i, w_i, and θ_i of the centers of the rigid links.

The free-body diagram of the ith vertebral body is shown in Fig. 13, where the forces and moments developed are given by the following:

$$T_7 Y_i = XK_i (AC_i - AC_{oi}) + C_i \dot{AC_i} \tag{1}$$

$$T_7 X_i = XK_{si} (BC_i - BC_{oi}) + C_{si} \dot{BC_i} \tag{2}$$

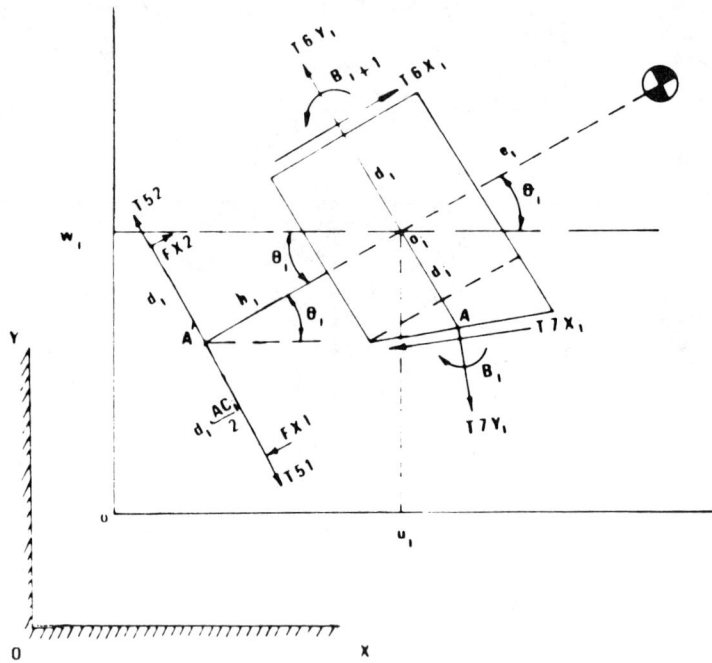

Fig. 13—Free-body diagram of the i th vertebral body

$$B_i = XKT_i \{(\theta_i - \theta_{oi}) - (\theta_{i-1} - \theta_{oi-1})\} - C_{ti} (\dot{\theta}_i - \dot{\theta}_{i-1}) \qquad (3)$$

$$T_6Y_i = XK_{i+1} (AC_{i+1} - AC_{oi+1}) + C_{i+1} \dot{AC}_{i+1} \qquad (4)$$

$$T_6X_i = XK_{si+1} (BC_{i+1} - BC_{oi+1}) + C_{si+1} \dot{BC}_{i+1} \qquad (5)$$

$$B_{i+1} = XKT_{i+1} \{(\theta_{i+1} - \theta_{oi+1}) - (\theta_i - \theta_{oi})\} + C_{ti+1} (\dot{\theta}_{i+1} - \dot{\theta}_i) \qquad (6)$$

$$T_{5i} = XKH_i \{A' B'_i - A' B'_{oi}\} \qquad (7)$$

$$T_{5i+1} = XKH_{i+1} \{A'B'_{i+1} - A'B'_{oi+1}\} \qquad (8)$$

where:

XK_i = stiffness of axial spring of ith disc
XK_{si} = stiffness of shear spring of ith disc
XKT_i = stiffness of torsional spring of ith disc

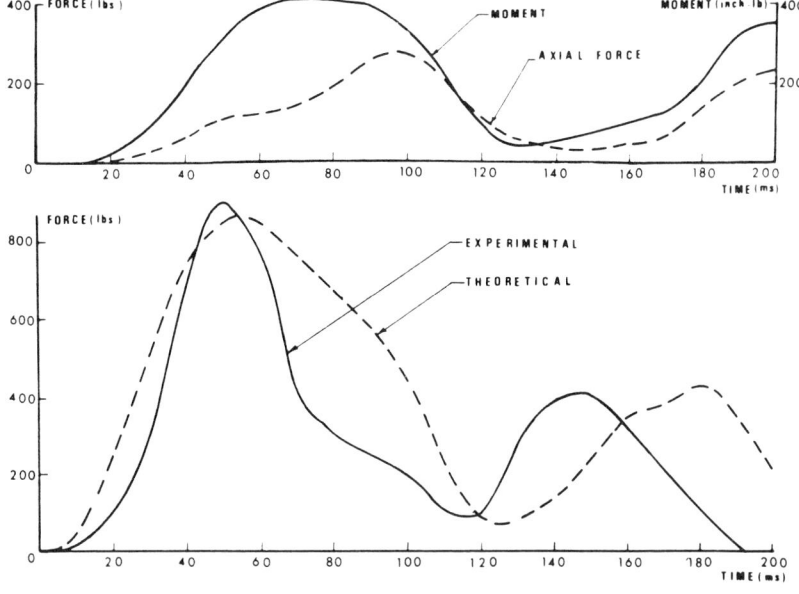

Fig. 14—Results from mathematical model and comparisons with experimental data

C_i = damping constant in axial loading of ith disc
C_{si} = damping constant in shear loading of ith disc
C_{ti} = damping constant in torsional loading of ith disc
XKH_i = stiffness of ith lamina and facets
o = initial configuration

Resolving the forces on the ith vertebra parallel to the u_i and w_i axes and taking the sum of moments about the c.g. and then using Newton's law of motion, we get the equations of motion of the ith vertebra

$$\Sigma F_{ui} = m_i \{\ddot{X} + \ddot{u}_i - e_i \dot{\theta}_i^2 \cos\theta_i - e_i \ddot{\theta}_i \sin\theta_i\} \qquad (9)$$

$$\Sigma F_{wi} = m_i \{\ddot{Y} + \ddot{W}_i + e_i \ddot{\theta}_i \cos\theta_i - \dot{\theta}_i^2 e_i \sin\theta_i\} \qquad (10)$$

$$\Sigma M_{gi} = I_g \ddot{\theta}_i \qquad (11)$$

where:

m_i = mass supported by i^{th} body
I_g = polar moment of inertia about c.g.

The above resulted in a system of 78 simultaneous, second order, nonlinear differential equations that were solved numerically using Hamming's predictor-corrector method on an IBM 360 digital computer.

Fig. 14 shows the axial force and bending moment developed in the intervertebral disc between L4 and L5 due to a 9 g trapezoidal acceleration pulse applied to a seated 120 lb cadaver. It should be noted that the peak compressive axial force and bending moment is reached at approximately 90 ms after the onset of the acceleration pulse. This time agrees with that for fracture of the spine during the experiments. A comparison was made of the predicted seat-pan load with that measured experimentally. This is also shown in Fig. 14. The material constants for the various model elements were selected from currently available data on the mechanical properties of tissue.

There is an abundance of data on axial stiffness. However, there is a lack of data on shear and rotational properties, for it can be seen from the model response that the parameters selected resulted in a lower-frequency response compared with the experimental results.

Discussions and Conclusions

The biodynamic response of the cadaveric torso subjected to $-G_x$ impact acceleration has been investigated with particular emphasis on the response of the vertebral column. The existence of an axial force along the spine and its manifestation as a load on the seat pan are re-reported. Spinal curvature appears to be an important factor in the generation of this spine load. In anthropometric dummies, the spine load does not exist.

There is no correlation between the load measured by the seat-pan load cell and that by the shoulder harness load cell. It can be seen from Figs. 4 and 5 that strap load is going up while the seat-pan load is dropping between 50-100 ms. Furthermore, the seat-pan load pattern is different for the dummy run during which the same shoulder belts were used.

A simple explanation of the spine load cannot be made at this time. However, the mathematical model tends to support the experimental evidence of the existence of a spine load. Further research is necessary to confirm this observation and to establish whether its magnitude should be of concern to designers of belt type restraint systems.

It may be argued that there is no field evidence of frequent occurrence of vertebral fractures in the thoracic or lumbar spine, as a result of automotive collisions. However, spinal injury data for occupants restrained by a lap and shoulder belt combination are sparse at present and are not indicative of the absence of a serious spinal problem with the use of such a restraint system. The results of a study on baboons by Clarke, et al., (16) indicate that they sustained compression vertebral fractures at high deceleration levels.

Acknowledgments

This work was supported in part by ONR Contracts N00014-69-A-0235-0003 and N00014-69-A-0235-0001 and by an NIH Career Development Award No. 5-K04-GM21145-02 (National Institute of General Medical Sciences).

References

1. J. R. Dehner, "Seat Belt Injuries of the Spine and Abdomen." Amer. Jrl. Roentgenography, Radium Therapy and Nuclear Med., Vol. 3, No. 4 (April 1971), pp. 833-843.

2. G. Q. Chance, "Note on Type of Flexion Fracture of Spine." Brit. Jrl. of Radiol., Vol. 21 (1948), pp. 452-453.

3. R. G. Snyder, et al., "Seat Belt Injuries in Impact." The Prevention of Highway Injury, Ed. by M. L. Selzer, et al., Highway Safety Research Inst., Univ. of Mich., 1967, pp. 188-210.

4. R. M. Steckler, J. A. Epstein, and B. S. Epstein, "Seat Belt Trauma of the Lumbar Spine: An Unusual Manifestation of the Seat Belt Syndrome." Jrl. Trauma, Vol. 9. No. 6, (1969), pp. 508-513.

5. J. W. Garrett and P. W. Braunstein, "Seat Belt Syndrome." Jrl. Trauma, Vol. 2 (1962), pp. 220-237.

6. J. F. Perry and R. J. McClellan, "Autopsy Findings in 127 Patients Following Fatal Traffic Accidents." Surg., Gynecology and Obstet., Vol. 119 (1964), pp. 586-590.

7. J. B. L. Hamilton, "Seat Belt Injuries." Brit. Med. Jrl. (1968), 485-486.

8. W. D. Nelson, "Lap-Shoulder Restraint Effectiveness in the United States." Paper 710077 presented at SAE Automotive Engineering Congress, Detroit, January 1971.

9. N. I. Bohlin, "A Statistical Analysis of 28,000 Accident Cases with Emphasis on Occupant Restraint Value." Paper 670925, Proceedings of Eleventh Stapp Car Crash Conference, P-20. New York: Society of Automotive Engineers, 1967.

10. L. M. Patrick, Personal Communication, June 1973.

11. P. Prasad, "The Dynamic Response of the Spine During +G_z Acceleration." Ph.D. Dissertation, Wayne State University, June 1973.

12. L. M. Patrick, "Airbag Restraints for Automobile Drivers." Final Report to Federal Highway Admin., National Highway Traffic Safety Admin., Washington, D.C., Contract FH-11-7067, September 1972.

13. J. A. MacKenzie and J. F. Williams, "The Dynamic Behavior of the Head and Cervical Spine During Whiplash." Jrl. Biomechanics, Vol. 4 (1971), pp. 477-490.

14. D. Orne and Y. K. Liu, "A Mathematical Model of Spinal Response to Impact." Jrl. Biomechanics, Vol. 4 (1971), pp. 49-71.

15. H. J. Mertz and L. M. Patrick, "Strength and Response of the Human Neck." Paper 720959, Proceedings of Fifteenth Stapp Car Crash Conference, P. 39, New York: Society of Automotive Engineers, Inc., 1972.

16. T. D. Clarke, D. C. Smedley, W. H. Muzzy, C. D. Gragg, R. E. Schmidt, and E. M. Trout, "Impact Tolerance and Resulting Injury Patterns in the Baboon: Air Force Shoulder Harness—Lap Belt Restraint." Paper 720974, Proceedings of Stapp Car Crash Conference, P. 45. New York: Society of Automotive Engineers, Inc., 1972.

741182

Results of 49 Cadaver Tests Simulating Frontal Collision of Front Seat Passengers

Georg Schmidt, Dimitrios Kallieris, Jurgen Barz, and Rainer Mattern
University of Heidelberg

Abstract

By an acceleration track operated through a falling weight (9, 11[*]) with a crash velocity of 50 km/h and a stopping distance of about 40 cm—corresponding to the crease region of many automobiles—the effect of three-point-retractor belts on 30 fresh cadavers and of two-point belts with kneebar on 19 fresh cadavers had been tested. The age of the cadavers ranged from 12-82 years. Qualitatively, almost all injuries known under the term "seat belt syndrome" could be reproduced. The dependence of the degree of injury in regard to the age was quite evident. It can be expected that persons over 40 years of age will suffer the same dangerous injuries as the tested cadavers, caused by the diagonal belts if the above mentioned crash conditions are existent. This will apply to both belt systems tested by us. The shoulder-belt-forces of all of our tests were between 340 hp and 1000 hp; but more serious injuries of the cadavers of older persons could be observed. To reduce the risk of injury, improvements of the now used restraint systems are necessary. To reach this aim, constructive changes on automobiles and seats have also become necessary to be carried out.

SINCE JANUARY 1974, the obligation exists in the Federal Republic of Germany that all newly-manufactured cars have to be equipped with three-point-safety belts. It is estimated that there will be the compulsion to wear safety belts starting in 1976, as it has been compulsary for Australia since 1971 and France since July 1973. In spite of many efforts to convince car drivers of the efficiency of safety belts, only a few are willing to wear them. In Germany, it is estimated that only 5-10% of the car drivers wear safety belts. In Sweden, 33% of the car drivers are wearing safety belts while driving on highways and 5% while driving in towns. In Victoria, Australia, 64-75% of the drivers in respectively metropolitan

---

[*]Numbers in parentheses designate References at end of paper.

areas are wearing seat belts. According to police figures for January–December, 1971, inclusive, the number of persons killed and injured in Victoria was reduced by 11.6% compared with the corresponding period of 1970 (J. Traffic Med. 1–2, 1973).

According to Williams (1) most accidents resulted in lethal injuries because of not wearing seat belts; but the injuries which occurred in spite of wearing a safety belt were often serious enough. In the analysis by Bohlin (2) 28,000 Volvo accidents have been described whereby the benefit of using safety belts has been further reinforced. The rarity of lethal injuries while wearing safety belts at a low wearing rate (25%) has shown the fact that in the whole series only three front seat passengers have been killed, although they were belted. McElhaney, et al. (3) indicate, by a variety of literature, the seriousness of injuries which directly occurred by wearing safety belts.

Simulated Crashes

Besides the statistical evaluation of road accidents, simulated crashes with belted and unbelted human cadavers have been carried out in the past years (4–8). So far, the number of simulated crashes with human cadavers is not extensive because the heterogenous and anisotropic human body is too small to give authentic evidence to all biomechanical questions.

Therefore, in order to obtain firmer statements, it is suggested that the test series be extended with mainly younger people because the other teams have used predominantly older people.

The Institute of Forensic Medicine of the Heidelberg University has been equipped with a deceleration sled since the end of 1972. The sled—occupied by a cadaver—is accelerated by an eightfold gear transmission ratio through a drop weight until it reaches a desired crash velocity (max 100 km/h). The kinetic energy is transformed according to the deflection of a flat-steel and therefore the deceleration of the sled is adjusted. The sheet metal strips defined by their size are plastically deformed (9). The time characteristic of the sled deceleration is that of a trapezium and meets the requirements of the European Economic Community's No. 16 regulation (10) concerning safety belt dynamic tests.

The following restraint systems (Fa. Repa, West Germany) were used when simulating frontal crashes of a belt-protected occupant—without using a dashboard.

1. Three-point belt, automatic retractor (with and without force limitor), torsion bar, and preloading device.

2. Diagonal shoulder belt, automatic retractor (with and without a force limitor and preloading device) combined with a kneebar.

In most cases, a 50 mm broad belt with an extension of 18%, only 6%

had been used. During some tests, a belt width of 100 mm had been used and 150 mm broad padded aluminium sheets and 100 mm broad padded leather plates have been put underneath the belt for a length of 45 cm.

The tests were carried out with 1-5 day old cadavers who had been preserved in a cold storage chamber at a temperature of 3°C. At the time of the tests, the body temperature of the cadavers ranged from 10-20°C. X-ray photographs of the thorax had been taken before the tests. If rigor mortis still existed, the cadavers were treated in such a manner to bring them to a seating position. Male and female cadavers in the age range from 12-82 years have been tested; the weights of the tested cadavers varied from 36-91 kg. Beside the crash velocity, the sled deceleration, the belt forces, and the head deceleration of the forehead—the cranium—(x-, z-direction; accelerometers fastened at the helmet) was recorded in dependence of the time of a light beam oszillograph during the tests (11).

The photographic coverage of each test consisted of high-speed 16 mm movies—side and frontal views. The high-speed movies were made with two Photosonic cameras and one Hitachi camera with nominal frame rates of 500 pictures/s and 1000/pictures/s.

Results

The results of 30 frontal crash tests with three-point automatic belts and 19 tests with diagonal-shoulder-belt kneebar systems are as follows:

1. The measured head acceleration peaks in the x-direction lay between 32-134 g; in the z-direction between 46-136 g. The investigation of the brain did not show any recognizable injuries and therefore a further discussion of the head acceleration was not necessary.

2. At a crash velocity of 50 km/h and a medium deceleration of 25 g shoulder-belt-forces between 340-1012 hp have been measured and are in dependence with the body weight of the tested person. Fig. 1 shows that, by a common dispersion experienced with biological testing material, a nearly linear increase of the shoulder-belt-forces was recorded by an increasing body weight. Hereby differences of the three-point-belt efficiency and the two-point-kneebar systems could not be noticed. The effect of the belt-force-limitor was not clear. The lap belt forces lay between 340-770 hp.

3. With the exception of younger tested persons (17-21 years), the following injuries of the upper part of the body have been recorded due to the safety belt: excoriations and under-skin bruises; fractures of the thorax skeleton, the clavicle and the spine; and injuries of the inner thorax organs like lung transfixings, pleura ruptures, heart injuries, and blood vessel ruptures. Dotzauer, et al. (7) and Tarrière et al. (12) observed similar injuries.

The distribution of the rib fractures on the right and left thorax showed

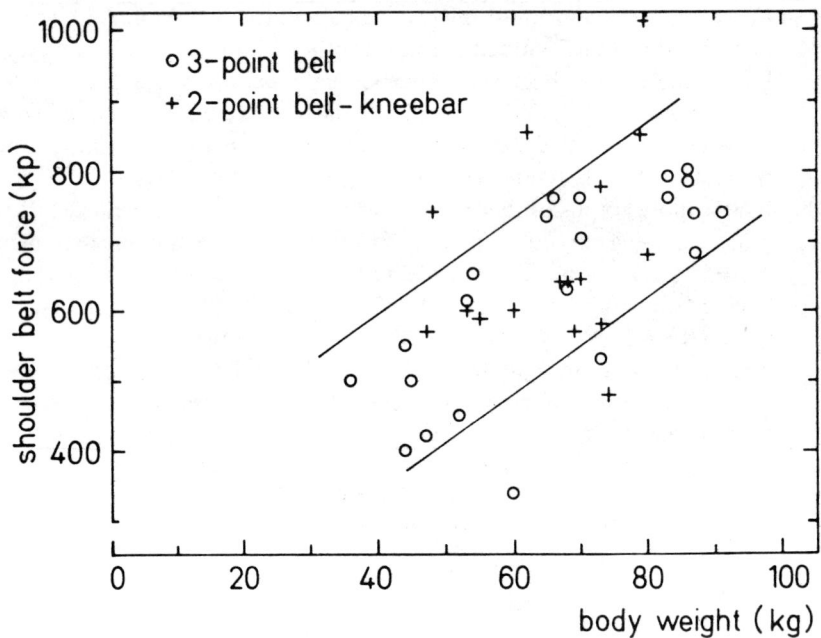

Fig. 1—Shoulder-belt-force dependent on weight of 38 crash tests (22 tests accomplished with 3-point-belts; 16 tests with 2-point-kneebar)

a typical injury pattern in regard to the belt direction; also the kind of sternum fractures—mostly diagonal sternum fractures from the right side above to the left side below—correspond to the bearing surface area of the belt on the thorax while in passenger position.

Most rib fractures are caused by a direct influence of the expanded belt as shear fractures—series rib piece fractures observed on older individuals often showed the width of the belt on the fracture pieces. Outside the bearing surface area of the belt, bending fractures have been noticed which in most cases pertained to the right below and the left upper thorax half; in rare cases, the paravertebral region was also covered.

According to the number of rib fractures, an approximate linear relation in regard to age was derived (Fig. 2). A possible explanation is osteoporosis coupled with a loss of elasticity increasing in old age, whereby a variable proceeding of these processes by advancing age effect a more intense dispersion of the results. Measurements in regard to the bending stability of single ribs of the tested persons are in accordance with our observations (13). The values of the bending stability of the sixth and seventh rib, related to a 8cm wide span, lie between 4 hp (female, 77 years old) and 90 hp (male, 21 years old) (13). The average hardness of the bones measured at the spot of the fracture (Vickers method) amount to 27

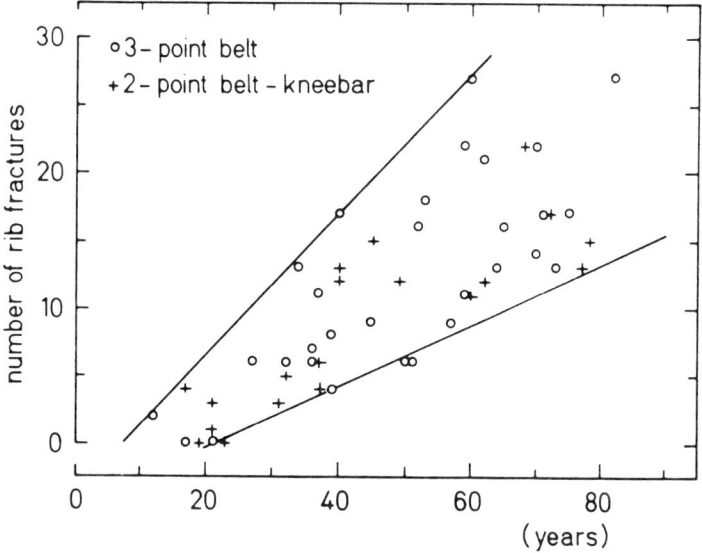

Fig. 2—Number of rib fractures dependent on age in 49 crash tests (30 tests accomplished with 3-point-belts; 19 tests with 2-point-kneebar)

hp/mm². Pathological hardness values in a sense of osteomalacia have not been observed with our tested cadavers. The bone hardness of the skeleton system of adults is in accordance with investigations of Kallieris (13) and Kallieris and Genser (14) not dependent upon the age (13, 14).

5. In nearly all cases where injuries of the inner organs of the thorax have been noticed, they were combined with numerous bone fractures of the thorax. These organ injuries, on the one hand, are possibly the result of a direct influence of the inward deformed thorax, as for example transfixing injuries of the lung or heart contusions. Table 1 gives a review of the frequency of thorax injuries observed in 49 tests. Williams (1) reported similar findings when evaluating clinical material of belt-protected vehicle occupants after road accidents. This report concerned the so-called seat-belt-syndrome so named by Garrett and Braunstein (16), which was caused by lap belts, diagonal shoulder belts and three-point-belts.

6. In 4 out of 49 tests, the clavicle was broken. Splinter fractures mostly occurred and were combined with extensive soft-tissue bruises and extravasations of the right regio colli lateralis and the right fossa supraclavicularis. Often also the plexus brachialis was concerned in one case, even a laceration of the right arteria carotis communis had been found. These injury pictures were especially noticed if the upper mounting point of the shoulder-belt had been kept low.

7. In the abdomen area, liver ruptures, spleen ruptures and kidney con-

Table 1—Frequency of Characteristic Injury Findings Of Upper Part of Body (thorax) in 49 crash tests
(30 tests with 3 point-belt, 19 tests with 2-point-kneebar)

Skin pocket formation at right of neck	8
Rupture of sternocleidomastoid muscle	2
Plexus brachialis-strains	5
Fractures of right clavicle	4
Rupture of right cartotid artery	1
Rib fractures	533
Fractures of sternum	35*
Mediastinal hemorrhage	1
Rupture of lung root	5
Transfixing of pleura	7
Rupture of pericardium	1
Rupture of epicard	1
Heart rupture	1
Rupture of thoracical below hollow vein	2

*29 cadavers had one and 3 had two fractures of the sternum.

Table 2—Frequency of Characteristic Injury Findings of Abdomen in 49 Crash Tests
(30 tests with 3-point-belt, 19 tests with 2-point-kneebar)

	3-point-belt	2-point-kneebar
Liver rupture	7	2
Spleen rupture	3	2
Kidney rupture right	1	0
Kidney rupture left	0	1
Rupture of small intestine	1	0
Mesentery rupture	4	0
Abdominal wall rupture	6	0
Peritoneum rupture	2	0
Fracture of right ilium	3	0

tusions caused by the diagonal shoulder-belt had been seen. Due to the lap belt, fat tissue and muscle tissue ruptures of the anterior abdomen; mesentery ruptures; intestinal ruptures, as well as os ilium fractures and, in rare cases, fractures of the process transverse of the lumbar vertebra had been caused. Table 2 shows the frequency of the abdomen injuries during 49 cadaver tests. Five out of 30 impact tests carried out with three-point-belts resulted in extensive bruises and lacerations of the posterior thigh muscular system caused by shear effects of the seat edges.

8. Five of the 19 tests with two-point-belt-kneebar systems resulted in injuries of the knee-joint and extremity bones, closely located to the knee, respectively. Single results can be noted from Table 3. So far, the knee

Table 3—Frequency of Characteristic Injury Findings of Leg at 19 crash tests with 2-point-kneebar

Fracture of trochlea of femur	2
Fracture of head of tibia	1
Rupture of ligamenta cruciata genus	6

impact forces have not been measured. But in the near future, test series with this kind of measurements are intended. According to Patrick and Mertz (17), both knees together can bear strains of up to 1271 hp. At our tests, fractures of the neck of the femur or coxofemoral diarthrosis injuries have not been observed so far.

Out of the 49 tests made with the cervical vertebra column and the thoracic vertebra column, bone injuries identified as throwing forward injuries of the cervical vertebra column skeleton occurred 12 times as corpus vertebrae fractures and fractures of the spinous and transverse processes; 6 times, these injuries were found at the thoracic vertebra column. At almost more than half of all cases, extravasations of the muscular system around the cervical vertebra column could be proven. Ligament and disc injuries occurred more rarely. However, the evaluation is not yet terminated.

9. Due to the test arrangement—passenger position without a dashboard—direct head impacts had been avoided. As a result of the head deceleration, tender bridge vein lacerations had been noticed in rare cases; in no case could a morphological noticeable damage of the brain tissue be established.

Evaluation

In case the injury grade is determined in accordance to the abbreviated ACIR-scale (0 = no injuries; 1 = slight injuries; 2 = no dangerous injuries; 3 = dangerous injuries; 4 = lethal injuries) it can be noticed (Fig. 3) that for 40 years on, in the test conditions mentioned above, dangerous to lethal injuries will occur at a crash velocity of 50 km/h. That applies especially to the two restraint systems used in our test series. Differences in the efficiency for the total injury grade could not be evidenced.

When evaluating the injuries of the internal organs inflicted upon and observed in the cadavers, it has to be taken into consideration, that, in any case, because of the low organ-turgor and the lacking of blood pressure in the blood vessels, possibly smaller injuries can be expected with regard to influencing forces. On the other hand, it is assumed that more serious injuries will be incurred by living persons under the same conditions.

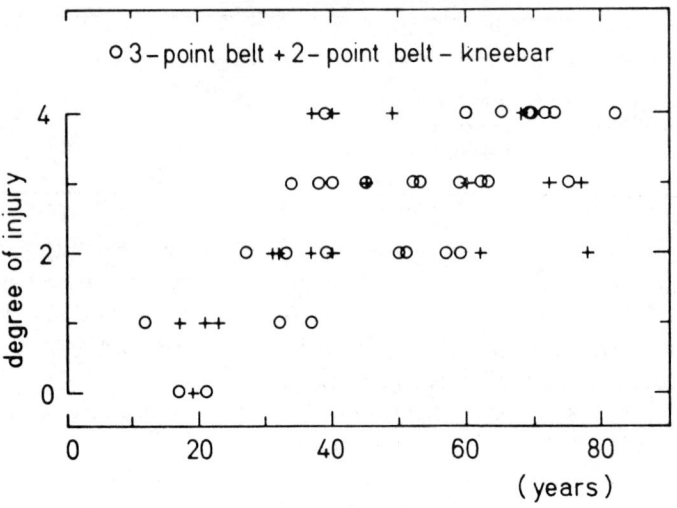

Fig. 3—Injury degree dependent on age in 49 crash tests (30 tests accomplished with 3-point-belts; 19 tests accomplished with 2-point-kneebar)

Summary

The examination of two belt restraint systems, which can be used in quantity, on 49 human cadavers by simulating a frontal impact of a car with 50 km/h shows injuries with mounting numbers and severities in accordance with age of cadavers. The results could be a base for the development of better restraint systems.

Acknowledgement

This work was sponsored in part by VDA (Verband der Automobil-Industrie e.V.), West Germany, with technical assistance by the Volkswagenwerk AG, for which we are grateful.

References

1. J. S. Williams, "The Nature of Seat Belt Injuries." Proceedings of fourteenth Stapp Car Crash Conference 1970, p. 44, Publ. by Soc. of Automotive Eng., Inc. New York

2. N. I. Bohlin, "A Statistical Analysis of 28,000 Accident Cases with Emphasis on Occupant Restraint Value." Paper 670925, Proceedings of the Eleventh Stapp Car Crash Conference P-20. New York: Society of Automotive Engineers, Inc., 1967.

3. J. H. McElhaney, V. G. Roberts, J. W. Melvin, W. Skelton, and A. J. Hammond, "Biomechanics of Seat Belt Design." Paper 720972,

Proceedings of Sixteenth Stapp Car Crash Conference P-45. New York: Society of Automotive Engineers Inc., 1972.

4. Ch. K. Kroell, and L. M. Patrick: "A New Crash Simulator and Biomechanics Research Program." Eighth Stapp Car Crash and Field Demonstration Conference 1964, p. 185, Detroit: Wayne State University Press, 1966

5. L. M. Patrick, H. J. Mertz, Jr. and C. K. Kroell: "Cadaver Knee, Chest and Head Impact Loads." Paper 670913, Proceedings of Eleventh Stapp Car Crash Conference P-20. New York: Society of Automotive Engineers, Inc., 1967.

6. L. M. Patrick and H. R. Trosien, "Volunteer, Anthropometric Dummy, and Cadaver Responses with Three and Four Point Restraints." SAE Transactions, Vol. 80, (1971), paper 710079.

7. G. Dotzauer, P. Hinz and W. Lange, "Das Verhalten Menschlicher Körper und Anthropometrische Puppen im Sicherheitsgurt bei der Simulation Von Schweren Frontalzudammenstössen." Z. Bechtsmed. 72, 8, 1973.

8. G. B. Voigt, W. Lange and G. Dotzauer, "Entstehunggeise der Verletzungen Von Fahrern und Beifahrern Frontal Kollidierender Kraftfahrzeuge. Z. Rechtsmed 73, 255 1973.

9. D. Kallieris, "Eine Fallgewichtsbeschleunigungsanlage zur Simulation von Aufpallunfällen." Prinzip und Arbeitsweise. Z. Rechtsmed 74, 25 1974.

10. D. Cesari, R. Qunicy and Y. Derrien: "Effectiveness of Safety Belts, Under Various Directions of Crashes." Paper 720973, Proceedings of Sixteenth Stapp Car Crash Conference P-45. New York: Society of Automotive Engineers, Inc., 1972.

11. D. Kallieris and G. Schmidt, "Belastbarkeit Gurtgeschützter Menschlicher Körper bei simulierten Frontalaufprallen." Z. Rechtsmed 74, 31 1974.

12. C. Tarrière, A. Fayon and G. Walfisch, "Human Tolerance to Impact and Protection Measures." C.C.M.C. Report 1974.

13. M. Theis, "Untersuchung der Dynamischen und Statischen Biegebelastung Frischer Menschlicher Rippen." Med. Diss. Heidelberg 1974.

14. D. Kallieris, "Härtemessungen an Frischen Menschlichen Knochen. Z. Rechtsmed 68, 164 1971.

15. D. Kallieris and J. Genser, "Härtemessungen an Frischen Menschlichen Femora. Z. Rechtsmed 71, 293 1973.

16. J. W. Garrett and P. W. Braunstein, "The Seat Belt Syndrome." J. Trauma 2, 220 1962.

17. L. M. Patrick and H. J. Mertz, "Human Anatomy, Impact and Injuries and Human Tolerances." Paper 700195, P-29, Presented at SAE Automotive Engineering Congress, Detroit, January 1970.

751144

Injury to Unembalmed Belted Cadavers in Simulated Collisions

L. M. Patrick and R. S. Levine
Wayne State University

Abstract

Unembalmed cadavers restrained with a three point harness were exposed to a deceleration environment of 20, 30 and 40 mph BEV.* Injuries were tabulated from detailed autopsies. The results indicate an AIS-1 injury at 25.5 mph, an AIS-2 injury at 31.5 mph and an AIS-3 injury at 34.5 mph. The AIS-3 injury level is recommended as the maximum acceptable injury.

The cadavers sustained the same types of injury that have been reported in medical literature including bruises, abrasions, lacerations, fractures and viscera ruptures, but injury severities were greater in the cadavers than in living humans at a given collision severity. Also, there is a wide spread in the degree of injury between cadavers due to differences in age and physical condition. The threshold of cadaver rib fracture is 30 mph and the threshold of cadaver vertebral fracture is between 30 and 40 mph for the environment utilized.

More numerous and severe abdominal injuries were observed. They were attributed to excessive submarining as a result of no restraint from the instrument panel and leg muscles of the cadavers. It is concluded that the cadaver is an excellent means of studying the types of injuries to be expected from a collision environment.

UNEMBALMED CADAVERS seated in a modified full size vehicle were subjected to decelerations and stopping distances corresponding to those of a barrier collision for a full size vehicle. Velocities of 20, 30 and 40 mph with corresponding stopping distances of 20, 30 and 40 inches were util-

---

*Program funded by Contract DOT-HS-146-3-753, National Highway Traffic Safety Administration, U.S. Department of Transportation.

ized in the program. Frontal force collisions were simulated with the instrument panel, windshield and steering assemblies removed to eliminate secondary injuries not directly attributable to the harness system. The experiments were conducted as soon after death as feasible, but not before rigor mortis had left.

The detailed objectives of the program include:

1. Delineation of the injuries sustained by the cadavers by visual observation, x-rays, palpation and autopsy as a function of BEV (Barrier Equivalent Velocity).

2. Determination of the HIC (Head Injury Criterion) for the cadavers and the dummy.

3. Measurement of chest acceleration and GSI (Gadd Severity Index) for the thorax.

4. Measurement of the belt load and maximum elongation of the belt during collision simulations.

5. Establishment of the maximum velocity for which protection is afforded including a definition of the degree of injury considered to be acceptable.

6. A record of the pressure-time history of the thoracic arterial pressure during collision simulation.

7. Extrapolation of the results of the cadaver experiments to living humans in similar collision environments.

In addition to the nine unembalmed cadavers used in this program, a Sierra 1050 Dummy was subjected to the same collision simulations to permit the cadaver reactions to be compared to those of the dummy. The injury criteria specified in MVSS 208 were calculated for the dummy and the cadavers with the exception of the femur loads which were not present due to removal of the instrument panel.

EXPERIMENTAL SET UP

The experimental program was conducted in a modified Chevrolet with modified 1974 three-point harnesses and standard anchor locations. Modification to the vehicle included removal of the engine, transmission, and other concentrated masses which do not affect the interior dynamics. The frame was reinforced to permit the modified vehicle to be subjected to high decelerations without damage. Transducer signals were transmitted from the vehicle to the electronic conditioning and recording equipment through trailing cables. Figure 1 is a photograph of the modified vehicle with the cadaver in position ready for a test.

Collision simulation was achieved by accelerating the vehicle to the desired velocity and stopping it with the deceleration pulse and stopping distance corresponding approximately to the barrier crash of the full size Chevrolet.

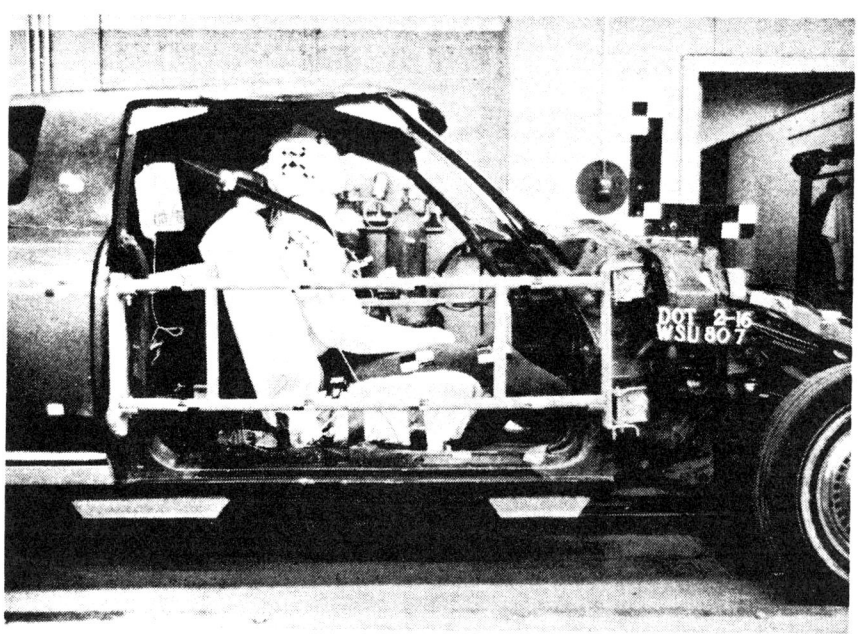

Fig. 1 - Cadaver in modified vehicle ready for test DOT 2-16

Instrumentation is summarized in Table 1 with the head accelerometer mount shown in Figure 2.

Cadaver preparation followed the protocol established at WSU for protecting personnel when working with unembalmed cadavers (1).* The cadavers were X-rayed and examined visually and by palpation to insure that there were no fractures or other abnormalities rendering them unsuitable for the program. The instrumentation was mounted on the head and elsewhere as required. The thoracic arterial system was pressurized by inserting a jejunostomy catheter through the femoral artery to a point just proximal to the diaphragm in the descending aorta. The bladder on the end of the catheter was inflated at that point to seal the vessel. Pressurization was achieved by forcing fluid into the system through the small tube in the catheter. Pressure transducers recorded pressure in the left ventricle and in the arch of the aorta. Before each experiment the cadaver was dressed in two layers of tight fitting leotards to simulate clothing.

The neck was wrapped in multiple layers of elastic bandage to provide approximately 1 g support. For this purpose, the cadaver was placed with the head extending

---

*Numbers in parentheses designate References at end of paper

Table 1 - Summary of Instrumentation for the Dummy, Cadavers, and Vehicle

ITEM	FUNCTION	TRANSDUCER TYPE	MODEL	NO. REQ'D	NO. OF RECORDER CHANNELS
1	Head Acceleration	Accelerometer	Endevco 2264	6	6
2	Chest Acceleration	Accelerometer	Endevco 2264	2	2
3	Head Acceleration C.G.*	Accelerometer	CEC Type 4-204	1	3
4	Chest Acceleration C.G.*	Accelerometer	CEC Type 4-204	3	3
5	Thoracic Arterial Pressure	Pressure	Kulite XQL 125-10 U.P.M. Model 150	2	2
6	Chest Deflection	Electromagnetic	DOT	1	1
7	Seat Belt Force	Tension Force	GSE T-2802	3	3
8	Seat Deflection	Potentiometer	WSU	1	1
9	Vehicle Acceleration	Accelerometer	Statham A6	2	2
10	Seat Belt Elongation	Potentiometer	WSU	2	2
11	Record Synchronization	Timing Generator	Custom	1	1
12	Head Displacement	Visual Targets			
13	Chest Deflection	Visual Targets			
14	Occupant Dynamics	Lateral Onboard Camera	Photosonic 1B		
15	Occupant Dynamics	Lateral Offboard Camera	Locam 164-5DC		
16	Occupant Dynamics	Front Offboard Camera	Photosonic 1B		

* USED WITH DUMMY ONLY

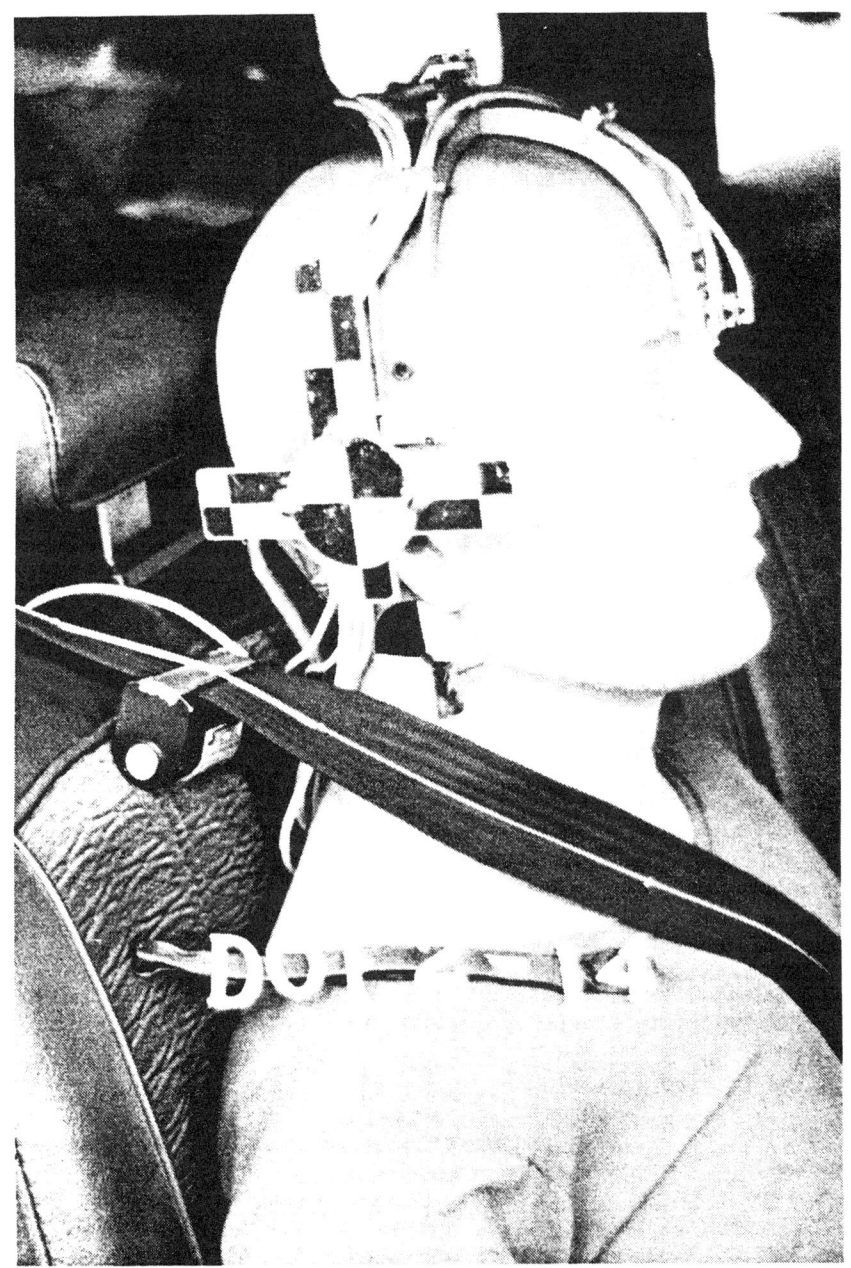

Fig. 2 - Nine component head accelerometer mount and seat belt load transducer

over the edge of the table and the neck wrapped until it remained in a normal position.

After the instrumentation was installed and the cadaver was ready for the experiment, it was placed in position in either the driver or passenger seat. The saline solution source was attached to the jejunostomy catheter through a solenoid valve. Just prior to the experiment the thoracic vascular system was pressurized to approximately 100 mm of mercury.

Set up photographs were taken just prior to the run and again immediately after the run. Post run visual and palpation examinations were made followed by X-rays and autopsy. Pertinent data on the experimental conditions and the cadaver are presented in Tables 2 and 3.

CADAVER INJURIES

Details of the cadaver injuries are provided in references (1,2). Nine unembalmed cadavers ranging in age from 32 to 61 years of age at time of death were subjected to barrier equivalent collision simulations at velocities of 20, 30, and 40 mph. C-1 (Cadaver No. 1) was subjected to two 20 mph simulations in the right front passenger and driver seats. The injuries after the two runs were AIS-1 with no skeletal or internal injuries. C-2 was subjected to one 20 mph and one 30 mph simulation. A single rib fracture was noted after the first run at 20 mph followed by multiple rib fractures at the 30 mph simulation. The cumulative effect of the 30 mph run following the 20 mph run with a single fracture resulted in an anomalous AIS-4 injury. This run was discarded as a result of the double exposure after skeletal damage in the first run.

Injuries at Simulated 30 mph Collision: Three cadavers were subjected to the nominal 30 mph barrier equivalent collision simulation. They resulted in an AIS-1 (DOT Run 2-12), AIS-1 (DOT Run 2-15) and AIS-3 (Cadaver Run 2-16). The AIS-3 injury consisted of segmental fractures of ribs 2 and 3 and single fractures of ribs 4, 5 and 6, all on the inboard side (Tables 2 and 3).

In the 30 mph simulation series there were no spinal fractures, thoracic organ injuries or abdominal organ injuries.

Injuries at Simulated 40 mph Collision: Four runs were made with cadavers at a nominal 40 mph barrier equivalent velocity. The injuries were AIS-3 for Run 2-19, AIS-7 for Runs 2-20 and 2-21, and AIS-8 for Run 2-22. The age at time of death ranged from 32 to 61 years (Tables 2 and 3).

The cadaver in Run 2-19 at 39.2 mph was 32 years old at time of death and died from carbon monoxide poisoning.

Table 2A - Summary of Cadaver Statistics, Experimental Exposure, and Injuries

Run(s) DOT/WSU	Cadaver DOT/WSU	Age Weight Height	Dates Death/Run/Autopsy	Cause of Death	Velocity Stop Dist. Position	Injury Summary	AIS
2-5 / 772	C-1 / 2742	53 yrs. 182 lbs. 5' 7"	11/22/73 12/06/73 None	Cardiac arrest; renal failure. Cirrhosis of liver, peptic ulcer disease	19.2 mph 21 in. RFP	No Fx - Palpation and x-ray examination. No organ examination no autopsy. Light belt marks.	1
2-6 / 775	C-1 / 2742	53 yrs. 182 lbs. 5' 7"	11/22/73 12/11/73 None		19.5 mph 21 in. DR	No Fx - Palpation and x-ray examination. No organ examination no autopsy. Light belt marks.	1
2-7 / 786	C-2 / 2775	58 yrs. 122 lbs. 5' 9 3/4"	12/27/73 01/05/74 None	Biliary cirrhosis	21.0 mph 21 in. DR	Single rib fracture suspected from palpation. No autopsy after this run since cadaver was used on Run DOT 2-8.	1
2-8 / 787	C-2 / 2775	58 yrs. 122 lbs. 5' 9 3/4"	12/27/73 01/16/74 01/17/74		29.2 mph 30 in. RFP	Bilateral mult. rib fx. starting at R-2 and running diagonally to R-9 at the mid-axillary line. Flail chest. No vertebral fx. Different belt system.	4
2-12 / 796	C-3 / 2771	61 yrs. 162 lbs. 5' 6 1/2"	12/24/73 01/31/74 02/07/74	Acute myocardial infarction, arteriosclerotic heart disease	29.2 mph 30 in. RFP	Bruise on right hip extending across belly - slight bruise on left hip. No skeletal fracture.	1
2-15 / 801	C-4 / 2823	41 yrs. 153 lbs. 5' 9"	02/10/74 03/05/74 03/06/74	Acute hepatic failure, arterial hypertension, alcoholism	29.0 mph 30 in. RFP	Abrasion on right side of neck. Bruise at about R-10 on mid-axillary line. No skeletal frac.	1
2-16 / 807	C-5 / 2862	57 yrs. 148 lbs. 5' 4"	03/17/74 03/21/74 03/28/74	Cerebral anoxia; cardiac arrest; acute myocardial infarction.	29.9 mph 30 in. RFP	Bruises and abrasions below left nipple. Segmental fracture R-2 and 3 (left). Single fracture R-4, 5 and 6 (left).	3

Table 2B - Summary of Cadaver Statistics, Experimental Exposure, and Injuries

Run(s) DOT/WSU	Cadaver DOT/WSU	Age Weight Height	Dates Death Run Autopsy	Cause of Death	Velocity Stop Dist. Position	Injury Summary	AIS
2-19 824	C-6 2892	32 yrs. 154 lbs. 5' 11 1/2"	04/30/74 05/08/74 05/09/74	Carbon monoxide poisoning. Inhaled automobile exhaust fumes.	39.2mph 40 in. DR	Abrasion over both hips and left shoulder. Rectus abdominis muscle torn. Central part of greater omentum torn. Bruise on interior peritoneum 2 1/2 cm dia. Three tears in mesentery. No skeletal fracture.	3
2-20 841	C-7 2906	56 yrs. 226 lbs. 6' 1/2"	05/19/74 05/29/74 06/03/74	Hypertensive Cardiovascular disease	40.1mph 40 in RFP	Bruises under lap and shoulder belts. Tear in fat over ribs under shoulder belt. Tear in fat, muscle and peritoneum in abdomen. Transection of small bowel. Rectus abdominis torn bilaterally. Tear in greater omentum. R-3, 4, 5, 6, 7, 8, and 9 fractured segmentally on the left side under shoulder belt mark. Fracture of body of C-6. Fracture of left superior aspect of body of L-1 at pedicle attachment.	7
2-21 846	C-8 2916	50 yrs. 158 lbs. 5' 6"	06/02/74 06/19/74 06/26/74	Cardiac Arrest Hypertensive Vascular disease	40.1mph 40 in. RFP	Severe laceration at right neck shoulder juncture. Bilateral bruises above superior rim of pelvis extending across abdomen. Laceration on chin from hitting chest instrumentation. Diagonal bruise from right side of neck to mid-axillary line at R-5 or 6 on left. Rib fracture under belt bruise on left side with Ribs R-1, 2, 3, 4, 5, 6, 8 fractured. Sternoclavicular joint dislocated on left side. R-1, 2, 3, 4, 5, 6, 7 fractured on right side. Fracture of atlas—both lateral processes fract. Posterior longitudinal ligament torn between L-1 and L-2. Subluxation between inferior facet of L-2 and superior facet of L-3. Bilateral tear in rectus abdorinis muscle. Tear in greater orentum 5 cm long. Transverse tear in abdominal wall. Tear in small bowel and the mesentery. Lacerated liver. Ruptured spleen. Fx posterior R-2, 3, 4, 5	7

Table 2C - Summary of Cadaver Statistics, Experimental Exposure, and Injuries

Run(s) DOT/WSU	Cadaver DOT/WSU	Age Weight Height	Dates Death Run Autopsy	Cause of Death	Velocity Stop. Dist. Position	Injury Summary	AIS
2-22/847	C-9/2912	61 yrs. 192 lbs. 6' 0"	05/27/74 06/21/74 06/27/74	Acute myocardial infarction; arteriosclerotic heart disease	40.0 mph 40 in. DR	Bruised left hip at superior iliac crest extending to navel. Bruise on right side under shoulder belt. Fracture of R-1 in super clavicular region and at the origin of R-1 on the left side. R-2 3, 4, 5 fract. on left side. Comminuted fracture of manubrium. R-1, 2, 3, 4, 5, 6, 7, 8 fractured on right side. Innominate artery transected. Transverse tear through abdominal wall including omentum. Tear in the mesentery. Mid portion of duodenum bruised. Psoas muscle bruised. Fractured tibia and fibula 4 cm below left tibial tubercle. Severe separation between C-5 and 6. Severe separation between T-12 and L-1. Liver badly lacerated on right superior dome. Poker spine from T-12 up. Superior end plate of C-7 sheared off with disruption of posterior ligaments and boney structure. Fracture of T-4 from inferior-anterior to superior-posterior of body. Fracture of anterior superior lip of T-11.	8

133

Table 3 - Cadaver Injury Rating with Range, Average, and Best Fit Valve for Each Nominal Velocity

VELOCITY MPH		DOT CADAVER NO.	DOT RUN NO.	ABBREVIATED INJURY SCALE (AIS)			
NOMINAL	MEASURED			INDIVIDUAL	RANGE	AVERAGE	SECOND ORDER BEST FIT*
20	19.2	C-1	2-5	1	1	1	0.9
	19.5	C-1	2-6	1			
	21.0	C-2	2-7	1			
30	29.2	C-3	2-12	1	1-3	1.7	1.52
	29.0	C-4	2-15	1			
	29.9	C-5	2-16	3			
40	39.2	C-6	2-19	3	3-8	6.3	6.1
	40.1	C-7	2-20	7			
	40.1	C-8	2-21	7			
	40.0	C-9	2-22	8			

* $AIS = 0.02V^2 - 0.94V + 11.72$
$R = 0.91$, $R^2 = .83$

The relatively minor AIS-3 injury (compared to the AIS-7 and AIS-8 injuries for the other 40 mph runs is attributed to the comparatively young age at time of death (32 years) and good health prior to death.

In Runs 2-20 and 2-21 the individuals both died from vascular disease and heart problems. These diseases often result in severely curtailed activities which tends to decrease the strength of the body tissues. Cadaver C-7 experienced rib fractures, cervical spine fracture, lumbar spine fractures and abdominal injuries.

Cadaver C-8 experienced injuries in the same body components as cadaver C-7 including fractured ribs, fractured cervical spine, fractured lumbar spine and abdominal organ injuries.

Cadaver C-9 suffered injuries that included fractured ribs, fractured cervical, dorsal, and lumbar spine and abdominal injuries. It should be noted that the X-rays and examination of the excised spine showed osteoarthritic changes resulting in a so-called poker spine from the twelfth thoracic vertebra upward. This condition probably contributed to the severe spinal injuries.

Injury Level as a Function of Velocity: Table 3 summarizes the injuries in terms of the Abbreviated Injury Scale at nominal velocities of 20, 30 and 40 mph. The AIS, the range of AIS values, the average AIS value at each velocity and the second order best-fit AIS injury at each vel-

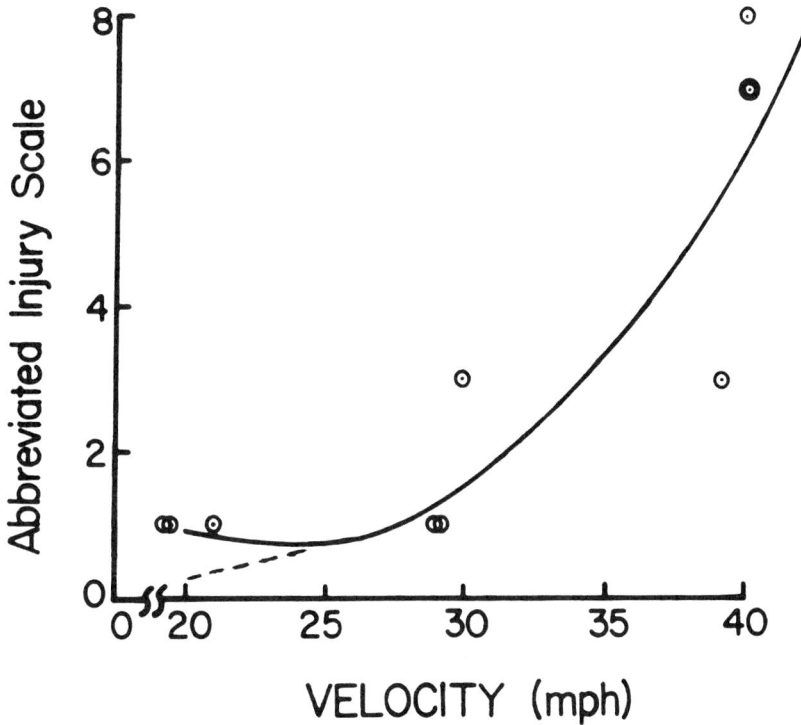

Fig. 3 - Cadaver injury as a function of BEV

ocity are included in the table. The best-fit, second order curve is shown at the bottom of Table 3. It results in an AIS-0.9 at 20 mph, AIS-1.5 at 30 mph, and AIS-6.1 at 40 mph. It should be noted that the fatal injury is the only one with gradations. These range from 6 through 8 in this series. If all fatals were listed as 6, or a single value, the second order best-fit curve results in an AIS of 5.4 at 40 mph instead of the 6.1 previously mentioned. Figure 3 shows the second order best-fit curve to the AIS vs. velocity data. The dashed portion of the curve below 25 mph is faired in with the direction leading to low injuries at lower velocities. The second order curve increases in degree of injury at velocities below the 25 mph which is obviously not representative of the true injury data. The results indicate that a finer scale is needed at the low velocities if the degree of injury is to be differentiated.

Types of Injury: The most prevalent skeletal injury consisted of rib fractures. Of the nine cadavers, there were five that suffered rib fractures of which one (C-2) had a single rib fracture while the others were multiple rib fractures. One out of three of the cadavers at the 30 mph simulations had multiple rib fractures. Three out of four of the cadavers at the 40 mph simulation had multiple rib fractures. Three out of four of the cadavers at the 40 mph simulation had multiple rib fractures while the fourth one had no rib fractures.

No spinal fractures were observed below 40 mph. In the 40 mph series, one cadaver (C-6) had no spinal fractures. Of the other three cadavers, two had cervical and lumbar fractures and the third (C-9) had cervical, dorsal and lumbar spine fractures.

There were no internal abdominal injuries below 40 mph. All four cadavers in the 40 mph series had abdominal injuries with three out of four having organ injuries and the fourth (C-6) having torn abdominal muscles, a torn greater omentum and three tears in the mesentery. The occupant in the first 40 mph simulation was 32 years old at time of death with damage to the abdominal muscles, mesentery and omentum, but no skeletal fractures and minimal submarining. In the other three 40 mph simulations, submarining was extreme with the lap part of the harness imbedded in the abdominal area and applying force to the inferior edge of the rib cage. The submarining is more prevalent in these simulations than observed in field data, probably due to the lack of muscle forces which tend to keep the pelvis in a normal position without rotation. Without muscle forces the pelvis rotates allowing the lap belt to slip over the anterior spines of the iliac crest into the vulnerable abdominal area.

HEAD INJURY CRITERION (HIC)

The HIC (3) is based upon the resultant acceleration at the CG of the head of the dummy. Since a triaxial accelerometer cannot be mounted at the CG of the head of the cadaver, a special mount shown in Figure 2 with six linear accelerometers was designed to mount on the exterior of the head of the cadavers and the dummy. A theoretical method for calculating the acceleration at the CG of the head based upon the six external accelerometer reading was developed. However, during the program it was found that the theoretical evaluation was not practical and consequently the CG acceleration could not be ascertained. The discrepancy was noted when the acceleration got so high that the computer program stopped.

An alternative method of approximating the acceleration at the CG was developed by using three of the acceleration components measured from accelerometers that were oriented to provide acceleration measurements along three orthogonal axes going through the CG. Comparison of the re-

Table 4 - Head Injury Criterion (HIC) Calculated from the Orthogonal Components and Resultant Acceleration at the CG of the Dummy Head and the Acceleration Measured on the Exterior of the Head of the Dummy and Cadavers

RUN NO. DOT	VEL (MPH)	OCCUPANT	MEASURED AT HEAD C.G. PEAK ACCEL (G's) AP	SI	LR	RES	HIC	CALCULATED USING FT-AP FT-AP AND SIDE SI PEAK ACCEL (G's) AP	SI	LR	RES	HIC★
2-1	20.9	Dum	18	11	5	20	58	24	11	15	25	103
2-2	19.8	Dum	15	7	5	16	47	16	9	8	18	80
2-2	29.1	Dum	28	24	6	33	227	37	19	12	40	359
2-4	29.6	Dum	35	21	9	38	415	-	-	-	-	-
2-5	19.2	Cad C-1						27	14	7	28	188
2-6	19.5	Cad C-1						26	22	11	33	259
2-7	21.0	Cad C-2						27	32	19	40	294
2-12	29.2	Cad C-3						47	36	21	51	646
2-15	29.0	Cad C-4						51	47	6	65	825
2-16	29.9	Cad C-5						57	34	22	64	1123
2-17	38.2	Dum	71	41	9	75	896	80	49	11	86	1003
2-18	39.9	Dum	83	47	7	85	1277	104	43	17	111	2097
2-19	39.2	Cad C-6						56	97	38	110	2187
2-20	40.1	Cad C-7						77	57	14	80	1591
2-21	40.1	Cad C-8						70	54		86	1727
2-22	40.0	Cad C-9						68	76	31	98	1916

* These values are approximately 50% too high and are presented only to permit a rough comparison of the HIC for different velocities and between dummy and cadaver.

sults, based upon the three external accelerometers and the three linear acceleration measurements at the CG, indicated a discrepancy due to the added acceleration at the exterior of the head caused by rotation. A discrepancy is obvious in Table 4 which summarizes the acceleration and the HIC for the measurements at the CG and the external components. The HIC measured from the external components is approximately 50% greater than the HIC measured from the resultant acceleration at the CG of the head.

Table 4 shows the HIC measured from the external acceleration components of the dummy and cadaver to be appreciably higher for the cadaver than for the dummy. This is apparently due to the lower resistance of the cadaver neck than the dummy neck to flexion. Although the cadaver neck was wrapped with elastic bandage to a 1 g stiffness, the reaction is considerably less than the Sierra 1050 dummy neck. It should be noted that the deceleration pulse plays an important role in the HIC value. In another program with a shorter stopping distance using the same dummy (4), the HIC measured at the CG of the dummy head is approximately twice the value found in this program.

The HIC measured from the external accelerometers on the cadaver head is over the allowable 1000 value even when reduced by the 1.5 factor relating the HIC measured from the external accelerometers and the CG accelerometers of the dummy head at 40 mph. At 20 and 30 mph, the HIC measured on the cadaver head appears to be well below the 1000 maximum specified in MVSS 208.

CHEST ACCELERATION AND GADD SEVERITY INDEX (GSI)

The Gadd Severity Index is based upon the resultant acceleration measured at the CG of the thorax of the dummy. Since the resultant acceleration cannot be measured at the CG of the cadaver, a comparison was made with the AP acceleration measured at the spine of the dummy and the cadaver. A summary of the results is shown in Table 5. While the GSI cannot be measured legitimately by the uniaxial spine accelerometer, a comparison of the results shows that it does give a reasonable measure of the Gadd Severity Index for the higher velocities. Most importantly, the table shows that the GSI is well below the allowable value of 1000 for all of the collision simulations including the 40 mph barrier equivalent collision. Even with a factor for the increased GSI measured with the resultant rather than the uniaxial acceleration, the values are well below the allowable limit.

Table 5 also shows the resultant acceleration measured at the CG of the thorax of the Sierra 1050 dummy. The accelerations are all well below the 60 g/3 ms criterion that has been considered as a thoracic injury criterion. DOT Runs 2-21 and 2-22 have an AP spine acceleration for the cadaver of 56 and 58 g peak respectively. These are approaching the 60 g limit and could possibly exceed the 60 g limit if a triaxial measurement had been made at the CG of the thorax.

BELT LOADS AND ELONGATION

The occupant was carefully positioned in the normal seated attitude with approximately 1.5 pounds of pre-load

Table 5 - Peak Components and Resultant Acceleration and Gadd Severity Index at Dummy Thorax CG and Peak Spine Acceleration and AP Gadd Severity Index for Cadavers

RUN NO. DOT	VEL (MPH)	OCCUPANT	OCCUPANT POSITION	PEAK DUMMY CHEST ACCEL. AT CG (g units) AP	SI	LR	RESULT	GADD CHEST INDEX AP	SI	LR	RESULT	PEAK SPINE ACCEL. (g's)	GADD SPINE INDEX
2-1	20.9	Dum	RFP	24	8	5	24	34	5	1	43	17	33
2-2	19.8	Dum	DR	19	6	9	19	30	2	1	34	17	37
2-3	29.1	Dum	DR	23	11	8	24	74	6	1	88	51	103
2-4	29.6	Dum	RFP	26	12	8	27	102	6	1	117	39	138
2-5	19.2	Cad C-1	RFP									16	12
2-6	19.5	Cad C-1	DR									14	15
2-7	21.0	Cad C-2	DR									32	34
2-12	29.2	Cad C-3	DR									38	73
2-15	29.0	Cad C-4	RFP									18	61
2-16	29.9	Cad C-5	RFP									20	42
2-17	38.2	Dum	RFP	30	29	14	40	184	51	9	282	32	192
2-18	39.9	Dum	DR	41	23	14	42	281	58	5	382	42	248
2-19	39.2	Cad C-6	DR									40	189
2-20	40.1	Cad C-7	RFP									36	148
2-21	40.1	Cad C-8	RFP									56	207
2-22	40.0	Cad C-9	DR									58	417

in the lap and shoulder belt. Belt load as a function of time during the simulation was obtained from inbelt load cells mounted on the belts near each of the three anchors. Peak belt loads are presented in Table 6 which also includes the peak force for the three load cells and the maximum sum. The sum of the loads is not the sum of the peak loads since the individual peak loads do not always occur simultaneously. The horizontal component of the peak belt load and the total load is also included in Table 6. The horizontal component was obtained by measuring the direction cosines from the high speed film and calculating the component of force parallel to the longitudinal axis of the vehicle.

Figure 4 shows the three belt forces and the sum of the three belt forces as a function of time for dummy run DOT 2-18 at 40 mph BEV. Figure 5 shows similar data for cadaver run DOT 2-21 at a 40 mph BEV collision simulation.

A composite graph showing the average total belt loads for the dummy and cadaver in the nominal 20, 30 and 40 mph runs is shown in Figure 6. Each curve in Figure 6 is for the average of all runs at each velocity for the dummy and the cadaver. The average of the cadaver runs at 20, 30 and 40 mph is shown by the dash lines, and the average of the dummy runs at each velocity is indicated by the solid

Table 6A - Summary of Belt Loads for DOT Injury Assessment of Belted Cadavers Study

Run No. DOT	Vel. (MPH)	Stop. Dist. (in)	Occupant	Pos./Belt Type	Peak Belt Loads (lbs) IBL	OBL	USH	Total	Horizontal Peak Belt Loads (lbs) IBL	OBL	USH	Total	Remarks
2-1	20.9	21	Dum*	RFP/ST'D	730	560	810	2100	610	380	670	1655	Belt elong.: 2 5/16" (lap), 2 1/2" (shoulder).
2-2	19.8	21	Dum	DR/ST'D	770	530	720	2000	670	390	550	1590	Lap belt elong.: 2 9/16".
2-3	29.1	30	Dum	DR/ST'D	1220	1080	1150	3250	1090	790	840	2540	Belt elong.: 2 7/8" (lap), 2 1/2" (shoulder).
2-4	29.6	30	Dum	RFP/ST'D	1140	n825	1210	3100	960	480	990	2360	Belt elong: 3 1/2" (lap), 3 1/4" (shoulder). Outboard belt load cell loose.
2-5	19.2	21	Cad C-1	RFP/ST'D	780	690	560	1970	635	435	440	1460	Belt elongations lost.
2-6	19.5	21	Cad C-1	DR/ST'D	640	650	750	2030	510	390	610	1500	" "
2-7	21.0	21	Cad C-2	DR/ST'D	590	520	710	1780	420	250	590	1220	Belt elong: 2 1/2" (lap), 7/8" (Shoud). Lap belt has slipped over the crest of Ilium. Occupant submarined.
2-12	29.2	30	Cad C-3	RFP/ST'D	1360	1120	1200	3660	1160	500	1030	2980	Belt elong: 3 1/8" (lap), 2 1/2 (Shoulder). Lap belt sensor cable broke at anchor pt. The shoulder belt was preloaded to 1.5 lbs. Occupant slightly submarined.

* Sierra 1050 Dummy

Table 6B - Summary of Belt Loads for DOT Injury Assessment of Belted Cadaver Study

Run No. DOT	Vel. (MPH)	Stop. Dist. (in)	Occupant	Pos./ Belt Type	Peak Belt Loads (lbs) IBL	OBL	USH	Total	Horizontal Peak Belt Loads (lbs) IBL	OBL	USH	Total	Remarks
2-15	29.0	30	Cad C-4	RFP/ST'D	1240	1070	1140	3400	1030	640	975	2600	All belts are preloaded to 1.5 lbs. Lap belt has 3 3/8" elong., shoulder belt 2 1/2". Occupant submarined with belt slipped over the crest and into the abdomen.
2-16	29.9	30	Cad C-5	RFP/ST'D	1020	570	1020	2600	830	320	900	2040	Belt elong: 2" (lap), 1 3/4" (Shoulder)
2-17	38.2	40	Dum*	RFP/ST'D	1440	1450	1550	4250	1330	1180	1310	3640	Occupant has outboard submarining. Chin hit chest. Belt elong.: 4 1/8" (lap), 4 1/4" (shoulder).
2-18	39.9	40	Dum	DR/ST'D	1520	1450	1520	4380	1420	1190	1230	3770	Belt elong.: 4" (lap), 4 1/8" (Shoulder)
2-19	39.2	40	Cad C-6	DR/ST'D	1260**	1260	1560	4066	1170	1040	1330	3520	Belt elong.: 2 7/8 (lap), 1 5/8 (shoulder). Inboard load cell failed to function.
2-20	40.1	40	Cad C-7	RFP/ST'D	1430	1640	1790	4840	1330	1440	1660	4380	Occupant submarined. Belt elong.: 5 1/4 (shoulder), 3 1/4" (lap).
2-21	40.1	40	Cad C-8	RFP/ST'D	1450	1660	1930	5040	1355	1460	1750	4560	Occupant submarined. Shoulder belt roll up on the neck under chin, lap belt pulled up into abdomen and abdomen distended over belt.
2-22	40.0	40	Cad C-9	DR/ST'D	1540	1720	1930	5170	1540	1540	1670	4680	Occupant submarined with stomach distended over belt off both hips.

* Sierra 1050 Dummy.
** Inboard load cell failed to function. Data were taken as those of outboard belt load.

141

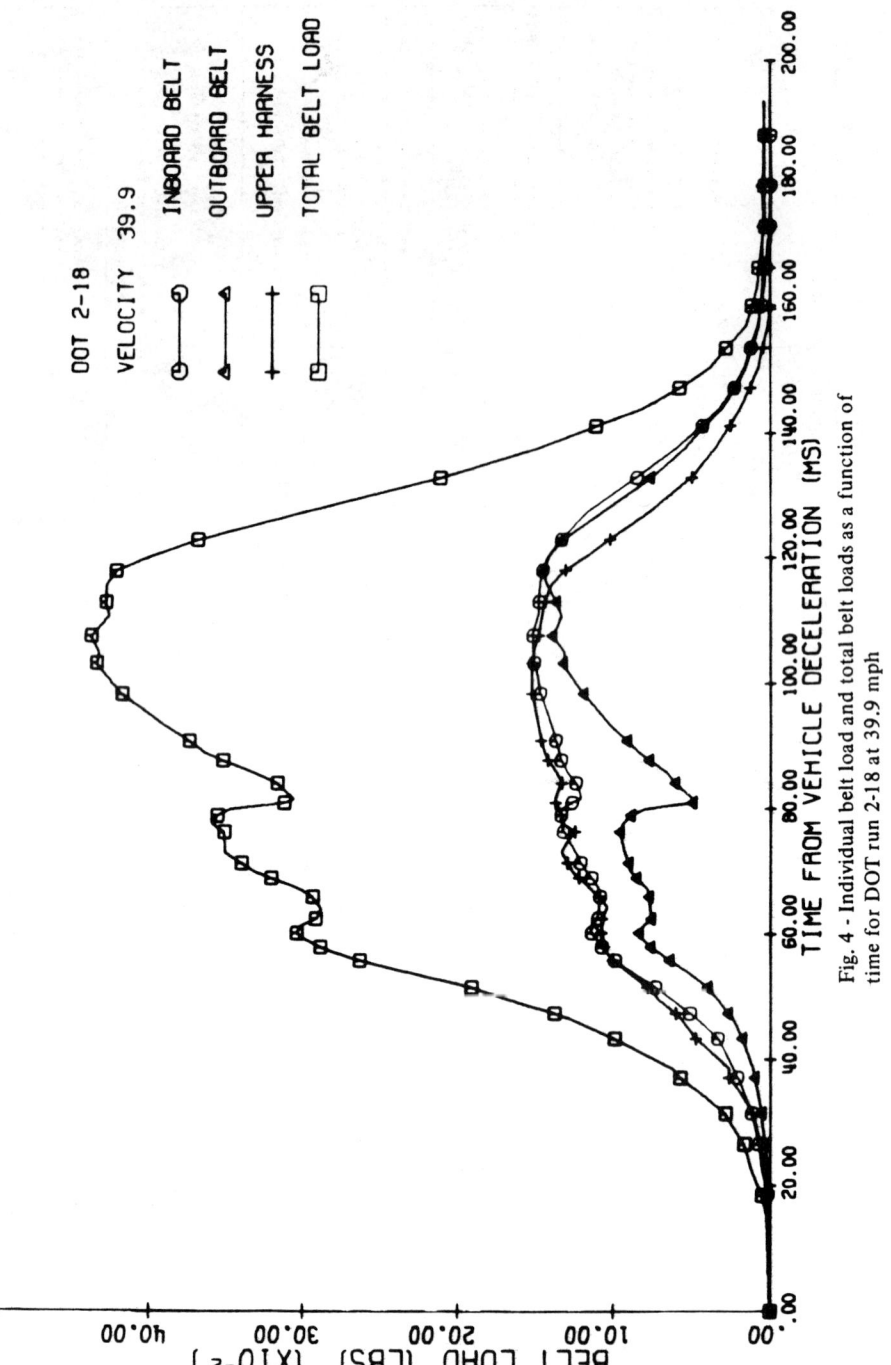

Fig. 4 - Individual belt load and total belt loads as a function of time for DOT run 2-18 at 39.9 mph

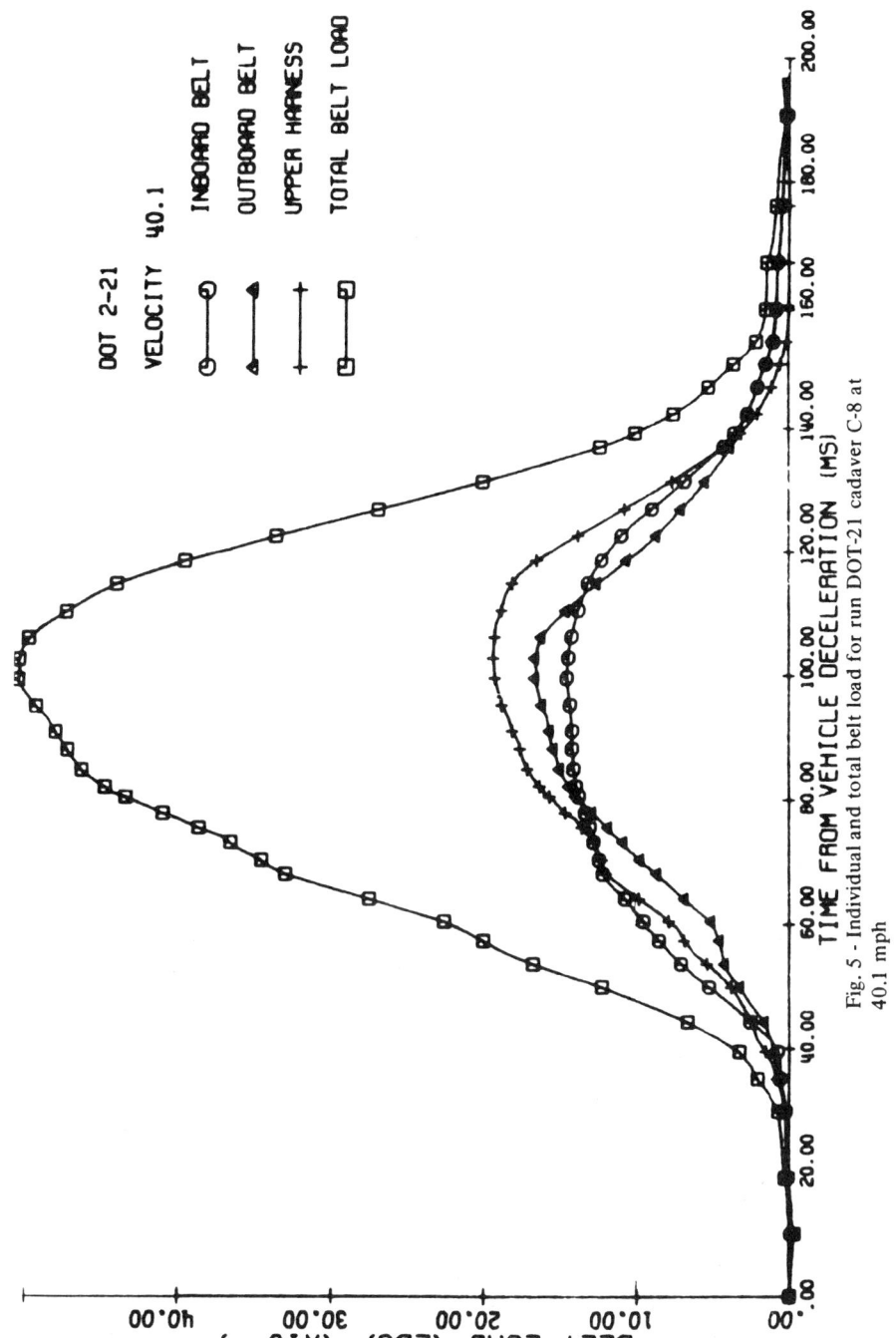

Fig. 5 - Individual and total belt load for run DOT-21 cadaver C-8 at 40.1 mph

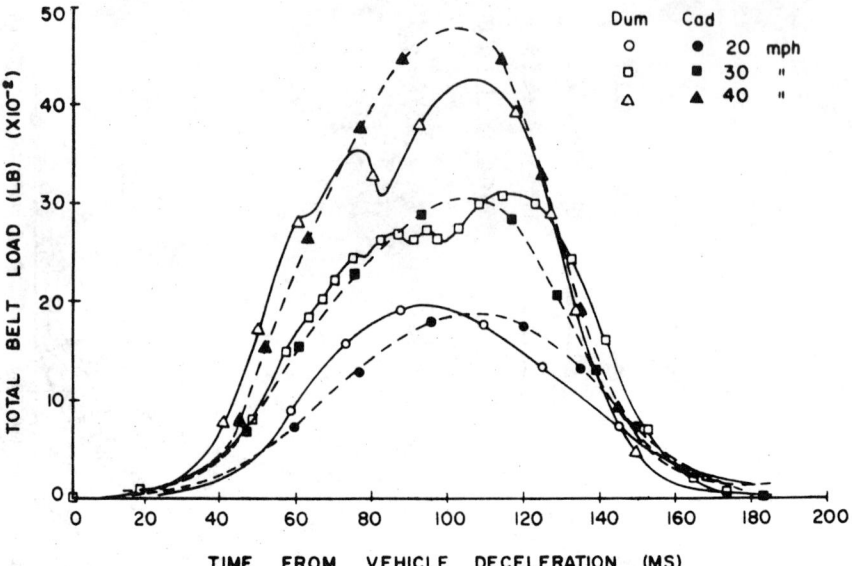

Fig. 6 - Average total belt load as a function of time at 20, 30, and 40 mph for the dummy and cadavers

lines. The cadaver curves are geometrically similar and approximate a half sine curve at each velocity. Each of the cadaver runs has about the same duration and approximately the same time to the peak force of about 105 ms from onset of vehicle deceleration.

The dummy graph of belt force as a function of time is similar to the cadaver curve in shape and magnitude at 20 mph BEV. There is a considerable difference in the shape of the dummy curves and the cadaver curves at 30 and 40 mph. The gross difference is caused by a dip in the curve for the dummy records which is not present in the cadaver records. The difference in geometry between the dummy and cadaver belt loads at 30 and 40 mph appears to be due to the submarining at these velocities. When the dummy submarines the belt slips over the iliac crest resulting in a momentary change in the loading condition. As the belt slides over the iliac crest the force decreases until it starts to load the abdominal area including the spine with a continued increase in the force level until the peak is reached after which the decrease in loads is similar to the cadaver records. The cadaver also submarines at 30 and 40 mph (in fact, more so than the dummy) but does not have the distinct change in the shape of the curve indicating a less precipitous change in loading condition.

Figure 7 is a graph showing the horizontal components of the total belt load for the 20, 30 and 40 mph velocities

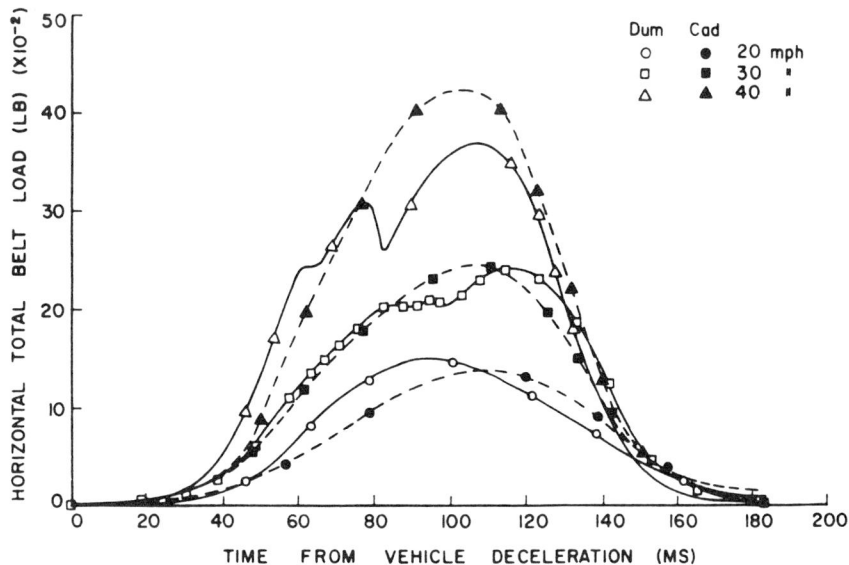

Fig. 7 - Horizontal component of average of total belt load as a function of time at 20, 30, and 40 mph for the dummy and cadavers

for the dummy and the cadaver. The general shape of the curve follows that of the total belt load of Figure 6. The horizontal component of the belt load is considered to be a better indicator of the forces applied to the body since the different angles of the different vehicle belt systems can affect the total forces without appreciably affecting the distribution and/or direct forces acting on the occupant. A comparison of the horizontal components of the total belt load for the cadavers and the dummy shows that there is a considerably greater range of peak values for the cadavers than for the dummies as would be expected due to the difference in weight and height.

Figures 8 and 9 are graphs of the maximum total belt load and the horizontal component of the maximum total belt load. Since rib fractures are the most prevalent injury, the maximum horizontal component of the upper shoulder harness force shown in Figure 10 is probably the most important indicator of injury potential.

The Belt Elongation of Table 7 was measured with a special transducer developed for that purpose. The elongation represents the total elongation over the lap and shoulder portion of the harness respectively.

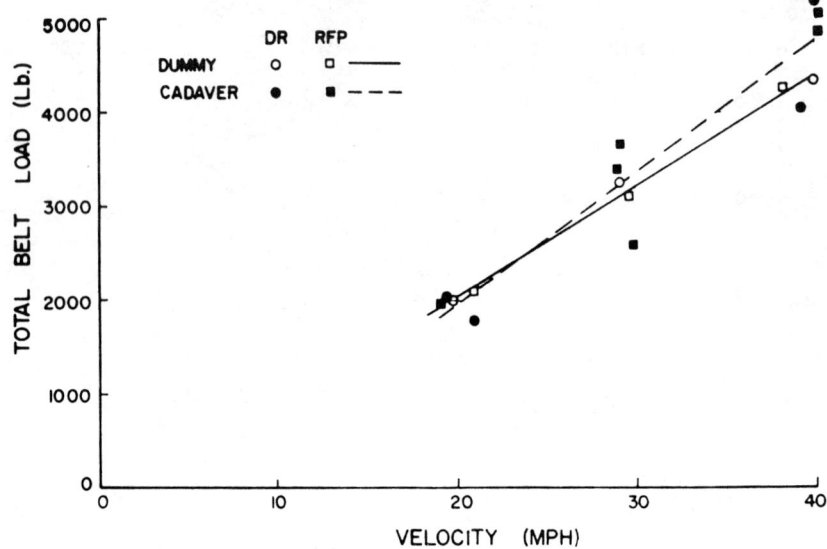

Fig. 8 - Total belt load as a function of velocity for the dummy and cadavers

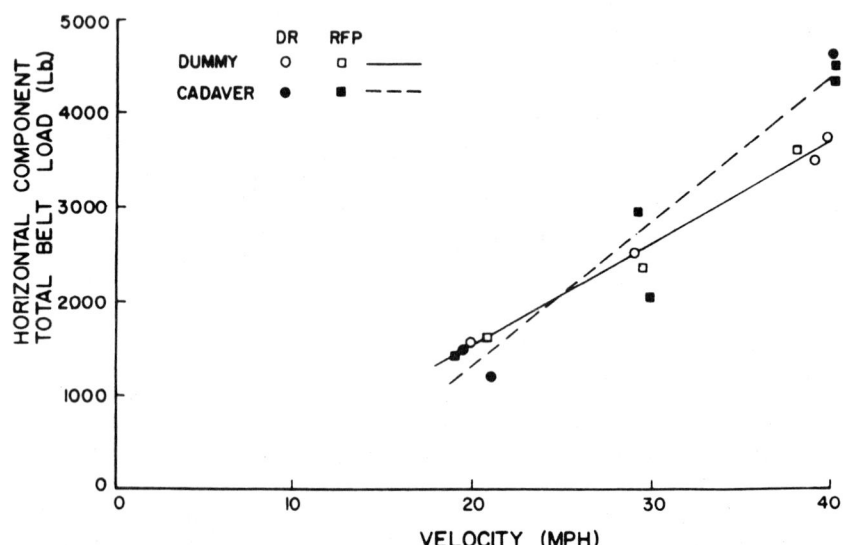

Fig. 9 - Horizontal component of the total belt as a function of velocity for the dummy and the cadaver

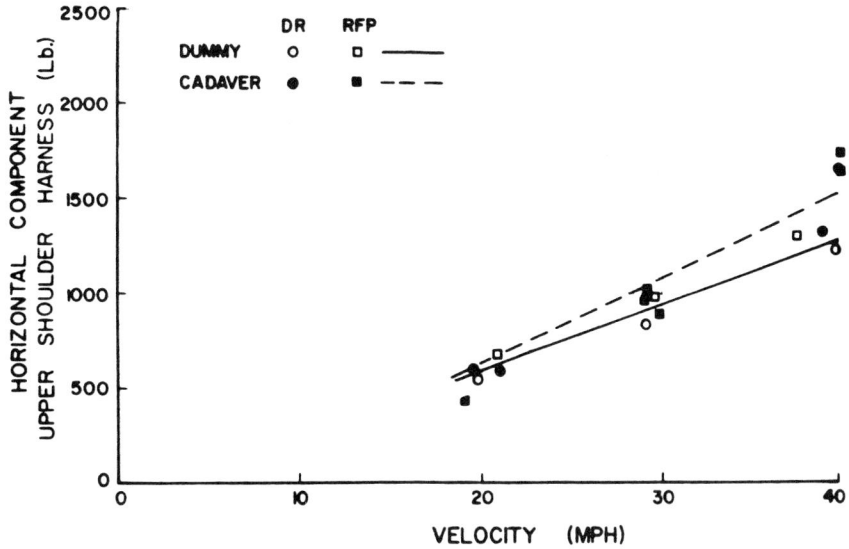

Fig. 10 - Horizontal component of upper shoulder harness load as a function of velocity for the dummy and the cadavers

THORACIC ARTERIAL PRESSURE

Prior to impact the thoracic arterial pressure was 100 millimeters of mercury which was achieved by inserting saline solution into the aorta through the jejunostomy catheter. The arterial system was sealed with a solenoid valve just prior to deceleration of the vehicle. Pressure transducers were inserted through the right carotid artery into the left ventricle and through the left carotid artery into the aortic arch above the heart.

Table 8 lists the peak thoracic pressure for the cadaver runs. There was no pressure reading on Cadaver C-1. Cadaver C-2 was the only cadaver for which a pressure reading was obtained at the nominal 20 mph simulation. In this exposure the peak pressure was 507 mm Hg (9.8 PSI). At the nominal 30 mph exposures the average of the peak pressures for the three experiments was 719 mm Hg (13.9 PSI). Pressure records were obtained for three cadavers at the nominal 40 mph simulation with an average peak pressure of 936mm Hg (18.1 PSI). There was no direct evidence that the pressure in the arterial system caused failure of any of the vessels. The only major artery damage occurred in Cadaver C-9 and consisted of the transected innominate artery at its insertion point in the aorta. The type of transection does not indicate that the failure was due to excessive pressure in the arterial system.

Table 7 - Summary of Belt Elongation

Run No. DOT	Vel. (MPH)	Stop. Dist. (in.)	Occupant	Position	Measured Lap	Measured Shoulder	From Visicorder Lap	From Visicorder Shoulder
2-1	20.9	21.	Dummy	RFP	2.3	2.5	2.5	2.5
2-2	19.8	21.	Dummy	DR	2.6	-	3	-
2-3	29.1	30	Dummy	DR	2.9	2.5	2.2	2.8
2-4	29.6	30	Dummy	RFP	3.6	3.2	3.5	4
2-5	19.2	21	C-1	RFP	-	-	-	-
2-6	19.5	21	C-1	DR	-	-	-	-
2-7	21.0	21	C-2	DR	2.5	0.9	-	-
2-12	29.2	30	C-3	RFP	3.1	2.5	3.2	2.4
2-15	29.0	30	C-4	RFP	3.4	2.5	3.6	2.4
2-16	29.9	30	C-5	RFP	2	1.8	-	-
2-17	38.2	40	Dummy	RFP	4.1	4.3	4	4.4
2-18	39.9	40	Dummy	DR	4	4.1	2.4	4
2-19	39.2	40	C-6	DR	1.3	4.4	2.6	-
2-20	40.1	40	C-7	RFP	-	2.8	3.2	5.2
2-21	40.1	40	C-8	RFP	2.3	6.4	-	-
2-22	40.0	40	C-9	DR	2.4	-	1.8	-

* Data taken from record.

MAXIMUM VELOCITY AND ACCEPTABLE INJURY FOR WHICH PROTECTION IS AFFORDED

In establishing a maximum velocity for which protection is afforded by the harness system in forward force collisions, the overall philosophy is to protect the maximum number of people from the maximum number and severity

Table 8 - Peak Thoracic Arterial Pressure for Cadaver Runs

Run No. DOT	Vel. (MPH)	Stop. Dist. (in.)	Gad. No.	Position	Peak Thoracic Pressure (PSI)	Remarks
2-5	19.2	21.	C-1	RFP	-	Pressure transducer failed to function.
2-6	19.5	21.	C-1	DR	-	"
2-7	21.0	21.	C-2	DR	9.8	
2-12	29.2	30.	C-3	RFP	15.2	
2-15	29.0	30.	C-4	RFP	13.6	
2-16	29.9	30.	C-5	RFP	13.0	
2-19	39.2	40.	C-6	DR	10.0	
2-20	40.1	40.	C-7	RFP	18.0	
2-21	40.1	40.	C-8	RFP	18.8	
2-22	40.0	40.	C-9	DR	17.5	

of collisions. Practically, this requires the acceptance of a certain degree of injury rather than elimination of all injury in the collision with the understanding that the goal is to eliminate all injury. To arrive at the velocity for which protection is available with a harness system it is necessary to establish the acceptable injury level and to base the maximum velocity on certain criteria regarding the occupants and the collision. These points will be covered in the following sections.

Recommended Acceptable Injury Level - AIS-3: When considering the degree of injury that is acceptable, it is necessary to establish certain criteria to maximize the benefits stated in the overall philosophy of minimizing the injuries and fatalities for the greatest number of occupants exposed to the greatest number and severity of collisions. In this particular study, only frontal force collisions are considered. Consequently, the following criteria are based upon frontal force collisions:

(1) Protection will be provided to the maximum number of occupants.

(2) Protection will be provided at the maximum possible collision severity.

(3) Some predetermined level of injury will be accepted to achieve the previous two criteria.

(4) The acceptable injury will be based upon the "average" individual.

These criteria will be discussed individually.

It is desirable to set acceptable injury levels as low as possible with zero injury under all conditions an optimum goal. This goal appears to be unattainable under the current state of the art of automobile crashworthiness at the maximum velocities at which collisions occur. It is axiomatic that the lower the acceptable injury, the lower will be the collision velocity or severity at which protection can be afforded. Therefore, from a practical standpoint it is essential to set the "acceptable injury level" as high as practical since there are some very high collision severities. Obviously, the goal of eliminating all injuries and the simultaneous desire to mitigate injury in all collisions provides opposing requirements.

Considering only the data in this program as summarized in Table 3, the BEV 20 mph collision simulations resulted in AIS-1 injuries in all three of the experiments. Therefore, if zero is to be the goal, the maximum velocity for which protection is afforded would have to be under 20 mph. The other extreme (which is unacceptable) is illustrated in Figure 3 in which the AIS-5 injury is reached at 38.5 mph for the best fit curve. Even the AIS-5 did not include the upper end of the collision severity range, but obviously is the highest possible acceptable injury level since if fatal injuries are acceptable there would be no need for improving the safety record.

The recommeded acceptable injury level is based upon:
(1) Nondangerous to life injuries.
(2) Injuries that are unlikely to become dangerous to life in the time required to obtain adequate medical attention.
(3) Tolerance of the "average" individual.

These criteria result in an acceptable injury level recommendation of AIS-3 of SEVERE (Not Life-Threatening) in which the following maximum injuries specified in the AIS-3 rating are pertinent according to the results of this program:

(1) Rib fracture without respiratory embarrassment.
(2) Cervical spine fractures without cord damage.
(3) Thoracic or lumbar spine fractures without neurological involvement.
(4) Contusion of abdominal organs.
(5) Single open long bone fractures.
(6) Major contusion of abdominal wall.
(7) Hemothorax or pneumothorax.

It is important to note that the "average" individual. concept means that 50% of the occupants may have injuries of less than AIS-3 and 50% may have injuries greater than AIS-3 at the collision severity in which the "average" individual sustains an AIS-3 injury. Another way of considering this is that those individuals least able to withstand the collision environment will have injuries greater than AIS-3 while those most able to withstand the collision environment will have injuries less than AIS-3.

The AIS-3 degree of injury for the cadavers utilized in this program was reached at 34.5 mph. Age, sex, weight, size and physical condition prior to death, all effect the resistance to injury. Muscle tone is another important factor in degree of injury. Consequently, the 34.5 mph is considered to be overly conservative and indicative of the greater propensity to injury to the cadavers used in this program than to the average population exposed to collisions.

EXTRAPOLATION OF CADAVER DATA TO LIVING HUMANS

The cadaver injuries are similar to those observed in humans involved in automobile collisions as evidenced by the reports in the literature (2). The Medical Literature (5 to 22) includes many references to injuries similar to those observed in the cadaver and listed in Table 2. It should be noted that most of the reported injuries are for occupants wearing only the lap belt. In general, it appears that the cadaver injuries are more severe than human injuries in collisions of the same severity.

Rib and sternum injuries are the most common injuries of severity greater than AIS-1 in cadavers and living humans. Vertebral and abdominal injuries appear to be more prevalent in the cadavers than in living humans subjected to the same deceleration environment. Muscle and other soft tissue damage is found at autopsy to a greater extent than diagnosed in living humans where such injury is often manifested as pain without pin pointing the exact cause. Therefore, many of the less severe injuries that are reported in this series of cadaver experiments may or may not occur in humans where it is not possible to examine the tissues in the same detail.

Bruises and/or abrasions occurred in all of the cadavers with or without skeletal or internal injury. Medical reports often do not record any such bruising. The lack of reported bruises on living humans could be because no bruising was present or it could be that the more serious injuries are noted and the minor bruises are ommitted as being inconsequential.

Extrapolation of the cadaver data to living humans will be based primarily upon injuries to living humans under known collision conditions compared with the cadaver data from the study. The primary comparison will be with the study by Patrick, et al (4) in which forward force collisions are duplicated in the laboratory with dummy occupants to compare the results with the 169 occupants wearing a three point harness that were involved in collisions at barrier equivalent velocities up to 53 mph.

Head Injury: The cadaver head vascular system was not pressurized, and the brain was not examined at autopsy so there is no brain injury recorded for the cadavers. With the steering assembly and instrument panel removed in this program, the cadaver did not hit the steering wheel which eliminated the fractured facial bones and facial lacerations observed in the field accident study. Correct posture and no belt slack further reduced the HIC and the head injury potential.

Of the 169 occupants wearing harnesses in the field study (4), there were no brain injuries greater than AIS-2 which is a moderate injury without post-traumatic amnesia. Of the nine occupants with head injury greater than AIS-1, eight were drivers and one was a right front passenger. The only AIS-3 head injury was a fractured mandible sustained by a driver when his head struck the steering assembly. Seven nasal fractures were reported at the AIS-2 injury level with five facial lacerations at the AIS-2 level. Several of the injuries from contact with the steering assembly included facial fractures and laceration to the same driver, with the overall injury at the AIS-2 level.

The Head Injury Criterion (HIC) calculated from the resultant acceleration at the center of gravity of the dummy head in this program is approximately 50 for 20 mph, 330 for 30 mph, and 1025 for 40 mph. These values are considerably lower than those for the same velocity in the Volvo automobile (4) in which the HIC was approximately 50 at 20 mph, 1000 at 30 mph, and 1850 at 40 mph. Since the same dummy was used for both studies, the greater HIC for the Volvo vehicle is caused by the more severe deceleration pulse and/or the driver's head hitting the steering assembly.

Schmidt, et al (23) found no evidence of brain damage in 49 unembalmed cadavers subjected to 30 mph (50 km/h) sled tests with 15.75 inch (40 cm) stopping distance. With the shorter stopping distance of 15.75 inches compared with the 30 inch stopping distance of this program, his environment was more severe which could correspond to a higher BEV for a U.S. full size car. Since no injuries occurred, it is not possible to establish the velocity at which injury will occur, but the peak deceleration for a similar pulse geometry will be 90% higher at the shorter stopping distance indicating a severity corresponding to a considerably higher velocity.

Based upon the accident data (4) there does not appear to be a need for calculating or using the HIC or any other criterion for indicating potential internal head injury for occupants wearing a three point harness unless the head hits the steering assembly or some other component. The HIC on the dummy at 53 mph was over 3000 with no brain damage to the occupants in the field study at that velocity. Therefore, the HIC corresponding to brain injury would be higher than 3000. It is concluded that brain damage to harnessed occupants is not likely at any collision severity up to at least 53 mph BEV for which the passenger compartment integrity is maintained unless the head hits an interior component or the occupant does not have normal resistance to injury from head acceleration.

Neck and Spine Injury: Hyperflexion occurring in severe frontal force collisions is a potential source of neck injury to occupants wearing a three point harness. In the current series of simulations there were no neck injuries at 20 and 30 mph BEV for the unembalmed cadavers, and the 32 year old cadaver had no neck injuries at 40 mph. The other three cadavers at 40 mph sustained cervical vertebrae damage. Cadaver C-7 had a fracture of the sixth cervical vertebra at 40 mph. Cadaver C-8 had a fracture of C-1. Cadaver C-9 had the most extensive damage to the cervical spine with severe separation between C-5 and C-6 and a fracture of C-7. Injuries to Cadaver C-9 were aggravated by the osteoarthritic changes with the so-called poker spine from T-12 upward which probably contributed to the spinal injuries.

The 1 g neck resistance that was simulated by wrapping the neck with ace bandage produced much less resistance or muscle simulation than the maximum muscle reaction which a living human can exert. Higher head accelerations and greater torque at the occipital condyles result when the neck muscles are relaxed than when tense for the same acceleration exposure. Mertz (24) has reported on the increased reaction (torque and force) at the base of the skull with the neck muscles relaxed as compared to the tense neck muscles. With the muscles relaxed or only partly tensed, the relative rotational velocity is higher during the collision deceleration than with the muscles tensed. When the end of rotational travel occurs, the head accelerations and neck reactions are greater with muscles relaxed than for the lower relative rotational velocity which results when the muscles are tensed.

In the field study (4) there were two cervical vertebra fractures resulting in an AIS-3 injury level. A fracture of C-2 occurred in a 76 year old female at a forward impact velocity of 15 mph. However, the vehicle was subjected to three impacts, including the final 15 mph forward force collision. The multiple impacts plus the advanced age of the individual contributed to the injury. The other cervical spine injury was a fracture of C-4 in a 12 year old male in a forward force collision of BEV 40 mph severity. In the same vehicle, the 25 year old driver sustained an AIS-1 injury without neck injury. The greater propensity for injury in the child has been noted by Burdi, et al (25). The head of the child is a greater part of his total weight than an adult. Furthermore, the neck musculature is less well developed, resulting in a greater likelihood of neck injuries.

Three of the occupants in the field study (4) sustained thoracic and/or lumbar vertebra fractures. A 35 year old male who had been sleeping with the seat back in a reclined position sustained a fracture of T-12 in a 28 mph collision He was awakened by a shout from the driver and sat up just before the collision occurred. With this sequence of events, the harness was probably grossly incorrectly located at the time of the accident which contributed to the injury. A 61 year old male sustained fractures of L-3 and L-4 in a 30 mph BEV frontal force collision. Fractures of T-12, L-1 and L-3 occurred to a 45 year old male in a 35 mph BEV frontal force collision. None of the three occupants with thoracic and/or lumbar vertebra or the two occupants with cervical vertebral fractures had any neurological deficit. Their injuries were all rated AIS-3 with complete recovery.

While the vertebral injuries to the occupants in the field occurred at velocities from 15 to 40 mph, it should be noted that they were not accompanied by the severe abdominal injuries that were observed in the three Cadavers, C-7, C-8 and C-9 or the less severe abdominal injuries of Cadaver C-6 at 40 mph BEV.

Lack of muscle reaction in the legs probably contributed to the aggravated injuries of the cadavers. The lack of muscle tone permits the cadaver to submarine, exposing the abdomen to injury from the lap belt. Thus, injury to the lumbar and thoracic spine in cadavers is probably greater than what would be expected in living humans. On the other hand, the occupants of vehicles are probably out of position with the harness not optimumly located in many of the accident situations which will aggravate the injuries. Of the nineteen occupants (4) in collisions at BEV 30 mph severity or greater, three sustained vertebral fractures: the 12 year old male at 40 mph and a 45 and 61 year old male both at 30 mph. Four male adults were involved in collisions of 40 to 53 mph BEV without any vertebral fractures.

It is concluded (4) that vertebral fracture is not a major problem at velocities up to 50 mph BEV unless the ocpants are at the extremes of the age range, they have some inherent spinal weaknes, they are not in a normal position, and/or they are not wearing the harness correctly. Cadavers receive greater injuries at 40 mph BEV than living humans at 50 mph BEV probably due to the excessive submarining resultint from lack of muscle tone.

Rib Cage Injury: Rib fracture is the most prevalent injury observed in the present study and in the study by Schmidt, et al (23) and Patrick, et al (4). At 30 mph with a more severe deceleration pulse, Schmidt found 533 rib fractures in 49 cadavers exposed or approximately eleven fractures per cadaver. In the present study, there were 39 rib fractures in 9 cadavers exposed for an average of 4.3 ribs fractured per cadaver for the 20, 30 and 40 mph runs or 5.6 ribs per cadaver for the seven cadavers exposed at 30 and 40 mph. In the 30 mph series, one out of three cadavers had rib fractures for an average of 1.7 per cadaver, and in the 40 mph series three out of four had fractures for an average of 8.5 per cadaver.

In the field study (4), there were 38 ribs fractured at velocities from 10 to 53 mph. Fourteen of the 169 occupants had rib and/or sternum fractures with eleven occupants with rib fractures and four with sternum fractures including one which had both rib and sternum fractures. At or above 30 mph there were 19 occupants, five of whom had rib and sternum fractures with 17 rib fractures and one sternum fracture. At 30 mph or greater BEV severity, the occupants sustained an average of 0.9 fracture per occupant. All rib fractures occurred on the inboard or belt side of the rib cage.

Summarizing the rib fracture data shows an average of eleven rib fractures per cadaver at 30 mph BEV with a severe deceleration pulse reported by Schmidt (23); 1.7 rib fractures at 30 mph BEV and 8.5 rib fractures at 40 mph BEV per cadaver for the WSU cadaver data (1), and 0.9 rib fracture per occupant at 30 mph BEV or greater in the WSU-Volvo field accident study (4). These data indicate that rib fractures are more prevalent in cadaver impacts than in humans involved in accidents of equal or greater severity.

It should be noted that Schmidt (23) found an increase in rate of rib fractures with age and that most of the cadaver studies have been performed on elderly cadavers. In the field study (4), there were no rib fractures to individuals less than 43 years of age, further indicating the importance of age on the susceptability of rib fracture.

Schmidt reported four clavicle fractures in the 49 cadavers exposed at 30 mph (23). In the present cadaver study there were no clavicle fractures and one sternoclavicular joint dislocation. No clavicle fractures to living humans occurred in the field study (4).

It is concluded that the cadavers suffer more rib fractures at a given severity of impact than do living humans. Age plays an important role with a larger number of ribs fractured in elderly people than in younger people both living and dead. There is a distinct increase in rib fracture incidence with collision severity and age in both living and dead with the cadavers sustaining several times the number of fractured ribs in the same collision severity In the living human, the fractures are on the inboard or shoulder belt side while they occur on both sides of the rib cage in the cadaver with a marked preference for the inboard side.

Abdominal Injuries: Abdominal injuries in the field study (4) were rare. There was one ruptured spleen representing the most severe injury from a life threatening standpoint of all of the injuries sustained by the 169 occupants. Other abdominal injuries were listed only as bruises or pain of short duration. Thus from the field study, abdominal injuries appear to be rare in frontal force collisions with the Volvo harness system.

In the present study, only superficial injuries such as bruises and abrasions to the abdominal wall were observed at the 20 and 30 mph exposures. The only major abdominal injury in the field study was a ruptured spleen in a 62 year old female at 25 mph.

Schmidt, et al (23) reports many abdominal injuries. Unfortunately, it is not possible from his publication to determine whether the abdominal injuries he reports are multiple injuries to a few cadavers or individual injuries to many cadavers. The incidence of abdominal injuries at 30 mph from the Schmidt study is greater than in the 30 mph simulations of the Wayne study where there were no serious abdominal injuries. Schmidt reports the following ruptures to abdominal organs: 9 liver, 5 spleen, 2 kidney, 1 small intestine, 4 mesentery, 6 abdominal wall, 2 peritoneum. None of these organs were injured in the Wayne study at 30 mph with the less severe deceleration pulse.

At 40 mph BEV in the Wayne study with four cadavers exposed, there were 2 lacerated livers, 1 ruptured spleen, 0 kidney injuries, 2 small intestine ruptures, 4 mesentery tears, and tears to the peritoneum or greater omentum.

More extensive abdominal injuries in both cadaver studies (1,2,3) than in the field study (4) indicate that the cadavers are more prone to injury to the abdominal region than living humans. In the present Wayne study, the gross submarining has been assumed to be the cause for the abdominal injuries. Submarining is probably aggravated in the cadaver studies by the lack of leg muscle reaction.

It is concluded that the abdominal injuries in the cadaver studies are more severe than those sustained by living humans in accidents of the same severity.

While the field study (4) with the three point harness in frontal force collisions did not result in a large number of abdominal injuries, there are isolated cases reported in the literature of injury to abdominal organs. Most of these have been found with only the lap belt worn and are reported as isolated cases. The cadaver injuries reported at Wayne (1) and by Schmidt (23) represent injuries that are seen occasionally in the field, but occur more frequently and with greater severity in the cadaver.

Factors Affecting Cadaver Results: Three factors that probably affect the cadaver results by increasing the likelihood of submarining and abdominal injuries are:

(1) Pretensioning of the shoulder belt
(2) Lack of muscle tone
(3) No instrument panel

These conditions are abnormal and distort the results toward greater injury as do the advanced age and poor physical condition prior to death of most of the cadavers.

The shoulder and lap belt retracting reels were removed and the belts were attached directly to the anchors with a tension of approximately 1.5 pounds in each belt. This resulted in both belts (lap and shoulder) starting to load simultaneously or the shoulder belt slightly ahead of the lap belt. With slack in the shoulder belt and some looseness in the webbing on the shoulder belt retracting reel in the standard installation, the lap belt starts to load before the shoulder belt. Also, the slack allows the torso to move forward as the lap belt applies a force to the pelvis. These actions result in the lap belt tending to remain in the correct position with the force applied to the pelvis without submarining.

As the shoulder belt tightens with the reel in the standard system, the spooled webbing tightens more gradually than the solid webbing which may reduce the maximum force applied to the torso. The phenomenon should be studied to verify whether the cushioning effect of tightening the webbing on the reel is beneficial or detrimental

Lack of muscle tone in the legs causes the inertial force of the lower limbs to be applied to the pelvis and femoral head at a point below the point of application of force of the belt to the pelvis with a resulting moment tending to rotate the bottom of the pelvis forward. The rotation of the pelvis causes the lap belt to ride over the iliac crest after which the restraining force is applied to the abdomen causing serious internal injuries if the force is high enough. Some means of simulating the muscle forces to realistically duplicate the leg forces would make the cadaver results more meaningful.

Elimination of the instrument panel and steering assembly insured that any injuries sustained by the cadaver would be from the harness rather than from striking interior components. Unfortunately, removal of the instrument panel aggravated submarining by eliminating the knee forces that limit the forward motion of the lower limbs. Knee forces accomplish the same results as tensing the leg muscles by reducing or eliminating the inertia forces of the legs that cause rotation of the pelvis.

Analysis of the high speed movies shows excessive submarining. The instrument panel would have definitely limited the submarining due to restriction of space for forward movement of the legs. Muscle tensing would probably have reduced the submarining, but must be investigated further before a definite conclusion on its effectiveness can be established accurately.

CONCLUSIONS

The following conclusions are based upon the results of this research program with its prescribed restrictions and comparison of the data with accident data. Extrapolation of the results and conclusions to other vehicles, directions of impact, and restraint systems may invalidate or modify the results and conclusions. Based upon these conditions it is concluded that:

(1) Injuries to cadavers are similar to injuries reported in the literature in accident cases (many of the reported injuries are with lap belts only).

(2) Injuries are more severe and occur with greater frequency at a given collision severity in cadavers than in living humans.

(3) Rib fractures are the most prevalent, but not necessarily the most serious injury.

(4) Bilateral rib fractures are more common in cadavers than in living humans with more fractures on the inboard than on the outboard belt side.

(5) The threshold of cadaver rib fracture is 30 mph corresponding to a horizontal upper shoulder belt force of about 1000 pounds (it is much higher for living humans) with one out of three cadavers sustaining rib fracture at 30mph.

(6) The threshold of cadaver vertebral fracture is less than 40 mph at which 3 out of 4 cadavers had vertebral fractures and greater than 30 mph at which no vertebrae were fractured.

(7) Abdominal injuries are more numerous in cadavers than in living humans.

(8) The threshold of cadaver abdominal injury is be-

tween 30 mph (no abdominal injury) and 40 mph (severe abdominal injury).

(9) Submarining is a major cause of the abdominal injuries in the cadavers. Since abdominal injuries are not as prevalent in real world accidents, submarining apparently does not occur as frequently to the living humans.

(10) There was no thoracic visceral injury attributable to the collision simulation.

(11) No gross arterial damage attributable to the pressures generated during the collision simulations were observed at peak pressures up to 18.8 psi (972 mm Hg.)

(12) The relationship between AIS and BEV for the cadavers in this study is:

$$AIS = 0.02V^2 - 0.94V + 11.72 \qquad (1)$$

with a correlation coefficient of R = 0.91. The equation results in an: AIS-1 at 25.5 mph, AIS-2 at 31.5 mph, AIS-3 at 34.5 mph, AIS-4 at 36.5 mph, AIS-5 at 38 mph, and AIS-6 at 40 mph.

(13) A maximum injury of AIS-3 is the most practical acceptable injury for an upper limit with a target of zero injury under all conditions.

(14) In this series the AIS-3 limit is reached at 34.5 mph BEV - the velocity is considerably higher for the general population in field accidents.

(15) Cadavers are a useful research tool for assessing possible injuries from restraint systems because the injuries are similar to those in living humans including: (1) Bruises (2) Abrasions (3) Lacerations (4) Fractures (5) Viscera Ruptures

(16) There is a wide spread in the degree of injury to cadavers at a given collision severity depending upon age, size, and pre-death condition as evidenced by an AIS-3 to AIS-8 range of injury at 40 mph.

(17) Difference in the physical properties of tissue at the low temperatures (1-5°C) may contribute to the increased injuries sustained by the cadavers. The effect of the temperature of the cadaver on the type and degree of injury in a given exposure should be investigated.

(18) The stopping distance and deceleration pulse shape are important factors in the degree of injury experienced at a given impact velocity.

REFERENCES

1. L. M. Patrick and R. S. Levine, "Injury Assessment of Belted Cadavers." Final Report to DOT under Contract NO. HS-146-3-753, May, 1975.

2. R. S. Levine and L. M. Patrick, "Injury Assessment of Unembalmed Cadavers Using a Three Point Harness Re-

straint." 1975 AAAM Conference Proceedings.

3. Motor Vehicle Safety Standard No. 208 "Occupant Crash Protection in Passenger Cars, Multipurpose Passenger Vehicles, Trucks, and Buses." Effective Date: August 15, 1973.

4. L. M. Patrick, N. Bohlin, A. Andersson, "Three Point Harness Accident and Laboratory Data Comparison." 18th Stapp Car Crash Conference, Ann Arbor, Michigan, December 4-6, 1974.

5. Peter Fisher, "Injury Produced by Seat Belts Journal of Occupational Medicine, Annual Meeting of the American Association of Automotive Medicine, Louisville, Kentucky, Oct. 1964.

6. W. S. Smith and H. Daufer, "Patterns and Mechanisms of Lumbar Injuries Associated with Lap Seat Belts." Department of Surgery, Section of Orthopaedic Surgery, University of Michigan Medical Center, Ann Arbor Mich. The Journal of Bone and Joint Surgery, March 1969.

7. David C. Burke, "Spinal Cord Injuries and Seat Belts." The Medical Journal of Australia, October 27, 1973.

8. Anthony G. Ryan, "A Study of Seat Belts and Injuries". SAE Paper No. 730965, 17th Stapp Car Crash Conference, November 1973.

9. D. F. Huelke and W. A. Chewning, "Comparison of Occupant Injuries With and Without Seat Belts." SAE Paper No. 690244, January 1969.

10. Harold W. Sherman, "Car Results of Some 1974 Passenger Car Crashes." Proceedings of 18th Conference of the American Association for Automotive Medicine, 1974.

11. Charles L. White, "Mesentery and Bowel Injury from Automotive Seat Belts." Annals of Surgery, Vol. 167, January-June 1968.

12. Maj. Janis Sube, Col. H. Haskell Ziperman, and Capt. William J. McIver, "Seat Belt Trauma to the Abdomen." American Journal of Surgery, Vol. 113, Jan.-June 1967.

13. James S. Williams, Bert Lies Jr. and Harry Hale Jr., "The Automotive Safety Belt: In Saving a Life May Produce Intra-Abdominal Injuries." The Journal of Trauma Vol.6, No. 3, 1966.

14. Samuel D. Porter and Edward W. Green, "Seat Belt Injuries." Archives of Surgery, Vol. 96, Jan-June 1968.

15. Wallace Ritchie, Robert A. Ersek, Wilton L. Bunch and Richard L. Simmons, "Combined Visceral and Vertebral Injuries From Lap Type Seat Belts." Surgery, Gynecology and Obstetrics, September 1970.

16. John R. LeMIre, Daniel E. Early and Chapin Hawley, "Intra-Abdominal Injuries Caused by Automobile Seat Belts." JAMA Vol. 201, No. 10, September 4, 1967.

17. J. H. MacLeod and D. M. Nicholson, "Seat - Belt Trauma to the Abdomen" The Canadian Journal of Surgery, Vol. 12, April 1969.

18. Lewis Wexler and James Silverman, "Traumatic Rupture of the Innominate Artery - A Seat Belt Injury." The New England Journal of Medicine, May 21, 1970.

19. William S. Smith and Herbert Kaufer, "A New Pattern of Spine Injury Associated with Lap-Type Seat Belts: A Preliminary Report." University of Michigan Medical Center Journal, 1967.

20. G. Q. Chance, "Note on a Type of Flexion Fracture of the Spine." British Journal of Radiology, Vol. 21, Sept. 1948.

21. Lee F. Rogers, "Injuries Peculiar to Traffic Accidents: Seat Belt Syndrome, Laryngeal Fracture, Hangman's Fracture." Texas Medicine, January 1974.

22. Barry D. Fletcher and Byron G. Brogdon, "Seat-Belt Fractures of the Spine and Sternum." JAMA Vol. 200 No. 2, April 10, 1967.

23. G. Schmidt, D. Kallieris, J. Barz and R. Mattern, "Result of 49 Cadaver Tests Simulating Frontal Collision of Front Seat Passengers." Proceedings of the Eighteenth Stapp Car Crash Conference, Ann Arbor Michigan, December 4-5, 1974

24. H. J. Mertz and L. M. Patrick, "Strength and Response of the Human Neck." Proceedings of the Fifteenth Stapp Car Crash Conference." Coronado, California, Nov. 17-19, 1971.

25. A.R. Burdi and D.F. Huelke, "Infants and Children in the Adult World of Automobile Safety Design:Pediatric and Anatomical Considerations for Design of Child Restraints." Jrl. Biomechanics, Vol. 2, London: Pergamon Press, 1969, pp. 267-280

751158

Static Bending Response of the Human Lower Torso

Gerald W. Nyquist
General Motors Research Laboratories

Clarence J. Murton
Wayne State University

Abstract

This report defines humanlike quasi-static bending response characteristics of the lower torso. Six volunteers were subjected to a total of 72 tests to define response characteristics for sagittal flexion and extension bending. The effects of muscle tensing and knee bend on the response are evaluated. Sixteen loading corridors of moment of applied force about the H-point axis versus thorax-pelvis and pelvis-femur angles are suggested. The significant differences between the relaxed and tensed muscles results illustrate the need for a philosophical decision regarding which of these conditions should be adopted to define lower torso bending response for the human surrogate used in automotive safety studies.

THE OBJECT OF THIS RESEARCH was to define humanlike quasi-static bending response characteristics for the lower torso to provide design criteria for anthropomorphic dummies and response definitions for mathematical modeling.

BACKGROUND

Since no appropriate response criteria have been available, the lumbar and pelvic regions of dummies have not been designed, a priori, to reflect biomechanical fidelity. Likewise, the lower torso response specifications used in mathematical modeling have been somewhat arbitrary. The Part 572 dummy (1)* currently required in connection with Motor Vehicle Safety Standard 208 (2) must satisfy a specific quasi-static bending response

---

*Numbers in parentheses designate References at end of paper.

requirement in flexion (forward bending); however, this specification is not based on biomechanical data. Furthermore, the specification deals only with the response of the lumbar region, leaving the characteristics of the hip joint region undefined. Since the kinematics of a vehicle occupant during a crash must be expected to depend significantly on the bending response of the lower torso, the pertinence of the study presented herein becomes obvious.

In this study, six volunteers were subjected to a total of 72 tests to define response characteristics for sagittal flexion (forward bending) and extension (rearward bending). The effects of muscle tensing and knee bend on the response were evaluated. Each test subject was positioned on his side with legs immobilized and upper torso supported by a dolly free to roll on the floor. Film analysis targets, potted and strapped to the subject, were referenced to the skeletal structure and monitored by an overhead camera during the test. A force applied near the shoulders provided a bending moment at the lower torso, causing lumbar bending and hip joint articulation. The data have been analyzed to provide sixteen loading corridors of moment of applied force about the H-point axis versus thorax-pelvis relative angle and versus pelvis-femur relative angle.

TEST SUBJECT CONSIDERATIONS

VOLUNTEER SELECTION - The test subjects consisted of six adult male volunteers as indicated in Table 1. They were selected to provide a range in height and weight, and are compared to the adult males in the 1962 HEW survey (3) in Table 1. The HEW sample 50th percentile* values are 74.5 kg (164 lb weight) and 173.5 cm (68.3 in) with standard deviations of 12.7 kg (28 lb weight) and 7.3 cm (2.85 in).

The data indicate that the mean of the sample used for this study was a bit taller [2.5 cm (1.0 in)] and less massive [1.8 kg (4 lb weight)] than the HEW 50th percentile. Likewise, the standard deviations of height and mass of the sample used for this study were, respectively, the same [both 7.3 cm (2.85 in)] and somewhat smaller [by 4.8 kg (10.6 lb weight)] than those of the HEW sample.

---

* The HEW data closely approximate a normal distribution; therefore, mean values and 50th percentile values are nominally equivalent.

Table 1 - Definition of Test Volunteers

Volunteer *	Age Bracket (Years)	Nude Mass (kg)	Nude Weight # (lb)	Nude Weight # HEW Percentile	Erect Standing Height (stocking feet) # (cm)	Erect Standing Height (stocking feet) # (in)	Erect Standing Height (stocking feet) # HEW Percentile
GWN	30-40	80.4	177	68	188.0	74.0	98
WEH	30-40	65.8	145	24	169.5	66.7	29
FJR	40-50	83.5	184	76	170.0	66.9	31
LMP	50-60	72.6	160	44	172.5	67.9	44
SAT	30-40	69.5	153	34	181.5	71.5	88
KWK	20-30	64.0	141	19	175.5	69.1	63
Mean:		72.6	160	44	176	69.4	67
Std. Deviation:		7.9	17.3	-	7.3	2.9	-

* All adult males.

\# Weights and heights rounded-off to nearest lb and half cm.

SUBJECT PREPARATION - Film analysis targets were installed after taking a series of anthropometric measurements. Targets were required at the thorax and the pelvis for photographically monitoring the angles during the bending experiment. Whereas targets can be attached to the skeletal structure of cadaver subjects efficiently using bone screws, this is obviously not acceptable in volunteer studies. The alternative is to tightly strap form-fitting target assemblies in a manner that minimizes target movement relative to the skeletal elements to be monitored. The target assemblies developed for this program are shown in Fig. 1.

Each target assembly had a long target bar with contrasting colors to clearly define a straight line. The target bar was coupled through a locking ball and socket adaptor to an aluminum plate which was, in turn, potted to the volunteer's skin with plaster of paris. Small screws extended through the aluminum plate into the plaster of paris to provide a mechanical locking function and to enable the removal and subsequent reattachment of the custom-contoured body/target interface. A coat of paste wax on the skin prior to application of the plaster of paris provided a mild adhesive effect to help preclude target motion relative to the skin.

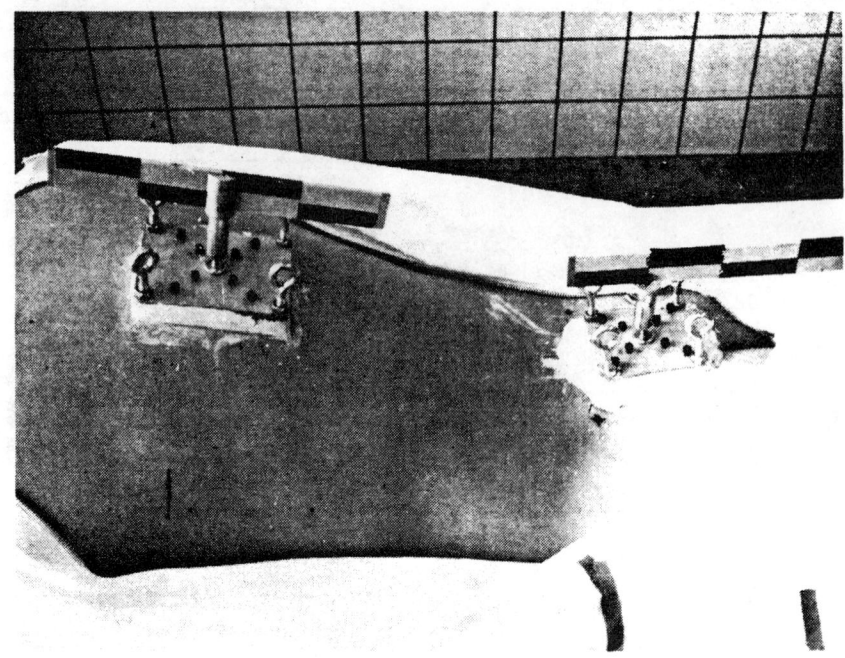

Fig. 1 - Thoracic and pelvic target assemblies

Criteria for locating the thoracic target assembly were threefold:

    i. Center of aluminum plate to be at the palpated location of the 8th thoracic vertebra (T8) spinous process;

    ii. Plane of aluminum plate to be parallel to a line tangent to the axis of the spine at T8 and to a lateral-medial line;

    iii. Target bar to be located in the midsagittal plane.

Reasonable approximations of conditions (i) and (iii) were achieved by eye without difficulty. Condition (ii) was approximated by orienting the aluminum plate parallel to midsagittal and lateral-medial skin surface tangent lines at the palpated T8 spinous process.

Criteria for locating the pelvic target assembly at the sacrum (the posterior aspect of the pelvis) were also threefold:

    i. Aluminum plate to be sufficiently inferior to the lumbar region to preclude target movement relative to the pelvis as a result of lumbar spine articulation;

    ii. Target bar to be located in the midsagittal plane;

    iii. Plane of aluminum plate to be parallel to a lateral-medial line and target bar to be at a known orientation relative to the pelvic skeletal reference line in the midsagittal plane.

Condition (i) was satisfied by mounting the target assembly sufficiently low on the buttocks that the superior-most portion of the aluminum plate was inferior to the posterior, superior iliac spines. Reference to an anatomy chart indicates that this criterion assures that the aluminum plate will not interfere with the 5th lumbar vertebra. Locating the plate in this manner positioned its inferior edge in proximity of the superior margin of the buttocks cleavage. This proved to be advantageous because potting of plaster of paris in this highly-contoured region led to added stability of the target assembly. Condition (ii) of the target assembly location criteria was approximated by eye without difficulty. Condition (iii) was met by locating the aluminum plate, by eye, nominally parallel to the skin surface and establishing the target bar orientation, relative to a pelvic skeletal reference line, after the target assembly was completely installed. The referencing procedure is described in the next section of the paper.

The thoracic and pelvic target assemblies were strapped in place using the four eyebolts in each aluminum plate (Fig. 1). Fabric straps (adjustable length) were attached to the eyebolts via swivel snaps and positioned as illustrated in Fig. 2 (the volunteer donned the disposable coveralls prior to initiation of the target installation procedure). Thoracic target straps extended laterally, around the thorax, from both the upper and lower pairs of eyebolts. In addition, a set of straps from the upper eyebolts passed crisscross over the shoulders. The lateral straps were coupled to elastic cords, which traversed the chest. The elastic action tended to facilitate breathing without loss of strap tension. The straps crossing over the shoulders terminated at the upper lateral strap/elastic cord juncture points. A similar arrangement was used to immobilize the pelvic target assembly. The two sets of pelvic lateral straps extended around the lower torso to elastic cords. Both elastic cords were hooked below the anterior, superior iliac spines and were under moderate, constant tension. A crotch strap extended from each of the lower eyebolts around and up to the upper lateral strap/elastic cord juncture points (the crotch straps did not crisscross left to right). The shoulder straps and crotch straps were not pulled taught but were pulled snug to hinder potential target movement.

THE PELVIC TRIANGLE - Location of an acceptable midsagittal reference line on the pelvis of a volunteer subject poses two problems. First, one must locate suitable landmarks on the pelvis to define the line. Second, the line must be sufficiently accessible to enable the establishment of its orientation relative to the axis of the pelvis

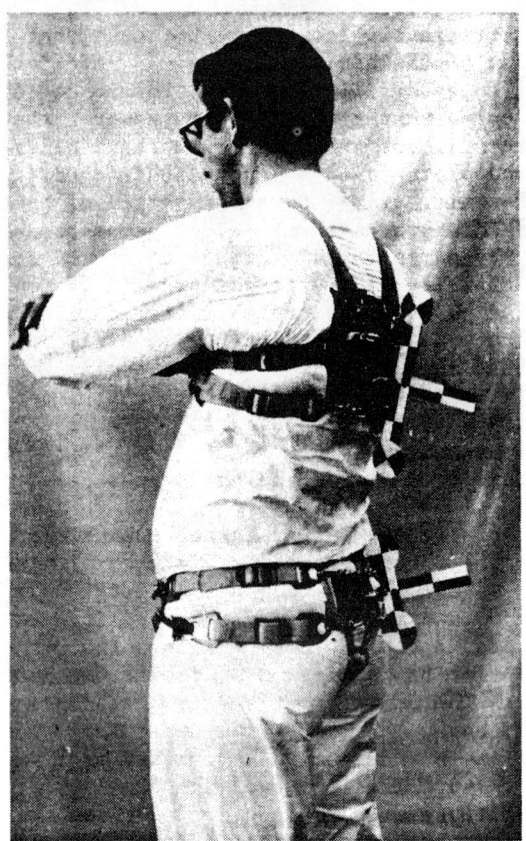

Fig. 2 - Fully installed target assemblies

target bar. X-ray radiography in the pelvic region of the volunteers could not be justified;* therefore, another noninvasive technique was developed.

Palpation of the anterior, superior iliac spines and the pubic crest is feasible and enabled establishment of a midsagittal plane reference line as illustrated in Fig. 3. The reference line is defined as the line, tangent to the pubic crest, that bisects the line joining the left and right anterior, superior iliac spines. The point of tangency and the bisection point constitute two specific points of reference for the pelvis. The H-point axis**

---

* X-ray radiation exposure of the genitalia could be justified only when used for medical diagnosis because of the sterilization hazard.

** The H-point axis is defined to be the straight line connecting the pseudocenters of rotation of the hip joints.

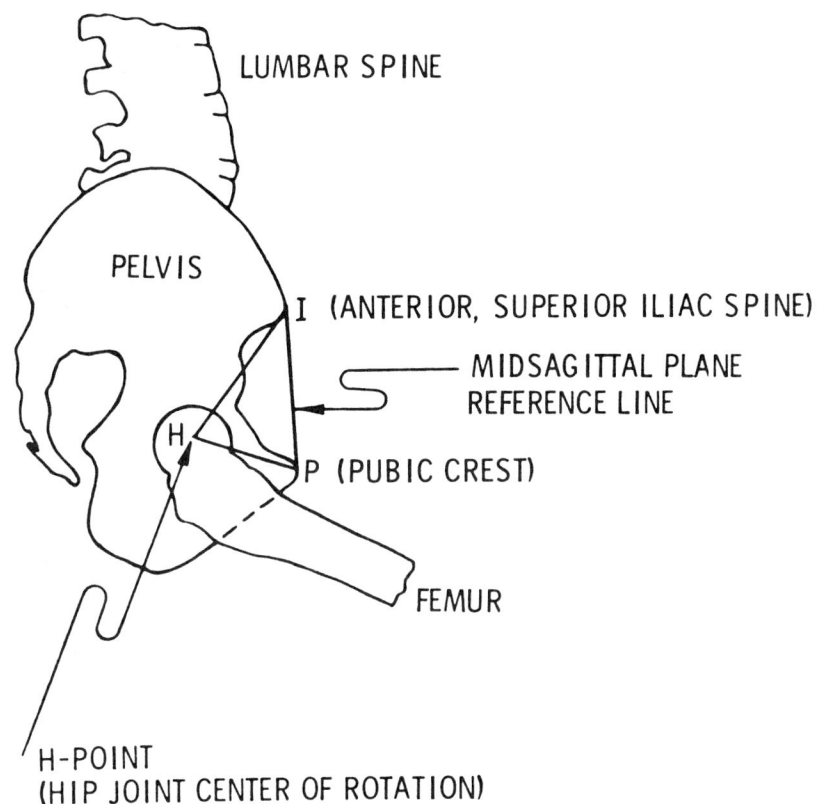

Fig. 3 - The pelvic triangle

location was required in the data reduction phase of the study to define the moments of the applied forces. H-point axis location techniques are discussed later. The intersection of the H-point axis and the midsagittal plane provided a third specific reference point for the pelvis. These three reference points are, by definition, the apexes of the pelvic triangle (Fig. 3).

PALPATION FIXTURE - Location of the pelvic reference line relative to the pelvic target assembly, utilizing palpation of the pelvic landmarks discussed above, was accomplished with the aid of a palpation fixture (Fig. 4). Whereas palpation is normally accomplished using the fingers, in this case palpation rods with hemispherical ends were utilized. The fixture had sufficient adjustability to enable the volunteer to palpate the left and right anterior, superior iliac spines, and the pubic crest, with the hemispherical ends of the three palpation rods. The palpation rods were locked in place, relative to the

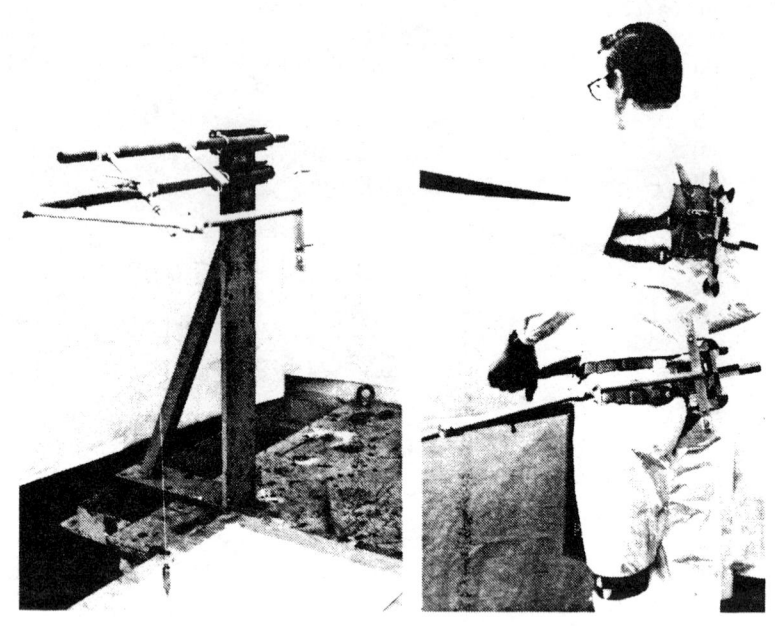

Fig. 4 - Pelvic landmark palpation fixture

fixture, when the volunteer indicated that proper palpation had been achieved.

An adjustable outrigger assembly attached to the palpation fixture enabled the position of the pelvic target assembly to be determined relative to the palpation rods. Two reference points on the outrigger assembly were positioned at two reference points on the target after the volunteer had assumed the palpated position. Upon locking the outrigger adjustments, the volunteer was carefully removed from the fixture without disturbing the fixture geometry. The target reference points and the palpated points were then located relative to one another by measuring their coordinates relative to reference axes. The volunteers were instructed to estimate flesh thicknesses at the palpated points, and the estimates were used to make corrections in the coordinates described above. These data enabled the location of two apexes of the pelvic triangle (points I and P of Fig. 3). Location of the third apex (point H in Fig. 3) is discussed next.

H-POINT LOCATION - The H-point axis was first located relative to the pelvic target bar using a graphical analysis of cinematrographic data. The technique enabled construction of the center of a quasi-circular arc generated by a point near the knee as the leg was flexed and extended relative to the pelvis. The volunteer reassumed his position in the palpation fixture for this procedure. The iliac spine palpation rods served to restrain the pelvis alignment such that the H-point axis remained parallel to, and nominally coaxial with, the optical axis of a 16 mm motion picture camera. The palpation fixture was mounted on an elevated bedplate such that the midsagittal plane of the volunteer coincided with the edge of the plate. This enabled the volunteer to stand on his right leg and swing his left leg without foot/plate interference. The leg and pelvis kinematics during full voluntary flexion and extension of the thigh were filmed, documenting the motion of a target point, tightly strapped just above the knee,* relative to the pelvic target. The film was analyzed to establish the arc, relative to the pelvis target, traced by the knee target. The arc was nearly circular; and on this basis, the center of the best circular approximation was taken to define the H-point axis.

The above procedure seemed reasonable but gave questionable results. Palpation of the greater trochanter appeared to give a more reasonable approximation. This procedure was accomplished using the previously described palpation fixture with an additional palpation rod extending from the outrigger assembly to the trochanter. Additional discussion on the H-point location problem is included under RESULTS and ANALYSIS OF RESULTS.

TEST DESCRIPTION

BENDING TEST FIXTURE - The experiment was conducted with the volunteer positioned on his side as indicated in Fig. 5. This was convenient because the test data include the moment of the applied force about the H-point axis, and in this configuration (H-point axis vertical) the force of gravity on the upper torso did not influence the moment, regardless of the state of bending of the volunteer.

The volunteer was immobilized by clamping the thighs to a rigid, vertical seatpan assembly (Fig. 5). The seatpan assembly included a padded, midsagittal support bracket between the thighs to properly align the subject and to provide some vertical support. The seatpan was sufficiently short to assure that there was no interference with the buttocks, thus enabling uninhibited articulation at the

---

* The volunteer was instructed to keep the knee in full extension (leg straight) while swinging the leg. This helped to minimize target motion, relative to the thigh, caused by flesh movement.

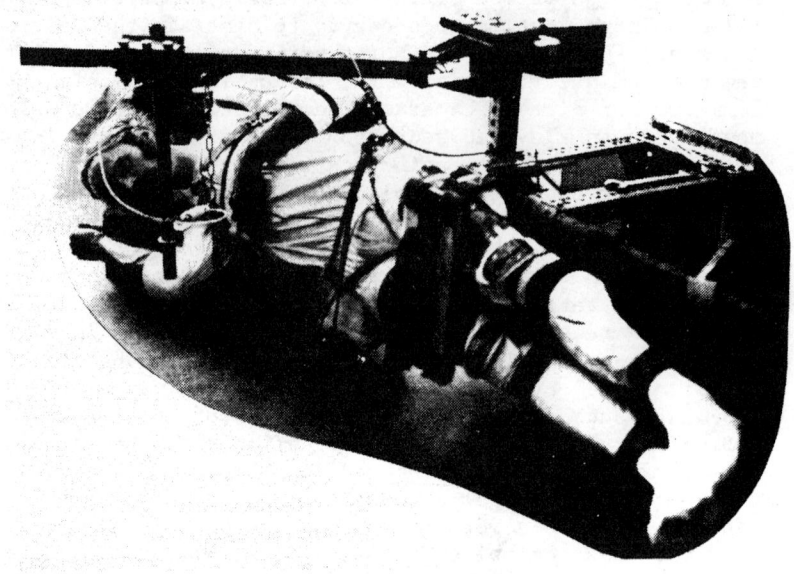

Fig. 5 - Bending test fixture with volunteer installed

hip joints. A panel hinged to the front edge of the seatpan, in conjunction with two sets of straps, provided lower leg restraint. Adjustments enabled the panel to be fixed coplanar with the seatpan (legs straight configuration) or fixed perpendicular to the seatpan [1.57 rad (90 deg) knee flexion configuration]. The seatpan assembly included provisions for a lap belt to further restrain the volunteer. The lap belt, used in some tests, limited the hip joint articulation and thereby assured that significant lumbar bending would be developed, irrespective of the pelvis/thigh stiffness.

The upper torso was supported by placing the right shoulder on a dolly that was equipped with precision casters and rolled on tempered Masonite (negligible rolling resistance). A similar, smaller dolly was placed under the pelvis of some volunteers to provide additional lower torso support, thereby affording an acceptable comfort level. The shoulders were lashed to a vertical post extending from the base of the larger dolly. This enabled a bending force to be applied to the volunteer as a somewhat distributed load because the force was applied to the dolly assembly rather than directly to the volunteer.

A lever arm assembly was provided for manually applying the bending force. The lever was located above the volunteer and had a vertical pivot axis nominally coaxial with the H-point axis. Since the bending force was to be applied to the volunteer in the midsagittal plane, and the lever arm was elevated above this plane, it was necessary to cantilever an outrigger downward from the lever arm. The outrigger was located radially outward from the lever arm pivot axis a distance nominally equal to the volunteer H-point-to-shoulder dimension. The shoulder dolly assembly was coupled to the outrigger through a force transducer located with its axis in the midsagittal plane. Clevis joints at each end of the transducer link assured that no bending moment was transmitted. The arrangement described above resulted in the application of a bending force nominally perpendicular to the thoracic spine and enabled a quantitative definition of the magnitude of the bending load--the moment of this force about the H-point axis. This moment was equal to the product of the tensile force in the transducer link by the perpendicular distance from the axis of the link to the H-point axis.

In flexion (forward bending) tests the force transducer link was coupled to the dolly assembly through a section of chain extending upward from the base of the dolly to a beam cantilevered out from the vertical post to which the shoulders were lashed (Fig. 5). This geometry enabled the force transducer link to be coupled to the dolly assembly, yet remain in the midsagittal plane, without interfering with the volunteer. In extension (rearward bending) tests the lever arm and outrigger assembly were behind the volunteer, and the force transducer link was coupled directly to the vertical post to which the shoulders were lashed.

A 1 300 N (300 lb) capacity force transducer was used to monitor the bending force. Honeywell Accudata signal conditioning equipment was utilized in conjunction with a Visicorder light beam oscillograph to record the force as a function of time. A Fastair 16 mm high-speed camera was mounted overhead to photograph the test event. The camera framing rate was nominally 100 pictures/sec--considerably higher than necessary to document a quasi-static test. The time bases of the film and the oscillograph record were synchronized by means of a light bulb flashing in the field of view of the camera. An oscillograph galvanometer was driven by a photoelectric cell adjacent to the bulb so that a trace deflection occurred simultaneously with the lighting of the bulb.

TEST PROTOCOL - The lower torso bending response of each volunteer was evaluated under twelve different test conditions. A test parameter matrix defining the

Table 2 - Test Matrix Description

Test Designation	Bending Direction Forward (Flexion)	Bending Direction Rearward (Extension)	Knee Angle Legs Straight	Knee Angle Right Angle	Muscle Tone Relaxed	Muscle Tone Tensed	Lap Belt No	Lap Belt Yes
A	x		x		x		x	
B		x	x		x		x	
C	x		x		x			x
D	x		x			x	x	
E		x	x			x	x	
F	x		x			x		x
G	x			x	x		x	
H		x		x	x		x	
I	x			x	x			x
J	x			x		x	x	
K		x		x		x	x	
L	x			x		x		x

* The symbol x implies the subject condition is in force.

experimental conditions is presented in Table 2. The experiments were designed to provide insights into several aspects of the lower torso bending response. Anatomical considerations lead one to expect that the response in forward bending (flexion) will differ from that in rearward bending (extension); therefore, it is pertinent to evaluate both conditions. Likewise, it is easily demonstrated that one can attain a greater degree of flexion if the legs are bent at the knees than if the legs are straight. Knee angle, therefore, is also a pertinent parameter to investigate. Accordingly, the tests were conducted with the legs straight and with the legs bent nominally 1.57 rad (90 deg) at the knee. One can tense his muscles and resist bending to a significant degree. A quantitative evaluation of this phenomenon was pursued by conducting each test with muscles relaxed and with muscles tensed. Each of the flexion experiments was conducted with and without a lap belt. The rationale was that if lower torso bending tended to occur primarily as a result of hip joint articulation, the lumbar region would perhaps never be forced far into flexion unless the pelvis was restrained in some manner from rotating relative to the thighs.

The initial position of the volunteers in all tests was determined by placing the thoracic spine axis approximately perpendicular to the seatpan (there was no effort to maintain close control of this variable). Upon completing a checklist, to insure the instrumentation was in proper order, the volunteer was informed of the test conditions, and the test followed immediately. The oscillograph/film synchronization light commenced flashing approximately two seconds after the oscillograph paper drive and high speed camera were actuated. The sound of the camera motor was the indicator used by the volunteer to sense that the bending force was to be applied. Bending commenced upon sight of the first light flash, at which time an operator manually began to push the lever arm assembly (described in the previous section of the paper) through its range of travel. In relaxed muscle tests the volunteer was instructed to simply follow passively and let his torso bend, whereas in tensed muscle tests he was instructed to strenuously resist the bending force and attempt to retain his initial configuration. The test proceeded until there was a command from the volunteer that he did not wish to tolerate further bending, which was defined as his utterance of any sound (it was difficult to actually speak while the muscles were tensed). Upon command, further bending stopped and the lever arm was backed-off somewhat to release the load.

The test durations were approximately 10 s. The tensed muscle tests proved to be tiring, both for the volunteer and the lever arm operator. However, since relaxed and tensed tests were run alternately, and there was a pause between tests to check instrumentation and change test conditions, both parties appeared to have had sufficient time to recover. At all times during the test sequence the welfare of the volunteer was the first priority, and he was questioned regularly regarding his condition. The team was prepared to quickly remove the volunteer from the fixture and strip-off the tightly-strapped target assemblies if the volunteer showed signs of distress.

RESULTS

The palpation fixture data and the cinematographic H-point location data were reduced to provide the pelvic triangle information of Fig. 6. The data reduction also defined the location and orientation of the pelvic target bar relative to the pelvic triangle. Accordingly, the orientation of the midsagittal plane reference line, relative to the pelvic target bar axis, became known. This enabled bending angles to be defined as illustrated in Fig. 7. The thoracic target assembly had been installed with its target bar axis nominally parallel to a tangent line at T8. X-ray radiograms of a cadaver leg strapped

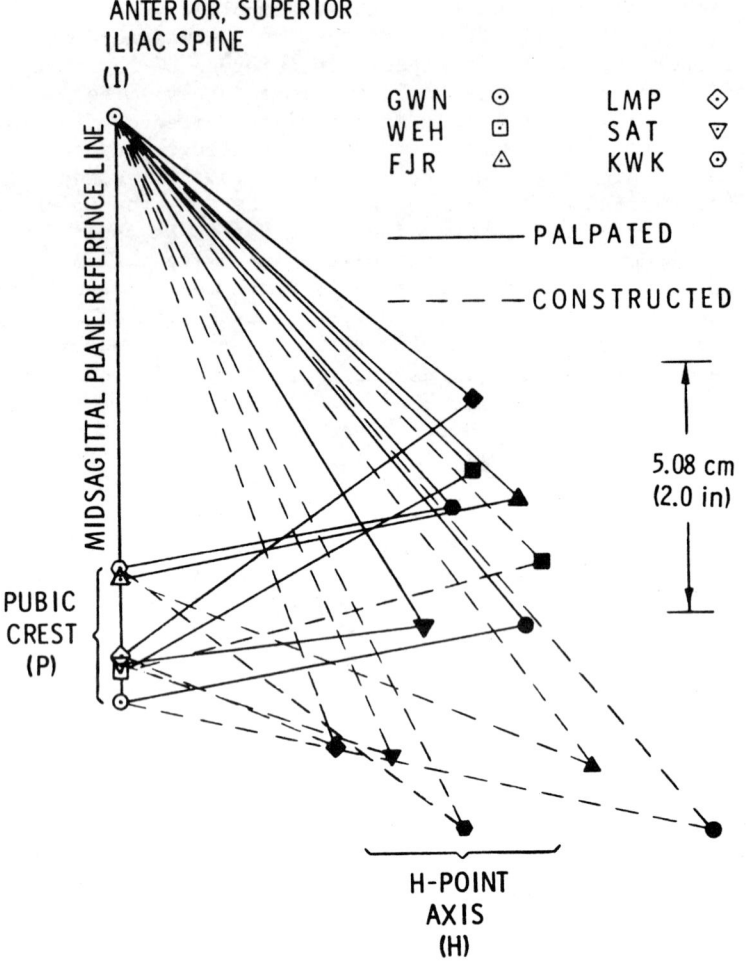

Fig. 6 - Volunteer pelvic triangles

into the test fixture indicated that it is a good assumption to consider the femur link axis to be parallel to the plane of the rigid seatpan assembly (which was well defined in the films of the test events). These conditions enabled analyses of the films, which led to the data points in Figs. 8-23. The loading corridors of these figures are discussed in the ANALYSIS OF RESULTS.

At each flash of the film/oscillograph synchronization light, the thorax-pelvis and pelvis-femur angles (Fig. 7) and perpendicular distance from the bending force line-of-action to the H-point axis were determined. The moment of the applied force about the H-point axis was defined

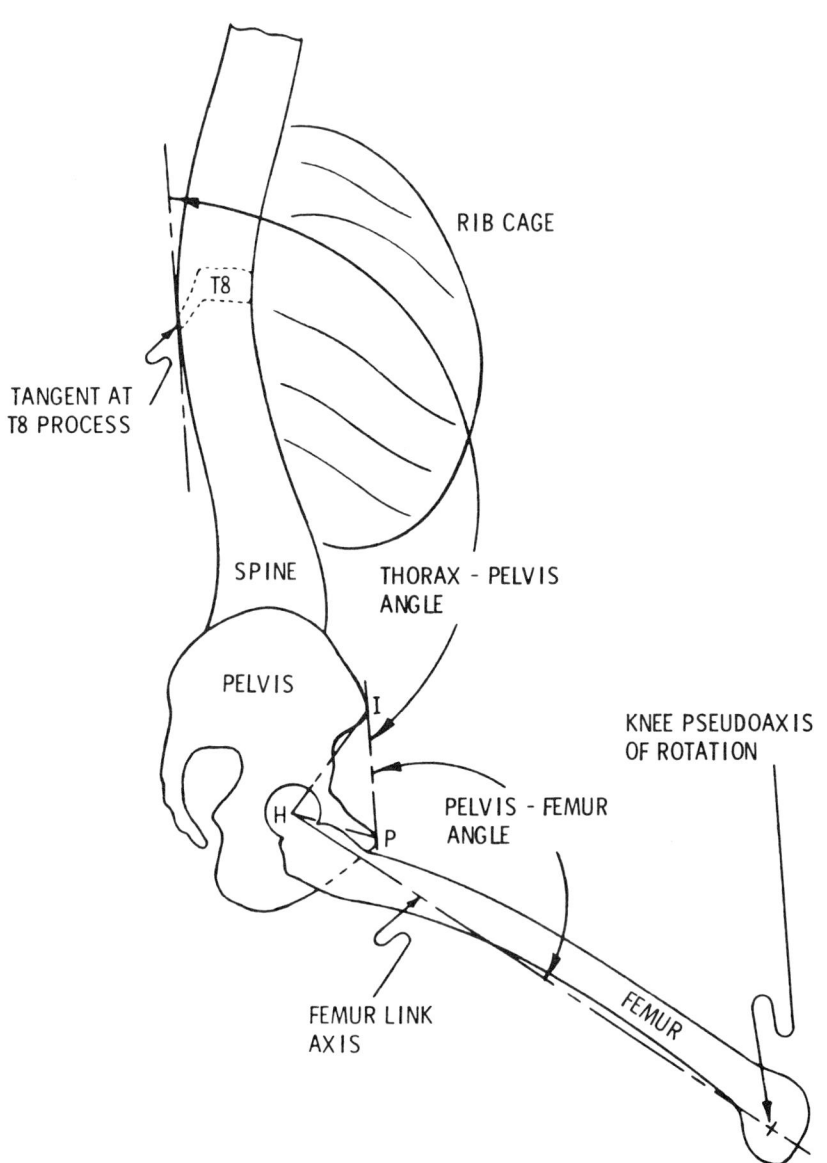

Fig. 7 - Definition of bending angles

at each step as the product of this lever arm distance by the force* scaled from the oscillograph record.

The thorax-pelvis response data are plotted in Figs. 8-15, and the pelvis-femur data are plotted in Figs. 16-23. In Figs. 8-11 the data sets for experiments A and C, D and F, G and I, and J and L have been paired and plotted--each pair on one figure.** The rationale is that the test conditions within each group were identical, except that one test included a lap belt, and the other did not. The lap belt was included only to insure that significant lumbar bending would occur, regardless of the degree of hip joint articulation. The bending moment distribution in the lumbar region was not affected by the presence of the belt; accordingly, the belted and unbelted data may be pooled.

Pooling of the pelvis-femur response data in the manner described above is not allowable because the actual moment at the H-point axis does depend on whether or not a lap belt is present. Accordingly, only the unbelted test data are used to define pelvis-femur responses in Figs. 16-19.

In utilizing the results of this study it is important to realize that the thorax-pelvis angle data are measured using a film target attached at the level of the eighth thoracic vertebra. The ranges of thorax-pelvis articulation indicated by the data, therefore, include the articulation of part of the thoracic spine (T8 through T12).

ANALYSIS OF RESULTS

Further comments are pertinent with regard to the volunteer pelvic triangle drawings of Fig. 6 and the moment-angle bending response data of Figs. 8-23.

PELVIC TRIANGLE DISCUSSION - It was noted earlier, in the H-Point Location discussion, that the cinematographic technique employed to locate the H-point axis gave questionable results. These results are plotted in Fig. 6 as the "constructed" legs of the pelvic triangles (dashed lines). In contrast, the solid-line triangles represent the results based on palpation of the greater trochanter. Note that the constructed points consistently fall below (inferior to) the palpated points. Also, note the skewed shape of the constructed triangles as compared with their

---

* The rolling resistance of the shoulder support dolly was sufficiently small to be neglected in this analysis.
** In the figures, the data points for belted tests are plotted with a plus sign (+) in the symbol to distinguish them from the unbelted data points.

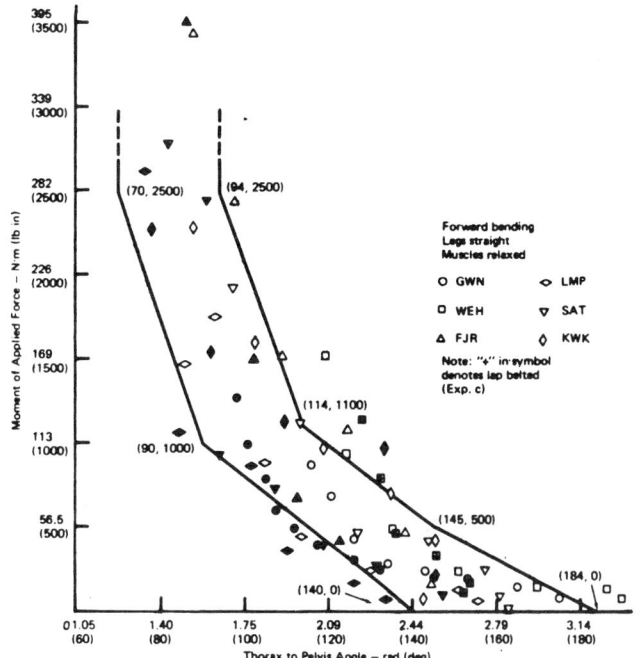

Fig. 8 - Thorax-pelvis response for experiments A and C

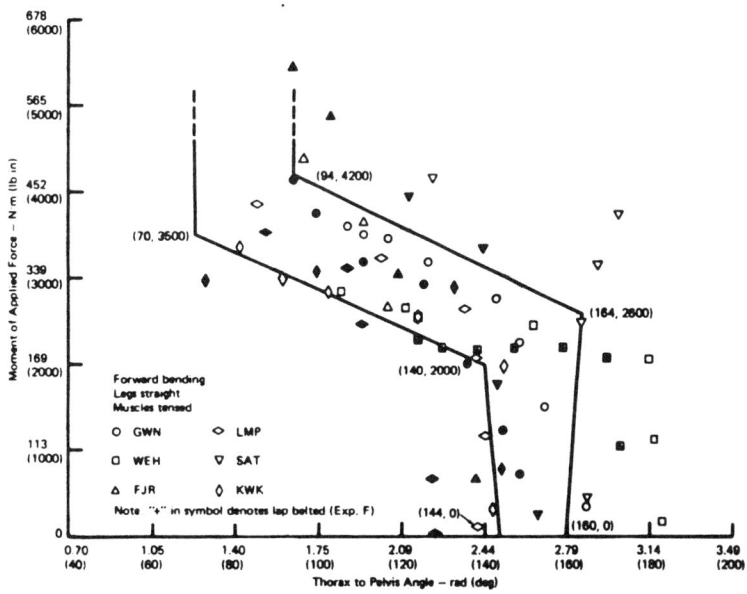

Fig. 9 - Thorax-pelvis response for experiments D and F

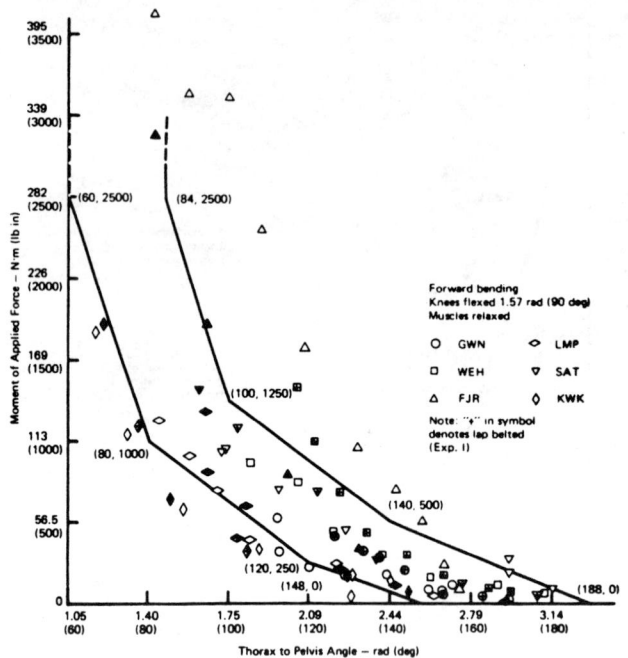

Fig. 10 - Thorax-pelvis response for experiments G and I

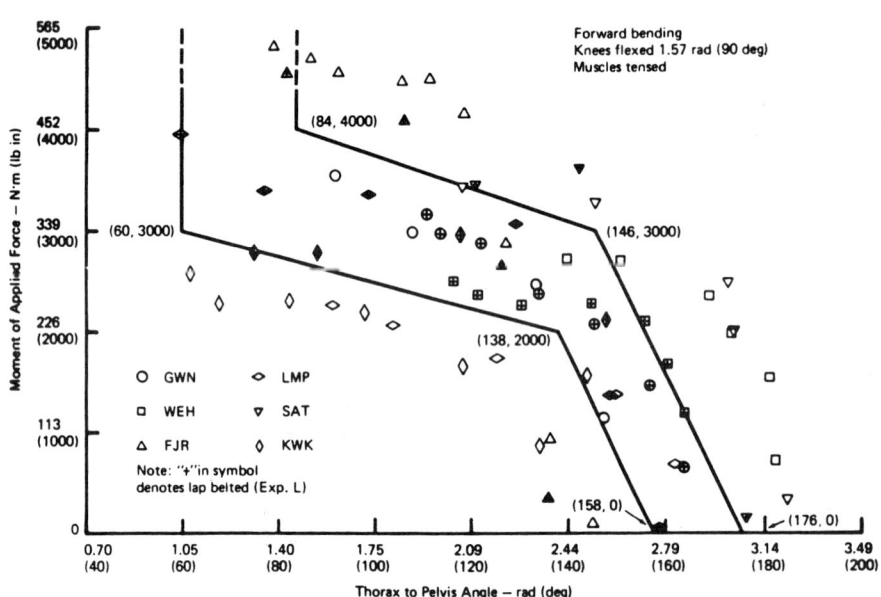

Fig. 11 - Thorax-pelvis response for experiments J and L

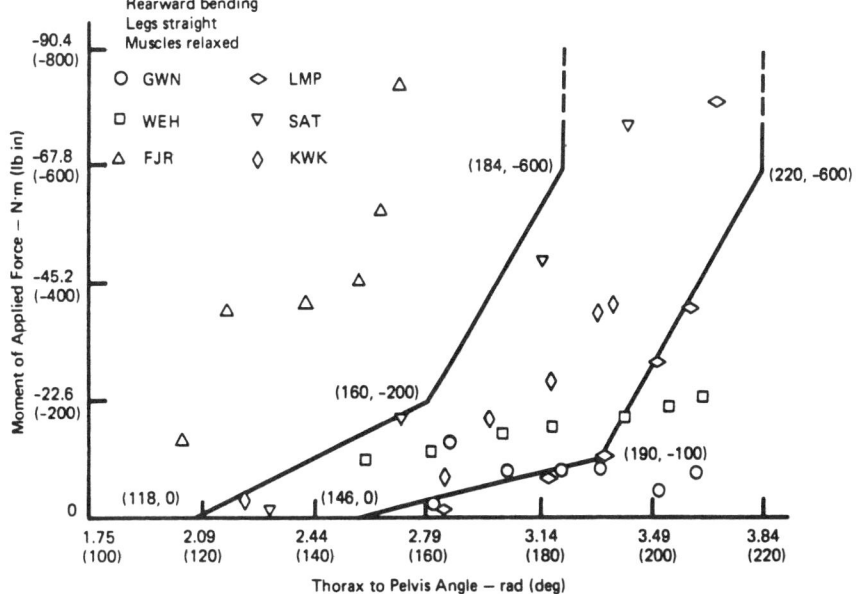

Fig. 12 - Thorax-pelvis response for experiment B

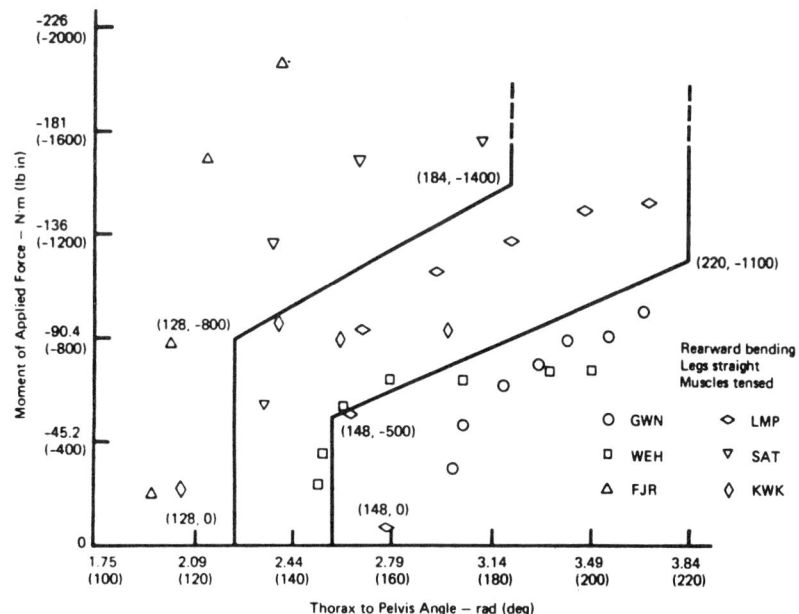

Fig. 13 - Thorax-pelvis response for experiment E

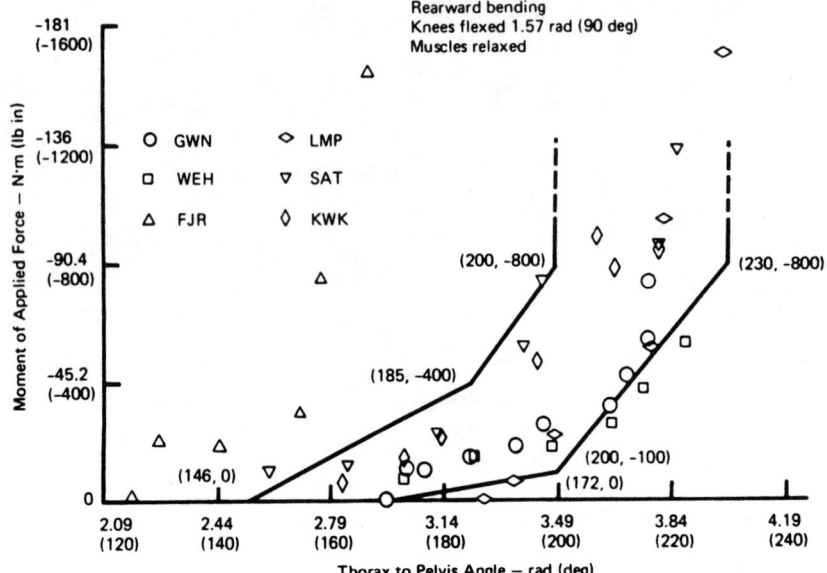

Fig. 14 - Thorax-pelvis response for experiment H

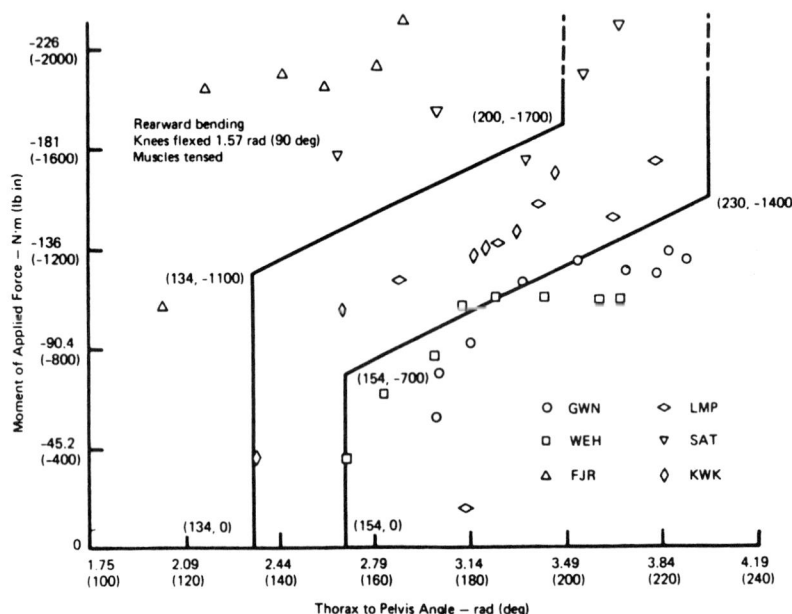

Fig. 15 - Thorax-pelvis response for experiment K

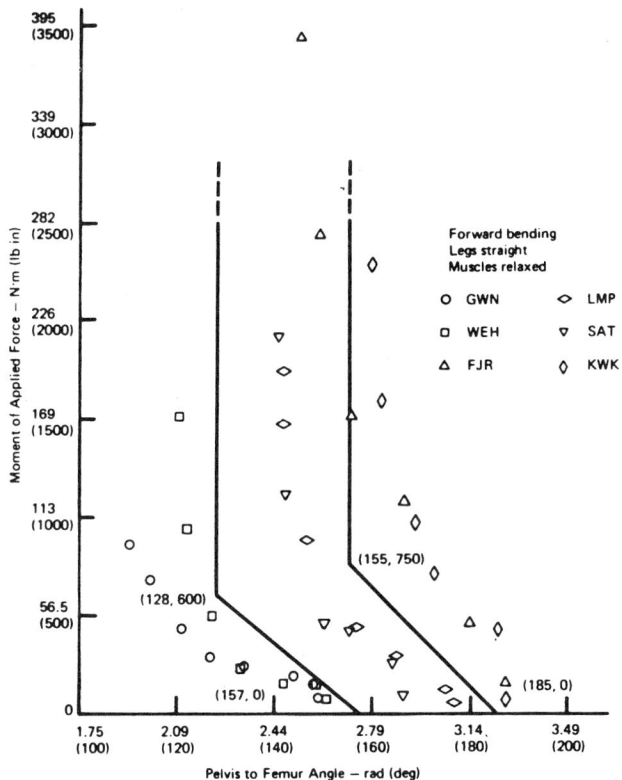

Fig. 16 - Pelvis-femur response for experiment A

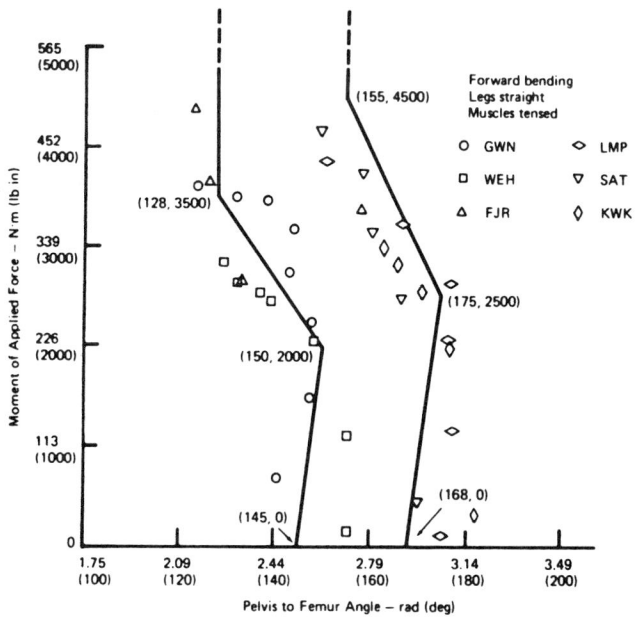

Fig. 17 - Pelvis-femur response for experiment D

183

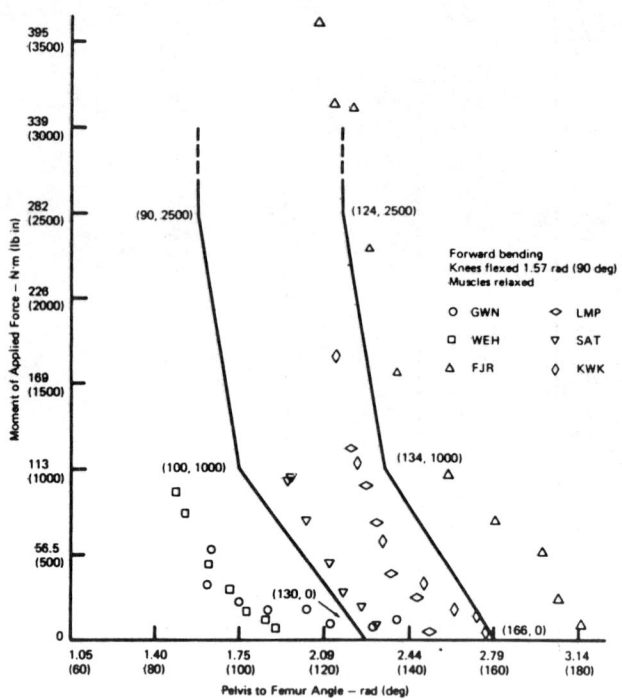

Fig. 18 - Pelvis-femur response for experiment G

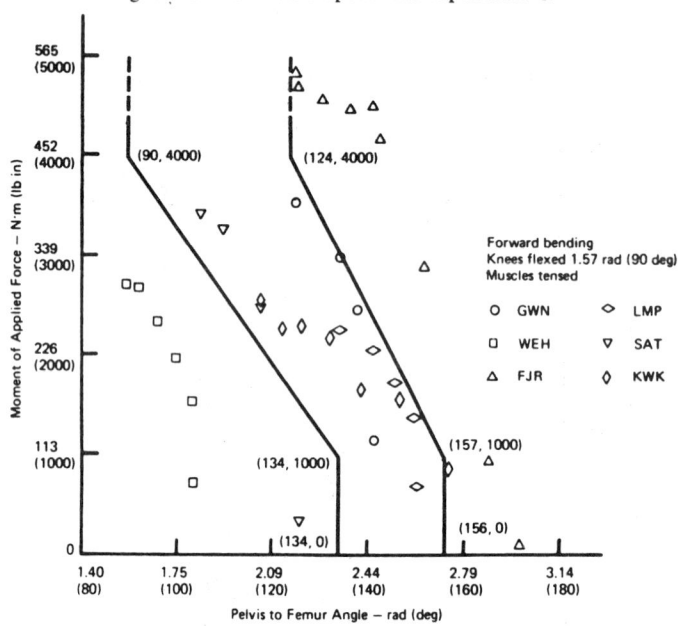

Fig. 19 - Pelvis-femur response for experiment J

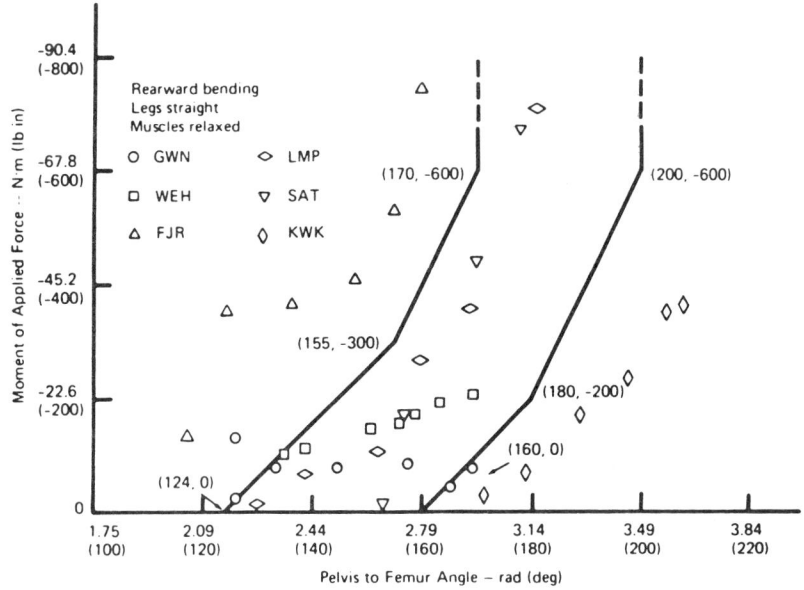

Fig. 20 - Pelvis-femur response for experiment B

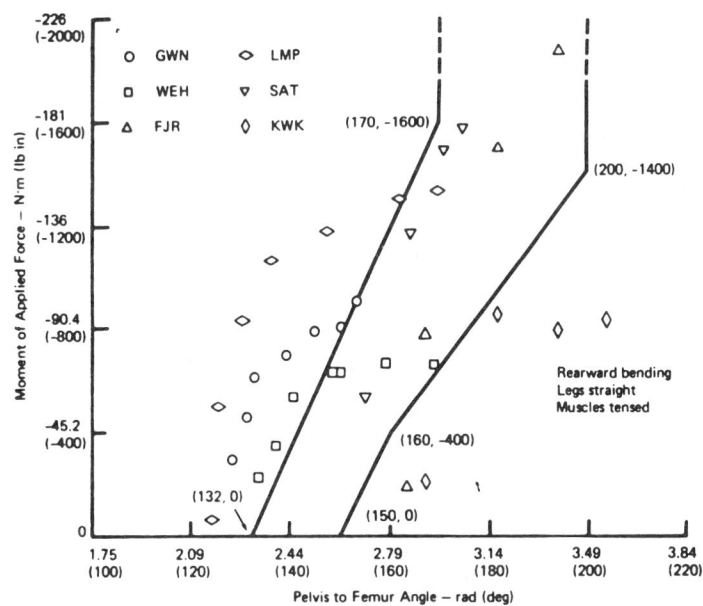

Fig. 21 - Pelvis-femur response for experiment E

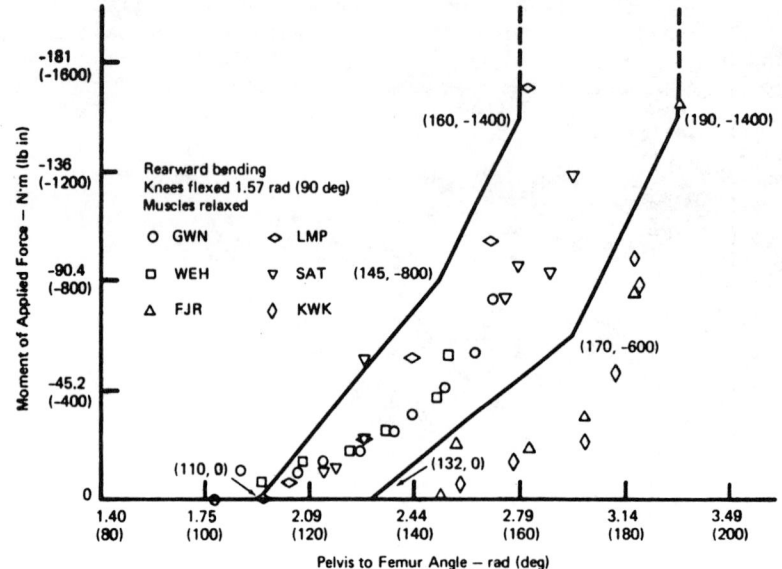

Fig. 22 - Pelvis-femur response for experiment H

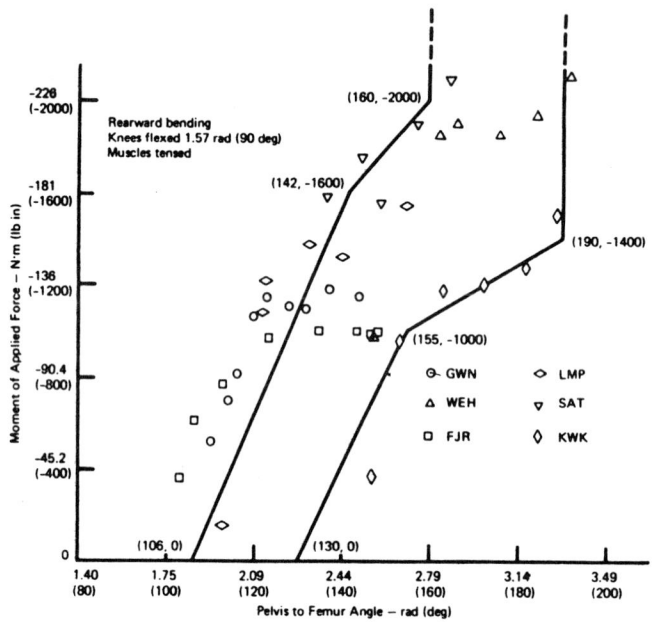

Fig. 23 - Pelvis-femur response for experiment K

palpated counterparts, which tend toward an equilateral configuration. Analyses of X-ray radiograms of cadaver pelves, an excised pelvis, and anatomy charts and drawings all indicate that the quasi-equilateral geometry is correct. To be more specific, it appears that a straight line erected through apex H of the triangle, perpendicular to the mid-sagittal plane reference line $\overline{IP}$, must always pass between points I and P on the adult male human pelvis. Accordingly, it is concluded that the palpated data of Fig. 6 are the better of the two approximations.

LOADING CORRIDORS - The loading corridors are plotted in Figs. 8-23. The intent of these corridors is not to define an envelope of the family of responses of the six volunteers, but rather to provide biomechanically sound criteria for defining the response of a 50th percentile adult male anthropomorphic dummy. The statistics of Table 1 indicate that the heights and weights of the volunteers produce HEW percentile numbers ranging from 19 to 98. Accordingly, one must expect a significant spread in the response data. However, the mean height and mean weight of the sample each approximate the HEW 50th percentile data; and on this basis the mean response may be considered appropriate for a 50th percentile dummy. The boundaries of the loading corridors "tend toward" a representation of mean response plus and minus one-half a standard deviation. Thus, a dummy providing smooth response curves, hugging the centers of the corridors, would be judged to have optimum performance with respect to the requirements suggested herein.

The loading corridors were constructed using straight line segments with the endpoint coordinates labeled, thereby enabling accurate reproduction by future users.

The corridors are open-ended at the top. When a subject "bottoms-out" at the ends of the ranges of articulation, the moment will continue to increase, but there will be little change in the angle. Accordingly, a proper interpretation of the open-ended corridor is that it extends upward indefinitely. If, in the course of usage of an anthropomorphic dummy, very large moments are applied, the angle should remain within the specified limits. The human, of course, has an injury tolerance moment value which when exceeded would result in injury and further articulation. These tolerances have not been defined.

It was noted in the TEST PROTOCOL section that there was no effort to maintain close control over the initial position of the volunteers. That is, among tests, there was some variation in the initial (zero moment) thorax-pelvis and pelvis-femur angles. This variation led to significant scatter in the tensed muscle tests because one can "lock-up" and resist the applied bending force to nominally the same degree, regardless of the initial angles involved. This phenomenon was accounted for in developing the tensed muscle corridors by computing the mean angle at zero moment, for the six volunteers, and adding a correction factor to the angles so that each volunteer's response curve initiated at a common point. The plotted data points do not reflect this correction factor; accordingly, the angular spreads appear quite large compared to the corridor widths in some of Figs. 8-23.

Definition of the limits of articulation is important information for use in dummy development. It was important, therefore, to define the upper, open-ended portions of the loading corridors. The "bottom-out" angles were most apparent in the relaxed tests and were defined from these data. This portion of the relaxed corridor was then incorporated into the tensed corridor counterpart as well.

Since the tensed muscle corridor shapes are a function of the particular initial angle configuration of the volunteers, it may not be appropriate to require a surrogate of the tensed vehicle occupant to conform to these specific requirements. The angles of the seated configuration are likely not equivalent to the zero-moment angles of the corridors. The corridors cannot simply be translated (shifted) along the angle axis because the upper "bottom-out" portion must be assumed invariant. It appears reasonable, instead, to adjust the bottom (zero-moment portion) of the corridors as necessary, and to redefine the intermediate corridor points using linear interpolation to define the angle shifts.

Some comments with regard to the criteria used in defining the loading corridors are pertinent. Statistical analyses utilized in evaluating trends in the response data included computer curve fitting programs defining least-squares regressions of moment on angle and of angle on moment. Also, means and standard deviations of moment data in finite angle increments and of angle data in finite moment increments were computed. In addition, some subjective decisions, based on studies of trends indicated by the responses of the individual volunteers, were necessary. Whereas the quantitative techniques offer rigorous, well-defined criteria for fitting the data points, they are not discriminating with regard to maintaining the unique features common among the individual volunteers' responses. This is where the subjective analyses became important. The bottom (zero-moment) portion of each corridor was established using linear extrapolation of the data on each volunteer to define angles at zero moment. The corridor width at the bottom is nominally the mean value plus and minus one-half a standard deviation.

Although most of the loading corridors are easily recognized to follow the data trends closely, some are not. It was felt, however, that corridors were necessary for each data set to enhance the usefulness of the data and to provide a unified basis for application of the results to dummy design problems, mathematical modeling, and/or further discussion.

One may note that at zero-moment the corridor boundaries for relaxed forward and rearward bending, under otherwise identical conditions, are not equivalent. Although the corridors overlap, there is a discontinuity. Since there is no justification for shifting the relaxed corridors, as explained for tensed corridors, it appears that there is a discrepancy in the data. It is postulated that the discrepancy is a result of shortcomings of the linear extrapolation procedure utilized in computing the mean angle at zero moment. In actuality, the moment-angle relationship is perhaps highly nonlinear near zero moment. The resolution of the data is insufficient to evaluate this situation with reasonable confidence; therefore, the corridors were not redefined to eliminate the zero-moment discontinuity. It is suggested, in using a forward-rearward pair of relaxed corridors in connection with dummy development, that the response be allowed to fall outside either one, but not both, of the two corridors for the first 310 N·m (200 lb in) of moment.

It was noted in the RESULTS that the thorax-pelvis data include the articulation of part of the thoracic spine (T8 through T12) in addition to lumbar articulation. Since a practical scheme for isolating only the lumbar articulation on a volunteer is not obvious, there was little choice in the matter. However, since current dummies, and probably the next several generations of dummies, utilize rigid thoracic spines, it is reasonable to add some of the thoracic articulation range to that of the lumbar region. It appears, therefore, that the thorax-pelvis corridors, without modifications, may be used to define response requirements for the dummy lumbar region.

Analyses of the loading corridors indicate that the thorax-pelvis and pelvis-femur articulations are influenced by the degree of knee flexion. One can evaluate the influence by observing midrange angles of the upper, bottomed-out portion of the response corridors of Figs. 8 through 23. From Figs. 8 and 12 it is evidenced that the thorax-pelvis range of articulation with legs straight covers angles from 1.44 rad (82°) to 3.53 rad (202°), whereas with the knees flexed 1.57 rad (90°), Figs. 10 and 14 indicate a range from 1.26 rad (72°) to 3.76 rad (215°). Thus, flexing the knees from the legs-straight configuration to the right-angle configuration increases the full extension-to-full flexion thorax-pelvis range of motion from 2.09 rad to 2.50 rad (120° to 143°) and enables greater degrees of flexion and extension. Similarly, from Figs. 16 and 20 it is evident that the pelvis-femur range of articulation with legs straight covers angles from 2.46 rad (141°) to 3.23 rad (185°), whereas with the knees flexed 1.57 rad (90°), Figs. 18 and 22 indicate a range from 1.86 rad (107°) to 3.05 rad (175°). Thus, flexing the knees from the legs-straight configuration to the right-angle configuration increases the full extension-to-full flexion pelvis-femur range of motion from 0.77 rad to 0.19 rad (44° to 68°) and enables a greater degree of flexion and a reduced degree of extension.

A scan of individual plotted data points in Figs. 8 through 23 indicates that the maximum moment of applied force tolerated in flexion was 616 N·m (5450 lb in). The maximum in extension was 240 N·m (2120 lb in). In each case these data refer to Volunteer FJR. The maximum flexion moment occurred in a legs-straight test (Fig. 9), whereas the maximum extension moment occurred in a test with the knees flexed 1.57 rad (90°) (Fig. 15).

CONCLUSIONS

The following conclusions may be drawn from this study:

1. The relaxed and tensed lower torso bending responses are significantly different from one another. The basic shapes of the loading corridors are not the same.

2. Flexing the knees from the legs-straight configuration to the right-angle configuration increases the full extension-to-full flexion thorax-pelvis range of motion from 2.09 rad to 2.50 rad (120 deg to 143 deg). The right-angle configuration affords both a greater degree of flexion and a greater degree of extension.*

3. Flexing the knees from the legs-straight configuration to the right-angle configuration increases the full extension-to-full flexion pelvis-femur range of motion from 0.77 rad to 1.19 rad (44 deg to 68 deg). The right-angle configuration affords a greater degree of flexion; however, the degree of extension is reduced.*

---

* These conclusions are based on the midrange angles of the upper, bottomed-out portion of the response corridors of Figs. 8-23.

4. The maximum moment of applied force tolerated by a volunteer in flexion was 616 N·m (5450 lb in). The maximum extension was 240 N·m (2120 lb in).

RECOMMENDATIONS

Recommendations based on this research program are as follows:

1. The loading corridors suggested herein should be considered preliminary guidelines for 50th percentile adult male anthropomorphic dummy performance for interim use until dynamic response data become available.

2. A decision should be made with regard to dummy design philosophy. Should the dummy respond as a relaxed or as a tensed human, or perhaps in accordance with some intermediate criteria? If an intermediate criterion is adopted, new loading corridors should be constructed using those defined herein as guidelines.

3. Dynamic experiments should be pursued to establish the significance of rate-dependent effects.

4. Static and dynamic experiments should be pursued to define the lower torso bending responses in the lateral direction and in oblique directions.

5. Torso torsion and shear biomechanical response requirements should be developed to complement the bending response definitions.

6. The lower torso bending responses of current dummy structures should be evaluated with respect to the performance requirements suggested herein.

ACKNOWLEDGMENT

The experimental data were generated at the Biomechanics Research Center of Wayne State University. Gratitude is expressed to L. M. Patrick and the Biomechanics personnel for their help in conducting the tests and volunteering as test subjects. Special thanks are extended to Mr. Roger Culver for his contribution.

REFERENCES

1. "Motor Vehicle Safety Regulation No. 572 Test Dummy Specifications." Federal Register, 38FR20449-56, August 1, 1973.

2. "Motor Vehicle Safety Standard No. 208 Occupant Crash Protection--Passenger Cars, Multipurpose Vehicles, Trucks, and Buses." Federal Register, 35FR1513, January 10, 1974.

3. "Weight, Height, and Selected Body Dimensions of Adults." Public Health Service Publication No. 1000, Series 11, No. 8, U.S. Department of Health, Education, and Welfare, Washington, D.C., 1965.

760821

Lumbar and Pelvic Orientations of the Vehicle Seated Volunteer

Gerald W. Nyquist
General Motors Corporation

Lawrence M. Patrick
Wayne State University

Abstract

   An X-ray radiographic study of two volunteers in a vehicle seated configuration was performed to gain insights into the lower torso skeletal geometry associted with this posture. A pseudo three-dimensional analysis of each radiogram was utilized to obtain quantitative results. The analyses provided indications of the pelvis and femur relative and absolute orientations. Further, the geometry of the lumbar spine and its location relative to the pelvis were defined. The relevance of the data from the standpoint of anthropomorphic dummy design is discussed, and recommendations are offered for further studies of vehicle seat/vehicle occupant interfacing biomechanics. Anthropometric data on each volunteer are included.

QUANTITATIVE DESCRIPTIONS of the human lower torso skeletal configurations for typical automotive seated postures have not been available. Accordingly, there has not been a suitable biomechanical basis for defining this portion of an anthropomorphic dummy design. The pelvic orientation of the vehicle seated dummy may be significantly different from that of the human. This would adversely affect the biomechanical fidelity of the dummy's performance. The initial orientation of the pelvis, and the manner in which it is coupled to the upper torso and femurs are obviously important parameters governing lap belt/pelvis interaction. This paper describes a study performed to gain some insights into the problem.

Two adult male volunteers served as test subjects. X-ray radiography was utilized to study their lumbar spine, pelvis, and femur configurations while in the seated posture. Whereas X-ray radiography appeared to be the technique offering the most complete documentation of the lower torso skeletal geometry, there were some problems associated with adapting clinical diagnostic procedures to this study. First, with the subject positioned in a soft seat, it was not possible to juxtapose the film cassette and the lower torso properly because of seat cushion interference. Second, it was not possible to X-ray the volunteer while seated in a complete veicle. It was necessary to obtain a representative seat, mount it properly, and attempt to position the volunteer as though he were in a complete vehicle.

The X-ray cassette/volunteer juxtaposition problem was solved by making a thin plaster cast of the volunteer/seat interface and constructing a narrow, wooden seat of proper contour to support the volunteer during the X-ray series. The narrow seat enabled the cassette to be located adjacent to the pelvis. Further descriptions and procedural details follow.

VOLUNTEER SELECTION

The test subjects consisted of two adult male volunteers. Volunteer LMP was near 50 years of age, and Volunteer CJM was near 60 years of age. Some anthropometric dimensions of the volunteers are summarized in Table I. Figure 1 defines the measurements. Volunteer LMP's stature and body mass approximate those of the USA 50th percentile adult male. Volunteer CJM is larger.

Table I-Volunteer Anthropometry

	VOLUNTEER			
	LMP *		CJM **	
MEASUREMENT	cm	in	cm	in
Erect Standing Height	173.2	68.2	180.2	70.9
Erect Seated Height	89.4	35.2	96.1	37.8
Seated Eye Height	78.8	31.0	83.2	32.8
Seat Height or Popliteal Height	45.1	17.8	45.9	18.1
Knee Height	53.9	21.2	65.9	25.9
Upper Leg Length or Buttock-Knee Length	59.9	23.6	59.1	23.3
Seat Length or Buttock-Popliteal Length	49.6	19.5	48.5	19.1
Seat Wdith or Seat Breadth	41.6	16.4	41.7	16.4
Shoulder Width	49.7	19.6	46.9	18.5
Upper Arm Length	37.6	14.8	39.8	15.7
Lower Arm Length	47.9	18.9	50.5	19.9

* Mass (weight) partially clothed: 363.4 kg (165 lb) = 48 percentile
**Mass (weight) partially clothed: 378.9 kg (172 lb) = 59 percentile

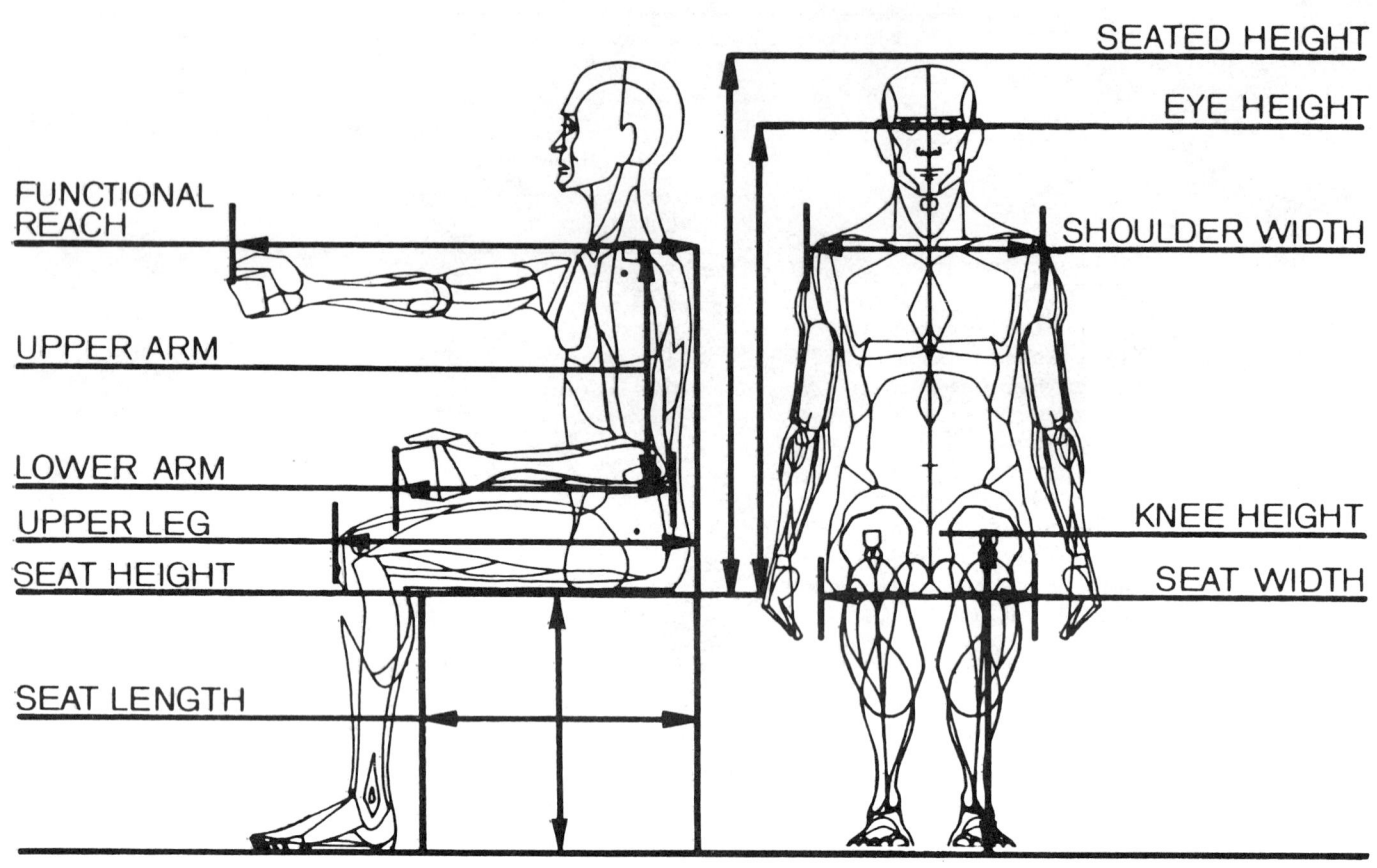

Fig. 1 - Anthropometric measurements

VEHICLE SEAT DESCRIPTION

The typical vehicle seat selected for this program was a 1971 Oldsmobile Delta bench seat*. Measurements were taken on a complete vehicle to enable proper orientation of the remotely mounted seat. In addition, a foot support block was utilized to simulate the vehicle floorpan, thereby enabling proper (vehicle-like) support for the feet. The seat was vinyl-trimmed.

The above description of the seat documents its design sufficiently to enable the procurement of design data from Fisher Body; however, there are significant variations in the characteristics of individual seats of the same design due to manufacturing tolerances. Accordingly, the specific seat utilized in this study was further evaluated following the procedure specified in SAE Standard J826a (1)** wherein a three-dimensional H-point machine (Fig. 2) is utilized to define an H-point*** location and seatback angle**** for the particular test seat. Whereas the seating drawings indicate a 0.445 rad (25.5 deg) seatback angle, the actual angle for the seat of this study was 0.358 rad (20.5 deg). Likewise, there was an H-point location discrepancy. The actual H-point location for this seat was 1.63 cm (0.64 in) above and 0.20 cm (0.08 in) aft of the design location.

In spite of the above discrepancies, the seat of this study was not judged to be atypical. Subjectively, it looked normal and felt normal.

---

*   Although this paper bears a 1976 date, the study was performed in late 1972. Accordingly, at that time, the 1971 seat design was not outdated. Further, current seats do not appear to differ significantly from the 1971 design.

**   Numbers in parentheses designate references at end of paper.

*** The H-point axis is a straight line connecting the left and right hip centers of rotation. From the left or right side it appears as a point--the H-point. The H-point is defined on the three-dimensional H-point machine. Part 571 Federal Motor Vehicle Safety Standards refer to the location of the H-Point, relative to the seat, as the "seating reference point."

****The seatback angle is, by definition, an angle measured on the H-point machine. This angle represents the angle, relative to the vertical, of a tangent line to the "small of the back" (loins).

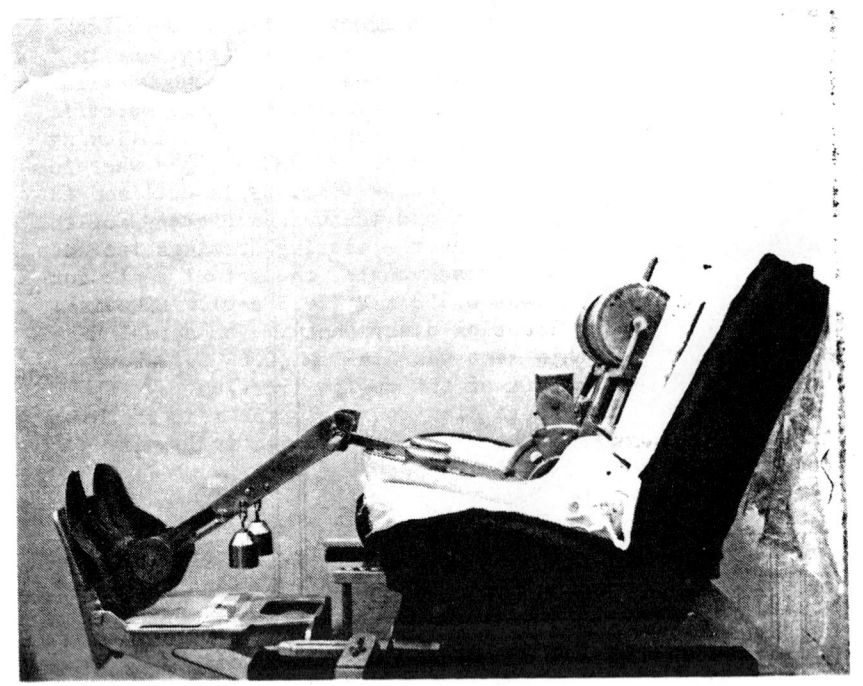

Fig. 2 - H-point machine installed on soft seat

SOFT-SEAT CONTOUR OF THE VOLUNTEER

Documentation of the contour of the interface of each volunteer with the soft seat was accomplished as illustrated in Fig. 3. A thin sheet (approximately 5 mm (0.2 in) thick) of plaster bandage of sufficient size to cover the interface was prepared and sandwiched between plastic sheeting. This preparation was positioned on the seat, after which the volunteer sat down and remained motionless during the curing cycle of the plaster. Careful removal of the volunteer 10 to 15 minutes later, followed by careful removal of the preparation from the seat, resulted in a thin casting documenting the interface contour (Fig. 4). The interface castings were used to prepare custom wooden X-ray seats (described in the next section of the report).

Defining a criterion for positioning the volunteer on the soft seat posed somewhat of a problem. Arbitrarily specifying and following some seating procedure would perhaps lead to a repeatable result, but it would not necessarily lead to a realistic result. On the other hand, it is also plausible that a given volunteer could assume many different postures in the same seat, since posture undoubtedly depends to some degree on the volunteer's kinematics during the seating process. For this X-ray study of only two volunteers, without test replications, it was not feasible to define and control the many pertinent seating parameters; therefore, the subjects were simply instructed to sit down in the driver location and "pretend that they were driving." A marker on the wall in front of the subject, at eye height, was provided to represent a typical object upon which a driver's eyes might fixate. The resulting postures are those shown in Fig. 3. (The arm was raised only momentarily to provide a better view of the torso.) It is obvious that the two volunteers assumed similar, but not the same, postures. The most significant difference appears to be that CJM had his legs drawn up closer to the torso than did LMP.

X-RAY SEAT PREPARATION

The volunteer/soft seat interface castings were sectioned as illustrated in Fig. 5 to obtain profile information for fabrication of wooden X-ray seats. The locations of the left and right thighs and the spine were clear from indentations left in the castings and served to define lines along which saw cuts were made. Poster board inserts through the saw cuts defined the midsagittal plane and left and right sagittal planes through the thighs. The poster board/contour casting intersection lines were traced onto the poster board for further analyses.

To facilitate straight-forward fabrication of the wooden seats, it was desirable to approximate the volunteer/soft seat interface by defining one representative profile

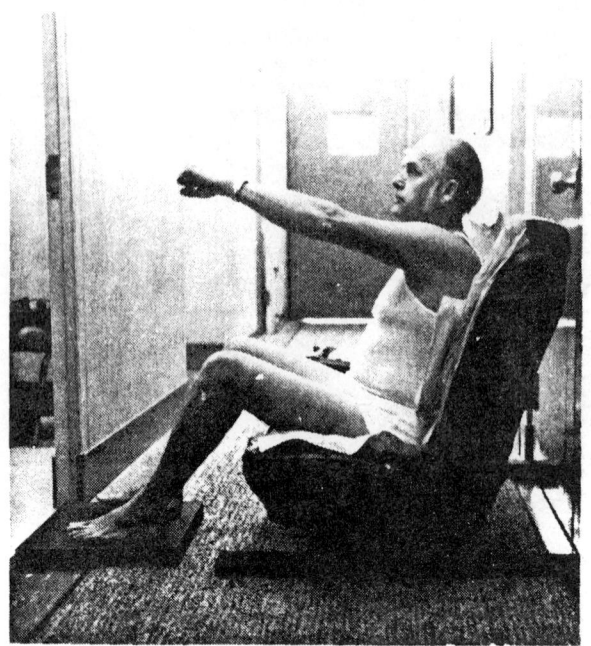 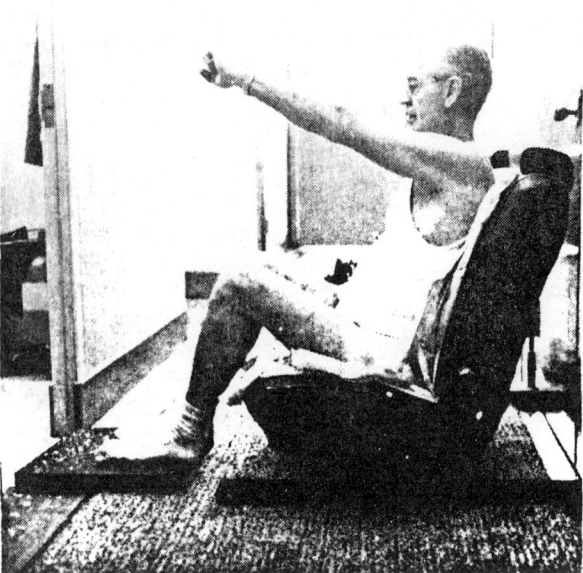

Volunteer LMP Volunteer CJM

Fig. 3 - Determination of volunteer/soft seat interface contour (Arms raised only momentarily to provide a better view of the torso)

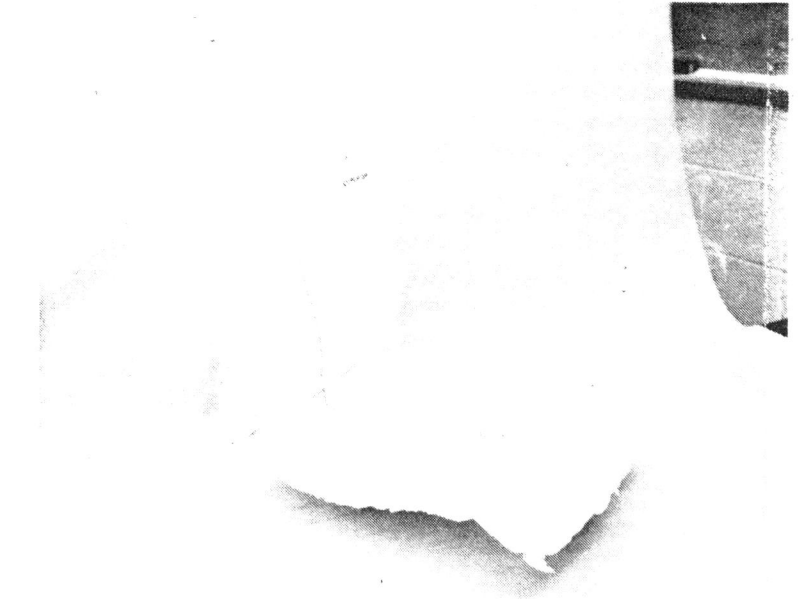

Fig. 4 - Volunteer/soft seat interface contour casting

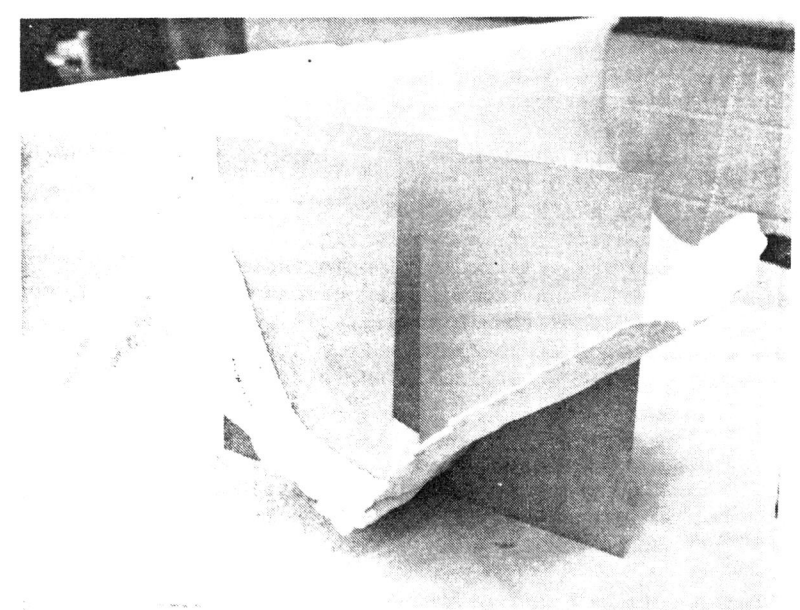

Fig. 5 - Sagittal and midsagittal planes through interface contour casting

line to approximate all sagittal section profile lines of the volunteer. That is, the contour of the wooden seat was to be of a two-dimensional nature, completely described by any one sagittal plane profile. Accordingly, the left and right thigh profiles were averaged and were used in conjunction with the spine profile to describe a single sagittal plane profile. The transition of profile definition from the thighs to profile definition from the spine was made in the region of the superior aspect of the buttocks.

The profiles established using the procedure described above were reproduced in wood, 30.5 cm (12 in) thick (left to right) as shown in Fig. 6. The seats were designed with a seatback angle* of 0.45 rad (26 deg), and the contours were adjusted vertically so that the lowest point (at the buttocks) was 10.2 cm (4.0 in) above the elevation of the surface supporting the feet. This vertical positioning was comparable to that of the three-dimensional H-point machine installation in the soft seat.

The seats were placed on a 1.04 m (41 in) high table for compatibility with the X-ray machine.

X-RAY PROCEDURE

The volunteers were X-rayed at the GM Technical Center Main Medical facility. The wooden seat and custom support table were positioned in the X-ray facility such that the film cassette was parallel to the midsagittal plane of the seated volunteer and was adjacent to his right side. The X-ray "point source" was nominally on a line from the center of the cassette, perpendicular to the film plane. For Volunteer LMP the X-ray source-to-cassette distance was 1.02 m (40 in), and the midsagittal plane-to-cassette distance was 27 cm (10.5 in). For Volunteer CJM these distances were 1.22 m (48 in) and 28 cm (11 in), respectively. The seated volunteers are shown in Fig. 7.

Acceptable skeletal definition in radiograms of the pelvic region produced from lateral exposures is difficult to achieve because of the large soft tissue thickness included in the paths of the rays. Four exposures were necessary to obtain a marginally satisfactory radiogram for the first subject, Volunteer LMP. Marginal success for Volunteer CJM was achieved on the first exposure. Although these radiograms may not have been optimum, it appeared that the desired information could be obtained. Accordingly, in the interest of mitigating the volunteer's radiation exposure, no additional optimization was pursued.

---

* As noted earlier, in the discussion of the three-dimensional H-point machine, the seatback angle is the angle, relative to the vertical, of a tangent line to the "small of the back." This tangent line was easily defined on the seat profiles. Seatback angles near 0.45 rad (26 deg) are widely used.

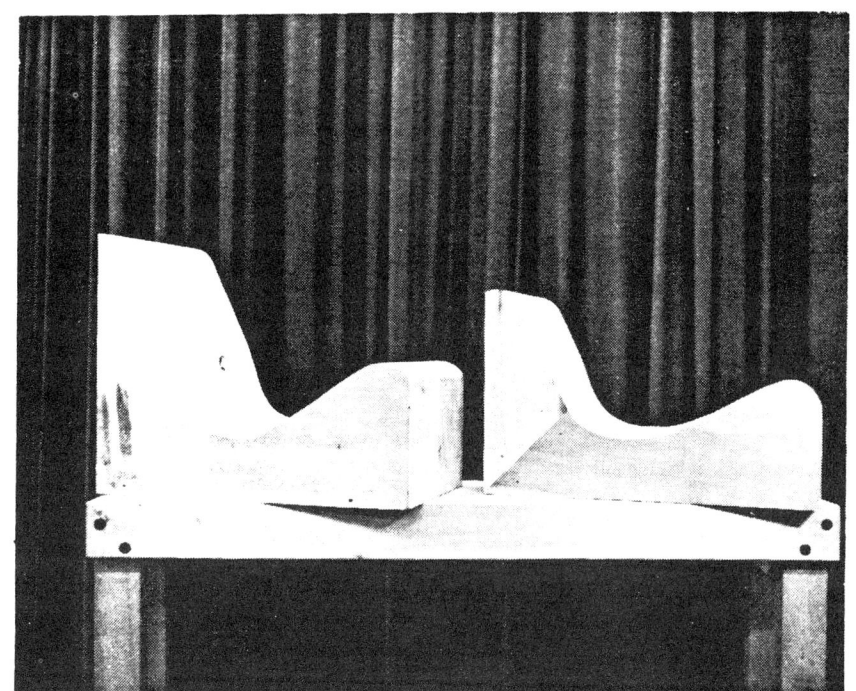

Fig. 6 - Wooden X-ray seats

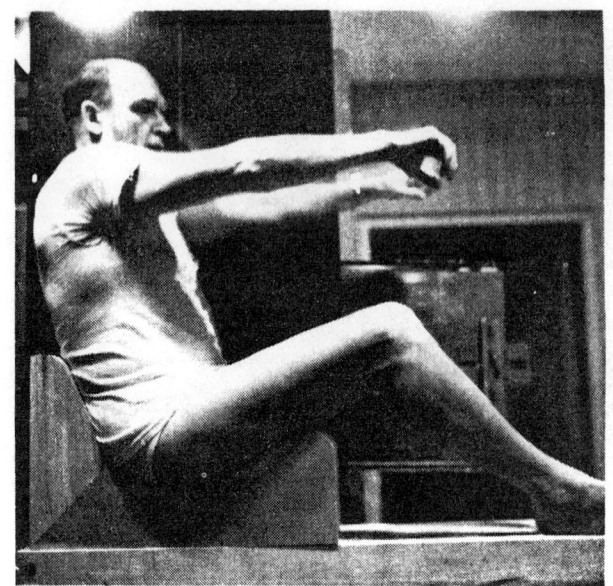 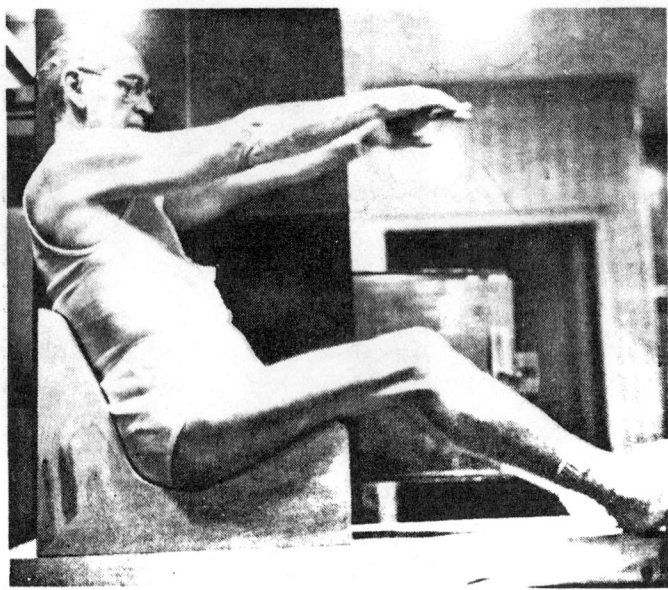

Volunteer LMP   Volunteer CJM

Fig. 7 - Volunteers on wooden X-ray seats (Arms raised only momentarily to provide better view of lower torso)

RESULTS

X-ray radiogram tracings for the two volunteers are shown in Figs. 8 and 9. The marginal contrast and clarity of the films precluded their reproduction as figures herein; however, with appropriate illumination, it was possible to accurately define the pertinent detail shown in these figures. Although the individual femurs could not be discerned clearly in the radiograms, an approximation of the longitudinal axis direction was made based on the image(s) of the anterior and/or posterior surface(s) of the proximal portion of the shaft.

The radiogram tracings of Figs. 8 and 9 also include indications of the vertical direction and the location of the center of the film. The tracings show double images for the anterior, superior iliac spine and the acetabulum. These represent left and right images, both of which appear on the radiogram because of the parallax present in the X-ray procedure.

ANALYSIS OF RESULTS

In order to define the position and orientation of the lower torso, it is necessary to establish a reference system on the pelvis. This topic has been treated in a recent study, "Static Bending Response of the Human Lower Torso" (1), where a pelvic reference system was established on volunteers. A pelvic triangle was defined as illustrated in Fig. 10. By definition, the triangle lies in the midsagittal plane. The three apexes of the triangle, labeled H, I, and P in Fig. 10, are defined as follows: Point H is the bisector of the line joining the left and right hip joint centers of rotation; point I is the bisector of the line joining the left and right anterior, superior iliac spines; and point P is the point of tangency, at the pubic crest, of a midsagittal plane line containing point I.

In the static bending response study referenced above, the pelvic triangle apexes were located by palpation. In contrast, for the program described in this report, X-ray radiography was utilized. A discussion regarding the scale factor of an X-ray radiogram is presented in Appendix A. With reference to Fig. A-1, one can define a scale factor S in accordance with equation (A-1), and it can be evaluated numerically using equation (A-5) if dimensions d_1 and d_2 of the setup are known. In summary, for a simple X-ray system geometry where the object is in a plane parallel to the X-ray film cassette, there is one unique scale factor S defined as:

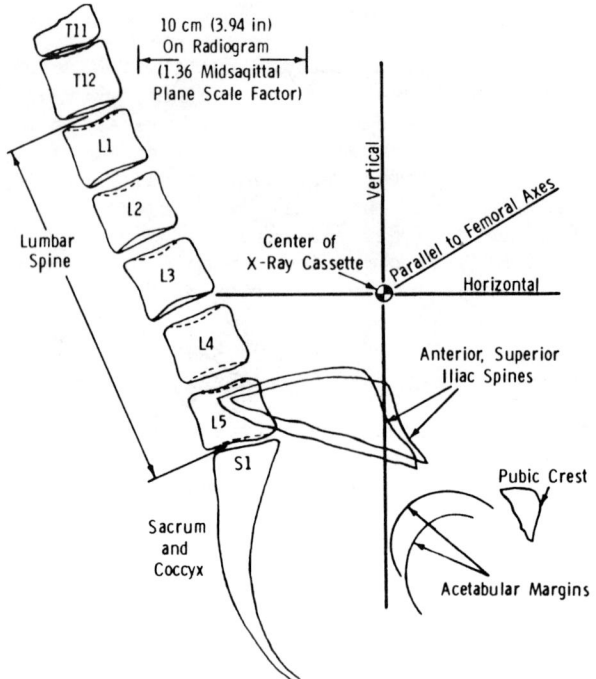

Fig. 8 - Radiogram tracing for Volunteer LMP

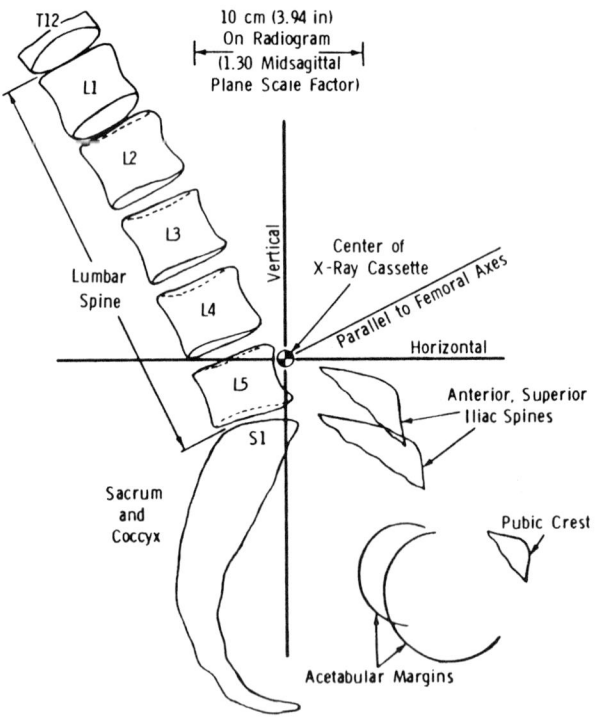

Fig. 9 - Radiogram tracing for Volunteer CJM

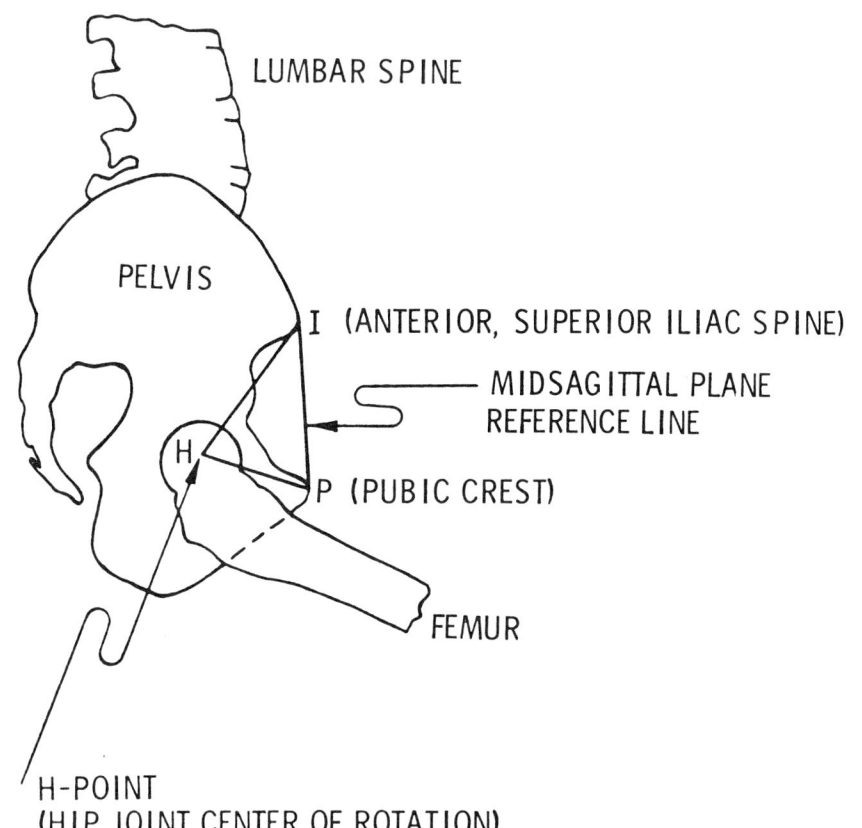

Fig. 10 - The pelvic triangle

$$S = \frac{\text{Image Length}}{\text{Object Length}} . \qquad (1)$$

Also,

$$S = \frac{d_1}{d_1 - d_2} \qquad (2)$$

where

d_1 = X-ray source-to-cassette distance, and

d_2 = Object plane-to-cassette distance.

Dimensions d_1 and d_2 for the volunteers were enumerated in the X-ray Procedure section of the report, where d_2 was referred to the midsagittal plane.

Using these numbers, the radiogram scale factors for the midsagittal planes are:

$$S_{LMP} = \frac{1.02}{1.02 - 0.27} = 1.36 \qquad (3)$$

$$S_{CJM} = \frac{1.22}{1.22 - 0.28} = 1.30 . \qquad (4)$$

Unfortunately, the left and right anterior, superior iliac spines and the left and right hip joint centers of rotation (which are points utilized in defining the pelvic triangle) do not lie in the midsagittal plane, and a more complicated analysis must be pursued. One's first thought may be that, on the radiogram, points H and I of the pelvic triangle lie midway between the associated left and right points. Actually, however, although this can be a reasonable first-order approximation, it is not the exact solution to the problem.

An analysis of the above problem, enabling an exact solution, is presented in Appendix B. In this analysis a factor K is defined to locate, along the straight line connecting the left and right images on the radiogram, a point representing the image of a (midsagittal) point midway between the actual left and right points on the subject. The analysis shows that the value of K depends on dimensions d_1 and d_2 used in computing the midsagittal plane scale factor and, in addition, one more dimension--the distance W between the left and right points.

The dimension W was evaluated by means of palpation for the anterior, superior iliac spines (W_I). It was 26.7 cm (10.5 in) for each volunteer. Dimension W for the hip centers of rotation (W_H) cannot be evaluated by palpation because the hip sockets are inaccessible. Accordingly, the value was extrapolated from the anterior, superior iliac spine W-dimension. Measurements on an excised human cadaver pelvis* indicated that:

$$W_H = \frac{3}{4} W_I . \tag{5}$$

Thus, the extrapolated value for the hip centers of rotation of the volunteers is:

$$W_H = \frac{3}{4} (26.7 \text{ cm})$$

$$= 20.3 \text{ cm } (7.9 \text{ in}). \tag{6}$$

The above values of W_H and W_I, used in conjunction with the X-ray setup dimensions d_1 and d_2 noted earlier, were substituted into equation (B-10) to obtain the K values of Table II. This information was used in conjunction with geometric data from Figs. 8 and 9 to plot the pelvic triangles. (The hip centers of rotation were assumed to be located at the centers of the circular acetabulum images.) The plots are presented in Figs. 11 and 12.

The vertebrae tracings of Figs. 8 and 9 were analyzed to provide the spine data plotted in Figs. 11 and 12. The centers of the vertebral interspaces and the centers of the vertebral bodies were established using the constructions illustrated in Fig. 13. In this figure points A through F are subjective approximations of the "corners" of the vertebral bodies as they appear in a lateral (left-right) radiogram. Point P is midway between points A and B, and point Q is midway between points C and D. The vertebral interspace center is midway between points P and Q. Likewise, the vertebral body center is taken as the intersection point of straight line segments through points C and F and points D and E.

Several pertiennt observations regarding the geometry and orientation of the volunteers' pelves and spines can be made from Figs. 11 and 12. A list of items is presented in Table III. These data are of a quantitative nature. A significant qualitative remark is with regard to the shape of the lumbar spine. The series of line segments connecting the vertebral body centers and/or vertebral interspace centers approximates a straight line.

---

* WSU Cadaver 2955, 184 cm (72.5 in) stature, 75.6 kg (166.5 lb).

Table II—Summary of Scaling Coefficients K'

Volunteer	Application	Dimensionless Scaling Coefficient K' *
LMP	Anterior, Superior Iliac Spine	0.70
LMP	Hip Joint Center	0.76
CJM	Anterior, Superior Iliac Spine	0.75
CJM	Hip Joint Center	0.81

* See Appendix B
Computed using equation (B-10)

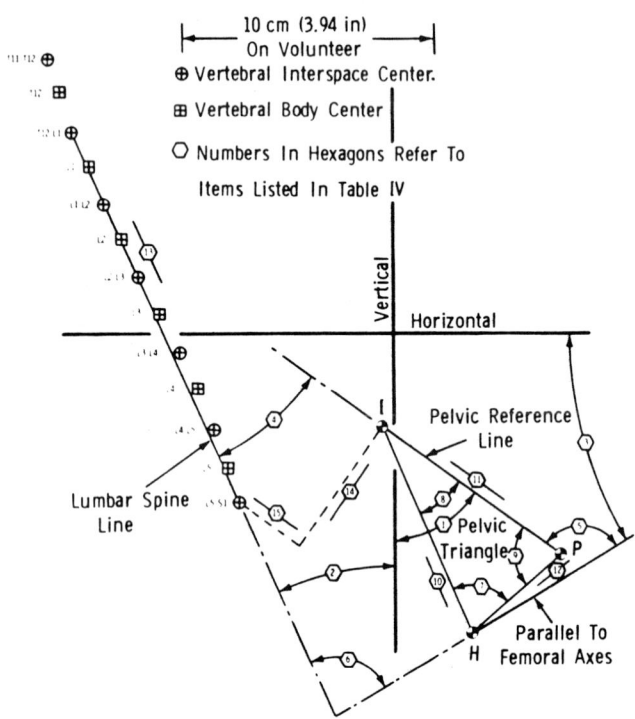

Fig. 11 - Spine and pelvis geometry and orientation--Volunteer LMP

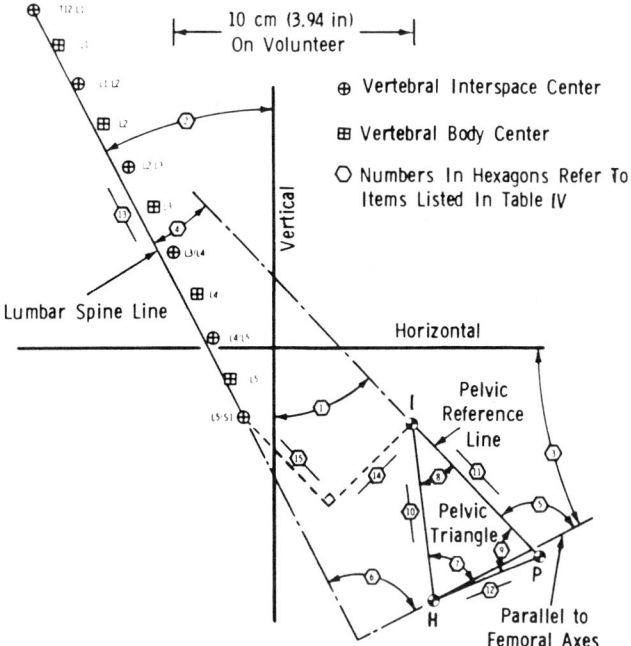

Fig. 12 - Spine and pelvis geometry and orientation--Volunteer CJM

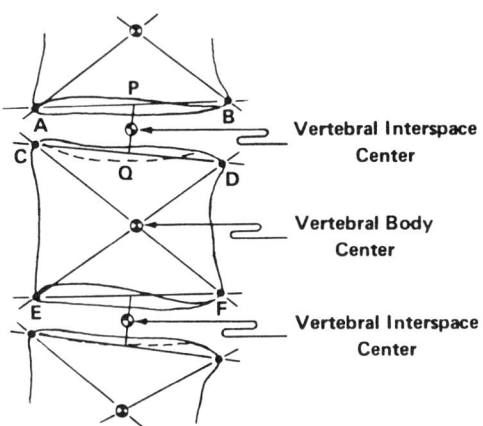

Fig. 13 - Definitions of vertebral body and vertebral interspace centers

Table III - Pelvis and Spine Geometry and Orientation

Item §	Description of Measurement	Dimension LMP	CJM
1	Pelvic reference line angle to vertical--rad (deg)	0.95 (54.5)	0.77 (44)
2	Lumbar spine line* angle to vertical--rad (deg)	0.43 (24.5)	0.47 (27)
3	Femur axis angle to horizontal--rad (deg)	0.54 (31)	0.47 (27)
4	Pelvic reference line/lumbar spine line relative angle--rad (deg)	0.52 (30)	0.30 (17)
5	Pelvic reference line/femur axis relative angle--rad (deg)	1.98 (113.5)	1.87 (107)
6	Lumbar spine line/femur axis relative angle--rad (deg)	1.46 (83.5)	1.57 (90)
	Pelvic triangle angles--rad (deg):		
7	Apex H:	1.27 (73)	1.31 (75)
8	Apex I:	0.54 (31)	0.65 (37)
9	Apex P:	1.33 (76)	1.19 (68)
	Pelvic triangle leg lengths--cm (in):		
10	Leg HI:	8.79 (3.46)	7.29 (2.87)
11	Leg IP:	8.64 (3.40)	7.59 (2.99)
12	Leg PH:	4.63 (1.82)	4.79 (1.88)
13	Lumbar spine length**--cm (in)	15.91 (6.26)	18.80 (7.40)
	Lumbar spine base # location relative to pelvic triangle--		
14	Posterior to I, measured along a perpendicular to IP--cm (in):	5.69 (2.24)	4.81 (1.89)
15	Superior to I, measured along a parallel to IP--cm (in):	2.97 (1.17)	5.10 (2.01)

§ Numbers refere to number in hexagons in Figures 11 and 12.
* Lumbar spine line defined as straight line-segment through T12/L1 and L5/S1 vertebral interspace centers.
** Lumbar spine length defined as length of line segment defined in preceding footnote (*).
\# Lumbar spine base defined as L5/S1 vertebral interspace center point.

CONCLUSIONS

1. The techniques utilized in the study proved to be practical for analyzing the lower torso skeletal geometry of the vehicle seated volunteer.

2. Sufficient resolution on a lateral pelvic radiogram, to enable definition of the pelvic triangle and femoral axes, requires careful control of exposure conditions.

3. For the particular typical seated configuration studied in this program, the volunteers' lumbar spine centerlines are nearly straight lines.

4. Accurate quantitative data can be obtained from X-ray radiograms, in spite of the inherent parallax problem, if the set-up geometry is carefully documented and proper geometrical principles are applied in reducing the raw data scaled from the film.

RECOMMENDATIONS

1. Skeletal geometric information of the type presented herein should be developed for a representative cross-section of volunteers seated in a representative cross-section of vehicle seats to evaluate the lower torso skeletal configuration on a statistical basis. Such a study should include a determination of the thorax-to-pelvis orientation in order to provide data compatible with the lower torso bending response study of Reference (2).

2. Palpation techniques should be considered for use in place of X-ray radiography for studies of the nature of that reported herein. The X-ray radiation hazard would be eliminated, and the volunteer's posture could be studied directly, without the need for fabrication of custom wooden seats. Definition of the pelvic triangle by palpation proved to be practical in the study of Reference (2).

ACKNOWLEDGMENT

The volunteer/soft seat interface contour casting technique described in this report was a technique recommended by Frank J. Biluk, M.D., Technical Center Medical Director. Dr. Biluk also directed the volunteer X-ray portion of the study. Volunteer Clarence J. Murton of Wayne State University deserves special thanks for participating in this program. Gratitude is expressed to Mr. Ron W. Roe of G.M. Design Staff for making arrangements with regard to the three-dimensional H-point machine evaluation of the soft seat and the anthropometric documentation of the volunteers.

REFERENCES

1. "Devices for Use in Defining and Measuring Motor Vehicle Seating Accommodation--SAE J826a," SAE Standard, SAE Handbook, Part 2, 1974.

2. G. W. Nyquist and C. J. Murton, "Static Bending Response of the Human Lower Torso," SAE Paper 751158, Nineteenth Stapp Car Crash Conference Proceedings, October, 1975.

APPENDIX A - X-RAY RADIOGRAM SCALE FACTOR

Images of objects on X-ray radiograms are always larger than full scale due to the geometry of the setup (object positioned between X-ray source and film). Therefore, in quantitative analyses of radiograms, to obtain anthropometric data, it is important that a scale factor be defined and evaluated for each radiogram to enable scaling of measurements to full size.

The geometry of a typical X-ray setup is illustrated in Fig. A-1. An X-ray point source is located a distance d_1 from the film plane of an X-ray cassette. Consider a radiopaque object of length ℓ located a distance d_2 from the film plane. Also, the object is located a radial distance R from the axis constructed through the X-ray source, perpendicular to the film plane. The shadow of this object on the film plane is the image, of length ℓ', recorded on the radiogram. It is obvious from Fig. A-1 that $\ell' \geq \ell$ for $d_2 \leq d_1$. It is convenient to define a scale factor S as:

$$S = \frac{\ell'}{\ell} . \qquad (A-1)$$

The scale factor is therefore a number always greater than unity for clinical type radiological studies.

A simple exercise in geometry enables the scale factor to be defined in terms of the dimensions of the setup. An analysis of similar triangles in Fig. A-1 enables one to write:

$$\frac{Q}{d_2} = \frac{R-\ell/2}{d_1-d_2} . \qquad (A-2)$$

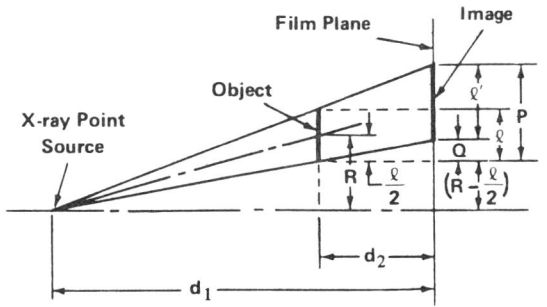

Fig. A-1 - X-ray setup geometry

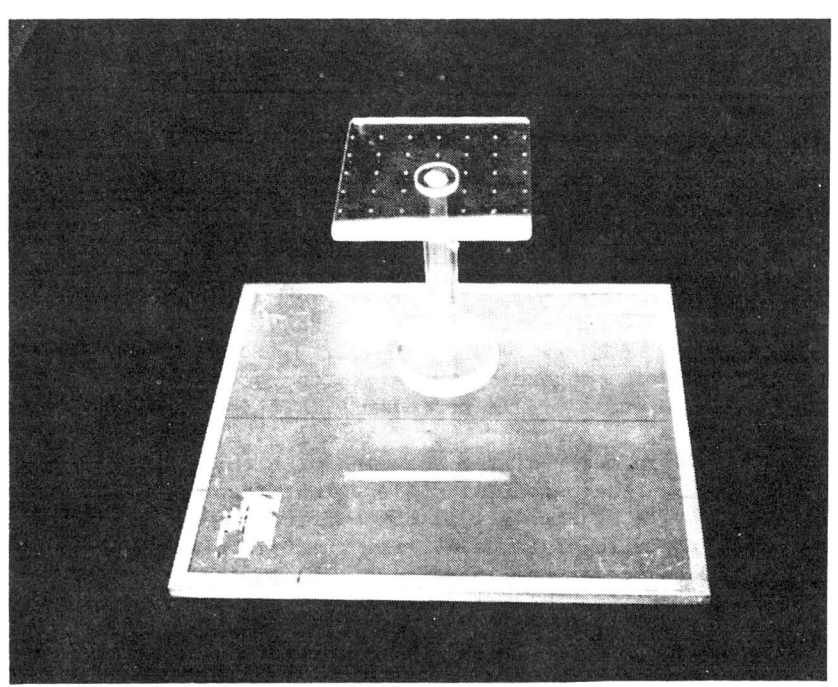

Fig. A-2 - Experimental setup for validating radiogram scale factor analysis

Likewise,

$$\frac{P + R - \ell/2}{d_1} = \frac{R + \ell/2}{d_1 - d_2} . \qquad (A-3)$$

Solving equations (A-2) and (A-3) for Q and P and noting that

$$\ell' = P - Q$$

enables one to obtain the following expression for the image length:

$$\ell' = \frac{d_1}{d_1 - d_2} \ell . \qquad (A-4)$$

Thus, using equations (A-1) and (A-4) gives the scale factor:

$$S = \frac{d_1}{d_1 - d_2} . \qquad (A-5)$$

It is interesting to note that the scale factor is independent of the radial distance R.

The validity of this analysis was checked experimentally by X-raying a 25 mm (one in) square grid pattern constructed of lead spheres embedded in a flat sheet of plastic (Figure A-2). Dimension d_1 was set to 1.02 m (40 in), and values of 20 and 30 cm (8 and 12 in) were utilized for dimension d_2. The difference between the theoretically and experimentally derived radiogram scale factors was negligible (less than 0.5 percent error).

APPENDIX B-RADIOGRAM ANALYSIS FOR THE PELVIC TRIANGLE

A discussion regarding the scale factor of an X-ray radiogram was presented in Appendix A. It is clear that equation (A-5) may be used when Fig. A-1 is adequate to describe the geometry of the setup. For a three-dimensional object such as the pelvis, it is apparent that the scale factor analysis of Fig. A-1 is not sufficient because one plane, at a single distance d_2 from the film plane, is inadequate to describe the location of all points on the object. For pelvic triangle determination, however, where it is reasonable to assume skeletal symmetry with respect to the midsagittal plane, one can define virtual (not actually present) radiopaque points, midway between the anterior, superior iliac spines and midway between the hip joint centers of rotation. Further, criteria can be defined for determining where the images, of these virtual points, would be located on the radiogram. These images, along with the image of the pubic crest, are images of the three apexes of the pelvic triangle (Fig. 10). Since the pelvic triangle lies in the midsagittal plane, and the midsagittal plane has one unique d_2 dimension (Fig. A-1), the geometry of Fig. A-1, and therefore the scale factor definition of equation (A-5), may be used to scale the radiogram pelvic triangle image back to full size. The criteria for determining where the images of the virtual points are located on the radiogram is developed in the following presentation.

Figure B-1 illustrates the geometry for a lateral pelvic X-ray setup. Pelvic points Q_ℓ and Q_r are symmetrically located relative to the midsagittal plane and may be thought of as either the left and right anterior, superior iliac spine points, or the centers of rotation of the left and right hip joints. They are located a radial distance R from the film plane normal through the X-ray source. The X-ray source is located a distance d_1 from the X-ray film plane, and the midsagittal plane-to-film plane distance is d_2. Point Q'_ℓ is the radiogram image of point Q_ℓ, and Q'_r is the image of Q_r. Likewise, point Q is the virtual radiopaque point midway between Q_ℓ and Q_r, and its virtual image is Q'. It is obvious from the figure that, although Q is midway between Q_ℓ and Q_r, the virtual image Q' is not midway between images Q'_ℓ and Q'_r; that is, the factor K' is not equal to unity. Concisely stated, the problem is to derive an expression to evaluate the factor K' in terms of the parameters of the X-ray geometry. This derivation follows.

In Fig. B-1, by analyzing similar triangles,

$$\frac{h}{W/2} = \frac{R + h}{d_1 - d_2} ;$$

therefore,

$$h = \frac{WR}{2(d_1 - d_2) - W} . \qquad (B-1)$$

Likewise, by similar triangles,

$$\frac{R - Kh}{d_1 - d_2} = \frac{R}{d_1 - d_2 + W/2} ,$$

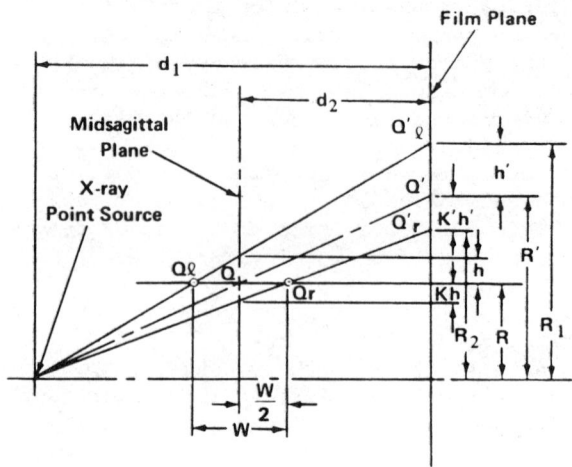

Fig. B-1 - Pelvic X-ray geometry

and therefore,

$$Kh = \frac{WR}{2(d_1-d_2)+W} \quad . \tag{B-2}$$

Combining equations (B-1) and (B-2) provides the factor K:

$$K = \frac{2(d_1-d_2)-W}{2(d_1-d_2)+W} \quad . \tag{B-3}$$

Additional similar triangles provide the relationships:

$$\frac{R'}{d_1} = \frac{R}{d_1-d_2} \quad ,$$

$$\frac{R_1}{d_1} = \frac{h}{W/2} \quad ,$$

and

$$\frac{R_2}{d_1} = \frac{R-Kh}{d_1-d_2} \quad .$$

Therefore,

$$R' = \frac{d_1}{d_1-d_2} R \quad , \tag{B-4}$$

$$R_1 = \frac{2hd_1}{W} \quad , \tag{B-5}$$

and

$$R_2 = \frac{d_1}{d_1-d_2} (R-Kh). \tag{B-6}$$

Next,

$$h' = R_1 - R'$$

and, using equations (B-4) and (B-5), this becomes:

$$h' = \frac{d_1}{W(d_1-d_2)} [2h(d_1-d_2)-WR]. \tag{B-7}$$

Also,

$$K'h' - R' - R_2$$

and, using equations (B-4) and (B-6), this becomes:

$$K'h' = \frac{d_1}{d_1-d_2} Kh . \qquad (B-8)$$

Dividing equation (B-8) by equation (B-7) yields:

$$K' = \frac{KhW}{2h(d_1-d_2)-WR} .$$

Finally, substituting h from equation (B-1) into this expression, and simplifying, the result is:

$$K' = K \qquad (B-9)$$

or, using equation (B-3):

$$K' = \frac{2(d_1-d_2)-W}{2(d_1-d_2)+W} . \qquad (B-10)$$

Note that equation (B-10) indicates K' is independent of the radial distance R. It depends only on the object and image distances d_1 and d_2 required for scale factor determination [equation (A-5)] and the width W separating the left and right anatomical points.

The radiogram produced under the conditions of Fig. B-1 contains image points Q'_ℓ and Q'_r. Accordingly, one can physically measure the distance $\overline{Q'_\ell Q'_r}$. Also, it is apparent from Fig. B-1 that

$$h'(1+K') = \overline{Q'_\ell Q'_r} .$$

Therefore,

$$h' = \frac{1}{1+K'} \cdot \overline{Q'_\ell Q'_r} , \qquad (B-11)$$

where K' is evaluated using equation (B-10). Equation (B-11) enables one to locate the desired virtual image point Q' of Fig. B-1. The distance h' is always measured <u>from</u> the image point most distant from the film plane normal through the X-ray source <u>toward</u> the image point nearest this normal. That is, in Fig. B-1, h' is measured from Q'_ℓ toward Q'_r to define point Q'. Note that the point where this normal intersects the film plane need not be known. It is only necessary that one establish which vector,

$$\overrightarrow{Q'_\ell Q'_r} \quad \text{or} \quad \overrightarrow{Q'_r Q'_\ell} \quad ,$$

points toward the normal.

The validity of this analysis was checked experimentally by X-raying a plastic mock pelvis constructed with small lead spheres representing the pubic crest and the left and right hip sockets and anterior, superior iliac spines (Figure B-2). Dimension d_1 was set to 1.02m (40 in), and values of 20 and 30 cm (8 and 12 in) were utilized for dimension d_2 (measured to the midsagittal plane). The pelvic triangle shapes derived from analyses of the radiograms were compared with the actual triangle geometry of the mock pelvis. Errors in the angles were within the limit of resolution of the measurements [less than 0.009 rad (0.5 deg)]. The maximum error in the triangle leg lengths was two percent.

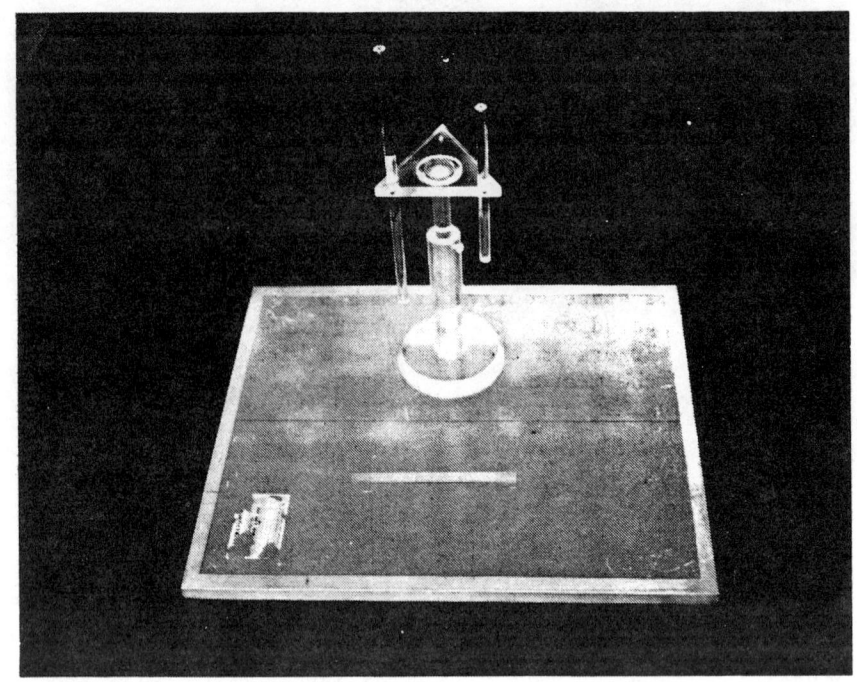

Fig. B-2 - Experimental setup with mock pelvis for validating radiogram analysis for pelvic triangle

770931

Biomechanical Experiments with Animals on Abdominal Tolerance Levels

E. Gögler and A. Best
Accident Research Surgical University

H.-H. Braess, H.-E. Burst, and G. Laschet
Research and Development Center Porsche (Germany)

Abstract

In order to improve the active safety and the aerodynamic drag a special rear end configuration was developped for the Porsche 911 (4)[+]. Typical sequences of movements were determined during impact tests in the course of which dummies were hit by various rear end variants. It was stated that some pedestrians and cyclists incurred direct abdominal impacts. To find out whether under real traffic situations and in a speed range of 16 through 24 km/h this type of collision results in intraabdominal injuries, 12 corresponding test series with Göttingen minipigs were carried through in the course of which the test animals were projected against various rear end variants. Measurements were made to determine the forces and accelerations acting on the respective rear end. The acceleration to which the animal was subjected was measured by means of an acceleration sensor sutured to the test subject's back. In addition the point of impact on the animal's body was determined. Immediately following the test, the animals were dissected and the interior organs microscopically examined. When impacting against a flexible rear end structure of a mass of 8.5 kg the limit between AIS grades 3 and 4 is located at approximately 1471.5 N for a duration of up to 5 ms. Under the given test conditions the tolerance limit between a subacute and an acute shock is at approximately 981 N for a duration of up to 2o ms. When hitting against non-flexible structures, the abdominal region incurred particularly severe injuries, which in two cases were only insufficiently recorded due to the monoaxial force measurement. With certain restrictions, the results obtained may be applied to an 8 to 12 year old child.

[+] Numbers in parentheses designate References at end of paper

REVIEW OF LITERATURE

MAYS (1966 (13)) carried out tests with human livers removed from dead bodies. The salt-solution filled organs were dropped from heights of 2.60 - 27.8 m, with capsula dehiscencies occurring at 27.5 Nm and liver ruptures taking place at 382 Nm - 480 Nm. GLENN (1963 (8)) also determined the limiting value for a liver rupture at 336.5 Nm when effecting corresponding tests with dog livers, filled with salt solution and dropped from heights of 2 - 8 m.

TROLLOPE (1973 (28)) et al. as well as MELVIN et al. (1973 (14)) surgically mobilised the livers of anesthetised monkeys and placed them on force sensors in order to submit them to impactor tests with varying velocities and impact surfaces (Fig. 1). The estimated severities of injuries ranged from "slight" (1), with subcapsular liver haematoma, over "mild" (2), corresponding to AIS 3, with small liver dehiscencies, and "moderate" (3), corresponding to AIS 4, with a spleen rupture and surigcal treatment of the liver, to (4), with liver resection and pancreas rupture, and (5) with death at the place of accident. The limiting value for AIS-4 injury to the liver is 303 kPa. The corresponding value for an injury of the kidney is higher, due to the greater tensile strength of the capsula.

The definition of ESI is given by:

$$ESI = \lg \frac{F \cdot t^2}{m \sqrt{A}}$$

where:

F = impact force
t = duration of impact
m = mass
A = impact surface

NICKERSON (1967 (18)) examined the longitudinal impact load limits of dogs by dropping the animals in upright position from heights of 10 - 200 cm. The decelerations to which the interior organs were submitted ranged from 7.1 through 58 g. No injuries occurred during these tests.

BAXTER and WILLIAMS (1961 (2)) carried out tests with 80 dogs using an impactor with 11.26 km/h and impact energies of 270 - 406 Nm. Lateral impacts against the right flank of the test dogs resulted in 5 times as many liver ruptures and 2 times as many kidney ruptures as occurred with impacts along the longitu-

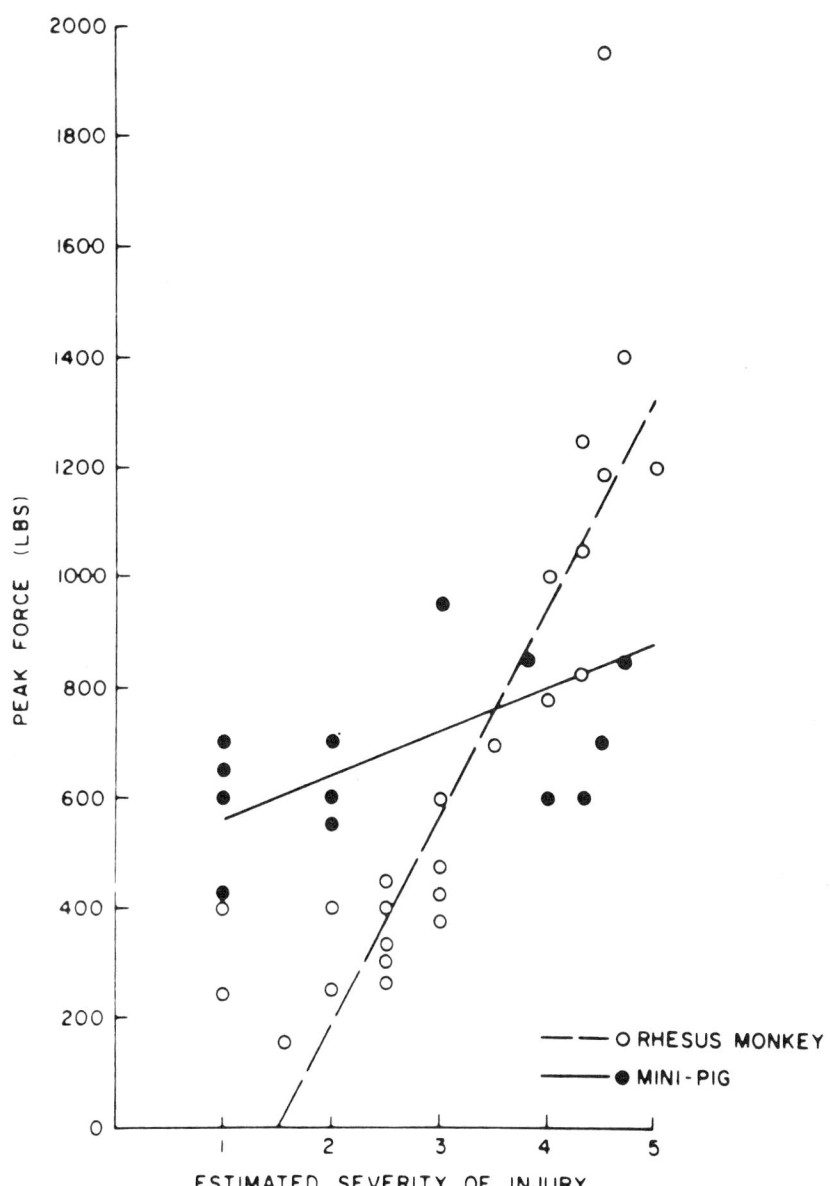

Fig. 1 - Peak contact force versus estimated severity of injury

dinal direction. Unfortunately there are no details available as concerns the impactor and the weight of the test dogs. The relation between impactor/dog appears to be similar to the relation between steering wheel and man.

HELLSTROM and GRIMELIUS (1966 (11)) carried out impact tests with 23 sitting dogs (13,15 - 34.9 kg), hitting their right flank with a pendulum ram of a weight of 15.4 kg and a surface of 9.61 cm^2. With an impact velocity of 9.3 km/h the pendulum ram generated forces of 533.6 - 1063.4 N resulting in lateral compressions of the animal body of 5o - 7o %. At an impact velocity of 15.8 km/h forces of 129o - 258o N led to lateral compressions of 7o - 8o %. Due to the body-inherent visco-elasticity, the maximum body compression occurred 3o - 45 ms later than the maximum force level.

Four of the dogs were subjected to one single impact test and dissected immediately afterwards. One impact occurring at a velocity of 9.3 km/h caused a severe liver rupture. Another impact effected at 15.8 km/h led to small capsular dehiscencies with superficial parenchyma lesions. No apparent reason was given for the difference in effects.

The essential factor for the lesions of the intestine was the traction at the organ attachment and the compression of the organs between the abdominal wall and the spinal column rather than the pressure on the organs themselves. When filled with liquid or gas, the intestine is much more vulnerable (KENNEDY 1960 (12)).

WINDQUIST et al. (1953 (31)) projected pigs against obstacles with various surfaces. The impact of a 47 kg pig against an obstacle of a surface of 64.51 cm^2 (9.06 cm dia.) at a velocity of 22.27 km/h produced a maximum load of 4797 N and a body compression of 3o % which resulted in only subpleural and subendiocardial haemorrhages (this is rather due to a shock than to a trauma (note by first author). Subseral, probably traumatical haemorrhages occurred at the colon (note by first author).

One test animal of a weight of 28.4 kg survived an acceleration sled test at an impact velocity of 21 km/h and a belt load of 3335.4N N. The animal had been attached by means of a 7.6 cm wide belt across the abdomen (no lap belt). The impact also caused subendiocardial haemorrhages (shock) and subseral haemorrhages of the jejunus. Another animal of a weight of 31.6 kg died when hitting the belt at an impact velocity of 48.4 km/h and a load of 2088.4 N using an identical test set up. The resulting fatal injuries were a diaphragm rupture and ruptures of stomach, colon, and spleen. The liver showed only capsula dehiscencies.

SNYDER and YOUNG (1968 (23)) carried out tests using chimpansees and submitting the animals to an abdominal belt load of 13616.3 N for a duration of 3 ms. The only resulting lesions were an acute hyperaemia of spleen, liver, heart, and kidneys indicating a general shock.

SCHMIDT et al. (1975 (22)), when carrying out tests with corpses, found good chances of survival at lap belt forces of 7112.2 N as well as multiple severe intraabdominal injuries without any chances of survival at a lap belt foce of only 3727.8 N. This leads to the conclusion that in the latter case the belt did not pass across the pelvic bones but across the soft part of the abdomen, and that in this case a load of 3727.8 N is sufficient to generate fatal intraabdominal injuries.

Based on reconstructions of accidental injuries, caused by wrongly attached belts, SNYDER (1972 (24)) assumes a tolerable speed range of 16 - 24 km/h, whereas MELVIN (1973 (14)) and FACEKAS (1971 (7)) indicate a value of only 392.4 N.

The blunt impact against the abdomen may lead to a shock of the entire body without causing lesions of the interior organs. When considering the dynamic load on the entire body, distinction must be made between hydraulical and biochemical effects (WISNER et al.) (1970 (32)). To create fluid movements in the human organism which are strong enough to produce general shock symptoms, the human body must be exposed to a deceleration of at least 80 g for more than 20 ms (Figures 2 and 3).

According to THOMPSON (1962 (27)) and KORNHAUSER (see (10)) the human body and organs behave like solid bodies with accelerations inferior to 70 ms; traction, thrust, and pressure forces cause structural failures. With decelerations exceeding 70 ms, the influence of fluid movements increases, and with impact durations of more than 2 s they cause patho-physiological reactions.

The biochemical effects lead to the destruction of a great number of body cells, releasing numerous biochemical substances the composition and effects of which are still largely unknown. This phenomenon occurs already with microscopical lesions. Thus the biomechanical investigation of the trauma - more precisely the blunt abdominal trauma - must be complemented by biochemical examinations of people hurt during accidents and surviving test animals. This type of research might possibly lead to a new classification of injury severity.

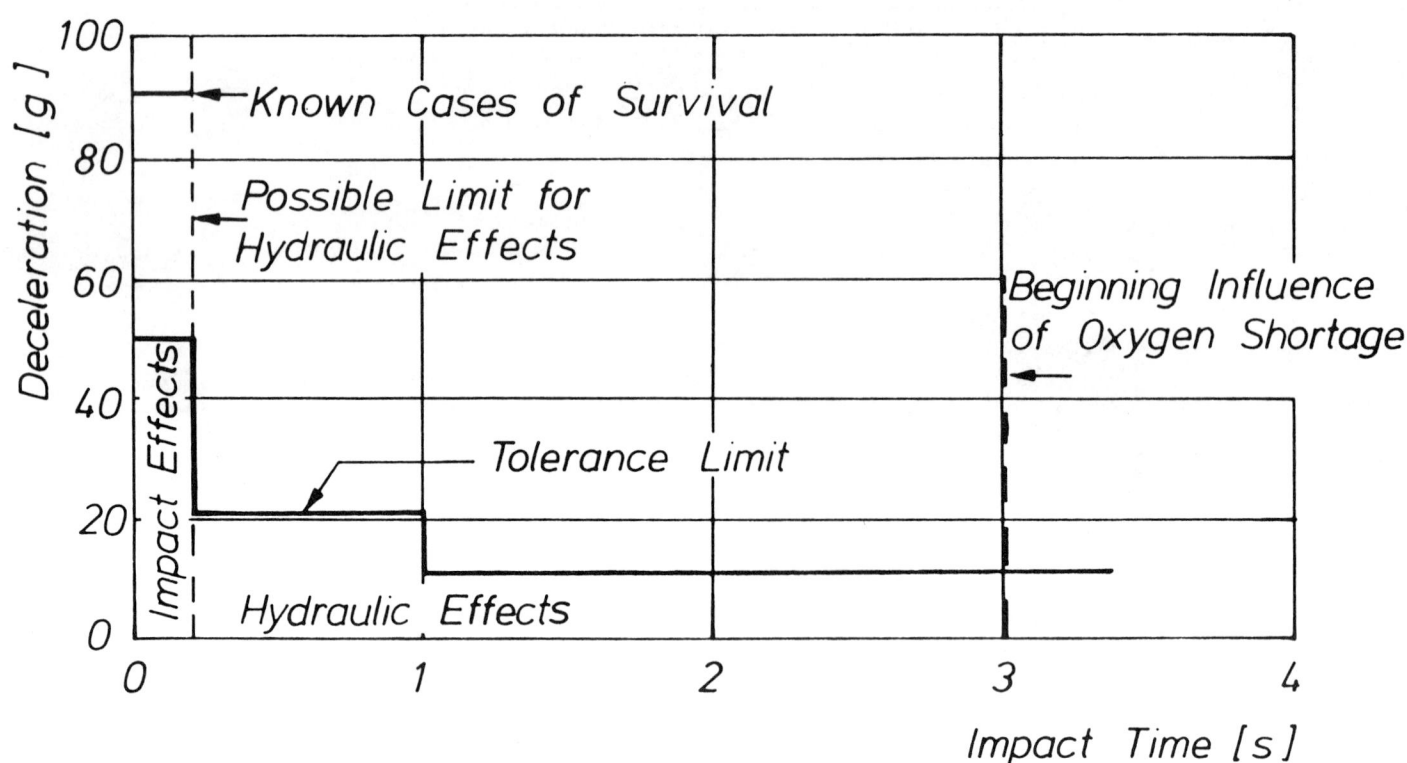

Fig. 2 - Deceleration tolerance levels versus impact time

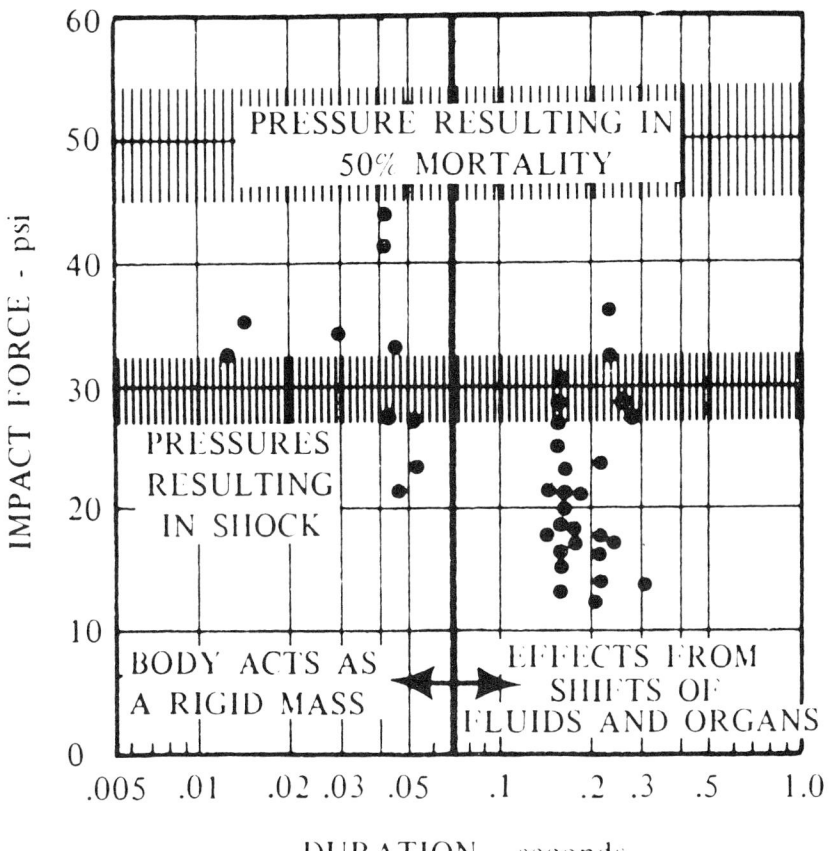

Fig. 3 - Impact force versus impact duration showing shock and mortality limits (literature from accidental falls and sled tests [23])

SUMMARIZING the pertinent literature furnishes little information about the biomechanical aspects of the blunt abdominal trauma. The papers available show considerable deviations and the results obtained are in part not comparable.

VEHICLE REAR END VARIANTS

The dummy as well as the animal tests were performed using the following variants of the Porsche 911 rear body configuration (Figures 4-7):
- standard version
- spoiler of fiber-reinforced plastic (GFR-configuration) with soft PUR-foam edge of 80 - 120 mm width
- spoiler of PUR-foam
- simulated rear trunk of sheet metal

The deformation curves characterizing the impact behaviour (static force-deflection/energy-deflection curves) were determined using the test set up of Figure 8. The results are shown in Figures 9 and 10.

Up to about 200 N, resp. 6 Nm, the deformation of about 30 mm is almost identical for both materials. In the intermediate range up to a deflection of 55 mm the PUR-spoiler proves to be more rigid: a deflection of 45 mm requires a force of 1140N with the PUR spoiler, in comparison to just 530 N with the GRP version. The deflection work increases correspondingly. Beyond a deflection of 57 mm the GRP spoiler was found to be stiffer. Under dynamic load only a slight increase of the force characteristic and the energy absorption occurs with the given spoiler configurations and test conditions. For the standard trunk configuration the deflection under these loads is almost nonexistent.

SLED AND SITTING POSITION OF TEST ANIMAL

See Figure 11

MEASURING AND PROCESSING EQUIPMENT (Fig. 12)

VEHICLE - When setting up the measuring equipment it was assumed that the injury relevant time domain of the animal impact against the vehicle rear end could be almost entirely defined by horizontal forces and movements. Thus only the horizontally acting impact forces generated during the impact of the animal against the vehicle were measured. For that purpose, three force

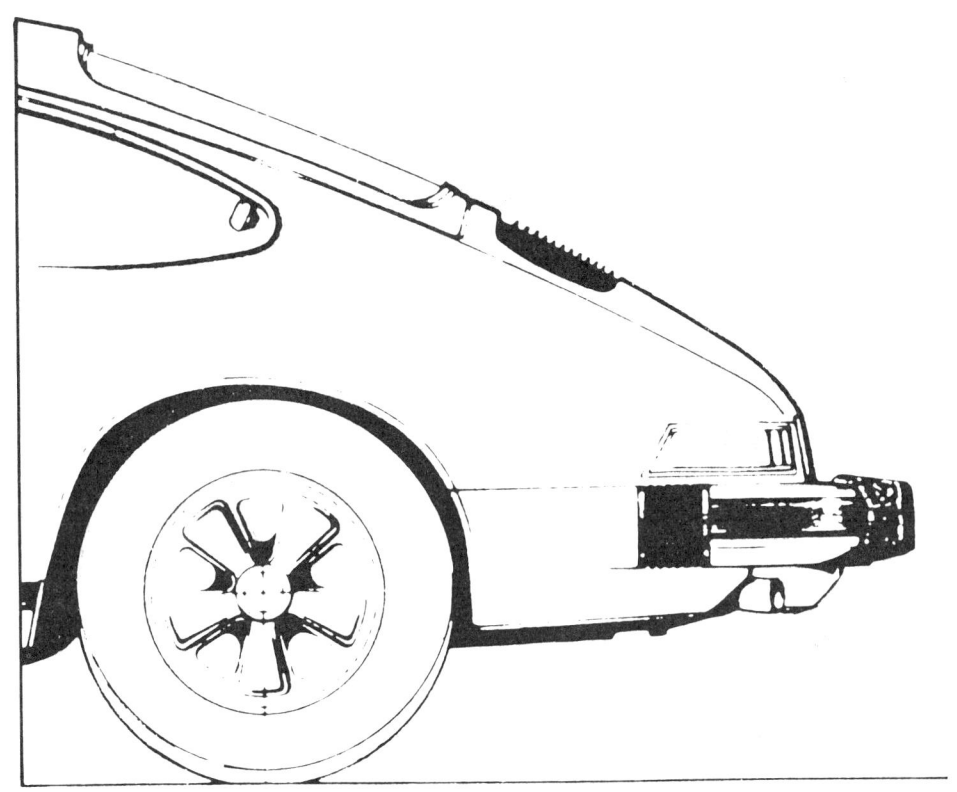

Fig. 4 - Vehicle rear (basic version)

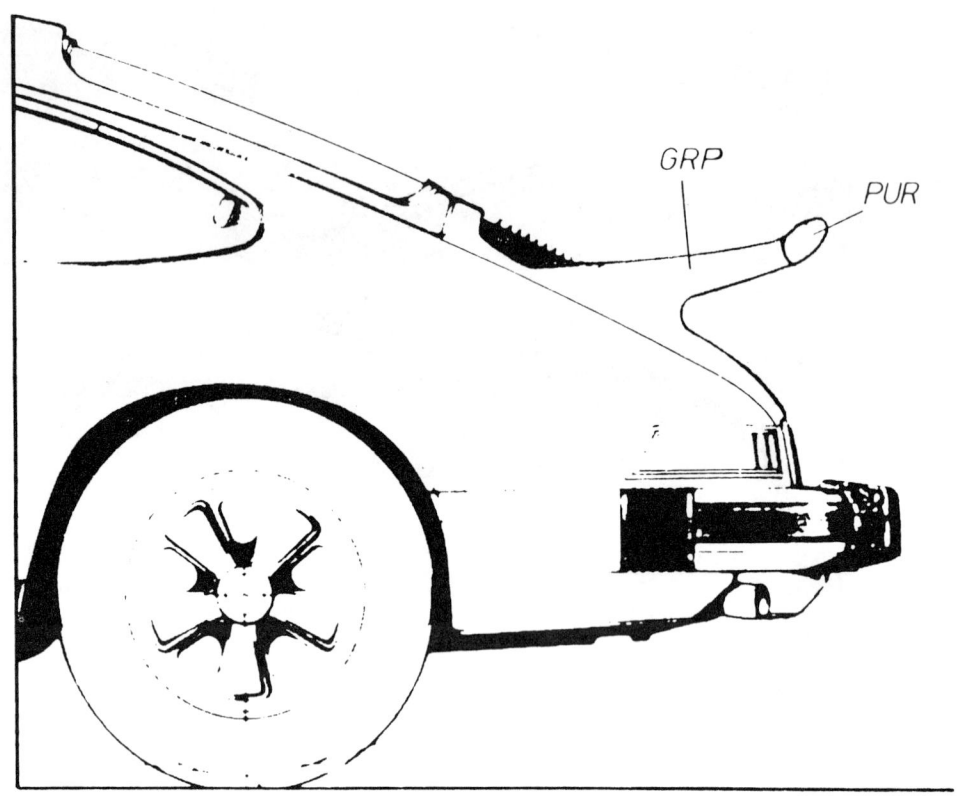

Fig. 5 - Vehicle rear (GRP-spoiler)

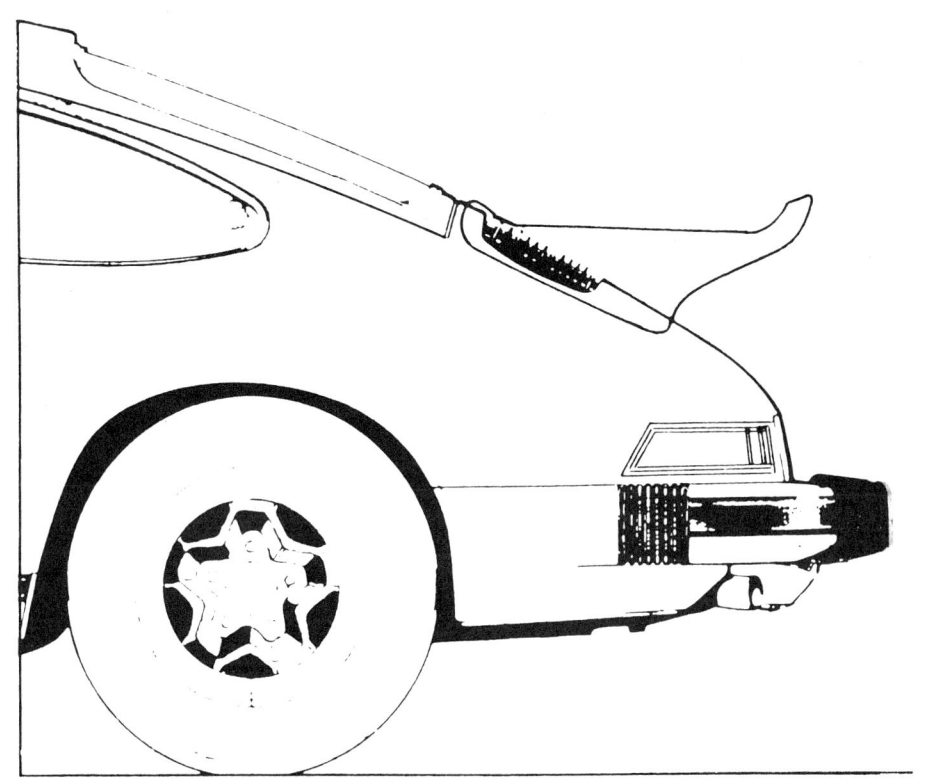

Fig. 6 - Vehicle rear (PUR-spoiler)

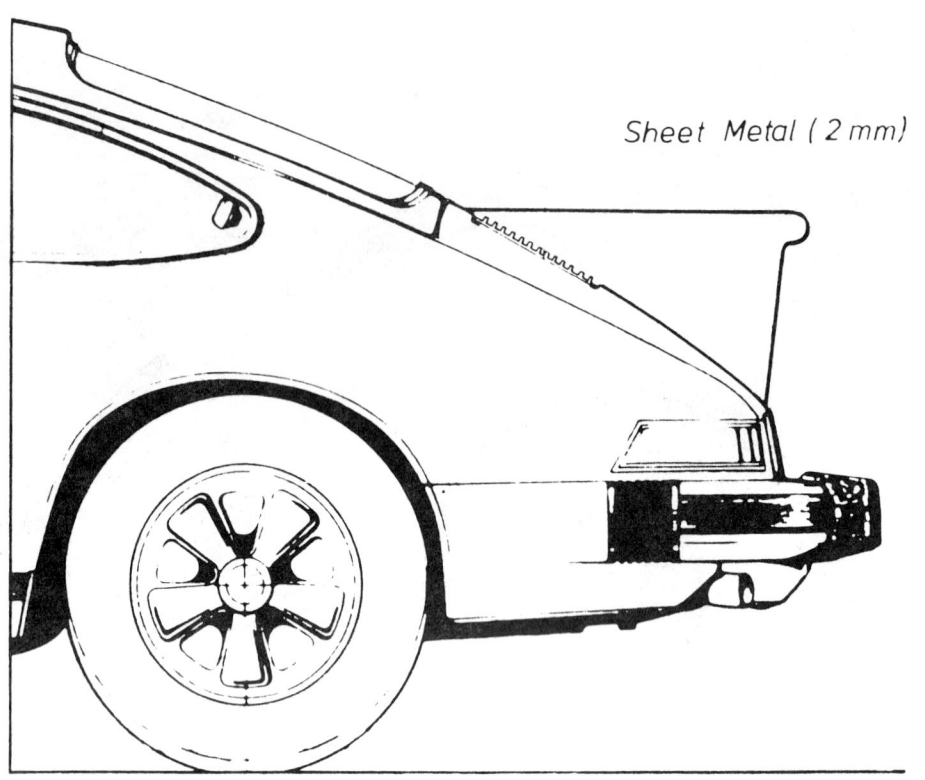

Fig. 7 - Vehicle rear (simulated standard trunk configuration)

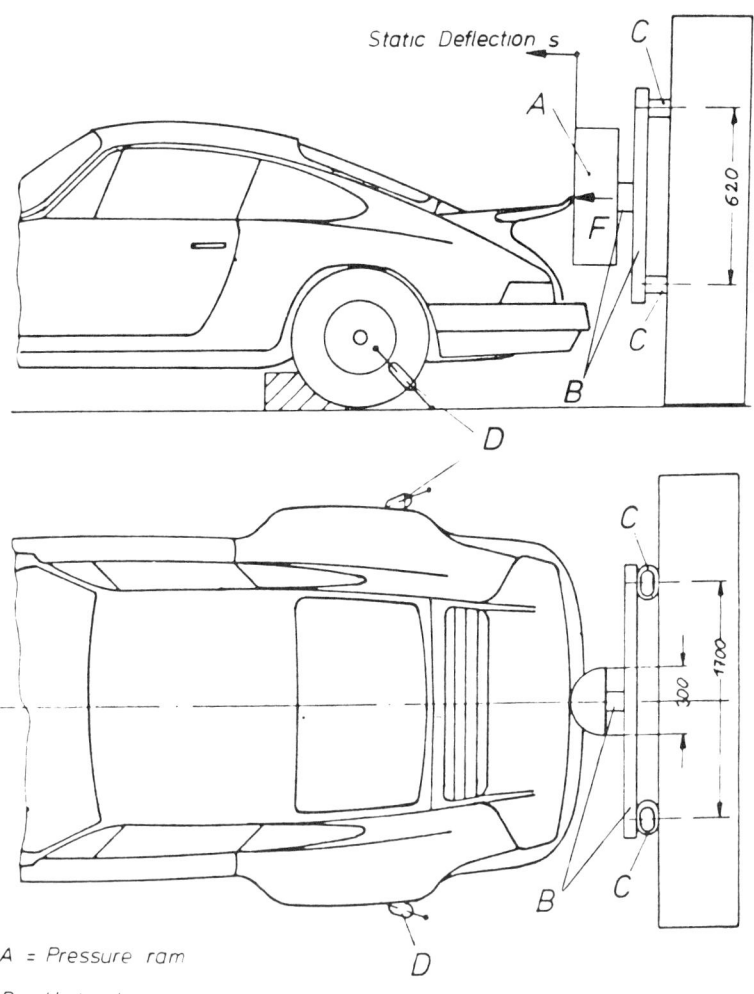

A = Pressure ram
B = Hydraulic ram apparatus
C = Force sensor
D = Turnbuckle

Fig. 8 - Force measurement apparatus of the spoiler flexibility

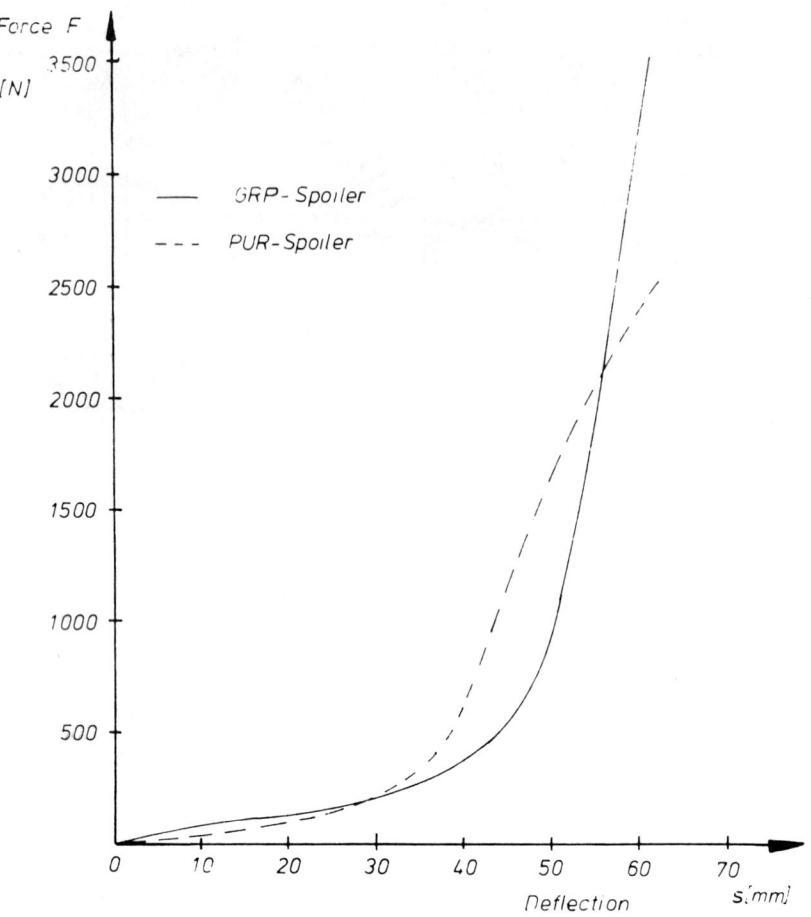

Fig. 9 - Static force-deflection-diagram of the spoiler (force application according to Fig. 8)

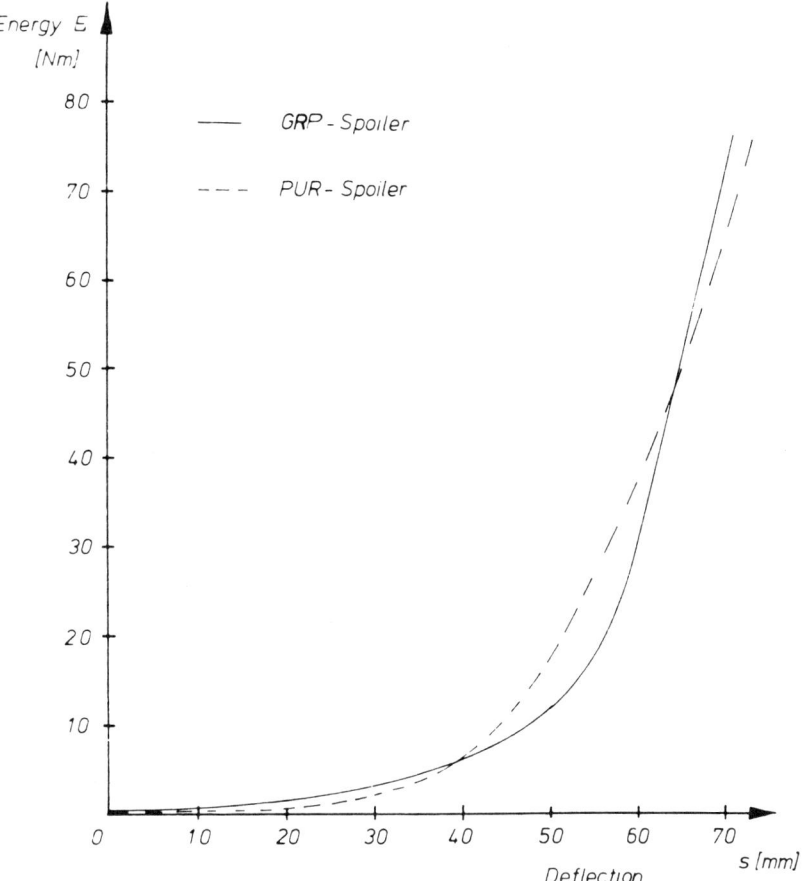

Fig. 10 - Energy-deflection-diagram of the spoiler

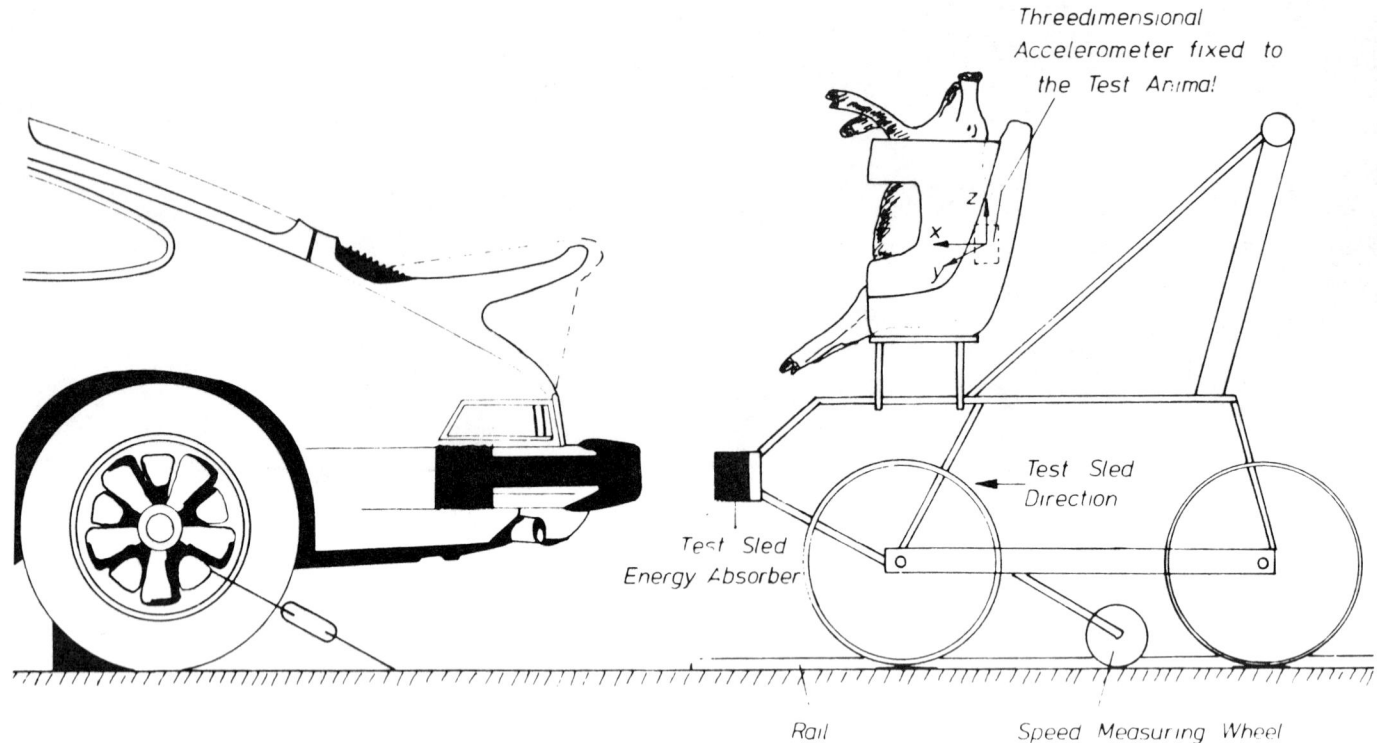

Fig. 11 - Test configuration

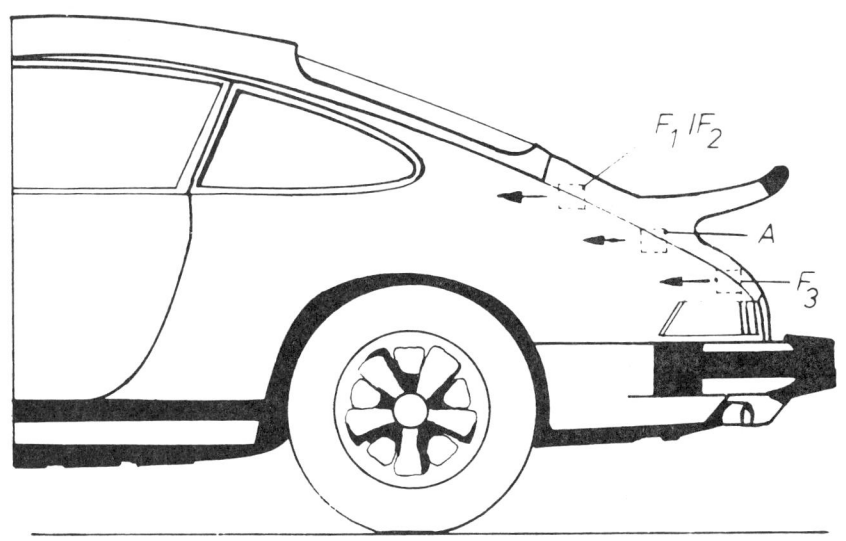

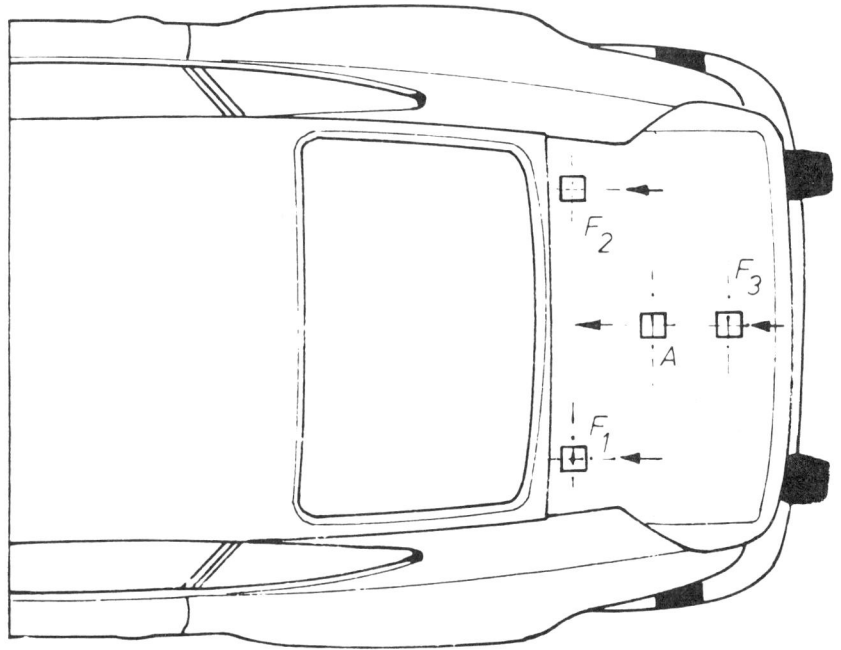

F_1, F_2, F_3 = Force Sensors

A = Acceleration Sensor

Fig. 12 - Location of sensors for forces and acceleration on the rear of the vehicle

sensors were mounted in the area between the engine lid and the vehicle body structure. In addition, it was necessary to take into consideration the forces resulting from the acceleration of the engine lid. This was calculated using the formula $F_4 = m \cdot a$, taken from the recordings of the acceleration sensor located at the mass center of the lid.

Thus, the resulting impact force acting upon the animal is:
$$F_R = F_1 + F_2 + F_3 + F_4$$
where the individual forces are:
- F_1 = force measured at the upper left sensor
- F_2 = force measured at the upper right sensor
- F_3 = force measured at the lower center sensor
- F_4 = mass force (see above)

The measured signals were recorded by a PCM system and displayed on an XY-recorder via a process computer.

ANIMAL - A triaxial acceleration sensor (Endevco, model 2262-2oo) was fastened to the back of the test animal. The individual acceleration values were processed by means of a computer which determined the resulting total acceleration curves.

FILM RECORDING - Three high-speed cameras (Stalex) and a video-recorder were used.

TEST ANIMALS

As test animals the so-called Göttingen minipigs were used, which in our experiments correspond to an 8-12 year old child (GLODECK, Personal Communication) as far as weight, height, and age are concerned.

RESULTS

The most important data obtained are summarized in Table 1. Selected tests are discussed in detail following the presentation of results.

ANALOGOUS to the WAYNE-STATE brain tolerance curve (23) according to which for impact durations of 3, 5, and 2o ms accelerations of 15o, 1oo, and 5o g are tolerable respectively, the impact forces of the present tests were evaluated for the same durations. The values obtained are given in Table 1.

The injuries determined in the course of the microscopical and patho-morphological examination of the organs were classified according to AIS. With all tests except test no. 7_2, the ge-

Table 1 - Summary of All Tests

Test No.	Spoiler Material	Spoiler Mass [kg]	Mass of Test Subject [kg]	Impact Velocity [km/h]	Maximum Spoiler Acceleration [g]	Maximum Total Force to Spoiler [N]	Maximum Impact Force to Test Subject [N]	Maximum Resulting Acceleration of Test Subject [g]	Typical Impact Forces (Duration) 3 ms [N]	5 ms [N]	20 ms [N]	Point of Impact+ [mm]	Maximum Horizontal Deformation Test Subject [mm]	Spoiler [mm]	Remarks	Injuries
1	GRP Spoiler	8.5	14	22.6	6.8	1620	1750	-	1550	1500	1400	+55	112	79	Tolerance limit just attained, AIS 3, camera 2 failed	Acute shock, shock organs, microscopic spleen rupture, haematoma at the abdominal wall
2	GRP Spoiler	8.5	15	23.2		≈2800			2750□	2720□	2250□	+60	119	68	Tolerance limit exceeded, AIS 4	Acute shock, shock organs, spleen rupture, blood release into the abdominal cavity
3	PUR Spoiler	16.5	12.5	21.7	6.2	1400	2300	19	2100	2100	500	-30	96	104	Animal was already dead when test was carried out	No histological examination, animal died prior to test
4	PUR Spoiler	16.5	14	22.6	9.0	2440	3750	23	3300	2700	900	+10	112	97	Tolerance limit slightly exceeded, AIS 3-4, multiple injuries	Acute shock, shock organs, microscopic rupture of spleen and kidney, haemorrhage of the suprarenal gland capsula
5	Simulated Notch Back	16.1	12.5	22.9	7.5	2300	3500	39	3250	2800	1800	+75	86	0	Large-area impact, hindlegs leaning against rear end, AIS 3-4, multiple injuries	Severe acute shock, shock organs, contusion of liver, kidneys and suprarenal glands, blood and fluid agglomeration in the abdominal cavity
6	GRP Spoiler	13.2	11.35	15.6	6.5	1435	1880	36	1580	1360	800	+60	No evaluation possible		Tolerance limit just attained, AIS 3; camera 1 and 2 failed, films failed	Acute shock, shock organs, microscopic spleen rupture
7₁	GRP Spoiler	13.2	12.55	15.2	6.1	1780	2480	54.5	2300	2160	1240	-	No evaluation possible		Animal fell under spoiler, camera 2 failed	
7₂	GRP Spoiler	13.2	12.55	16.3	4.6	1150	1540	29	1220	1060	860	+60	125	56	Below tolerance limit, AIS 2-3, haematoma at the abdominal wall	Subacute to acute shock, shock organs, haematoma at the abdominal wall
8	PUR Spoiler	16.7	13.05	13.5	2.0	760	960	11.7	950	920	610	+10	118	76	At tolerance limit, AIS 3, camera 2 failed	Acute shock, shock organs, contusion of the kidneys, perirenal haemorrhage
9	PUR Spoiler	16.7	15.45	14.1	2.0	900	1180	18.4	1080	960	740	+20	117	89	At tolerance limit, AIS 3, camera 2 failed	Subacute to acute shock, shock organs, microscopic spleen rupture, kidney contusion, haematoma at the abdominal wall
10	without Spoiler	16.7	13.55	14.4	2.86	230	450	10.7	300	160	160	-	No evaluation possible		Radial acceleration, tolerance limit exceeded, not recorded, AIS 3-4, camera 2 failed	Severe acute shock, shock organs, incomplete rupture of the aorta wall, kidney contusion
11	without Spoiler	7.7	13.95	16.8	4.48	610	960	25.4	820	700	200	-	No evaluation possible		At tolerance limit, AIS 3, camera 2 failed	Acute shock, shock organs, contusion of the suprarenal gland cortex, contusion of the stomach wall (heart contusion?)
12	Simulated Notch Back	19.7	11.65	14.1	2.85	1440	1940	24.5	1700	1440	960	+75	79	0	At tolerance limit, AIS 3, camera 2 failed	Acute shock, shock organs, contusion of kidneys, spleen and (heart?)

Remark: The impact forces acting upon the test subject were ascertained using the following equation:

$$F_R = F_1 + F_2 + F_3 + F_4$$

+ Distance at impact between penis attachment point and upper edge of spoiler (Positive: Upper edge of spoiler above penis attachment)

□ Forces to Spoiler $F = F_1 + F_2 + F_3$

$10 \text{ N} \triangleq 1.02 \text{ kp}$

neral shock symptoms and the morphological state of the shocked organs correspond to AIS-classification 3: "severe" without danger to life. In the same category belong the organ contusions, i.e. traumatical tissue haemorrhages in the organ, mostly subcapsular drip haemorrhages, and microscopically small (no macroscopical) dehiscencies of the organ capsule. The macroscopical spleen rupture (test no. 2) belongs to AIS-category 4. Cases with extremely severe morphological shock symptoms of all shocked organs and wi th category-3 injuries to several intra-abdominal organs (liver, kidneys, spleen, suprarenal glands), however, without macrsocopical organ ruptures and subsequent release of blood into the abdominal cavity, were attributed AIS category 3-4.

Taking these criteria into consideration the tolerance limit of test no. 1 as compared to test no. 2 is located between AIS 3 (tolerable) and AIS 4 (with danger to life). According to the film evaluation, tests 1 and 2 were similar to each other: in both cases the forelegs were hanging down at the moment of impact against the GRP spoiler, and there was a difference of only 5 mm between the impact height on the animal bodies.

Unfortunately, during both tests the acceleration sensors fixed to the animal body failed, so that the resulting animal acceleration could not be evaluated. In addition, during test no. 2 the acceleration sensor mounted to the spoiler failed, and so the overall impact forces acting upon the animal could not be determined. Thus the only comparable value was the total horizontal force on the spoiler, while neglecting the additional force resulting from the spoiler acceleration, which in test no. 1 with a maximum value of $F_1 + F_2 + F_3$ amounted to 13o N.

According to these results, the tolerance limit for an impact against a GRP spoiler with defined deformation characteristics and mass is situated between a 5 ms impact load of 15oo N and a 5 ms impact load of 2943 N. The differing impact loads with identical test conditions might be due to the somewhat higher impact vel ocity and the higher animal weight in test no. 2.

Test no. 4 with a total impact force on the spoiler of 2o8o N for a duration of up to 5 ms corresponds to test no. 2. The injury severity of both tests is comparable (AIS 4 with test no. 2; AIS 3-4 with test no. 4). The tolerance limit for life-threatening injuries had been just exceeded. This was demonstrated by multiple microscopical organ ruptures, which had occurred at 27o1 N for a duration of up to 5 ms.

This tolerance limit is also valid for test no. 8, which despite the lower animal weight, the 4o % lower velocity, and an impact load of only 92o.5 N for up to 5 ms (as compared to 27o1 N in test no. 4), resulted in a kidney contusion and must be classified into AIS category 3. While in test no. 4 the spoiler acceleration, the total forces at the spoiler, as well as the resulting impact force curves, followed by the time-lagged animal acceleration, showed distinct peaks, test no. 8 was characterized by an extremely flat curve.

Obviously a tolerance limit had been reached for these test parameters (v + m of the animal). The energy absorption took place mainly at the relatively soft spoiler edge, contrary to test no. 4 where the spoiler was deformed due to the higher impact velocity. The curves also show that tolerance cannot be defined using the criteria of impact force and duration only, but that the different deformation characteristics and masses of the various rear end configurations result in highly differing recordings.

The maximum deceleration at the animal's back was time-lagged as compared to the spoiler readings. The animal's body was impressed down to the spine and during this phase the abdominal injuries were caused. However, it is only at the moment of impact against the spinal column that the deceleration at the animal's back reached a maximum value.

As compared to the GRP spoiler the force increase is much more rapid during a 22.6 km/h impact against the PUR spoiler of approximately double the mass. This conclusion is also confirmed by test no. 3. As the animal had died during the anesthesia, the test was carried out using the cadaver. Prior to the test, an additional acceleration sensor was surgically installed into the animal's body in front of the spine, and the abdominal wall was closed. During the impact of the abdominal wall and organs against the spoiler, the surgically sutured wall burst open, releasing the intestines. When the impact finally reached the spinal column, the acceleration sensors showed their maximum values as did the spoiler sensors, whereas the maximum recordings of the acceleration sensor at the animal's back was slightly lagging behind.

In other words, immediately upon the impact, the impact force first increased during the impression of the abdominal wall, it then decreased while the abdominal wall burst and the intestines welled out, to increase steeply again when hitting the spinal column.

In test no. 5, the tolerance limit was overstepped resulting in severe shock symptoms and multiple organ contusions (AIS 3-4), when the test animal was projected against a simulated practically rigid rear trunk configuration with an impact force of 2801 N for a duration of 5 ms. The impact against the rigid simulated rear trunk resulted in a profound impression of the animal body and, as compared to the previous test, the recordings showed pronounced peaks. It must be noted that the deceleration of 30 g in X-direction remained constant for 9.5 ms. Thus the impact forces up to 5 ms and 20 ms were specially high, despite the fact that the hindlegs were forced against the cross panel above the bumper. Due to the impact against the overall body surface, however, the force was widely distributed. This caused very severe shock symptoms and multiple organ contusion but in neither case did the injury severity overstep AIS category 3.

As far as tests 10 and 11 are concerned, the measured values do not correspond to the forces acting at the moment of impact. With test no. 10 e.g., the hindlegs hit the engine lid immediately above its lower edge, the entire animal body was subjected to a radial acceleration and then fell heavily onto the slanted surface of the engine lid, having an inclination of 30 degrees. Thus only part of the forces acting in horizontal direction could be registered by the force and acceleration sensors which picked up horizontal movements only. The partial rupture of the abdominal aorta was the result of the considerable blunt force acting upon a wide region of the animal body.

TEST NO. 1 - (Measured data can be taken from Table 1 and Figure 13)

Film Evaluation - The safety belts were released too early. The forelegs were hanging down at the moment of impact so that the spoiler first hit the forelegs and then the abdomen about 55 mm above the penis attachement. The animal slid over the horizontal surface of the spoiler until the inguinal region reached the rear spoiler edge. With the upper part of its body still on the spoiler surface, the lower portion then raised with stretched hindlegs, executing a counterclockwise turn of 180 degrees and dropped down to the spoiler in a transverse direction with its head to the left and its back first to the rear and then turned upwards.

The Autopsy revealed neither blood in the abdominal cavity nor haemorrhages or ruptures of abdominal organs; there was only a haematoma at the left flank below the 12th rib.

The Histological Examination of heart, liver, kidneys, spleen lungs, muscles, subcutane fatty tissues and a small mesenterial lymphatic ganglion revealed that all organs were in a state of acute shock. The organ changes had occurred immediately before the dissection. The spleen showed so-called pulpa haemorrhages which are also a typical shock symptom. In some places, however, small ruptures were found on the spleen capsula which led to slight drip haemorrhages. Sporadically disseminated intravascular clots of blood were found in the kidneys. They are rather to be attributed to a vascular-neurotic shock than to a lesion caused by mechanical contusion. Of great interest in the framework of the general shock symptoms was the beginning hypoxic lesion of the myocardial parenchyma.

Summary - The application of a maximum load of 175o N resp. of 15oo N for a duration of 5 ms led to a haematoma at the left abdominal wall and to microscopically small ruptures of the spleen with subsequent drip haemorrhage. Thus the level had just reached the tolerance limits of a spleen rupture. The overall impression is that of general shock symptoms accompanied by moderate organ shocks.

TEST NO. 2 - (Measured data can be taken from Table 1 and Figure 14)

The maximum impact force acting upon the animal could not be evaluated due to a technical defect. As the maximum horizontal force acting upon the spoiler was about 28oo N, the impact force to which the animal was subjected must therefore in any case have been higher.

Film Evaluation - As in test no. 1 the retaining belts were once again released too early. The forelegs were hanging down at the moment of impact so that they hit the spoiler edge first, followed by the abdomen. The secondary impact hit the animal at about 6o mm above the penis attachment which is somewhat lower than with test no. 1. With the front part of the body lying on the spoiler surface, the rear body part rose with stretched hindlegs, describing a steep spiral followed by counterclockwise turn. The animal's head executed a similar movement in the same direction with the front body part still lying on the spoiler. The rear body part then fell vertically pulling the front part down from the spoiler edge with the animal's back turned to the left side. Finally the animal fell onto its hind part and then backwards into the hollow between the two rubber foam pads on the sled guiding rail.

The Autopsy revealed a spleen rupture with a haemorrhage in the abdominal cavity.

The Histological Examination showed general pathological and morphological symptoms of an acute to subacute shock. The subcutaneous tissue of the abdominal wall showed small streaky

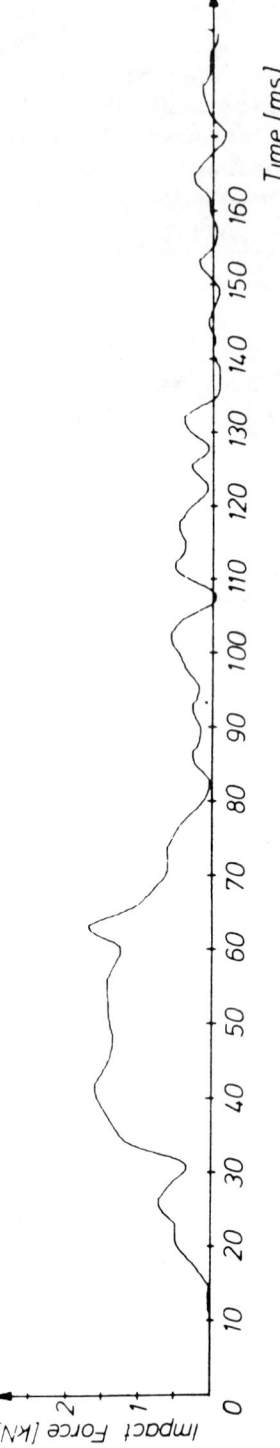

Fig. 13 - Force-time history from test 1, GRP-spoiler

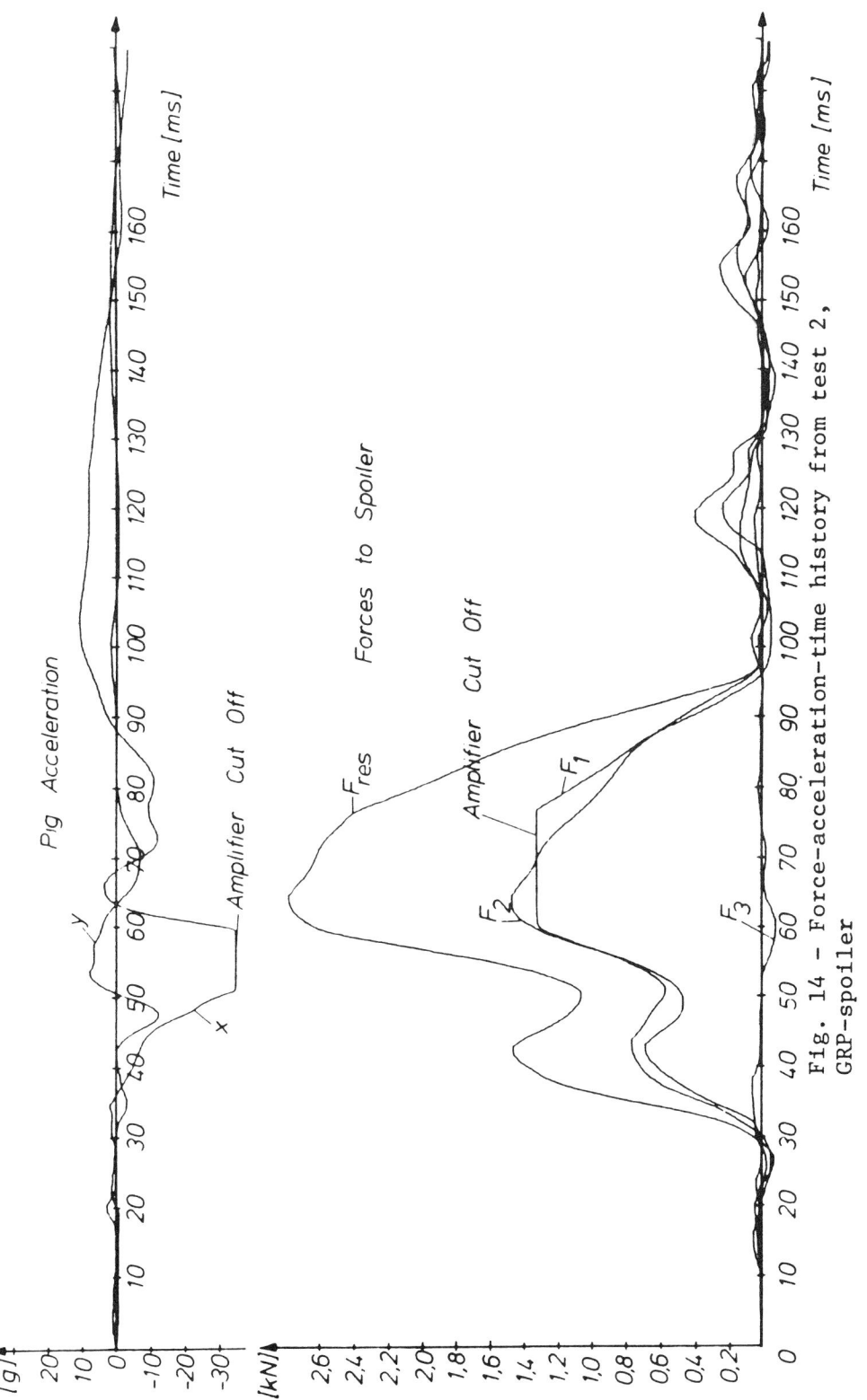

Fig. 14 - Force-acceleration-time history from test 2, GRP-spoiler

traumatic haemorrhages.

Summary - Unfortunately, the measured values of the impact forces acting upon the animal could not be evaluated with sufficient accuracy. Their lower limit of 2750 N, however, should have exceeded the values of test no. 1 by about 981 N. Again the forelegs were hanging down at the moment of impact. The point of maximum deformation of the animal's abdomen is located somewhat lower than with test no. 1. The biomechanical load not only caused general shock symptoms accompanied by organ shocks but also an unequivocal spleen rupture with haemorrhage into the abdominal cavity. The tolerance limit which had been just approached in test no. 1 was clearly overstepped in test no. 2

TEST NO. 4 - (Measured data can be taken from Table 1 and Figures 16 and 17)

Film Evaluation (Figure 15) - In the first phase following the animal's impact against the spoiler edge, its upper body part stretched horizontally on the spoiler surface. The animal hit the rear window with its snout and its lower body part rose describing a steep spiral movement. The whole body turned around and remained lying on the spoiler.

The Autopsy revealed no signs of tissue contusion of the abdominal wall and the interior organs.

The Histological Examination of the left kidney showed several microscopical dehiscencies and an almond-shaped drip haemorrhage in the area of the capsula. The same applied to the spleen, while the left suprarenal gland showed a surface haemorrhage of the outer capsula. All three organs suffered traumatic consequences. In addition, microscopic signs of an acute shock were found.

Summary - Test no. 4, as compared to test no. 8, proved that greater forces and decelerations result in more severe injuries. The injured organs showed microscopical signs of contusion with capsula bursts and haemorrhages, but no severe ruptures with blood in the abdominal cavity. The admissible tolerance limit had been just overstepped.

TEST NO. 8 - (Measured data can be taken from Table 1 and Figure 18)

Film Evaluation - The point of impact was located approximately 10 mm above the penis attachment. The impact resulted in a deep impression of the abdomen an d a distinct deformation of the spoiler edge. Upon the impact, the animal's upper body part fell onto the horizontal spoiler surface with the snout hitting

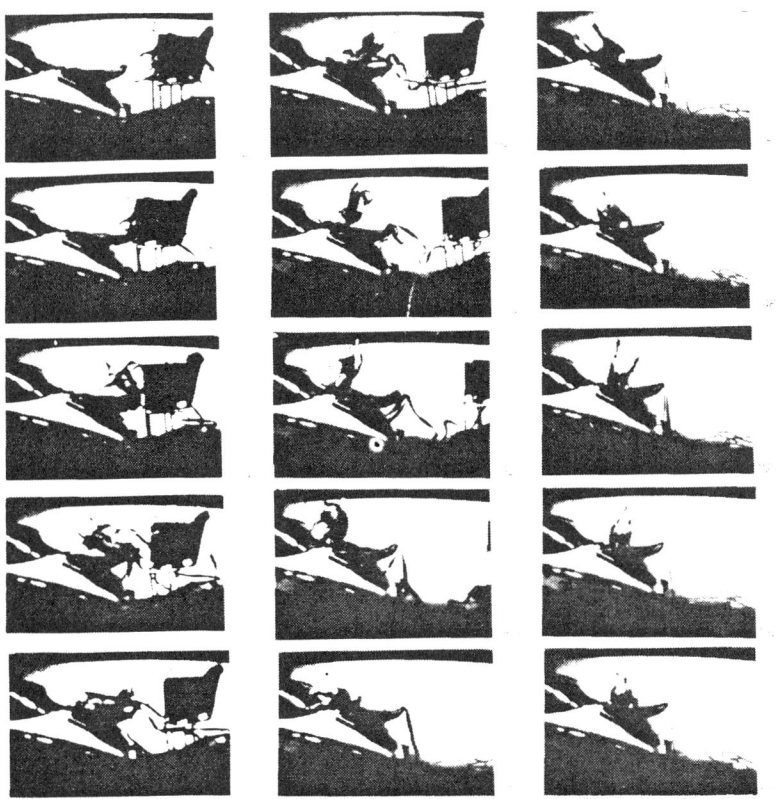

Fig. 15 - Motion sequence from test 4, PUR-spoiler

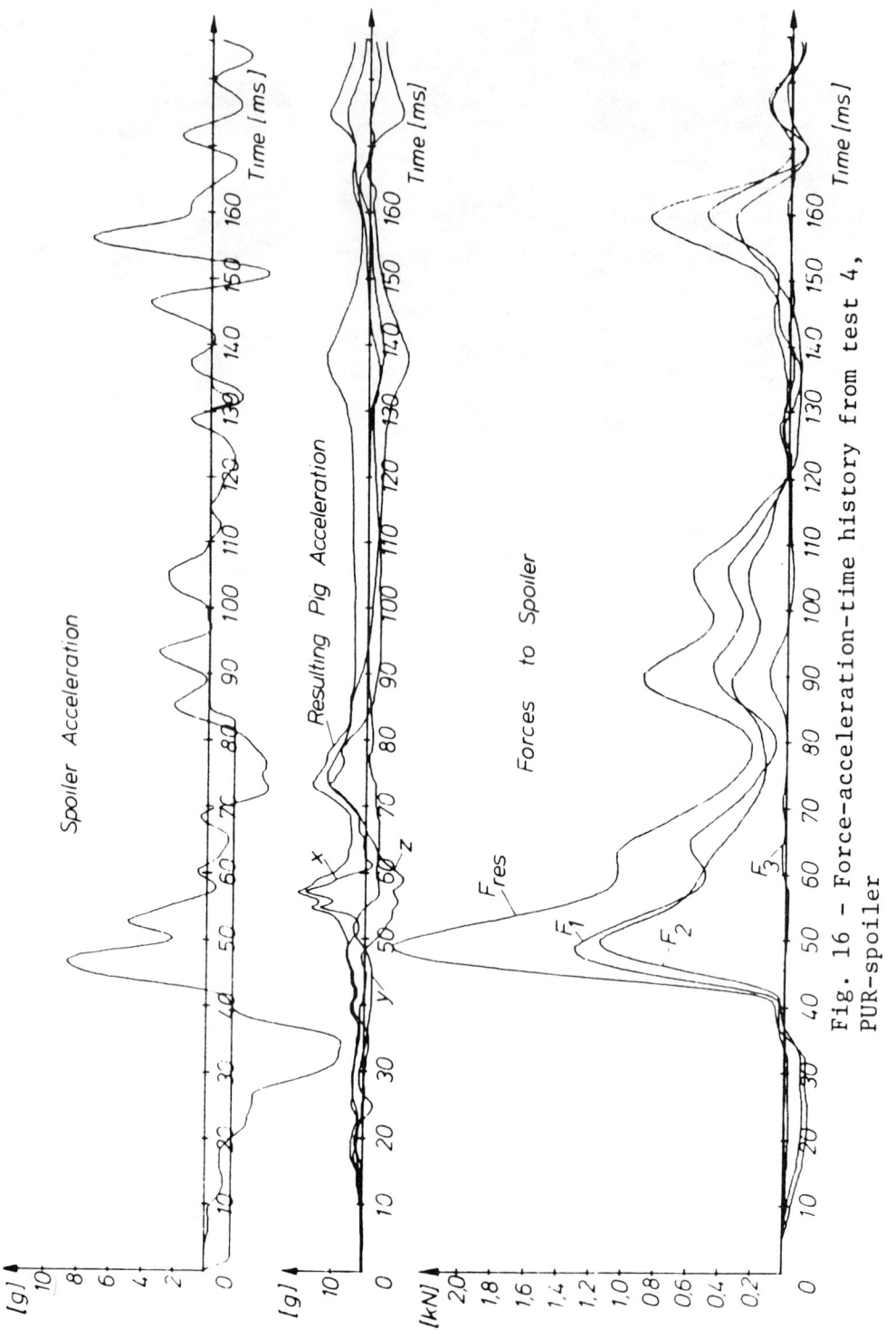

Fig. 16 - Force-acceleration-time history from test 4, PUR-spoiler

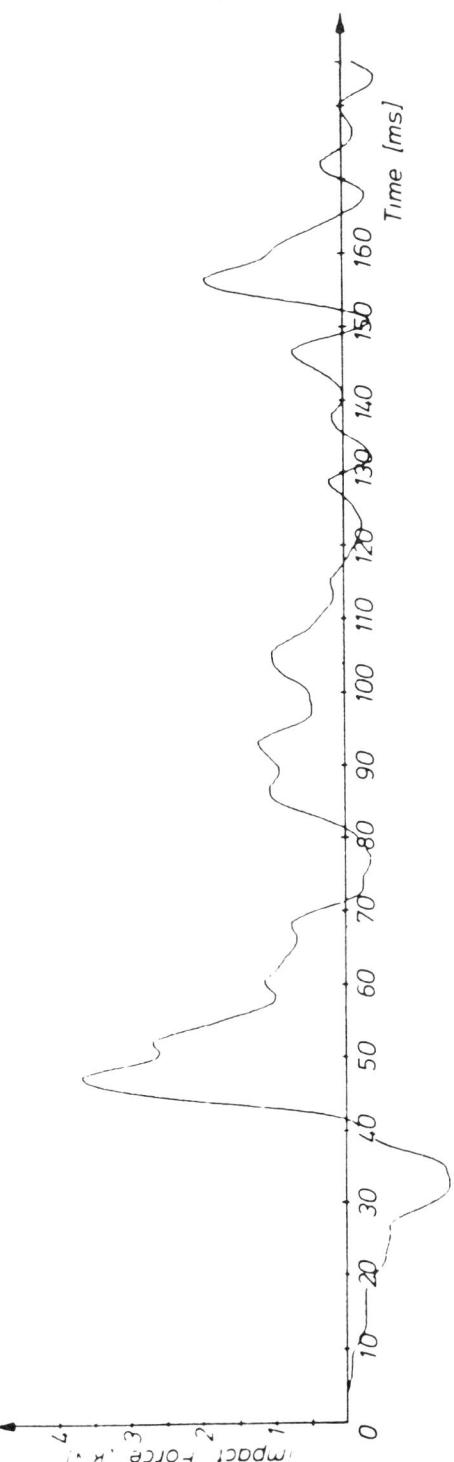

Fig. 17 - Force-time history from test 4, PUR-spoiler

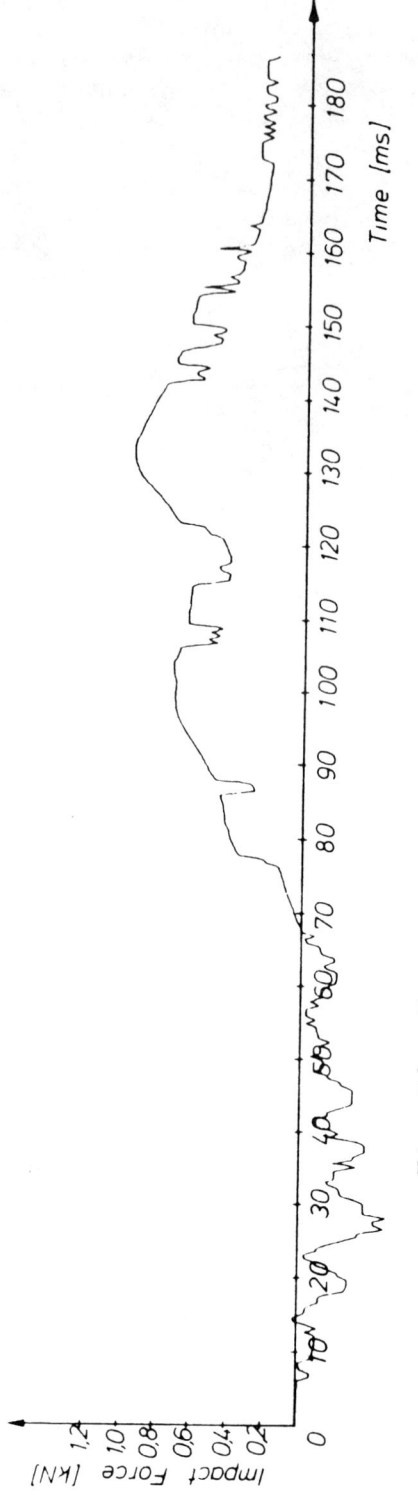

Fig. 18 - Force-time history from test 8, PUR-spoiler

against the air inlet grill of the engine lid. The head was slightly turned to the right and the lower part of the body fell slowly to vertical position. The upper body portion remained on the spoiler surface with the rear part hanging down over the spoiler edge. This position caused the rather deep impression of the animal's abdomen.

The Autopsy revealed neither organ lesions nor interior haemorrhages.

The Histological Examination revelaed signs of an acute shock for all examined organs. In one kidney, a diffuse haemorrhage had occurred, while a haematoma had formed under the mucous membrane of the renal pelvis, and the adjacent perirenal fatty tissue was interspersed with fresh haemorrhages. The cardiac muscle showed subendocardial haemorrhages which number among the histological shock symptoms but may also be caused by an accident trauma. No injuries were found at the point of impact on the abdominal wall.

Summary - As compared to the other examinations and the resulting diagnosis, the measured values were below the threshold. Nevertheless, no bursting but an unequivocal contusion of the kidney had occurred. The comparison between this test and test no. 4 with PUR spoiler and an impact velocity of 22.6 km/h led to an astonishing result. While with test no. 4 the spoiler acceleration as well as the total force showed several peaks, followed by time-lagged corresponding animal accelerations, test no. 8 was characterized by an extremely flat curve. It is assumed that with the parameters v and m of the animal a certain tolerance limit had just been reached as far as the injury symptoms are concerned. The energy absorption was mainly effected by the relatively soft spoiler edge, whereas with test no. 4 a much greater deformation of the spoiler took place, due to the higher impact velocities.

TEST NO. 5 - (Measured data can be taken from Table 1 and Figure 2o)

Film Evaluation (Figure 19) - The deep impression of the animal body was followed by a recoil movement caused by the impact against the rigid rear trunk configuration. The lower body part first rose, describing a spiral movement, then dropped down and hit the ground with its bottom.

The Autopsy showed slightly bloody ascites but no macroscopic organ bursts were found. However, a pronounced hyperaemia of the entire mesentery region was noticed with a subcapsular haematoma (2 cm) situated centrally on the convex side of the

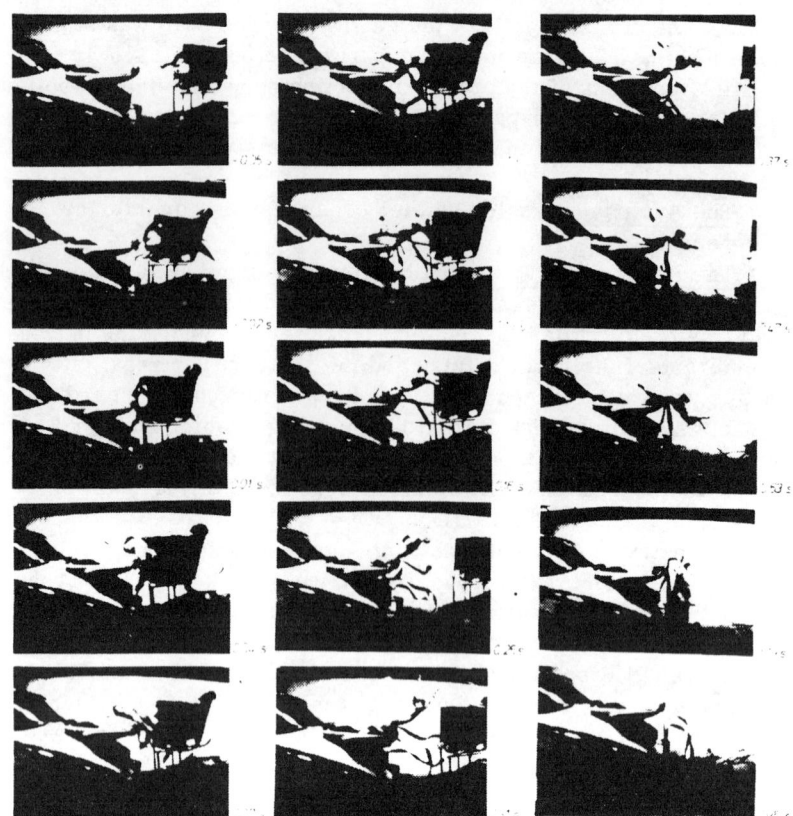

Fig. 19 - Motion sequence from test 5, simulated standard trunk configuration

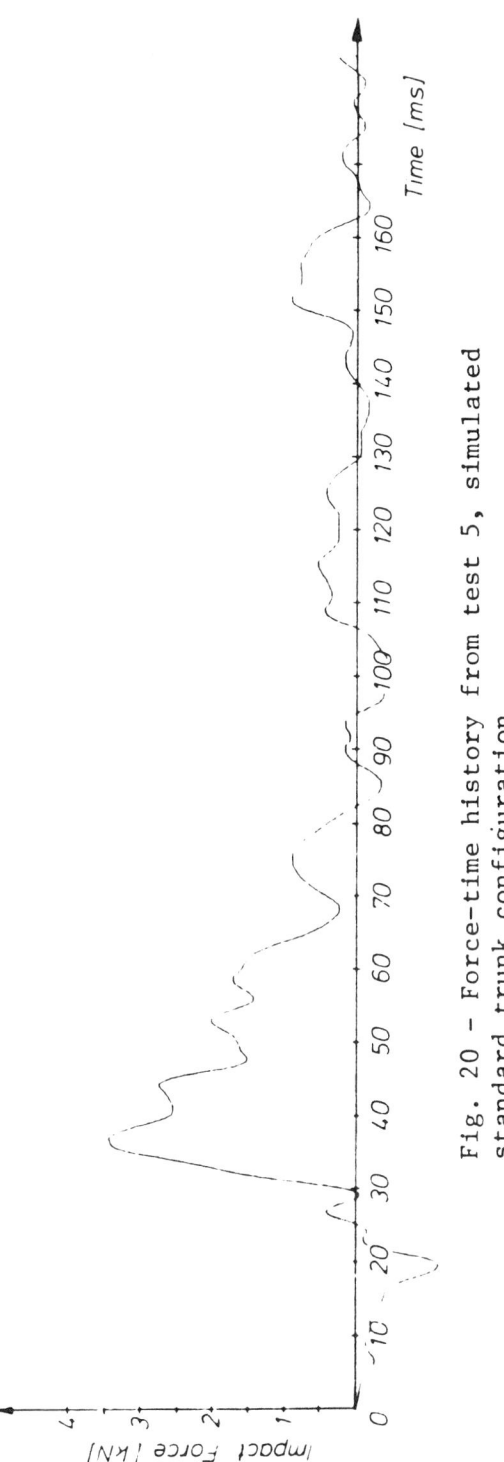

Fig. 20 - Force-time history from test 5, simulated standard trunk configuration

left kidney.

The Histological Examination revealed small capsular drip haemorrhages of the liver, indicating a liver contusion but no rupture. Streaky haemorrhages were found in the vicinity of the suprarenal glands as well as in its subcutaneous tissue and also in the suprarenal pulpa cortex. While the subcutaneous haemorrhage was certainly due to a trauma, the cortex haemorrhage might also have been caused by shock, showing the same symptoms. The overall histological examination revealed that the abdominal region had suffered a considerable blunt force. The shock symptoms were more pronounced than with the previous tests.

Summary - The considerable forces which were experienced during the impact against the simulated rear trunk, caused severe general shock symptoms. Due to the distribution of forces to the animal body and the energy absorption influenced by the hindlegs and the pelvis, only slight signs of contusion were found on the liver, the left kidney and the left suprarenal gland.

DISCUSSION OF RESULTS

With all tests, the intensity and duration of the impact forces reached a level which caused general shock symptoms. The mechanical phenomena generating these shock symptoms are fluid movements in the organism, caused by loads of a duration of at least 2o ms. According to the present test results, the limiting values for these shock symptoms, occurring during an impact duration of up to 2o ms, are located between 588.6 N and 981 N. Tests no. 7_2 and 9 (86o N resp. 74o N , duration of 2o ms) led to slight subacute shocks. Comparable values were obtained with tests no. 6 (8oo N), no. 8 (61o N), and no. 4 (9oo N), however, with distinctly acute shock symptoms. Thus, it might be concluded, that with consideration of the deviations of the measured results and the physiological differences, the tolerance limit between a subacute and an acute shock is situated in this range (Figure 21).

In the case of the severe shock ascertained in test no. 5, the impact force was 18oo N for a duration of 2o ms. Tests no. 1o to 12 must be neglected, the recording of the measured values being incomplete.

The measured values concerning the abdominal organ injuries correspond to the investigation results obtained by TROLLOPE et al. (28), who state an impact force of 1549.9 N on the abdomi-

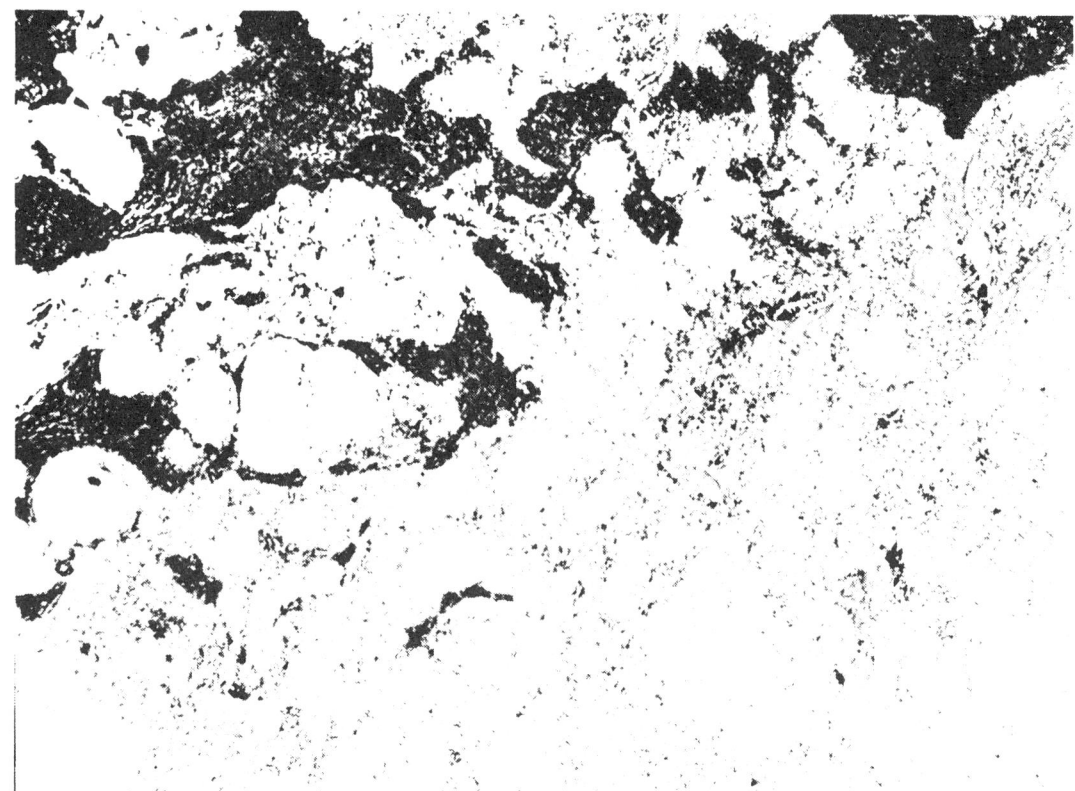

Fig. 21 - Microscopic slide of the spleen: diffuse hemorrhage into the pulp of the spleen as morphological evidence of a subacute shock syndrome. This is not caused by direct impact against the spleen

nal wall, needed to create an injury of ESI-grade 1, i.e., a small dehiscency of the kidney capsula without major haemorrhage or else a subcapsular haematoma. HELLSTROM and GRIMELIUS carried out tests using dogs of a weight of 13 - 34 kg. The animals were subjected to lateral loads of 1290 - 2580 N at 15.8 km/h provoked by a pendulum ram with a small ram surface. The results were small capsular dehiscencies with superficial parenchyma lesions.

The investigations carried out by WINDQUIST (31) using much heavier domestic pigs of weights of 28 - 89 kg show certain parallels to the present tests in the case where a 28 kg animal survived a 3335.4 N impact at 21 km/h against the 7.5 cm wide abdominal belt. The animal showed signs of a general shock and slight subserosal haemorrhages of the small intestine. As these animals have a much thicker abdominal wall and double the weight of the minipigs used in the present tests, a reduction of the impact load by 50 % with identical impact surface and velocity results in loads and injury degrees comparable to the present test results.

With test no. 12, the measured values are low, not only because of the reduced impact velocities but also due to the fact that during the impact the animal was top-heavy. Thus it was hit below the mass center of its body, and as it fell heavily on the rear trunk configuration, sliding along the horizontal surface, part of the essential horizontal forces were not recorded.

CONCLUSIONS

When projecting the Göttingen minipigs (weight range of 12.5 - 16.0 kg) at a velocity of 13.5 - 23.2 km/h against an obstacle, hitting the animal body at a 10 cm wide zone across the abdomen, the tolerance limit for an impact duration of 5 ms is located between AIS injury levels 3 (approximately 981 N) and 3-4 (approximately 1471.5 N).

The tolerance limit for the shock symptoms under determined test conditions is also approximately 981 N, for a duration of 20 ms however. With certain reserves, these data may be applied to an 8 - 12 year old child.

The impact against rigid structural elements (tests no. 5, 12, 10, 11) resulted in excessive values for durations of 3, 5 and 20 ms (test no. 5) with correspondingly severe injuries of AIS category 3-4 and extremely severe shock symptoms. The large surface impact resulted in multiple organ lesions, but did not cause ruptures of the individual organs (see Trollope (28)).

ACKNOWLEDGEMENTS

Medical staff: Mr. FINKENBEIN (medical assistant), Mr. STEINBERG

The patho-morphological tissue examinations were done by head physician Dr. med. A. TSCHAHARAGANE of the Pathological Institute of the University of Heidelberg (directed by Prof. Dr. med. DOERR).

The test animals were provided by the experimental station for livestock breeding, the Relliehausen domain of the University of Göttingen.

REFERENCES

1. "Technologien für die Sicherheit im Straßenverkehr" Study published by the Federal Department of Research and Technology, Bonn 1976.
2. C.F. Baxter, R.D. Williams, "Blunt Abdominal Trauma" J. Trauma 1961: 241
3. H.-H. Braess, "Konzeption künftiger Personenkraftwagen" Fortschrittsbericht VDI-Z, Reihe 12, No. 25 (1975)
4. H.-H. Braess, H. Burst, H. Hamm, R. Hannes "Verbesserung der Fahreigenschaften durch Verringerung des aerodynamischen Auftriebs", ATZ 1975, page 119/124
5. F. Ellendorf, F. Elsaesser, N. Parvizi, D. Smidt "Das Göttinger Miniaturschwein - Ein Laboratoriumstier mit weltweiter Bedeutung" 1. Mitteilung Züchtungskunde 49, 33 (1977)
6. E. Faerber, E. Gülich, H.A. Heger, G. Rüter "Biomechanische Belastungsgrenzen" Unfall- und Sicherheitsforschung Str. V. Heft 3, 1976, Bundesanstalt für das Straßenwesen BRD
7. G.Y. Fazekas, F. Kosa, G. Jobba, E. Meszaros, "Die Druckfestigkeit der menschlichen Leber mit besonderer Hinsicht auf die Verkehrsunfälle" z.Rechtsmed. 68, 2o7 (1971)
8. F. Glenn, Z. Mujahed, W.R. Grafe, "Trauma in Liver Injuries", J. Trauma 3, 388 (1963)
9. P. Glodeck, E. Bruns, B. Oldigs, W. Holtz "Das Göttinger Miniaturschwein - Ein Laboratoriumtier mit weltweiter Bedeutung" 1. Mitteilung, Züchtungskunde 49, 21 (1977)
1o. E. Gögler, "Chirurgie und Verkehrsmedizin" Handbuch Verkehrsmedizin, Springer-Verlag, 1968, BRD
11. L. Grimelius, G. Hellstrom, "Patho-Anatomical Changes After Closed Liver Injury: An Experimental Study on

Dogs" AF chir. Schnd. 131, 485 (1966)

12. R.H. Kennedy, "Nonpenetrating Injuries of the Abdomen" Springfield Thomas, 1960

13. E.T. Mays, " Bursting Injuries of the Liver" Arch Surg. 93, 92 (1966)

14. J.W. Melvin, R.L. Stalnaker, V.L. Roberts, M. Trollope, "Impact Injury Mechanism in Abdominal Organs" SAE Paper no. 730968 (1973), 17th Stapp Car Crash Conference

15. J.W. Melvin, D. Mohan, R.L. Stalnaker, "Occupant Injury Assessment Criteria" SAE Paper no. 750 914 (1975)

16. H.J. Mertz, Ch-K. Kroell "Tolerance of Thorax and Abdomen" in Impact Injury and Crash Protection

17. Gurdjian et al. :"Impact Injury and Crash Protection" Thomas Springfield, Ill 1970

18. J.L. Nickerson "Study on Internal Movements of the Body Occurring on Impacts" 11th Stapp Car Crash Conference

19. L.M. Patrick, H.R. Lissner, E.S. Gurdjian "Survival by Design - Head Protection" 7th Stapp Car Crash Conference

20. V.L. Roberts "Experimental Studies in Thoracic and Abdominal Injuries", the Prevention of Highway Injury, Highway Research Institute, University of Michigan, USA 221-215

21. G. Rüter, M. Hofmann "Beanspruchungsgrenzen des Menschen beim inneren Aufprall" Batelle-Institut Frankfurt/Main Brd, 1975

22. G. Schmidt, D. Kalliers "Dynamische Versuche mit Versuchspuppen und menschlichen Leichen zur Untersuchung von Verletzungsmöglichkeiten gut geschützter Fahrzeuginsassen während einer Frontalkollision" Der Verkehrsunfall, 1975, 40

23. R.G. Snyder "Human Impact Tolerance" SAE Paper no. 700398 (1970)

24. D.J. Snyder "Bowel Injuries From Automobile Seat Belts" Am J. Surg. 123, 312 (1972)

25. J.P. Stapp "Human Tolerance to Deceleration" Am. J. Surg. 93 (1957)

26. J.D. States, D.F. Huelke, L.H. Hames "The abbreviated Injury Scale (AIS)" 18th Stapp Car Crash Conference (1974)

27. A.B. Thompson "A Proposed New Concept of Estimating The Limit of Human Tolerance to Impact Acceleration" Aerospace med. 33, 1349 (1962)

28. M.L. Trollope, L.R. Stalnaker, Mc Elhaney, J.H.; R. Frey "Injury Tolerance Levels in Blunt Abdominal Trauma" IRCOBI, Amsterdam 1973

29. J. Unselm "Konstitutionskriterien bei Schweinen verschiedener Rassen" Habil-Arbeit, Landwirtschaftliche Fakultät Göttingen, 1970

3o. J. Versace "A Review of the Severity Index" 15th Stapp Car Crash Conference 1971, SAE Paper 1972

31. P.G. Windquist, P.W. Stumm, R. Hansen "Crash Injury Experiments with the Monorail Decelerator" AF techn. Report, no. AFFTC 53-7 April 27, 1953

32. A. Wisner, J. Leroy, J. Bandet "Human Impact Tolerance" SAE Paper 7oo399 (197o)

780889

Dynamic Characteristics of the Human Spine During $-G_x$ Acceleration

Naveen K. Mital, Richard Cheng, Robert S. Levine, and Albert I. King
Wayne State University

Abstract

Spinal kinematics and kinetics of human cadaveric specimens subjected to $-G_x$ acceleration are reported along with an attempt to design a surrogate spine for use in an anthropomorphic test device (ATD). There were a total of 30 runs on 9 embalmed and 2 unembalmed cadavers which were heavily instrumented. External photographic targets were attached to T1, T12 and the pelvis to record spinal kinematics. The subjects were restrained by upper and lower leg clamps attached to an impact seat equipped with a six-axis load cell.

A rigid link 486 mm long and pinned at both ends was proposed for use in an ATD as a surrogate spine. An optimization method was used to obtain the location and length of a linkage which followed the least squares path of T1 relative to the pelvis.

STATIC BENDING CHARACTERISTICS of the human spine were recently reported by Nyquist and Murton (1)* who used human volunteers as test subjects. Additional static data were provided by Mallikarjunarao et al (2) for the purpose of defining loading corridors during flexion, extension and lateral bendint. Cadaveric and living human volunteer data were acquired.

---

* Numbers in parentheses denote references at end of paper.

These studies were motivated by the need to obtain information on spinal kinematics for the design of a human-like surrogate spine. This spine should be adaptable to existing anthropomorphic test devices (ATD) which are currently equipped with a rigid 'thoracic' spine and a relatively flexible 'lumbar' segment. Since ATD's are used in an impact environment, it is necessary to study the dynamic response of the human spine. This paper provides kinematic data of cadaveric spinal response during $-G_x$ acceleration. The relative rotation of T1, T12 and the pelvis was measured along with seat pan loads and moments. These data were used to establish the relative flexibility of the thoracic and lumbar spines and to quantify resistance to flexion as a function of a hip-joint moment.

EXPERIMENTAL PROCEDURES

COORDINATE SYSTEMS - The design of a surrogate spine requires the definition of body-fixed anatomically related coordinate systems to describe the location of the spine relative to known anatomical landmarks. An ad hoc Committee of the International Workshop on Human Subjects for Biomechanical Research made recommendations for coordinate systems for the head, T1 and the pelvis. That for the head and T1 were first described by Ewing and Thomas (3).

Figure 1 shows the T1 coordinate system taken from (3). Its positive x-axis is a directed line segment connecting the midpoint of the superior and inferior corner of the posterior spinous process of T1 to the anterior-superior border of the vertebral body where the origin is located. The positive z-axis extends superiorly and is normal to the x-axis in the mid-sagittal plane which contains the above three points. The positive y-axis is directed laterally and to the left, forming a right-handed coordinate system. It is normal to the x-z plane. The same system can be used for T12.

The pelvic coordinate system has been described in detail by Padgaonkar (4) and is shown in Figure 2[†]. To locate this system with respect to the pelvis, it is necessary to define a triangular plane with vertices at the right and left anterior superior iliac spine and the midpoint of the upper edge of the public symphysis. Its positive x-axis is normal to the plane and passes through the origin which is located at the midpoint of the line joining right and left anterior superior iliac spine. The positive y-axis is along this line directed leftward, and the positive z-axis is perpendicular to the x-y plane, directed approximately in the inferior-superior direction.

[†]Courtesy of Dr. Daniel J. Thomas, NAMRL, New Orleans. Dr. Thomas is chairman of the ad hoc Committee of the IWHSBR.

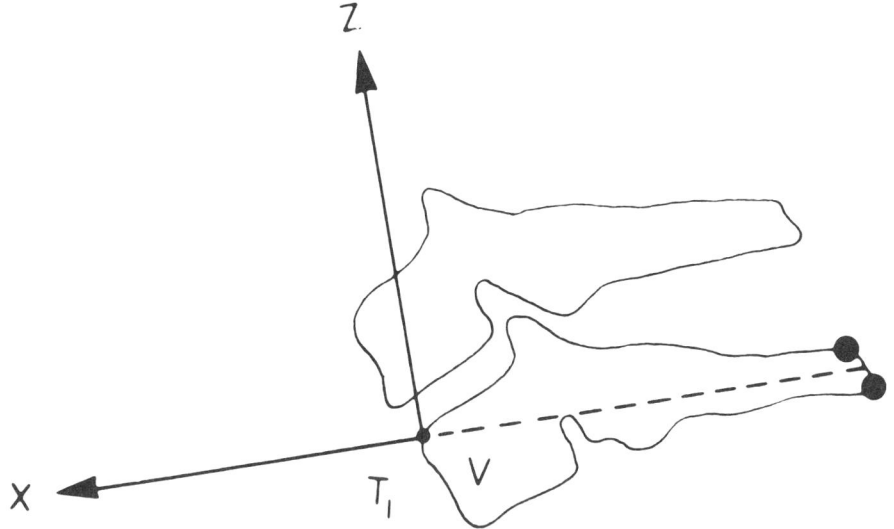

Fig. 1 - T1 anatomical coordinate system

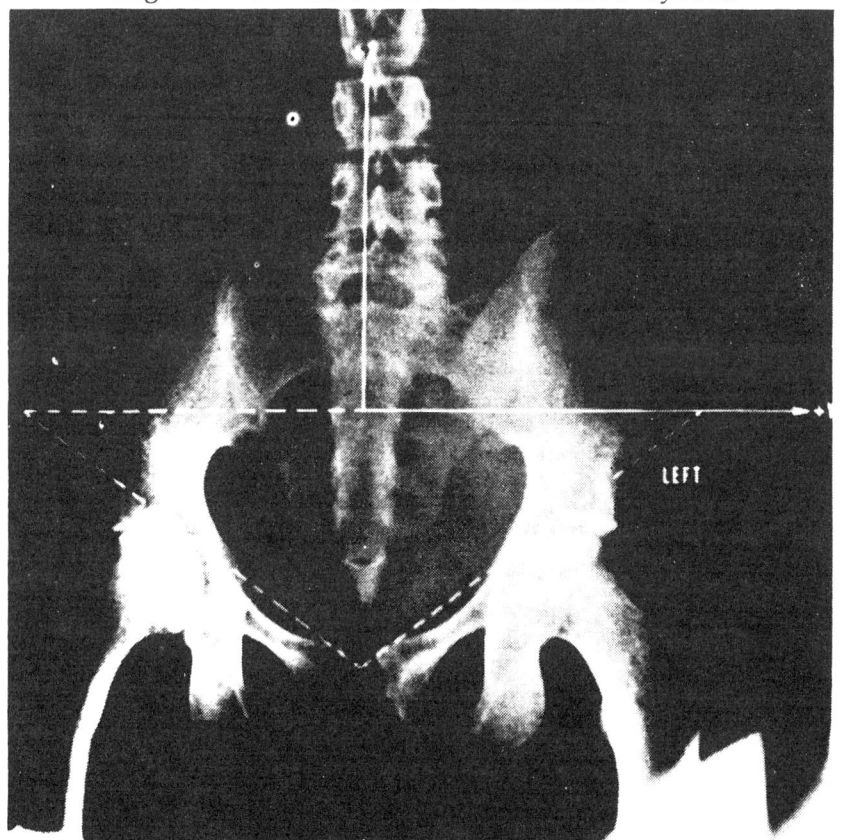

Fig. 2 - Pelvic anatomical coordinate system

The sled reference frame is also a right-handed coordinate system with the x-y plane parallel to the flat bed surface of the sled. Its positive x-axis is directed forward, in the direction of motion of the sled and the positive z-axis is directed upward, perpendicular to the x-y plane. For a forward-facing seated subject, the x-axis of the sled is approximately along the posterior-anterior direction. The inertial reference frame is assumed to have coordinate axes parallel to those of the sled reference frame. For the nine-accelerometer modules, the coordinate system described by Padgaonkar et al (5) is used. When a module is mounted on a body segment, an attempt is made to designate the axis closest to the inferior-superior direction as the z-axis.

TEST SUBJECTS - Eleven cadaveric specimens were used in this experimental test series. Nine of them were embalmed and two were unembalmed. Pertinent information regarding these cadavers is given in Table 1. There were 5 male and 6 female cadavers, with an age range of 52 to 74 years. Anthropometric measurements were made on each subject, using a predetermined list. Whole body x-rays were taken to ensure that there were no pre-existing fractures and to identify the vertebrae to be instrumented.

Radio-opaque markers in the form of thumb tacks were placed near T1 and T12 along the mid-sagittal plane to pinpoint the location of the laminae of these vertebrae on x-ray. A threaded Steinmann pin was then inserted into each lamina of T1 and T12 to act as anchors for the instrumentation mount. The same technique was used for the pelvic mount which was located opposite S2. This method of installing instrumentation mounts was found to be simple, fast and reliable. The cadaver could be lifted off the table via the T1 Steinmann pins without slippage. There was thus reasonable assurance that the motion of the mount reflected that of the vertebra on which the mount was located.

INSTRUMENTATION - Each test subject was instrumented with a nine-accelerometer module at T1, T12 and the pelvis, using Steinmann pins as anchors. A photographic target in the form of a cube was attached to each module. A typical T1 mount is shown in Figure 3. The configuration of the nine accelerometers was given by Padgaonkar et al (5) for the measurement of angular acceleration and velocity. High speed cameras were located laterally, posteriorly and overhead the seated subject to monitor motion of the targets. Other instrumentation included a sled accelerometer, a six-axis seat pan load cell, a sled velocity transducer and a time synchronization indicator to match film data with transducer data.

SLED FACILITY - All experiments were carried out on WHAM III (Wayne Horizontal Accelerator Mechanism), a flat bed sled which was accelerated to the desired speed at low acce-

Table 1 - Pertinent Data on Cadavers Used

Cadaver No.	Body Mass (kg)	Age (yrs)	Sex	Cause of Death
1	76.1	54	M	Respiratory arest
2	68.9	62	F	Coronary thrombosis
3	81.2	70	M	Cerebral infarction
4	66.7	62	M	Pulmonary carcinoma
5	70.3	62	F	Cerebral vascular thrombosis
6	107.7	52	M	Brain tumor
7	78.0	65	F	Subarachnoid hermorrhage
8	105.9	60	M	Pneumonitis
9	79.4	59	F	Cardio-respiratory failure
10*	53.8	74	F	Massive cerebral-vascular accident
11*	81.2	55	F	Respiratory arrest

* Unembalmed cadaver. All others are embalmed.

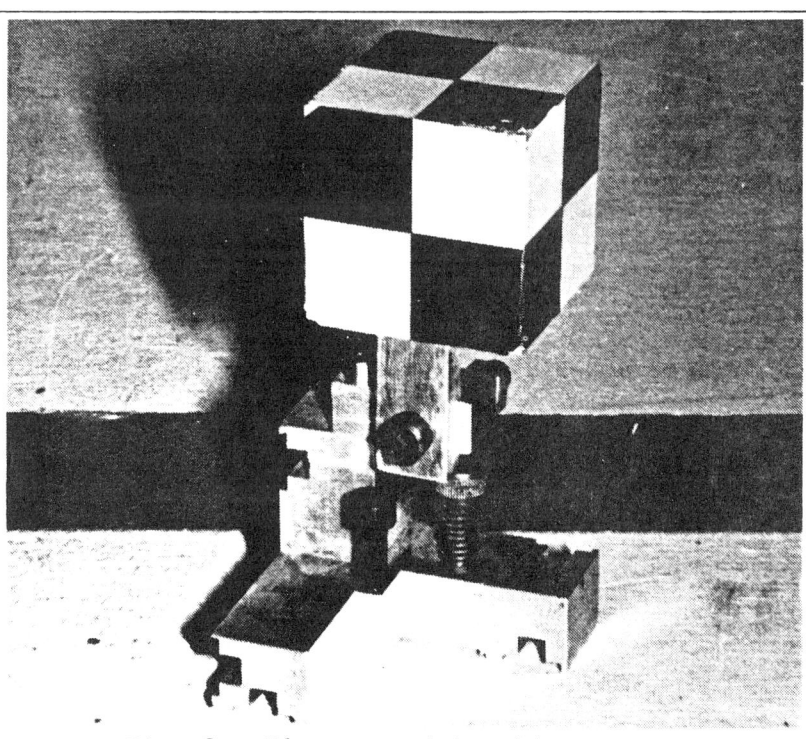

Fig. 3 - T1 mount with cubic target

leration levels and was made to impact a programmable hydraulic snubber. The impact seat and associated equipment are shown in Figure 4. The subject was seated upright and restrained by clamps which held its upper and lower legs firmly to the seat. A lapbelt was added to restrain the pelvis after several femoral fractures resulted from relatively low levels of impact. A piece of 140 mm thick urethane foam was placed above the lap of the test subject to cushion the impact of the torso on the thighs and to prevent excessive flexion of the torso. It was necessary to avoid skeletal fractures for repeated runs, generally at increasing g-levels. Furthermore, these cadaver runs were a prelude to living human volunteer runs which were scheduled for this study. The net and belts behind the subject were designed to prevent rearward rotation of the torso during rebound, without causing any injury to the test subject or damage to the accelerometer mounts.

TEST PROCEDURES - Upon completion of all preparatory work on a cadaver, it was seated on the sled and restrained by the leg clamps and the lapbelt. All transducers were balanced and calibrated before each run was made. After each run, whole-body x-rays were taken to determine any fractures that might have occurred. If no fractures were found, a second run at a predetermined higher g-level was made. Fracture of a major bone, such as the femur of a vertebra, terminated the test series. Occasionally, a cadaver would 'survive' a high g-level run and was used at lower g-levels in subsequent runs to fill out the test matrix.

RESULTS

ANTHROPOMETRIC DATA - Anthropometric data of interest consist of the lengths of the thoracic and lumbo-sacral spines. They were measured by palpation of the coccyx and the spinous processes of T12 and C7. The subjects were in a prone position. These dimensions were required to determine the length of a surrogate spine which was representative of this sample. The spinal data are shown in Table 2. The total length ranged from 515 to 698 mm. The mean and standard deviation were 596.3 and 57.8 mm respectively. A normalizing factor was computed for each spine by dividing its length by the average length. The factors are shown in the last column of Table 2.

EXPERIMENTAL DATA - The g-levels experienced by each cadaver are shown in Table 3 which divides the runs into 3 broad groups. The 12 low g runs were made at a nominal level of 5g with the exception of one run which was made at 3g. There were 8 runs in the intermediate 10g group (7-13 g) and 10 runs in the 15 - 30 g group. The peak g-levels of those

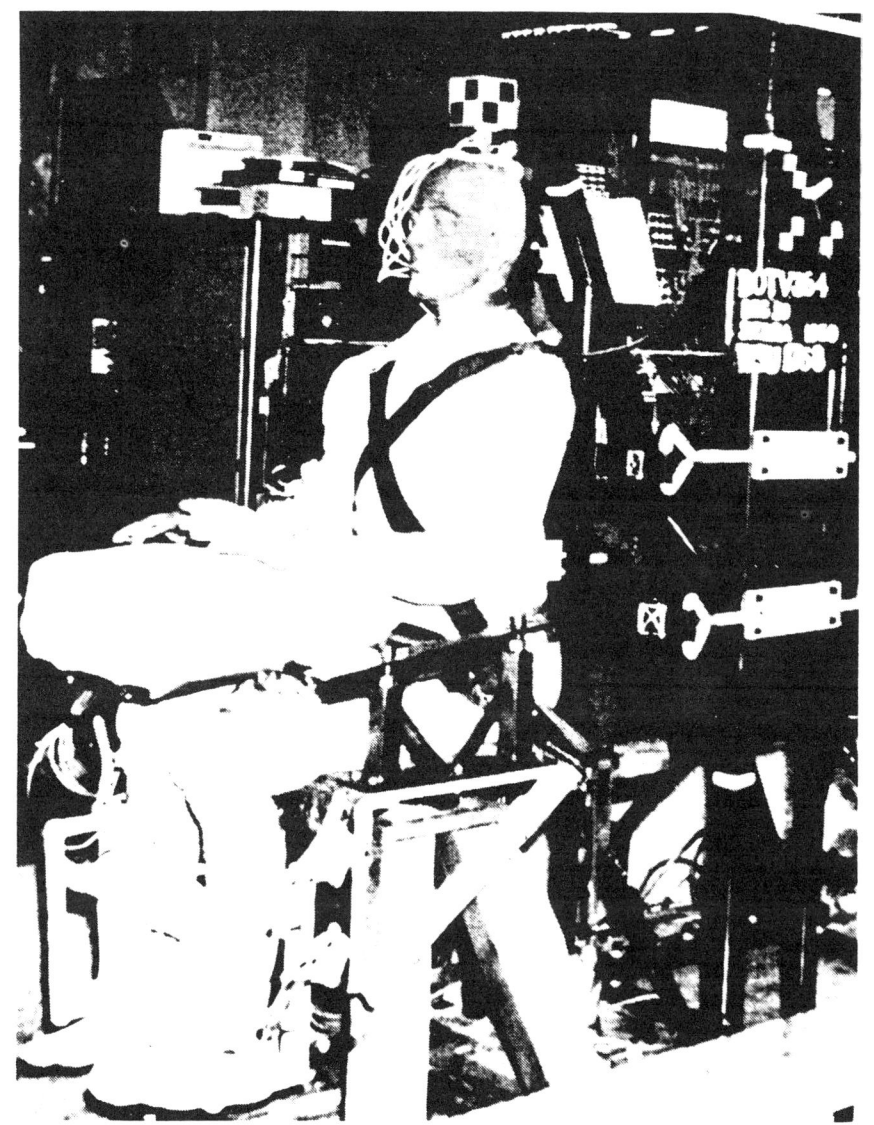

Fig. 4 - Sled setup on WHAM III with an ATD as test subject

Table 2 - Anthropometric Data on Cadaveric Spines

Spinal Length (mm)

Cadaver No.	Thoracic C7-T12	Lumbo-sacral T12 - Coccyx	Total	Normalizing Factor
1	260	315	575	0.96
2	280	296	576	0.97
3	288	315	603	1.01
4	315	336	651	1.09
5	280	315	595	1.00
6	345	353	698	1.17
7	259	402	661	1.11
8	193	322	515	0.86
9	283	299	582	0.98
10	239	267	506	0.85
11	265	332	597	1.00

Average Total Length $\pm$S.D. = 596.3 $\pm$57.8mm
Normalizing Factor = Total Length/Average Total Length

Table 3 - Summary of Experimental Runs

Cadaver No.	5g	Run Number 10g	15-30g
1	226	232	233(20g)
	231		234(15g)
2	305	303	304(15g)
3	309	305	310(24g)
		306	
4			312(16g)
5		313	314(25g)
6	316		317(25g)
7	318(3g)		
	319		
8	320		321(26g)
9	332		333(30g)
10	342		343(20g)
	344	345	
11	353	354	
		355	

in the last group are indicated next to the run number. Figure 5 shows a typical sled deceleration profile, filtered digitally at 100 Hz.

ACCELEROMETER DATA - During each run, the acceleration of T1, T12 and the pelvis was measured using a nine-accelerometer module. The z-axis accelerometer of T1 (AZ0) usually registered the largest peak acceleration. Figure 6 shows a combined plot of 7 runs on 7 different embalmed cadavers impacted at a nominal deceleration of 5g. Reproducibility of the data can be considered good, particularly during the first 150 ms of the impact, at which time the torso interacts with the lap cushion and more variation in the traces is to be expected. For the nominal 10g runs on embalmed cadavers, the acceleration traces are shown in Figure 7. The corresponding data for embalmed cadavers are shown in Figure 8.

FILM DATA - The rotation and displacement of cubic film targets were measured from high-speed film using a Vanguard film analyzer. A computer program analyzed the data and plotted the position and rotation of the T1, T12 and pelvic target with respect to an inertially-fixed frame or with respect to each other. The data can also be transformed to a specified body-fixed reference frame. The program checks for errors in the film data, thus improving their accuracy. Figure 9 show target motion of T1, T12 and the pelvis relative to the inertial reference frame, for a run made on a male embalmed cadaver. The targets are represented by solid lines during flexion and by dotted lines during extension. Figure 10 shows the motion of T1 and T12 relative to each other as well as to that of the pelvic target. It indicates that the T12/ pelvis motion is much smaller in comparison with that of T1/T12 or T1/ pelvis. Figure 11 and 12 show the target motion for an unembalmed female cadaver. If Figures 8 and 12 are compared, it is seen that for an unembalmed cadaver, the relative motion of the targets is much larger than that of an embalmed cadaver. Figure 11 also shows that for an unembalmed cadaver, the target motion during rebound or extension did not follow the flexion trajectory as closely as that of an embalmed cadaver.

LOAD CELL DATA - A six-axis load cell was used to measure seat pan forces and moments. A typical output of the load cell during impact is shown in Figures 13 and 14. The sled-fixed coordinate system was used to define the components of forces and moments measured by this load cell. Since the impacts were principally two-dimensional, F_x and F_z in Figure 13 and M_y in Figure 14 were used in data analysis. It can be seen from these figures that F_y, M_x and M_z are all small.

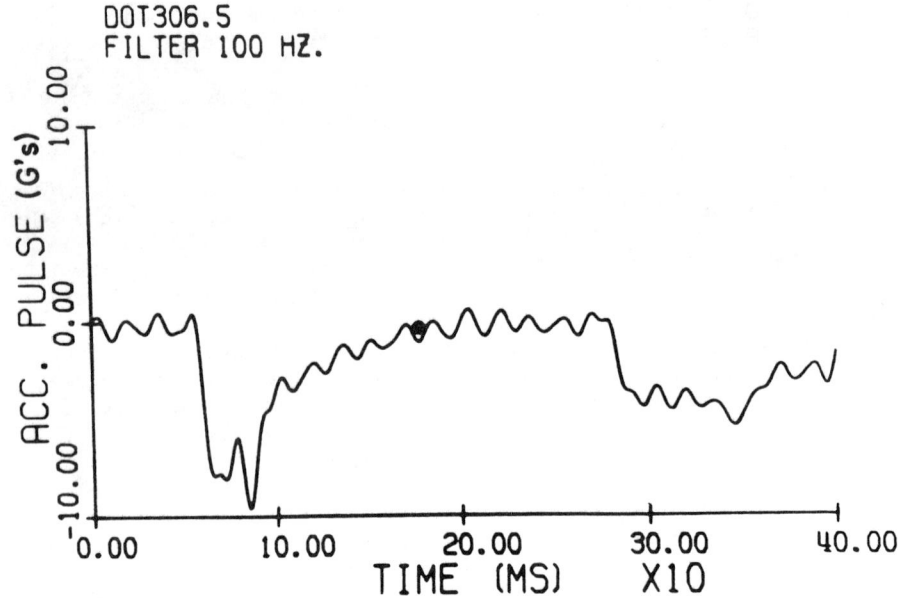

Fig. 5 - Sled deceleration profile for Run 306

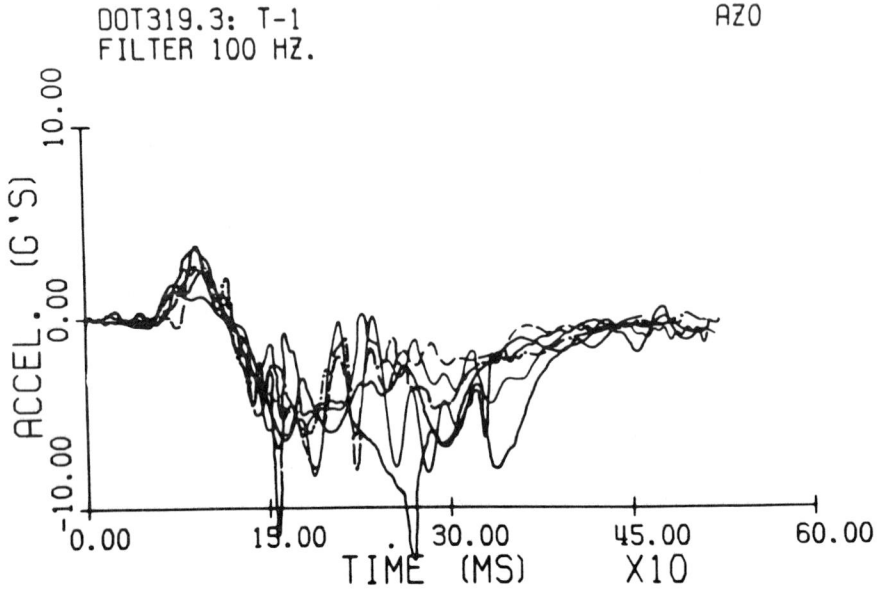

Fig. 6 - Z-axis acceleration for 10g embalmed cadaver runs

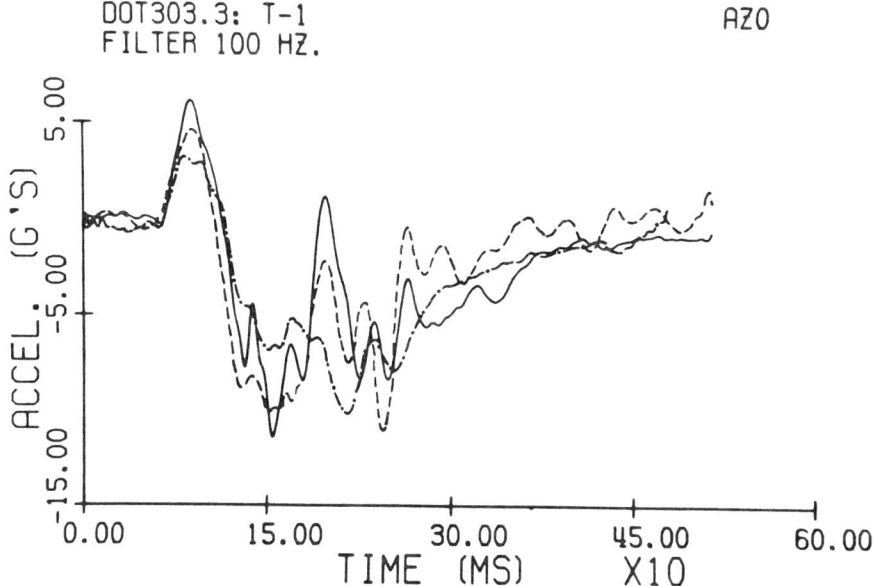

Fig. 7 - Z-axis acceleration for 10g embalmed cadaver runs

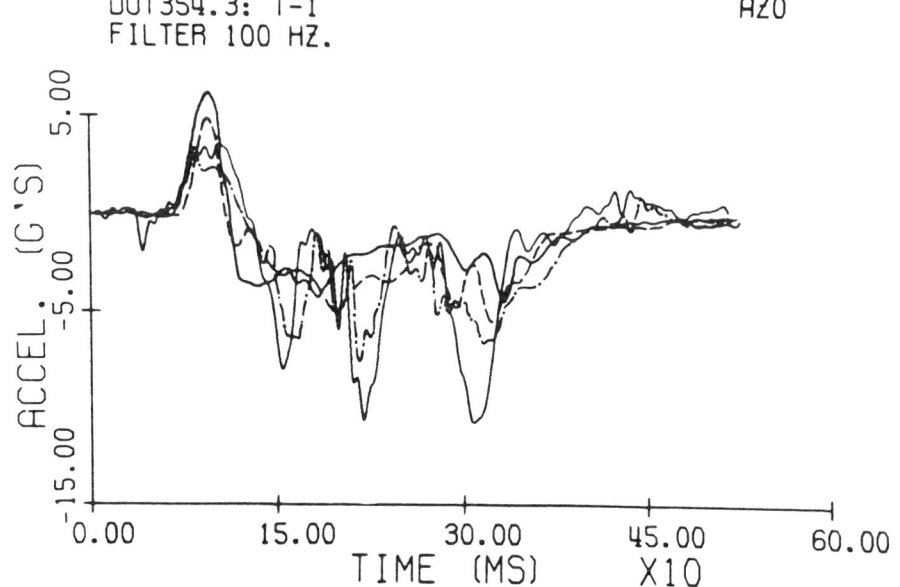

Fig. 8 - Z-axis acceleration for 10g unembalmed cadaver runs

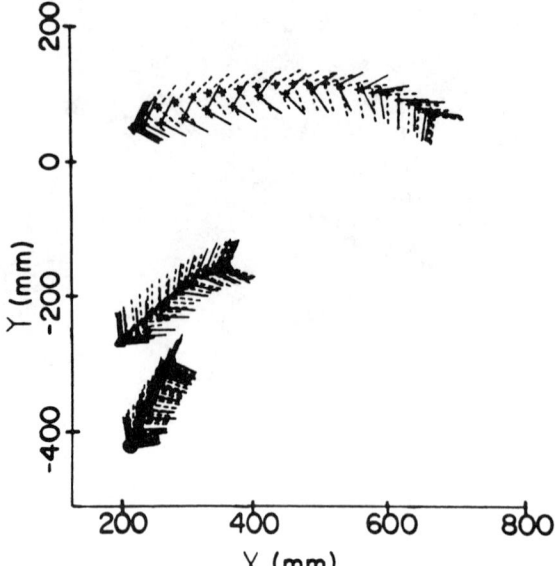

Fig. 9 - Motion of the T1, T12 and Pelvic target relative to the inertial reference frame for Run 306

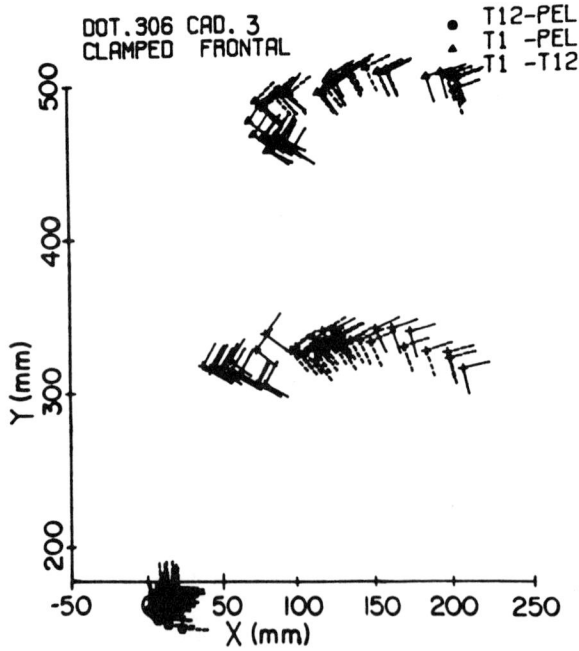

Fig. 10 - Relative motion of T1 and T12 with respect to the pelvis and T1 with respect to T12 for Run 306

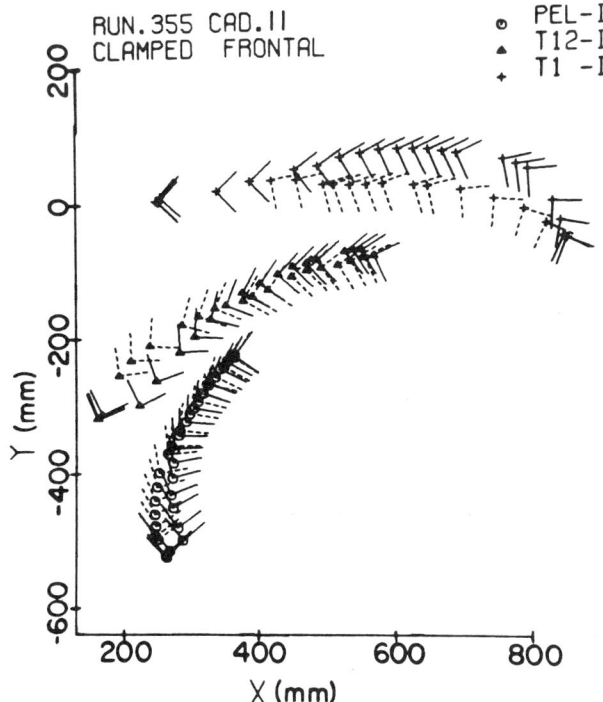

Fig. 11 - Motion of the T1, T12 and Pelvic target relative to the inertial reference frame for Run 355

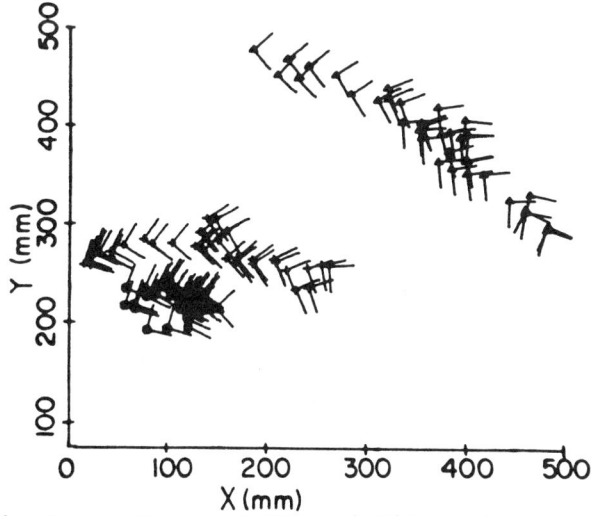

Fig. 12 - Relative motion of T1 and T12 with respect to the pelvis and T1 with respect to T12 for Run 355

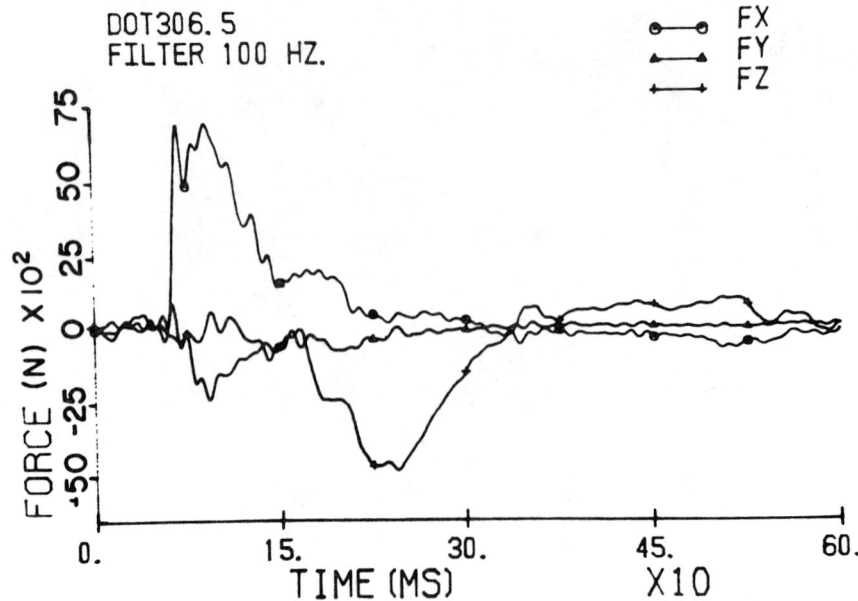

Fig. 13 - Force measurements from a six-axis seat pan load cell

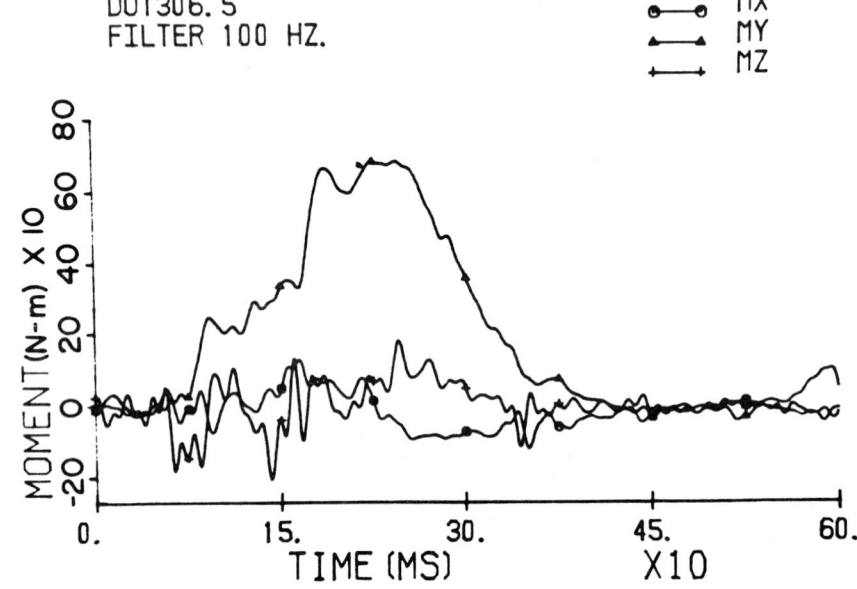

Fig. 14 - Moment measurements from a six-axis seat pan load cell

DATA ANALYSIS

SPINAL FLEXIBILITY - In order to design a surrogate spine which simulates the kinematics of cadaveric spines, it is necessary to delineate the principal characteristics of vertebral motion during impact. One of the obvious parameters is relative rotation of the targeted vertebrae with respect to each other and to the pelvis. It was found that the thoracic spine underwent an initial extension due to inertial loading. This occurred before extensive torso flexion took place. The total relative rotation of T1 with respect to T12 was taken to be the sum of maximum extension and flexion. Data for 19 runs are shown in Table 4. The lumbar spine showed less extension and generally had a smaller total relative rotation of T12 with respect to the pelvis. Thus, the thoracic spine is apparently more flexible than the lumbar spine. However, the measured relative rotation is the sum of the rotations of individual vertebrae at the intervertebral joints. The true flexibility of each segment should reflect the number of joints in each segment. A unit rotation is defined as the average rotation of each joint required to attain the total relative rotation and is computed by dividing the total rotation by the number of joints involved, 6 for the lumbar segment and 11 for the thoracic spine. The values for the unit rotation are comparable for the two segments, in the case of the embalmed cadavers. However, the lumbar spines of the two unembalmed cadavers tested are more flexible than the thoracic spine.

RESISTANCE TO FLEXION - While the sled is in motion, an analysis of the forces and moments at the hip joint during forward flexion can only be made with the aid of complex mathematical models, such as the crash victim simulators. However, after the sled has come to rest, the analysis is greatly simplified. Although the torso is still undergoing flexion and extension, providing seat pan loads and moments, an equation of static equilibrium can be written for that portion of the body which is firmly strapped to the seat; that is, the lower torso, below the hip joint. With the aid of Figure 15, an expression for the resultant hip joint moment, M_R, can be derived:

$$M_R = M_y - F_z \cdot X_L - F_x \cdot Z_L$$

where

M_y = seat pan moment about the sled fixed z-axis

F_x and F_z = seat pan loads along the sled fixed x- and z-axis

X_L and Z_L = moment arms as shown in Figure 15

Table 4 - Relative Rotation of T1 with respect to T12 and T12 with Respect to the Pelvis

Nominal g-Level	Run No.	Rotation of T1 with Respect to T12 (deg) Max. Ext.	Max. Flex.	Tot. Rot.	Unit Rot.	Rotation of T12 with Respect to Pelvis (deg) Max. Ext.	Max. Flex.	Tot. Rot.	Unit Rot.
Embalmed Spine									
3	318	9.0	- 5.0	14.0	1.3	0.0	-12.0	12.0	2.0
5	226	0.0	-11.4	11.4	1.0	0.0	-15.9	15.9	2.6
	319	17.0	-13.0	30.0	2.7	4.0	-14.0	18.0	3.0
	332	16.0	- 8.0	24.0	2.2	0.0	-12.0	12.0	2.0
10	303	5.0	-56.0	61.0	5.5	38.0	- 4.0	42.0	7.0
	305	9.0	-42.0	51.0	4.6	30.0	0.0	30.0	5.0
	306	5.0	-45.0	50.0	4.5	9.0	0.0	9.0	1.5
15-30	312	20.0	-20.0	40.0	3.6	11.0	-11.0	22.0	3.7
	310	0.0	-21.0	21.0	1.9	0.0	-12.0	12.0	2.0
	314	20.0	- 6.0	26.0	2.4	6.0	-17.0	23.0	3.8
	333	56.0	0.0	56.0	5.1	23.0	-19.0	42.0	7.0
Unembalmed Spine									
5	342	28.0	0.0	28.0	2.5	0.0	-44.0	44.0	7.3
	344	22.0	- 4.0	26.0	2.4	0.0	-29.0	29.0	4.8
	353	2.0	-15.0	17.0	1.5	6.0	0.0	6.0	1.0
10	345	29.0	0.0	29.0	2.6	0.0	-32.0	32.0	5.3
	354	54.0	- 9.0	63.0	5.7	0.0	-14.0	14.0	2.3
	355	47.0	- 6.0	53.0	4.8	6.0	-25.0	31.0	5.2
20	343	30.0	- 8.0	38.0	3.5	0.0	-30.0	30.0	5.0

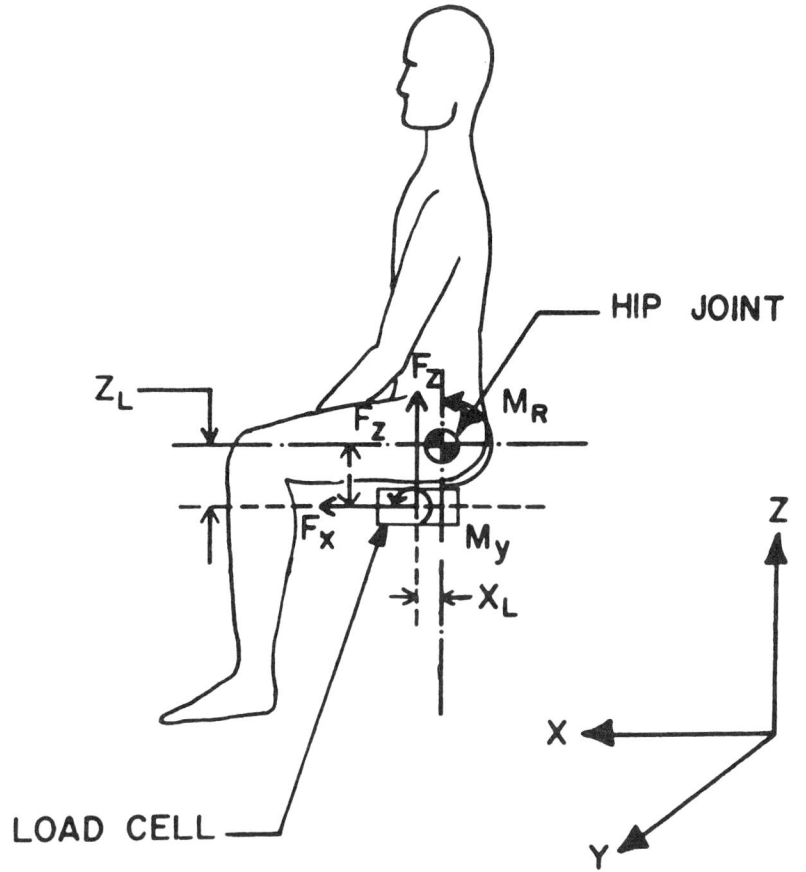

Fig. 15 - Free body diagram for computing the resisting moment of the spine at the hip joint

Calculation of this moment can begin at approximately 125 ms after the initiation of impact, as shown in Figure 5, for a 10g run (Run No. 306). The point is marked in Figure 5 at about 180 ms along the abscissa. The resultant moment, M_R, and the other terms in the static equilibrium equation are shown in Figure 16 for Run No. 306. The corresponding rotation of T1 with respect to the pelvis (Angle θ) as a function of time, for the same run, is shown in Figure 17. Plotting M_R against θ results in a curve defining the stiffness of the spine. For Run No. 306, the curve is shown in Figure 18 for an embalmed spine. A cubic spline interpolation program was required to obtain equally spaced film data samples compatible with the digital load cell data before a cross-plot could be made. The anomaly in the form of a 'reversed' hysteresis loop near the maximum values of M_R and θ is presumably due to the cross-plotting of the noise in the two signals and to errors in the film data. This curve was filtered at 100 Hz. It is possible to eliminate the 'reversed' hysteresis loop by using a 10 Hz filter but there is a severe degradation of peak amplitudes at this frequency. The hysteresis loop is very large for an unembalmed cadaver, as shown in Figure 19. The energy dissipated is estimated to be approximately 200 N-m.

A DESIGN APPROACH FOR A SURROGATE SPINE

The data acquired from these experiments can be used to make an initial design of a surrogate spine suitable for installation in an existing ATD. One of the constraints is the requirement for a rigid thoracic spine in an ATD to facilitate the design of a more human-like rib cage. However, both the thoracic and lumbar spines show considerable flexibility and in the case of the embalmed cadavers, the same degree of flexibility. There is also the over-riding consideration that surrogate spines must satisfy the dual requirements of repeatability and reproducibility. It must, therefore, be simple in design yet realistic in response. A method for the synthesis of a planar linkage joining two rigid bodies was developed by Sarkisyan et al (6) who proposed a means to determine the length and locations of the pivot points of a rigid link which will enable one body to move relative to the other along a predetermined path. The method minimizes the error between the actual and desired path in the least squares sense. This procedure can be applied to the design of a surrogate spine. One of the rigid bodies is the pelvis while the other is the upper torso, defined relative to the T1 coordinate system, as shown in Figure 20. An optimization procedure is required to minimize the error between the path taken by the surrogate spine and that measured during the experimental runs. The ninth order equation developed by

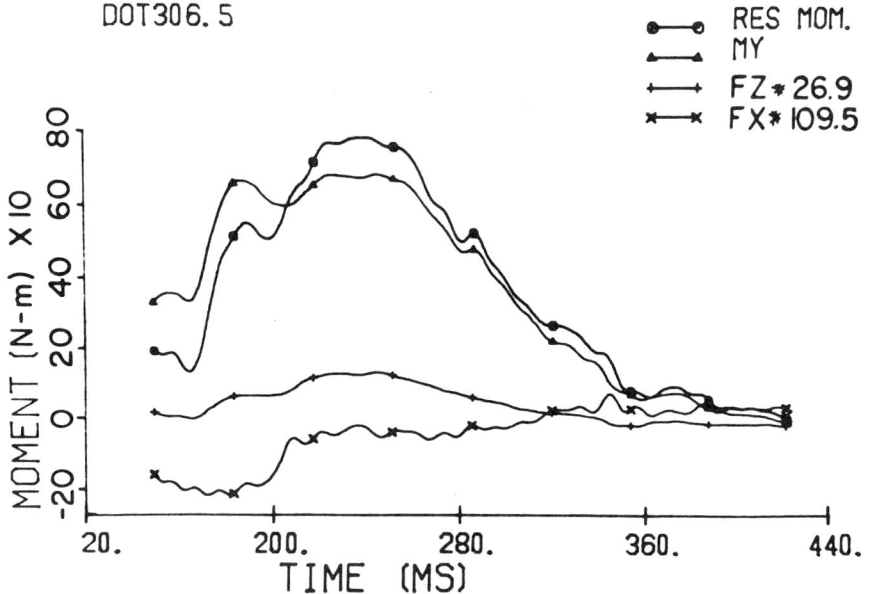

Fig. 16 - Hip joint resisting moment and values of terms in static equilibrium equation for the Run 306

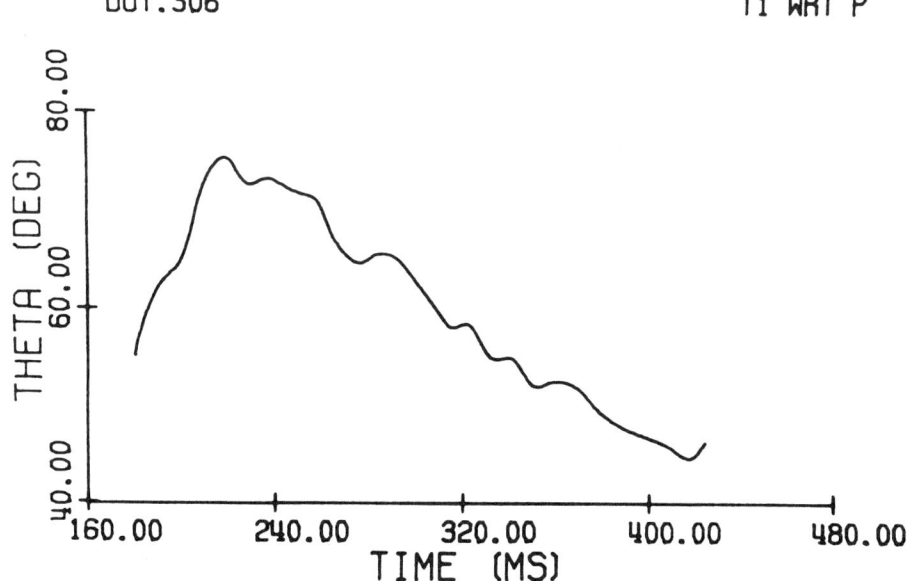

Fig. 17 - Rotation of T1 with respect to the pelvis as a function time for Run 306

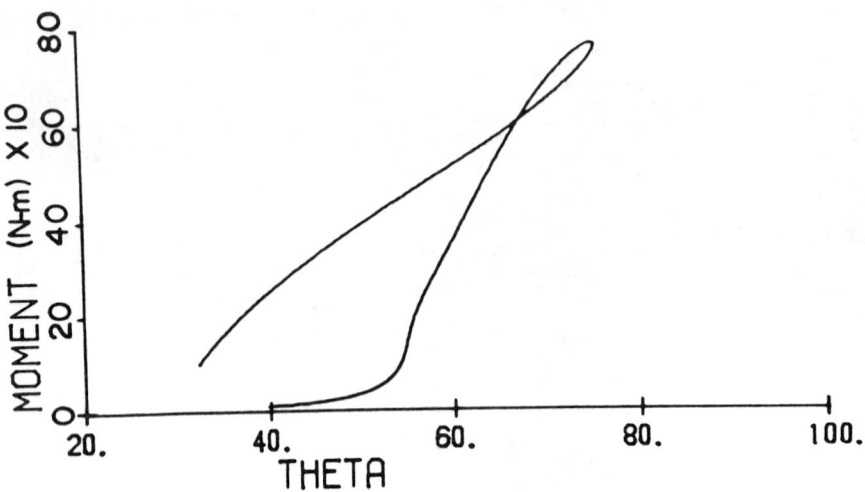

Fig. 18 - Resisting moment as a function of relative rotation of T1 with respect to the pelvis for Run 306

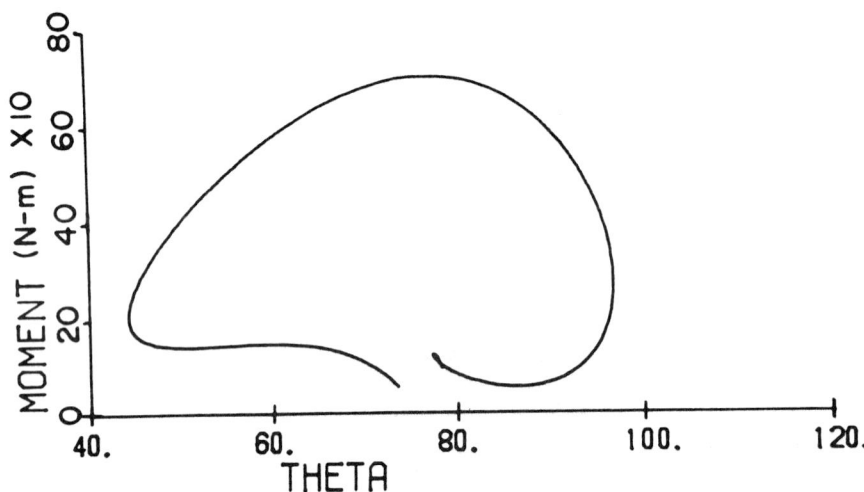

Fig. 19 - Resisting moment as a function of relative rotation of T1 with respect to the pelvis for Run 355

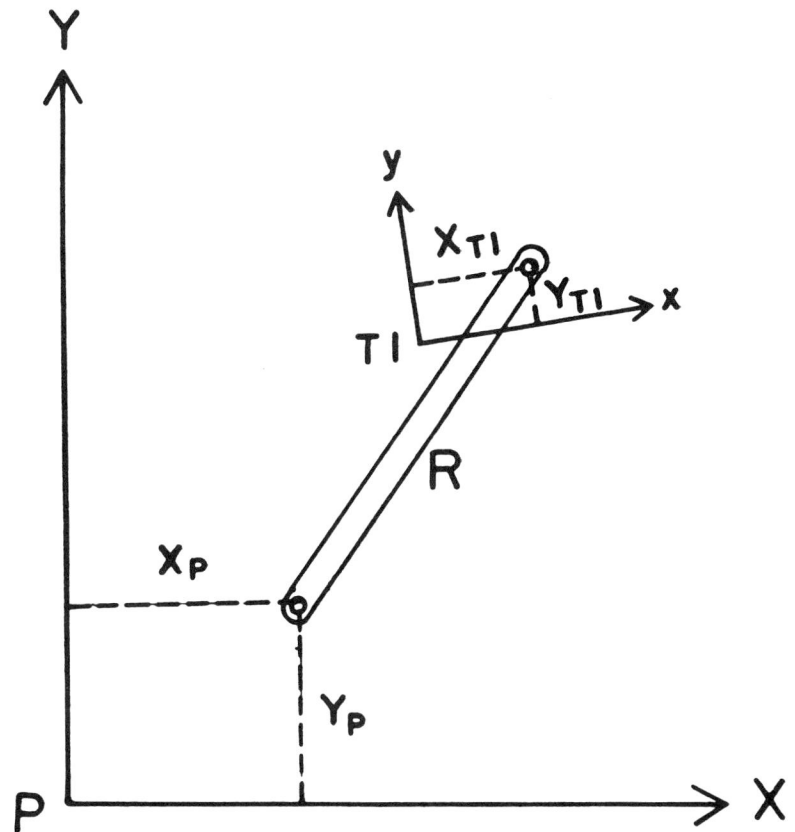

Fig. 20 - Diagram for a planar linkage

Sarkisyan et al (6) can have a maximum of 9 possible links for a given path of T1 relative to the pelvis. An efficient Nelder-Meade optimizer developed by Wong et al (7) was used to determine the optimal link. It finds the length of the link, R, and the coordinates of the pivot points on each body, X_P and Y_P in the pelvic coordinate system and X_T and Y_T relative to the origin of the T1 coordinate system, as shown in Figure 20. In view of the possibility of multiple solutions, it is essential to make intelligent guesses for the initial values of these 5 quantities. Differences in spinal column length was accounted for by obtaining a normalized desired path, using the normalizing factors computed in Table 3. Normalized data from 20 runs were put through the optimizer and the results are shown in Figure 21 and Table 5. The average link was obtained by averaging the values of X_P, Y_P, X_T, Y_T and R for the 20 sets of data points. This link was found to be 486 mm long. Its pelvic pivot is located 208 mm behind and 8 mm below the origin of the pelvic coordinate system, along the x- and y-axis respectively. The upper torso pivot is located 127 mm behind and 80 mm above the origin of the T1 coordinate system, along the x- and y-axis respectively. It is seen from Figure 21 that the link as computed from the optimization program lies outside the profile of a 50th percentile ATD. A proposed feasible link can be located within the dummy as shown by the dotted line by translating both pivot points anteriorly 100 mm as shown in Figure 21. A scaled paper model for the proposed feasible link was constructed to check for its ability to track the motion of T1 relative to the pelvis, measured from film data. The link performed satisfactorily.

CONCLUSIONS

1. Cadaveric data on the range of spinal motion during $-G_x$ impact acceleration have been acquired.
2. Kinematic data useful for the design of a surrogate spine included relative rotation of T1 and T12 with respect to the pelvis and to each other and acceleration of T1, T12 and the pelvis.
3. The dynamic flexural resistance for the spine was also measured, using a six-axis seat pan load cell.
4. The total relative rotation of the thoracic spine was generally larger than that of the lumbar spine. However, the flexibility of the two segments, defined in terms of an average rotation at each vertebral joint, was comparable for embalmed spines. The unembalmed lumbar spine was more flexible than the thoracic spine but this conclusion is based on 7 runs and 2 cadaveric subjects. Living human volunteer data will be required to determine whether the embalmed or the un-

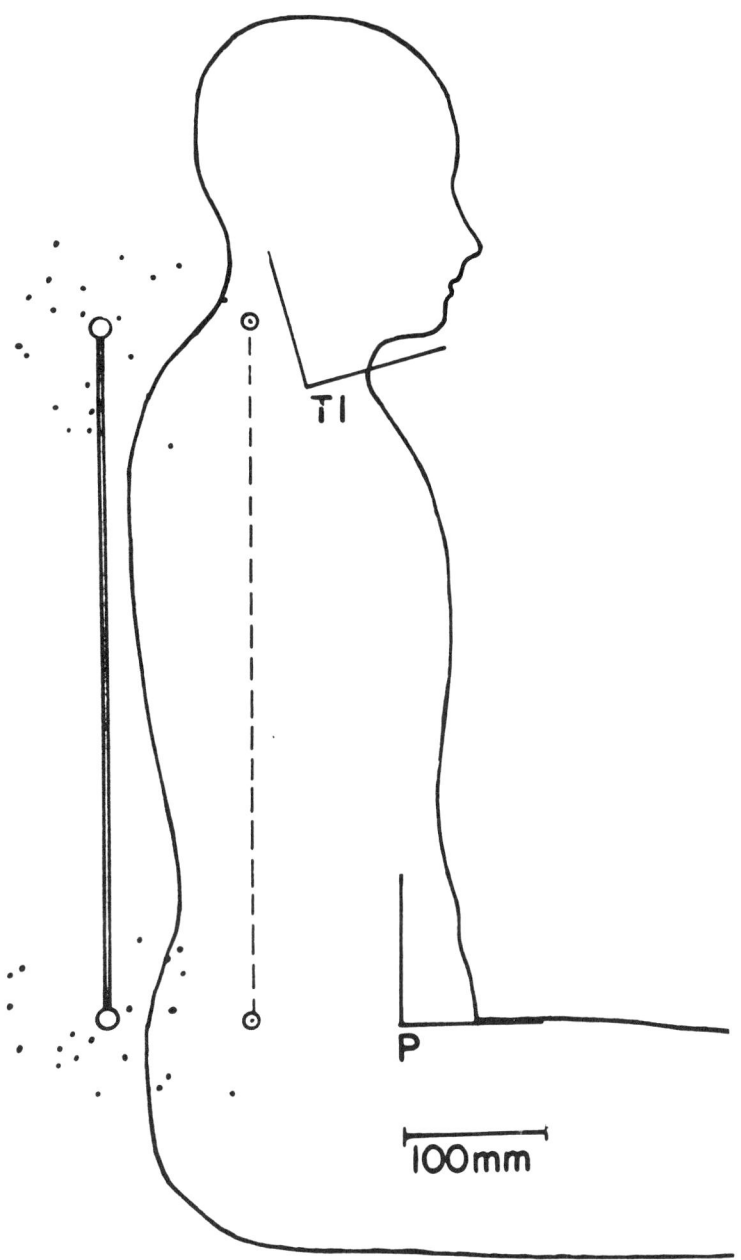

Fig. 21 - Optimized planar linkage representing an ATD spine-solid line by Nelder Meade method, dotted line by proposed feasible link

Table 5 - Planar Linkage Data for a Proposed Surrogate Spine

Cadaver No.	Run No.	Nominal G-Level (g)	Pelvic Coordinates X_P (mm)	Y_P (mm)	T1 Coordinates X_T (mm)	Y_T (mm)	Link Length (mm)
1	226	5	-218.4	- 2.5	17.8	27.9	464.8
1	231	5	-172.7	-35.6	135.4	83.8	513.1
2	303	10	-193.0	17.8	38.1	76.2	492.8
3	305	10	-233.7	2.5	- 83.8	106.7	495.3
3	306	10	-243.8	- 7.6	- 61.0	106.7	497.8
3	309	5	-195.6	-15.2	-139.7	150.0	508.0
3	310	24	-243.8	-17.8	- 96.5	127.0	475.0
4	312	16	-269.2	- 5.1	-111.8	86.4	487.7
5	314	25	-162.6	17.8	134.6	99.1	500.4
7	318	3	-215.9	-38.1	-154.9	124.5	497.8
7	319	5	-231.1	-17.8	-132.1	111.8	459.7
9	332	5	-165.1	-33.0	-170.2	116.8	502.9
9	333	30	-121.9	-40.6	-160.0	160.7	497.8
10	342	5	-154.9	43.2	-167.6	17.8	452.1
10	343	20	-165.1	53.3	-154.9	15.2	454.7
10	344	5	-160.0	58.4	-147.3	27.9	447.0
10	345	10	-185.4	63.5	-170.2	35.6	490.2
11	353	5	-276.9	43.2	-111.8	55.9	480.1
11	354	10	-269.2	48.3	-144.8	45.7	467.4
11	355	10	-276.9	22.9	-182.9	78.7	530.2
Average			-207.8	7.9	-126.5	80.0	485.8
Standard Deviation			46.6	34.6	52.3	40.6	22.5

embalmed spinal data are more human-like. Both types of spines lack muscle tone but the rigidity of the embalmed spine may be able to simulate some muscular action.

5. A design approach to a surrogate spine for an existing ATD was proposed. Using a planar linkage synthesis method, the proposed spine was found to be 486 mm long and was located along the posterior aspects of the ATD torso. A complete design requires the incorporation of joint resisting torques and joint stops to simulate the actual motion of T1 relative to the pelvis.

ACKNOWLEDGMENTS

This research was supported by DOT Contact No. DOT-HS-5-01232. The technical assistance of Ms. A. Mital, Drs. S. Sinha, A. J. Padgaonkar and S. A. Tennyson and Messrs. L. Matthews and C. Mallikarjunarao is gratefully acknowledged.

REFERENCES

1. Nyquist, G. W. and Murton, D. J., "Static Bending Response of the Human Lower Torso", 19th Stapp Car Crash Conference, 1975, pp. 513-541.
2. Mallikarjunarao, C., Padgaonkar, A. J., Levine, R. S., Gurdjian, E. S., and King, A. I., "Kinesiology of the Human Spine Under Static Loading", Proc. of the 1977 Biomechanics Symposium, 1977, pp. 99-102.
3. Ewing, C. L. and Thomas, D. J., "Human Head and Neck Response to Impact Acceleration", NAMRL Monograph 21, 1972.
4. Padgaonkar, A. J., "Validation Study of a Three-Dimensional Crash Victim Simulator for Pedestrian-Vehicle Impact", Ph.D. Thesis, Wayne State University, 1976.
5. Padgaonkar, A. J., Krieger, K. W. and King, A. I., "Measurement of Angular Acceleration of a Rigid Body Using Linear Accelerometers", J. of Applied Mechanics, 1975, pp. 552-556.
6. Sarkisyan, Y. L., Gupta, K. C. and Roth, B., "Kinematic Geometry Associated with Least-Square Approximation of a Given Motion", J. of Engineering for Industry, 1973, pp. 503-510.
7. Wong, Y. Y., Twigg, D. W., Erickson, R. A., Southall, R. M., OPTREG - an Interactive Computer Program for Optimization and Regression, Tech. Rept. #BCS-G0792, NHTSA Contract No. DOT-HS-356-3-719, 1975.

791027

Biodynamics of the Living Human Spine During $-G_x$ Impact Acceleration

R. Cheng, N. K. Mital, R. S. Levine and A. I. King
Wayne State University

SPINAL RESPONSE TO $-G_x$ IMPACT ACCELERATION was quantified by Mital et al (1)* recently. Cadaveric data were provided to demonstrate the relative motion of the spinal segments and the flexibility of the thoracic and lumbar spine. A surrogate spine in the form of a rigid link pinned at both ends was designed for use in a current anthropomorphic test device (ATD), the Part 572 dummy. The basis for a rigid link was the dual requirement of repeatability and reproducibility in an ATD. These conditions would be difficult to satisfy if a multi-segment spine were used. A preliminary physical model of this surrogate spine was fabricated and tested by Mital et al (2). It was found to perform satisfactorily. Its T1 kinematics relative to the pelvis fell within the corridor of cadaveric data upon which the spine was designed.

In this paper, human volunteer data on spinal kinematics are reported. Both male and female subjects participated in this experimental test series. It describes the experimental instrumentation packages applied to these subjects for consistent data without

*Numbers in parentheses designate References at the end of the paper.

discomfort. The data are compared with those obtained from cadaveric tests.

METHODS OF PROCEDURE

INSTITUTIONAL REVIEW BOARD APPROVAL - All procedures involving the use of human subjects were submitted to the Wayne State University Committee on Human and Animal Investigation (the Institutional Review Board for the University) for review and approval. Detailed protocols and assurances were submitted along with the appropriate forms for informed consent. All experiments were carried out within the limitations of the approved procedures and additional tests of procedures required separate approvals from the same board.

EXPERIMENTAL DESIGN - The objective of this study is to acquire data for the design of an ATD spine which has human-like responses. To achieve this, it is necessary to quantify living spinal response to $-G_x$ acceleration in terms of the kinematics of selected spinal segments and the kinetics of resistance to flexion and extension. Moreover, a restraint system needs to be specified to protect the

---

ABSTRACT

Spinal kinematics of the living human volunteers undergoing $-G_x$ impact acceleration are described along with the experimental procedures followed to acquire such data. There were 4 male and 3 female volunteers who were subjected to impacts in the tensed and relaxed mode from 2 - 8 g, in 1-g increments. Their lower extremities were tightly clamped to the impact seat and the pelvis was restrained by a lapbelt. The biodynamic response of the living spine is quite similar to that of the cadaveric spine, particularly in terms of T1 displacement, acceleration at T1 and flexural resistance. Female volunteers tend to withdraw from the test program at lower g-levels than males due to transient neck pain.

test subject during the impact test.

The experimental plan called for 2 modes of restraint. The first is called the clamped mode in which the lower extremities are tightly clamped to the impact seat and the pelvis is restrained by a lap belt. The upper torso is free to flex forward but is protected from impacting the thighs by a cushion placed across the lap. This mode permitted substantial flexion of the spine without inordinate risk to the test subject. The second mode utilizes the standard three-point belt system which yields a set of norms for spinal kinematics that the ATD spine is expected to match.

The deceleration pulse shape should be representative of an automotive collision. However, the measurement of spinal resistance to bending requires the sled to be brought to rest as quickly as possible. in this way, a static analysis of seat pan loads and moments results in a resisting moment which can be expressed as a function of spinal flexion.

The magnitude of peak deceleration exposure is set at 8 g. It can be lower if the volunteer refuses to go on with the test or if it is deemed by the medical officer that the subject should not go on. The first run is to be made at a level of 2 g to acclimate the subject to the acceleration environment. The incremental level is 1 g and at each g-level, the subject makes 2 runs, first with the muscles tensed and then relaxed.

SUBJECT SELECTION - All subjects were recruited from a pool of over 50,000 students at Wayne State University. Their age range is from 18 to 25. The primary requirement is good health. Individuals with a history of bone fractures or other injuries are disqualified. They can also be disqualified by the examining physician for a variety of pre-existing conditions. The medical examination is scheduled for each volunteer to minimize unnecessary tests in the event that the subject is disqualified during the process. Thus, the x-ray exam is taken last. The medical evaluation consists of the following:
1. Complete history
2. Complete physical
3. ECG
4. Stress ECG
5. Laboratory tests, including
   a) SMA 1260
   b) Electrolytes
   c) Complete hemogram
   d) Urinanalysis
6. Ophthalmologic exam with fundus photography
7. Orthopedic exam
8. X-rays of the skull, spine and chest

The subjects were covered by workmen's compensation as they were hired as student assitants and performed other laboratory tasks in addition to volunteering for the sled runs. A medical insurance policy was purchased for the group from the Continental Casualty Insurance Co. as additional protection.

INSTRUMENTATION - Accelerometer clusters were mounted on the spinous process of T1 and T12 and on the pelvis. Each cluster consisted of 9 uni-axial accelerometers arranged in the configuration described by Padgaonkar et al (3) for the purpose of measuring three-dimensional linear and angular acceleration. The mounts were custom-made to fit the spinal contours at each vertebral level. They were held onto the spinous process by means of a series of elastic straps and belts. Figure 1 shows the T1 mount which is most complex in design. A cubic photographic target is attached rigidly to the mount. Although it is a 7.6 mm cube, it is extremely lightweight, being made out of

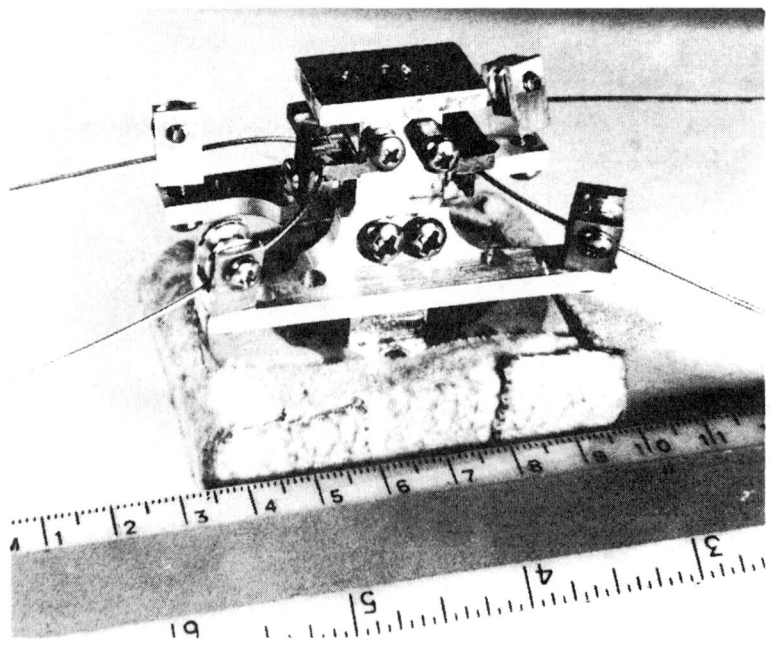

Fig. 1 - T1 accelerometer mount for human volunteers

urethane foam. Figure 2 shows an instrumented volunteer subject with all mounts attached to his spine.

There was photographic coverage from three high-speed cameras placed along 3 orthogonal axes. Other instrumentation included a sled accelerometer and velocity transducer, a six-axis seat pan load cell, an on-board ECG monitor and a time synchronization indicator to match film and transducer data. Belt load cells were used during runs involving the three-point belt restraint system.

SLED FACILITY - All runs were carried out on WHAM III (Wayne Horizontal Accelerator Mechanism), a flat bed sled which was slowly accelerated to a speed of 16 to 17 km/h and was made to impact a programmable hydraulic snubber. The deceleration distance varied from 240 mm to 585 mm. Figure 3 shows a subject seated upright in the impact seat and restrained in the clamped mode. The thighs and legs were held firmly to the seat by clamps which could be released rapidly for emergency egress from the sled. A lapbelt was used to prevent excessive lifting of the pelvis. It was found during the cadaveric experiments that femoral fractures occurred without a lapbelt and were prevented by means of a lapbelt. A piece of 140 mm thick urethane foam was placed over the lap as a cushion to prevent excessive spinal flexion and to protect the rib cage. Head contact with the cushion did not occur. Because of the accelerometer mounts on the back of the subject, two pieces of seat belt webbing were used as a seat back. They were positioned to avoid interaction with the targets and mounts.

Before each run, at least two responsible investigators, including a physician go through a detailed check-list, as required by the test protocol. An ambulance and crew are required to stand-by for transport of the test subject to a predesignated nearby hospital, in the event of an injury. The emergency ward of the hospital was also notified in advance of the scheduled tests. The snubber length, accumulator pressure and all on-board equipment were checked by at least two people. The subject's blood pressure and pulse rate were measured immediately before and after each run and at regular intervals. After each series of runs, the subject was asked to report any pain or discomfort to the physician. Such reports were usually received on the following day but they were all minor and short-lived.

RESULTS

ANTHROPOMETRIC DATA - Table 1 shows the weight, age, sex and sitting height of the seven subjects who participated in this study. There were 3 female subjects and 4 male subjects. Data used for the computation of percentiles were taken from 1962 HEW data (3). Anthropometric data of interest consist of the length of the thoracic and lumbo-sacral spines. They were measured by identifying the coccyx

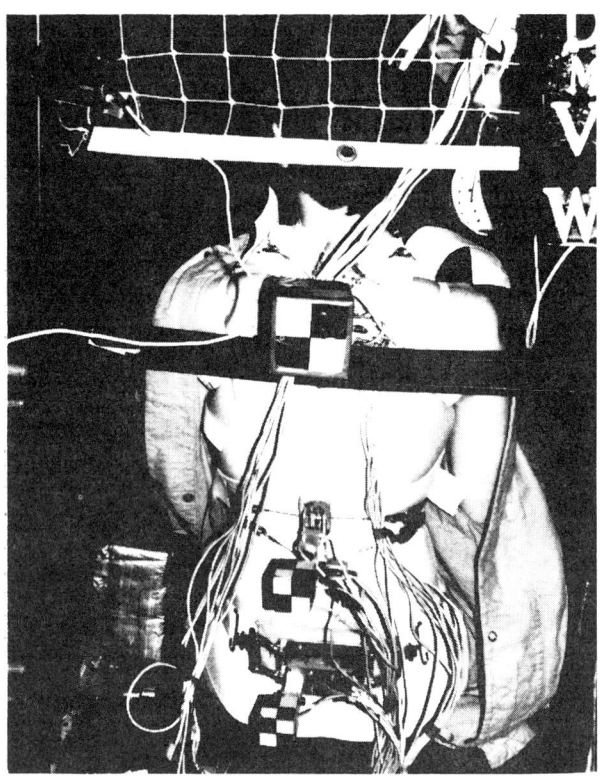

Fig. 2 - Volunteer instrumented with accelerometer mounts

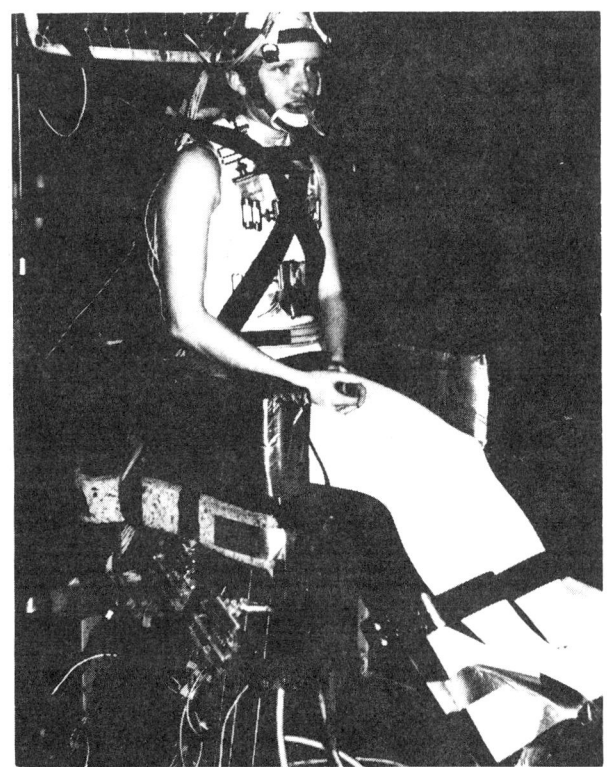

Fig. 3 - Volunteer in impact seat

and spinous process of T12 and C7. The volunteers were measured in a standing position. These dimensions were required to compare the length of the spine of volunteers to the length of the spines of cadavers reported by Mital et al (1). As shown in Table 2, the spine length of volunteers ranged from 440 mm to 592 mm. The mean and standard deviation were 497.7 and 51.3 mm respectively. A normalization factor was computed by dividing the average length of cadaveric spines by the spine length of the individual volunteers as shown in the last column of Table 2.

EXPERIMENTAL RUNS - The volunteer runs were divided in 4 broad groups according to mode and g-level. Runs at 2-4 g (2-3 g for females) were placed in the low-g category and those at 5-8 g (4-8 g for females) were considered as the high-g group. Table 3 summarizes the number of runs conducted on each volunteer in different modes and g-levels. The total number of runs was 88 (25 female runs and 63 male runs). There were a total of 36 belted runs (24 male and 12 female) and 52 clamped runs (39 male and 13 female). Approximately half of the clamped runs were conducted with muscles tensed and the other half with muscles relaxed.

The data presented in this paper are taken from the clamped runs during which there is substantial spinal flexion and extension and with which cadaveric data from (1) can be compared.

ACCELEROMETER DATA - During each run, the acceleration of T1, T12 and the pelvis was measured by a nine-accelerometer module. With these data, the acceleration at the origin of a body-fixed anatomical system can be computed. Using the coordinate system defined by Ewing et al (4) for T1, the resultant acceleration of T1 for runs made at 4-7 g by a male subject is shown in Figure 4. A peak acceleration of approximately 20 g is recorded. The angular acceleration and velocity about the lateral or Y-axis at T1 are shown in Figures 5 and 6 respectively for these runs by the same volunteer. The axis is normal to the mid-sagittal plane and is positive towards the left. The acceleration values are largest about this axis due to the predominately two dimensional motion of the clamped mode. The peak angular acceleration is of the order to 700-900 rad/s^2 for the 7-g case. Figures 7, 8 and 9 show the data from a parallel sequence of tests for a female volunteer.

In terms of data reproducibility, it was found that the corridors for X-axis and Z-axis acceleration (relative to the mount) were quite narrow for each group of runs. The X-axis acceleration at T1 is shown in Figures 10 and 11 for male high-g runs and female low-g runs respectively. There is a similarity in the two negative peaks between these two sets of runs. The Z-axis accelerations are shown in Figures 12 and 13 for the same groups of volunteers. There is again good reproducibility and a characteristic positive peak followed by a negative one. The only difference between the male and female data is the extended duration of the negative peak for the female runs. The Z-axis pelvic acceleration are 2 positive peaks separated by a negative one.

FILM DATA - The rotation and displacement of the cubic film target were measured from high-speed film using a Vanguard film analyzer. A computer program analyzed the data and plotted the position and rotation of T1, T12 and pelvic target with respect to an inertially-fixed frame or with respect to each other. The data can also be transformed to a specified body fixed reference frame. Figure 16 shows target motion of T1, T12 and the pelvis relative to the inertial reference frame for a high-g male volunteer run in the tensed mode. Relative displacement data for the same run are shown in Figure 17. Figures 18 and 19 show the data for the same volunteer in the relaxed mode. The motion in the relaxed mode is usually larger than that in the tensed mode for the same g-level. Film data for a

Table 1 - Pertinent Data on Volunteers

Volunteer No.	Body Weight (kg)	Age (yrs)	Sex	Sitting Height (mm)	Percentile
1454	40.8	22	F	840	30
1156	50.0	24	F	820	11
1760	45.8	18	F	878	60
2953	59.0	23	M	880	30
1555	60.1	21	M	880	30
0159	71.2	19	M	960	92
0252	61.2	24	M	920	55

Table 2 - Anthropometric Data on Volunteer Spines

Volunteer No.	Thoracic C7-T12	Lumbo-sacral T12-Coccyx	Total	Normalization Factor
F 1454	245	220	465	1.28
F 1156	280	200	480	1.24
F 1760	300	185	485	1.24
M 2953	265	175	440	1.36
M 1555	321	161	482	1.24
M 0159	370	222	592	1.01
M 0252	280	260	540	1.10

Average Total Length ± S.D. = 497.9 ± 51.3 mm

Normalizing Factor = $\frac{\text{Average Cadaveric Spine Length (596.3)}}{\text{Volunteer Spinal Length}}$

Table 3 - Summary of Experimental Runs

Vol. No. Male	Belted 2-4g	5-8g	Clamped 2-4g	5-8g
2953	6	2	2	7
1555	7			
0159	5	4	6	8
0252			6	12

Vol. No. Female	Belted 2-4g	5-8g	Clamped 2-3g	4-5g
1454	4	8		
1156			4	3
1760			6	

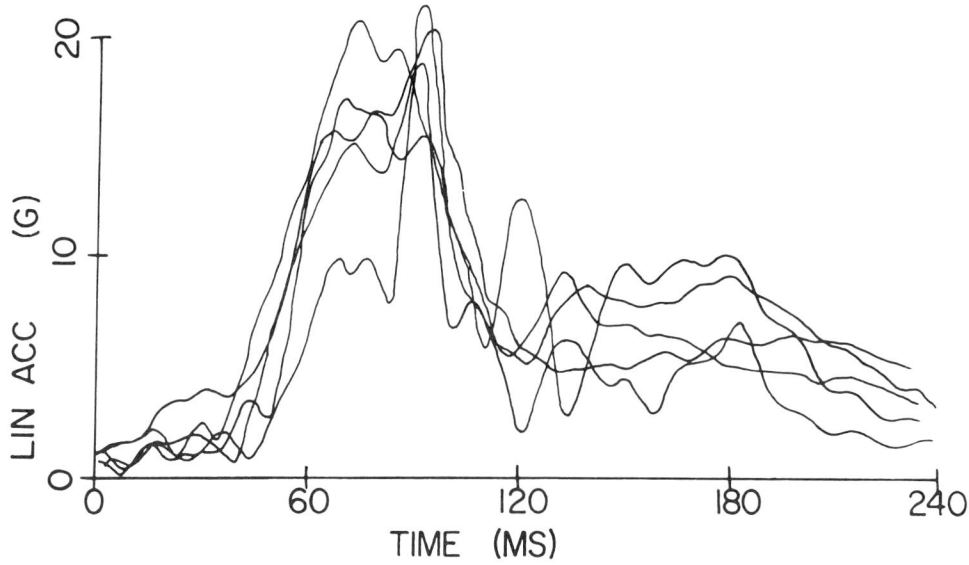

Fig. 4 - Resultant acceleration of T1 at the origin of the T1 coordinate system - male subject (4-7g runs)

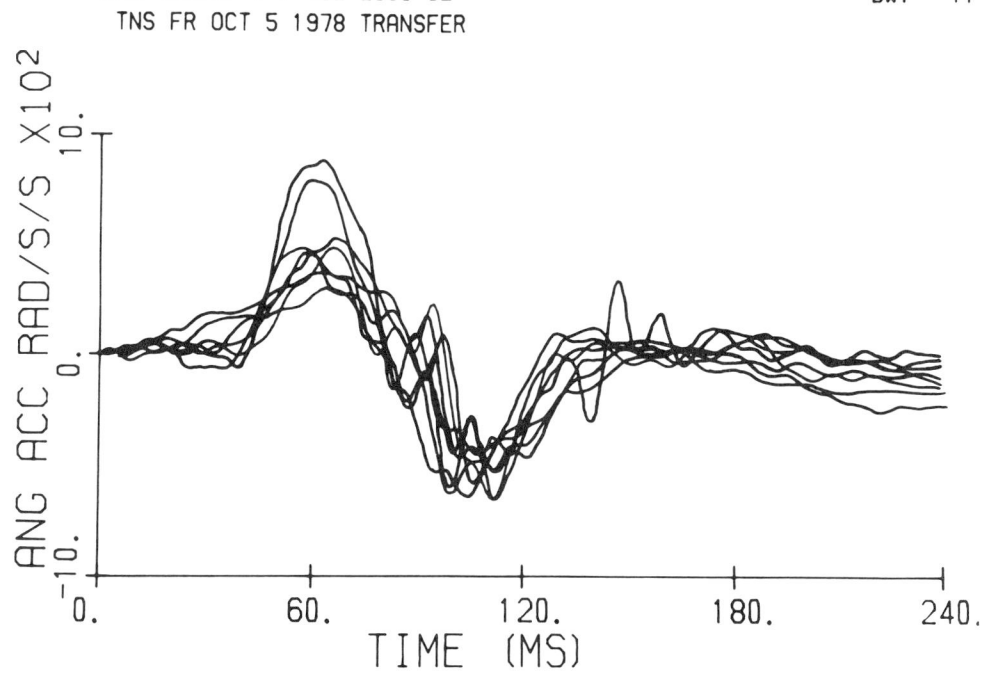

Fig. 5 - Angular acceleration of T1 about the Y-axis - male subject (4-7g runs)

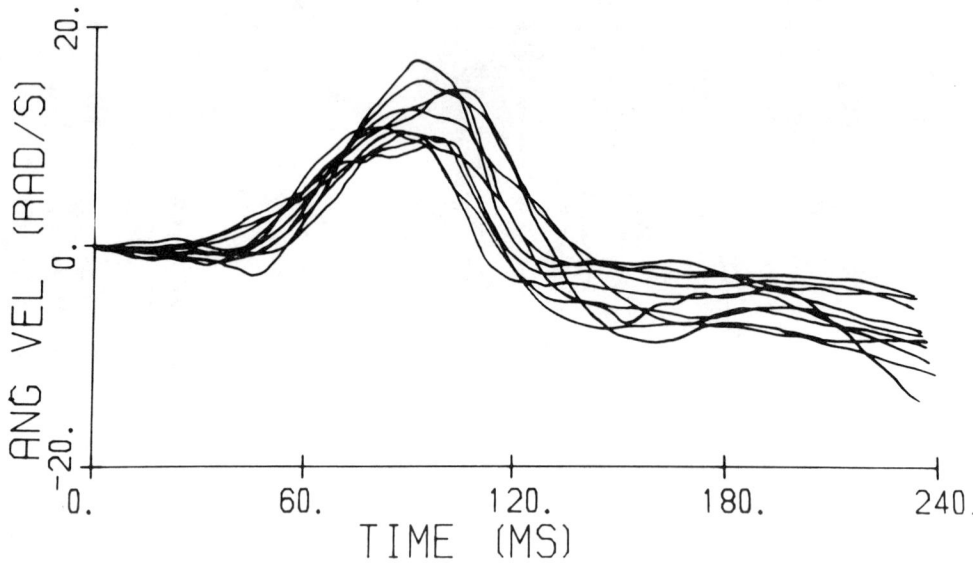

Fig. 6 - Angular velocity of T1 about the Y-axis - male subject (4-7g runs)

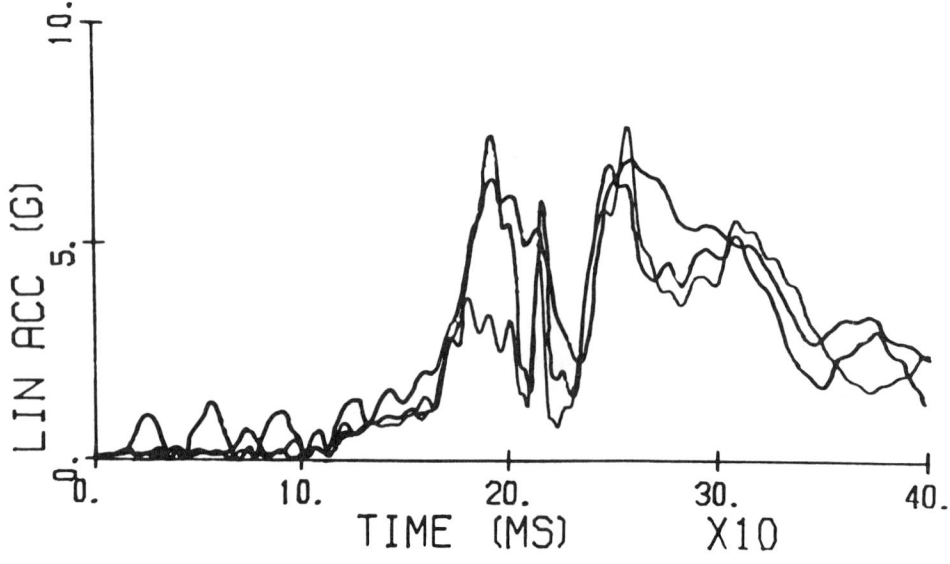

Fig. 7 - Resultant acceleration of T1 at the origin of the T1 coordinate system - low-g runs (female subject)

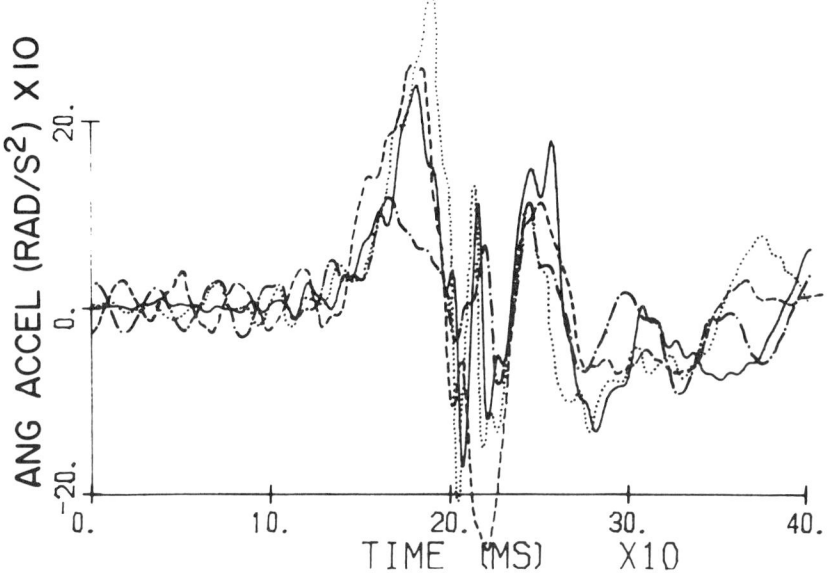

Fig. 8 - Angular acceleration of T1 about the Y-axis - low-g runs (female subjects)

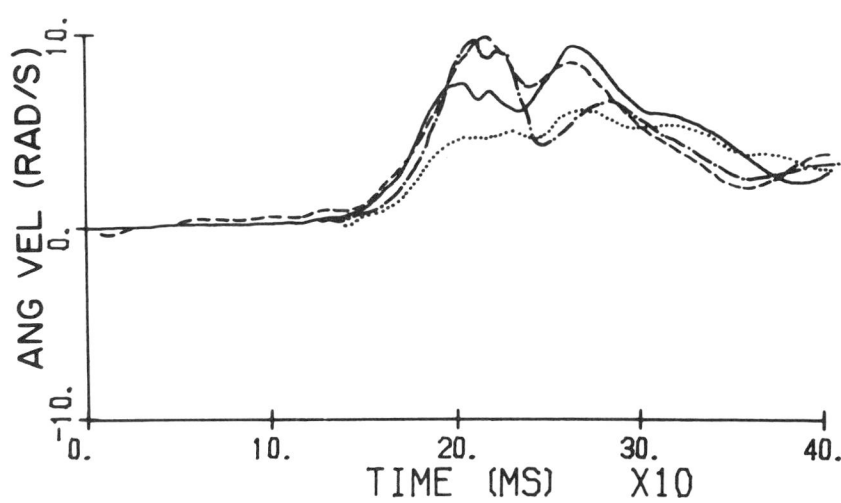

Fig. 9 - Angular velocity of T1 about the Y-axis - low-g runs (female subjects)

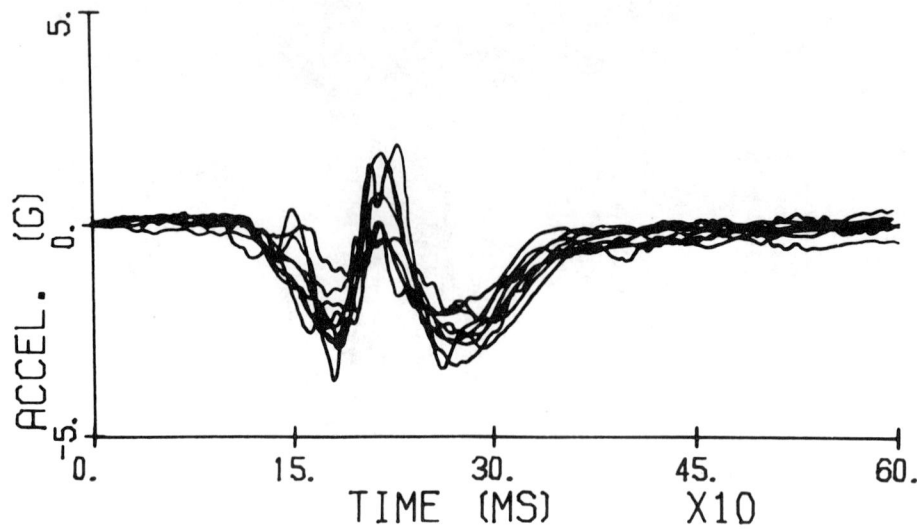

Fig. 10 - T1 X-axis acceleration corridor - male high-g runs

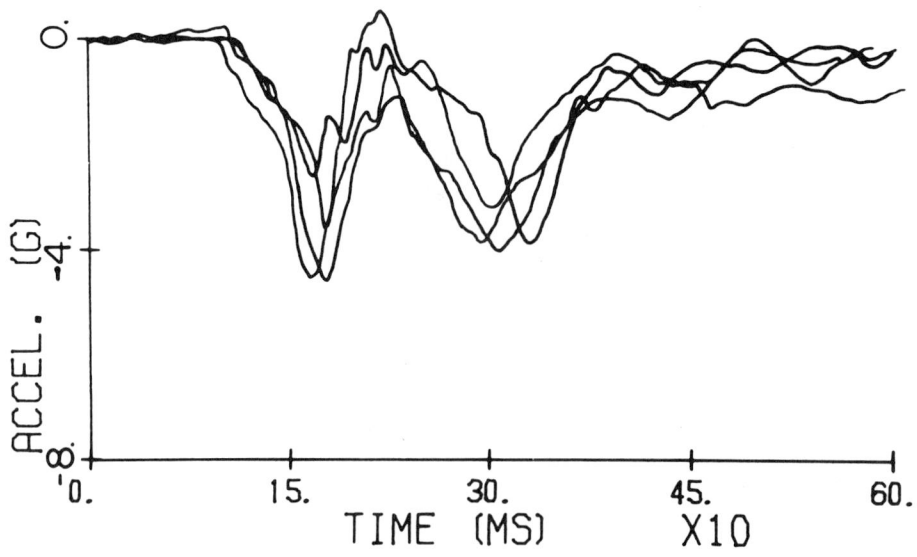

Fig. 11 - T1 X-axis acceleration corridor - female low-g runs

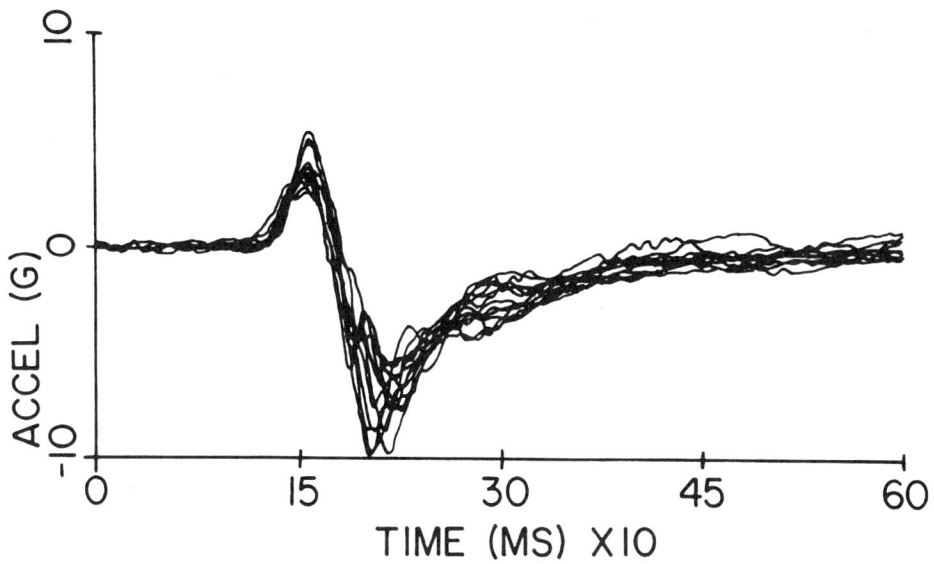

Fig. 12 - T1 Z-axis acceleration corridor - male high-g runs

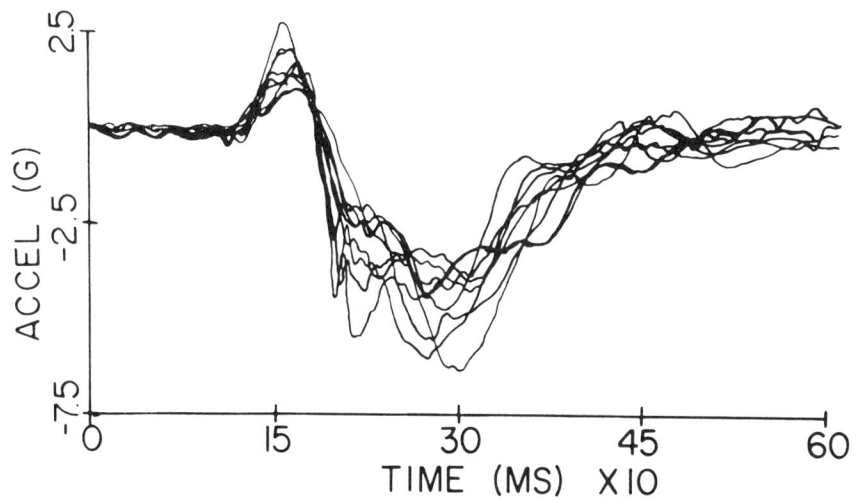

Fig. 13 - T1 Z-axis acceleration corridor - female low-g runs

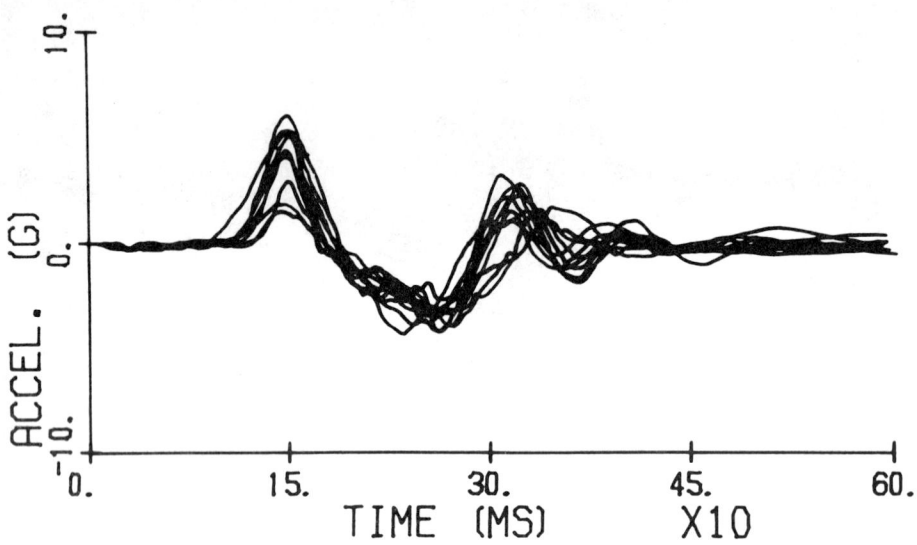

Fig. 14 - Pelvic Z-axis acceleration corridor - male high-g runs

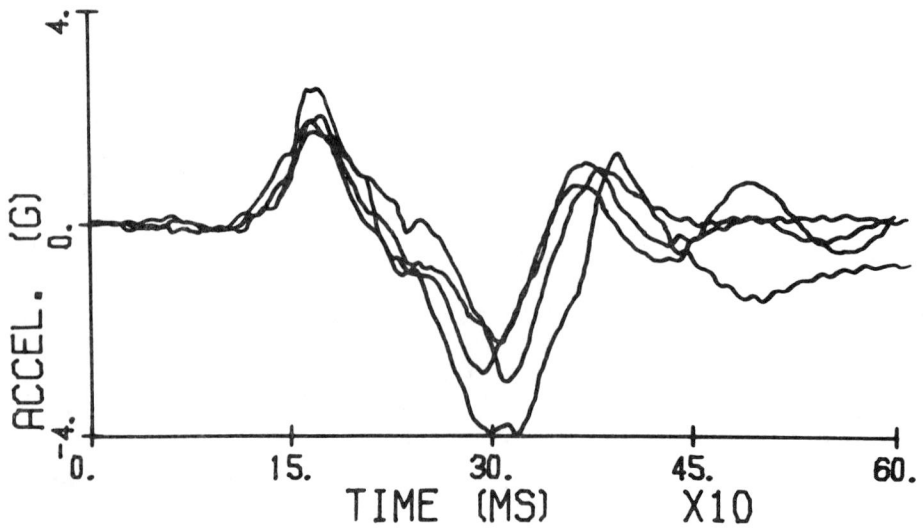

Fig. 15 - Pelvic Z-axis acceleration corridor - female low-g runs

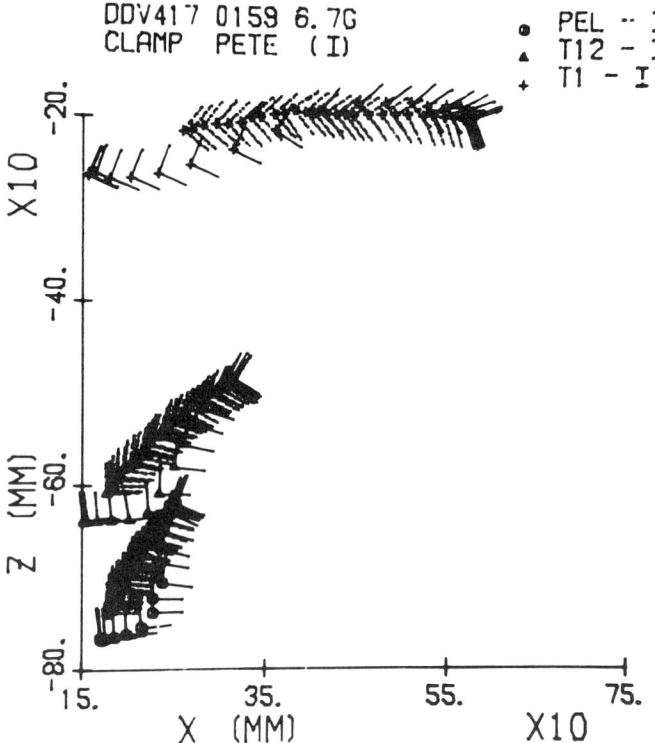

Fig. 16 - Position of T1, T12 and pelvic targets relative to the inertial frame - tensed male volunteer run

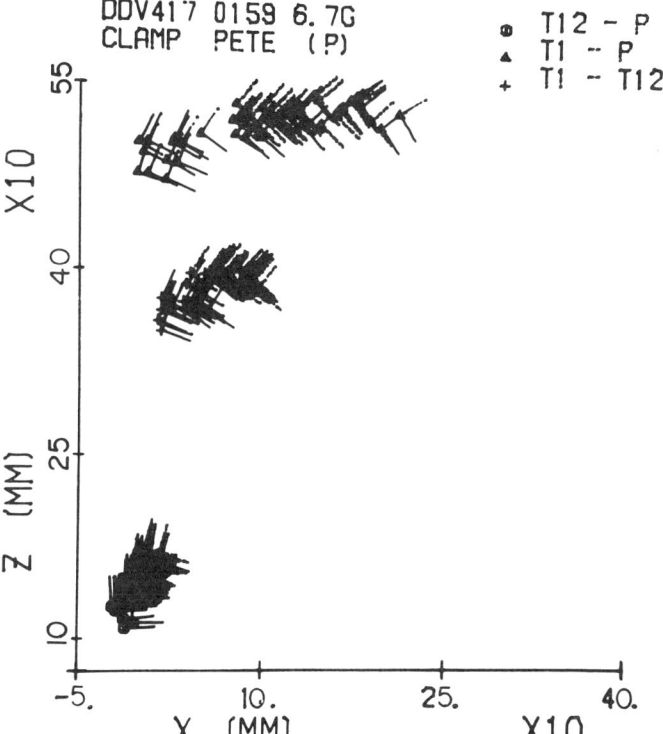

Fig. 17 - Position of T1 and T12 relative to the pelvis and position of T1 relative to T12 - tensed male volunteer run

female volunteer run in the tensed mode are shown in Figures 20 and 21.

LOAD CELL DATA - A six axis load cell was used to measure seat pan forces and moments. A typical output of load cell for a high-g female volunteer run is shown in Figures 22 and 23. The sled-fixed coordinate system was used to define the components of forces and moments measured by this lead cell. Since the impacts were principally 2-dimensional, F_X and F_Z in Figure 22 and M_Y in Figure 23 were used in data analysis. It can be seen from these figures that F_Y, M_X and M_Z are all small.

DATA ANALYSIS

SPINAL FLEXIBILITY - In order to design a surrogate spine which simulates the kinematics of cadaveric spines and volunteer spines, it is necessary to delineate the principal characteristics of vertebral motion during impact. One of the obvious parameters is relative rotation of the targeted vertebra with respect to each other and to the pelvis. The total relative rotation of T1 with respect to T12 was taken to be the algebraic sum of maximum extension and maximum flexion. This represented the total bending of the thoracic spine. A similar rotation was also computed for the lumbar spine; that is the rotation of T12 with respect to the pelvis. A unit rotation is defined as the average rotation of each joint required to attain the total relative rotation and is computed by dividing the total rotation by the number of joints involved, 6 for the lumbar segment and 11 for the thoracic spine. Data for male volunteer run (stensed and relaxed) are listed in Table 4 and for female volunteer runs in Table 5.

RELATIVE ROTATION - Volunteer data of the motion of T1 relative to the pelvis can be compared with cadaveric data reported by Mital et al (1). The corridors in Figure 24 envelope the cadaveric data reported previously. The position plots within the corridors are representative data taken from a large pool of data.

RESISTANCE TO FLEXION - The mathematical formulation to compute the resistance of the spine to flexion was given by Mital et al (1). The free body diagram from computing the resisting moment of the spine at the hip joint is reproduced in Figure 25. The expression for the resultant hip joint moment M_R is given by:

$$M_R = M_Y - F_Z X_L - F_X Z_L$$

where,

M_Y = seat pan moment about the sled fixed Z-axis

F_X and F_Z = seat pan loads along the sled fixed X- and Z-axis

F_L and Z_L = moment arms as shown in Fig. 25

Figure 26 shows the resisting moment and its components for a high-g female volunteer run. The corresponding rotation of T1 with respect to pelvis (Angle θ) as a function of time is generated from the film data. A cubic spline

299

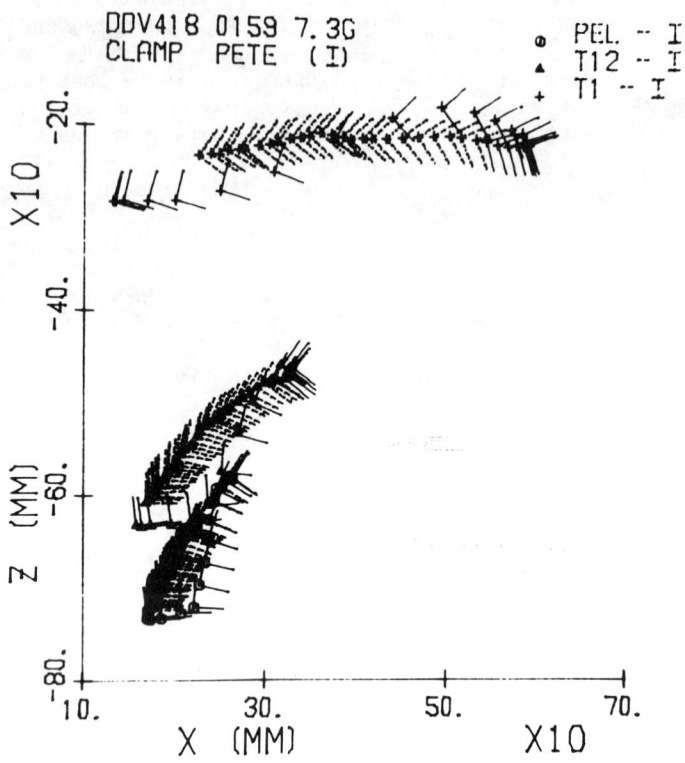

Fig. 18 - Position of T1, T12 and pelvic targets relative to the inertial frame - relaxed male volunteer run

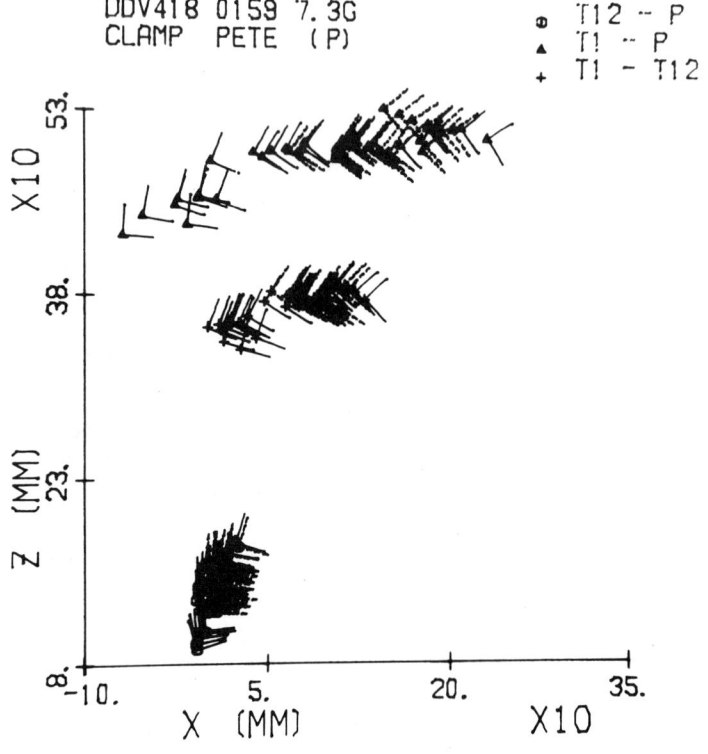

Fig. 19 - Position of T1 and T12 relative to the pelvis and position of T1 relative to T12 - relaxed male volunteer run

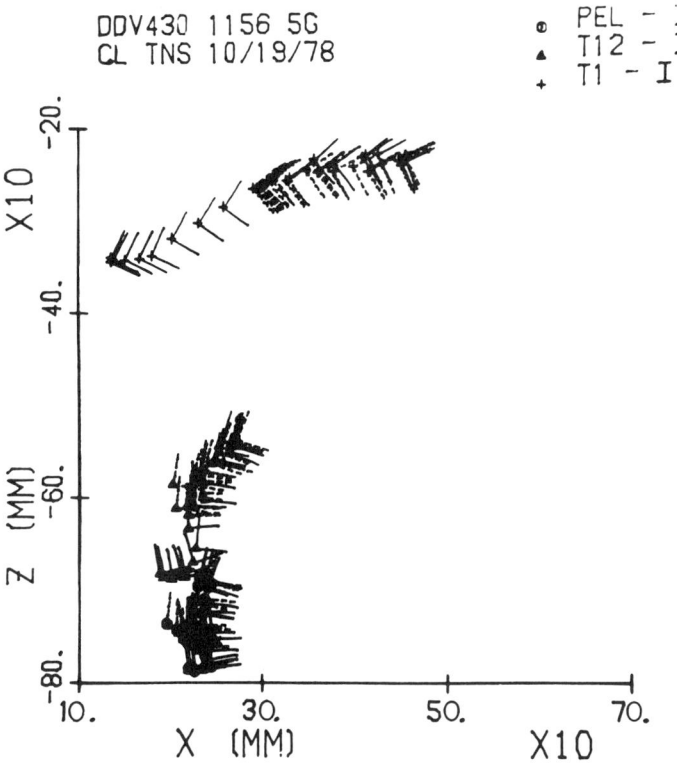

Fig. 20 - Position of T1, T12 and plevic targets relative to the inertial frame - tensed female volunteer run

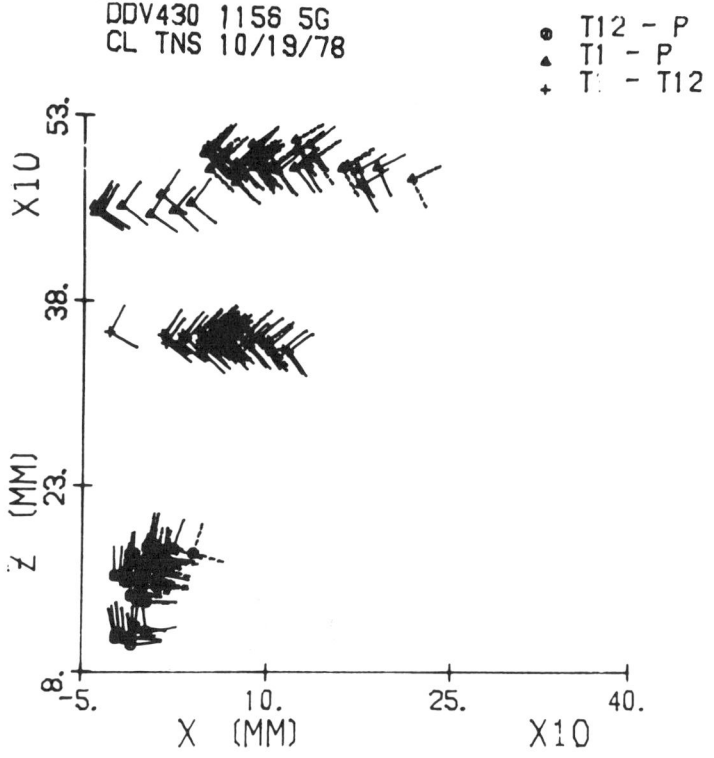

Fig. 21 - Position of T1 and T12 relative to the pelvis and position of T1 relative to T12 - tensed female volunteer run

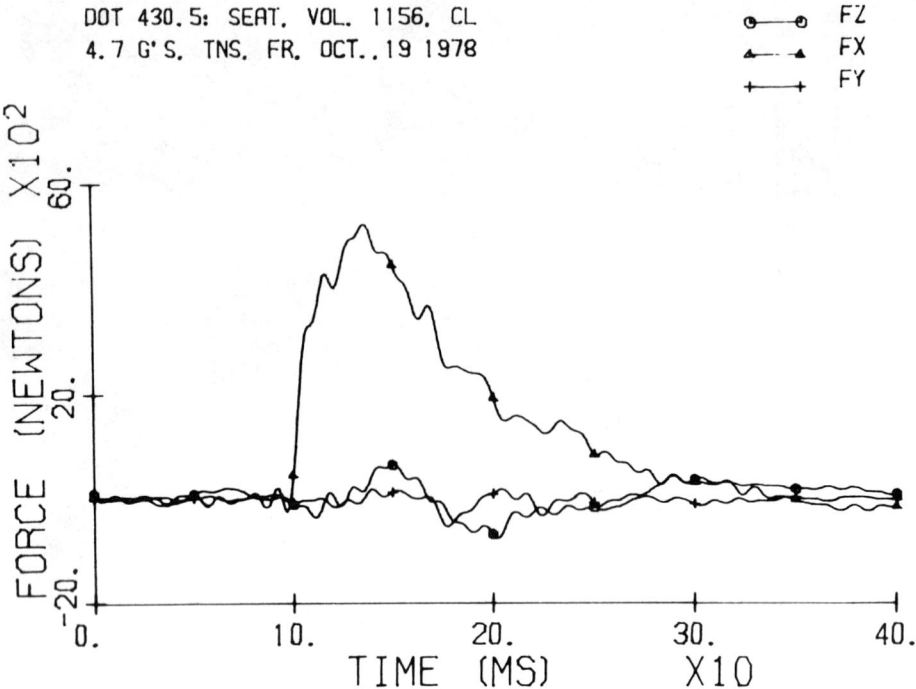

Fig. 22 - Seat pan load cell force output - female 5-g run

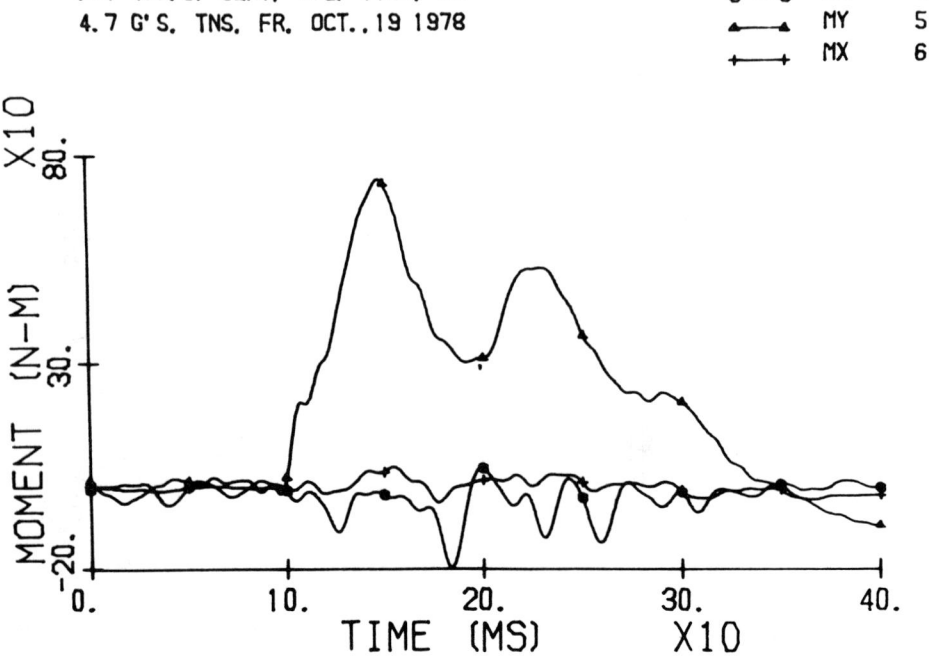

Fig. 23 - Seat pan load cell moment output - female 5-g run

Table 4 - Relative Rotation of T1 with respect to T12 and T12 with Respect to the Pelvis

Nominal g-Level	Run No.	Rotation of T1 with Respect to T12 (deg)				Rotation of T12 with Respect to Pelvis (deg)			
		Max. Ext.	Max. Flex.	Tot. Rot.	Unit Rot.*	Max. Ext.	Max. Flex.	Tot. Rot.	Unit Rot.†
Male Tense
1.8	403	-33.2	-59.1	25.9	2.35	1.1	-28.3	29.3	4.88
2.8	433	-34.4	-63.1	28.7	2.60	10.0	-17.6	27.6	4.60
3.2	405	-41.3	-61.4	20.1	1.83	14.8	-10.9	25.7	4.30
3.5	407	-38.4	-55.8	17.4	1.58	25.4	4.7	20.7	3.45
4.0	435	-36.0	-65.6	29.6	2.69	2.8	-25.4	28.1	4.60
4.4	419	-18.9	-39.9	21.0	1.90	11.4	-16.7	28.1	4.68
4.8	409	-23.4	-60.9	37.5	3.40	8.4	-3.6	12.0	2.00
5.0	437	-30.6	-60.3	29.7	2.70	9.4	-21.6	31.0	5.10
5.4	421	-17.4	-47.3	29.9	2.71	7.2	-17.5	24.7	4.12
5.7	453	-32.5	-63.2	30.7	2.79	-55.5	-31.4	24.1	4.01
5.7	455	-34.3	-58.8	24.5	2.22	-1.5	-29.1	27.6	4.60
6.1	411	-17.4	-36.3	18.9	1.72	2.3	-18.6	13.7	2.28
6.5	457	-11.7	-50.3	38.6	3.50	-1.5	-32.1	30.6	5.10
6.6	424	-31.4	-61.6	30.2	2.75	4.8	-26.8	31.6	5.27
6.7	417	-19.4	-45.8	26.4	2.40	4.9	-16.0	10.9	1.81
8.1	426	-24.9	-51.3	26.4	2.40	4.6	-26.9	31.5	5.25

* Average Unit Rotation ± S.D. = 2.47 ± 0.54 † Average Unit Rotation ± S.D. = 4.1 ± 1.15

Male Relax

1.5	404	-54.9	-100.0	45.1	4.10	-2.9	-23.3	20.4	3.40
2.0	432	-36.3	-75.7	39.4	3.58	3.9	-22.8	26.7	4.45
2.8	434	-33.0	-83.0	50.3	4.57	-13.0	-31.2	18.2	3.03
3.1	406	-36.1	-64.3	28.2	2.56	10.1	-8.2	18.3	3.05
4.0	436	-33.3	-70.0	36.7	3.33	-2.5	-35.9	33.4	5.56
4.2	408	-35.8	-94.8	59.0	5.36	18.8	-11.7	30.5	5.08
4.4	420	-24.1	-79.5	55.4	5.03	6.8	-16.2	23.0	3.80
4.9	410	-23.4	-82.7	39.3	3.57	2.7	-27.7	30.4	5.06
5.0	438	-41.3	-84.9	43.6	3.96	-2.7	-20.2	17.5	2.92
5.6	422	-21.9	-60.3	38.4	3.50	11.2	-16.6	27.8	4.63
5.7	454	-40.7	-63.2	22.5	2.05	3.2	-30.7	33.9	5.65
5.8	412	-26.9	-50.7	23.6	2.14	6.3	22.2	28.5	4.75
6.2	458	-44.2	-82.0	37.8	3.43	-24.8	-0.4	24.4	4.06
6.6	425	-22.9	-63.4	40.5	3.68	2.7	-28.2	30.9	5.15
7.0	456	-28.9	-60.6	31.7	2.88	-1.7	-33.2	31.5	5.25
7.3	427	-24.3	-54.9	30.6	2.78	9.1	-16.8	25.9	4.32

* Average Unit Rotation ± S.D. = 3.51 ± 0.89 † Average Unit Rotation ± S.D. = 4.4 ± 0.95

Table 5 - Relative Rotation of T1 with respect to T12 and T12 with Respect to the Pelvis

Nominal g-Level	Run No.	Rotation of T1 with Respect to T12 (deg)				Rotation of T12 with Respect to Pelvis (deg)			
		Max. Ext.	Max. Flex.	Tot. Rot.	Unit Rot.*	Max. Ext.	Max. Flex.	Tot. Rot.	Unit Rot.†
Female Tense
2.0	443	-40.9	-68.6	27.7	2.51	8.4	-3.8	12.2	2.03
2.3	413	-24.7	-55.6	30.9	2.80	2.3	-18.6	20.9	3.48
3.2	415	-34.1	-54.4	20.3	1.84	1.2	-21.9	22.9	3.81
4.7	428	-30.1	-48.2	18.1	1.64	2.2	-26.3	28.5	4.75
4.7	430	-28.6	-56.0	27.4	2.49	8.4	-20.4	28.8	4.80

* Average Unit Rotation ± S.D. = 2.25 ± 0.49 † Average Unit Rotation ± S.D. = 3.77 ± 1.13

Female Relax

2.0	444	-50.7	-85.1	34.4	3.12	13.7	-16.3	30.0	5.00
2.4	414	-42.7	-67.4	24.7	2.24	-3.9	-30.0	26.1	4.35
3.2	416	-34.5	-59.5	25.0	2.20	-7.6	-29.1	21.5	3.58
4.0	452	-39.0	-65.9	26.9	2.44	8.2	-21.4	29.6	4.90
4.7	429	-28.6	-57.3	28.7	2.60	5.7	-26.9	32.6	5.43

* Average Unit Rotation ± S.D. = 2.52 ± 0.37 † Average Unit Rotation ± S.D. = 4.6 ± 0.37

interpolation program was required to obtain equally spaced film data samples compatible with digital load cell data before a cross plot could be made. This cross plot of M_R against θ shows a curve defining the stiffness of spine and in most cases is a hysteresis loop which is indicative of energy dissipation. Figure 27 shows several $M_R - \theta$ curves for male volunteer data at different g-levels in the tensed and relaxed modes. Figure 28 shows $M_R - \theta$ curves for female data. The volunteer curves are all within the unembalmed cadaver curve reported by Mital et al (1).

DISCUSSION

The Z-axis acceleration corridors shown in Figures 12, 13 and 14 match well with cadaver data (1). There is similarity in the first positive peak and the second negative peak which occur approximately at the same time. Beyond this time the cadaver torso interacts with the lap cushion and more variation is observed in the cadaver data as compared to volunteer data. In most cases, volunteer data showed only 1 or 2 negative peaks. Load cell data for cadaver and volun-

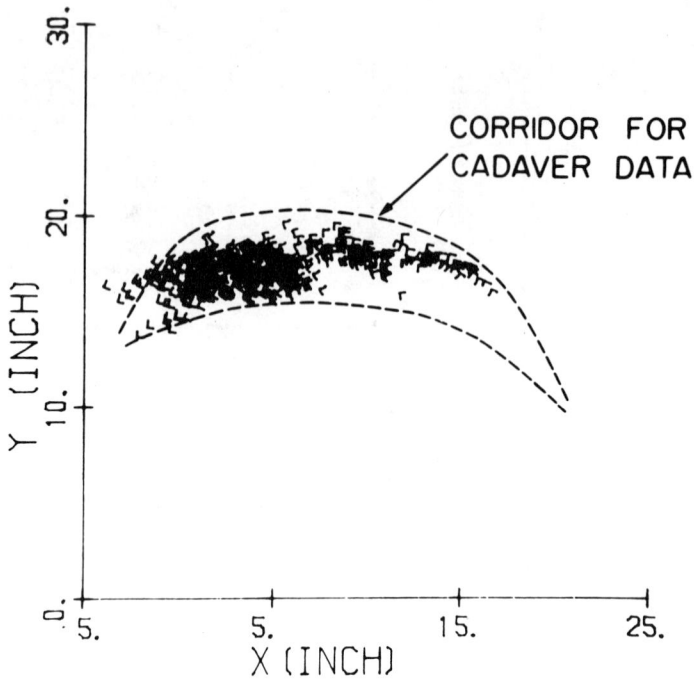

Fig. 24 - T1 motion relative to the pelvis - volunteer data within cadaver data corridors

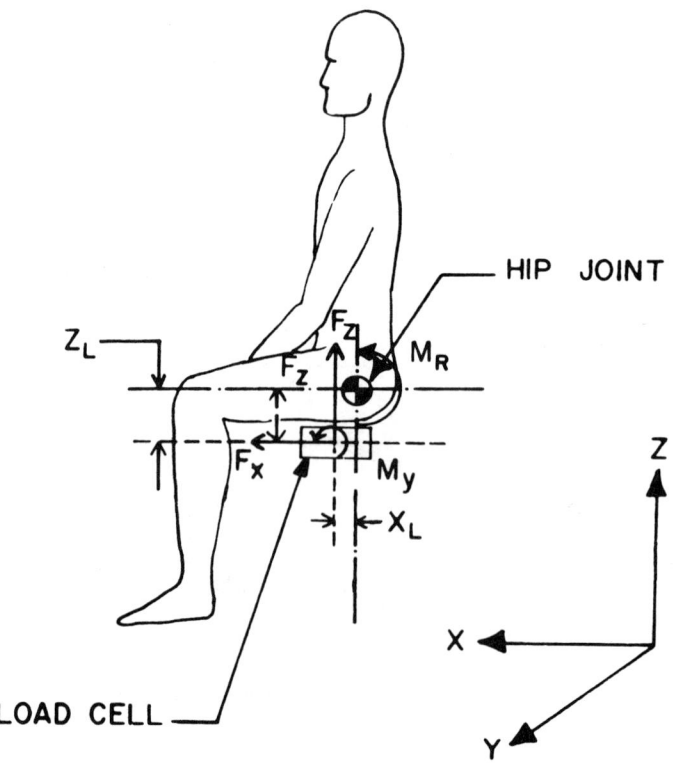

Fig. 25 - Free body diagram for computing resisting moment at the hip

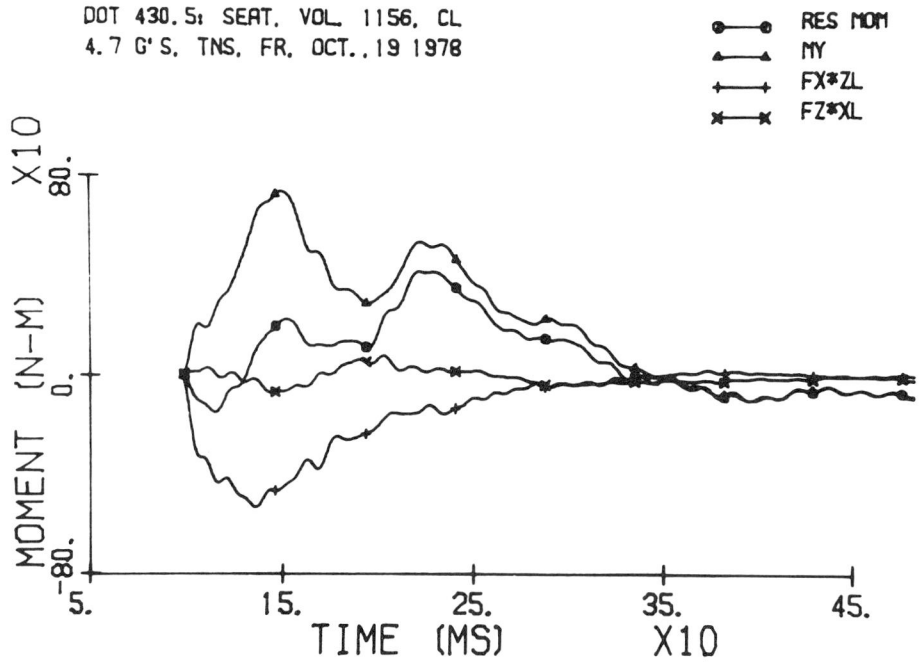

Fig. 26 - Resultant moment computed from seat pan load cell data

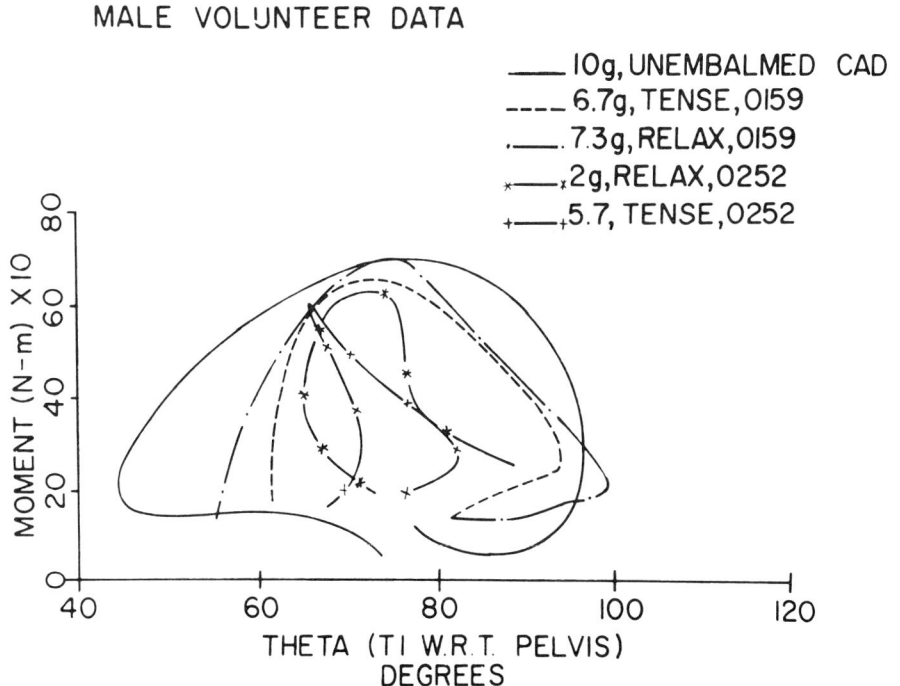

Fig. 27 - Moment - angle curves for spinal flexion - male data

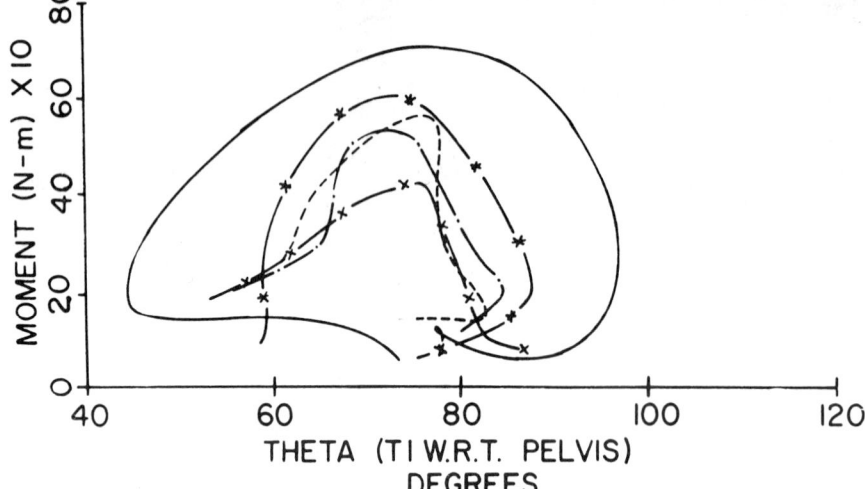

Fig. 28 - Moment - angle curves for spinal flexion - female data

teer runs are also comparable. F_x and M_y are the major components for force and moment and are in the order of 6000 N and 700 N-m, as shown in Figures 27 and 28, are comparable to those plotted from cadaver data. The energy dissipated is less due to the lower g-level of impact. In general, it can be observed from these figures that there is more dissipation with increased g-level and in the relaxed mode in comparison with that for the tensed mode.

The total relative rotation of the thoracic spine appeared to be generally larger than that of the lumbar spine. However, in terms of the flexibility of the two segments, defined as an average or unit rotation at each vertebral joint (Tables 4 and 5) the lumbar spine is apparently more flexible than the thoracic spine for both male and female subjects. As far as cadaver data are concerned, the unit rotation for the thoracic and lumbar segments is comparable for embalmed cadavers. That for the unembalmed cadaver is similar to the data reported for volunteers in this paper. In the relaxed mode, the unit rotation is larger than that in the tensed mode. Male and female unit rotations are comparable. It should be noted, however, that none of the observed differences were found to be statistically significant as determined by the t-test.

The use of a lapbelt to prevent excessive rotation and lifting of the pelvis was the result of cadaveric tests made prior to the human volunteer runs. Bilateral femoral fractures were observed at relatively low g-levels in cadavers due to the excessively high moments applied to the femurs. These moments were reduced by the lapbelt which eliminated femoral fractures up to 20 g. The value of cadaver testing as a prelude to volunteer testing cannot be overemphasized and should be incorporated in all protocols involving human experiments of this type.

Female subjects were more likely to withdraw from the test program than males. Only one of the three females completed an entire sequence of runs up to 8 g. The other two stopped at 4 or 5 g because of transient neck pain. One of the five male subjects was disqualified by the medical officer after 2 runs at 2 g. He had a precipitous rise in blood pressure and pulse rate and was visibly in fear. The data from these 2 runs were not reported and he was not considered as one of the subjects for this experiment.

CONCLUSIONS

1. Spinal kinematics of living human subjects during $-G_x$ acceleration have been quantified up to 8 g.
2. Displacement data of T1 relative to the pelvis are comparable to those of cadaver runs.
3. There is also a qualitative similarity in T1 acceleration between volunteer and cadaver data.

4. Flexural resistance of the spine in human subjects exhibit similar characteristics to that of unembalmed cadavers. There is appreciable dissipation of energy.

5. Cadavers are a valuable tool in human volunteer experiments of this kind. They point out possible sources of injury to the volunteer and should be used, if available.

6. Female subjects have a weaker neck musculature and are likely to withdraw from the program before reaching the maximum level of 8 g. the principal reason is transient neck pain.

ACKNOWLEDGMENTS

This research was sponsored in part by the National Highway Traffic Safety Administration (NHTSA), under Contract No. DOT-HS-5-01232. Opinions expresed in this paper are those of the authors and are not necessarily of NHTSA or of Wayne State University.

REFERENCES

1. Mital, N.K., Cheng, R., Levine, R.S. and King, A.I. Dynamic Characteristics of the Human Spine During $-G_x$ Acceleration, Proc. 22nd Stapp Car Crash Conf., pp. 141-165, 1978.

2. Mital, N.K., Cheng, R., and King, A.I., A New Design for a Surrogate Spine, Proc. 7th ESV Conf., Paris, France, June, 1979 (In Press).

3. Department of Health, Education and Welfare, Weight, Height and Selected Body Dimensions of Adults, National Center for Health Statistics, June 1965.

4. Ewing, C.L., Thomas, D.J., Lustick, L., Becker, E., Willems, G. and Muzzy, III, W.H., The Effect of the Initial Position of the Human Head and Neck to $-G_x$ Impact Acceleration, Proc. 19th Stapp Car Crash Conf., pp. 487-512, 1975.

801312

Biodynamic Response of the Musculoskeletal System to Impact Acceleration

P. C. Begeman, A. I. King, and R. S. Levine
Wayne State University

D. C. Viano
General Motors Technical Center

A LARGE PROPORTION OF EXISTING KNOWLEDGE on human response to impact acceleration is based on experiments for which the human cadaver was the principal test subject. The proprioceptive response of the living human subject has not been fully investigated. Armstrong et al (1968) have provided experimental evidence to show that muscular restraint can significantly alter body segment kinematics for impact acceleration levels up to 16g, when a restraint system is used. Hendler et al (1974) also showed that a three point restraint system can protect a human volunteer up to 30 mph (20g) with an active muscular response and preloaded lap belt.

The physiology of human muscular response during impact acceleration is not well understood. There is very little information available on electromyographic (EMG) response to impact. Tennyson et al (1977) developed recording techniques for monitoring EMG signals during impact, using sled-borne preamplifiers which are resistant to shock. Unanesthetized canines were used to obtain data on the delay of EMG response and the time-history of the EMG derived muscle force during low level impact accelerations of 5g or less. The generation of mechanical force by the muscles has a delay of approximately 80 ms relative to the initiation of the EMG derived force. This was determined by Hannan

---ABSTRACT---

The effect of muscular response on occupant dynamics was studied in human volunteers exposed to low level impact acceleration. The study includes identification of muscular response, correlation of electromyographic activity with reaction force, and investigation of the effects of muscular restraint during impact. Human volunteers were subjected to $-G_x$ impact acceleration in a simulated automobile environment while EMG activity of various lower extremity muscles was monitored. The seat and floor pan were supported on load cells which measured all restraining forces. Nine-accelerometer modules and high-speed photography were used to measure kinematics. Identical runs were made with an embalmed cadaver and dummy for comparison.

Static EMG and force traces as well as dynamic results for various acceleration levels are presented. Differences between tensed and relaxed states are compared and discussed as to EMG response, force levels, and head kinematics.

It was found that reflex responses of the relaxed volunteer are too slow to have a significant effect on loads and accelerations sustained. However, the voluntary pre-impact contracted musculature in a volunteer can reduce certain acceleration levels and change the restraint load distribution so that significantly more load goes through the legs to the floor board with a concomitant lowering of seat and belt loads. Although a similar load distribution was seen in dummy and cadaver tests, the response of the relaxed or tensed volunteer was substantially different from either surrogate.

et al (1975) for jaw closing force in man. However, a similar evaluation of delays during impact have not been measured.

The principal aim of this research is to investigate the response of the human musculoskeletal system to impact acceleration. Inclusion of the muscular system necessitates the use of living subjects and is an attempt to render the experimental simulation of vehicular collision more realistic. In particular the objectives of the research are:

1. Identification of muscular response before, during and after an impact acceleration of short duration.
2. Investigation of beneficial and detrimental effects of muscular restraint during impact acceleration.
3. Correlation of electromyographic activity with contractile force, by direct measurement.
4. Comparison of human volunteer response with those of the cadaver and the anthropomorphic test dummy.

METHODS OF PROCEDURE

All impact tests were made on WHAM II (Wayne Horizontal Accelerator Mechanism) which was run in the acceleration mode. The test subject was positioned in a rearward-facing conventional automotive seat and was restrained by a three-point lap-shoulder belt system with retractor. A knee bolster was in place as a back up for the lap belt. An overall view of the system is shown in Figure 1. Foot loads were measured by a triaxial load cell under each foot. The foot plate was at 45° from the horizontal. The seat was mounted on the sled at three points through biaxial load cells. Thus the subject was isolated from the sled through load cells. Inertial correction due to fixture acceleration was subtracted from reported loads. Foot loads were resolved along sled-fixed coordinate axes: + x being a horizontal axis in the posterior-anterior direction of the subject and + z being normal to sled surface in the caudocephalad direction. Four belt webbing load cells were used at each end of the lap and shoulder belts to measure restraint forces.

Nine-accelerometer modules were attached to the head and pelvis to determine head and pelvic kinematics. The pelvic module was strapped on to the iliac crest through a molded mounting pad. The head module was originally a strapped-on mount but was changed to a more rigid attachment using a molded upper jaw mount which incorporated a 9-accelerometer mounting bracket. Photographic targets for film analysis were attached to various body segments and were viewed by an on-board lateral high speed camera, an off-board frontal high speed camera, two TV cameras and a sequence cameras for immediate analysis.

EMG activity was measured using surface electrodes on various muscles. Usually, the following muscle groups were monitored: the tibialis anterior of each leg, the vastus medialus of each thigh, the rectus adominus, and the spinous longissimus of the torso. ECG of the volunteer was also monitored by

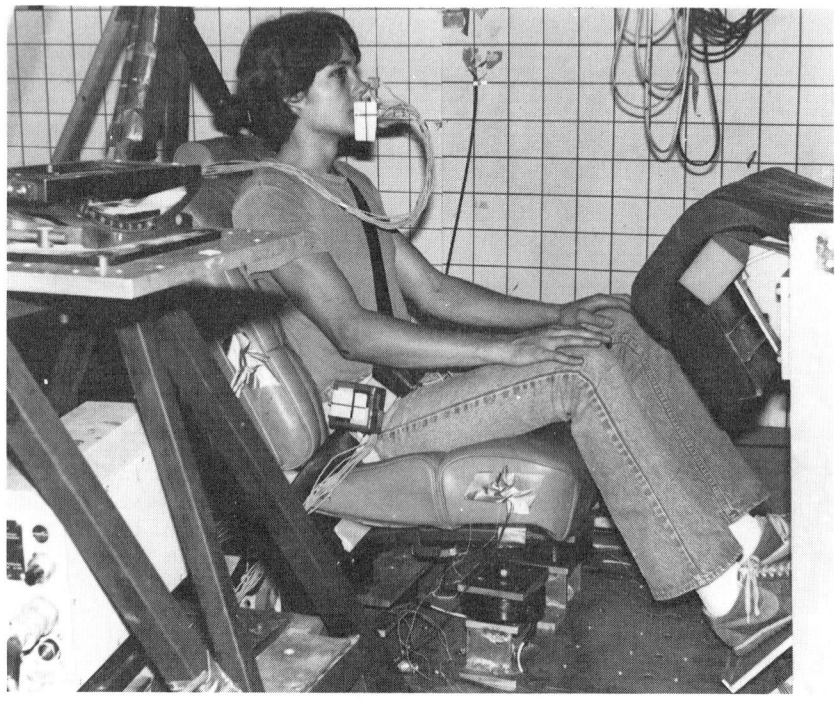

Fig. 1 - Testing configuration

the medical officer.

Healthy male volunteers between 18 and 25 years of age were recruited from the student population of Wayne State University. They were qualified under a volunteer test protocol which was described by Cheng et al (1979). Anthropometric measurements were taken from each subject for use in computer simulations. Cadavers were examined radiographically before and after a testing sequence.

Volunteer testing consisted of a static and a dynamic part. Static tests were done either just prior to or just after a series of dynamic runs, with the volunteer seated on the sled as in the dynamic runs. The volunteer was asked to push with his feet as hard and as quickly as possible on the foot load cells when a light was flashed. Loads and EMG were monitored to obtain reaction times as well as peak forces. Dynamic runs were done in pairs, first tensed and then relaxed, for each g level. Each volunteer started at approximately 2 g. The incremental g-level was 1 g. The maximum g-level sustained by a volunteer was 6.5 g. Cadaver and dummy (Part 572) tests were dynamic runs starting at 2 g and attaining 14 g in 2 g increments. A total of 99 runs were made.

RESULTS

Static tests - Figure 2 shows the results of one test involving the vastus medialis. Muscular reaction had a considerable delay of 900 ms and there was a gradual build up of force. The correlation between the EMG derived force* and actual force is apparent, although there was a delay between the onset of EMG activity and the development of force. Results of other muscles of the same volunteer during the same experiment are shown in Figures 3-5 for the gastrocnemius, tibialis anterior and quadriceps. These demonstrate that there are different levels of activity in different muscles. Responses for the tibialis anterior and gastrocnemius of another volunteer are shown in Figures 6 and 7. Here the reaction time is much shorter and the buildup of force is much quicker. Note that short bursts of EMG are not reflected as bursts of reaction force but do indi-

---

* 'Integrated' EMG has been recognized as a qualitative measure of muscle force. To obtain this derived force, the EMG signal was rectified and smoothed. The rectification was done by means of a root mean-square (RMS) analysis:

$$E_{RMS} = [(1/N) \sum_{i=1}^{N} e^2 \, dt]^{\frac{1}{2}},$$

where e = instantaneous value
      N = number of points in the window.

The rectified data were smoothed with an FFT filter. EMG derived force plots are labeled RMS.

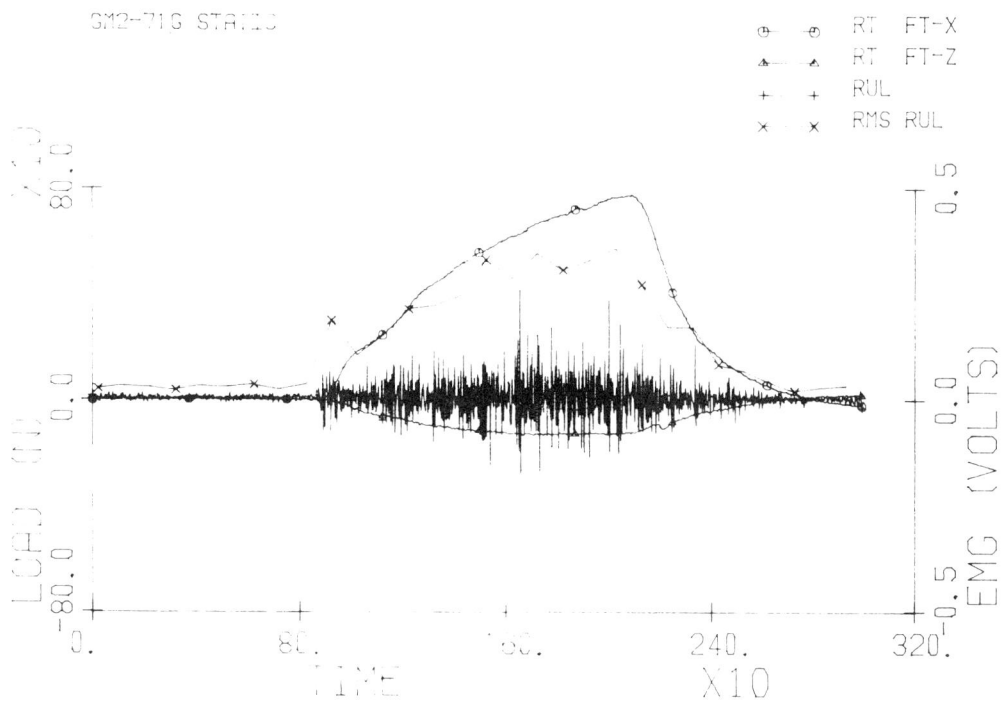

Fig. 2 - Response of right foot loads and the corresponding EMG of the right vastus medialis during static testing

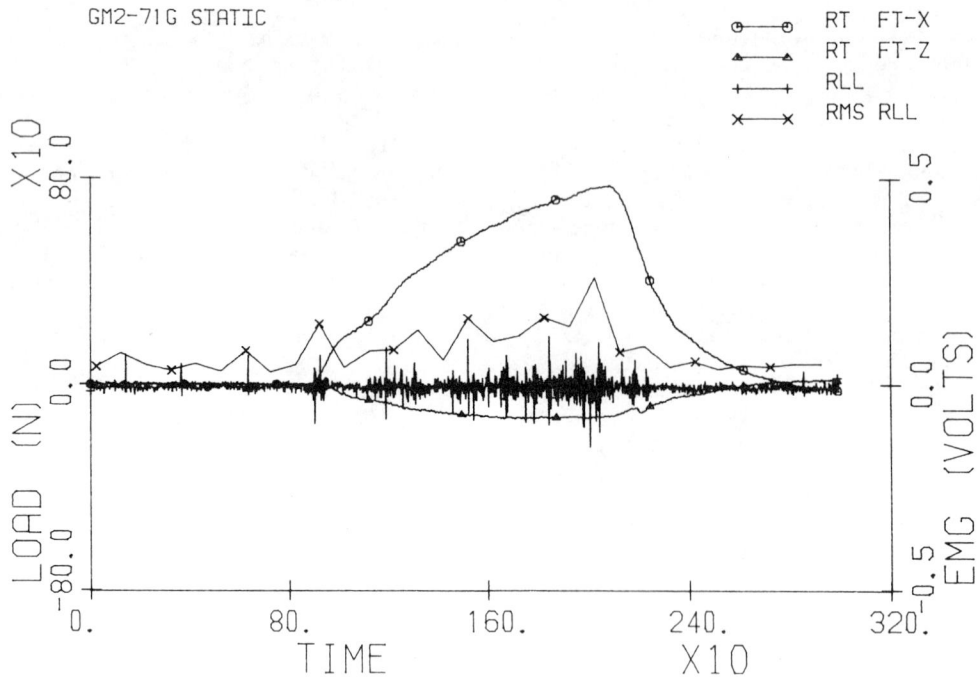

Fig. 3 - Response of right foot loads and the corresponding EMG of the right gastrocnemius during static testing

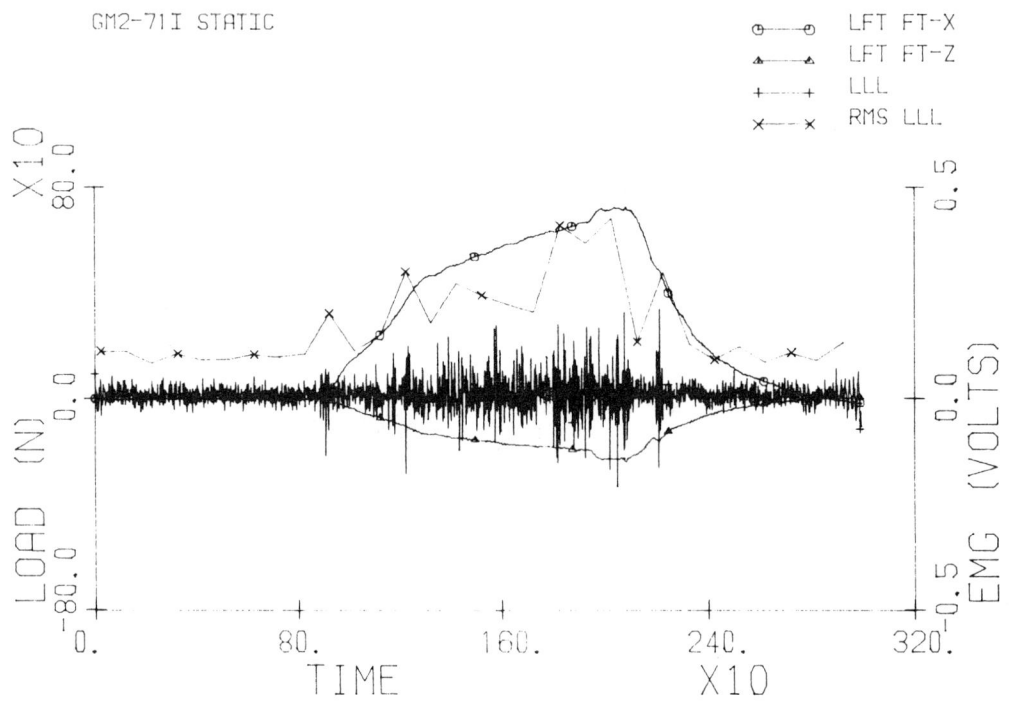

Fig. 4 - Left foot loads and EMG of the left tibialis anterior during static testing

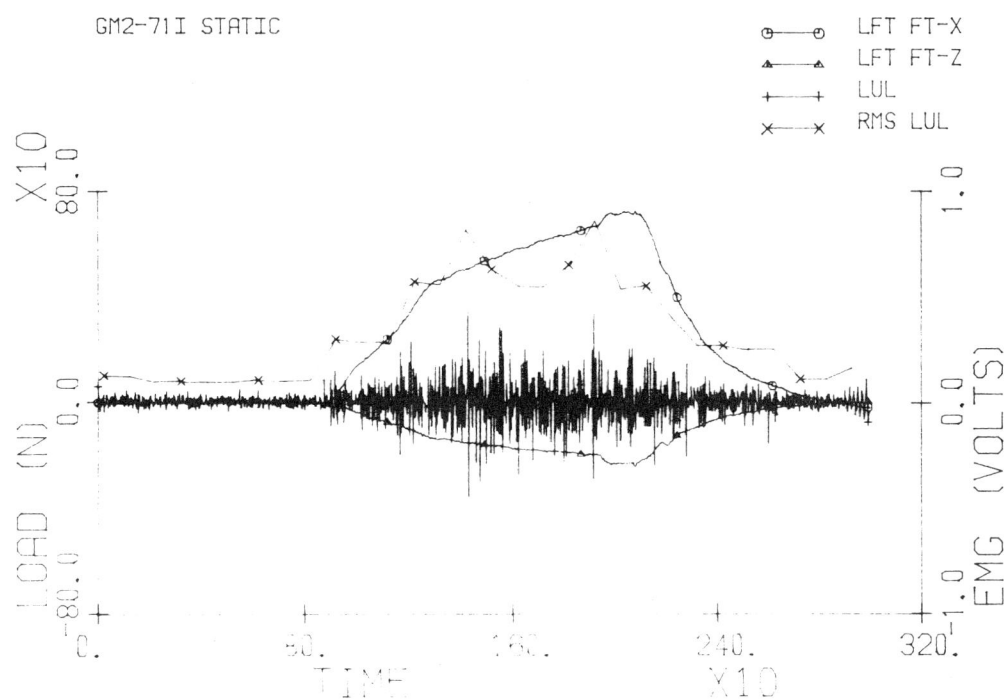

Fig. 5 - Left foot loads and EMG of the left quadriceps during static testing

cate an RMS equivalent force.

In general, reaction delays varied from 200-900 ms and the start of force development from the onset of EMG activity occurred after 80-150 ms. The attainment of peak force after its start could occur within 75 ms and peak forces ranged from 200 to 1000 N per foot. A static balance of forces exerted by the volunteer on the foot rest and seat was successfully made indicating that the data had been accurately acquired. Note that time delays to force generation were considered in several components: the time from stimulus to onset of EMG activity, the time from EMG activity to onset of force development, and the time for the development of peak force. There is consider able variation in the reaction times and peak forces developed between different volunteers as well as for the same volunteer in different tests.

Dynamic Tests - The sled acceleration pulse, as shown in Figure 8, was similar for relaxed and tensed volunteer experiments. The acceleration profile was of the same form for all runs. In dynamic runs the foot loads are characterized by three peaks as shown in Figures 9 and 10. The first occurs at approximately 100 ms and shows a correlation to g-level. It is concluded that this peak is due to the inertial weight of the foot and part of the lower leg only. The second peak occurs at approximately 200 ms and shows a correlation to g-level and the tensed or relaxed state. This peak is considerably higher in the tensed mode and is attributed to the inertia of other body parts transferring their load to the feet. The amount of force applied through the feet depends on the stiffness of the legs or their muscle tone. The joint torque generated by volunteers was not controllable and had a wide range of variation, as was evidenced from the static tests. Foot loads varied from 100 to 1300 N per foot. The inertia of the rest of the body is restrained by the belts and the seat. The time of the restraint peak forces coincides with the time of the second foot force peak and there is an inverse correlation in magnitude. The magnitude of the difference of second peak force levels between tensed and relaxed modes ranges between 100-1300 N and does not appear to be a function of acceleration, but rather a constant effect. Thus, at higher g-levels, as the inertial forces became higher, the significance of the effect of muscles on foot loads decreases.

The third peak is a broad peak of 100-500 N occurring around 400 ms or later and is due to muscular action. Figures 11 and 12 show foot loads and EMG response for two muscles. The estimated delay time from the onset of EMG to the onset of force is 80-150 ms. The root mean square (RMS) EMG signals generally do not show a correlation to force levels except perhaps for the quadriceps response and the third peak. Cadaver and dummy foot loads in the x-direction are shown in Figure 13 along with tensed and relaxed volunteer response. These loads do not have a substantial third peak and the first two peaks

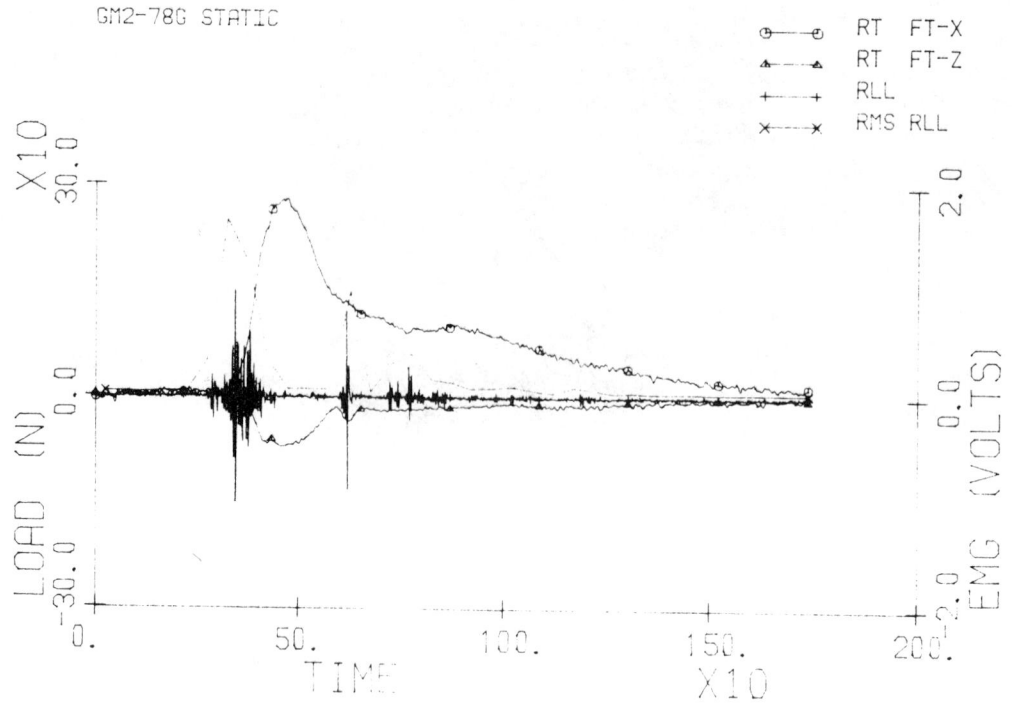

Fig. 6 - Static test response for right foot loads and EMG of the right tibialis anterior

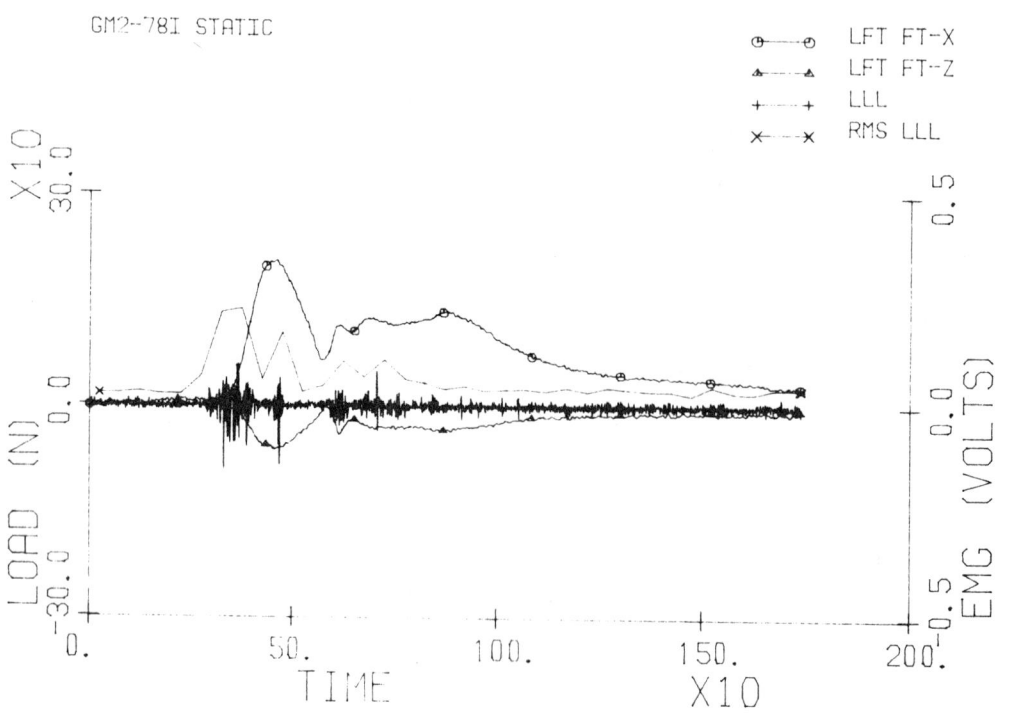

Fig. 7 - Static test response for left foot loads and EMG of the left gastrocnemius

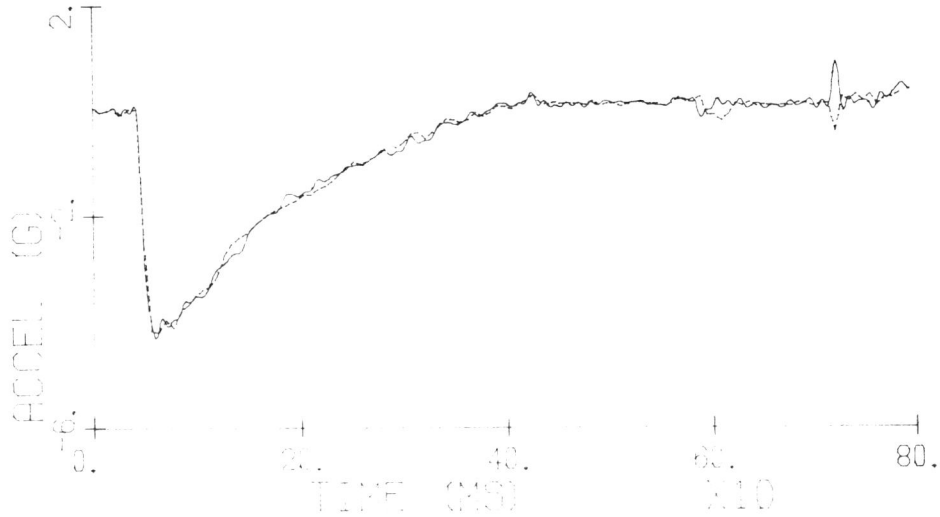

Fig. 8 - Typical sled acceleration pulse

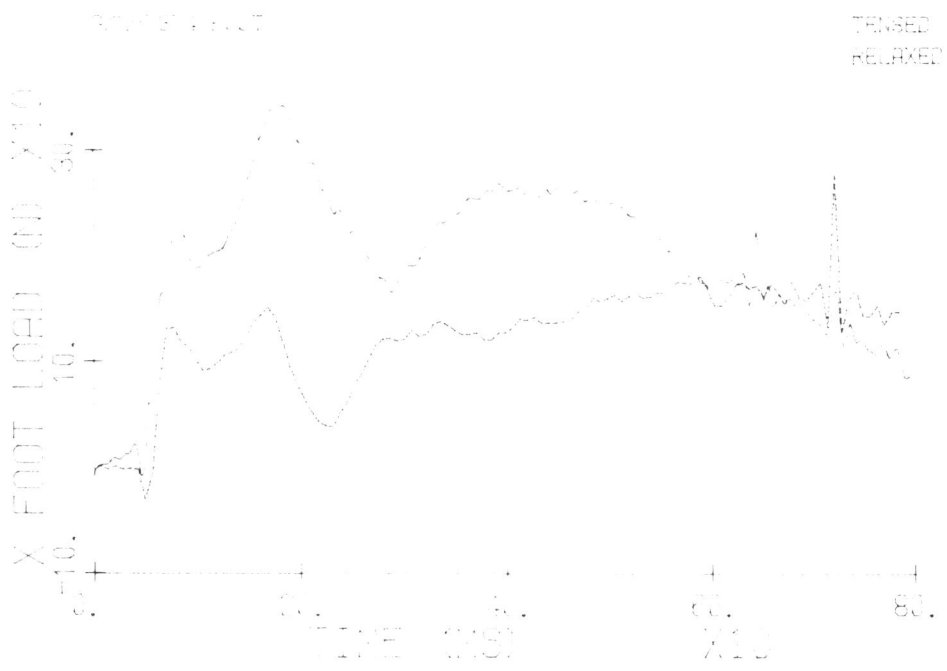

Fig. 9 - Foot loads in the forward direction for 4g volunteer runs

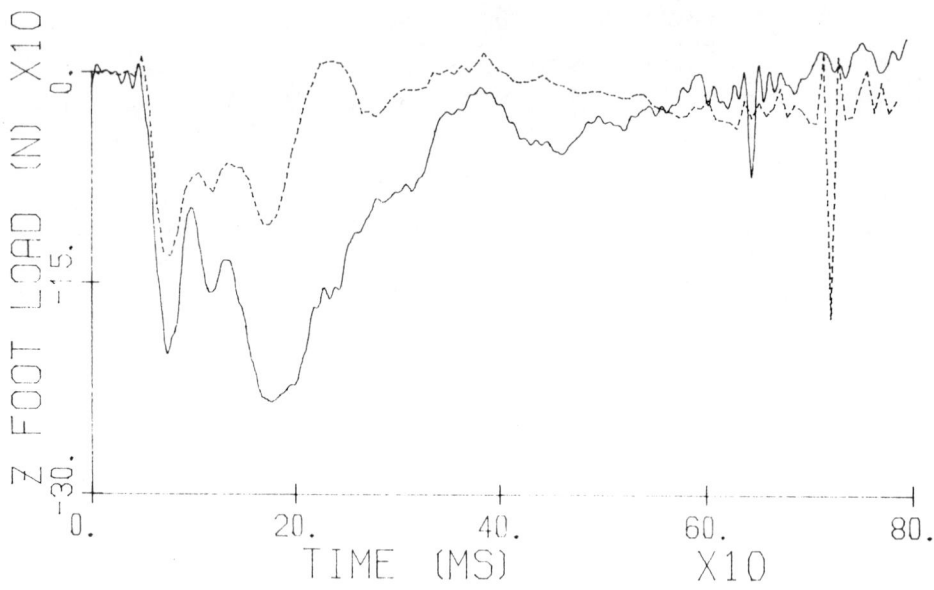

Fig. 10 - Foot loads in the vertical direction for 4g volunteer runs

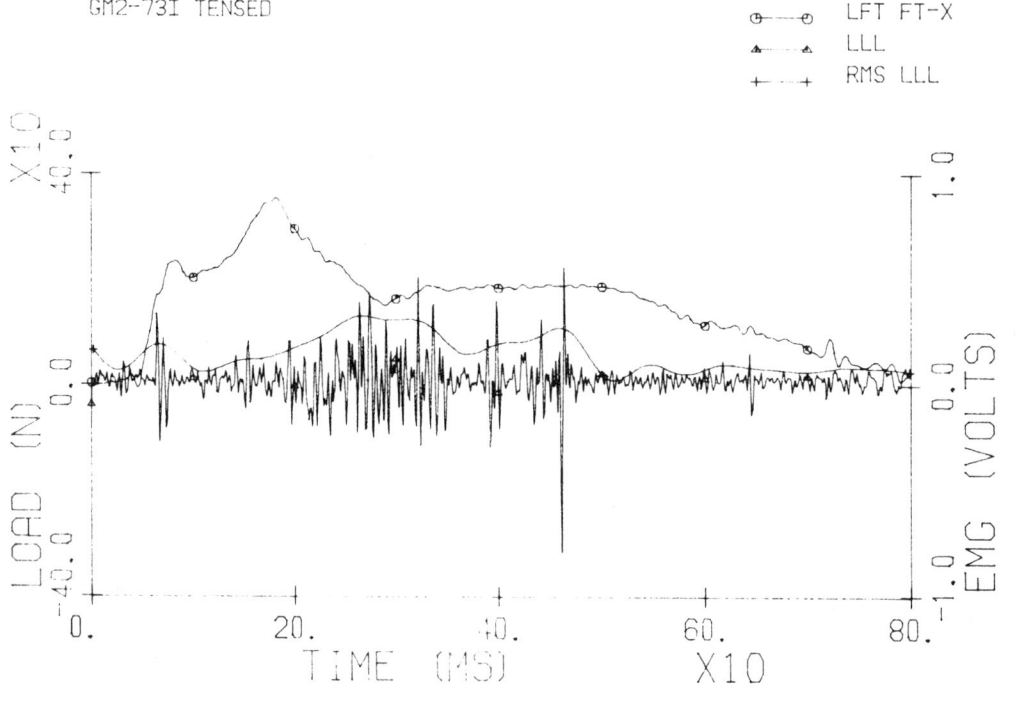

Fig. 11 - EMG response of the left tibialis anterior during a 4g tensed volunteer run

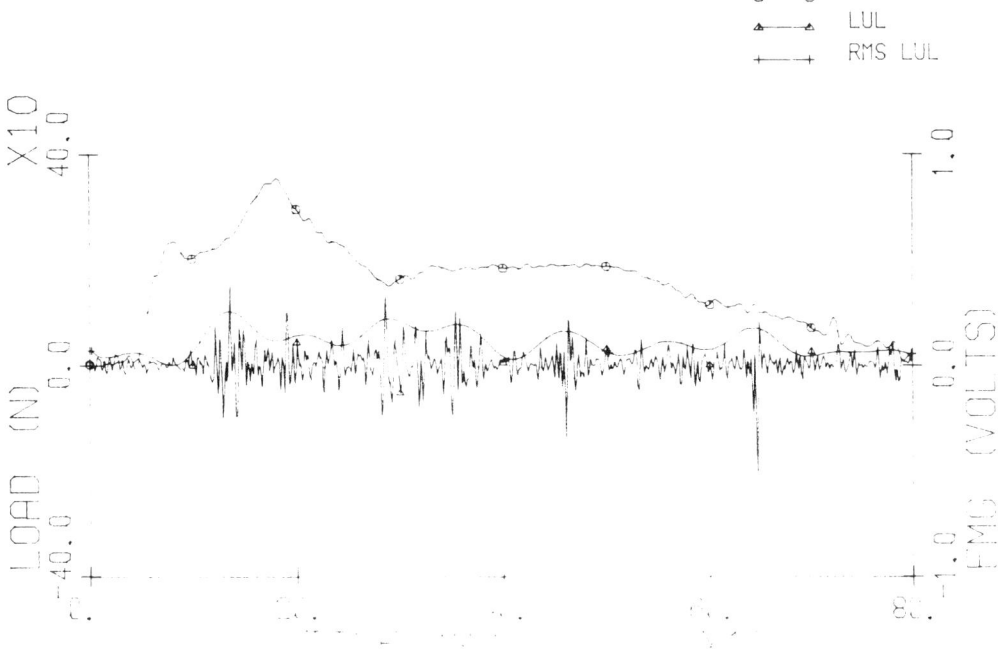

Fig. 12 - EMG response of the left quadriceps during a 4g tensed volunteer run

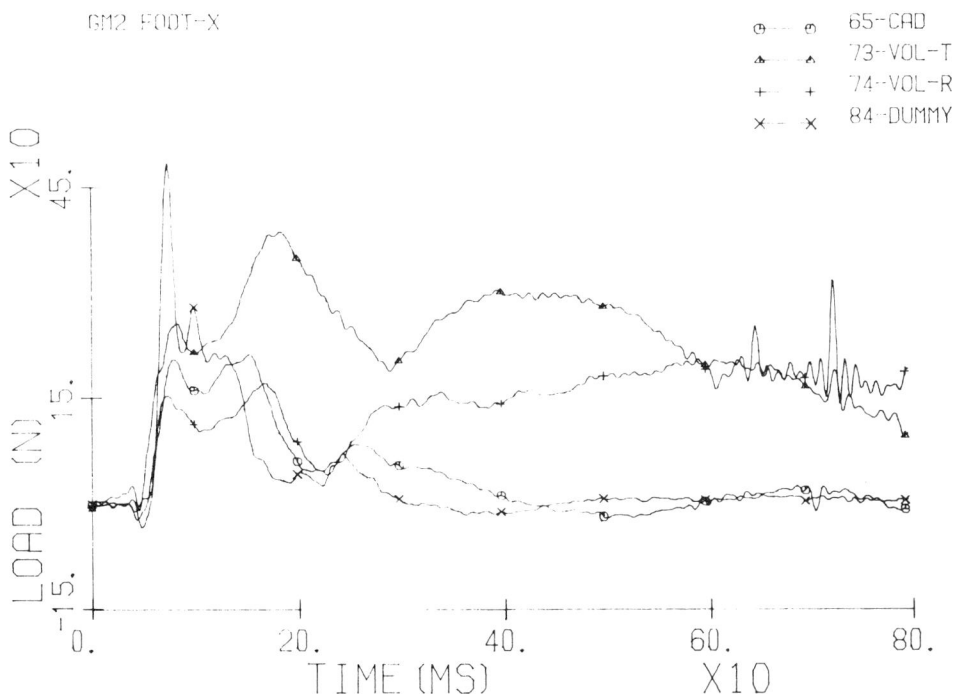

Fig. 13 - Comparison of forward foot loads for 4g acceleration

are always about equal.

Seat loads are shown in Figures 14 and 15. There is a decrease in peak load in the tensed mode. Peak head and pelvic accelerations decrease in magnitude in the tensed mode as does head rotation. Signal characteristics are essentially not changed.

A comparison of various responses as a function of sled acceleration is shown in Figures 16-22 for a tensed and relaxed volunteer, an embalmed cadaver and a Part 572 dummy. All forces have been normalized to a subject weight of 734 N. The difference in volunteer responses between tensed and relaxed modes is clear. Cadaver and dummy data generally fall in between. Joint stiffnesses affect the distribution of loads. Figure 23 show foot loads for 4-g cadaver runs with and without knee springs to simulated muscle tension. Foot loads are substantially higher with knee springs.

DISCUSSION

EMG signals were taken from six different muscle groups during each test. Exact placement of the electrodes over any muscle on different days cannot be assured. It was noticed that the same muscle could have different activities on different runs. Some of the variation could be due to electrode placement, but large differences in activity were noticed for each muscle group during the same series of runs. In general, EMG responses in the tensed mode were greater. Usually the tibialis anterior gave a good response for both relaxed and tensed test modes. The vastus medialis gave the weakest response. The gastrocnemius and quadriceps gave either strong or weak responses.

The large bursts of EMG activity appear to occur at or after the instant of peak loads (i.e., second force peak) and are apparently not a contributory factor in providing proprioceptive restraint until later in the occupants dynamics. From the static tests the time to force generation from the onset of EMG activity was at least 80 ms. Therefore, reflex (or voluntary) muscle forces could not be generated early enough in these tests to mitigate the first and second peak in restraint forces. However, the third force peak and all of the pretensed volunteer responses were significantly influenced by muscle action.

Although the stimulus is different in the dynamic situation, there is still a delay in response. If the stimulus is the stretch reflex, the muscle spindles cannot be stimulated until approximately the time of generation of restraint forces. These delays would put the development of a reflex force at the time of the third foot load peak, at which time the primary kinematics would be over and the restraint loads would have essentially returned to zero. The third peak shows an increase in force level in the tensed state but it cannot be determined

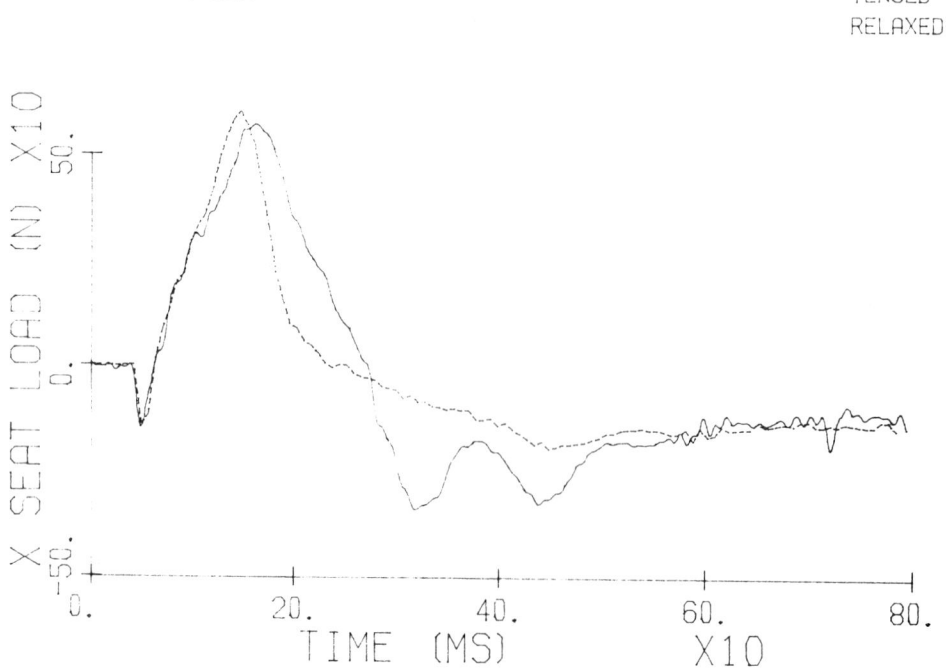

Fig. 14 - Forward seat forces during 4g volunteer run

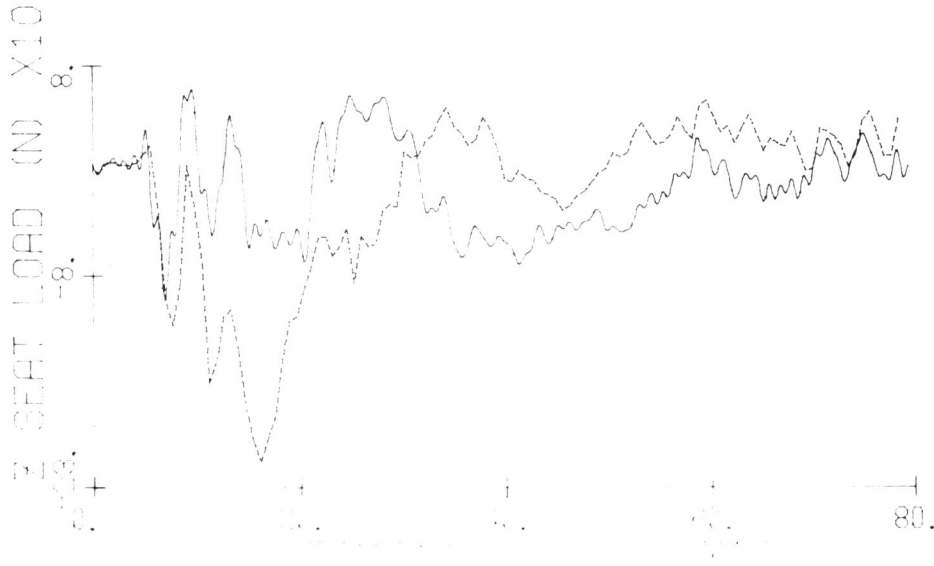

Fig 15 - Vertical seat forces during 4g volunteer run

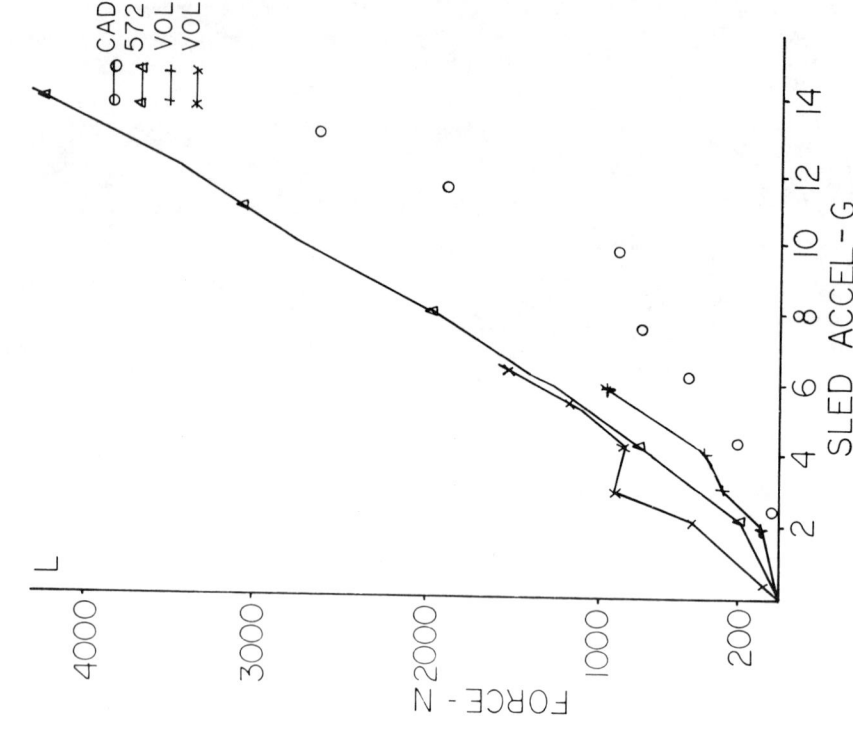

Fig. 17 - Comparison of lap belt forces

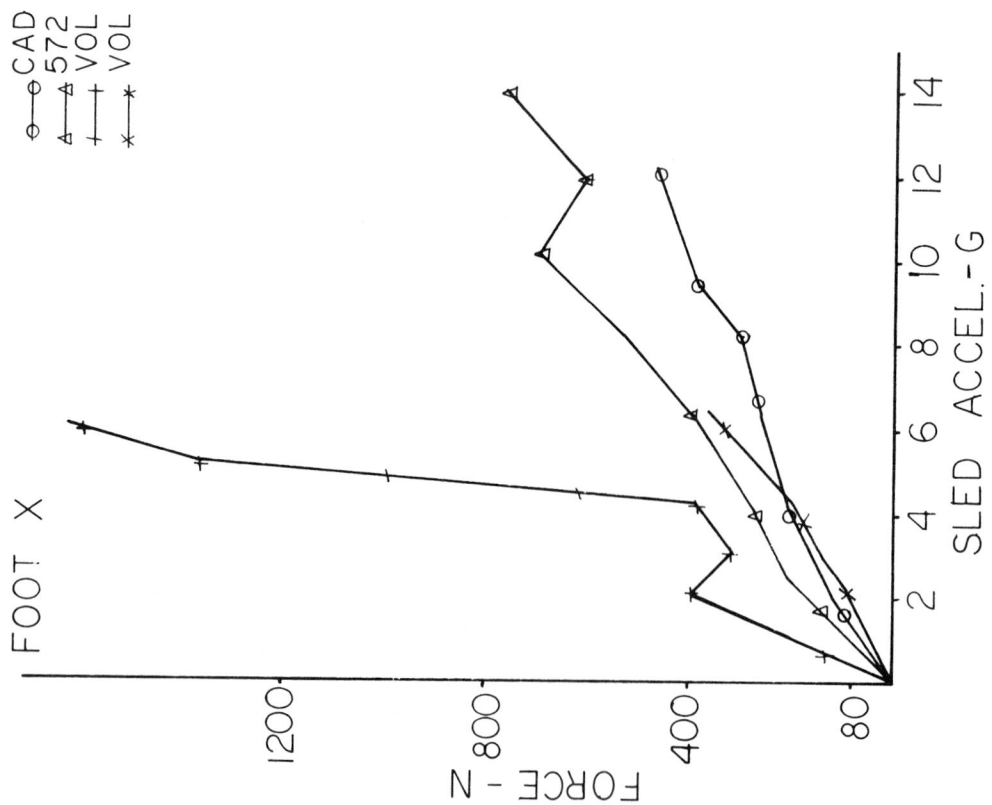

Fig. 16 - Comparison of forward foot forces

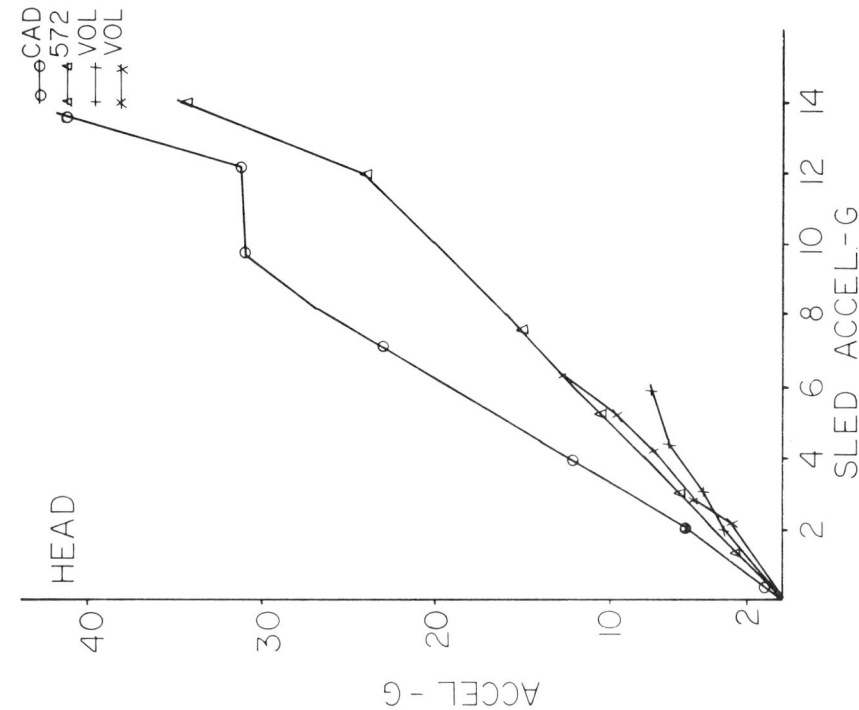

Fig. 19 - Comparison of head accelerations

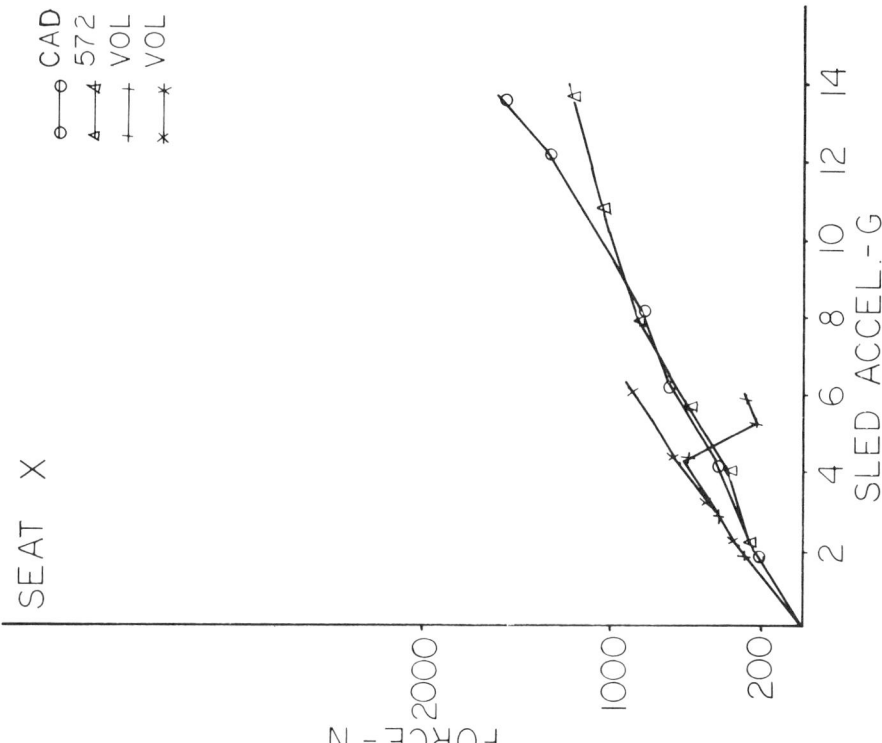

Fig. 18 - Comparison of forward seat forces

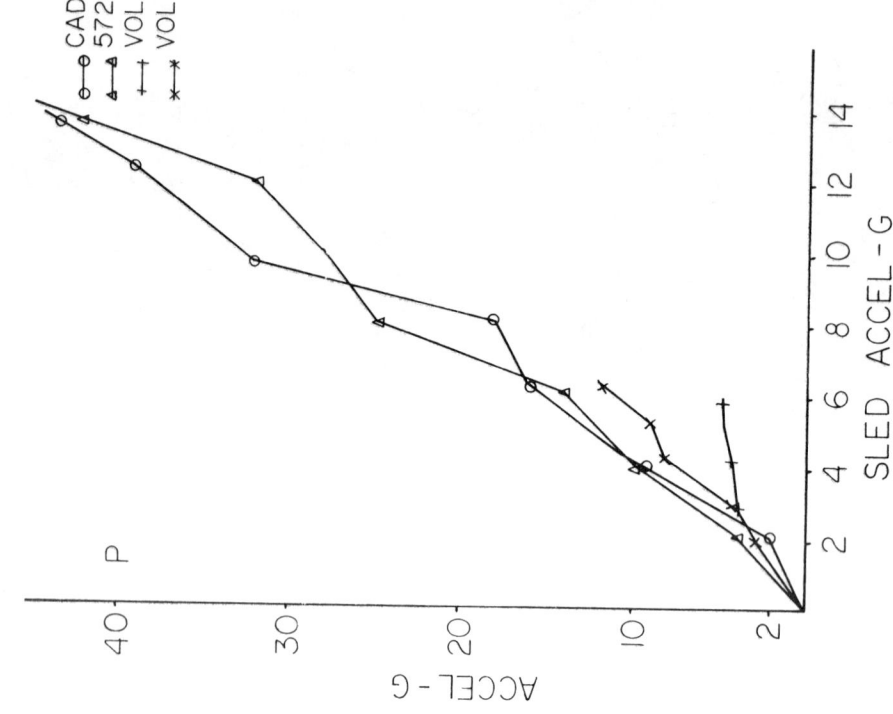

Fig. 21 - Comparison of pelvic accelerations

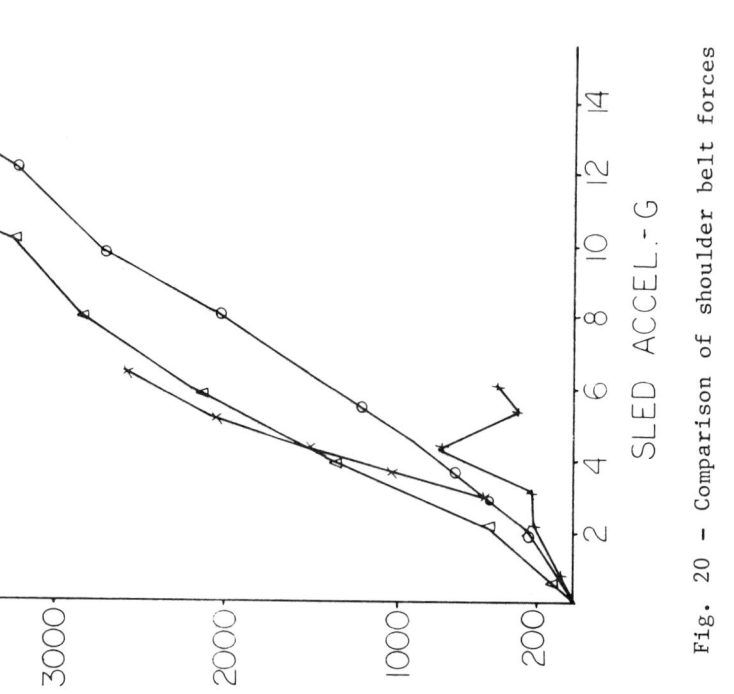

Fig. 20 - Comparison of shoulder belt forces

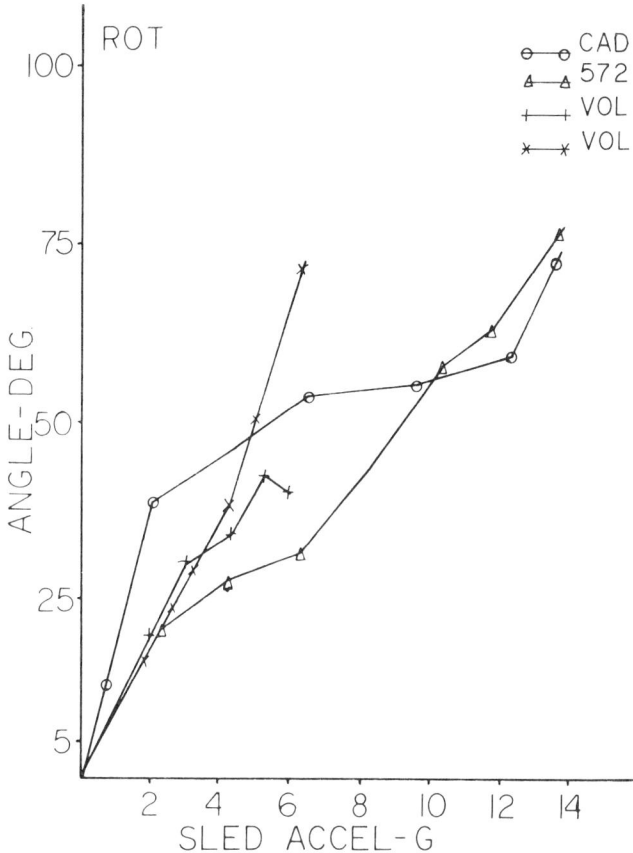

Fig. 22 - Comparison of head rotations

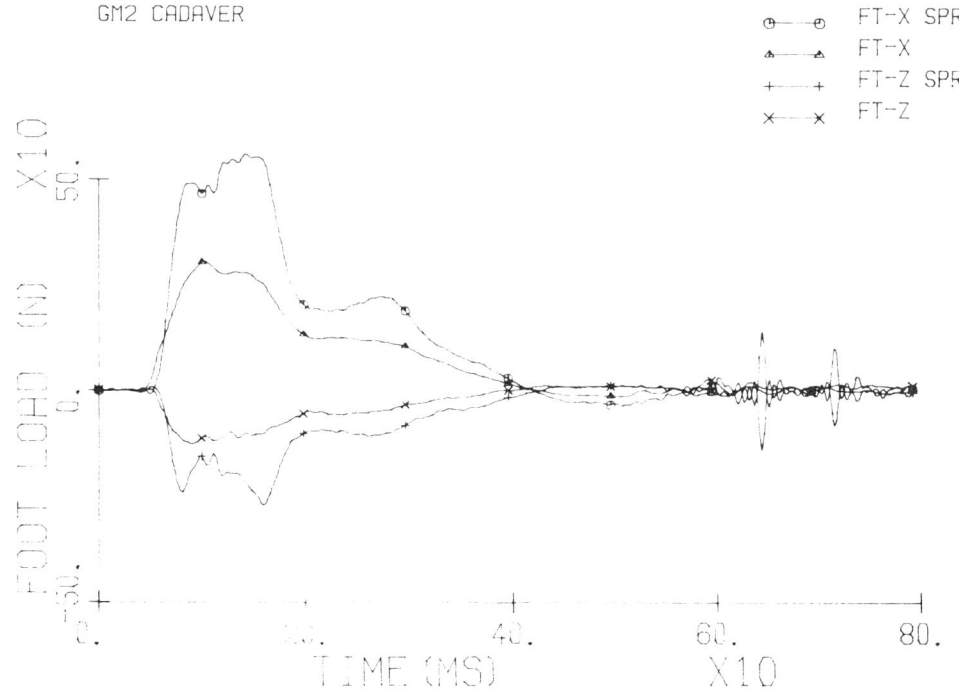

Fig. 23 - Forward and vertical foot forces of 4g cadaver runs with and without knee springs

whether this force is reflex or voluntary action.

CONCLUSIONS

It is concluded that the tone of the lower extremity muscles changes the occupant's dynamics and restraint force distribution. With muscular contraction the body becomes more rigid and transmits more load through the legs to the floor. Using friction type knee braces to simulate muscle tone, Levine et al (1978) were able to prevent submarining in cadaver tests. The maximum strength of voluntary muscle tension is limited. Therefore, the difference in restraint force between tensed and relaxed states is relatively constant so that at higher accelerations the influence of muscle tone on occupant dynamics diminishes. Comparison of responses of volunteers, cadavers and dummy show substantial differences in the distribution of restraint loads and dynamic response. It is clear that the stiffness, or muscle tone, affects the response of the various occupants.

EMG delay varied from 50-150 ms. A difference in response time between the tensed and relaxed mode could not be ascertained. Forces generated by muscular response (reflex or voluntary) in the dynamic situation were small, less than 300 N per foot, although statically, they could be as high as 1300 N.

REFERENCES

1. Levine, R. S., Patrick, L. M., Begeman, P. C., and King, A. I., "Effect of Quadriceps Function on Submarining." Proc. 23rd Annual Conference of AAAM, pp. 319-329, 1978.

2. Cheng, R., Mital, N. K., Levine, R. S. and King, A.I., "Biodynamics of the Living Human Spine During -Gx Impact Acceleration." Proc. 23rd Stapp Conf. SAE, Warrendale, pp 723-726, 1979.

3. Armstrong, R. W., Waters, H. P. and Stapp, J. P., "Human Muscular Restraint During Sled Decelaration." Proc. 12th Stapp Conf., SAE, NY, pp 440-462, 1968.

4. Hendler, E., O'Rourke, J., Schulman, M., Katzeff, M., Domzalski, L. and Rodgers, S., "Effect of Head and Body Position and Muscular Tensing on Response to Impact." Proc. 18th Stapp Conf., SAE, Warrendale, pp 303-338, 1974.

5. Patrick, L. M. and Trosien, K; Volunteer, "Anthropometric Dummy and Cadaver Responses with Three and Four Point Restraints." SAE Paper No. 710079, 1971.

6. Tennyson, S. A., Mital, N. K. and King, A. I., "Electromyographic Signals of the Spinal Musculature During +Gz Impact Acceleration." Orthopedic Clinics of North America, 8(1):97-119, 1977.

7. Hannan, A. G., Inkster, W. C. and Scott, J. D., "Peak EMG Activity and Jaw Closing Force in Man." J. of Dental Research, 54(3):694, 1975.

821158

Submarining Injuries of 3 Pt. Belted Occupants in Frontal Collisions— Description, Mechanisms and Protection

Y. C. Leung, C. Tarrière, and D. Lestrelin
Laboratory of Physiology and Biomechanics

J. Hureau
Faculty of Medicine, University of Paris

C. Got, F. Guillon, and A. Patel
I.R.B.A. Raymond Poincaré Hospital

ABSTRACT

Accidentological studies show, firstly, what kind of injuries are sustained by seatbelt wearers in frontal collisions, to abdomen, lumbar spine and lower members and, secondly, how to determine their frequencies and severities. Corresponding data are presented.

Then, a synthesis is made, in which the results of extensive cadaver testing - more than 300 human subjects - are examined with particular emphasis on the abdominal injuries, and on the association of injuries, such as lumbar spine injuries. Causation is particularly looked at. This experimental survey is completed by the results of specialized testing in abdominal tolerance when submarining occurs.

These two surveys enable the development of protection.

Finally, former attempts for defining an abdominal protection criterion are reviewed and a final definition for such a criterion is presented and justified.

ABDOMINAL PROTECTION IN AUTOMOBILE ACCIDENTS IS A SUBJECT WHICH HAS NOT BEEN FULLY EXPANDED UPON IN LITTERATURE ON ACCIDENTOLOGY AND BIOMECHANICS.

It is true that the head, thorax and lower members were the areas where those sustaining multiple injuries were the most frequently and most severely injured. Injuries in these areas were often evident (coma, breathing problems and fractures of long bones) whilst the possible share of abdominal injuries is more difficult to ascertain. In fatal accidents in particular, the autopsy is too often incomplete and only indicates the main injuries which are enough to account for the cause of death. Here again, abdominal injuries are often ignored in the same way as spinal injuries which require long and tedious research work before they can be detected.

In the 1970's, the wearing of seatbelts became general practice, especially in Europe. A new approach to regulation from the USA is gradually making headway. It is known as the global approach and sets out to appraise the secondary safety provided by a car, by simulating the most frequent and most deadly accidents and by measuring performance on one or more anthropomorphical dummies.

The first proposal for this type of regulation dates back to 1971. The American Administration wishes to appraise the protection provided by the vehicle in a frontal collision. The performance to be measured on the dummy concerns acceleration of the head and thorax and the load through the main axis of the thigh bone.

It is not surprising that the head, thorax and lower members are privileged areas we wish to protect. Indeed, methodological tools exist which we are not challenging. It is easy to measure the resultant acceleration of almost rigid models (head and thorax) by installing a three directional accelerometer at their centre of gravity.

Difficult research work is being conducted to determine the thresholds beyond which occupant protection cannot be ensured (to eliminate, for example, the risk of irreversible injuries). These thresholds must be based on human impact tolerance.

For 30 years, data have been progressively gathered and refined,
Curiously, the abdomen was overlooked. Until 1979, the first tolerance values (load-deflection) of a human abdomen loaded by a seatbelt in static test conditions was presented(1). Because the tolerance could not be measured by accelerometer techniques, a specific methodology was used to define abdominal tolerance and translated into a measurable performance on a dummy. To make the distinction between values which are specific to the human being and their applications to a dummy, we employ the term "tolerance" for the former and "protection criterion" for the latter. The protection criterion may be different if the dummy itself changes definition.

The purpose of this publication is to establish a consolidated version of the most recent work devoted to abdominal protection in frontal collisions(xx) for belted occupants and to attempt to ascertain whether the protection criterion currently available would be sufficient to avert the great majority of abdominal injuries. Because submarining is the most involved mechanism, the analysis is enlarged to all injuries induced, by submarining that is to say lumbar, lower members, pelvic as well as abdominal injuries.

An analysis is presented for the abdominal injuries observed in a sample of 1542 subjects wearing 3-point seatbelts and involved in frontal impacts. This is followed by a corresponding analysis of abdominal injuries observed in the tested cadavers which were divided-up into two independent samples groups, one composed of 70 subjects, and the other 211 subjects, corresponding to the observations supplied by different research groups.

After having specified the relative importance of the risk of lumbar, lower members and abdominal injuries, the study goes on to analyze and consider the prevention of abdominal injuries caused by the mechanism the most often involved, well-known under the name of "submarining" (factors which influence the occurrence of submarining and in particular the definition of a protection criterion to eliminate the risk of submarining by means of principles of a well-designed vehicle).

By discussing all available information, it is possible to estimate the extent of protection provided by currently available criterion.

(x) Numbers between parentheses are references at the end of paper
(xx) Other publications cover a similar study on abdominal protection in side impacts.

SUBMARINING INJURIES IN REAL-LIFE ACCIDENTS

The accident survey file contains 1017 frontal impacts in which drivers wearing three-point seatbelts were involved.

The impacts are selected based on the following body injury criterion ; at least one of the occupants involved in the accident was taken to the hospital.

SEVERITY OF SUBMARINING INJURIES IN RELATION TO OVERALL RISK - The population of seriously injured among the 1017 drivers (M.AIS 3, 4 or 5) is slightly less than that observed among the 525 passengers. Respective proportions of those killed are not significantly different. (Table 1). (See also Appendix I)

From among the severely injured front occupants, 1 driver out of 5 and 1 passenger out of 3 sustained severe injuries to abdomen and dorso-lumbar spine fractures (Table 2).

Table 2 - Proportion of AIS $\geqslant$ 3 to Abdomen and Dorso-Lumbar Column Among Severely Injured Drivers and Passengers (M.AIS $\geqslant$ 3) wearing 3-pt belt.

Thoracic-lumbar spine and Abdomen AIS

	$\leqslant 3$	$\geqslant 3$	Total
Drivers	69 (79%)	18 (21%)	87 (100%)
Passengers	37 (64%)	21 (36%)	58 (100%)
Total	106 (73%)	39 (27%)	145 (100%)

SEVERITY OF ABDOMINAL INJURIES IN RELATION TO OTHER BODY AREAS - The abdomen, with the head and thorax, is, for belted drivers, the body area most exposed to critical injury (AIS $\geqslant$ 4). Injuries to lower members very largely dominate at level 3. (Table 3).

One of the advantages of the adoption of retractor belt systems which are fitted to cars produced since 1978 has been to reduce the slack with which static belts were habitually worn. Further, their geometrical lay-out in the car is a great improvement; the central mounting systems do, in particular, eliminate any further risk of initial contact of the adjusting buckle against the abdomen.

This progress accounts for the very great difference in the risk of abdominal injury between those wearing static and those wearing retractor belts (Table 4).

The improvement to seat belt has, therefore, approximately halved the share of abdominal injuries

However, they are still dangerous and some progress should be made. A precise description of the injuries and their most probable mechanisms may help to throw some light on the subject.

Table 1 - Severity of Frontal Impacts for Front, Belted (3-point) Drivers and Passengers.

	M.AIS 0-1-2	3-4-5	$\geqslant 6$	Total
Drivers	892 (87.8%)	87 (8.5%)	38 (3.7%)	1017 100%
Passengers	451 (86%)	58 (11%)	16 (3%)	525 100%

Table 3 - Severity of Injuries by Body Area Sustained by Belted Drivers and Passengers During Frontal Impact (Excluding Those Killed and not Subjected to Autopsy).

DRIVERS   Frontal Impacts (11.12.01 o'clock)

	Head/Face	Neck	Thorax	DL. Spine	Abdomen	Pelvis	L. Members
AIS - 0	651	917	762	968	948	938	670
1	225	75	207	24	31	40	229
2	96	1	16	6	3	6	50
3	16	4	2	1	4	15	50
4	2	1	11	-	11	-	-
5	9	1	1	-	2	-	-
	999	999	999	999	999	999	999

RIGHT FRONT PASSENGERS

	Head/Face	Neck	Thorax	DL. Spine	Abdomen	Pelvis	L. Members
AIS - 0	395	456	326	492	477	498	366
1	90	61	159	27	30	23	123
2	33	4	28	4	1	1	19
3	4	3	7	3	5	4	18
4	3	1	6	-	13	-	-
5	1	1	-	-	-	-	-
	526	526	526	526	526	526	526

Table 4 - Proportions (%) of Occupants Sustaining Severe Abdominal Injuries (AIS ≥ 3) and/or Dorso-Lumbar Fractures (AIS ≥ 3) Among the Seriously Injured Drivers and Passengers (M.AIS 3, 4 or 5).

	Static Belt	Retractor Belt
Drivers	22.6%	12 %
Passengers	37.5 %	16.7 %

THE RISK OF SUB-MARINING INJURIES INCREASES WITH THE VIOLENCE OF IMPACT - This relationship, which can be seen in Table 5 allows us to rule out the assumption, occasionally put forward, whereby the risk of injury to the abdomen is primarily governed by malfunctions or by the presence, in the population studied, of dangerous and badly designed systems, irrespective of the violence. The mechanisms which sometimes cause the abdomen to be subjected to excessive loading, resulting in injury, are not easy to describe for the accidentologist. A number of factors do, however, allow us to state, with a good degree of certainty, that each case matches up with one of the following configurations :

1- Restraint is achieved by the most resistant bone segments, including and more especially- the pelvic region, but the abdominal mass undergoes a deceleration beyond the level of tolerance, It results in tears, wounds or rupture of viscera which certain authors thought could be described by specific features (2).

2 - A variant of these cases on which the seatbelt firmly fastens the pelvis and where we could still observe abdominal injuries, would correspond to another mechanism, that is a very important flexion of the trunk around the pelvis. This flexion can be clearly observed in experimental impacts (Figure 1), and the head can come into contact with the knees. A great kinematics was produced possibly within the certain car models, in which the superior anchorage was very behind that favored the sliding of the shoulder under the shoulder belt. Abdominal injuries would not be the result of the deceleration of the viscera in relation to the belt restrained skeletal frame, but would be induced by very high pressure in the viscera, and even compression between the trunk and thighs. The stout persons are more exposed than others to this type of compression. If here is a submarining process, the lap-belt still increases the pressure in viscera.

3 - The belt is worn in such a way that, when the slack is taken up, the lap-belt presses against the abdomen, penetrating through even as far as the spinal column when deceleration is high (Table 6). This second configuration, where play is a major factor, is frequent when the seat belt anchorage installation is faulty. Its consequences are aggravated when the restraint system on the oldest static belt models includes a buckle for adjusting belt tension, located on the end of a flexible stalk anchored to the centre of the car. This system has significantly deteriorated seat belt performance in numerous accidents which have occurred over the past ten years.

4 - The lap-belt is correctly positioned against the pelvic bone but, when the occupant is displaced forward, loading conditions of the restraint system are such that the lap-belt, under tension, runs up over the iliac crests and compresses the abdomen. This is submarining in the strict sense of the term.

The last two configurations have the most adverse effects on the abdomen. The injuries they cause have no specific typology whereby it would be possible, from a review of the medical file, to determine whether the case in point falls into configuration 3 or 4. Amongst the relevant indications capable of distinguishing between them, we can name the presence of cutaneous erosion in the pelvic region, particularly below or above the anterior superior iliac spines : the distance over which the belt shows signs of friction compared to occupant stopping distance.

In the last two configurations, the pressure exerted on the abdomen is the risk to be avoided. Whether it be at the just beginning of occupant displacement or after slipping from the pelvis, that in no way obviates the need to design restraint systems and their installation in such a way that restraint acts only against the pelvis throughout the whole of the occupant's deceleration phase. The share of the shoulder belt as a direct cause or aggravating factor in injuries to tissues or organs in the upper abdomen region (liver, spleen, in particular) is not negligible but the results of an analysis indicated in Table 7 show that, when it exists, it is most often accompanying the preponderant action from the lap-belt.

Table 5 - Proportion of Occupants With Severe Abdomen Injuries and Dorso-Lumbar Fractures and Proportion of Severely Injured (M. AIS $\geqslant$ 3) in Each ΔV Category.

ΔV (kph)	$\leqslant$35	36-45	46-55	56-65	$\geqslant$65
AIS abdomen $\geqslant$ 3	0.3%	2.4%	13.3%	13.5%	46.2%
M.AIS $\geqslant$ 3		2% 16.0%	48.0%	59.5%	92%

Likewise, drivers sometimes strike against the steering unit which contributes to the injuries or is the sole cause of them, but this is a rare occurrence, since we have seen (above) that the abdominal risk is lesser for driver than for passenger.

The 26 drivers and 21 passengers who sustained severe submarining injuries (AIS $\geqslant$ 3) were equipped with seatbelts almost half of which had a geometrical defect and were worn too loose. The presence of one or other of these two factors or both combined, was noted in more than two out of three cases (Table 8).

CONCLUSIONS

1. The process described by the term of submarining of the lower part of the trunk (pelvis-abdomen-lumbar-spine and the lower thorax) under the lap-belt is a mechanism fairly frequently encountered among belted occupants in frontal impact.

Submarining is considered to be the mechanism most probably at cause in the vast majority of cases involving the seriously injured (AIS $\geqslant$ 3) sustaining injuries to the abdomen, the lower members, the pelvis or the dorso-lumbar column.

One of the original aspects of this in-depth cases analysis is that it shows how submarining can cause severe injuries to the lower members (legs-knees-femurs), the pelvis and the dorso-lumbar column (fracture-compression of the first lumbar vertebraes or fracture of the transverse processes) as well as to the abdomen. There are besides often combinations of these different injuries.

Other injuries may more exceptionally be combined, such as wounds or injuries to the neck and occasionally rib fractures.

2. The lap-belt is certainly the cause of 68% (32/47) of cases of victims of abdominal (AIS $\geqslant$ 3) and/or dorso-lumbar column (AIS $\geqslant$ 2) injuries.

Table 6 - Dorso-Lumbar Spine Injuries (AIS ⩾ 2) - N = 14 Cases

LEVEL OF FRACTURES	INJURIES' MECHANISMS					
	SUBMARINING			DIRECT REAR IMPACT (rear passenger or object)		
	Sure	Probable	Uncertain	Sure	Probable	Uncertain
D9 - D11			1*			
D 12	1	1	1			
L 1	4					
L 2	2					
Lumbar vertebrae process-transverse:	1	2*	1			
L5 process transverse:				1		

(*) aggravating influence of the rear passenger

Table 7

SYNTHESIS OF SUBMARINING - ANALYSIS OF INJURIES' MECHANISMS

PARAMETERS	LAP-BELT Sure	LAP-BELT Probable	LAP-BELT Uncertain	SHOULDER BELT Sure	SHOULDER BELT Probable	SHOULDER BELT Uncertain	OTHER DIRECT IMPACTS (steering-system for example) Sure	Probable	Uncertain
POOR GEOMETRY OF THE RESTRAINT	14 43%(A)	6	1	1	0	2	0	0	0
BELT WORN WITH SLACK	13 36%	4	2	0	0	1	0	0	0
FRONT SEAT TRACK DAMAGE	13 38%	5	1	0	1	2	0	0	0
ADDITIONAL LOADING	7 21%	3	0	0	0	1	0	0	0
NECK CONTUSIONS OR ABRASIONS BY SHOULDER-BELT	6 19%	3	0	0	1	1	0	0	0
LOWER MEMBERS IMPACT AGAINST LOWER PANEL	30 83%	9	5	1	1	4	0	2	1
CRASH VIOLENCE $\Delta V \geq 50$ km/h mean $\gamma \geq 10$ g	19 58%	6	2	0	1	3	0	1	1
ABDOMINAL INJURIES SUB-MESOCOLIC	25 64%	5	2	0	1	3	0	1	0
ABDOMINAL INJURIES ABOVE MESOCOLIC	8 21%	2	1	1	1	3	0	1	0
DORSO-LUMBAR FRACTURES	8 23%	3	1	0	0	0	1	0	0
LOWER MEMBERS FRACTURES	17 45%	4	2	1	1	2	0	0	0
PELVIC INJURIES	3 8%	1	2	0	0	1	0	0	0
RIB FRACTURES	14 32%	1	1	1	0	1	0	0	0
AGGRAVATING INFLUENCE OF RIB FRACTURES	3 8%	1	0	1	0	0	0	0	0

IMPORTANT REMARKS:

(A) This percentage corresponding to the two first columns means that the parameter involved plays for x% of all cases where lap-belt submarining is sure or the most probable. For example, "Poor geometry..." plays in 20 cases out of 47 where submarining is sure or the most probable.
(B) The total in each ROW could overpass the number of involved people because, for some cases, two mechanisms could play simultaneously (ex.: lap-belt submarining and abdominal injury induced by shoulder-belt (rib fracture).

Its rôle is very probable in 19% of the other cases; only in 13% of cases it is absent or doubtful.

The rôle of the shoulder belt is unquestionable in 1 out of 47 cases as complementing the action of the lap-belt and is possible in one other case. In 4 cases there is some doubt.

3. It is difficult to strictly specify the mechanism causing abdominal injuries as it means taking into consideration all the medical, anthropometric and technical data in the accidentology files. Two analysis grids have been established and they are given in Appendices I and II.

Submarining is evident when contributory factors such as poor geometry of the restraint system and (or) slack in the belts (one or other or both these factors combined are present in 74% of cases) are observed with the following:

a) Seat-tracks damages in 38% of cases

b) Knee or leg impact under the instrument panel with very obvious deformation of the latter in 83% of cases.

c) Violent impact ($\Delta V \geqslant$ 50kph and $\gamma \geqslant$ 10g in 58% of cases where submarining is certain or very probable).

4. It should be noted that apart from submarining and the auxiliary rôle played by the shoulder belt, the responsability of the instrument panel and/or the steering unit is exceptional in the occurrence of abdominal or lumbar injuries (one probable case and one doubtful).

5. The additional load from the rear passengers is an aggravating factor (in 21% of cases where submarining is certain or probable).

6. Fractures of the pelvis are seldom but could be the result of submarining (8% of cases where submarining is certain or probable) whether by knee impact or by direct action of the lap-belt.

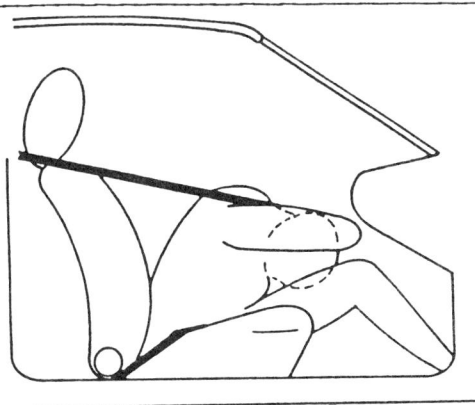

FIG. 1 . DIAGRAM OF A CADAVER TEST.

7. Another Sub-marining consequence already noted in a previous publication (2) is the great frequency (23%) of dorso-lumbar vertebraes fractures (D12-L1-L2) by direct impact of the lap belt or (and) hyperflexion of the trunk around the lap-belt penetrated in the abdomen.

8. The lower members injuries (legs, knees and femurs fractures) are not specific ; however they are observed in 45% of cases of sub-marining sure or most probable and could be considered as another consequence of this process.

ANALYSIS OF ABDOMINAL INJURIES OBSERVED IN EXPERIMENTS CONDUCTED ON HUMAN CADAVERS FOR 281 FRONTAL IMPACT TESTS.

Two test samples with cadavers simulating frontal collisions with three-point seatbelts provide a total of 281 observations. All the subjects were fresh cadavers conserved at a temperature of around 0° and experiments were conducted a few hours or days following their death.

An initial sample known as "APR" groups 70 subjects. A second one, the "Heidelberg" sample groups 211 subjects.

ABDOMINAL INJURIES OBSERVED IN THE "APR" SAMPLE - The most frequent injuries are fractures of the rib cage and litterature already exists on this subject.

In this paper, the injuries indicated are only the abdominal injuries or the lumbar vertebra injuries which can be produced by the same mechanism, in particular submarining.

Out of the 70 frontal impact tests using cadavers, there were 47 cases with injuries, 23 with lap-belt submarining and 24 without lap-belt submarining. The rest were cases where no injury was sustained and there was no evidence of submarining. The appended Table 9 illustrates which of the tested cadavers sustained only the injuries observed in the liver, the spleen, the lumbar vertebra and other abdominal injuries, including the intestines, mesentery, colon, iliac crest and abdominal muscles. Cases with only iliac crest fracture or abdominal muscle injury are also presented in this Table which contains 24 cases, 6 of which are non-submarining and 18 submarining.

Table 8 - Quality of Restraint System Geometry and Belt Wearing Among Victims of Abdominal injuries and Dorso-Lumbar Fractures

		POOR GEOMETRY		
		YES	NO	TOTAL
EXCESS SLACK	YES	8	8	16
	NO	12	13	25
	UNCERTAIN	3	3	6
	TOTAL	23	24	47

Table 9 - Abdominal and spine injuries observed in frontal impact tests with cadavers (APR sample).

Test N°	Seat N°	Submarining	Liver	Spleen	Lumbar vertebra	Other abdominal injuries and pelvic bones fractures
2	1	yes	yes		L4 sacrum	colon, mesentery
4	1	no	yes			
6	2	yes				
8	2	no		yes		ilium, diaphragm
10	1	no	yes			ilium
12	2	yes				mesentery
16	2	no		yes		diaphragm
25	2	no				mesentery, ilium (*)
44	2	no				
127	4	yes			L1	
154	4	yes	yes		L2	iliac crest
170	1	yes			L4,L5	
182	2	yes			L1	
183	1	yes	yes			
184	1	yes	yes			
185	2	yes				mesentery
189	4	yes			L5,S1	abdominal muscle, mesentery
231	2	yes	yes	yes		mesentery
243	4	yes				colon, abdominal muscle
244	4	yes				left ilium crest
245	4	yes				abdominal muscle
246	4	yes			T6,T7	abdominal muscle
247	4	yes				abdominal muscle
255	2	yes		yes		

Seat N°. 1 : driver
Seat N°. 2 : front passenger
Seat N°. 4 : right rear passenger

(*) very light injury

Table 10 - Abdominal injuries observed in Frontal Impact tests with cadavers ("Heidelberg" sample).

	Mean $\gamma \leq 16$ g		Mean $\gamma > 16$ g	
	Drivers	Passengers	Drivers	Passengers
Size of sample	81	0	46	84
Liver	0	0	2	14
Spleen	0	0	0	5
Kidneys	1	0	1	3
Mesenterium	2	0	4	11
Intestines	1	0	3	4
Vessels	0	0	2	4

The following comments can be made :

1. No lumbar vertebra fracture was found in non-submarining cases but lumbar vertebra fractures occurred frequently in submarining cases (5 cases out of 14).

2. No injuries observed in intestine, colon, and mesentery were found in non-submarining cases (except for N° 25 who sustained a light mesentery injury). These injuries were frequently observed in the submarining cases (6 cases out of 17).

3. 5 drivers sustained liver injuries, 2 of which were non-submarining cases.

4. 2 passengers sustained liver injuries with submarining.

5. All four "spleen injury" cases were observed only on front passengers, 2 of which were non-submarining cases, three were submarining cases

ABDOMINAL INJURIES OBSERVED IN THE "HEIDELBERG" SAMPLE - An ISO document based on experimental data from the University of Heidelberg which have appeared in numerous past publications presents the following summary as shown in Table 10.(3)

Except for spleen injuries, there is no preferential distribution of injuries between drivers and passengers. Liver is injured in 16% of cases for the passenger and 3.5% for the driver. The mean sled deceleration was exceeding 16g.

These results confirm the absence of specificity regarding liver injuries which would, as for spleen injuries, seem to be sustained more often by the passenger. This does, therefore, consolidate the findings of the APR sample analysis.

DISCUSSION

1. Out of 23 cases of liver injuries, 7 were drivers. 2 of them were non-submarining cases, 5 were submarining cases. This is not sufficient to ascertain that the shoulder belt is responsible for liver injuries in non-submarining cases, as we could see similar results for the front passenger. 16 cases of liver injuries were observed among front passengers (or right rear passengers), and they were submarining cases. The possible effect of the shoulder belt on liver injuries was relatively small in this group of the sample.

2. All of 5 spleen injury cases were observed in the front passengers. Two of them occurred in submarining cases.

3. As observed for the spleen, or for the liver, any sustained injury cannot be automatically due to the shoulder belt. It would be more suitable to say that the shoulder belt favours submarining on the buckle (interior)side. In certain cases, the shoulder belt could play a role in provoking such injuries without the occurrence of submarining.

4. No intestine, colon, mesentery injuries were found in non sub-marining cases (except one case where a light mesentery injury occured).

5. In our previous submarining studies (4), it was found that submarining began, in most cases on the interior side, for both cadaver and dummy tests. Two cases were found where submarining was limited to the interior side only, This illustrates the statement made in 3. to the effect that "the shoulder belt favours submarining on the buckle (interior) side".

CONCLUSIONS

1. Abdominal injuries occurred rarely in non submarining cases.

2. Dorso-lumbar vertebra fracture was never found in non-submarining cases. But lumbar vertebra fractures are often associated with submarining and, sometimes, without abdominal injury.

3. Spleen and lever injuries are possible consequences of lap-belt sub-marining. Liver injuries are not specific to anyone occupant seat. Spleen injury is found particularly to the right passenger (front or rear).

4. The possible effect of shoulder belt is rather low. The shoulder belt could favour the submarining process on the buckle interior side.

5. All sub-mesocolic injuries (except one) are consequences of lap-belt sub-marining.

DEFINITION OF SUBMARINING (MECHANISM)

A definition problem regarding the word"submarining" was experienced on several occasions these last years, in particular with I.S.O. (ISO TC22/SC12/GT 6).

Corresponding to a personal communication of G.M. NYQUIST, several types of submarining referred to by various authors in the past are :

- Lap-belt submarining
- Shoulder belt submarining
- Air bag submarining
- Instrument panel submarining.

He stressed the fact that abdominal injuries are not the only consequences of a submarining and that knee injuries due to impact following submarining should be considered as submarining injuries. We also agree with this point of view. One should note that, in practice if lap belt submarining is avoided, the risk of knee impact is very much reduced.

For the wearer of a three point safety belt, submarining is reduced to the relative movement of the body in relation with the belts. The submarining can only take place through release of the iliac crests passing under the lap belt. A slanting displacement of the pelvis takes place downwards and frontwards. This movement of the pelvis corresponds to a simultaneous movement of the whole trunk which could be named thoracic submarining relating to the thoracic belt. However, no thoracic syndrome specific to submarining has yet been described. Some cervical injuries could be due to this whole trunk submarining as we have seen in our accidentological sample.

So as not to complicate things, at least as regards the wearer of a three point safety belt, one should avoid talking of submarining regarding the body as a whole. To make things clear one should talk about pelvis submarining relating to the pelvis belt. This usually causes abdominal injuries, injuries of the dorso-lumbar vertebra, of the knee-femur-pelvis axis, all these injuries which can either be isolated or associated.

It is difficult to distinguish, within this category, the difference of the submarining occurred with the initial positioning of the lap-belt on abdomen and with the initial positioning on the pelvis. In real accidents, in most cases, it is impossible to know exactly the initial positioning. This depends on the care taken by the wearer in placing correctly the safety-belt (however does the wearer know that the lap-belt, sometimes called "abdominal", should really restrain the pelvis ?) The placing of the belt depends firstly on the restraint geometry but also of the posture and slack in the belt.

FACTORS INFLUENCING THE OCCURRENCE OF LAP-BELT SUBMARINING

"Submarining" is a complicated problem because its occurrence is associated with many parameters, for example the geometry of the seat-belt system, orientation of the pelvis, dynamic characteristics of the seat and vehicle, impact velocity, etc... These are the external parameters determined by test conditions. An internal parameter is the pelvis shape; the area in question is the upper half of the notch below the Anterior Superior Iliac Spine (A.S.I.S.). Here as in previous publications (4)(5), this pelvic area situated just below the ASIS is given the name "Sartorius" and has a length of A1A2 (see figure 2).

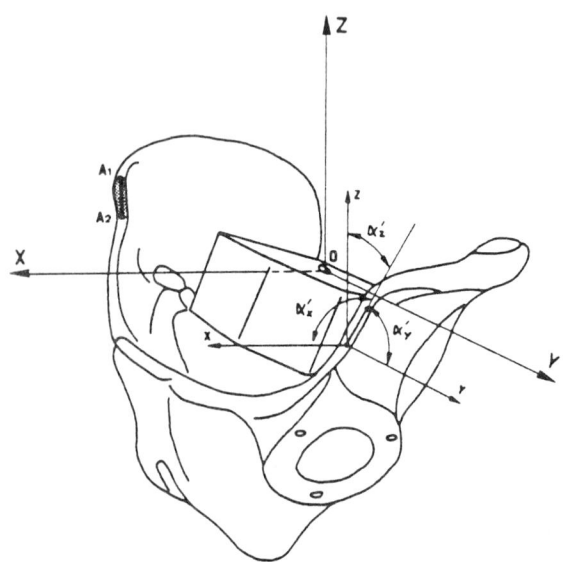

FIG. 2 . DIRECTION OF THE UPPER HALF NOTCH (A1A2)"SARTORIUS" DEFINED IN THREE DIMENSIONS.

In fact, to avoid any confusion, it is necessary to state that Sartorius is the original name given to the muscle attached to this referred bone area in Gray's Anatomy (pp. 228, 492).

INFLUENCE OF LAP-BELT ANGLES - During frontal impact, the load applied to the "Sartorius" on one side of the pelvis is the resultant of lap-belt tensions on the corresponding side. This load can be resolved into two components: one is parallel to the "Sartorius", the other is perpendicular. The parallel one orients downward and backward along the "Sartorius"; it can be defined as a load to keep the pelvis in a favorable position necessary to prevent the process of submarining. This load is related to the orientation of the "Sartorius" and the geometry of the lap-belt as well as to lap-belt tension. The coefficient of the load can be used as an indicator of the efficiency in reducing the submarining tendency. A brief technical term referring to "anti"-submarining scale was used in a previous paper (4).

If the orientation of the Sartorius is considered as a constant, the anti-submarining scale is only a function of the geometry of the lap-belt defined in three dimensions. Since some experimental results cannot be explained by the traditional geometry definition of the lap-belt given in two dimensions, a complete geometrical definition of the lap-belt determined in three dimensions was developed.

Thanks to the anti-submarining scale curves established on the basis of the present theory and the submarining tendency as a function of lap-belt angles β_1, β_2, determined in experimental results, an anti-submarining scale $\xi = 0.63$ is proposed for a limit of submarining risk on lap belt geometry. Hence, this paper shows that the graphs of the anti-submarining scales can be used for checking the submarining risk in the seat-belt system.

Theoretical study: using a geometrical model of the lap-belt during impact (Fig. 3), the following equations can be found:

$F_3 = F \cos \theta$
$F_4 = F \sin \theta$

where load F is the resultant of lap-belt tension applying to the "Sartorius" (A1A2) on one side.

When the magnitude of F is known, F_3 and F_4 depend only on the angle θ which is formed between the direction of Sartorius and the resultant load F. F_3 is a load parallel to the Sartorius, preventing the lap-belt from riding-up over the A.S.I.S, and keeping the pelvis in a correct position. Therefore, it is a load that plays an important role in reducing the submarining tendency. In contrast, F_4 is a load which rotates the pelvis backward and downward, i.e. it increases the risk of submarining. F3 could be used as an indicator of the efficiency in reducing the submarining tendency.

By a mathematical study (4), load F_3 is given by another expression,

$F_3 = \xi F_1$

Lap-belt tension in this equation depends on collision velocity, seat and vehicle dynamic characteristics, mass of the belted occupants, etc... If F1 is determined, F3 is a function of the coefficient ξ. Since F3 is defined as an indicator of the efficiency in reducing the submarining tendency, the coefficient ξ can be designated as an anti-submarining scale indicating the efficiency to prevent the process of submarining for a given configuration.

The coefficient ξ depends, on one part, on the direction cosines of the "Sartorius" and, on the other part, on the lap-belt geometry designated by angles β_1, β_2. It is presented precisely by the following equation:

$$\xi = \cos\beta_1 . \cos[\tan^{-1}(\cos\beta_1 . \tan\beta_2)] . \cos\alpha'_x + [\cos 1/2 \tan^{-1}(\cos\beta_1 . \tan\beta_2) - \sin 1/2 \tan^{-1}(\cos\beta_1 . \tan\beta_2)]^2 . \cos\alpha'_y + \sin\beta_1 . \cos[\tan^{-1}(\cos\beta_1 . \tan\beta_2)] . \cos\alpha'_z$$

Since α'_x, α'_y and α'_z were three-dimensions defined previously for the "Sartorius" of an occupant within a car (5), anti-submarining scale could be determined as a function of lap-belt angles β_1, β_2.

By using above equation, the relationship between the coefficient ξ and the lap-belt angles (β_1, β_2) can be obtained, as illustrated in Figure 4 for human subject (male) and for Part 572 dummy (Figure 5).

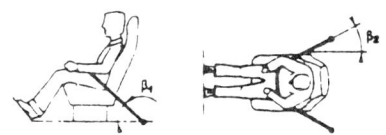

ANTI-SUBMARINING SCALE ξ

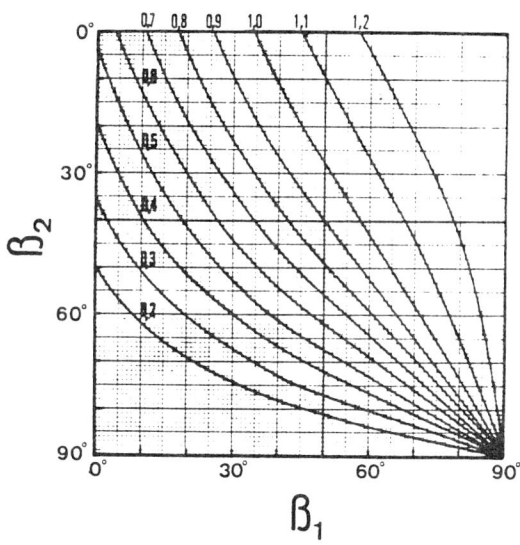

FIG. 4 . ANTI-SUBMARINING SCALE ξ CURVES AS A GUNCTION OF LAP-BELT ANGLES β_1, β_2 DERIVED FOR HUMAN SUBJECTS (MALE).

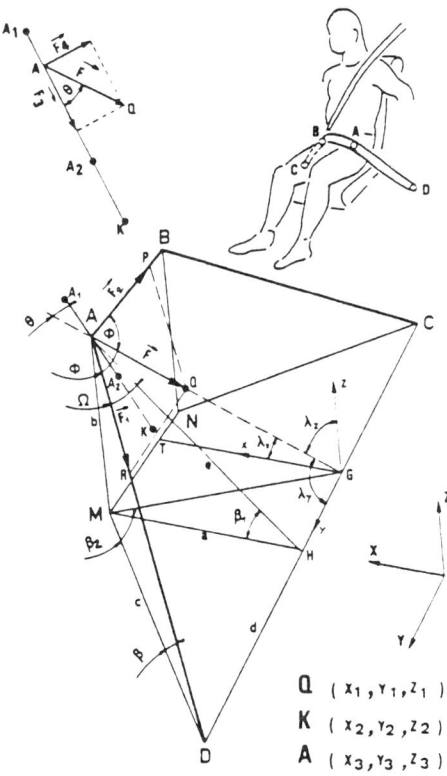

FIG. 3 . GEOMETRICAL MODEL OF THE LAP-BELT DURING IMPACT.

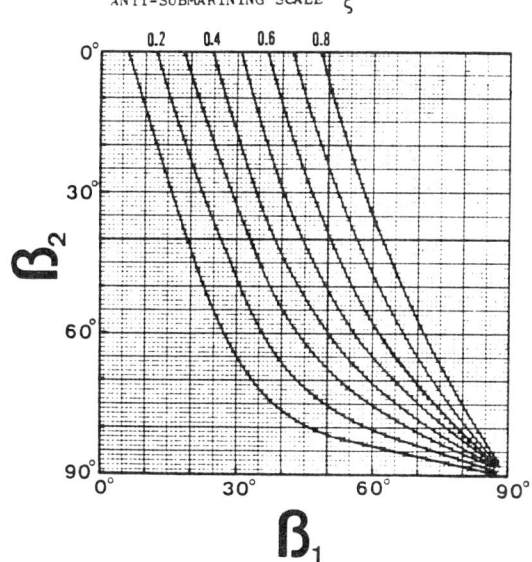

FIG. 5 . ANTI-SUBMARINING SCALE ξ CURVES AS A FUNCTION OF THE LAP-BELT ANGLES β_1, β_2 DERIVED FOR PART 572 DUMMY.

Experimental study - In order to put into practice and examine this theoretical study and the results, a series of sled tests was performed with human cadavers, the Part 572 dummy and the modified dummy. Three different bodies of European car models were used and mounted on the sled for the tests.

The lap-belt angles β_1, β_2 were measured with the tested subjects in the initial position, the test conditions and the complete experimental results were given in reference (4).

The details of the conservation of human cadavers can be consulted in reference (6). Briefly, the cadavers were fresh and non-embalmed. Death occurred less than 4 days before the test. They were put in a cold box and then taken out a few hours before the test.

Following the experimental results, submarining consequences in relation to the lap-belt angles β_1, β_2 are illustrated generally in Fig. 6 for the human subjects, Part 572 dummy and modified dummy.

Based on both the theoretical study and experimental results, the anti-submarining scale ξ can be traced between the groups of submarining data points corresponding to the 0.66 curve on Figure 4. It can be found in this figure: firstly that the submarining data points locate at the area which is formed by the smaller angles β_1 and the greater angles β_2 corresponding to the lower anti-submarining scale zone. Secondly, non-submarining data points locate inversely at the other area where β_1, β_2 are respectively greater and smaller, corresponding to the higher anti-submarining scale zone. Thirdly, two non-submarining data points for a cadaver test and a modified dummy test are situated in the submarining zone. This may be explained once more by the fact that the cadaver and the modified dummy are less inclined to submarine than the Part 572 dummy.

The figuration and location of the curve indicate that for the same anti-submarining scale, the decrease of β_1 should be associated with the decrease of β_2, i.e. if angle β_1 is favorable to submarining (smaller), it is necessary to associate a good angle β_2 (smaller) to reduce the submarining tendency if other conditions remain unchanged. This case corresponds to the highest data points (circle). On the other hand, while angle β_1 is great enough, according to previous beliefs, it seems to be unfavorable to submarining. Unfortunately, the submarining process occurred. In Figure 6, the three or four lowest black data points correspond to this case and it can be explained by the fact that these data points have greater angles β_2. Experimental results reveal that the geometrical definition of the lap-belt designated only by angle β_1 is insufficient to define its submarining tendency.

The traditional geometrical definition is used in two dimensions given as the angle formed by the lap-belt and the X-axis from side view, specified as angle β_1. A wide range of this angle had been proposed as an unfavorable angle to submarining by the previous researchers. There were, for example, 45-50° proposed by Haley (7), 45° by Patrick (8), 50-70° by Adomeit (9), Hontschik (10), and 69° by Billault (11). These reference angles are represented in Figure 6 for a comparison.

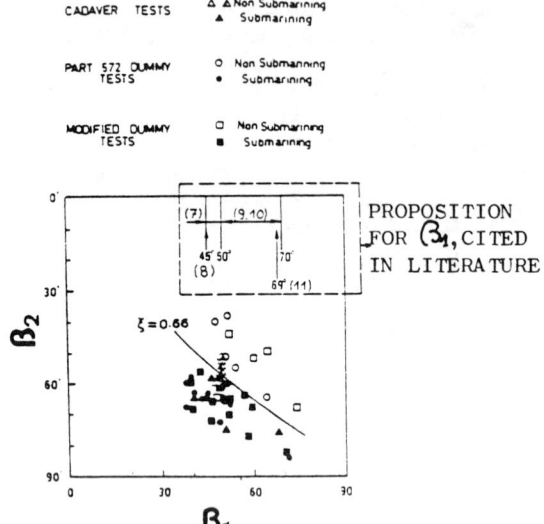

FIG. 6 . ANTI-SUBMARINING SCALE DETERMINED IN CADAVER, PART 572 AND MODIFIED DUMMY TESTS. THE RESULTS GIVEN IN THREE DIMENSIONS (β_1, β_2) ARE COMPARED WITH THOSE GIVEN IN TWO DIMENSIONS (β_1) PROPOSED IN LITERATURE.

Angles β_1 proposed in the above references cover almost all the submarining and non-submarining data points in the Figure 6. This variation was caused certainly by the variable angles β_2 which had been used but not observed by the authors of the references. Indeed, it is difficult to state what is the unfavorable angle β_1 to submarine if angle β_2 is not given.

Actually, the submarining tendency cannot be indicated when using the traditional definition of the lap-belt geometry as determined by angle β_1 alone. It is according to our theoretical and experimental study.

INFLUENCE OF SEAT DESIGN - Seat design is another parameter influencing the submarining consequence. Necessary motions of the pelvis are the forward and downward displacements which provoke probably a lap-belt submarining. To limit these two displacements, there is the conception for the creation of an "anti-submarining" seat.

Adomeit and Heger (9) proposed an energy-absorbing seat constructed with the front wall of the seat metal pan. On the forward area of the seat pan, a density of foam of 53 kg/m³ was used (Figure 7).

Lundell et al. (12) presented a seat which had a contourned floor pan with a pronounced ridge at the front end. The seat cushion had a greater thickness which decreased gradually to the front edge of the cushion (Figure 8). In comparison with their flat seat tests, it showed that the new seat design gave both reduced injury criteria and low risk of submarining.

On the previous study (4), a comparison of submarining tendency was taken for the front occupant in the passenger seat and rear occupant in the bench. It was shown clearly that the rear occupant submarined more easily than the front occupants.

It can be explained by, firstly, a bad fixation system of the lap-belt on the interior side, corresponding to a smaller anti-submarining scale; secondly, no ridge support under the rubber foam at the front end of the bench.

These two parameters played together a role in the greater submarining tendency of rear occupant.

INFLUENCE OF "INTERNAL" PARAMETERS - Seat-Belt geometry, seat design, impact violence are external parameters. Others could be called "internal" parameters, such as anthropomorphic data (size and weight, relative bigness and shape of the pelvic bone, volume and stiffness of soft tissues in front of the "Sartorius", direction in space of "Sartorius" and direction of the pelvis in sitting position.

As indicated in the anti-submarining scale equation, if the lap-belt angles (β_1, β_2) are determined, we can see how the direction of "Sartorius" affects the submarining tendency. A comparison of the anti-submarining scales can be shown in Figure 9 and Figure 10 for human sub-

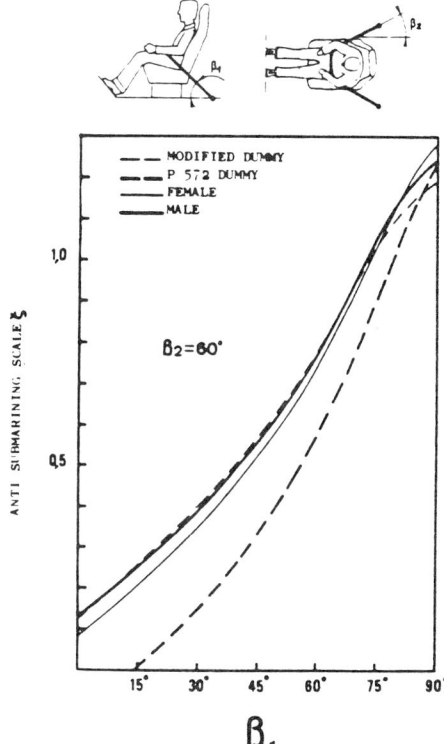

FIG. 9. COMPARISON OF THE ANTI-SUBMARINING SCALE CURVES BETWEEN THE DIFFERENT SUBJECTS STUDIED AS A FUNCTION OF β_1 WHEN $\beta_2=60°$.

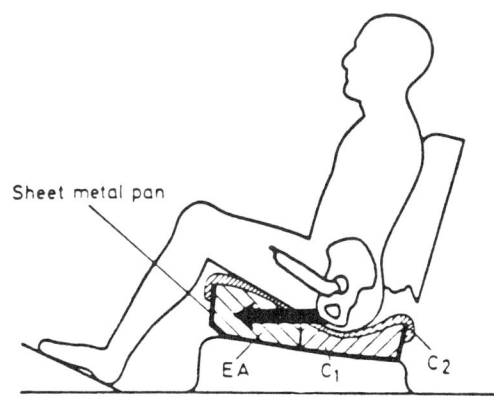

FIG. 7. DIAGRAM OF A SEAT DESIGN GIVEN BY ADOMEIT ET AL.(9).

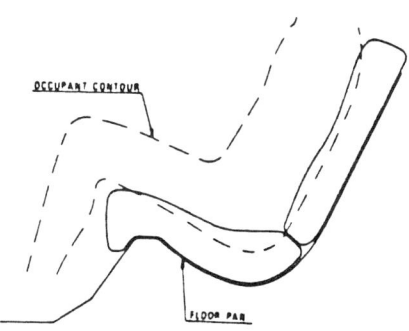

FIG. 8. DIAGRAM OF A SEAT DESIGN GIVEN BY LUNDELL ET AL.(12).

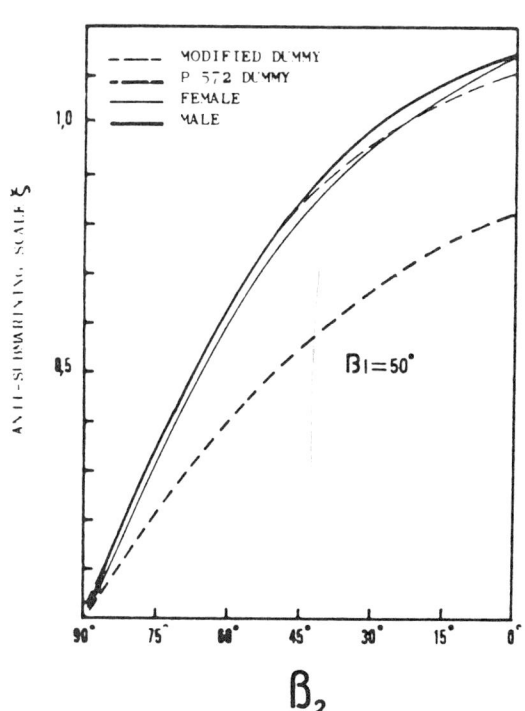

FIG. 10. COMPARISON OF THE ANTI-SUBMARINING SCALE CURVES BETWEEN THE DIFFERENT SUBJECTS STUDIED AS A FUNCTION OF β_2 WHEN $\beta_1=50°$.

jects (male and female), Part 572 dummy and modified dummy.

In (5), it was shown that the direction of the Sartorius varies with the sex of the individual and with the different pelvic models. For example, the angle $\alpha'x$ (Fig. 2) is the most critical angle for indicating the tendency to submarine. This angle varies from 85° for males to 79° for females and to 109° for Part 572 and 83° for the FAA-USAF-NHTSA pelvic model. The submarining tendency is stronger when this $\alpha'x$ is higher (4)(5).

Flexibility of the soft abdominal tissue is greater for human subjects than for Part 572 dummy (5). An attempt was made in order to have a more human-like dummy. A Part 572 dummy modified at the level of "Sartorius" and abdominal tissue was defined (Fig. 11) and evaluated (4).

The theoretical approach still applies to these evaluations and experiments already widely described (4) have shown that the frequency of submarining is very similar for the modified dummy and the cadavers (65 % and 62.5 % respectively), smaller than for Part 572 (75 %). It was also observed that submarining occurs in a shorter time for the Part 572 (67.8 ms against 74.5 and 73.5 ms for the human subject and the modified dummy). This constitutes another reference for the justification of submarining tendency.

The direction of the "Sartorius" depends not only on the pelvic shape of the individual but also on the orientation of the pelvis in sitting position. It is known that the lap-belt submarining performance depends significantly on pelvic orientation. The submarining tendency increases with the rearward rotation of the pelvis. This rotation was defined for a sitting position within a car in relation to a standing position. An angle of 36.7° was recommended by Nyquist (13); it was determined an X-ray-radiograms-study on the basis of two volunteers from his study (14) and 5 volunteers from reference (5).

STUDIES BY MATHEMATICAL MODEL OF THE INFLUENCE OF CERTAIN OCCUPANT PARAMETERS ON THE RISK OF SUBMARINING OCCURRING.

A study by mathematical model of occupant related factors was conducted in 1979 with the financial backing of the French Government, as part of the Programmed Thematic Action "Vehicle Safety - Submarining Criterion". The purpose of this study was to evaluate the influence of parameters such as stiffness of the lumbar column, hips and knees, or mass distribution adjacent to the pelvis, on the tendency of a dummy to submarine (15).

MODEL - The model used, "Prakimod", is a two-dimensional one. It has ten degrees of freedom and offers the advantage of being a sophisticated and tried method of simulating a belt restraint system (16).

REFERENCE TEST - An experimental test - 50th Percentile Part 572 dummy in front passenger position, restrained by a 3-point-inertia-reel-belt type on a sled (Renault 5 configuration without instrument panel), catapulted at 50 kph against a 30° inclined rigid wall - was reproduced by mathematical modelling, to act as a reference.

OUTPUT PARAMETERS - Actual submarining is not simulated by the model, but it does provide, at each moment, an output of the angle formed by the inboard and outboard webbings of the lap-belt with the pelvis projected along the sagittal plane (Figure 12). The maximum value of this angle during impact, together with its value when maximum forces in the lap-belt occur, make it possible to identify the risk of submarining. Maximum head, thorax and pelvis accelerations are also recorded as well as the maximum tensions of the different webbings and resultant forces applied to the dummy.

SIMULATIONS FOR COMPARISON PURPOSES - After the reference simulation, eleven other simulations were carried out using the same set of data but modidying each time the value of one of the input parameters to be tested.

RESULTS (Table 11) - Stiffening of the lumbar-column would greatly reduce the risk of submarining which is natural. A major increase in head accelerations would be observed simultaneously, along with a significant decrease in the longitudinal displacement of the centre of the head.

Stiffening of the hips generally heightens the risk of submarining, reduces head and pelvis accelerations and increases thorax accelerations. Moderate stiffness of the knees is of very little consequence.

Significant stiffening tends to slightly reduce the risk of submarining, as well as diminishing all maximum accelerations and belt forces. Transferring load from the thigh to the trunk tends to reduce the risk of submarining, especially if the load is transferred to the abdomen and not to the pelvis. Furthermore, a reduction in forward movement of the head and maximum acceleration of the pelvis and an increase in shoulder belt loading were recorded.

FINDINGS OF STUDY - Two possible orientations emerged from this study to reduce the tendency of the Part 572 dummy to submarine, independently of any change to the shape of the pelvis:

-Pending accurate accurate and reliable anthropometric data, displace load from the thighs to the pelvis, or better still, to the abdomen. This would entail modidying the dummy build.

-Or simply modify the adjustment of hip and knee friction torques, by requiring that these torques balance not the weight of the members as specified in Standard 208 (Figure 13A) but the weight of the whole body, realistically positioned in line with the working of the muscles of these members (Figure 13 B). This gives a smaller hip torque (61Nm against 100Nm for both hips), but a knee torque more than seven times greater (146Nm against 20Nm).

Two further simulations confirmed the accuracy of this solution regarding the change in output parameters (risk of submarining, accelerations..) but also showed that excessive blocking of the

Table 11 - Part of Mathematical Simulation Results

TEST No.	REFERENCE 1	HIP STIFFNESS DIVIDED BY 3 — 2	MULTIPLIED BY 3 — 3	MULTIPLIED BY 9 — 4	KNEE STIFFNESS DIVIDED BY 3 — 5	MULTIPLIED BY 3 — 6	MULTIPLIED BY 9 — 7	LUMBAR STIFFNESS DIVIDED BY 3 — 8	MULTIPLIED BY 3 — 9	MASSES DISPLACEMENT −4kg from upper legs +4kg onto pelvis — 10	−4kg from upper legs +2kg onto pelvis +2kg onto lumbar segment — 11	−4kg from upper legs +4kg onto lumbar segment — 12
MAX. HEAD ACCELERATION (G)	71.00	70.38	57.51	53.59	71.12	70.64	67.85	42.16	75.50	72.04	64.18	50.81
HEAD G.S.I.	511.75	521.09	397.71	371.35	514.13	504.84	473.78	281.06	568.40	535.11	417.17	371.35
H.I.C.(*1)	408.17	417.15	327.41	298.28	410.38	401.64	373.87	242.50	465.93	416.61	380.61	315.55
MAX THORAX ACCELERATION (G)	46.32	47.75	47.14	50.02	46.64	45.37	42.37	49.01	53.10	46.55	49.27	51.35
THORAX G.S.I.	262.28	260.97	269.15	325.80	265.11	253.70	228.97	297.28	354.94	249.76	258.16	276.90
MAX PELVIS ACCELERATION (G)	71.30	74.27	70.36	63.21	71.42	70.88	69.53	69.83	69.27	68.90	67.40	65.97
MAX FORCE 1 (*2) (N)	12813	13266	13117	13509	12833	12750	12523	13082	13529	13251	13669	14025
MAX FORCE 2 (*2) (N)	9589	10163	9532	9937	9624	9482	9133	10974	10550	9961	10522	11148
MAX FORCE 3 (*2) (N) AT TIME (ms)	15713 50	16177 50	15753 52	16329 63	15809 50	15423 51	14484 51	14569 66	17848 51	16089 50	15876 50	15590 50
θ ANGLE WHEN FORCE 3 IS MAX. (°)(*2)	127.97	124.73	132.67	138.03	128.13	128.93	127.14	158.15	123.30	126.42	125.64	124.88
MAX. θ ANGLE (°)	152.14	149.92	147.44	138.04	152.35	151.47	148.91	165.02	134.59	150.54	149.39	148.16
HEAD x-DISPLACEMENT (cm)	51.78	50.33	51.22	50.18	51.76	51.86	51.78	51.24	43.72	51.41	49.92	48.07

(*1) Not significant because of absence of head impact

(*2) see Figure 12

knees could significantly increase the horizontal displacement of the head.

-It can be clearly seen that the study to reduce the severity of head impacts cannot be carried out separately from the controlling of submarining.

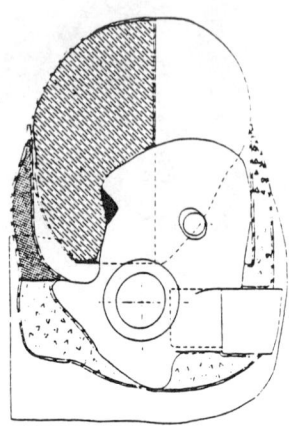

 Silicone foam RTV 5370
Density 0.20 instead of 0.26

 Silicone foam RTV 5370
Density 0.16 instead of 0.20

 Removed portion of the pelvis

To provide a human like three dimentional direction of "Sartorius" in sitting posture

FIG. 11 . PELVIC MODIFICATIONS.

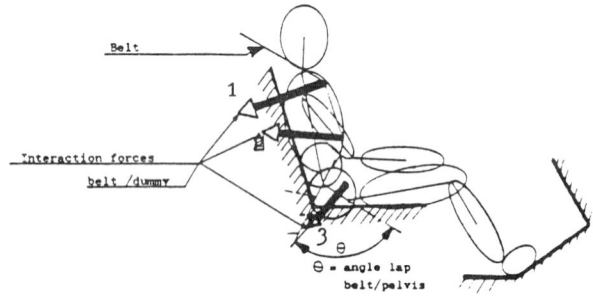

FIG. 12 . INITIAL POSITION OF THE DUMMY.

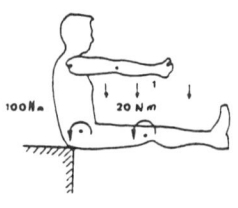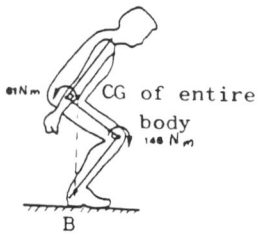

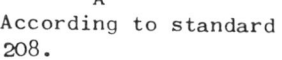
A — According to standard 208. B — According to a more natural position.

FIG. 13 . TORQUES APPLYING TO DUMMY'S LOWER LIMB JOINTS.

DEFINITION OF AN ABDOMINAL PROTECTION CRITERIA

Past publications have described the complexity of the factors influencing the occurence of submarining and concluded that it was impossible to avert it by a single geometrical criterion as exists in Regulation 14, for example. That is why a great deal of work had been carried out with the object of seeking an abdominal protection criterion.
These different approaches have in common the determination to eliminate the risk of abdominal injuries induced by submarining under the lapbelt.

AN ACCOUNT OF THE DIFFERENT ATTEMPTS MADE TO DEFINE AN ABDOMINAL PROTECTION CRITERION

To our knowledge, the first attempt at defining a protection criterion for abdominal organs was published in 1973 (17). It stated that the "protection of abdominal will be satisfactorily guaranteed if any rising of strap -in dynamics- (during test) above anatomical reference marks materializing the limit compatible with a satisfactory rest on pelvis is forbidden"(Figure 14)
"Compliance with the criterion is checked by cinematographic observation".
This first method successfully used in research could not be retained for the regulation test as the presence of doors -and unmodified doors- precludes filmed observation of the pelvis.

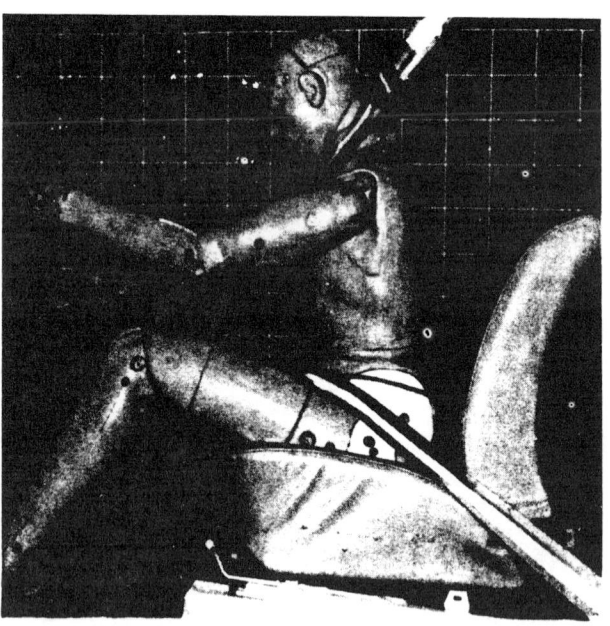

FIGURE 14.

The following year, in June 1974, at the ESV Conference in London, Citroen proposed fitting the dummy with optical transducers located on the pelvis beneath the Anterior Superior Iliac Spine (A.S.I.S.). These transducers would allow movement of the lap belt in relation to the A.S.I.S. to be detected. (18)
In the same year, a Ford patent dated 15th October 1974, proposed an almost identical system of detec

340

tion in which the optical transducer was replaced by force transducers. (19) .This solution was also to be retained by Citroen in 1977 (20).
A criticism which can be levelled against two above solutions is that abdominal danger cannot be stated to exist by the mere fact of the belt running up over the iliac crests.Indeed,the belt may be positioned against the abdomen at the end of impact without there being the risk of the occupant sustaining abdominal injury,if belt load is zero or low.Experimental work on human subject showed that certain cases of submarining proved to be of little danger provided that belt penetration into the abdomen as well as belt load -these two variables are obviously interdependent- were lower than a given limit.Moreover,the abdominal tolerance which justifies the abdominal protection criterion presented in following chapter is based on such values.
Three other ideas were formulated which would enable the detection of submarining:
 —measure the angle of rotation of the pelvis (21)
 —measure the pressure in the abdominal air bag with which dummy Part 572 is equipped (22)
 —measure the pressure exerted on a set of pressure transducers arranged over the anterior face of the dummy (abdomen and thorax) (23).
These ideas are still in the early proposal stage. With the lack of experiments on dummies and references to the tolerance of human beings,they have not been able to be transposed into a protection criterion determining a limit which must not be exceeded if the non-occurence of abdominal injuries is to be guaranteed.

EXPERIMENTAL WORK CONDUCTED ON CADAVERS TO DEFINE THE ABDOMINAL TOLERANCE IN THE SUBMARINING CASE.

To define this abdominal tolerance in the event of submarining under the lap-portion of a three-point belt,10 cadaver tests were performed. Results have already been published as an ISO document (24).

METHODOLOGY USED IN CADAVER TESTS
Ten human cadaver tests were first and last performed with a current Renault 18 and Renault 20 car body mounted on a sled.The maximum sled deceleration and impact velocity were 21-30g and 50 kph.The fresh cadavers were placed on the front passenger seat (Nb 2) or on the rear bench seat at the right side (Nb 4).Three-point retractor belts were used.Because the car occupant is more likely to submarine in the rear seat than in the front seat,owing to different seat-belt geometry (4), most of the fresh human cadavers were placed on the rear bench seat at the right side (seat Nb 4). Eight cameras (velocities 500 or 1000 pictures/second) were used for this study.The positions of these cameras are shown in figure 15.
For two subjects (Nb 246 and 247),accelerations were recorded for the thorax at D1,D4,D7,D12,the ribs and the pelvis (on sacrum).No head deceleration recordings were taken because of recording capacity.Two shoulder belt loads (upper and lower) two lap-belt loads (inboard and outboard) were also recorded.
Autopsies on the human cadavers were carried out after tests by the specialist of IRBA under the direction of Pr. C.GOT.

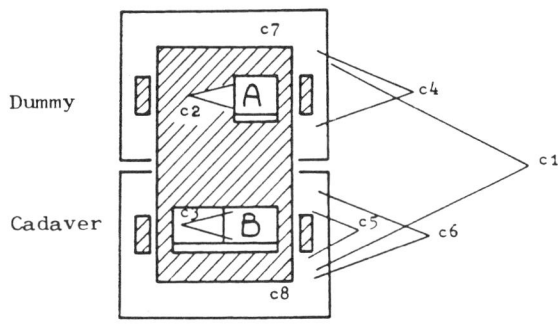

Cameras C1,C4,C5,C6:Placed at the right side of the sled.
Cameras C2,C3:Placed at the left side of the sled.
Cameras C7,C8:Placed at the top of the sled.

FIG. 15 . POSITION OF THE CAMERAS USED IN THE TESTS.

RESULTS AND DISCUSSION
The acceleration recordings are presented in Table 12.The anthropometrical data of the human cadavers and the results of the dissections are shown in Tables 13 and 14.
In five recently conducted tests ,Nb 244 and Nb 245 were normal cases of submarining.This means that the lap-belt firmly restrained the pelvic bone region below the Anterior Superior Iliac Spines.It then rode-up over the iliac crests and penetrated into the abdomen.In this case,the tension time curve appeared as a distinct "saddle shape".In precise terms,the first peak of lap-belt tension was always greater than that of the second peak which corresponded to a lower compression load penetrating into the abdomen(Fig.16). That is why no dangerous abdominal injuries were found.Heavy submarining occured in the remaining tests.The lap-belt rode-up rapidly over the ASIS and tension increased continuously(Fig.17).The tension was usually greater at the second peak applied to the abdomen than at the first peak, to the pelvic bone region.Therefore,abdomen AIS$\geqslant$3 were found in the cadavers.
Penetration of the lap-belt into the abdomen was measured using the same method as described in reference (1).By means of kinematical studies, this penetration was taken into account together with the fact that the lap-belt rode-up over ASIS. Because no significant difference in abdominal injuries between left and right hand sides was observed,either in the autopsies or in the real-life traffic accident,the severity of the abdominal injuries is specified for the whole abdomen as given by the anatomo-pathologists.The average lap-belt tension was taken from both sides.
In order to compare the dummy tests,lap-belt ten-

TABLE 12 - DECELERATIONS RECORDED - TESTS WITH HUMAN CADAVERS

Test N°	Seat N°	Sled decel. γ (g)	Sled speed (km/h)	Thorax D1	$[\gamma(g)/SI]$ D4	D7	D12	Sacrum $\gamma(g)/SI$	Shoulder belt (N) upper	lower	1st peak lap-belt (N) int.	ext.	2nd peak lap-belt (N) int.	ext.
127	4	23	50.9	-	-	-	-	86/1501	6800	8500	4000	9100	3900	9000
148	2	21	50.1	-	-	-	-	50/563	7700	2250	7600	4100	4200	2000
148	4	21	50	-	-	-	-	53/340	6000	5000	8600	4500	6500	2800
154	4	37	50.7	-	82/620	147/8064	-	71/779	6400	10050	5400	7400	5400	6700
182	2	24	47.5	39/171	36/76	81/555	107/437	45/272	5200	5500	6450	3900	7750	4300
243	4	27	47.4	-	-	-	-	93/471	4200	4600	600	700	4900	5100
244	4	34	50.1	-	-	-	-	63/334	5000	2800	3400	3900	1800	2200
245	4	22	49.8	-	-	-	-	52/859	5000	1800	3000	3700	2800	3700
246	4	30	50.1	56/521	82/678	81/774	79/637	153/1070	6600	4500	1500	4800	6000	7200
247	4	30	50.5	67/622	76/683	79/723	65/494	133/1067	8900	5800	5000	5200	6800	8600

TABLE 13 - NORMALIZED LAP-BELT TENSIONS FOR THE SECOND PEAK (AFTER SUBMARINING)

Test N°	Mass Kg	Coefficient for normalized tension	Average 2nd peak tension of 2 sides (N)	Normalized lap-belt tension (N)	Abdomen AIS	Relative bigness x 10^{-6}
127.4	41	1.49	6450	9610,5	3	10,2
148.2	59	1.17	3100	3627	0	13,9
148.4	67	1.08	4650	5022	0	13,2
154.4	42,5	1.46	6050	8833	5	8.5
182.2	62	1.14	6025	6868,5	3	11,4
243.4	74	1.01	5000	5050	4	14,5
244.4	54	1.24	2000	2480	0	12.0
245.4	62	1.14	3250	3705	1	16.0
246.4	52	1.28	6600	8448	3	11.5
247.4	58	1.19	7650	9104	4	13.3

Table 14 - Injuries of the Tested Human Cadavers

Cadaver No.	Sex	Age	Size (m)	Weight (kg)	Thorax (Rib fractures)	Injuries and Corresponding AIS Abdomen	
127-4	M	57	1.59	41	28 ribs, AIS 4	L 1 fracture	AIS 3
148-2	F	65	1.62	59	8 ribs, AIS 3		AIS 0
148-4	M	62	1.72	67	12 ribs AIS 3		AIS 0
154-4	M	63	1.71	42.5	40 ribs+sternum AIS 4	liver + L2 fracture	AIS 5
182-2	M	57	1.76	62	8 ribs AIS 3	L 1 fracture	AIS 3
243-4	M	61	1.72	74	7 ribs AIS 3	colon + break of rectus	AIS 4
244-4	F	57	1.65	54	24 ribs AIS 4	fractures of left ilium crest	AIS 3
245-5	M	56	1.57	62	7 ribs AIS 3	fissure of adipose tissue	AIS 1
246-4	M	62	1.65	52	12 ribs AIS 3/T6-T7 AIS 3	break of rectus	AIS 3
247-4	M	42	1.63	58	8 ribs+sternum AIS 3	break of rectus	AIS 4

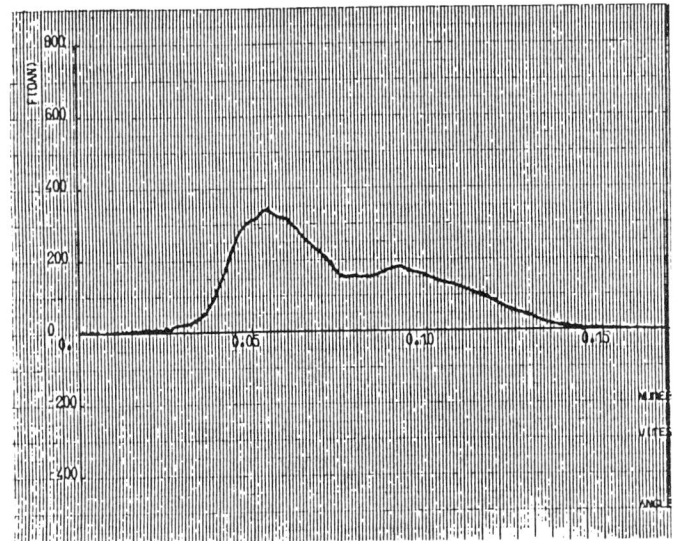

FIG. 16 . LAP-BELT TENSION/TIME HISTORY RECORDED AT THE INTERIOR SIDE OF CADAVER N°244

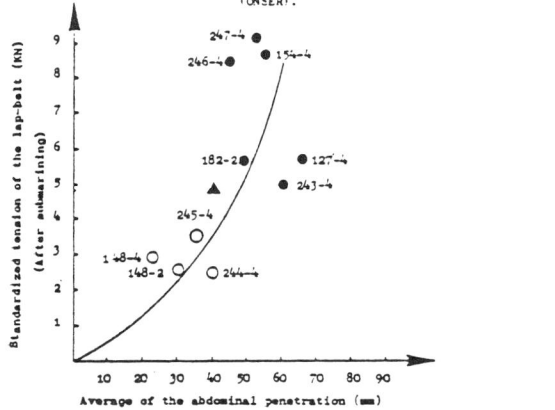

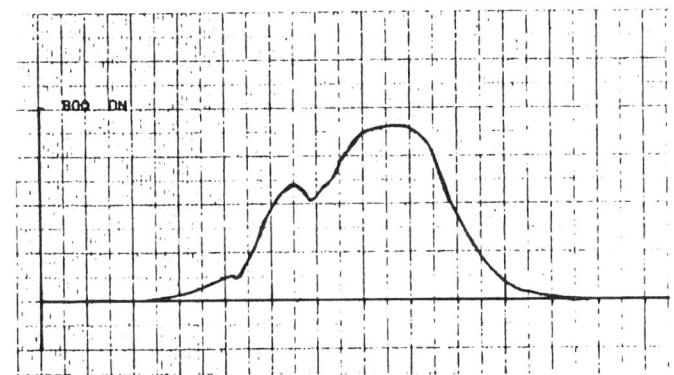

FIG. 17 . LAP-BELT TENSION/TIME HISTORY RECORDED AT THE EXTERIOR SIDE OF CADAVER N°246.

Test N°	Mass	Size	AIS
127-4	41kg	150cm	3
148-2	59kg	161cm	0
148-4	67kg	172cm	0
154-4	42.5kg	171cm	5
182-2	62kg	176cm	3
243-4	74kg	172cm	4
244-4	54kg	165cm	0
245-4	62kg	157cm	1
246-4	52kg	165cm	3
247-4	58kg	163cm	4

Previous results — 127-4 through 182-2
Recent results — 243-4 through 247-4

FIG. 18 . ABDOMINAL TOLERANCE TO THE SUBMARINING.

sion recorded in the cadaver tests should be standardized with respect to the mass of the Part 572 dummy (75kg).A formula given by Eppinger is used in this study,which has been described in references (24)(25).
In figure 18,a parabolic curve can be drawn as a relationship between the standardized tension of the lap-belt and abdominal penetration.The scatter of the data points is due to the differences in the anthropometric data of the cadavers.A similar curve can be found also in figure 19 for the standardized lap-belt tension (after submarining) and the abdomen AIS.Previous results are also presented in these figures.It can be seen that Nb 243-4 is the lowest point (5KN) in the new group with dangerous injuries.This value is smaller than that (5.7KN) of Nb 182-2, the lowest one in the old group of previous results.One datum point (without test number) given by ONSER is also presented in these two figures.
Specific comments on the severity of abdominal injuries (AIS) concerning cadavers Nb244 and 245 are given below:

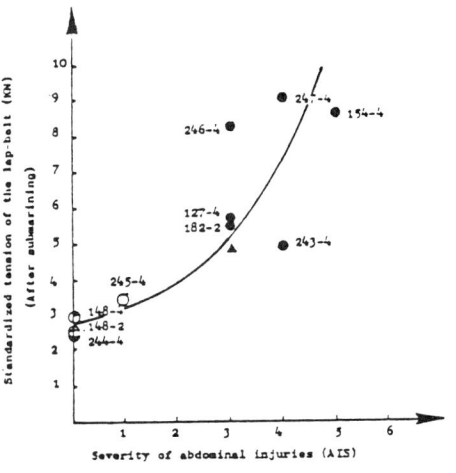

FIG. 19 . RELATIONSHIP BETWEEN THE STANDARDIZED TENSION OF THE LAP-BELT (AFTER SUBMARINING) AND THE ABDOMEN AIS.

Nb 244 sustained only pelvic fracture with an AIS=3 but no abdominal injuries.An abdominal AIS=0 was given to this case.It implied that if no pelvic fracture has occured,the lap-belt would probably have penetrated into the abdomen,with greater force and caused abdominal injuries,which in real-life could be a dangerous situation. It is an ambigous case difficult to interpret and we prefer to avoid underestimating the abdominal risk.

-Nb 245 sustained abdominal AIS=1 and was the only subject situated between the group with dangerous injuries (AIS ≥ 3) and the group with injuries (AIS=0). Since the severity of the abdominal injuries due to submarining is probably influenced by the "relative bigness" defined as "weight/height^3" (kg/cm^3) in reference (24), a further study of this factor is described here. The "relative bigness" of the human cadavers versus their abdomen AIS is illustrated in figure 20 where the previous results are also presented. Cadaver Nb 245 had the greatest "relative bigness" in all results. We made the assumption that this subject would sustain a greater AIS if his bigness had been so to speak, smaller. It may be for this reason that the only fissure of the abdominal adipose tissue was found in this subject.

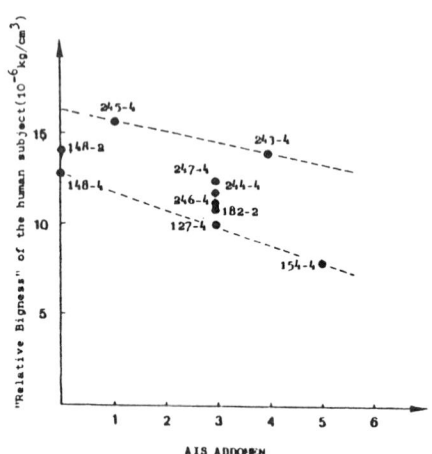

FIG. 20 . "RELATIVE BIGNESS" VS SEVERITY OF THE ABDOMINAL INJURIES (AIS).

The abdomen AIS is certainly influenced by other parameters, for example rib cage strength, which are not discussed in this study. In general, no big difference can be found between previous and recent results. But the limits between the groups with and without injuries are closer due to the recent results; therefore the latest determination of the abdominal tolerance will be more accurate. The determination of critical lap-belt tension should be considered more carefully. As just mentionned above, the case with Nb 244 cadaver produced no injuries, yet it is nevertheless a dangerous situation. On the other hand, Nb 243 (5KN) produced the lowest datum point in the group with injuries in recent results; Nb 182-2 (5.7KN) was the lowest one in previous results. Based on previous and recent available data points presented in figure 18 and figure 19, the critical standardized lap-belt tension was reconsidered. A value of 3 KN can be contemplated, which is smaller than the previous value of 4.4 KN which had been proposed (25,26,27).

EXPERIMENTAL WORK WITH DUMMIES INSTRUMENTED WITH "ILIAC CREST TRANSDUCERS"

SCHEDULE OF RECENT RESEARCH PROGRAMS FOR DUMMY TESTS

-First series - Dummy tests with a Renault 20 car body and seat -
The same car body and sled used in cadaver tests were employed for the dummy tests. The sled deceleration and impact velocity were similar to those registered in cadaver tests. The Part 572 dummy was equipped with short (40mm) or long (55mm) APR submarining transducers and placed in the front passenger seat (Nb 2) or in the rear bench seat on the right side (Nb 4). Three-point retractor seat belts (60mm width) and different positions of lap-belt were used in these tests. Standard recordings were made. Test conditions were similar or more severe with respect to test Nb 5 given in reference (28).

-Second series - Dummy sled tests with Renault 20 seat directly on the sled -
This series of tests was performed by T.N.O. The test conditions were similar to those used in reference (28). Some tests were performed under excessive test conditions (with the seat back set at an angle of about 30° from the vertical for example. Classical recordings were taken.

-Third series - Dummy sled tests with Citroen Visa seat directly on the sled -
This series of tests was the reconstruction of test NB 10 in reference (29). Briefly, the test conditions were:
-front passenger Citroën Visa seat
-Part 572 dummy without fore-arms
-3-pt static seat belts (50mm width)
-sled deceleration and impact velocity about 20g and 50kph respectively
-inclination of seat back 28°
-weakened seat frame
-slack of the lap-belt and shoulder belt about 25 mm
Recordings were made for pelvic deceleration, shoulder belt tensions (upper and lower) and lap-belt tensions (inboard and outboard). Citroën transducer and APR short or long transducers were used.

RESULTS

-First series - Dummy tests with Renault 20 seat.
The results of this series of tests are presented in Table 15. The first three tests (Nb 1013,1014, 1015) are cases of non-submarining with the lap-belt positioned correctly. Tests Nb 1018,1019 and 1021 are submarining cases with the lap-belt positioned 1 cm higher than in the first three tests. The compression loads recorded by the submarining transducer are in the range between 463N and 798N. Tests Nb 1016,1017 and 1020 are cases of excessive submarining in which the lap-belt rode up over the submarining transducers. Nb 1016 and 1017 are tests in seat Nb 2 with the worst position of the lap-belt. Nb 1020 is a test performed in seat Nb 4 with a correct position of the lap-belt and using short transducers (Figure 21). The recorded loads range from 805N to 1116N and it serves as an exam-

TABLE 15 - DUMMY TESTS WITH RENAULT 20 SEAT

Test N°	Seat N°	Submarining transducer	Position of lap-belt with relation to ASIS from side view (cm)	Lap-belt tension after submarining Int (N)	Ext (N)	Transducer (N) Int.	force Ext.	Remarks
1013	2	short	+ 4	-	-	-	-	no submarining
1014	2	"	+ 3	-	-	-	-	"
1015	2	long	+ 2	-	-	-	-	"
1016	2	"	- 1	2200	2240	1030	994	Lap-belt rode-up over transducers
1017	2	"	+ 1	1940	1550	869	805	"
1018	2	"	0	1667	4520	798	614	Transducers worked correctly
1019	2	"	0	1117	1620	638	521	"
1020	4	short	+ 4	5237	-	1116	-	lap-belt rode-up and touched direct submarining transducers
1021	2	"	+ 1	1122	-	463	-	transducers worked correctly

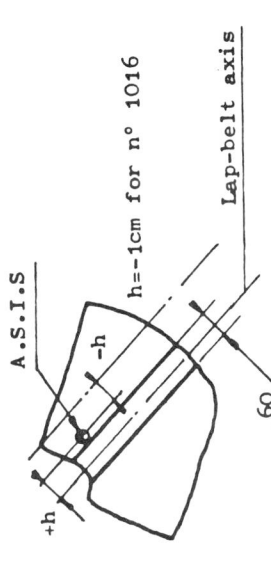

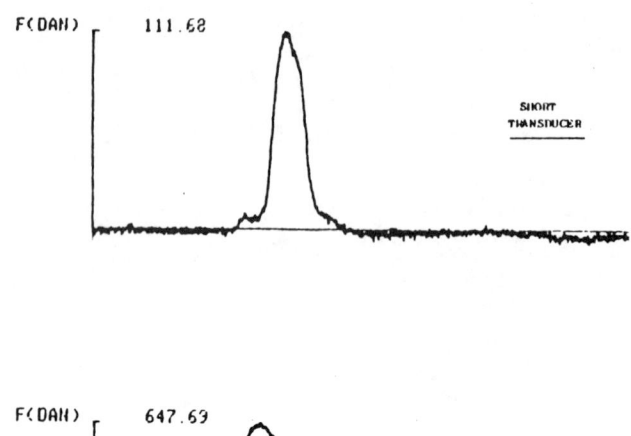

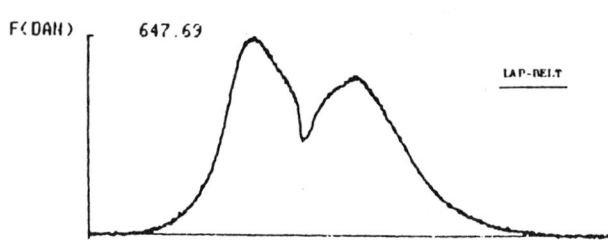

FIG. 21 . TENSION (T) AND FORCE (F) CURVES OF TEST N° 1020 (INTERIOR SIDE).

ple where the short transducer works correctly and records a greater load under test conditions more favorable to submarining in seat Nb 4 (rear bench) than in seat Nb 2 (front individual seat) (4).
In order to make a comparison with cadaver tests, a new research program is being prepared to perform the dummy tests under these same conditions. It can be recognized from the above analyses that the responses of the transducer to the submarining process were in accordance with the different test conditions.

-Second series - TNO sled dummy tests -
The results of this series of tests are presented in Table 16.No submarining occurred in the first three out of a total of nine tests,even with the lap-belt located 15 mm higher than the correct position.In the rest of the tests,a submarining phenomenon could only be obtained by placing sheets of double plastic foil between the dummy and the car seat in combination with a 25 mm "higher than correct" position of the belt on the pelvis.Excesive submarining in tests Nb 454,456 and 457 could only be obtained by additionally inclining the seat back to about 30° from the vertical.The excessive submarining cases all resulted in a short peak loading of the transducers (duration 6 ms),followed by an over-riding of the transducers.Consequently,the lap-belt was loaded again by the lumbar spine.In all tests,a reasonable symmetrical loading of left and right lap-belt and transducers was found.

-Third series - Dummy tests with Citroën Visa seat
In table 17 tests Nb 5363 and 5364 correspond to non-submarining cases.The lap-belts were positioned correctly.Tests Nb 5360,5361 and 5365 are normal submarining cases.Their descriptions are simi

lar to the ones given for the first series of dummy tests.The positions of the lap-belts are relativively worse than in the non-submarining group.Both short and long transducers work correctly in these three tests.The long transducer is used in test Nb 5361;the lap-belt tension and transducer load as function of time for the outboard side are illustrated in Figure 22.

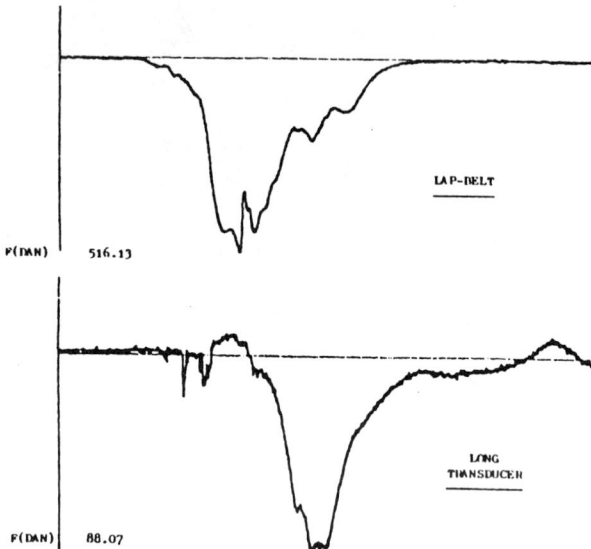

FIG. 22 . TENSION (T) AND FORCE (F) CURVES OF TEST N° 5361 (EXTERIOR SIDE).

Test Nb 5362 corresponds to a submarining case in which the lap-belt rides-up over the transducer. The position of the lap-belt was the least desirable one observed in this series of tests.However, a significant load of 2531N was recorded by the short transducer.This sample again illustrates how the submarining transducer can provide a correct response:when the test is performed under more severe submarining conditions,a greater compression load can be recorded by the transducer, so indicating that it would be a more dangerous submarining case.The lap-belt tension (t) and transducer load (f) for outboard side in the test Nb 5362 are illustrated in Figure 23.

RELATIONSHIP BETWEEN LAP-BELT TENSION AND THE SUBMARINING TRANSDUCER LOAD

All data points obtained from the recent results of dummy tests are illustrated in Figure 24 The two parameters are the maximum transducer load and the corresponding lap-belt tension at the same points in time.The previous results are also presented.A linear correlation between lap-belt tension and transducer load can be proposed.
Since the standardized critical lap-belt tension (3000N) is already determined in Figures 18 and 19 a corresponding transducer load of 800N can be found in Figure 24.
Based on previous and recent results obtained from cadaver and dummy tests,a submarining transducer load of 800N is proposed as an abdominal protection criterion in the dummy tests.

CONCLUSIONS

TABLE 16 - T.N.O. SLED TEST EVALUATION OF APR SUBMARINING TRANSDUCERS ON PART 572 DUMMY WITH RENAULT 20 SEAT

Test No.	Submarining transducer	lap-belt position upper ASIS (cm)	Seatback	Max. seat belt tension after submarining (N) Int.	Ext.	Transducer force (N) Int.	Ext.	Remarks
449	long	correct	25°	-	-	-	-	no submarining
450	"	1	25°	-	-	-	-	"
451	"	1.5	25°	-	-	-	-	"
452	"	2.5	25°	1500	1300	900	1000	submarining
453	"	2.5	25°	2000	1100	1130	1100	"
454	"	2.5	35°	2200	1000	1100	1000	excessive submarining
455	short	2.5	25°	-	-	-	-	no submarining
456 *	"	2.5	>25°	(?)	3200 (?)	750	450	excessive submarining
457	long	2.5	>25°	3600	2100	1100	820	" "

* In this test, there were the problems found in the recordings.

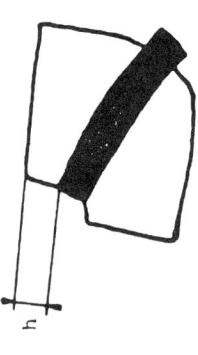

349

TABLE 17 - DUMMY TESTS WITH CITROEN VISA SEAT

Test No.	Seat No.	Submarining transducer	Position of lap-belt (cm) *	Seat	Lap-belt tension after submarining Int (N)	Lap-belt tension after submarining Ext (N)	Transducer force (N) Int.	Transducer force (N) Ext.	Remarks
5360	2	short	2	weaken	2627	1564	-	607	transducer worked
5361	2	"	1	"	-	2198	-	880	"
5362	2	"	0	"	-	4050	-	2531	lap-belt rode-up over transducer
5363	2	"	3	weaken+flexible	-	-	-	-	no submarining
5364	2	long	3	"	-	-	-	-	"
5365	2	"	3	"	4506	-	1239	-	transducer worked

* Definition is same as given in the diagram presented in Table 2.

1. A standardized critical lap-belt tension of 3000N is determined, based on available values from previous and recent submarining cadaver tests.
2. In human cadaver submarining tests, a relationship between abdominal injury (AIS) and "relative bigness" of the subject can be found: abdomen AIS increases as "relative bigness" decreases.

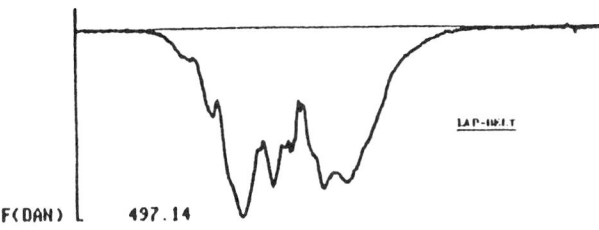

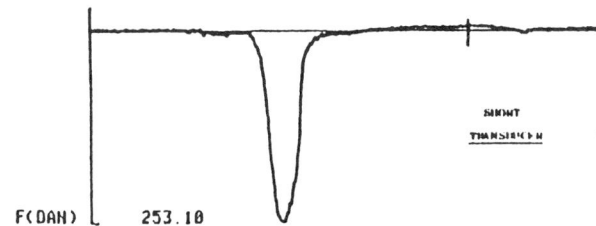

FIG. 23 . TENSION (T) AND FORCE (F) OF TEST N°5362 (EXTERIOR SIDE).

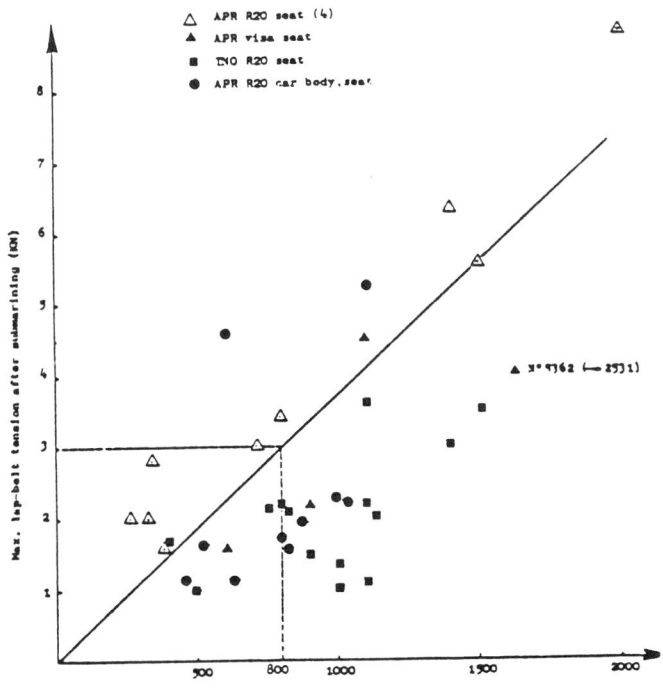

FIG. 24 . RELATIONSHIP BETWEEN THE LAP-BELT TENSION AND THE COMPRESSION LOAD RECORDED BY THE TRANSDUCERS.

3. With a dummy in the front passenger seat (Nb 2) and a correctly positioned lap-belt, non-submarining cases were usually obtained.
4. Submarining cases were obtained at the front passenger seat (Nb 2) by deliberately positioning the lap-belt at an excessive level on the abdomen or by increasing backrest rake, only weakening the seat frame.
5. In all submarining cases, the short (40 mm) and long (55 mm) transducers were able to detect the submarining phenomenon.
6. The values recorded by the short or long submarining transducers corresponded to the different conditions used in the dummy tests.
7. Based on recent critical lap-belt tension determined from the cadaver tests and, also the data points concerning a relationship between the lap-belt tension and the transducer load found in dummy tests, the abdominal protection criterion of 800N is proposed for dummy tests.
8. The short transducer can usually be used in submarining tests for the abdominal protection criterion; the long transducer can be used successfully in tests performed particularly under excessive submarining conditions.

GENERAL CONCLUSIONS

1. LAP-BELT SUBMARINING in real-life accidents is a process inducing severe injuries in a relatively high proportion of severe frontal crashes (27%) - but it is too often underestimated in previous studies-. Reasons of underestimation were for example that dorso-lumbar spine fractures, or lower members fractures, or above mesocolic injuries were not often considered as submarining consequences. Present findings constitute an attempt to clarify the whole pattern of such lap-belt submarining.
From a whole sample of 1423 three-point belted front occupants involved in 958 frontal car crashes, a sub-sample of 45 cars have been selected in which, at least one of the 77 front occupants sustained either a severe abdominal injury (AIS $\geqslant$ 3) or a dorso-lumbar column fracture (AIS $\geqslant$ 2). Among this survey sample, 47 injured people sustained a lap-belt submarining which was sure or most probable (61%). These submarinings induced three main types of injuries:
    -abdominal injuries (sub-mesocolic but also above mesocolic) (AIS $\geqslant$ 3)
    -dorso-lumbar spine fractures (mainly T12, L1, L2) (AIS $\geqslant$ 2)
    -lower members fractures (mainly legs, knees and femurs fractures) (AIS $\geqslant$ 2)

2. Among submarining cases, 68% of cases of abdominal injuries (AIS $\geqslant$ 3) and (or) dorso lumbar spine fractures (AIS $\geqslant$ 2) were SURELY induced by the lap-belt section. The percentage reached 94% if we considered the cases where the lap-belt influence was sure or only MOST PROBABLE.

3. The influence of shoulder-belt plays only as an

aggravating factor - complementary to the lap-belt- for less than 10% of cases.

4. Poor geometry and (or) slackly worned belts were present in 74% of submarining cases.

5. Most of the submarining cases were observed in high violence crashes ($\Delta V \geq 50$ kph and mean $\gamma \geq$ 10g occured in 58% of cases).

6. In real-life accidents, the most frequent severe consequences of lap-belt submarining are according to a decreasing order:
   - sub-mesocolic injuries
   - lower members fractures
   - dorso-lumbar spine fractures
   - above-mesocolic injuries
   - pelvic fractures

7. Taking into account the severity of above-mesocolic injuries (liver and (or) spleen), it is noticeable that 3/5 of such victims sustained a lap-belt submarining which is sure or most probable (of course these lesions are often associated to sub-mesocolic injuries).

8. In cadaver tests (with blood pressure restored at normal level), submarining process is checked by special in-board camera which shows then all these above described injuries which could be induced by lap-belt submarining, even for above-mesocolic injuries (liver or spleen injuries) or dorso-lumbar spine fractures. These experiments also confirm the possible aggravating influence of shoulder-belt section.

9. Abdominal or dorso-lumbar spine TOLERANCE to lap-belt submarining is low. Injuries are observed for lap-belt tension higher than 3000N.

10. A PROTECTION CRITERION - ANTI-LAP-BELT SUBMARINING CRITERION - has been proposed. It consists in the record of lap-belt loading against specific ILIAC-CREST TRANSDUCERS symetrically installed on the pelvis of the dummy. Based on recent critical lap-belt tensions determined from specific cadaver tests and - also - the data points concerning a relationship between the lap-belt tensions and the Iliac-Crest-Transducer loads found in dummy tests, the LAP-BELT-SUBMARINING PROTECTION CRITERION of 800N is proposed for dummy test.

REFERENCES

(1) G. Walfisch, A. Fayon, Y.C. Leung, C. Tarriere; C. Got, A. Patel "Synthesis of Abdominal Injuries in Frontal Collisions with Belt-Wearing cadavers Compared with Injuries Sustained by Real-Life Accident Victims. Problems of Simulation with Dummies and Protection Criteria." in Proceedings of IRCOBI GOETEBORG, Sweden, 7-9 Sept. 1979.

(2) J.S. Dehner, "Seat Belt Injuries of the Spine and Abdomen." American J. Roentgen, VIII, PP833-843, April 1971.

(3) Document ISO/TC 22/SC 12/GT6 N107.

(4) Y.C. Leung, C. Tarrière, A. Fayon P. Mairesse, P. Banzet. "An Anti-Submarining Scale Determined from Theoretical and Experimental Studies Using Three-Dimensional Geometrical Definition of the Lap-Belt " SAE Paper n°811020, in the Proceedings of 25th Stapp Car Crash Conference, San Francisco, Sept. 28-30, 1981.

(5) Y.C. Leung, C. Tarrière, A. Fayon, P. Mairesse, A. Delmas and P. Banzet, "A Comparaison Between Part 572 Dummy and Human Subject in the Problem of Submarining." in the Proceedings of 23rd Stapp Car Crash Conference, San Diego Calif., Oct. 17/19, 1979, SAE Transaction Paper N°791.026.

(6) A. Fayon, C. Tarrière, G. Walfisch C. Got, A. Patel "Thorax of 3-Point Belt Wearers During a Crash (Experiments with Cadavers)" in the Proceedings of 19th Stapp Car Crash Conference, SAE paper 751148, San Diego, Calif., Nov. 17/19, 1975.

(7) J.L. Haley Jr., "Fundamentals of Kinetics and Kinematics as Applied to Injury Reduction "in "Impact Injury and Crash Protection ", C.C. Thomas Publisher 1970.

(8) L.M. Patrick and A. Andersson "Three-Point Harness Accident and Laboratory Data Comparaison". SAE Paper N°741.181, in the Proceedings of the 18th Stapp Car Crash Conference, Ann Arbor Michigan, Dec. 4th, 1974.

(9) D. Adomeit and A. Heger, "Motion Sequence Criteria and Design Proposals for Restraint Devices in order to Avoid Unfavorable Biomechanic Condition and Submarining". SAE Paper N°751.146 In the Proceedings of 19th Stapp Car Crash Conference, San Diego, Calif. Nov. 17th 1975.

(10) H. Hontschik, E. Müller and G. Rüter, "Necessities and Possibilities of Improving the Protectice Effect of Three-Point Seat-Belts ", in the Proceedings of the 21st Stapp Car Crash Conference, New Orleans, Louisiana, Oct. 19/21st 1977.

(11) P. Biilaut, C. Tisseron, M. Dejeammes, R. Biard, P. Cord, P. Jenoc, "The Inflatable Diagonal Belt "7th

Internatinal Technical Conference on the Experimental Safety Vehicles, Paris June 5/9, 1979.

(12) B. Lundell, H. Mellander, I. Carlson, "Safety Performance of a rear Seat Belt System with Optimized Seat Cushion Design", SAE Paper N°810.796, Passenger Car Meeting Dearborn, Michigan, June 8 12, 1981

(13) G.W. Nyquist "Comparaison of Vehicule-Seated Volunteer Pelvic Orientations Determined by Leung et al, and by Nyquist et al .Document ISO /TC22/SC12/WG5?April 10, 1980.

(14) G.W. Nyquist et al ., "Lumbar and Pelvic Orientations of the Vehicle Seated Volunteer" SAE 760821, 20th Stapp Car Crash Conference 1976.

(15) D. Lestrelin "Etude par modele Mathematique de l'Influence de quelques Paramètres du Mannequin Part 572 sur sa Propension au sous-Marinage ".Rapport Interimaire N°2 Contrat N°78043 "Critères de Sous-Marinage" dans le Cadre des Actions Thematiques Programmees Françaises, 1979.

(16) D. Lestrelin, A. Fayon, C. Tarrière "Development and use of a Mathematical Model Simulating a Traffic Accident Victim" Proceedings of 5th International IRCOBI Conference, Birmingham, Sept. 1980.

(17) C. Tarrière "Proposal for a Protection criterion as Regards Abdominal Internal Organs" P371 Proceedings of Conference of A.A.A.M., Oklahoma City, Oklahoma, Nov.14/17, 1973.

(18) M. Clavel "Restraint Systems Improvement " Proceedings of 5th International Technical Conference on Experimental Safety Vehicles, London, June 4-7 1974.

(19) R.P. Daniel "Test Dummy Submarining Indicate in United States Patent, 3.841.163 Oct. 15, 1974.

(20) Citroën, "Methode de Detection de Depassement des crêtes Iliaques" Document ISO/TC 22/SC 12/GT6(F3)21F, 1977.

(21) D. Adomeit "Seat Design -A Significant Factor for Safety Belt Effec-tiveness " SAE Paper N°791004, in Proceedings of 23rd Stapp Car Crash Conference, San Diego, Calif., Oct.17-19 1979.

(22) Bröde, Personal Communication Nov.24, 1980.

(23) Fiat "Development of a Device to Evaluate the Abdominal Injuries in Submarining", Document ISO /TC 22/SC 12/GT 6(Italie 1)N 71, Sept.1980.

(24) Y.C. Leung, C. Tarrière, J. Maltha "A Review for the Abdominal Protection Criterion" Document ISO/TC 22/SC 12/WG6 N97 October 1981.

(25) "Experimental Elements for the Definition of Abdominal Protection Criterion in a Submarining Possibility" July 27th, 1980. ISO/TC 22/SC 12/WG. 6 N°72

(26) "Proposal for an abdominal Protection Criterion ", March 1980. ISO/TC 22/SC 12/WG. 6 N°58

(27) Y.C. Leung, P. Mairesse, P. Banzet "Submarining Criterion "Sept. 1980. ISO/TC 22/SC 12/WG N°77.

(28) R.L. Stalnaker "Submarining sled Testd Part 572 Pelvis with and without PSA/Renault Submarining Transducers and PSA/Renault modified Part 572 Pelvis with Submarining Transducers" TNO, October 8th, 1980.

(29) M. Dejeammes, R. Biard, Y. Derrien "Factors influencing the estimation of Submarining on the Dummy". ISO/TC 22/SC 12/WG.6-96, August 1981.

APPENDIX I - CHARACTERISTICS OF SAMPLE - FRONTAL IMPACTS WITH 3-POINT-BELTED FRONT OCCUPANTS ONLY

	WHOLE SAMPLE	SURVEY SAMPLE	VICTIMS WITH ABDOMEN AIS ⩾ 3 AND/OR DORSO-LUMBAR SPINE ⩾ 2	SUBMARINING PROBABLE OR SURE
N. Front Occupants	1423*	77	47	47
N. cars	958	45	45	39
[1] Abdomen AIS ⩾ 3		33	33	30
[2] Lumbar Spine AIS ⩾ 2				
[3] [1] + [2]		1	1	1
[4] Dorsal Spine AIS ⩾ 2		3	3	1
[5] Submarining Without [1] or [2]		6	-	6
[6] Other Cases		24	-	-
Male Drivers	791 (55 %)	37	19	18 (38 %)
Female Drivers	167 (12 %)	8	3	3 (7 %)
Male Right Front Passengers	155 (11 %)	13	9	8 (17 %)
Female Right Front Passengers	310 (22 %)	19	16	18 (38 %)
	100 %			100 %

(*) 119 cases are not included in this table because there are no available data concerning them about sex

APPENDIX II - SECTION OF THEBELT (LAP OR SHOULDER-BELTS) PRODUCING ABDOMINAL INJURIES
(Analyzis Process Based Upon Medical Data)

LAP-BELT			SHOULDER BELT	
ALMOST SURE	MOST PROBABLE	UNCERTAIN MECHANISM	MOST PROBABLE	ALMOST SURE
Two Above-Mesocolon Injuries At the Same Horizontal Level Exemple: Liver + Spleen PLUS at Least One Sub-Mesocolon Injury Or Symmetrical Rupture of Sheath of Rectus Or Horizontal Abrasions Above Antero-Superior Illiac Spine	Two Above-Mesocolon Injuries At the Same Horizontal Level Or One Above-Mesocolon Injury PLUS One Sub-Mesocolon Injury	Absence of Typical Pattern of Injuries Or Discordances (Technical Data Can Clear-Up Misunderstandings.)	One and Only One Above-Mesocolon Injury Close to Buckle (Example: Spleen for Right Front Passengers or Liver for Drivers	One and Only One Above-Mesocolon Injury Close to Buckle PLUS Rib Fractures Close to the Injury

Plus, Possibly:

- Wound, or Abrasion of the Neck Due to the Shoulder-Belt
- High Rib Fractures on the Buckle Side
- Lower Members Injuries
- High Lumbar or Low Dorsal Vertebrae Fractures

APPENDIX III - ACCIDENTOLOGICAL SIGNS OTHER THAN MEDICAL ONES WHICH HIGHLIGHT SUBMARINING UNDER LAP-BELT

[1] BELT

1.1. POOR GEOMETRY: . ANGLE $B_1 \leqslant 50°$
. ANGLE $B_2 \geqslant 100°$

[THE GEOMETRY IS THE WORSE WHEN B_1 IS LITTLE AND WHEN B_2 IS HIGH.]

. BUCKLE ABOVE THE SEAT (ADJUSTABLE BUCKLE ON THE WEBBING AT MIDDLE-ANCHORAG.) (THE HIGHER THE BUCKLE, THE WORST IT IS).

AS A WHOLE, 20 CASES OF CERTAIN OR PROBABLE SUBMARINING OUT OF 47 (43 %).

1.2. BELT WORN WITH SLACK: 17 CASES OF CERTAIN OR PROBABLE SUBMARINING OUT OF 47 (36 %)

[2] ASSOCIATED FACTORS

2.1. IMPACTS OF GREAT VIOLENCE ($\Delta V \geqslant 50$ KPH AND MEAN $\gamma \geqslant 10$ G): 25 CASES OF CERTAIN OR PROBABLE SUBMARINING OUT OF 47 (53 %).

2.2. IMPACTS OF THE KNEES UNDER THE PANEL: 39 CASES OF PROBABLE OR CERTAIN SUBMARINING (83 %)

2.3. FRONT SEAT TRACK DAMAGE OR FAILURE: 18 CASES OF PROBABLE OR CERTAIN SUBMARINING (38 %)

2.4. REAR OVERLOAD: 10 CASES OF PROBABLE OR CERTAIN SUBMARINING (21 %)

REMARKS (See the Bottom of Appendix I):

(1) Right Front Passengers Are Statistically Significantly More Involved in Submarining Than Drivers

(2) There is a tendency for Women to Be More Involved Than Men But This Difference Is Not Quite Significant From a Statistical Standpoint.

APPENDIX IV

Details of soft tissue injuries observed in the tested human cadavers.

Cadaver n°	Descriptions of the injuries
2	-Multiple wounds : superior and inferior part of the liver AIS 5 ☆ -Perforation of the low part of the descendant colon AIS 5 -Rupture of the mesentry (length of 8 cm) near to posterior AIS 4 -Fracture of L4 transverse process AIS 2 -Fracture of left lateral sacral crest AIS 3
4	-Wound of 2 cm of the right diaphragm AIS 3 -Wound of superior face of the liver AIS 4
8	-Rupture of the left diaphragm AIS 3 -Bruise of the spleen AIS 4 -Fracture of 2 ilium crests AIS 2
10	-Wound of the liver (little fissure of the vascular bad) AIS 4 -Fracture of the anterior part of 2 ilium crests AIS 2
12	-Fissure of the mesentary root without blessure of the artery AIS 3
16	-Rupture of the left part of the diaphragma AIS 3 -Irregular wound of the superior part of the spleen AIS 4
25	-Little fissure of the mesentary root without blessure of the artery AIS 3 -Fracture of the anterior part of 2 ilium crests AIS 2
127-4	-Compression of L1 vertebra body (centrum) AIS 2
154-4	-Wound of the liver (anterior exterior face of right lobe) AIS 4 -L2 fracture with marrows' elongation (no rupture) AIS 5
170	-Compression of L4 and L5 vertebra body AIS 2
183	-Fissure of superior part of the liver AIS 4
185	-Erosion of the skin in front of the A.S.I.S. AIS 1 -Wound of the gashed muscle at the level of abdomen AIS 3 -Rupture of the mesentery (10 cm) AIS 3
189-4	-Dislocation of L5-S1 AIS 4 -Fracture of the right lateral sacral crest AIS 3 -Fissure of the mesentary AIS 3
231	-Depth wound of the liver (anterior board of 2 lobes, superior face of the right lobe) AIS 5 -Wound of the spleen (superior part) AIS 4 -Bruise of the mesentery (without rupture) AIS 3
255	-Wound of the spleen (exterior face) AIS 4

☆ AIS numbers are referred from "1980 AIS"

821160

Impact Response and Injury of the Pelvis

Guy S. Nusholtz, Nabih M. Alem, and John W. Melvin
University of Michigan

ABSTRACT

Multiple axial knee impacts and/or a single lateral pelvis impact were performed on a total of 19 cadavers. The impacting surface was padded with various materials to produce different force-time and load distribution characteristics. Impact load and skeletal acceleration data are presented as functions of both time and frequency in the form of mechanical impedance. Injury descriptions based on gross autopsy are given.

The kinematic response of the pelvis during and after impact is presented to indicate the similarities and differences in response of the pelvis for various load levels. While the impact response data cannot prescribe a specific tolerance level for the pelvis, they do indicate variables which must be considered and some potential problems in developing an accurate injury criterion.

INTRODUCTION

Pelvis injuries of varying type and severity have been found to occur in a significant number of automotive accidents (1-5). Investigations of trauma of the pelvis resulting from impact in an automotive environment have been documented primarily through accident investigation methods. There have only been a limited number of biomechanical studies attempting to research pelvis impact trauma under laboratory conditions. One of the earliest of these studies was conducted by Evans and Lissner in 1955 (6), and consisted of impacts to the denuded pelvis in the inferior-superior direction. Although no fracture tolerance data were obtained, it was concluded from this study that the pelvis exhibited elastic behavior and failed due to tensile stresses in various structural members. Ten years later a study of the behavior of the knee-femur-pelvis complex in an automotive impact environment was reported by Patrick et al. (7) In this series of tests, an impact sled was used to apply femoral-axis impacts to the knee of embalmed cadavers. The lowest applied load found to cause pelvis injury was 7.1 kN, and loads ranging from 8.5 kN to 17 kN were found to cause multiple fractures of the pelvis. It was suggested that a maximum force criterion (of about 6.2 kN) should be the threshold level for injury for the patella/femur/pelvis complex. A similar study using unembalmed cadavers was reported by Melvin and Nusholtz in 1980. A single pelvis fracture was found to occur at an applied load of about 20 kN, however loads up to 26 kN were applied with no resulting pelvis injury.

A recent biomechanical study of pelvis impact in an automotive environment was documented first in 1979 (9) and more completely in 1980 (10) by Cesari and Ramet. The goal of this research was to supply data for design of side door padding by impacting cadavers laterally in the pelvis and recording the force/injury relationships observed. It was suggested from this study that the response to impact is characterized by velocity of impacts, maximum force, and impulse. Admissible force tolerance for females was documented as 5-7 kN (1100-1600 lb) and for males as 7-13 kN (1600-2900 lb). These studies essentially characterize pelvis injury tolerance using maximum force and impulse indicators.

To further investigate the kinematic and injury response of the pelvis in automotive-environment impacts, a series of tests involving indirect impacts to the pelvis have been conducted by the Biomechanics Deprtment at HSRI. The tests were conducted using unembalmed cadavers and two types of impact facilities: a pendulum impactor and a pneumatic impactor. Indirect loads were delivered to the acetabulum of the pelvis by impacting the femur either axially or laterally. This allowed loads to be delivered to the acetabulum in either anterior-to-posterior or right-to-left directions. The cadavers were instrumented to measure pelvic triaxial accelerations in all tests, while in some tests three-dimensional motion of the pelvis was recorded with nine accelerometers. Additionally, triaxial accelerations of the femur and the thoracic vertebrae (T8) were measured. Photographic targets on the pelvis and femur were used for photokinemetric analysis of motion due to the impact.

ANATOMICAL OVERVIEW

The bony pelvis (Figure 1) consists of two large, flat irregular shaped hip (coxal) bones that join one another at the pubic symphysis on the anterior midline. Posteriorly the wedge shaped sacrum completes the pelvic ring forming a relatively rigid structure.

In the adult, each hip bone is formed by the fusion of three separate bones, the ilium, ischium, and pubis, which join at the acetabulum. The ilium forms the broad upper lateral part of the hip bone and the upper portion of the acetabulum. Its upper curved edge is the iliac crest. The most commonly refered to prominence on this crest is the anterior-superior iliac spine. Posteriorly the crest ends in the posterior iliac spine, adjacent to its articulation with the sacrum, the sacroiliac joint. The ischium forms part of the acetabulum and has a superior ramus that ends below in the ischial tuberosity. From there the inferior ramus ascends to join with the inferior ramus of the pubic bone. Together this bar of bone is frequently referred to as the ischio-pubic ramus or inferior pubic ramus. The body of the pubic bone forms the anterior part of the acetabulum. From here the superior pubic ramus passes to the midline where it joins its fellow of the opposite side through the pubic symphysis. Below the inferior pubic ramus joins the inferior ischial ramus. The posterior-lateral bony pelvis is covered by multiple muscle layers, buttock fat and skin. The iliac crest is relatively free of heavy musculature. The rounded head of the femur articulates wih the acetabulum and is held within the socket by ligaments. Laterally, on the upper femur is a large bony prominence, the greater trochanter, for the attachment of muscles.

SUBJECT PREPARATION

Following transfer to HSRI, the cadaveric subjects were stored at 4° C until subsequent use. The cadavers were sanitarily prepared and were examined radiologically prior to the installation of accelerometer hardware and after the test.

IMPACT TESTING

Impact tests were conducted using HSRI's pendulum and pneumatic impacting devices. A total of 19 cadavers were used in three series of tests. Multiple left knee impacts (described below) and a single lateral impact were performed on a group of eight cadavers, instrumented with triaxial accelerometer clusters on the pelvis and right trochanter of the femur. A second group of eight cadavers was subjected to knee impacts along the direction of the femoral axis of each side. Of these eight subjects, four had triaxial accelerometer clusters on both trochanters, one was instrumented with a nine-accelerometer plate on the pelvis, and three had no instrumentation. Finally, three cadavers were subject to left-side lateral impacts, each instrumented with a pelvic nine-accelerometer plate.

Acceleration Measurement -- Accelerations were measured in three orthogonal directions at two different sites (trochanter and pelvis) with Endevco 2264-2000 piezoresistive accelerometers by securing a triaxial accelerometer cluster to a mounting platform at each site. Three-dimensional motion determination was made possible by affixing three triaxial clusters of accelerometers to a lightweight magnesium plate which was in turn rigidly attached to the pelvis. The location of the center of gravity, the coordinate system of the triaxial clusters, and the nine accelerometer array are shown in Figure 2. The figure is divided into four sections. The top half of the figure shows the location of the instrumentation for those tests in which the response of both trochanters were obtained. The lower left hand corner shows the location of triaxial clusters in those tests in which both trochanter and pelvis response were measured. The lower right hand corner shows the location of the triaxial cluster or nine accelerometer array for those tests in which only pelvis response was measured. The location and mounting of the accelerometer platforms were as follows:

Trochanter: An incision was made below the greater trochanter and several short self-

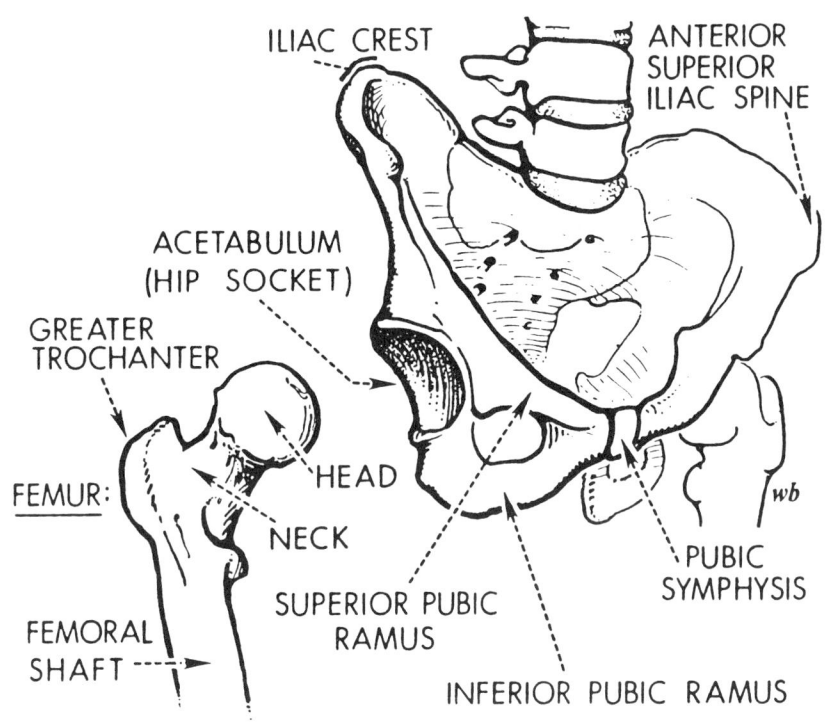

Fig. 1 - Anatomical overview of pelvis (5)

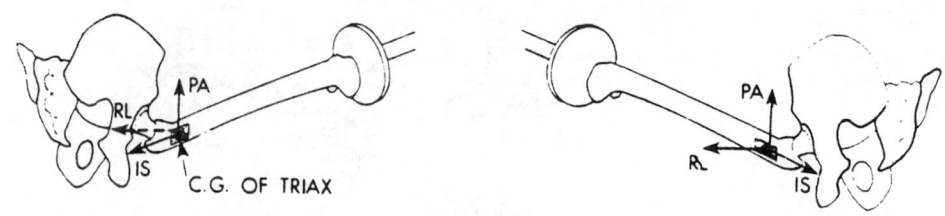

BI-TROCHANTERION RESPONSE

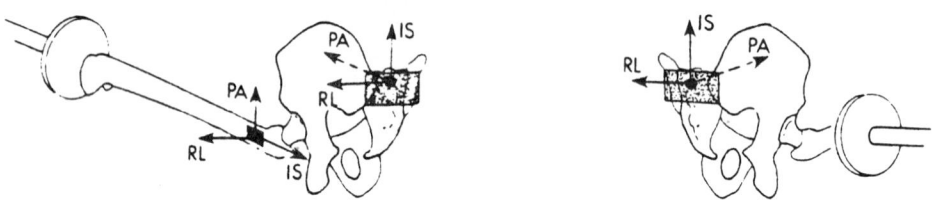

LEFT TROCHANTER AND/OR PELVIC RESPONSE

Fig. 2 - Instrumentation and phototarget location

tapping screws using a multi-point attachment scheme secured the mounting platform to the femur. The platform was then anchored with acrylic to insure rigidity.

Pelvis 9-Accelerometer: Four lag bolts were screwed into the pelvis near the posterior-superior iliac spines. Acrylic was applied, encasing both the bolts and the mounting plate, with the CG of the instrumentation plate midway between the posterior-superior iliac spines.

Pelvis Triax: Two lag bolts with tapped heads were screwed into the posterior-superior iliac spines. A lightweight magnesium plate spanned the bolts and was secured by two screws anchored into the tapped heads of the lag bolts.

Pendulum Impacts -- The pendulum impact device consists of a free-falling pendulum as an energy source which strikes either a 25 kg or a 56 kg impact piston. The impactor, guided by a set of Thompson linear ball bushings, was brought to impact velocity prior to impact and traveled up to 25 cm before being arrested. Axial loads were measured with either a GSE biaxial load cell or a Setra model 111 accelerometer. Shear loads were measured (when relevant) with the GSE biaxial load cell. Impact conditions between tests were controlled by varying impact velocity (up to 8.5 m/s), and the type and depth of padding on the impact piston surface. The piston excursion and the distance the piston traveled from the point of contact to the point of arrest ranged from 3 to 20 cm. The velocity of the piston was measured by timing the pulses from a magnetic probe which sensed the motion of targets on the piston at 0.89 cm intervals. A specially designed timer box was used to control and synchronize the events of a test, such as the release of the pendulum and activation and deactivation of lights and high speed cameras.

For tests conducted with this device, the subject was placed in a restraint harness and suspended in a seated position. Indirect impacts to the acetabulum in the anterior-to-posterior direction were delivered by impacting the knee along the direction of the femoral shaft axis ("axial knee impacts"). Indirect lateral impacts to the acetabulum were delivered by impacting the trochanteric region of the femur, along the axis of the neck of the femur.

Pneumatic Impacts -- The pneumatic impact device consists of an air reservoir which is connected to a honed steel cylinder. A driver piston is propelled down the cylinder by the pressurized air in the reservoir. The driver piston contacts a striker piston which is fitted with a piezoelectric accelerometer (Kistler 904A) and a piezoelectric load washer (Kistler 805A) to allow the determination of acceleration-compensated contact loads applied to the test subject. The mass, velocity, and stroke of the striker piston can be controlled to provide the desired impact conditions for a particular test. The velocity of the impactor is measured by timing the pulses from a magnetic probe which senses the motion of targets on the impactor at 1.3 cm intervals.

For the pneumatic impactor tests, the subject was suspended by a body harness and an overhead pulley system and in addition was seated on a block of balsa wood. Impacts were delivered indirectly to the pelvis through loading of the femur at the knee, as described above.

THREE-DIMENSIONAL MOTION DETERMINATION

The HSRI method used for measuring the three-dimensional motion of the pelvis is based on a technique used to measure the general motion of a vehicle in a simulated crash (11). In the current application, three triaxial clusters of Endevco 2264-2000 accelerometers are affixed to a light-weight magnesium plate which is then rigidly attached to the pelvis. With this method it is possible to take advantage of the physical and geometrical properties of the test subject as well as the site of impact in the design of a system for measurements of 3-D motion.

The nine acceleration signals obtained from the three triaxial clusters are used for the computation of the pelvis motion using a least-squares technique, the details of which are described elsewhere (12,13). The method takes advantage of the redundancy of nine independent acceleration measurements to minimize the effect of experimental error.

PHOTOKINEMETRICS

Each subject underwent two radiologic examinations, one prior to and one following the test. High-speed photographic coverage of the test consisted of two lateral views. A Hycam camera operating at 3000 frames per second provided a close-up view of the pelvis, while a Photosonics 1B camera operating at 1000 frames per second was used to obtain an overall view of the test subject. The motion of the subject was determined from the film by following the motions of five-point phototargets. The targets were affixed to the rigid accelerometer mounts located on the pelvis, trochanter, and spine. Since the resulting film provided a lateral view of the test, the motion observed was two-dimensional and restricted to the plane of the film.

INITIAL CONDITIONS AND POSITIONING

For all tests, the subject was placed in a restraint harness which was in turn suspended from the ceiling. For the axial knee impacts, the subject was positioned as in Figure 3 with the impactor initially 8 to 10 cm from the knee. These tests used as padding either 2.5 cm of Ensolite, 2.5 cm of styrofoam, or a combination of 2.5 cm Ensolite and 2.5 cm styrofoam. The lateral pelvis impacts required that the subject be positioned as in Figure 4, with the impactor initially centered 8 cm anterior to the greater trochanter. For these tests, the impactor was either rigid, padded with 2.5 cm Ensolite, or a combination of 2.5 cm Ensolite and 2.5 cm styrofoam.

PELVIS IMPACT RESPONSE

One method for analyzing the motion of a material body is to analyze the motion of a point on that body. In the case of the tests performed in this study, the point chosen is midway between posterior-superior iliac spines (PSIS). The motion is then analyzed using the concept of a moving frame discussed elsewhere (13) and briefly summarized here.

A vector field is a function which assigns a uniquely defined vector to each point along the path generated by the moving point. Similarly, any collection of three mutually orthogonal unit vectors emanating from each point on the path is a frame field. Thus any vector defined on the path (for example, acceleration) may be resolved into three orthogonal components of any well defined frame field.

In biomechanics research, frame fields which are frequently used are defined based on anatomical reference frames. The anatomical reference frames used here are shown in Figure 2. The frames are based on the anatomical orientation of a standing test subject. Therefore, the I-S direction of the trochanter is roughly equivalent to the minus A-P direction of the pelvis for a seated subject. Other frame fields such as the Principal Direction Triad (14) or Frenet-Serret frame (13), which contain information about the motion embedded in the frame field, have also been used to describe motion resulting from impact.

The Frenet-Serret frame consists of three mutually orthogonal vectors T, N, B. At any point in time a unit vector can be constructed that is co-directional with the velocity vector. This normalized velocity vector defines the tangent direction T. A second unit vector N is constructed by forming a unit vector co-directional with the time derivative of the tangent vector T (the derivative of a unit vector is normal to the vector). To complete the orthogonal frame, a third unit vector B (the unit binormal) can be defined as the cross product T x N. This then defines a frame at each point along the path and resolves the acceleration into two distinct types. The tangent acceleration (Tan(T)) is always the rate of change of speed (absolute velocity) and the normal acceleration (Nor(N)) contains acceleration information about the change in direction of the velocity vector. The binormal direction contains no acceleration.

In the case of a single triaxial accelerometer, the use of the Frenet-Serret frame is impractical but it has been found (14) that in many cases during direct impacts it is possible to find the most significant component of acceleration, therefore the principal direction of motion can be obtained.

One method of determining the principal direction of motion and constructing the Principal Direction Triad is to determine the direction of the acceleration vector in the moving frame of the triaxial accelerometer cluster and then prescribe the transformation necessary to obtain a new moving frame that would have one of its axes in the principal direction. A single point in time at which the acceleration is a maximum was chosen to define the directional cosines for transforming from the triax frame to a new frame in such a way that the resultant acceleration vector (AR) and "principal" unit vector (A1) were co-directional. This then can be used to construct a new frame rigidly fixed to the triax, but differing from the original one by an initial rotation. After completing the necessary transformation, a comparison between the magnitude of the principal direction and the resultant acceleration is performed. In the case of the impacts presented here, there was only a slight difference between the two quantities during the most significant part of the impact. However, for responses occurring after impact this was not always the case.

FORCE-TIME DURATION DETERMINATION

In order to define the pulse duration, a standard procedure was adopted which determines the beginning and end of the pulse. The procedure is to determine first the peak and the time at which it occurs. Next, the left half of the pulse, defined from the point where the pulse starts to rise to the time of the peak, is

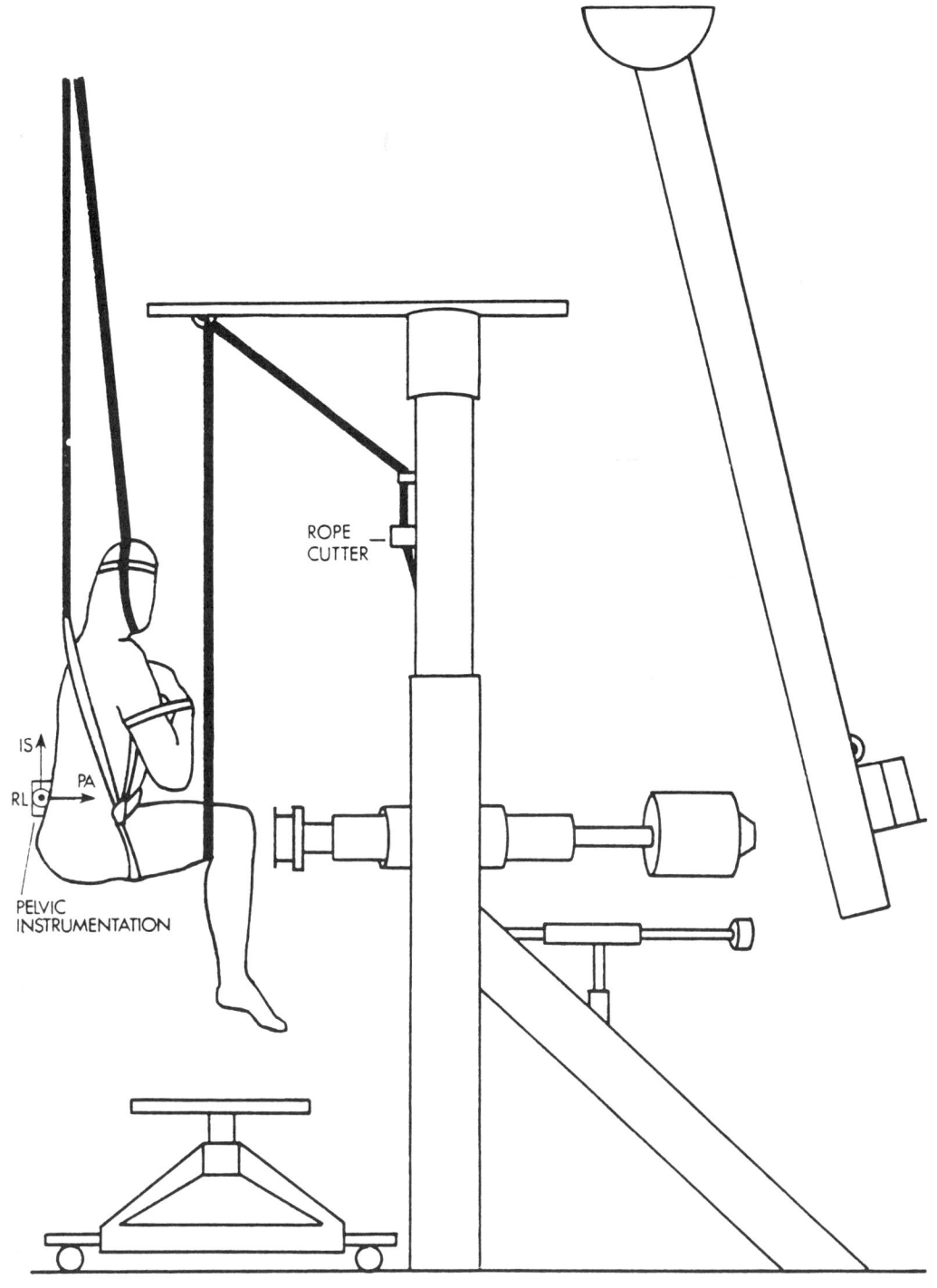

Fig. 3 - Schematic pendulum test setup — right leg impact

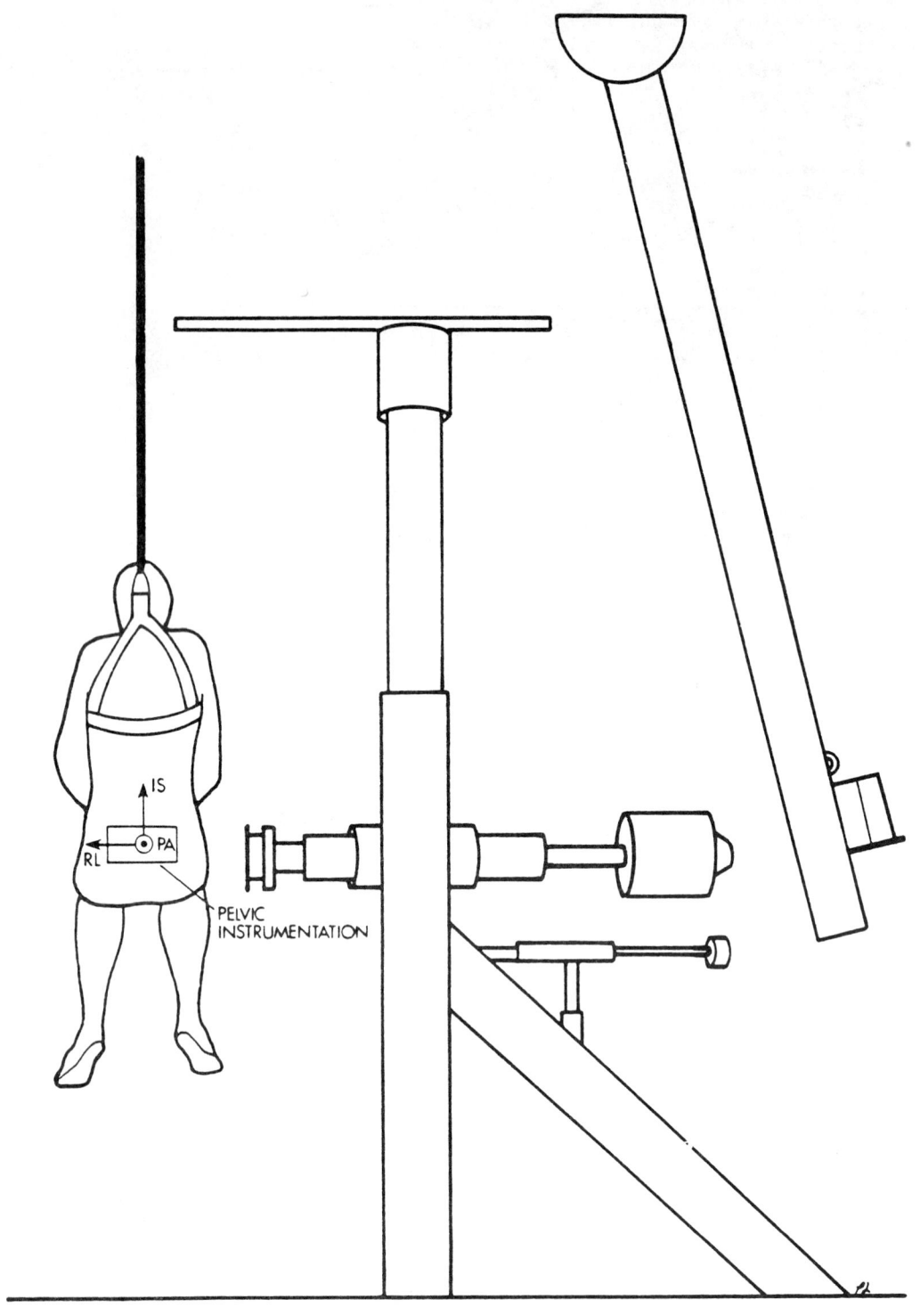

Fig. 4 - Schematic pendulum test setup — pelvis impact

least-squares fitted with a straight line. This rise line intersects the time axis at a point which is taken as the formal beginning of the pulse. For those tests which exhibit multimodal signals, the least-squares line is fitted from where the pulse starts to the time of the first significant peak. A similar procedure is followed for the right half of the pulse, i.e., a least squares line is fitted to the fall section of the pulse which is defined from the peak to the point where the first pulse minimum occurs. The formal end of the pulse is defined then as the point where the fall line intersects the time axis. In many cases, however, the formal end of the pulse (as defined above) is not the end of contact between the impactor and the subject. In these instances, two durations are used; one to indicate the end of the most significant aspect of the force-time history and one to indicate the end of the contact.

IMPACT TRANSFER FUNCTION ANALYSIS

With blunt impacts, the relationship between impact force and the motion resulting at various points of the impacted system can be expressed in the frequency domain through the use of a transfer function. A fast Fourier transformation of simultaneously monitored transducer time histories can be used to obtain the frequency response functions of impact force and accelerations of remote points. Once obtained a transfer function of the form

$$Z(i\omega) = \omega * \frac{F(F(t))}{F(A(t))}$$

can be calculated from the transformed quantities where ω is the given frequency, and $F(F(t))$ and $F(A(t))$ are the Fourier transforms of the impact forces and acceleration of the point of interest, at the given frequency. This particular transfer function is closely related to mechanial transfer impedance which is defined as the ratio between simple harmonic driving force and corresponding velocity of the point of interest. Mechanical transfer impedance (15) is a complex valued function which for the purpose of presentation will be described by its magnitude and its phase angle.

RESULTS

The tables and graphs presented on the following pages represent the data considered most pertinent in discussing the test results. Table 1 contains biometric data of all test subjects, as well as the test numbers corresponding to each subject (since most subjects received multiple knee impacts as well as a lateral pelvis impact, one subject will have several corresponding test numbers). The initial conditions for all knee impact tests and all lateral impact tests are presented in Tables 2 and 3, respectively.

A summary of gross autopsy results for the lateral impact tests is presented in Table 4. The series of knee impacts produced only one injury. All pelvic injuries were sustained on the impacted side of the pelvis.

Impact test summaries containing force and three-dimensional motion information for axial knee impacts to each cadaver appear in Table 5, and in Table 6 for lateral pelvis impacts. Summaries for force and triaxial acceleration are presented in Tables 7 and 8 for the axial knee impacts, and in Table 9 for the lateral impacts.

DISCUSSION

The results presented in this paper have been obtained from a series of pelvis injury research programs conducted during the past five years. The data is presented in abbreviated form to represent the trends which are felt to be important factors in pelvis impact response.

PELVIS RESPONSE FROM AXIAL KNEE IMPACTS

The response of the pelvis as characterized by the time history of various accelerations and velocities (both angular and linear) in addition to the force time history, is dependent on the impactor surface padding, mass and initial velocity as well as variations between individual test subjects. This is arrived at from analysis of three dimensional motion obtained from nine accelerometers, triaxial accelerometer clusters (affixed to the pelvis, the impacted femur and the femur opposite the impactor), as well as high speed photokinemetric documentation.

<u>Three-Dimensional Motion</u> -- Tests 79A243-79A248 represent six impacts to a single test subject. The six tests are divided into three groups with similar impacts on each knee. The three groups are: low velocity (3.5 m/s and 2.5 cm Ensolite impactor surface padding), medium velocity (5.0 m/s with 2.5 cm Ensolite impactor surface padding), and high velocity (8.5 m/s with rigid impactor surfaces). The time history of the three dimensional motion of the pelvis obtained from the nine accelerometer array is summarized in Table 5. The maximum impact force ranged from 4kN to 20kN with the duration of impact ranging from 12 ms to 30 ms.

Table 1. Biometrics

Cadaver No.	Height (cm)	Weight (Kg)	Age	Cause of Death
1	173	29.0	64	Differentiated lymphoma
2	160	57.2	73	Pneumonia
3	175	99.5	76	Cardiac arrest
4	178	106	63	Myocardial infarction
5	176	35.3	67	Cardiac resp. arrest intractible congestion
6	169	65.9	89	Cardiac arrest
7	176	68.1	76	Coronary occlusion
8	174	91.7	76	Myocardial infarction
9	179	41.6	66	Amyotrophic lateral sclerosis
10	174	61.9	73	Terminal pneumonia
11	180	91.2	56	Cardiac arrest
12	175	100	62	Cardiac arrest
13	--	88.0	61	Cardiac arrest
14	--	--	52	Cardiac arrest
15	184	52.0	60	Cardiac arrest
16	180	76.9	67	Cardiac arrest
17	169	86.5	65	Myocardial infarction
18	--	--	--	Cardiac arrest
19	174	68.3	40	Cardiac arrest

Table 2: Summary of Initial Conditions for Knee Impacts

Test No.	Cadaver No.	Impactor Velocity (m/s)	Impactor Mass (Kg)	Padding
77A204	18	15.2	10	10 cm Ensolite
77A205	13	12.2	10	10 cm Ensolite
77A206	13	15.2	10	10 cm Ensolite
77A207	12	18.3	10	10 cm Ensolite
77A208	12	21.3	10	10 cm Ensolite
79A243	14	3.4	25	2.5 cm Ensolite
79A244	14	3.4	25	2.5 cm Ensolite
79A245	14	5.0	25	2.5 cm Ensolite
79A246	14	5.0	25	2.5 cm Ensolite
79A247	14	8.6	25	Rigid
79A248	14	8.5	25	Rigid
79L081	1	5.5	56	2.5 cm Ensolite+ 2.5 cm Styrofoam
79L082	1	5.5	56	2.5 cm Ensolite+ 2.5 cm Styrofoam
79L085	2	5.5	56	2.5 cm Ensolite+ 2.5 cm Styrofoam
79L086	2	5.5	56	2.5 cm Ensolite+ 2.5 cm Styrofoam
79L089	3	5.5	56	2.5 cm Ensolite+ 2.5 cm Styrofoam
79L090	3	5.5	56	2.5 cm Ensolite+ 2.5 cm Styrofoam
80L094	4	5.9	56	2.5 cm Ensolite
80L097	5	5.5	56	2.5 cm Ensolite
80L098	5	5.9	56	Rigid

Table 2: Summary of Initial Conditions for Knee Impacts (continued)

Test No.	Cadaver No.	Impactor Velocity (m/s)	Impactor Mass (Kg)	Padding
80L102	6	5.5	56	2.5 cm Ensolite
80L103	6	5.8	56	Rigid
80L109	7	5.5	56	2.5 cm Ensolite
80L110	7	5.9	56	Rigid
80L114	8	5.9	56	2.5 cm Ensolite
80L115	8	5.8	56	Rigid
80L118	9	4.1	56	Rigid
80L119	9	4.2	56	Rigid
80L120	9	5.9	56	Rigid
80L124	10	4.1	56	Rigid
80L125	10	5.9	56	Rigid
80L129	11	4.0	56	Rigid
80L130	11	5.9	56	Rigid
80L135	19	4.0	56	Rigid
80L135	19	6.0	56	Rigid
80L135	19	4.0	56	Rigid
80L136	19	6.0	56	Rigid

Table 3. Summary of Initial Conditions for Lateral Impacts

Test No.	Cadaver No.	Impactor Velocity (m/s)	Impactor Mass (Kg)	Padding
80L095	4	5.1	56	2.5 cm Ensolite
80L099	5	5.7	56	2.5 cm Ensolite
80L104	6	5.8	56	Rigid
80L111	7	5.8	56	Rigid
80L116	8	5.7	56	Rigid
80L121	9	5.9	56	Rigid
80L126	10	5.8	56	Rigid
80L131	11	5.5	56	Rigid
80L137	19	5.9	56	Rigid
82E008	15	8.4	25	2.5 cm Ensolite+ 1.3 cm Styrofoam
82E028	16	8.4	25	0.5 cm Ensolite
82E049	17	8.6	25	2.5 cm Ensolite+ 2.5 cm Styrofoam

Table 4. Summary of Autopsy Results

Test No.	Results
80L095	No observed injuries.
80L099	No observed injuries.
80L104	Vertical separation fracture of superior pubic ramus approximately one inch from pubic symphysis.
80L111	Horizontal separation fracture of ilio-pubic ramus, connected to a horizontal fracture of the acetabulum.
80L116	No observed injuries.
80L121	Vertical stellar fracture on outer aspect of ilium extending from iliac crest to anterior-inferior iliac spine.
80L126	Non-separational fractures of superior and ischio-pubic ramus.
80L131	Horizontal fracture of ilio-pubic ramus.
80L137	No observed injuries.
82E008	No observed injuries.
82E028	Vertical Separation fracture of ischio-pubic ramus. Horizontal fracture of acetabulum extending two inches into superior pubic ramus.
82E049	No observed injuries.

Table 5. 3-D Motion Knee Impact Test Summary

Test No.	Peak Force (N)	Impulse (N.s)	Duration (m/s)	Peak Linear Acceleration (m/s/s)				Peak Angular Acceleration (rad/s/s)			
				P-A	R-L	I-S	TAN	P-A	R-L	I-S	RES
79A243 @ ms=	3750 11	58	30	-95 7	-150 6	70 6	160 6	-150 4	-670 5	1200 5	1180 6
79A244 @ ms=	3750 11	59	30	-90 5	200 5	75 5	250 5	430 3	-380 5	-1130 5	1050 5
79A245 @ ms=	5750 12	80	30	-120 7	+300 7	115 6	320 6	530 4	-800 5	-1750 5	2000 6
9A246 @ ms=	6000 11	75	32	-150 4	-260 4	160	340 8	-600 3	-1440 8	2000 5	2200 4
79A247 @ ms=	20000 3	120	12	-1750 2	-2600 2	100 3	3200 2	-1700 3	-30000 3	20000 2	31000 3
79A248 @ ms=	21000 2	135	12	-1050 2	2750 2	1600 2	3200 2	19000 1	-20000 2	-17500 1	25000 1

Table 6: Padded Knee Impacts

Test No.	Force Maximum (N)	Duration (ms)	Impulse (N-s)	Energy (N-M)	Acceleration Troch. Maximum (m/s)	Acceleration Opposite Troch. Maximum (m/s)	Velocity Troch. Maximum (m/s)	Velocity Opposite Troch. Maximum (m/s)
79L081= @ ms=	1550 11	25 (35)	22	5	43 4	16 35	4.9 22	2.8 60
79L082= @ ms=	1750 13	26 (31)	25	6	34 12	19 27	5.0 22	2.8 56
79L085= @ ms=	900	30	10	1	21 12	8 25	4.0	2.4 60
79L086= @ ms=	1100	30	12	1 +	7.5 15	10 20	4.3	2.5 65
79L089= @ ms=	5200 17	31 (43)	65		48 13	9 23	4.5 30	2.5 65
79L090= @ ms=	4600 17	34 (44)	60	32	33 (13)	13 27	4.0 30	2.2 65

Table 7: Knee Impacts

Test No.	Force 1st Peak (N)	Force Maximum (N)	Force Duration (ms)	Force Impulse (N-s)	Force Energy (N-m)	Accel. Troch. Maximum (g's)	Accel. Pelvis Maximum (g's)	Vel. Troch. Maximum (m/s)	Vel. Pelvis Maximum (m/s)
80L094 @ ms=		5850 8	27 (73)	88	69	80 8	60 12	3.7 22	3.4 15
80L097 @ ms=		3950 9	20 (5)	45	18	115 9	80 8	6.2 16	5.2 1
80L098 @ ms=		2475 2	12 (36)	21	3.9	450 1	250 2	5.5 4	6.2 6
80L102 @ ms=		7000 8	24 (46)	100	88.8	140 7	95 8	4.8 11	4.0 10
80L103 @ ms=		7550 3	15 (40)	56	28.4	400 2	120 4	5.9 3	3.2 5
80L109 @ ms=		8100 9	25 (61)	98	85.2	200 9	70 8	5.3 8	3.4 9
80L110 @ ms=		9500 3	20 (44)	89	0.9	700 2	190 3	5.7 6	3.7 5
80L114 @ ms=		10000 7	35 (55)	107	102	230 6		6.2 7	3.1 28
80L115 @ ms=		12000 2	24 (34)	100	92	675 2		5.9 3	3.4 16
80L118 @ ms=	5200 1	6000 2	12 (66)	36	11.6	220 1	115 1.5	3.9 8	3.2 7
80L119 @ ms=	4500 1	5750 2	13 (70)	45.7	18.7	300 2	155 3	4.2 4	3.2 8
80L120 @ ms=	5250 1	8900 3	15 (55)			500 3	150 (3.5)	4.9 3	4.0 10
80L124 @ ms=	1	7500 2	20 (77)	46.9	19.6	390 2	115 4	4.4 4	3.0 7
80L125 @ ms=	5600 1	9700 3	20 (57)	88	70	400 2	175 4	5.2 3	3.5 6
80L129 @ ms=		8750 3	20 (27)	74.4	49.5	205 1	140 2	4.1 6	3.5 15
80L130 @ ms=	8900 2	9750 3	16 (29)	105	100	650 2	185 2	5.6 6	5.1 14
80L135 @ ms=	5000 2	8700 4	17 (28)	75	51	1750 1	135 2	3.9 7	3.4 10
80L136 @ ms=	9700 6	11800 6	16 (58)	105	101	900 2	240 3	5.4 8	4.1 9

Table 8. Lateral Pelvis Impact

Test Number	Force Maximum (N)	Force Duration (ms)	Acceleration 1st Peak	Acceleration Maximum (g's)	Velocity Maximum (m/s)
80L095 @ ms=	10700 10	44		38 10	4.4 44
80L099 @ ms=	3200	42	23 5	50 11	4.6 38
80L104 @ ms=	5900 9	49		40 11	4.7 42
80L111 @ ms=	7600	50		100 4	4.7 40
80L116 @ ms=	7700 9	51		57 11	4.3 48
80L121 @ ms=	3300 15	30	105 2	110 4	4.3 56
80L126 @ ms=	7400 5	44	50 4	135 11	4.3 40
80L131 @ ms=	8500 7	40	50 6	135 11	4.3 52
80L137 @ ms=	9200 5	22	40 3	48 6	4.8 50

Table 9. Lateral Impacts

Test No.	Peak Force (N)	Impulse (N-s)	Duration (ms)	Peak Linear Acceleration (m/s/s) P-A	R-L	I-S	Tan	Peak Angular Acceleration (rad/s/s) P-A	R-L	I-S	Res
82E008 @ ms=	14000 13	190	29	300 18	840 11	-340 14	831 14	-2270 14	-6910 14	-4600 16	6010 11
82E028 @ ms=	13000 7	190	21	350 6	710 6	550 11	650 6	3620 4	10100 8	8190 5	10250 8
82E049 @ ms=	14000 14	206	26	127 15	360 14	-100 14	370 14	2700 13	-3480 13	-1990 16	3750 16

Several distinct events occurred in all the force time histories and could be used as event markers. They are: the beginning of impact noted as E1, the peak force noted as E2, and the end of impact noted as E3. Both angular and linear accelerations begin at the E1 event and reach maximums at or before the E2 event. Even though there is significant angular acceleration during this interval, the primary acceleration is in the tangent direction (with a smaller component in the normal direction) indicating that the direction of motion changes slowly with time. In addition, the angular acceleration during this interval differs in magnitude and direction for each of the three sets of tests. For tests 79A243 and 79A244 (Figures 5 and 6) the angular acceleration was found to be primarily in the I-S direction (although lesser components occurred in the R-L and P-A directions). In tests 79A245 and 79A246, the magnitude of the angular acceleration is greater and is to a greater degree in the R-L and P-A direction. In tests 79A247 and 79A248 (Figures 7 and 8), the magnitude of the angular acceleration in the R-L and P-A direction is similar in magnitude to that of the I-S direction. Along with the changes in magnitude and direction of the angular acceleration with changing impact velocity, there is an increasing ratio of angular acceleration to peak force as well as a change in the relative phasing of the angular acceleration time history to force time history during the E1-E2 interval. In addition to changes in angular acceleration with increasing impactor velocity, there were also changes in the linear acceleration; its magnitude, direction, and phasing with respect to the E2 events. For tests 79A243 and 79A244, the linear acceleration was primarily in the RL-PA plane during the E1-E2 event interval. As the magnitude of the loading increased (as in tests 79A245 through 79A248), a significant component of linear acceleration in the I-S direction developed.

Physically, this implies that the response of the pelvis can be interpreted as the response of one material body (the pelvis) in contact with other material bodies (the femur, spine, abdominal organs, and soft tissue). The degree to which each of the material bodies interacts with the pelvis is dependent upon the amount of available impactor energy and how it is transmitted to the pelvis.

Triaxial Bitrochanteric Response -- Although the padding on the impactor surface was different, the loading in tests 79L081 through 79L090 (Table 7) is similar to that of the the previous tests. The response is measured with two triaxial accelerometer clusters located near each trochanter. Using the same event markers on the force time history as in the previous tests, some information about the response of the pelvis from the trochanteric response may be obtained. Near the E1 event the acceleration of the trochanter of the impacted side begins, however the accelerometer of the opposite trochanter displays little or no motion until near or after the E2 event. Acceleration of the impacted side peaks before the E2 event, whereas the acceleration response of the other trochanter reaches a maximum near the E3 event. The motion indicated by this type of response is somewhat similar to test 79A243 and 79A244 (for the pelvis) with the greatest rotation in the I-S direction. However, it is clear from the accelerometer data and high-speed movies that although the pelvis seems to behave as it were rotating about a fixed point near the trochanter of the opposite femur during the E1-E2 interval, motion after the E2 event is considerably more complex, with the peak velocity of the opposite femur more than half of that of the impacted femur.

Pelvis and Trochanteric Response -- Tests 80L094 to 80L136 (Table 8) represent similar loading to that of the previously mentioned tests (79A243-248 and 79L081-090). The response is measured by the use of triaxial accelerometers located on the pelvis and trochanter on the side of impact, as well as photokinemetric documentation. The peak forces range from 6 to 12 kN.

In some of these tests, the force time history is similar to that of 79L081 through 79L090 with one peak and a well defined beginning and end, however a few of the tests have a more complex force time history. They exhibit several local maxima and/or continuing impactor contact after the initial part of the pulse occurs. Although the response of the trochanter as interpreted by the principal direction acceleration and resulting acceleration time-history waveforms is similar to some of the previous heavily-padded tests, others display damped oscillatory motion (Figure 9). This response is generally observed during the first section of the pulse and unobservable shortly after the E2 event. In addition the peak acceleration generally occurs around the time of the first significant maximum of the force time history. Other researchers using finite element modeling of the femur (16) have shown that various modes of bending and torsion can occur. Potentially both the oscillatory nature of the trochanteric response and the multimodal nature of the force time histories for these tests are a result of the bending of the femur.

Although in these tests only triaxial acceleration is measured and the force time history varies from test to test in a very

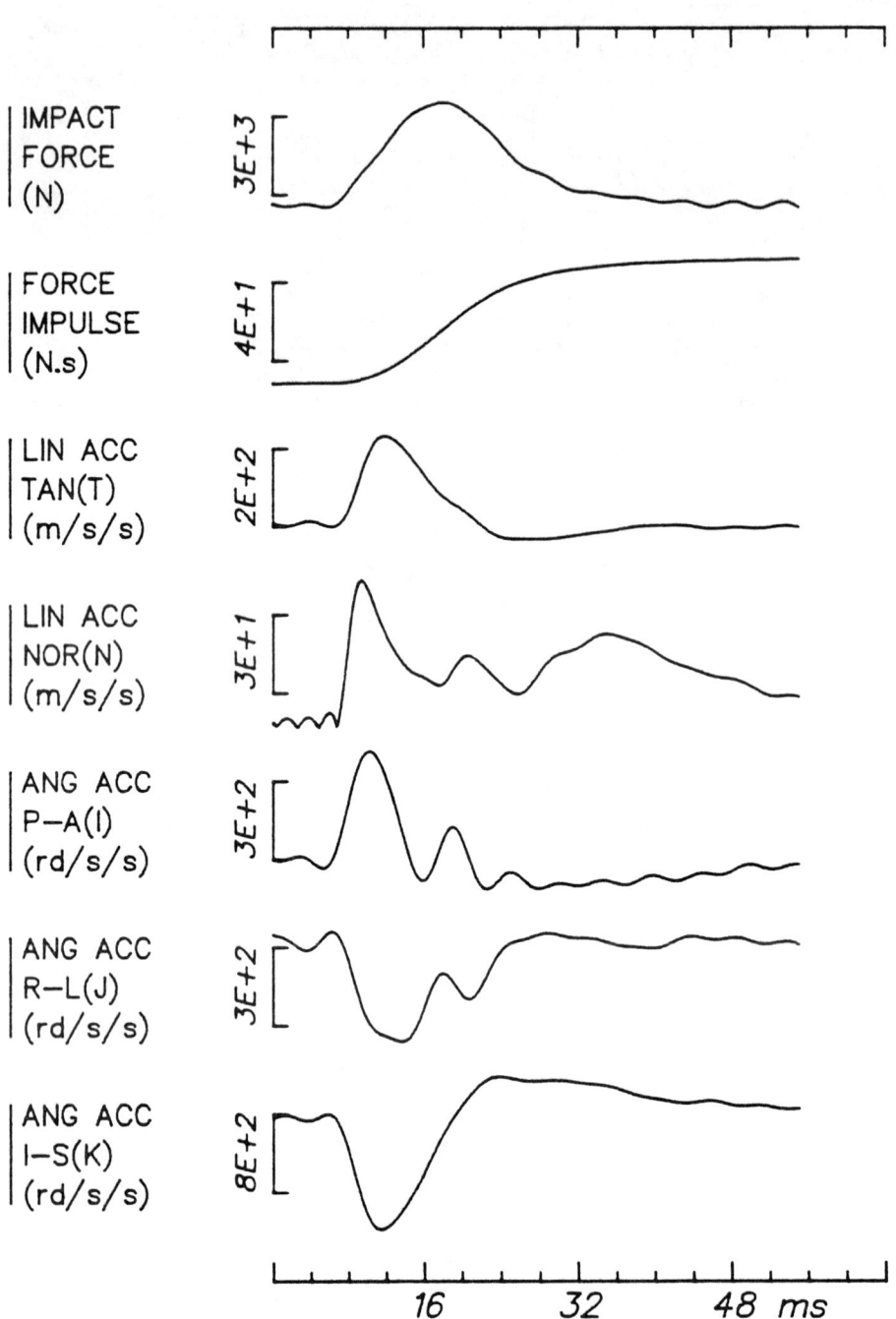

Fig. 5 - Test 79A244

Run ID: 79A244

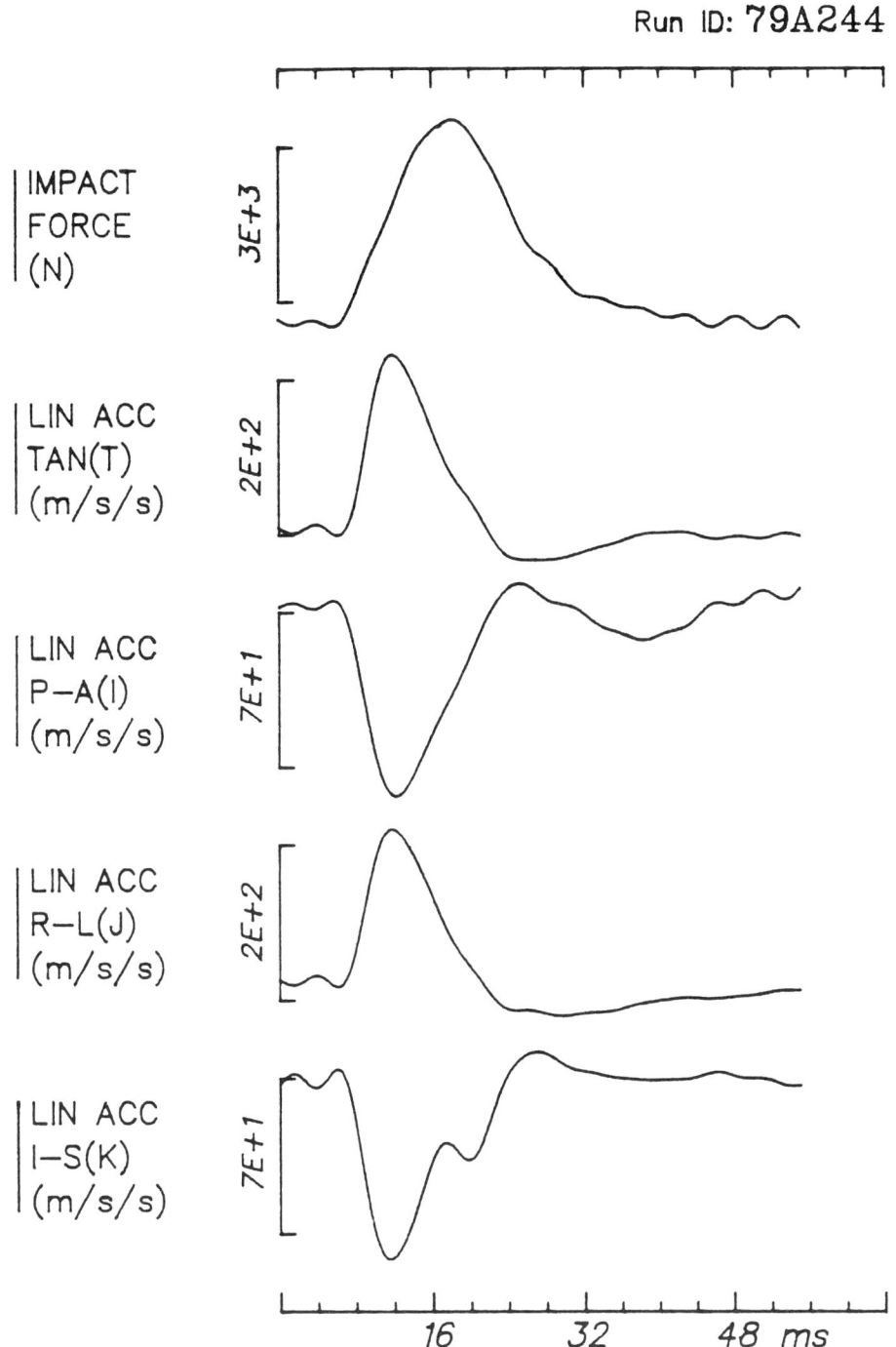

Fig. 6 - Test 79A244

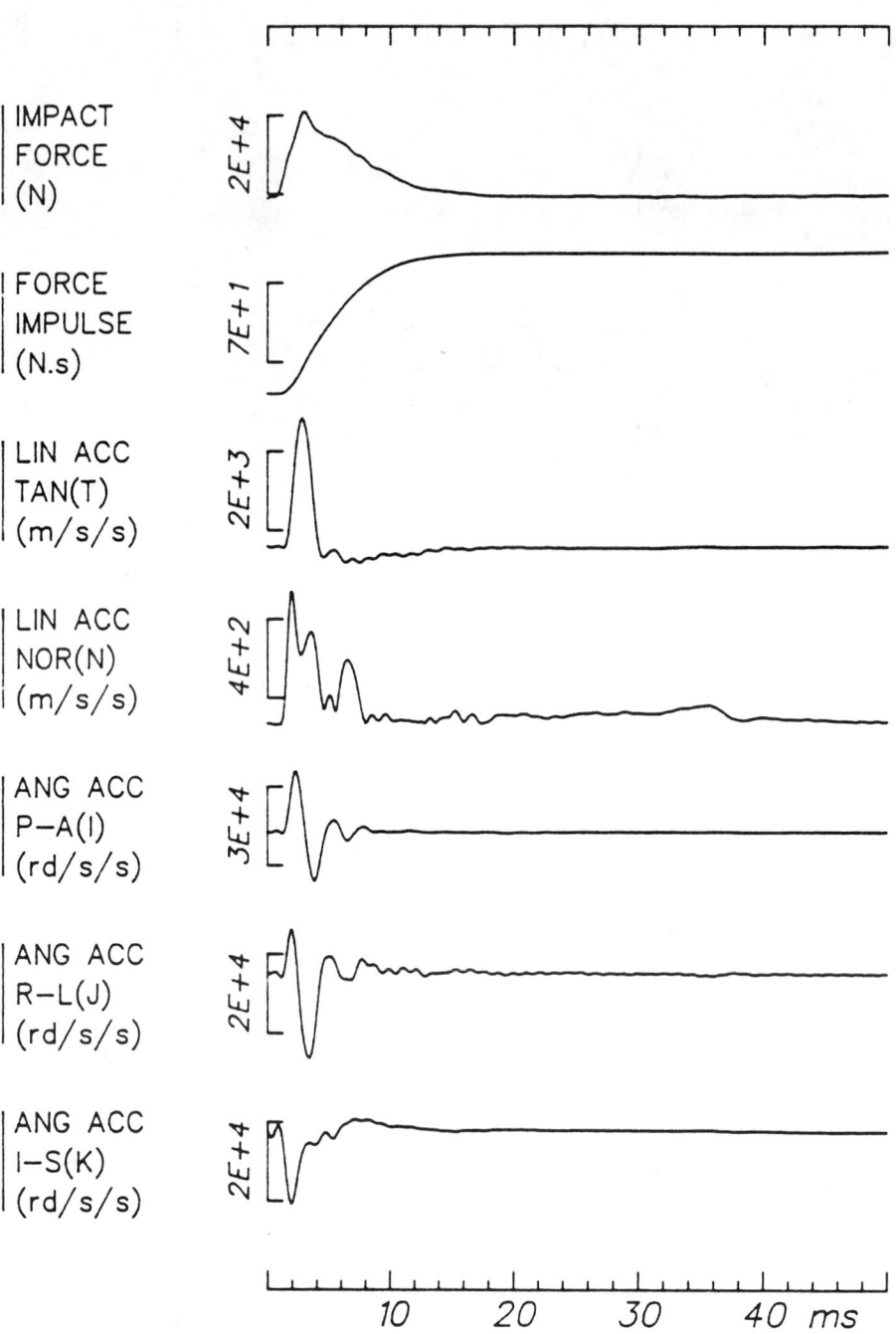

Fig. 7 - Test 79A248

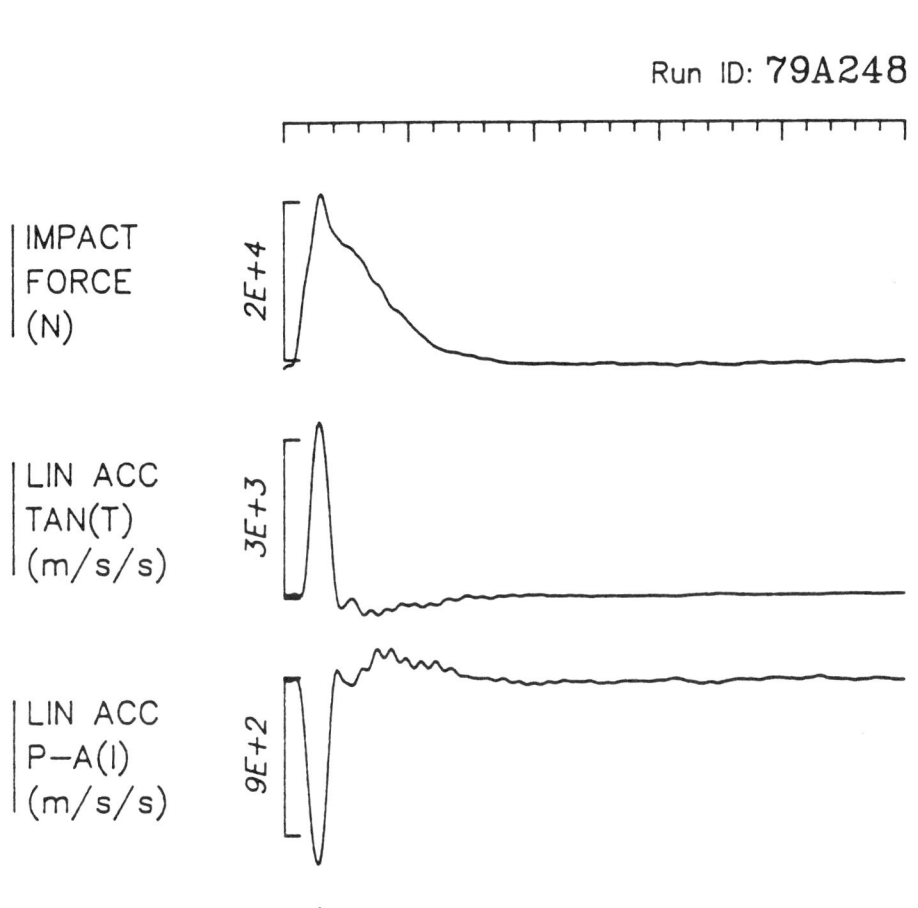

Fig. 8 - Test 79A248

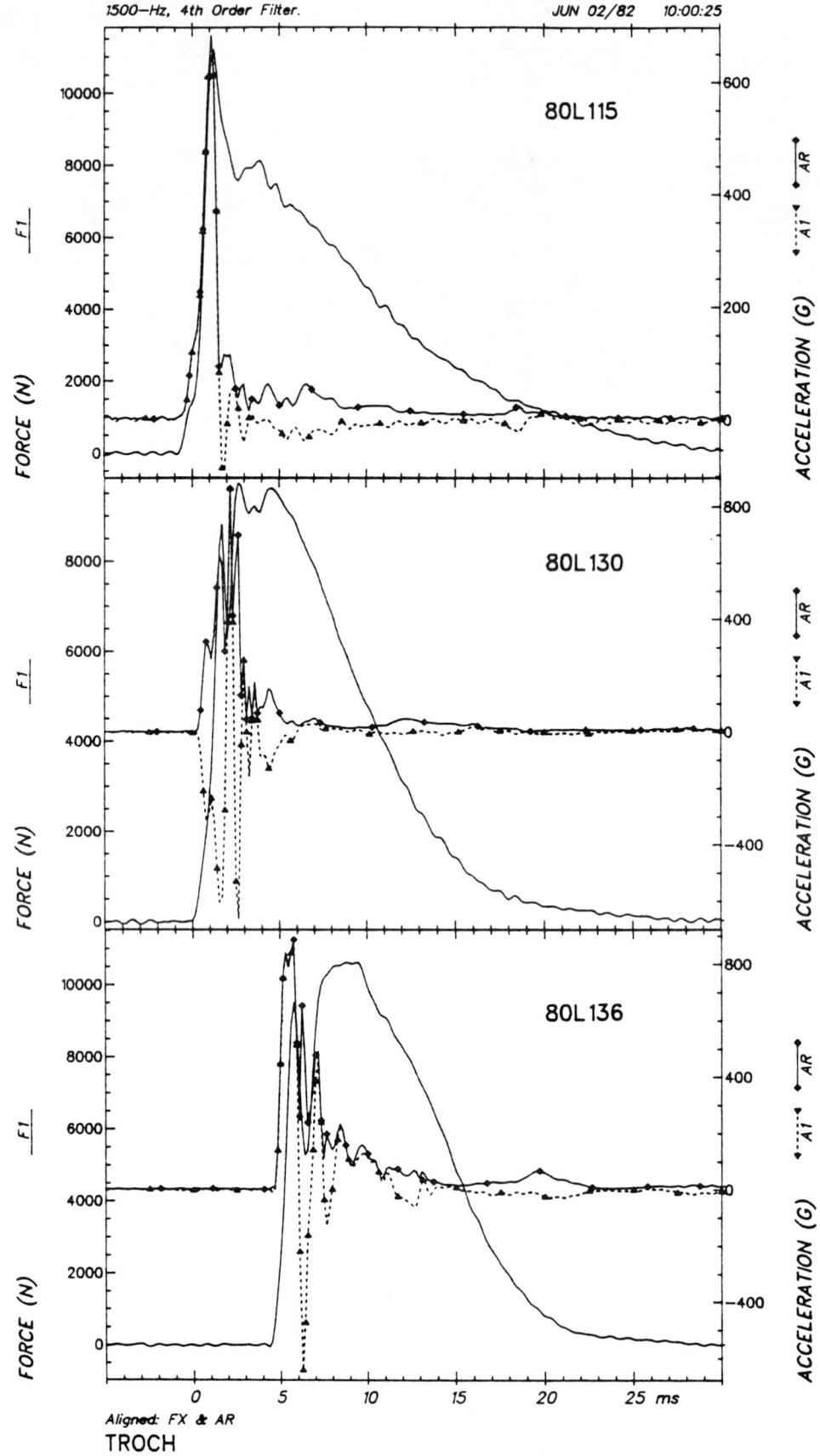

Fig. 9 - Trochanter impact response

general way the response of the pelvis, as interpreted by the principal direction accelerations, is similar in these tests to that of the response interpreted by tangential acceleration in tests 79A247 and 79A248. Table 8 compares the acceleration time history of the pelvis to that of the force time history and acceleration time history of the trochanter. In general, the peak acceleration of the pelvis is less than and lags behind that of peak trochanteric accelerations. In addition, the resultant peak velocity of the trochanter is greater than and precedes the pelvis peak velocity, and is primarily in the I-S direction (of the femur).

Transfer Functions -- The transfer function formed from the impact force and acceleration includes the effects of padding and subject response. A corridor for transfer functions formed from the impact force and tangent acceleration for tests 79A243-79A248 is shown in Figure 10.

For tests 79A243 and 79A244 the transfer function is included in the corridor to 100 Hz. For test 79A245 and 79A246 the transfer function is included to 150 Hz, and for tests 79A247 and 79A248, it is included from 10 to 400 Hz. The corridor representing pelvis response (interpreted by mechanical impedance for force and resulting velocity) shows that all six tests are similar to 100 Hz. Four tests are similar to 150 Hz and two are similar to 400 Hz. This seems to be true despite the different impact conditions (different padding, different initial velocity, opposite side impacts), and different time history responses. This would seem to indicate that the responses for this subject are repeatable, symmetric (same response for opposite sides) and linear to at least 100 Hz.

The mechanical impedance for tests 79A081 - 79A090 (Figure 11) is generated from force and principal direction acceleration, and is considered valid between 10 and 100 Hz. In the frequency range between 10 and 30 Hz it is somewhat similar to the impedance of tests 79A243 through 79A248. Above this range, however, there is a continual decline in the value of the impedance. This is believed to be a result of the styrofoam padding used in these tests.

For pelvis tests 80L094 - 80L136, the mechanical impedance obtained from the principal direction acceleration was significantly less than those calculated from the accelerations in the two directions normal to it above 25 Hz in all tests. For the trochanter, the mechanical impedance was valid for regions below this range however for comparison purposes it is presented down to 25 Hz. The upper limit for the validity of the pelvis impedance was 400 Hz and therefore the trochanteric upper limit is chosen as 400 Hz. To obtain information about the repeatability of the response of different test subjects, multiple impacts (at a subinjurious level) were performed on each subject (Table 8) with each subject in the same initial postural configuration while the impactor surface padding and velocity were varied. The transfer function formed from the principal direction acceleration and force-time history for both the pelvis and trochanter are shown in Figures 12 and 13 for tests 80L114 and 80L115, respectively, and in Figures 14 and 15 for tests 80L135 and 80L136, respectively.

It was observed that the acceleration response of the trochanter is primarily in the same direction as that of the force while the acceleration of the pelvis is not. Despite this and the fact that impact conditions varied between impacts to the same side, observation of these transfer function waveforms (and others not presented) show that the transfer functions for repeated tests on the same side are similar for both the pelvis and trochanter. The transfer function for the pelvis and the trochanter of the same subject are similar in waveform up to 200 Hz, although they differ in magnitude -- values for the mechanical impedance of the pelvis are generally two to four times that of those for the trochanter. The amount of scatter between subjects is addressed in Figures 16 and 17, which represent the corridor for impacts that did not result in injury for both the pelvis and trochanter, respectively. Although the two corridors look similar (differing only in magnitude below 100 Hz), they cover a wide range of possible responses, particularly above 200 Hz. This magnitude indicates that although the response of a single subject is similar for repeated impacts, there is wide scatter between subjects.

In addition to the above observations on the transfer functions, in some of the tests (e.g., 80L135 and 80L136) a resonance was observed between 180 and 280 Hz, which is within the band in which others have observed a resonance (16,17). This resonance (which is observed in both the pelvis and trochanter, although it is more pronounced in the trochanter transfer function) is potentially related to the oscillatory behavior mentioned above and also to the predicted first mode bending (16). Although most of the test subjects did not display this resonance, it does occur in a few of the tests which may help to explain some of the scatter observed.

Damage to the Pelvis and Femur -- Many of the tests involved loads above 10 kN, with only one resulting injury (test 80L103 resulted in a

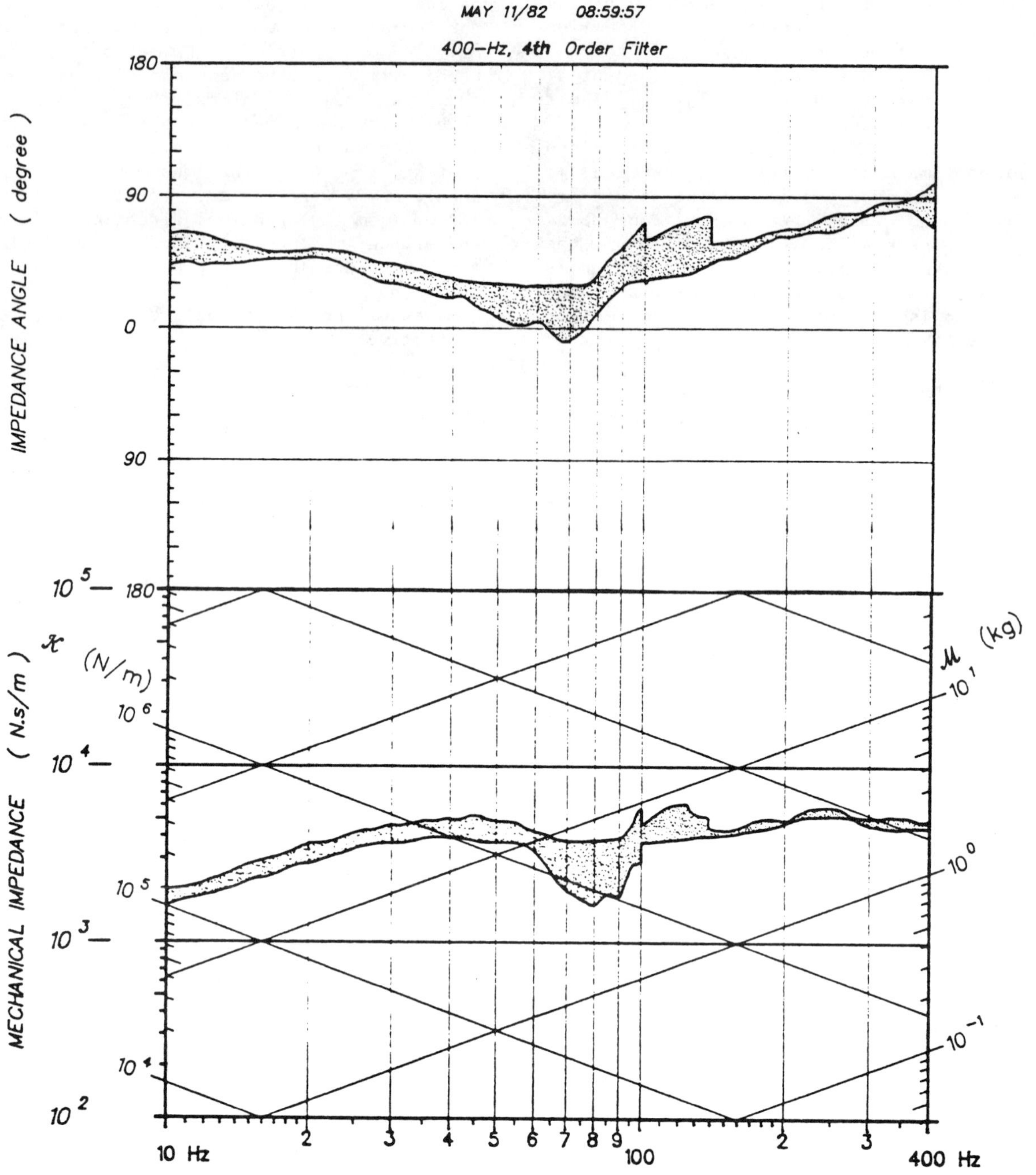

Fig. 10 - Corridor for pelvis impacts, 79A243-79A248

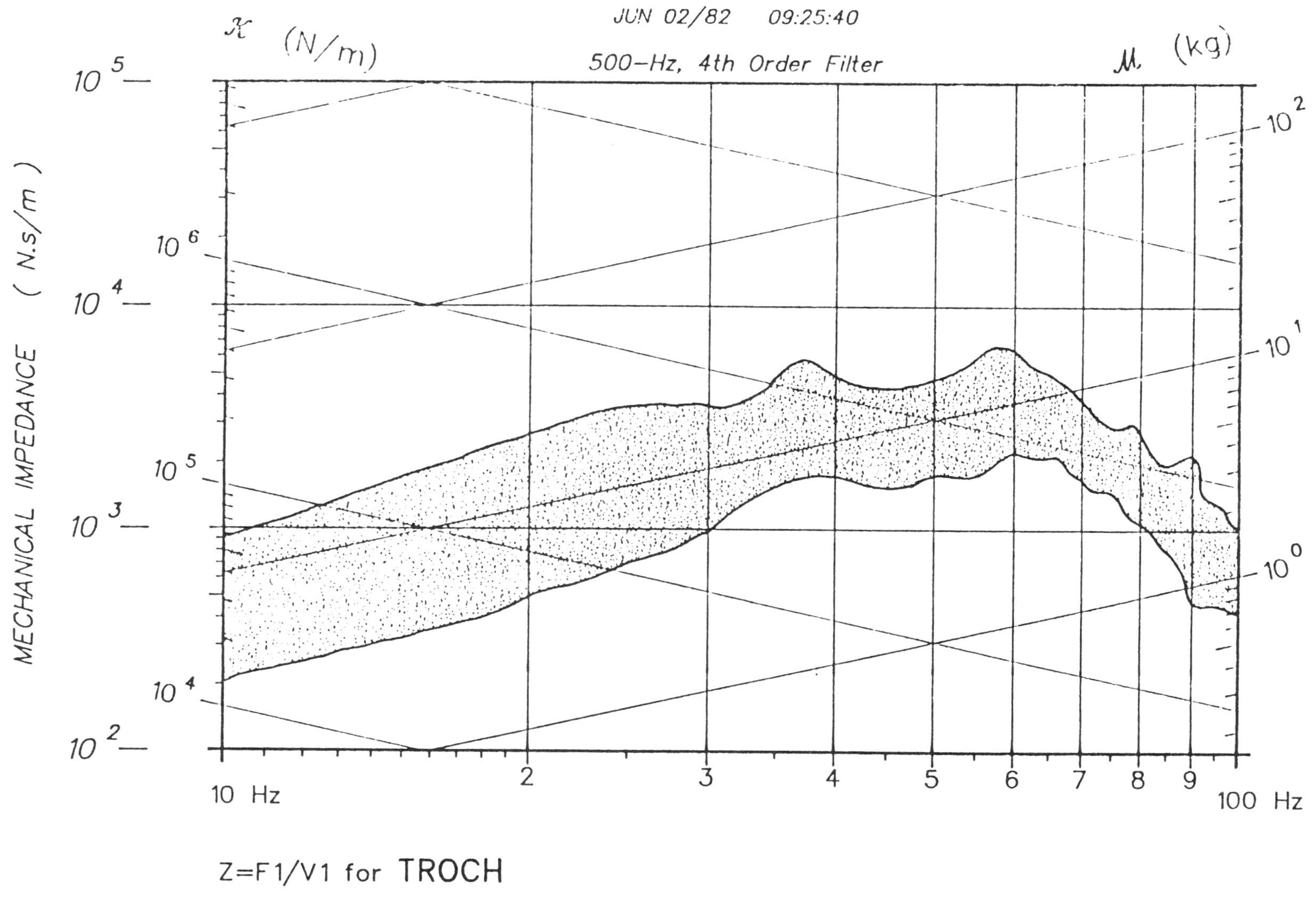

Fig. 11 – Trochanter corridor for axial knee impacts, 79L081-79L092

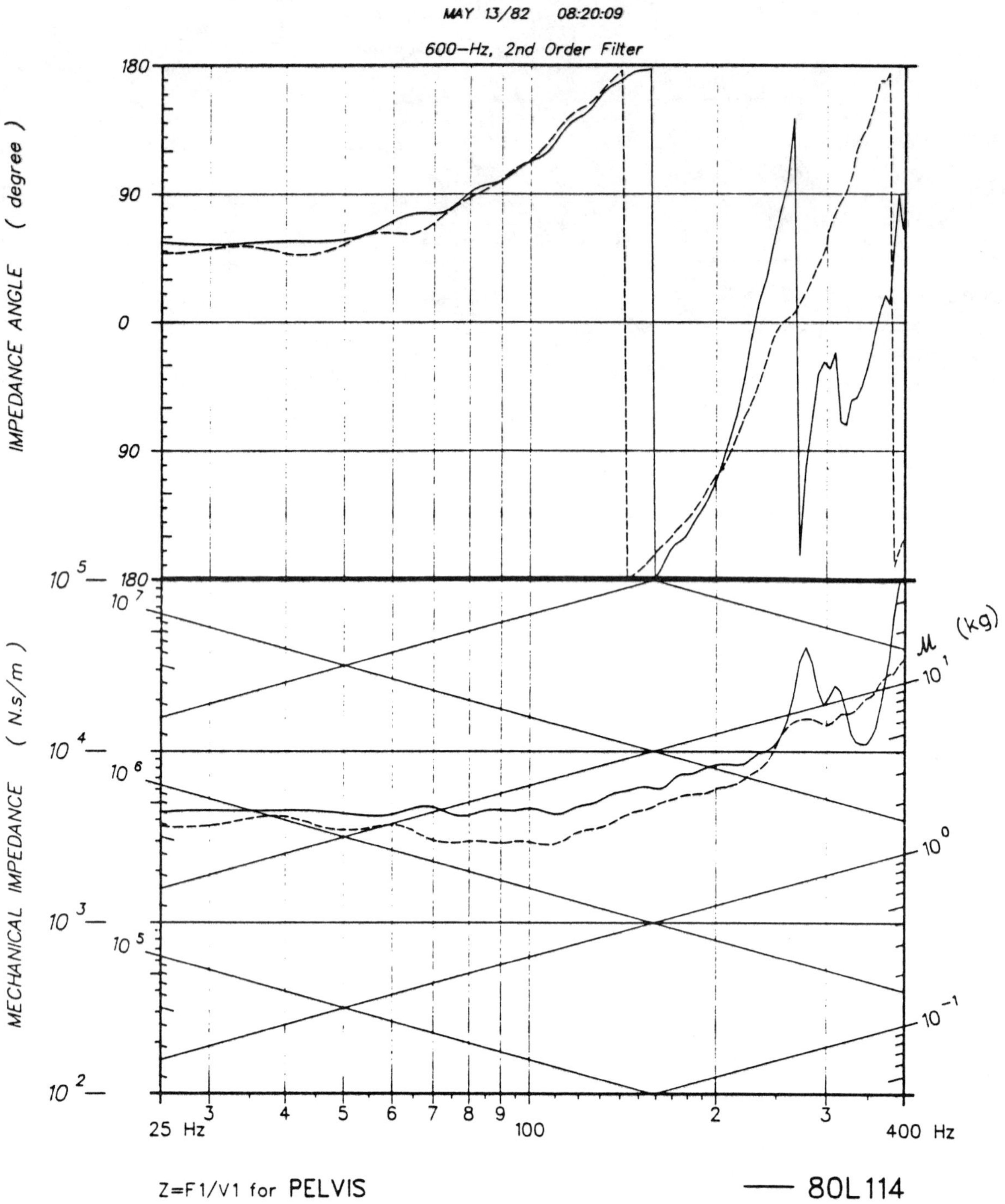
MAY 13/82 08:20:09
600–Hz, 2nd Order Filter
IMPEDANCE ANGLE (degree)
180
90
0
90
180
MECHANICAL IMPEDANCE (N.s/m)
10 5
10 4
10 3
10 2
10 7
10 6
10 5
M (kg)
10 1
10 0
10 −1
25 Hz
3
4
5
6
7
8
9
100
2
3
400 Hz
Z=F1/V1 for PELVIS
80L114
80L115

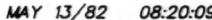

Fig. 12

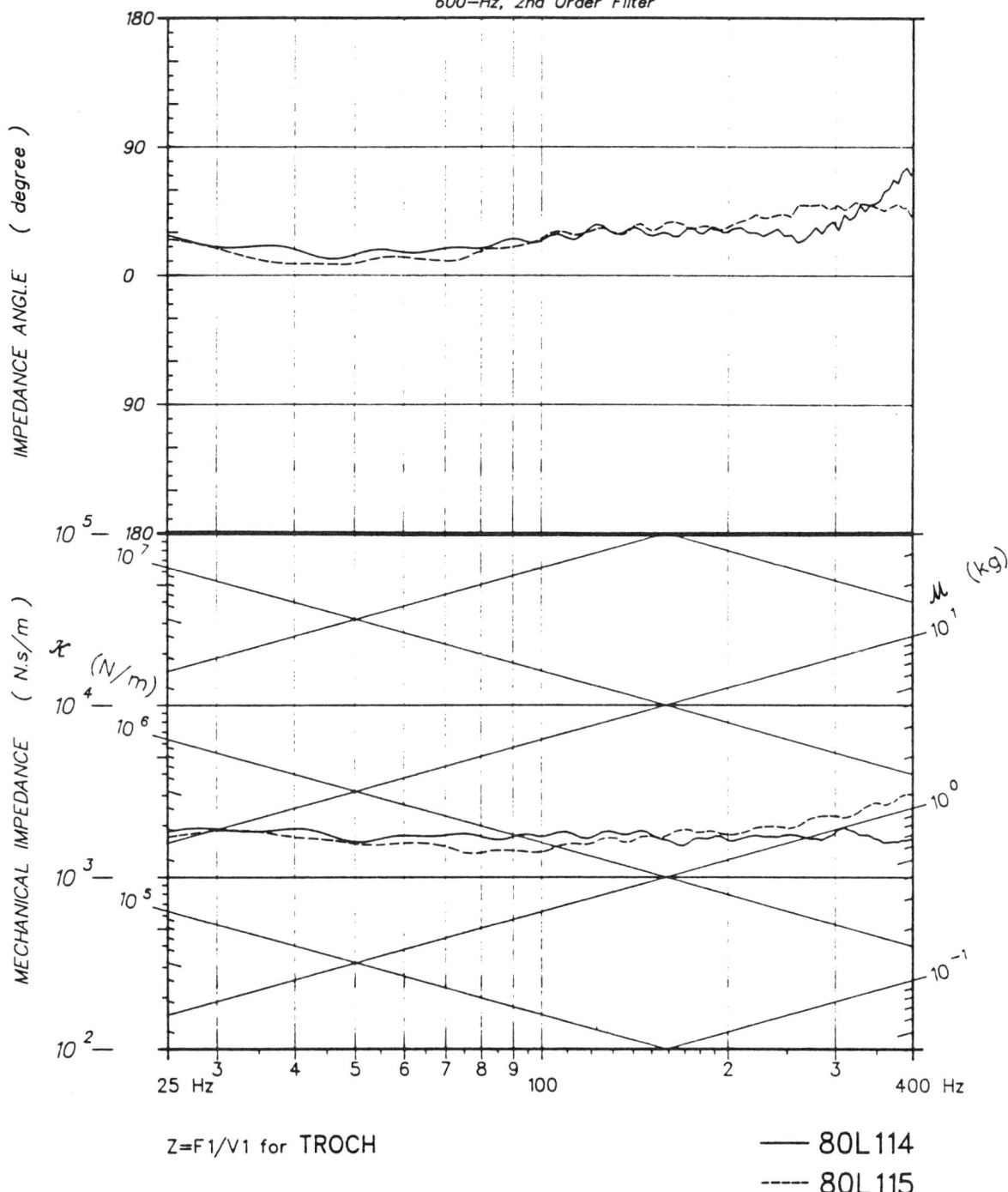

Fig. 13

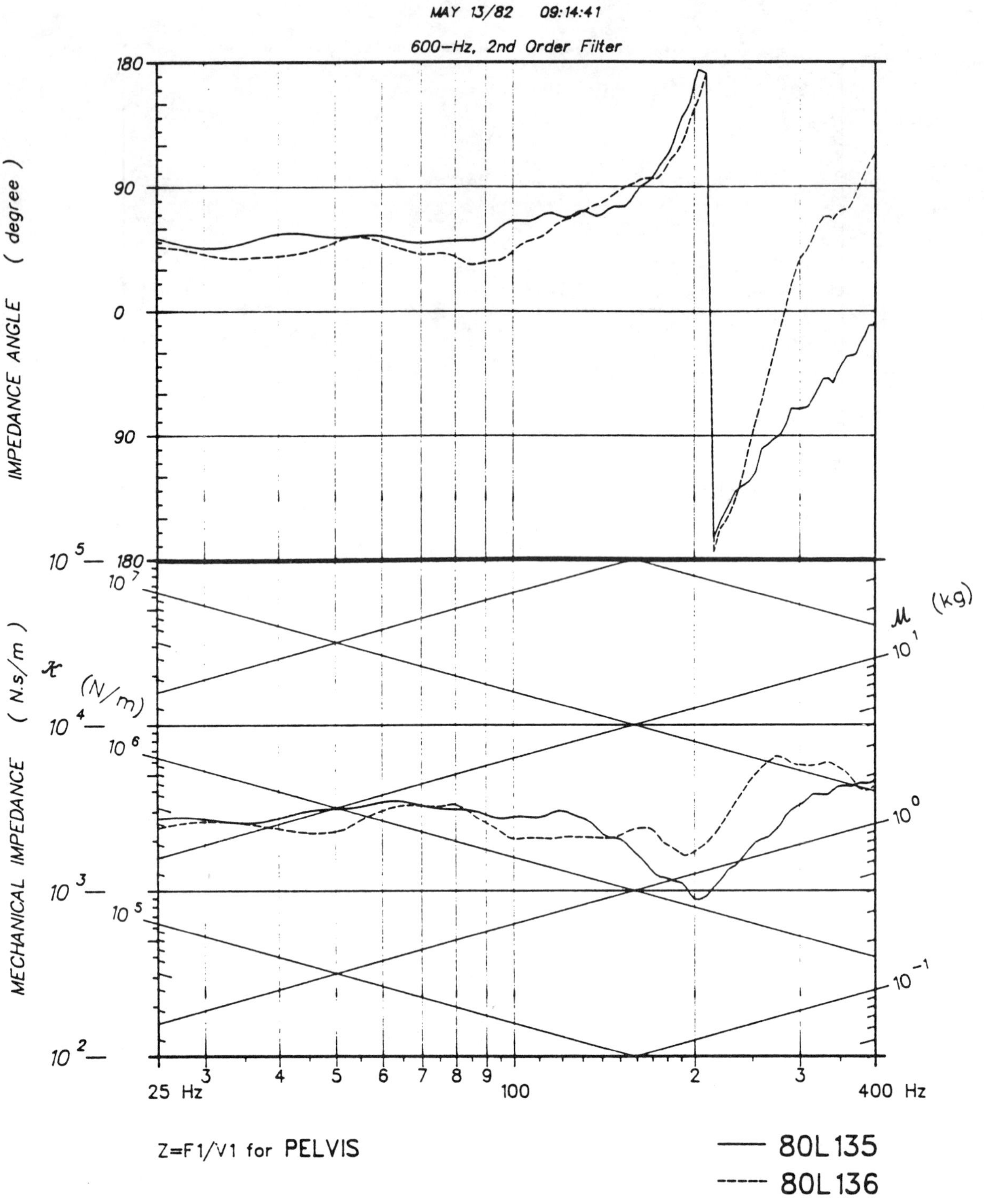

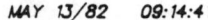

Fig. 14

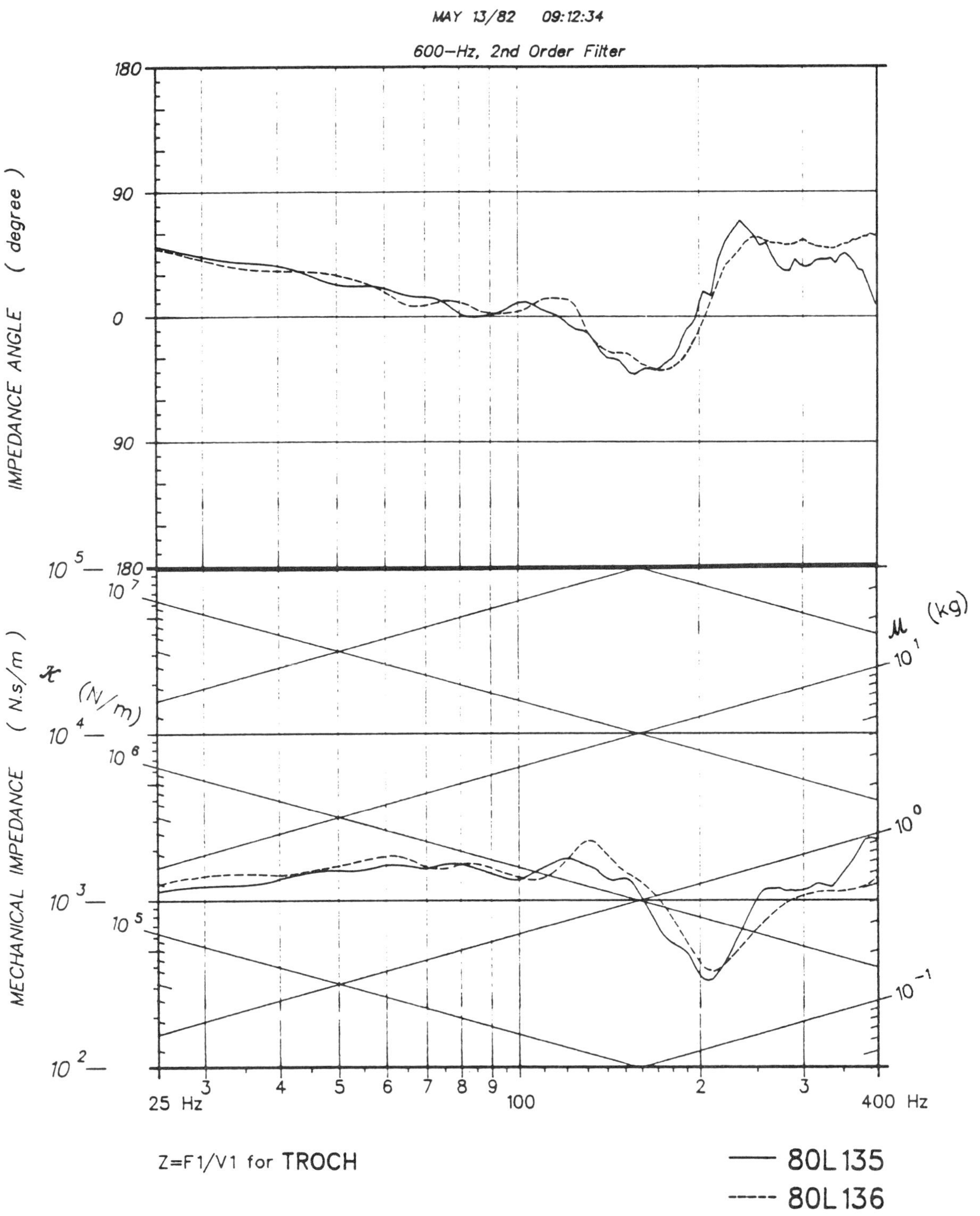

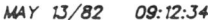

Fig. 15

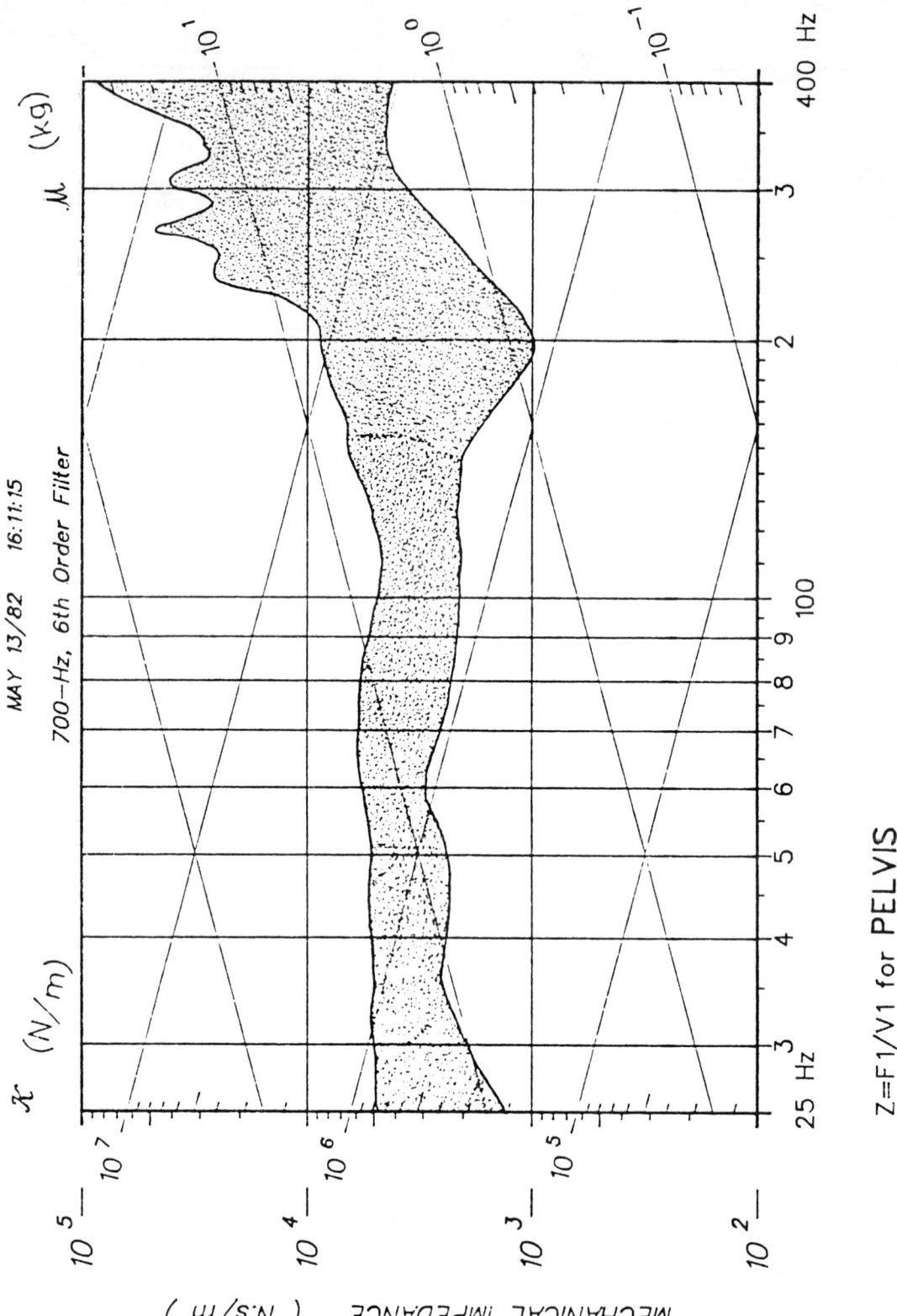

Fig. 16 - Pelvis corridor

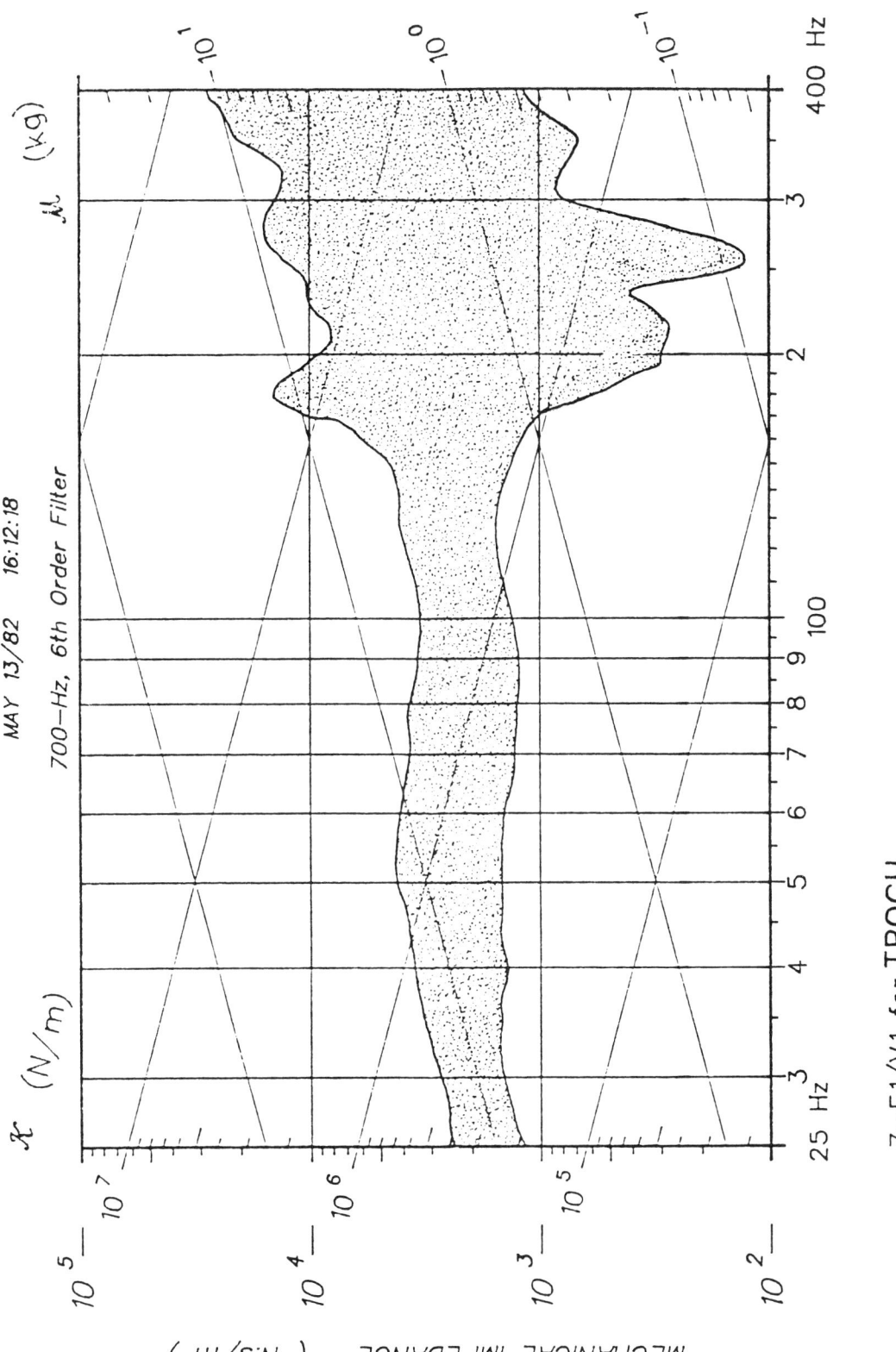

Fig. 17 – Trochanter corridor

commuted fracture of the femoral condyles). In this regard, tests 79A204 to 79A208, with loads from 20 to 37 kN, resulted in no injury to the femur or pelvis. Therefore, with respect to setting tolerance levels, the indication is that either much higher impact velocities (for a given mass) than have been used in these tests must be considered, or else other factors not addressed in this study influence the injury response of the pelvis. In these tests, the subject's initial configuration was held constant and the impactor padding, mass, and initial contact velocity were varied. Possibly, the tolerance level could be influenced by the orientation of the pelvis and/or femur before contact. In addition, no consideration was given to the interaction of the pelvis with a seat, which could be an important factor given the complexity of the pelvis response shown in this study. Therefore, the information generated in these knee impact tests cannot be used to set tolerance levels in and of themselves. The complex nature of the response and the scatter between test subjects emphasize the difficulty of this task.

LATERAL IMPACTS

The response of the pelvis under dynamic lateral loads requires the description of several material bodies: the impactor, the femur, the soft tissue and the pelvis. The ball and socket nature of the interface of the acetabulum and the head of the femur as well as the difficulty of impacting through the effective center of mass of the pelvis-femur complex suggest that in general an instability will result as asymmetric loading of the acetabulum occurs during impact. This type of interaction as well as the effects of damage produced during loading can lead to a wide range of responses. In this regard the accelerometer mounting platform, which is anchored to the pelvis through the use of lag bolts, may add to the lateral stiffness of the pelvis by reducing the differential movement between the two coxal bones during impact, and consequently simplifying the gross whole body motion of the pelvis. However, although the degree to which the accelerometer plate stiffens the pelvis is undetermined. No damage was observed as a result of the lag bolts indicating that the accelerometer platform was not a significant load path. The tests represented in Tables 6 and 9 describe the results of lateral acetabulum loadings through the trochanteric area. Only in test 80L121 was the pelvis loaded directly near the iliac crest. The force time-history from these tests can be described in a manner similar to that of tests 79A243 through 79A248 (Table 5) and 79L081 through 79L090 (Table 7) using the same event markers. The peak forces for the tests ranged from 3 to 19 kN with durations from 30 to 50 ms.

Table 6 summarizes the three-dimensional motion for the pelvis of 82E008, 82E028, and 82E049. In these tests the direction, magnitude, phasing, and waveform of the motion descriptors obtained from the nine accelerometer analysis did not follow a consistent pattern. These differences occur primarily in both angular acceleration and linear accelerations in those directions perpendicular to the impactor motion. Examples are Figures 18 and 19 for 82E049, and Figures 20 and 21 for 82E028. Both the linear and angular variables differ significantly during the E1 to E2 interval even though the gross overall motion as obtained from both the nine accelerometer analysis and the high-speed movies are the same. Variables representing this trend are the relative magnitude and phasing of the resultant and principal direction acceleration for tests 80L095 to 80L137 (depicted in Table 9), with no clear relation between peak force and acceleration as well as when it will occur in the force time history. This is consistent with the results from the acceleration data presented in (10). Figure 22 depicts some of the waveforms observed in these tests.

The response of the pelvis to impact is complicated not only by dynamic instabilities of the femur-pelvis complex, but also by the variability between subjects. Since load is distributed to the pelvis through both soft tissue and the femur, variations in these physical aspects between subjects can lead to varied stress levels on the acetabulum for a given impact force. For those subjects with large amounts of soft tissue, a longer E1 to E2 interval was observed.

Because of the complex nature of the response of the pelvis to lateral impacts, it becomes difficult to generate a transfer function for these experiments. However, for some tests in which a triax was used a transfer function could be obtained that generated mechanical impedance values significantly less than those calculated for the two directions normal to the principal direction above 10 Hz. In addition a transfer function was generated from the tangental acceleration for those tests in which the nine accelerometer plate was used (Figure 23). The transfer function shows that in these tests for low frequencies (from 10 to 40 Hz) the pelvis behaves as a mass of about 25 kg indicating that the gross overall motion of the pelvis may be simply modeled.

Damage -- The pelvic bone damages observed in these tests are similar to those observed in the automotive environment as reported in (1-5);

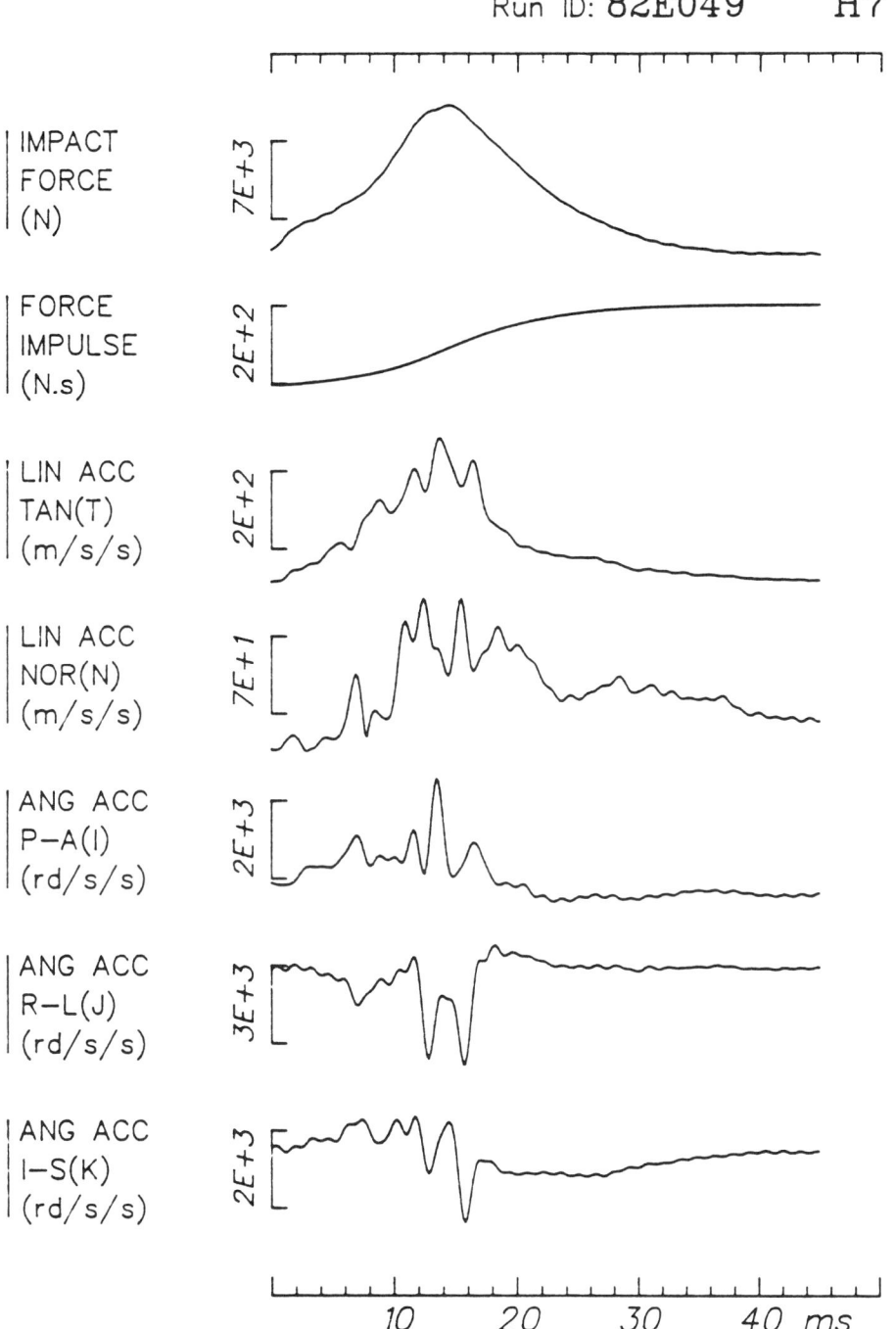

Fig. 18 - Test 82E049

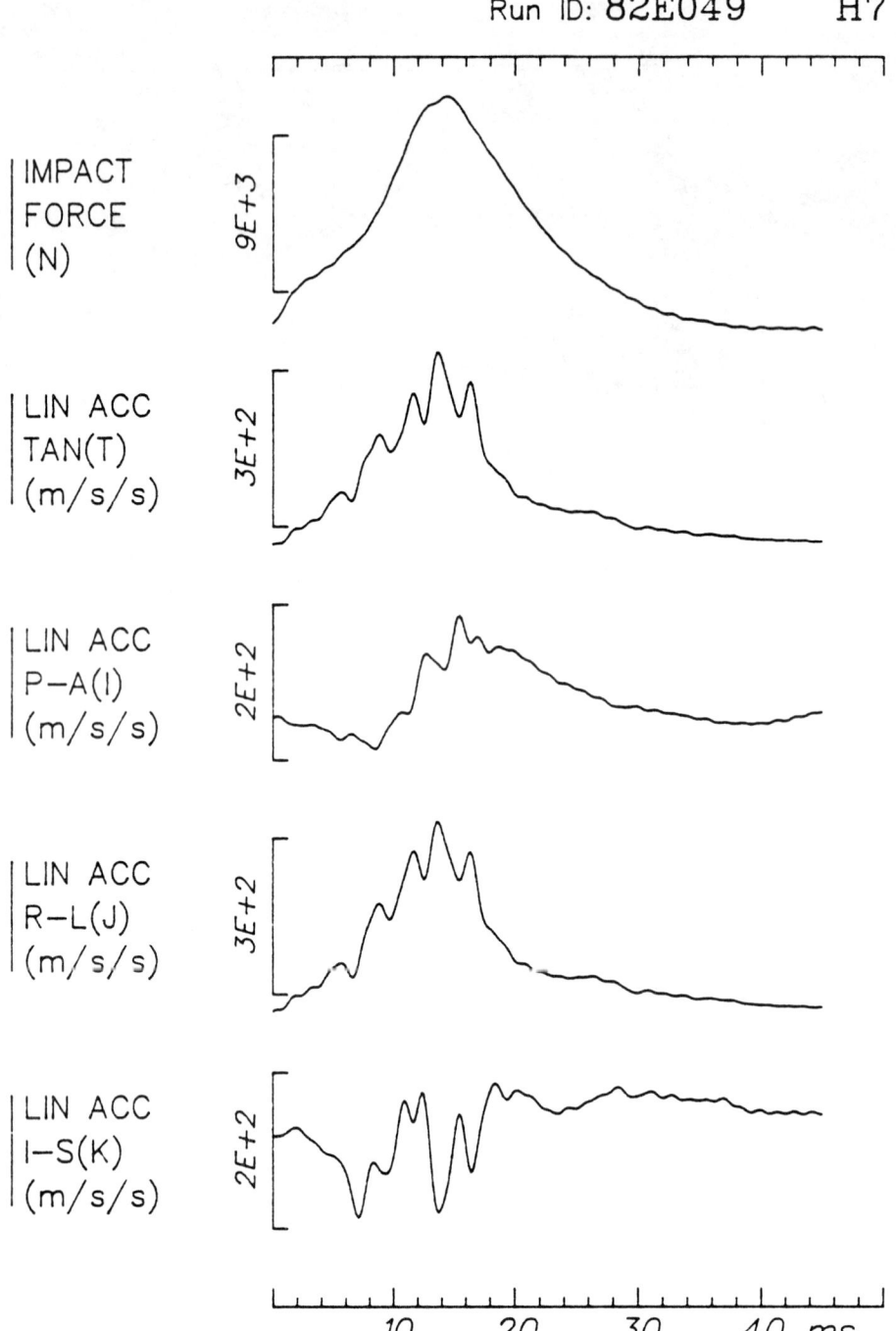

Fig. 19 - Test 82E049

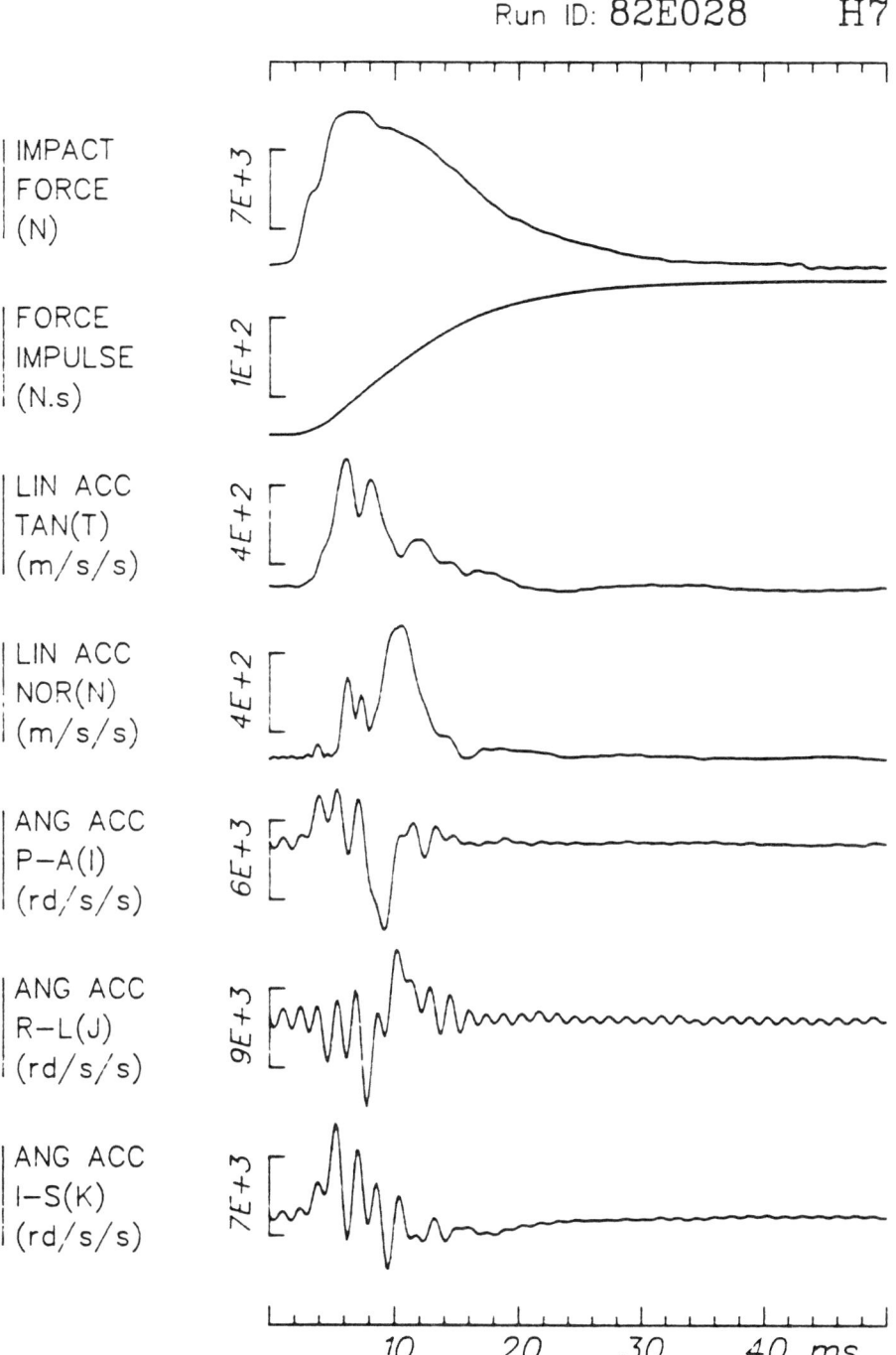

Fig. 20 - Test 82E028

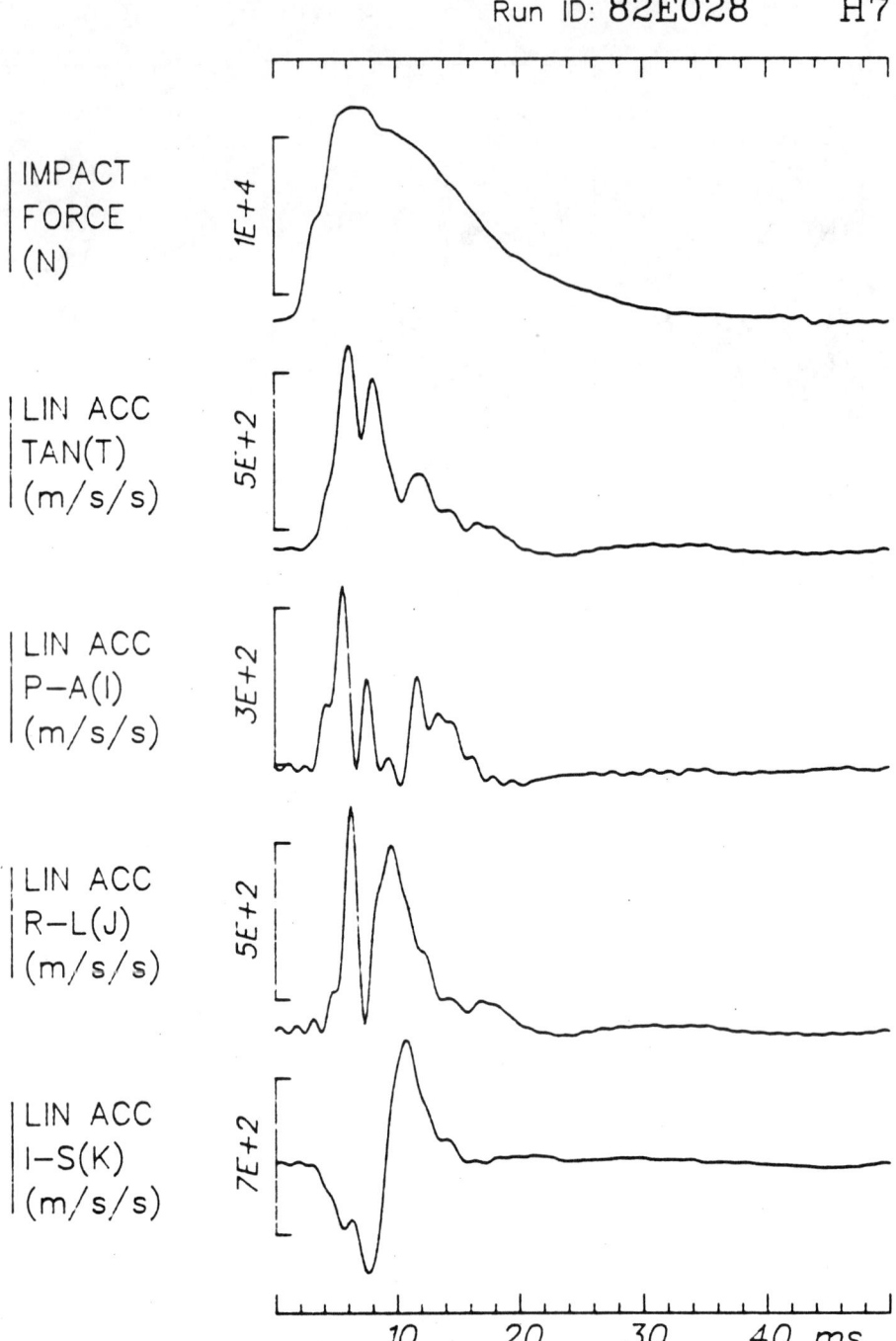

Fig. 21 - Test 82E028

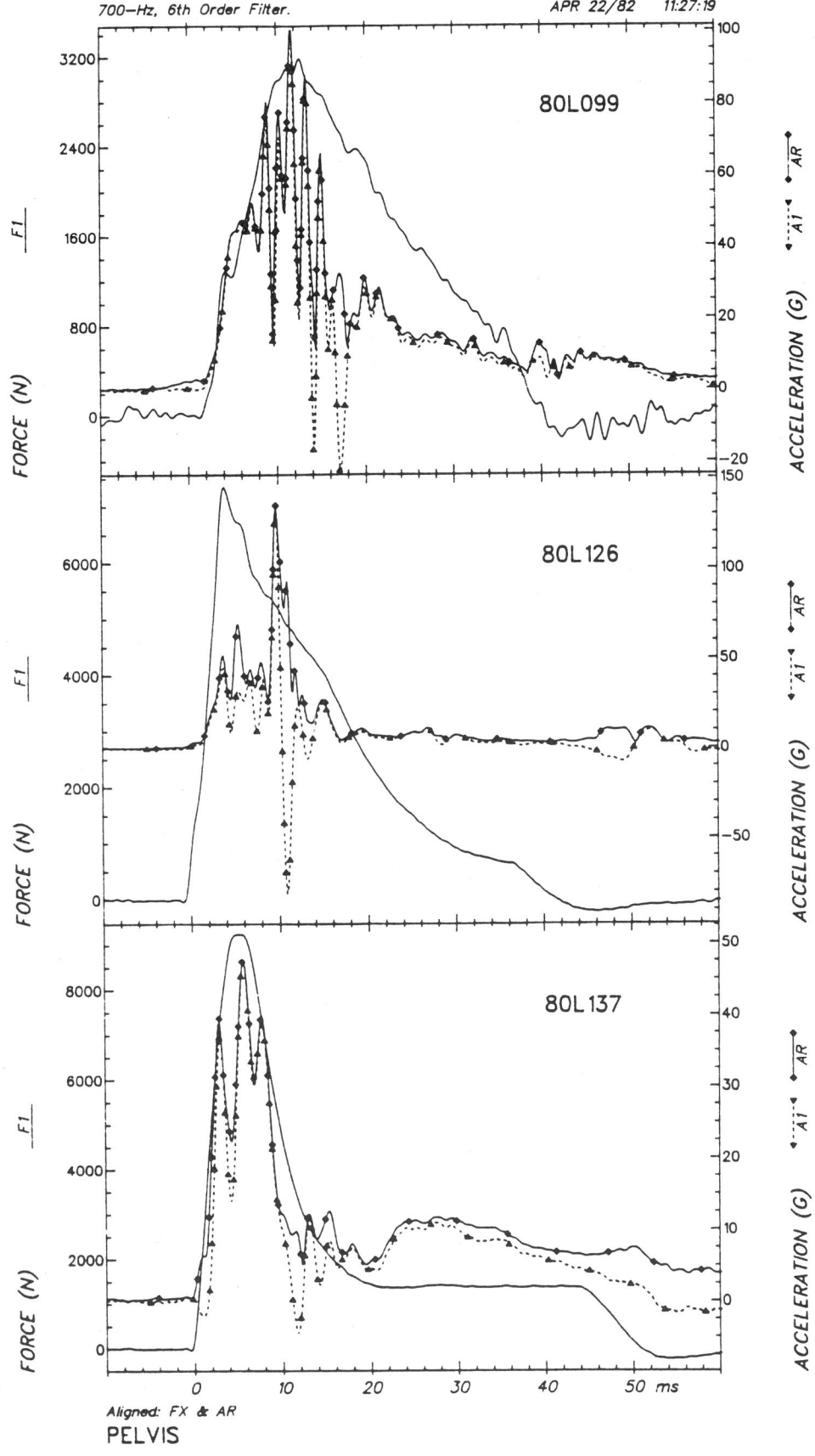

Fig. 22 - Pelvis impact response

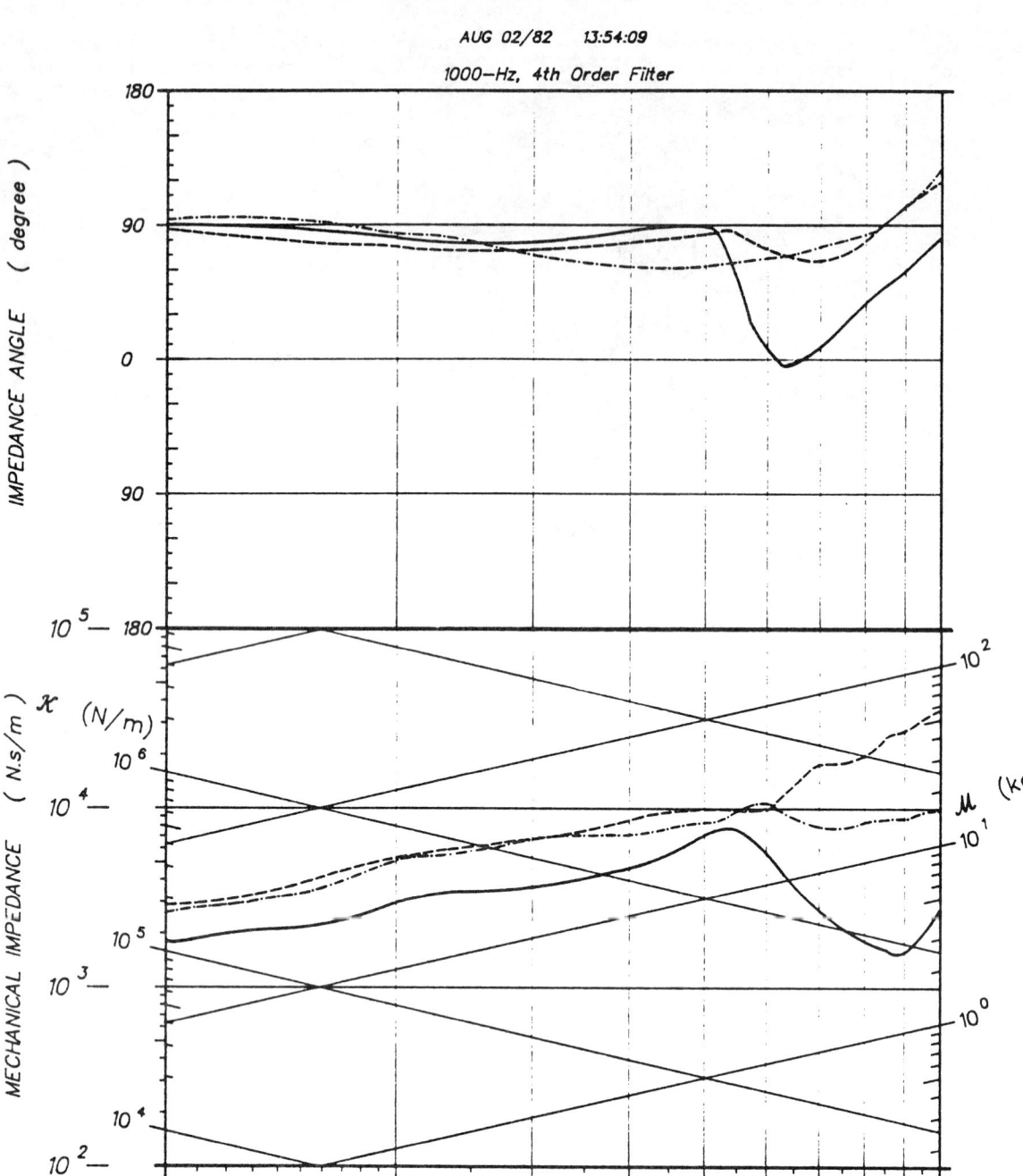

Fig. 23

however, no bilateral fractures occurred. The complex nature of the response of the pelvis to lateral loads may preclude the determination of a single tolerance criterion. This is arrived at by comparing the results in Tables 4 and 9 as well as the above discussion. In this regard, peak force does not relate to the damage produced. This is believed to be a result of the interactions of the padding, impactor surface shape, and/or the soft tissue between the impactor and the pelvis. With additional padding and soft tissue the load can be distributed over a larger area of the pelvis, and therefore less of the available impact energy is concentrated on the acetabulum. The maximum force tolerable seems to increase with an increase in load-distributing padding for similar available impact energy.

Based on differences in the initial conditions of the tests performed at HSRI and those described in (10), it is not readily verifiable that peak force and impulse are accurate pelvis injury criteria. The test methods described in (10) employed a subject seated in an upright position and impacted by an unpadded 17.3 kg impactor with a hemispherical surface. It was found in this series of tests performed at HSRI (which employed an unconstrained subject and flat impactor surface) that variations in impactor padding, mass, and load path may result in large differences in the peak force and impulse of the impact which do not necessarily correspond to the injuries produced. Additional test parameters, such as subject configuration, also affect comparisons between test series results in an unknown manner. For example, the fact that in one research program the subject is seated in a fixed position may result in subject-seat interactions thus producing different injuries for an otherwise similar impact.

CONCLUSIONS

This has been a limited preliminary study of some important kinematic factors and damage modes associated with indirect loading of the pelvis through the femur.

Because of the complex nature of the pelvis-femur interaction during an impact event, more work is necessary before these kinematic factors can be generalized to describe pelvis response. However, the following conclusions can be drawn:

(1) The complete description of three-dimensional motion is invaluable to the understanding of pelvis response.

(2) The response of the pelvis of a single test subject to axial knee impacts as given by mechanical impedance is linear from 10 to 100 Hz, repeatable, and symmetric (the same for each side).

(3) The complex nature of the response of the femur/pelvis/soft tissue system, between-subjects variability, and damage patterns produced may preclude the determination of a single tolerance criterion such as maximum force or peak acceleration response.

(4) Energy-absorbing and load-distributing materials are effective methods of transmitting greater amounts of energy to the pelvis without damage being produced in lateral impacts.

(5) The nature of the impactor/femur/pelvis interaction as well as the biometrics of the population at large are critical factors in understanding the response of the pelvis to impact and subsequent damage patterns.

ACKNOWLEDGEMENTS

The results presented in this paper have been obtained from a series of independently funded research programs conducted during the past five years. The funding agencies were: The Biomedical Science Department of General Motors, the Motor Vehicle Manufacturer's Association, and the United States Department of Transportation, National Highway Traffic Safety Administration.

The authors wish to acknowledge the contributions of Jean Brindamour, Don Huelke, Marv Dunlap, Jodi Blank, Valerie Moses, Paula Lux, Miles Janicki, Jeff Pinsky, and Carol Sobecki in completion of this work.

REFERENCES

1) States, J., and States, D., "The Pathology and Pathogenesis of Injuries Caused by Lateral Impact Accidents", Proceedings of the Twelfth Stapp Car Crash Conference, Society of Automotive Engineers, Inc., 1968.

2) Ryan, F., "Traffic Injuries of the Pelvis at St. Vincent's Hospital, Melbourne", Medical Journal of Australia, Vol. 1, 27 Feb. 1971.

3) Knudsen, P., "Pelvis Fraktur Ved Sidekollision" Ugeskrift for Lager, Vol. 143, No. 16, 13 April 1981.

4) Huelke, D., and Lawson, T., "Lower Torso Injuries and Automobile Seatbelts", SAE Paper 760370, 1976.

5) Huelke, D.F., O'Day, J., States, J.D., and Lawson, T.E. "Lower extremity injuries in automobile crashes." HSRI, Jan. 1980, 65 p. Report No. UM-HSRI-80-10. Sponsored by the National Highway Traffic Safety Administration.

6) Evans, F., and Lissner, H., "Studies on Pelvic Deformations and Fractures", Anatomical Record, Vol. 121, No. 2, Feb. 1955.

7) Patrick, L., Kroell, C., and Mertz, H., "Forces on the Human Body in Simulated Crashes", Proceedings of the Ninth Stapp Car Crash Conference, 1965.

8) Melvin, J., and Nusholtz, G., "Tolerance and Response of the Knee-Femur-Pelvis Complex to Axial Impacts", Final Report to the Motor Vehicle Manufacturer's Association, UM-HSRI-80-27, June 1980.

9) Ramet, M., and Cesari, D., "Experimental Study of Pelvis Tolerance in Lateral Impact", International IRCOBI Conference on the Biomechanics of Trauma, 4th Proceedings, Bron, 1979.

10) Cesari, D., Ramet, M., and Clair, P., "Evaluation of Pelvic Fracture Tolerance in Side Impact", Proceedings of the Twenty-Fourth Stapp Car Crash Conference, Paper No. 801306, Society of Automotive Engineers, Inc., 1980.

11) Bartz, J., and Butler, F., "Passenger Compartment With Six Degrees of Freedom", Auxiliary Programs to "Three Dimensional Computer Simulation of a Motor Vehicle Crash Victim", Final Technical Report on DOT Contract No. FH-11-7592, 1972.

12) Alem, N., et al., "Whole-Body Human Surrogate Response to Three-Point Harness Restraint", Proceedings of the Twenty-Second Stapp Car Crash Conference, Paper No. 780895, Society of Automotive Engineers, Inc., 1978.

13) Nusholtz, G., Melvin, J., and Alem, N., "Head Impact Response Comparisons of Human Surrogates", Proceedings of the Twenty-Third Stapp Car Crash Conference, Paper No. 780895, Society of Automotive Engineers, Inc., 1979.

14) Nusholtz, G., et al., "Response of the Cervical Spine to Superior-Inferior Head Impact", Proceedings of the Twenty-Fifth Stapp Car Crash Conference, Paper No. 811005, Society of Automotive Engineers, Inc., 1981.

15) Hixson, E., "Mechanical Impedance", Shock and Vibration Handbook, ed. C. M. Harris and C. E. Crede, McGraw-Hill Book Co., New York, 1976.

16) Khalil, T., Viano, D., and Taber, L., "Vibrational Characteristics of the Embalmed Human Femur", General Motors Research Laboratories, Publication #GMR-3270 29 Apr., 1980.

17) Melvin, J., et al., "Impact Response and Tolerance of the Lower Extremities", Proceedings of the Nineteenth Stapp Car Crash Conference, Society of Automotive Engineers, Inc., 1975.

831629

Study of "Knee-Thigh-Hip" Protection Criterion

Y. C. Leung, B. Hue, A. Fayon,
C. Tarrière, and H. Hamon
Peugeot-Renault Association (France)

C. Got and A. Patel
I.R.B.A. Raymond Poincaré Hospital

J. Hureau
University of Paris

ABSTRACT.

A series of fresh human cadaver and Part 572 dummy tests was performed under different conditions which were comparable to those of real-world accidents. A European car model mounted on a sled was used; a pair of knee-targets was fixed directly to the car body in front of the passenger knees. Test conditions are summarized as follows: human-3-pt-belted cadaver with a sled impact velocity of 50 or 65 kph; 2-pt (thoracic)-belted-cadaver with a velocity of 65 kph, the legs being positioned normally or in an oblique manner.

Since the knee-thigh-hip tolerance is related to the shape and duration of the impact pulse, these interactions were the subject of a study.

The tolerance to fractures depends to a great extent on the subject's bone condition. In order to predict the risk of fracture for the whole population from the tolerance found in the tested subjects, studies of mineralization and bone strength were carried out on the compact-bone-sections taken from the femurs of the tested cadavers.

Tests were conducted also, using a Part 572 dummy, which enabled to predict a criterion for the knee-thigh-hip protection matched to this surrogate.

Discussion of similar attempts, such as F.I.C. (Femur Injury Criterion) and K.T.H.I.C. is included.

THE FEMUR TOLERANCE and the corresponding protection criterion in frontal collisions have long been a controversial topic. There are great discrepancies between the values proposed by different countries and organizations. As mentioned in a recent paper (1)*, criteria ranging from 4 KN in United Kingdom to 10 KN were proposed. A reason for these differences could

be the test conditions. This led the authors to contemplate establishing a knee-thigh-hip protection criterion from experiments performed under realistic conditions. Besides, the analysis of the results had to pinpoint the effect of duration on the tolerance and criteria, according to existing literature.

A survey of available papers concerning the femur tolerance, and particularly the Femur Injury Criterion (F.I.C.) (12) yields the main facts. It can be summarized that the femur fracture tolerance depends on the methods and materials used in the tests. Two principal groups may be classified as follows:

- firstly, a set of important values for the compression forces sustained by the femur; they are associated with the shorter impact pulse durations. An impactor was used for striking the knees; it was actuated by free fall (2), air gun (3)(4)(5); a pendulum was also utilized (6)(7)(8). Peak knee forces up to 25 KN were recorded: the pulse duration was shorter than 20 ms.

- secondly, a set of reduced tolerable forces, associated with the longer impact pulse durations. These data were obtained from sled tests with impact targets for the knees, fixed onto the sled (9)(10)(11). In this group, the tolerable femur compression force was about 6 KN (9) or 7 KN (10), and the pulse durations were evaluated at about 30 ms. To achieve a sensible protection criterion requires a realistic approach as regards the test conditions, on the one hand, and an in-depth analysis of the force-time history on the other hand.

For realism, tests with belted fresh cadavers were performed in a current car body mounted on a sled.

Concerning the influence of the force-time history, several researchers have already done some interesting work. Cooke and Nagel (2) concluded that the peak force must be associated with the energy absorbed. Melvin et al. (3) suggested that the peak force could be used in conjunction with the impulse. Viano (12) studied

---
*Numbers in parentheses designate references at end of paper.

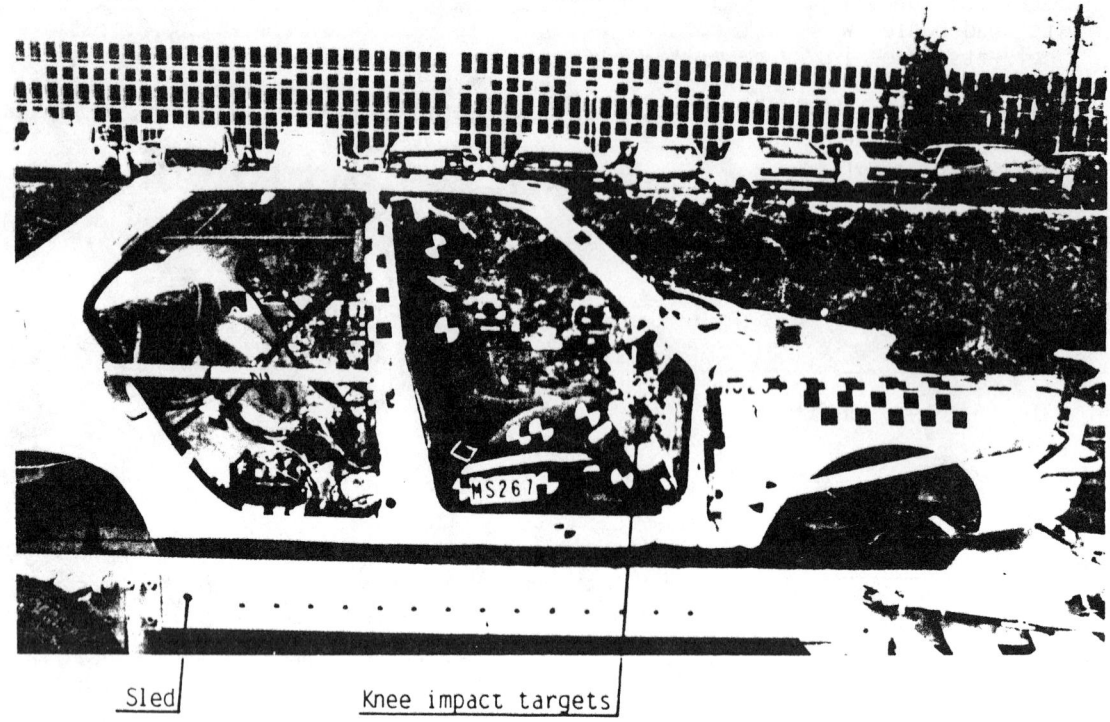

Figure 1 - Position of the Cadaver (or Dummy) Inside the Vehicle Body

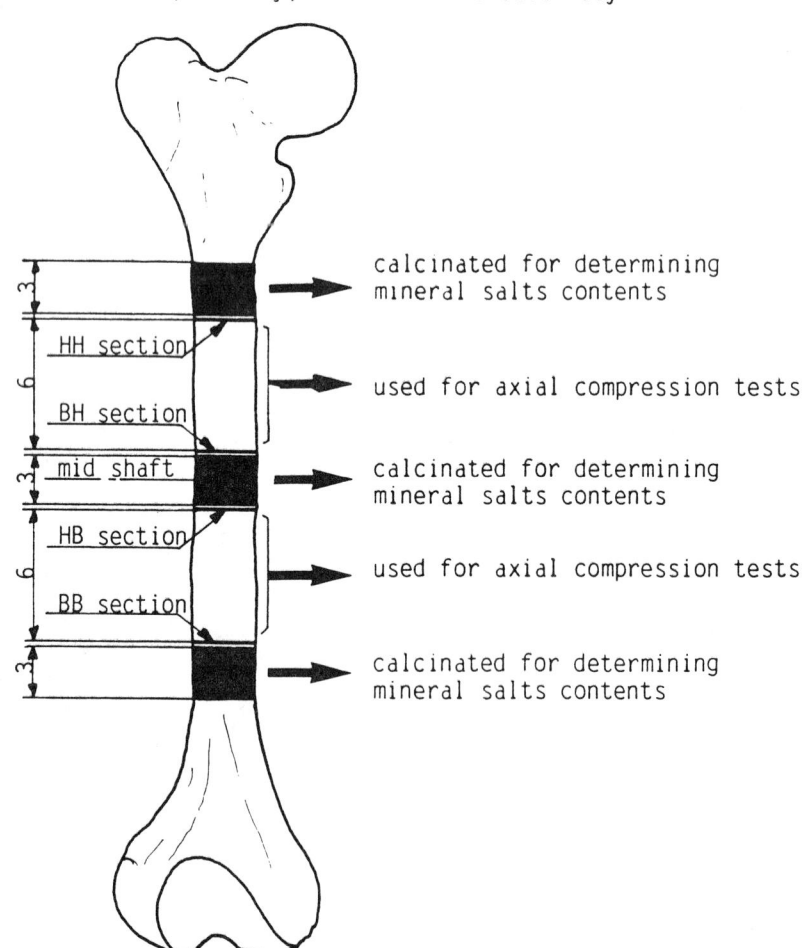

Figure 2 - Location of the Specimens Cut From a Femur for Calcination and Compressive Test.

402

TESTS AND TEST CONDITIONS - A first series of tests with dead bodies was performed at 50 kph with 3-pts belts. Knee impact severity proved to be insufficient, due to the efficiency of the restraint provided by the 3-pts belts. The belt slacks and the collision severities were therefore increased in the later tests.

A second series was consequently performed at 65 kph. In a third series, only a diagonal belt restrained the body. The fourth series consisted in reproductions of the previous runs with P. 572 dummies. Test conditions are summarized in Table 1 below.

peak force would be a reasonable mean for the estimation of the injury potential.

In 1977, Viano (12) studied in-depth, on the basis of the available results, how the force femur tolerance depended on the pulse duration. It can be easily understood that the peak force tolerable by a femur depends not only on the pulse duration but also on the impulse. It would be interesting, if a conventional factor could be derived together from the total pulse duration and impulse. Such a factor called "conventional pulse duration" is defined as follows:

Table 1 - Dynamic Test Conditions.

Subject No. or A.T.D.	Belt	Impact Velocity (kph)	Sled Deceleration max. (g)	Stopping Distance (cm)	Leg Position	Knee-Target Distance (mm) L	R
224	3-pts-belt	50.7	29	57	normal	85	85
231	" " "	50.7	30	58	"	105	100
232	" " "	50.7	31	58	"	110	80
233	" " "	50.1	30.5	60	"	90	85
254	" " "	49.5	31	54	"	52	50
255	" " "	50.9	31	57	"	54	50
1598-P. 572	" " "	48.7	32	55	"	90	90
2215-P. 572	" " "	48.9	26		"	100	105
257	" " "	67.1	39	100	"	85	80
258	" " "	65.1	38	108	"	86	83
267	" " "	60	34	67	"	75	75
268	" " "	66.8	42	87	"	85	85
276	" " "	65	72	100	"	80	85
277	" " "	67.7	31	98	"	75	80
2166-P. 572	" " "	65.7	35	76	"	91	80
280	diagonal belt	69	45	69	"	85	92
281	" "	65.7	45	58	"	82	80
294	" "	68.4	37	82	"	96	90
2167-P. 572	" "	64.3	39	70	normal	90	87
2216-P. 572	" "	50.3	24		"	90	90
296	" "	64.4	38	69	oblique	83	82

Conventional Pulse Duration - As mentioned at the beginning of the paper, it has been recognized by the researchers that load level alone is not a sufficient indicator of fracture conditions.

Cooke and Nagel in 1969 (2) from their drop weight impact tests on unembalmed cadavers, observed that the femur tolerance depended on both the peak force and the energy transmitted to the knee.

Using an impactor actuated by an air-gun Melvin et al. conducted in 1975, impact tests on the legs of seated unembalmed human cadavers. They suggested that the impulse computed with the force/time history, in conjunction with the

Corresponding to cadaver knee-impact tests, a general peak force-time profile is shown in figure 4.

The impulse (I) can be calculated as time integral of whole force-time profile:

$$I = \int_0^T f(t) \, dt \qquad (1)$$

where T is total pulse duration.

For defining the "conventional pulse duration", the same value of the impulse is expressed by the product of the peak force (F max) and the "conventional pulse duration" (T_ε); that is:

the relationship between the permissible knee force and the primary pulse duration. Another attempt made in this paper is to relate the force to the pulse duration and the impulse. Further, in order to predict the occurrence of femur fracture for the population at risk, correction factors have to be applied. Muscle tension effect (3)(13)(14)(15)(16) and the anthropometrical data of the tested subjects have to be taken into account. For comparing the dead bodies used in the tests and the population at risk, studies concerning the mineralization and the strength of the femurs were performed.

In order to define a femur protection criterion, runs with a Part 572 ATD were carried out. The method - a priori- was to make a comparison between the knee force-time history measured on dead bodies and axial femur-time history measured by transducers fit to the upper legs of the dummy. Other factors had to be taken into consideration.

METHODOLOGY.

Runs were performed with dead bodies and dummies. The human surrogate is placed in the front passenger seat of a vehicle body mounted on a sled. Retarder tubes allow a car deceleration to be simulated. A belt system is provided for the restraint, and the knee impact forces are recorded. Two plane rigid disks are mounted on a bracket in front of each knee. They are covered with a 2.5 cm thick polyurethane padding, the density of which is equal to .115. The position of the disks may be that of a knee bolster in a car body. Its height can be adjusted. Spacing of the centerlines of the 2 disks corresponds to the distance between the knees of a Part 572 dummy placed according to the procedure in FMVSS 208. Independent measurements of impact loads against each knee are obtained by means of half-bridge gauges. The measurement device is sensitive to the normal component of the impact load. However, due to the seat and disk height adjustments, the angle between the thigh axis and the perpendicular to the impacted disk remains small. Figure 1 shows a general lay-out of the test materials.

Human subjects used are fresh unembalmed cadavers which undergo for other purposes special treatment before the test, already described (17). The experiments take place less than four days after death, the bodies having been stored in the meantime in a cold room at 2° C. For the subjects, a preliminary selection was made based on bone quality: subjects who were involved in accidents involving lower members, or who suffered from bone diseases were not submitted to tests. Autopsies were carried out, with particular emphasis on the knee-thigh-hip complex. Measurements made, beyond the usual ones, were of pelvis decelerations and restraint forces. These measurements added to the femur loads for the dummy and to the knee impact forces enable one to perform a better analysis of the results. This analysis is facilitated by the aid of films and by the bone characterization of the subjects, explained later-on.

CHARACTERIZATION OF THE SUBJECT'S LEG SKELETON - If the tolerance level of the population at risk is aimed at, this characterization must be made as far as possible. The number of dead bodies considered here is still insufficient for statistic processings; however, data are gathered as regards mineralization and mechanical resistance of the femurs submitted to runs.

1./ Bone Mineralization Analyzes - After the test, parts of the femur were taken from different areas and calcinated in the oven at 700° C. The location of the samples is shown on Figure 2. They consist of:
- A 3 cm fragment taken from the middle of the femur,
- an upper fragment of 3 cm, taken near the lower limit of the trochanter minor,
- a lower fragment, 3 to 4 cm long, the upper end of which is located at the start of the lower widening zone of the diaphysis; its lower end is supracondylar.

The calcination yields the average weight of ashes per unit of volume, noted C/V.

2./ Mechanical Tests - They encompass compression and bending tests.

For the compression tests, two tubular parts of the femur were taken. They are actually located between the parts used for the calcination, and shown in Figure 2. Their length is about 8 cm, with a length/diameter ratio close to 5/1. The specimen is compressed longitudinally between parallel planes. The plunger velocity is 5 mm/mn. Pictures of the surfaces of the cortical areas are taken before the tests. Ultimate compression force is recorded.

For the bending tests, the specimens were undamaged femurs; they are loaded transversaly, as shown in Figure 3. Simple computations yield the ultimate bending stress.

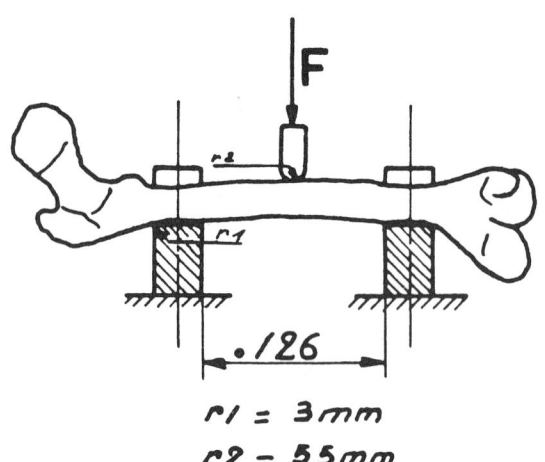

Figure 3 - Bending Test Diagram.

$$I = F_{max} \times T_\varepsilon \quad (2)$$

where T_ε is homogeneous to a duration. The quantity T_ε determined from the association of (1) and (2) is given as:

$$T_\varepsilon = \frac{\int_0^T f(t)\,dt}{F_{max}} \quad (3)$$

The value of the peak force (F max.) is used for defining a criterion, when associated with impulse (I) and with pulse duration (T), as described respectively in (3) and (12). It would be appealing and preferable when defining the femur tolerance, if peak force as a function of "Conventional Pulse Duration" (T_ε) could be used because T_ε links the impulse (I) and the total pulse duration (T). The analysis of the available results will indicate if the tolerance definition is improved in this way.

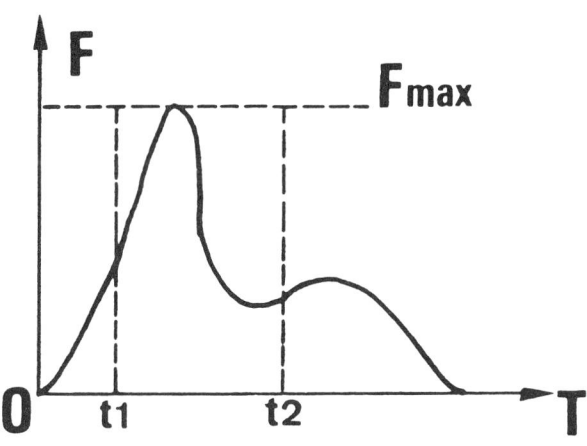

Figure 4 - General Peak Force Time Profile in Cadaver Knee Impact Tests.

RESULTS.

HUMAN SUBJECTS AND TEST CONDITIONS - The anthropometrical data of the tested human cadavers are presented in Table 2. The autopsies were conducted by the anatomist for all subjects after knee-impact tests. Descriptions of the injuries are also presented in Table 2, only for the knee-thigh-hip system. The injuries found in other corporal parts and organs are not presented here. The legs of each subject were positioned normally, excepting one (296) positioned in an oblique manner. The reason for testing this one is to obtain more information on the different injury severities between the legs positioned normally and obliquely.

The test conditions such as restraint belt system, impact velocity and sled deceleration are presented in table 1. They can be summarized as three different groups:
- first group: subjects with 3-pt-belts at impact, V = 50 kph;
- second group: subjects with 3-pt-belts at impact, V = 65 kph;
- third group: subjects with 2-pt-belts (shoulder belt), V = 65 kph.

KNEE-IMPACT TESTS WITH HUMAN CADAVERS - The results of knee-impact tests are given in Table 3. The peak knee-impact loads were recorded respectively for each femur by the knee targets. They were normal components applied to knee targets. With the aid of mechanical analysis and motion picture studies, these loads can be considered to be the axial forces passing through the femur.

The impulse (I) is calculated with the integration of knee-impact force time profile ($I = \int_0^T f(t)\,dt$). The conventional pulse duration (T_ε) developed in this paper, as described above, is a factor associated with the impulse and peak force. Total pulse duration (t) is the period during knee contact with target.

Peak knee-impact loads of human cadavers (F max.) versus conventional pulse durations (T_ε) are illustrated in Figure 5.

It is shown clearly in this figure that the fracture and non-fracture data points locate respectively at the right-upper corner and left-lower corner of the figure. The limit of the potential load to produce the femur fracture can be expressed by a line passing through 280L, 294R and 281R, and then turning at 281R, parallely to axis T. This line supplies basic values for defining femur injury tolerance. This formula is given as below:

$$F = a - bT \quad \text{and where} \quad T_\varepsilon = \frac{\int_0^T f(t)\,dt}{F_{max}}$$

where a = 23.4 KN, b = 0.72 KN/ms when $T_\varepsilon <$ 21ms, and F = 8.3 KN when $T_\varepsilon \geq$ 21 ms.

Its "shape" looks like the Viano's FIC (12) but the time definition is different. The accuracy of this limit is discussed later on.

PART 572 DUMMY TESTS - Surrogate tests were performed with a Part 572 dummy. The test conditions corresponding to those used in three series of cadaver tests are presented in Table 1. Results are presented with cadaver test ones in Table 3. This table illustrates the discrepancies between the cadaver and the Part 572 ATD responses in that type of test.

AXIAL COMPRESSION TESTS - They seek to characterize the bone condition as presented in "the methodology" part.

The results presented in Table 4 are the results obtained in the specimens cut from the proximal part as indicated in Figure 2. The initial lengths between HH and BH sections were

405

Table 2 - Anthropometrical Data of the Tested Human Cadavers and Description of the Observed "Knee-Thigh-Hip" Injuries.-

Cadaver No.	Sex	Age	Weight	Size	U	I + J	M	P	"Knee-Thigh-Hip" Injuries
224	M	34	40	161	88.5	64.1	44.6	54	-
231	M	60	61	165	82.5	68	48.9	56.1	-
232	M	57	49	163	90	62.5	-	-	-
233	M	56	63	173	90.8	66.6	56	59	F* right knee-cap, right iliac wing
254	M	63	52	162	-	-	-	-	-
255	M	68	56	165	89.5	69	52.5	57	-
257	F	42	53	155	85.5	62.5	46.5	53.5	-
258	M	42	64	164	91	69	49	56	-
267	M	68	71	164	89	66	48	55	-
268	M	62	66	172	92	67	50.5	55.7	-
276	M	55	82	180	-	-	-	-	-
277	M	52	50	164	-	-	-	-	-
280	M	62	78	175	93	68	55	52	Right and left knee-caps, right cotyle F*
281	M	73	63	164	85	60	59	50	F* of the neck of right femur, of right and left knee-caps
294	M	71	69	166	87	63	55	53	F* of the distal part of right femur
296	M	55	68	169	90	68	57	52	F* of the right part and sub-condyle of left femur.

N.B.: F* = fracture

Table 3 - Knee Impacts. Results From Cadaver and Dummy Tests.

Test No.	Knee-Peak Impact Load (KN) L	R	Impulses (Ns) L	R	Conventional Duration T_ℓ (ms) L	R	Loading Duration T(ms) L	R	Femur Force (Dummy Tests) L	R	Knee Impact Speed* (m/s) L	R
224	3.00	1.40	43.6	14.6	14.6	10.4	-	-	-	-	-	-
231	3.30	6.70	46.2	92.4	14	13.8	37	44	-	-	-	4.43
232	3.60	7.20	43.8	111	12.2	15.4	40	42	-	-	8.01	6.56
233	8.30	7.80	100	115	12.5	14.3	35	50	-	-	3.02	5.54
254	7.45	6.60	65.2	65.6	8.8	9.9	35	46	-	-	7.64	3.52
255	7.60	9.00	121.4	166	16	18.4	61	56	-	-	-	4.69
1598*	16.20	17.50	182	138.4	11.2	7.9	38	31	1530	1330	-	7.25
2215*	-	15.00	-	90.0	-	6.0	-	30	840	1810	9.58	5.98
257	3.50	2.60	36	18.6	10.3	7.2	50	38	-	-	4.98	4.84
258	6.60	7.70	94	133.2	14.2	17.3	44	47	-	-	3.52	3.51
267	6.00	8.50	79.8	159.4	13.3	18.8	38	62	-	-	4.06	5.77
268	6.20	-	109	-	17.6	-	64	-	-	-	4.29	4.66
276	6.00	7.80	146.6	83.6	24.4	10.7	46	66	-	-	2.81	3.89
2166*	14.40	-	176.6	-	12	-	39	-	1060	>1700	10.65	9.43
280	12.30	12.70	195	369	15.9	29.1	38	76	-	-	-	7.91
281	10.40	8.30	230	177	22.1	21.3	52	43	-	-	7.07	6.11
294	12.50	11.80	401	194	32.1	16.4	98	76	-	-	6.51	5.86
2167*	15.40	13.30	180	378.6	11.7	28	80	71	1660	1750	10.47	10.24
2216*	14.00	15.60	200	180	14	12	75	40	1410	1490	-	-
296	5.60	11.00	100.6	97.6	18	8.9	53	45	-	-	6.51	5.86

(*) Last tests of each series consist of a run with dummy.

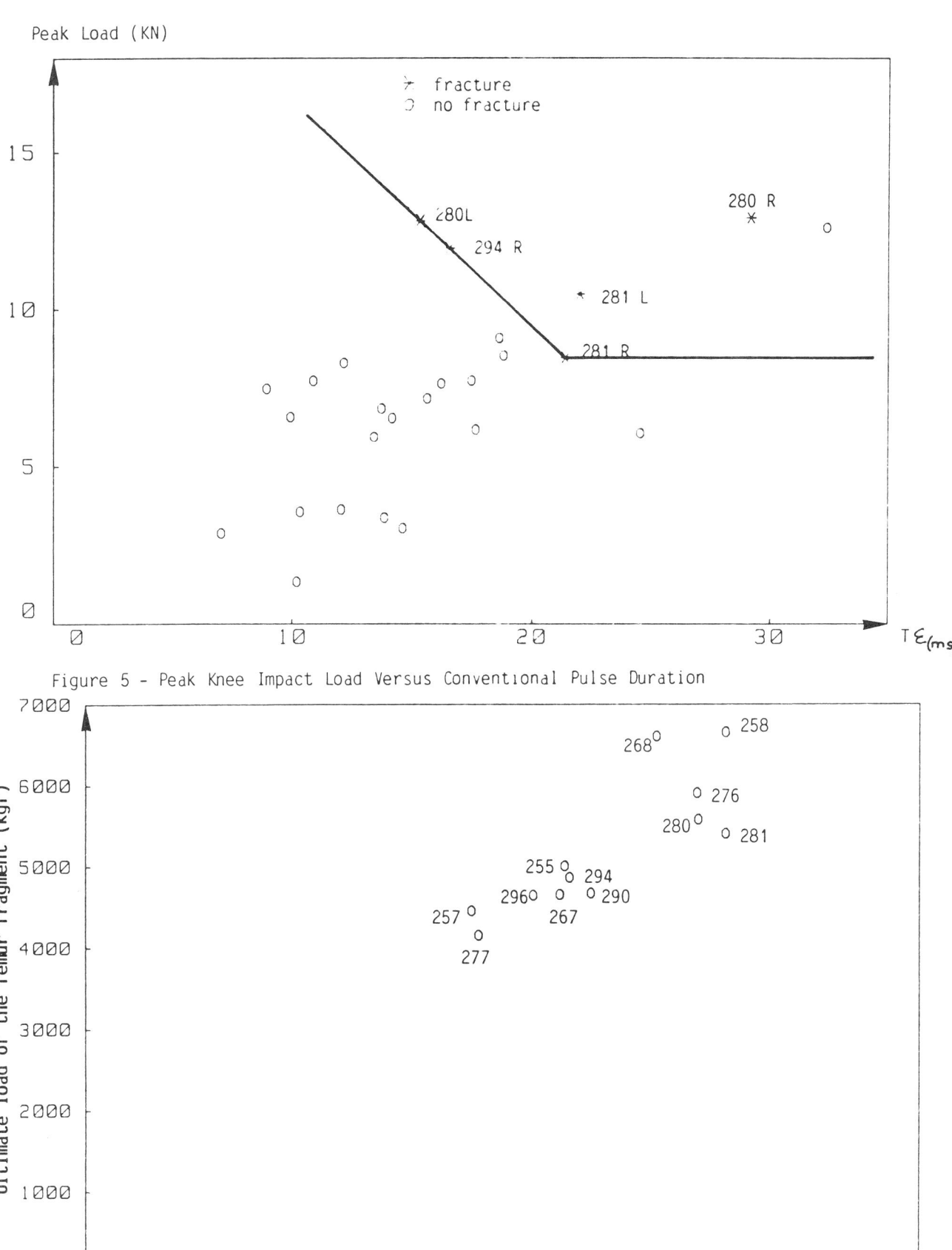

Figure 5 - Peak Knee Impact Load Versus Conventional Pulse Duration

Figure 6 - Ultimate Load of Femur Fragments Versus Corresponding Compact Bone Area.

6 cm. The area of the impact bone corresponding to the broken end during the compressive tests, were measured at BH section before tests.

The ultimate load is a peak load varied from 4150 to 6600 kgf, with a mean value of about 5.4 KN. The mean strain and the mean ultimate compressive strength are about 1.9 % and 12.13 kgf/mm2. The compact bone area is the area measured at the middle section of the femur, about 490 mm2.

Smaller strength found in this femur part, when compared to the intact bone result is due to the open ends of the compressed specimen. The ends of the femur, on the contrary, are closed. However that may be the two kinds of tests are not similar.

BENDING TESTS - The specimens were the intact femurs taken from the knee-impact tested cadavers. The experimental method was used with a 3-point bending test, illustrated in Figure 3. The results are in Table 4. No significant correlation was found between the ultimate loads in compression and in bending tests.

CALCINATION - The locations of the specimens are shown in Figure 2. The ash content C was obtained after calcination. The volume V of the compact bone was measured before calcination. The unit (ash content), defined by C/V (g/cm3), varied from 0.99 to 1.27 g/cm3. Because the broken ends of all proximal specimens occurred at the lower end (BH section), the results of the calcination presented in Table 5 were for the middle femur specimen (between BH and HB section) which was adjacent to the broken end of the compressive test specimens.

DISCUSSION.

Complementary studies aimed at determining tools for a better estimation of the tolerance of the population at risk. They are discussed firstly as follows.

ULTIMATE LOAD AND COMPACT BONE AREA - Based on the available results presented in Table 4, the ultimate load of the femur versus the compact bone area is shown in Figure 6. A good correlation between these two parameters can be found. The ultimate load of the femur increases with the increase in compact bone area at the midpoint of the femur. This fact draws attention to the need to adjust the femur fracture tolerance. Actually, the difference in ultimate load between maximum and minimum already exceeds 60 % caused by different bone areas. From the view of general knowledge, it would appear that the potential load to produce the femur fracture is related with ultimate load which is a function of the compact bone area. Consequently, it is necessary to find a parameter, such as an anthropometric parameter of the subject which connects with compact bone area. Due to a lack of this knowledge, we are attempting to establish here a relationship between the compact bone area and subject weight. However, the relationship of compressive strength between a segment specimen and an intact femur will be also investigated.

COMPACT BONE AREA AND WEIGHT OF SUBJECT - From available results, the compact bone areas at mid-femur versus the weights of the subjects are illustrated in Figure 7. It seems that the compact bone area correlates somewhat with the weight of the subject. The latter is an anthropomorphic parameter found easily from the tested subject. The mean weight of the tested subjects is about 60 kg with a relative compact bone area of 400 mm2. Corresponding to 75 kg, a relative area is about 500 mm2. An adjustment for ultimate load of the femur segment is to make a 20 % increase from 5000 kgf to 6000 kgf.

Assuming a uniform increase in strength, the adjustment for the peak knee-impact load would be taken parallely with the rate, the minimum fracture load found here would approach 10 KN (from 8.3 KN of the subject 281 R). This is just a hypothesis given here, further study for confirmation is necessary. In this case, the conventional pulse duration (T_ϵ) should be also normalized using the dimensional analysis.

ASH CONTENT AND ULTIMATE COMPRESSIVE STRENGTHS (U.C.S.) - As described previously by researchers (19, 20), the ultimate compressive strength (U.C.S.) relates strongly with ash content. Results support this statement. In Figure 8, one can also find this relationship, excepting point 281 beyond the cluster of points. Explanation for this point is that this subject had sustained relatively severe femur injuries during the knee-impact test. Consequently, the ultimate compressive strength was diminished in the axial compressive test.

However, the results encourage us to continue conducting the mineralization analysis of the bones which should be associated with the car crash test programs using dead bodies. Actually, the mineralization analysis justified to eliminate No. 233 from our list in the knee-impact results program because of a very poor bone condition, as described in a previous paper (17).

Average unit ash content is about 1.14 g/cm3 obtained from our specimens, corresponding to a value of 60 % for a normal bone with density of 1.9 (19) in air-dried conditions. Robinson (21) gave this value between 54.5 to 62.1 %.

Mean ultimate compressive strength (U.C.S.) and strain are 12.13 kgf/mm2 and 1.9 %. The ultimate compressive strength of 17.7 kgf/mm2 cited in reference (22) for Calabrisi (1951).

The specimens were hollow cylindrical fragments in an unembalmed or fresh condition. Our specimen conditions were dry. U.C.S. of 14.8 kgf/mm2 and strain 0.018 for age group of 60-69 are given in reference (23). The specimen conditions have not been given. Since mechanical properties of the bone depend on the specimen and test conditions, the difference between our results and the others would be acceptable.

ACCURACY OF THE TOLERANCE LIMIT DRAWN IN THE (F, T_ϵ) PLANE - Analysis of the results shows that the data points of the three series of human cadaver tests locate as follows: for the first and second series of tests, corresponding

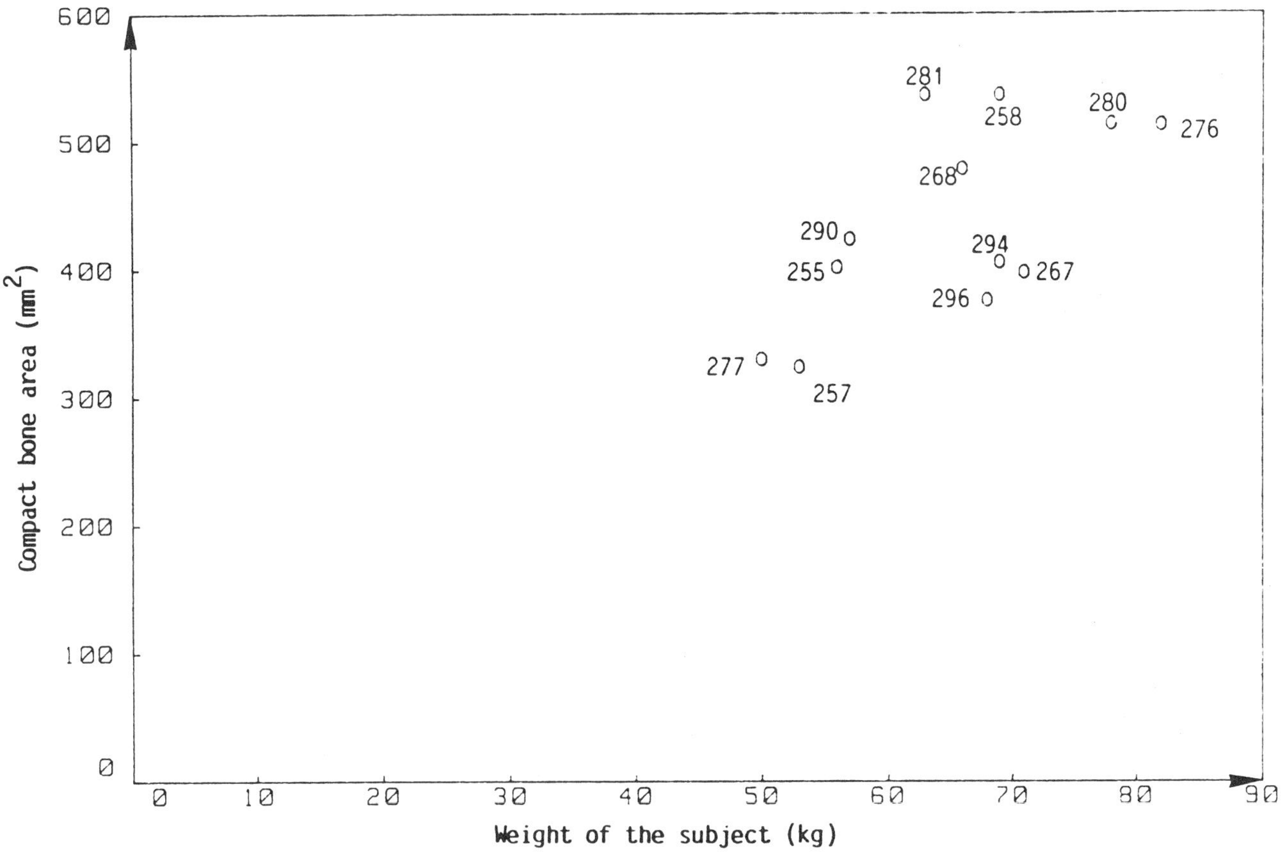

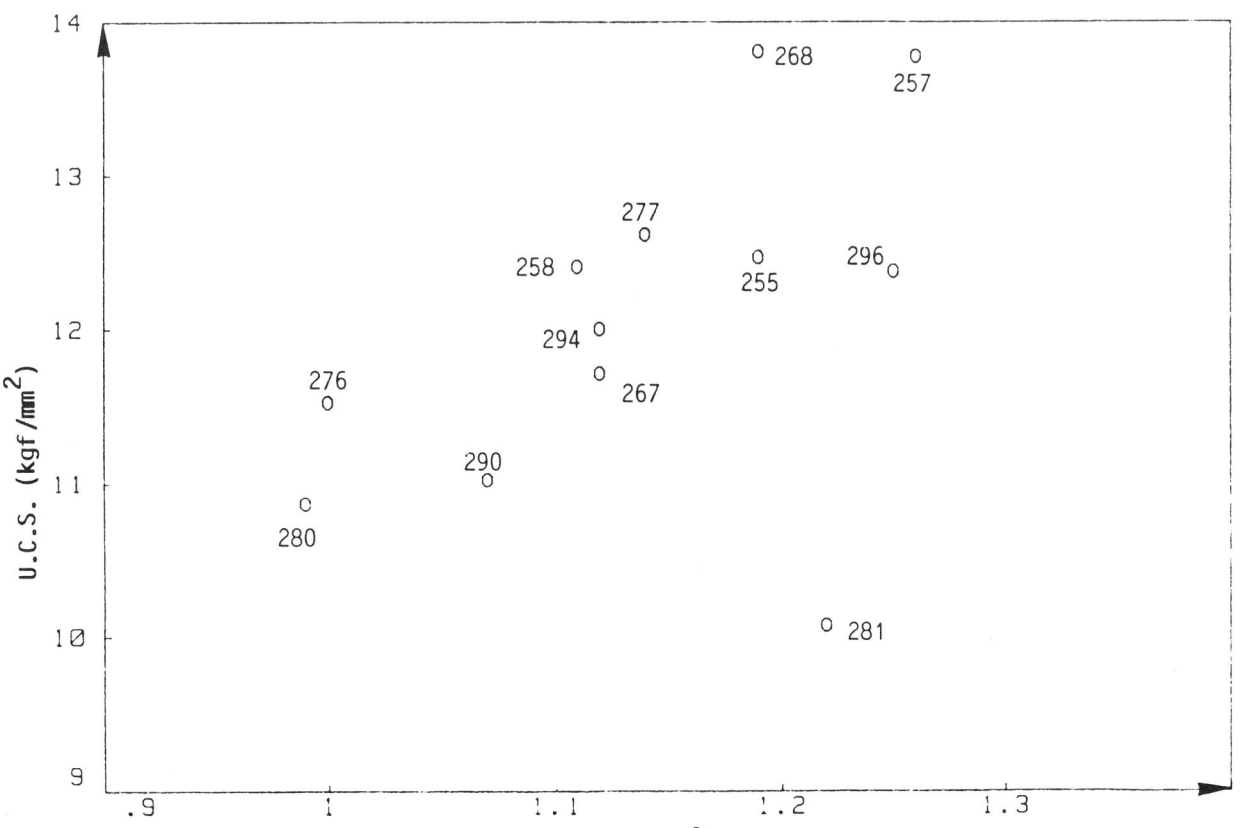

Figure 7 - Compact Bone Area at the Mid-Femur Section (BH) Versus Weight of the Subject

Figure 8 - Ultimate Compressive Strength Versus Ash Content.

Table 4 - Mechanical Tests Performed on Femurs

Subject No.	Overall Length (mm)	Cortical Bone Surface (mm2) HH	BB	HB	BH	Ultimate Compression Load (kgf) Lower Sample	Upper Sample	Initial Length (mm)
255	460	42.7	45.6	33.3	40.1	4175	5000	60
257	400	39.9	43.1	30.1	32.3	4100	4450	60
258	423	50.1	46.7	51.8	53.6	5675	6650	60
267	424	52.4	51.8	41.1	39.7	2525	4650	60
268	447	57.4	39.7	45.8	47.8	4150	6600	60
276	484	59.4	60.3	46.3	51.2	2490	5900	60
277	444	39.4	32.2	32.2	32.9	1800	4150	60
280	530	47.5	40.0	47.6	51.3	4400	5575	60
281	453	52.4	34.1	42.8	53.6	5150	5400	60
290	450	34.7	35.1	32.0	42.3	2340	4665	60
294	441	39.4	43.7	42.9	40.5	4145	4860	60
296	447	36.7	28.9	32.6	37.5	3555	4640	60

Table 4 - (Continued)

Subject No.	Deformation (mm) (U. Sample)	Strain (%) (U. Sample)	U.C.S. kgf/mm2 (Upper Sample)	Bending Breaking Load (E_b) (kgf)	Ultimate Deflection (δ_b) (mm)
255	1.25	2.08	12.46	686	5
257	0.80	1.33	13.77	738	4.7
258	1.20	2	12.4	1012	4.25
267	1.20	2	11.71	866	3.4
268	0.96	1.6	13.8	1072	3.3
276	1.14	1.9	11.52	860	3.85
277	1.04	1.73	12.61	267	2.15
280	1.14	1.9	10.86	606	2.25
281	1.34	2.23	10.07	476	4
290	1.22	2.03	11.02	-	-
294	1.23	2.05	12.0	1131	4.2
296	1.20	1.9	12.37	-	-

Table 5 - Results of Calcination of the Tested Cadaver Femurs.

Cadaver No.	Ash C(g)	lc (cm)	AC = (HB + BH):2 (cm2)	V = Ac x lc (cm3)	Ash (C/V) (g/cm3)
255	12.39	2.83	3.67	10.38	1.19
257	11.27	2.87	3.12	8.95	1.27
258	16.73	2.85	5.27	15.01	1.11
267	12.53	2.75	4.05	11.13	1.12
268	15.87	2.85	4.68	13.33	1.19
276	13.23	2.70	4.87	13.14	1.00
277	10.79	2.90	3.25	9.42	1.14
280	15.38	3.15	4.94	15.56	0.99
281	18.36	3.10	4.82	14.94	1.22
290	13.50	3.40	3.71	12.61	1.07
294	20.92	4.45	4.17	18.55	1.12
296	16.04	3.65	3.50	12.77	1.25

to a 3-pt belted condition, all data locate in the no-fracture area. For the third series of tests, all data points locate in the "fracture" area, excepting 294 L. The most femur fractures occurred in this area. Actually, five fracture points are found out of six. It is easily understandable, because the test conditions with a 2-pt (shoulder belt) and at 65 kph are more severe than for the first two series using a 3-pt-belt and at 50 or 65 kph.

A peak knee-impact load of 8.3 KN sustained by 281 R is the lowest value among the fracture points. It is considered as a static test value shown by a line parallel to $T\varepsilon$ axis: a value of 8.4 KN was used by Viano (12), it is found that three non fracture points have a greater load value and shorter $T\varepsilon$ in relation to 281 R. This case with the present criterion corresponds to a limit, as indicating that load value decreases as $T\varepsilon$ increases (Figure 5). When load value is determined, $T\varepsilon$ is a function of impulse. From this analysis, one can recognize again that peak load level alone cannot indicate femur fracture risk. Present conventional pulse duration might complement this insufficiency.

The tolerance limit of figure 5 consists of two parts, one horizontal and one oblique. As previously mentioned, the horizontal part closely corresponds to static tolerance values, already published, and is not deeply questionable. On the contrary, the oblique part is drawn from only a few points. No. 281 excepted, the corresponding subjects have a weight and a bone condition which suggests no particular remarks.

One can observe the similarity between the limit of the Viano's criterion (FIC)(12) and the limit proposed here when the impact duration diminishes until zero. This similarity is due purely to chance; however, it supports the proposed values for the femoral complex tolerance.

Remark: Muscle Effect - As described above, because of the estimates based on compact bone area, the load to regularly produce femur fracture would reach 10 KN. The authors of the paper believe that this value is sometimes and to a certain extent a conservative one for predicting the femur injury tolerance in a real accident. It has been recognized by research workers (22, 23, 4, 24) that the hip muscular effect would diminish the tensile stress in the femoral shaft when a force is applied from the knee to the head of the femur.

Because of the eccentricity of the femoral head and neck from the long shaft axis, great bending stresses were concentrated at the lateral region at the proximal part. This fact was demonstrated by the investigation in the knee-impact tests with human cadavers (22). In the living subject, muscular contraction occurs particularly in the tensor faciae latae. Consequently, the tensile stress would be reduced by the equilibrium of the muscular force action.

Although no references can be found to prove and qualify this muscular effect allowing to predict a greater femur tolerance level for the living, but the fact of muscular action leads us to believe that the present proposed femur injury tolerance is conservative for "active" victims.

PROBLEM OF THE CRITERION TO BE MET WHEN USING A DUMMY - At this step, let us assume that sufficient knowledge is got concerning femur complex tolerance, and let us consider the corresponding criterion for a given A.T.D. submitted to the same test. The correction factor depends largely on the type of test. As an example, 2 identical blows can be performed by means of a pendulum against the knee of a seated ATD or cadaver and a correction factor is easily given by such a method for such a type of experiment. On the contrary, in a car body, the restraint, the differences in trajectories, in position, in distance between the knees and their stopping areas, make the point very different; concerning the tests reported here, the knee-impact speeds against the targets, estimated by film analysis, are reported in Table 3. It appears clearly that the knees of the dummies strike the targets at higher speeds than cadaver knees. The mechanical response of the dummy knee is not the primary cause, according to Figure 9. This figure is a plot of the forces exerted on the knee targets as a function of the quantity body mass x knee impact speed (as a matter of fact, the normal component of the speed to the target). The main difference between the forces exerted by Part 572 and cadavers on the targets is due to the knee-impact velocities. This is true even if the weights of the cadavers are close to the weight of a Part 572 ATD. Reasons for so important differences have to be analyzed.

Presently, it is not sound to use the calibration factors obtained in tests where the knee impact speeds were similar for ATD and cadavers, due to the test conditions which concerned unrestrained human surrogates.

A first calibration factor defined by the ratio:

$$\frac{\text{dummy target force}}{\text{cadaver target force}}$$

could be infinite if the dummy reaches the targets and cadavers do not.

No restraint was used in the tests reported in (8) and (25), the results of which were utilized for defining calibration factors.

On the contrary, the second necessary calibration factor:

$$\frac{\text{Dummy target force}}{\text{Dummy femur force}}$$

can be roughly estimated (1).

Available data are not sufficient to clarify the problems related to the first calibration factor. Consequently, two questions have to be answered:

- Have different injury criteria to be defined for the restrained and unrestrained dummies?
- Is it possible to design an ATD, kinematics and impact response of which well duplicate

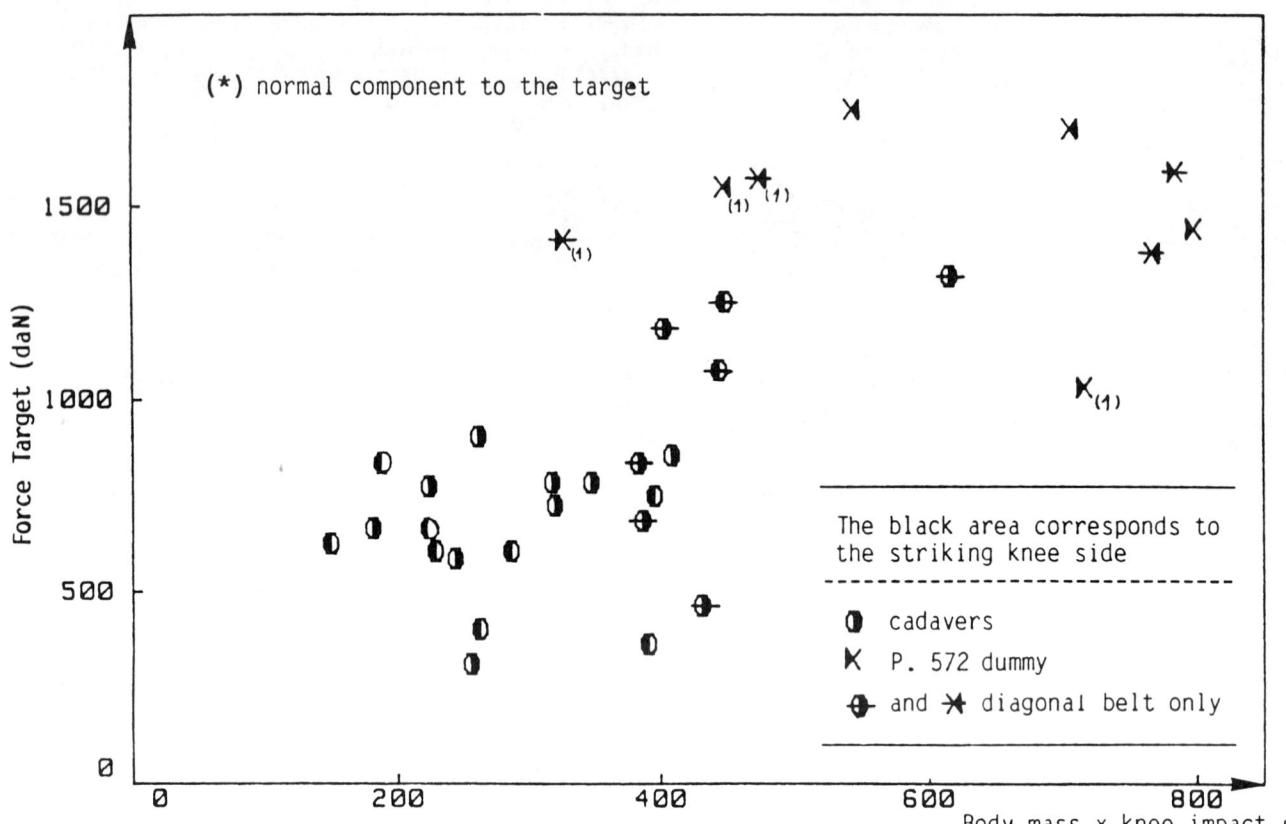

Figure 9 - Maximum Forces Exerted on the Knee Targets as a Function of Body Mass x Knee Impact Speed

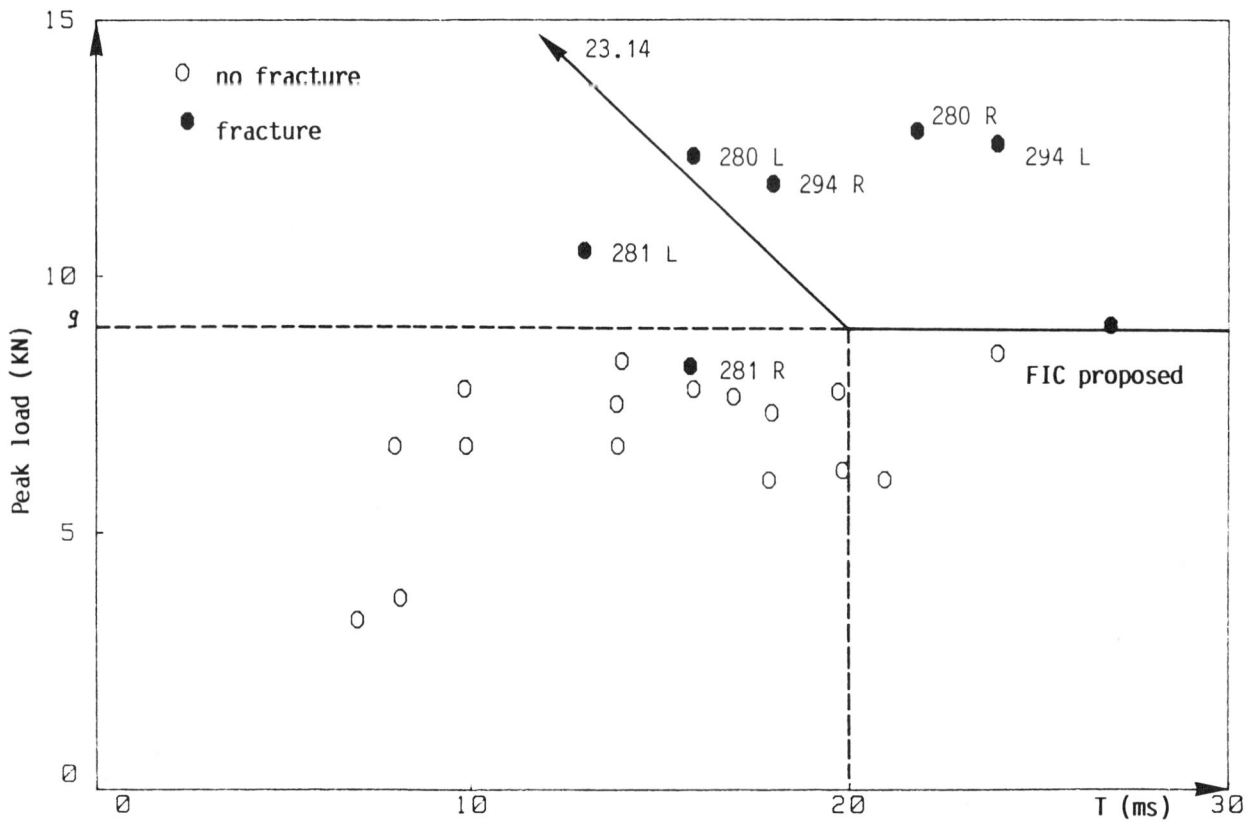

Figure 10 - Peak Knee-Impact Loas Versus Primary Pulse Duration (Viano)

the human beings' corresponding features ?

Presently, due to the huge differences in knee-impacts of restrained P. 572 and cadavers in frontal collisions, a criterion based on tolerance estimates, corrected for the femur response of the dummy at the same knee impact speed is highly conservative. The tolerance limit proposed here could constitute a protection criterion when associated to a really human-like ATD.

TESTING THE VALIDITY OF THE VIANO FEMUR INJURY CRITERION (F.I.C.) USING CURRENT BIOMECHANICAL DATA - In the femur injury criterion developed by Viano (12), the duration of the primary force exposure and the peak applied load are simultaneously taken into account. A permissible peak knee load dependence upon the duration of the primary force exposure is given following the formula (in which KN and ms are used for units):

F = 23.14 - 0.71 T   T < 20 ms
F = 8.90 KN   T ≥ 20 ms

In figure 10, the limit corresponding to this femur injury criterion is shown in a force versus pulse graph duration. The points representing the present test results are distributed on both sides of the criterion limit. Two points corresponding to two fractured femurs are situated in the "uninjured" area and so are at variance with the criterion. These two subjects have a normal bone condition (Table 4). Therefore it seems that the complete set of biomechanical data shows that the FIC is somewhat optimistic; nevertheless its principle can be kept for other studies and comparisons, regardless of the dummy problem.

One can recall the similarity between the limit of FIC for T = 0, and the limit proposed here (Tε = 0) drawing through.

TESTING THE KTHIC VALIDITY BY MEANS OF PRESENT DUMMY TESTS AND BIOMECHANICAL DATA - A comparison, for two test series, of the results obtained in the dummy tests with the results of the cadaver tests, with reference to the injuries sustained by the cadavers in these tests, enables the testing of the validation of the KTHIC, the knee-thigh-hip injury criterion developed by G. Nyquist (1).

For the two Part 572 dummy tests, the available recorded femur forces exceed the 8450 N threshold, proposed by Nyquist, as a limit for the appearance of injuries. The Femur Number (FN) was computed for each force pulse, according to the KTHIC definition, with peaks in excess of 8450 N. Only for the tests with a diagonal belt system does the FN exceed the proposed $3.0 \; 10^9 \; lb^{3.5}.s$ tolerance limit. That means:

- the first series of tests with a 3-pt belt system is considered as non injurious, according to KTHIC.

- the second series (65 kph-diagonal belt system) is considered as injurious, according to the same criterion.

If the injuries sustained in the corresponding cadaver tests are considered, the indications given by the KTHIC regarding the severity of the two series of test conditions are confirmed (see Table 1) in these cases. However, the correction factors between tests with ATD and dead bodies are a questionable matter.

Therefore, the "calibration factors" used for establishing the KTHIC have to be examined more closely. We have the possibility to analyse our cadaver data in terms of KTHIC. This method was developed with existing biomechanical data (4)(24)(25), for which the bone condition and anthropometry of the subjects were not available. If this method is used for our cadaver data, the direct computation of the C and K (Nyquist's correction parameters) does not confirm the previous indications regarding the severity of the two different series of tests. The second series of tests seems in this case non injurious.

Besides, it seems that, among the biomechanical data used by Nyquist, some are matched to those human subjects with a poor bone condition, the latter induce an increased scatter in the data of a same set. Further, it is recalled that Nyquist used the center of gravity of the data set minus 2/3 standard deviation of peak force.

CONCLUSIONS

1. A good agreement as regards the order of magnitude is found between the tolerance levels when the femur is axially compressed by external blows on the one hand and under realistic car crash conditions on the other hand.

2. Based on the available experimental results, the Femur Tolerance can be defined as: F = 23.4 - 0.72 T when T < 21 ms, F = 8.3 KN when T ≥ 21 ms. Where T is the conventional pulse duration.

3. This conventional pulse duration is defined by:

$$T_\varepsilon = \frac{\int_0^\tau f(t)dt}{F.\max}$$

when F. max is determined, Tε is a function of impulse. Using F. max associated to impulse enables to obtain a satisfactory explanation of the present results.

4. This tolerance is probably a conservative one, anthropometric parameters, muscle tension effect and age are reserved for the necessary corrections.

5. Analysis of mineralization and more gerenally the bone characterization is necessary for the utilization of cadaver tests, and particularly for the femur.

6. A good correlation between the mid-femur shaft area and the weight of the dead body was found. The latter may be a useful parameter, when used for the correction of the criterion.

7. A good correlation between ash contents and ultimative compressive strength was found in the specimens obtained from latter knee-impact tested subjects.

8. Part 572 dummy yields knee impact speeds much higher than cadavers do, when restrained in frontal collisions. It makes conservative present femur injury criteria under similar conditions.

ACKNOWLEDGEMENTS

This research has been made thanks to the results obtained within the framework of a contract with the French Administration (Institut de Recherche des Transports). Opinions are the authors'.

REFERENCES

1. G.W. Nyquist, "A pulse-shape dependent Knee-Thigh-Hip injury criterion for use with the Part 572 dummy", ISO/ TC 22/SC 12/WG. 6 [USA-12] No. 117, June 1982.

2. F.W. Cooke and D.A. Nagel, "Biomechanical analysis of knee impact", Proceedings of 13rd Stapp Car Crash Conference. S.A.E. 690800, Dec. 2-4, 1969, pp. 117-133.

3. J.W. Melvin, R.L. Stalnaker, N.M. Alem, J.B. Benson and D. Mohan, "Impact response and tolerance of the lower extremities", Proceedings of 19th Stapp Car Crash Conference, S.A.E. 751 159, Nov. 17-19, 1975.

4. J.W. Melvin and R.L. Stalnaker, "Tolerance and response of the knee-femur-pelvis complex to axial impact", HSRI report UM-HSRI 76-17, MVMA project No. 4.18, 1976.

5. D.C. Viano, C.C. Culver, R.C. Hant, J.W. Melvin, M. Bender, R.H. Culver and R.S. Levine, "Bolster impacts to the knee and tibia of human cadavers and an anthropomorphic dummy", proceedings of 22 nd Stapp Car Crash conference, Oct. 24-26, 1978.

6. W.R. Powell, S.H. Advani, R.N. Clark, S.J. Ojala and D.J. Holt, "Investigation of femur response to longitudinal impact", Proceedings of 18th Stapp Car Crash Conference, S.A.E. paper 741190, December 4-5, 1974.

7. W.R. Powell, S.J. Ojala, S.H. Advani, R.B. Martin, "Cadaver Femur Response to Longitudinal Impacts", Proceedings of 19th Stapp Car Crash Conference, S.A.E. paper 751 160, 1975.

8. W.E. Hering and L.M. Patrick, "Response Comparisons of the Human Cadaver Knee and a Part 572 Knee Impacts by Crushable Materials", proceedings of 21st Stapp Car Crash Conference, SAE paper 770939, Oct. 19-21, 1977.

9. L.M. Patrick, C.R. Kroell, H.J. Mertz Jr., "Force on the Human Body in Simulated Crashes", proceedings of 9th Stapp Car Crash Conference, Oct. 20-21, 1965.

10. L.M. Patrick, H.J. Mertz Jr., C.R. Kroell, "Cadaver Knee, Chest and Head Impact Loads", Proceedings of 11th Stapp Car Crash Conference, SAE paper 670913, Oct. 1967.

11. C.K. Kroell, D.C. Schneider and A.M. Noham, "Comparative Knee Impact Response of Part 572 Dummy and Cadaver Subjects", proceedings of 20th Stapp Car Crash Conference, SAE paper 760817, Oct. 18-20, 1976.

12. D.C. Viano, "Consideration for a Femur Injury Criterion", proceedings of 21st Stapp Car Crash Conference, SAE paper 770925, Oct. 19-21, 1977.

13. E.F. Rybicki, F.A. Simonen and E.B. Weiss, "On the Mathematical Analysis of Stress in the Human Femur", J. Biomechanics, 1972. vol. 5, pp. 203-215.

14. J.J. King, W.R.S. Fan and J.R. Vargovick, "Femur Load Injury Criteria - A Realistic Approach", proceedings of 17th Stapp Car Crash Conference, SAE paper 730984, Nov. 12-13, 1973.

15. S.L. Gordon, P.N. Orticke and J. Prince, R. Mc Meekin, "Dynamic Characteristics of Human Leg Joints", proceedings of 21st Stapp Car Crash Conference, SAE paper 770924, Oct. 19-21, 1977.

16. P.M. Calverale, A. Garro, G.L. Lorenzi, "Car Accident Mathematical Model, Femur and Pelvis Stress Analysis", proceedings of IRCOBI 1979, pp. 418-428.

17. F. Brun-Cassan, Y.C. Leung, C. Tarrière, A. Fayon, "Determination of Knee-Femur-Pelvis Tolerance from the Simulation of our Frontal Impacts", proceedings of IRCOBI 1982.

18. R.H. Eppinger, "Prediction of Thoracic Injuries Using Measurable Experimental Cadavers", proceedings of the 6th ESV Conference, Washington, USA, Oct. 1976.

19. J.D. Currey, "The Mechanical Consequences of Variation in the Mineral Contents of Bone", J. Biomechanics, pp. 1-11, 2, 1968.

20. G.P. Vose, A.L. Kubala, Hum. Biol. 31, 261 - 1959.

21. R.A. Robinson, "An Electron-Microscopic Study of the Crystalline Inorganic Component of Bone; its Relationship to the Organic Matrix", J. Bone and Joint Surgery., pp. 389-435, 34 A, 1952.

22. F.G. Evans, "Stress and Strain in Bones", C.C. Thomas Publisher, Springfield, ill., 1957.

23. H. Yamada, "Strength of Biological Materials", Edited by Evans F.G., the Williams and Wilkins Co.

24. C.K. Kroell, D.C. Schneider, A.M. Nahum, "Comparative Knee Impact Response of the Part 572 Dummy and Cadaver Subjects", proceedings of 20th Stapp Car Crash Conference, SAE paper 760817, 1976.

25. J.D. Horsch and L.M. Patrick, "Cadaver and Dummy Knee Impact Response", SAE 760799, Oct. 1976.

851724

Mechanism of Abdominal Injury by Steering Wheel Loading

John D. Horsch, Ian V. Lau, David C. Viano, and Dennis V. Andrzejak
GM Research Laboratories

ABSTRACT

The introduction of energy absorbing steering systems has provided a substantial reduction of occupant injury in car crashes. However, the steering system remains the most important source of occupant injury. Injury associated with steering assembly contact is due to high exposure; energy absorbing steering systems reduce the risk of injury for drivers when compared to the injury risk of right front passengers. Our investigation addressed loading of the upper abdominal region by the steering wheel rim using a physiological model for study of soft tissue injury.

Injury to the liver was related to the abdominal compression response associated with rim loading. Although liver injury correlated somewhat with peak abdominal compression, a better correlation was found when the rate of compression was also considered. Force limiting by the steering wheel, not by column compression, most strongly influenced the outcome of abdominal injury. The force generated by wheel-rim compression of the abdomen was insufficient to cause either column compression or significant whole-body motions. Subjects loaded by "stiff" steering wheels (having rim deformation forces greater than the abdominal compression force) exhibited greater abdominal compression, rate of compression and resulting extent of injury than did subjects loaded by "softer" wheels which deformed more and thus reduced abdominal compression.

ENERGY ABSORBING STEERING SYSTEMS introduced in 1967 were designed with a compressible element as a primary feature for occupant protection. The systems also controlled the amount of steering assembly rearward displacement in the occupant compartment in a frontal collision. Analysis of crash data by NHTSA (1)* has concluded that the energy absorbing steering system reduced the annual fatalities in frontal impacts by 12% and the critical to fatal injuries associated with steering system contact by 38%. Despite the reductions, the steering system remains the most frequent source of injury to car occupants. NHTSA (2,3) attributes more than 25% of the total automobile occupant "Harm" to steering system contact, Fig. 1.

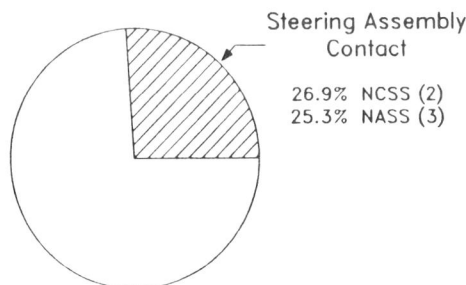

CAR OCCUPANT "HARM"

Fig. 1 Percent of car occupant "Harm" associated with steering assembly contact (2,3).

The presence of the steering system does not increase and may even reduce the injury risk for drivers (4) when compared to the injury risk of right front passengers. The relatively high incidence of injury associated with steering assembly contact is due to high exposure. Most car occupants are drivers -- many times the only occupant. Due to the driver's proximity with the steering assembly, the driver is more likely to interact with the steering assembly than other vehicle components -- particularly in frontal crashes -- and there is a greater risk of

---

* Numbers in parentheses designate references at end of paper.

injury since frontal crashes tend to be more severe than the general spectrum of crashes.

Driver interaction with the steering system has been the subject of many investigations which have substantially improved our understanding of driver protection by the steering system (1,5-11). With a compressible column system, the column plays the major role in force limitation and energy absorption when the driver is aligned with the steering assembly. The steering wheel also plays a major role since it is the component contacted by the occupant, and it determines the force distribution on the occupant. The steering wheel provides additional force limiting and energy absorption by deformation, particularly in situations where the driver is off-set or off-axis (6). Thus relative deformation of the wheel and compression of the column are highly dependent on the impact alignment of the occupant with the steering assembly (5,6). Crash data indicate that both column compression and steering wheel deformation are important occupant protection aspects (6). Efforts to further improve built-in occupant protection by the steering system must consider both the range of crash situations in which occupants are exposed and injured, and the response and tolerance of the various body regions contacting the steering assembly.

Injury ("Harm") related to steering assembly contact has been identified by body region (2,3), Fig. 2. The thorax has the highest portion of "Harm", followed by the abdomen (24% to 35%), and the head, which primarily involves facial injury. Injury is somewhat uniformly distributed across the range of impact severities as measured by the vehicle change of velocity (ΔV), from below 20 mph to at least 40 mph, (2,3), Fig. 3. Although the "Harm" per exposed occupant is greater at high ΔVs, the exposure frequency is greatest at lower ΔVs (3), resulting in nearly equivalent injury "Harm" over a large ΔV exposure range, Fig. 4. This suggests that high, moderate and low severity crashes

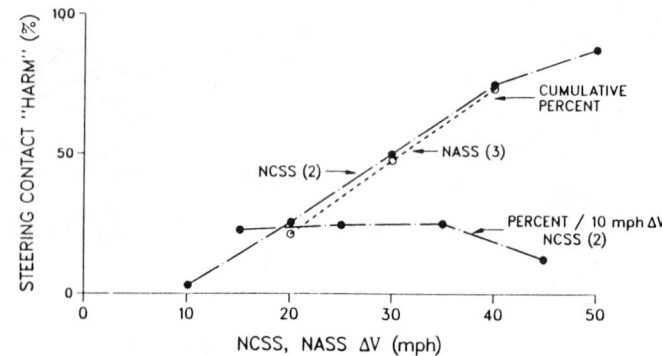

Fig. 3 Distribution of "Harm" associated with steering assembly contact as a function of vehicle velocity change (ΔV) (2,3).

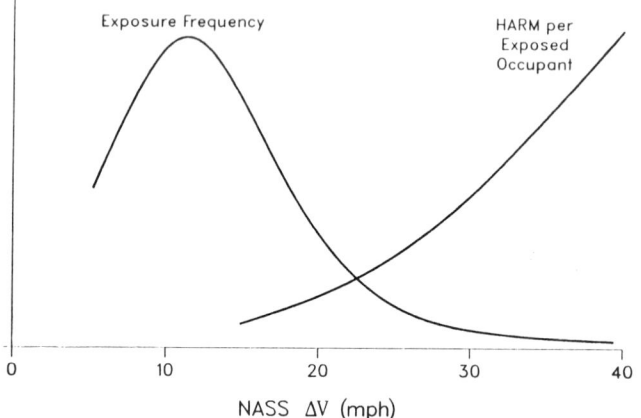

Fig. 4 NASS exposure frequency and "Harm" per exposed occupant (all sources) as a function of ΔV (3). "Harm" for each ΔV is the product of exposure frequency and "Harm" per exposed occupant.

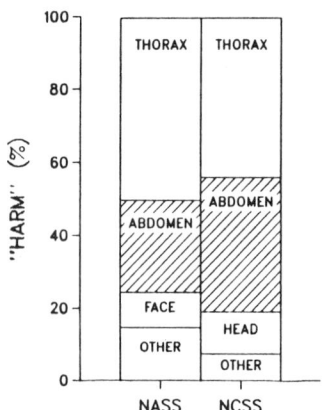

Fig. 2 Distribution of "Harm" associated with steering assembly contact by body region (2,3).

should be considered in analysis of occupant protection systems.

In the laboratory, the response of the steering assembly depends on construction and impact stiffness of the test dummy used for the evaluation (7). Additionally, trends associated with changes in steering assembly characteristics are strongly dependent on which dummy and response is used for the evaluation (7). The Hybrid III dummy was judged to be the best of the current mechanical surrogates to study the steering system in the laboratory based on its more human-like construction and frontal impact response, and its expanded instrumentation capacity -- chest compression being an important response for study of an unrestrained driver interacting with the steering assembly (7).

In spite of gains in understanding of driver protection and in laboratory evaluation tools such as the Hybrid III dummy, abdominal injury associated with steering contact is less well understood than thoracic trauma because current anthropomorphic dummies are not instrumented to assess injury potential for frontal abdominal loading. The steering column is elevated from the horizontal and its elevation may increase during vehicle deformation in a crash. The lower rim of the wheel can contact the driver first, depending on occupant kinematics. The liver is only partially protected by the rib cage and is a potential loading site for the lower rim.

We used an anesthetized animal to study the mechanics of upper abdominal injury from steering wheel rim contact in sled tests. 50-Kg swine,* were chosen for these experiments based on the need for a physiological model for soft tissue injury and human-like approximation of the torso and organ mass, and midtorso dimensions of the 50th percentile male. However, because of differences in the head, shoulder and pelvic regions, the swine may not be a representative human surrogate for other studies of the steering system. The swine has been successfully used as a physiological model for the study of injury mechanisms for vital organs in the torso in previous impact studies (12-16).

We investigated force, acceleration and compression response parameters in this study. The compression parameter included a "viscous" response defined as the time varying product of amplitude of the percent compression [C(t)] and the velocity of compression [V(t)]. The maximum value of the "viscous" response [V(t)*C(t)]max was previously shown to correlate with soft tissue injury for frontal thoracic (17-19), lateral abdominal (20), and frontal abdominal (21) impact, where it biomechanically correlated with liver injury (19,21).

METHODOLOGY

The test fixture consisted of a steel frame mounted on the Hyge sled carriage (Fig. 5). The fully anesthetized subject was supported by a suspension suit attached to a trolley at four corners. The position was adjusted to result in the lower rim loading directly in line with the liver (5 cm below the xyphoid). The trolley system consisted of four wheels suspended on two parallel rails. Slots were machined in the rails for the trolley to drop prior to subject contact with the wheel. During the impact, the surrogate was unrestrained by the tethers. To retain the subject on the sled fixture, the trolley had secondary restraints which came into play following the impact. Kinematics of the lower torso were controlled by belt restraints around each leg and anchored to a force limiter with a yield force of 2 kN. The belts did not interfere with abdominal loading by the wheel.

A sled velocity of 32 km/h was used for all the tests. The sled acceleration pulse and separation between the lower rim and the abdomen allowed the sled to reach test velocity before significant interaction of the subject with the wheel.

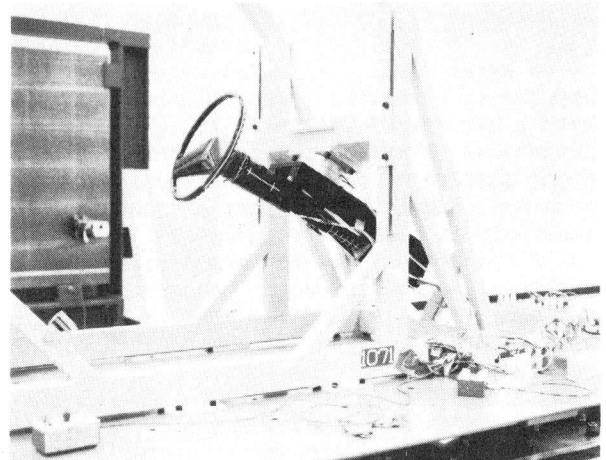

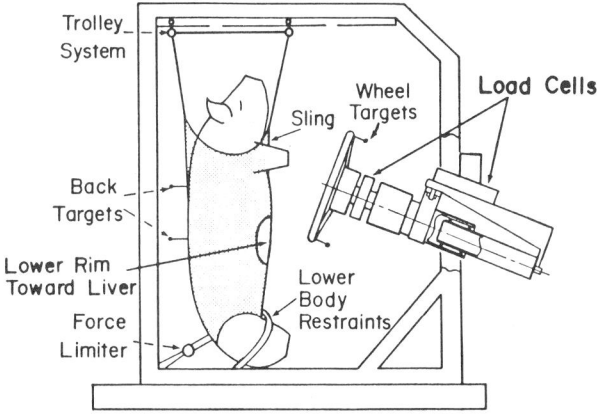

Fig. 5 Sled fixture showing mounting of steering assembly and a schematic of the sled test configuration.

---

* The rationale and experimental protocol for the use of an animal model in this program have been reviewed by the Research Laboratories' Animal Research Committee. The research follows procedures outlined in publications by the U.S. Department of Health, Education, and Welfare, 'Guide for the Care and Use of Laboratory Animals,' or the U.S. DHEW National Institute of Health (NIH), 'Guidelines for the Use of Experimental Animals,' and complies with U.S. Department of Agriculture (USDA) regulations as specified in the Laboratory Animals Welfare Act (PL 89-544), as amended in 1970 and 1976 (PL 91-579 and PL 94-279).

THE STEERING ASSEMBLY - The steering assembly consisted of a standard compressible column and modified wheels. Column angle was 20° or 30° compared to the horizontal. The column was mounted on a bracket which was rigidly attached to the sled fixture by a triaxial force transducer. Instrumentation of the steering assembly consisted of a triaxial force transducer located between the wheel and the column and a displacement transducer for column compression.

Several steering wheels were used in this study. A simulated wheel, Fig. 6a, and two experimental versions of a two-spoke wheel, Fig. 6b, provided several levels of wheel deformation stiffness for rim loading, Fig. 7. The simulated wheel provided a relatively rigid deformation characteristic. A "stiff" version and a "soft" version of the two-spoke wheel provided two deformation stiffnesses without changing other characteristics of the wheel. Additional variations of steering assembly characteristics were studied by alternating between wheel spoke across and vertical positions for tests with the modified two-spoke wheel. Table 1 provides the test matrix for this study.

ANIMAL PREPARATION FOR THE SLED TEST - Seventeen swine weighing 49.5 ± 2.0 Kg, were restrained without excitement by an injection of ketamine (20 mg/Kg, IM) and acepromazine (200 µg, IM) followed by atropine (0.08 mg/Kg, IM). The swine were then induced to a surgical plane of anesthesia with a mixture of fentanyl (40 µg/Kg, IM) and droperidol (2 mg/Kg, IM) and maintained on an equal mixture of oxygen and nitrous oxide with 1-1.5% halothane. They breathed spontaneously in a dorsal recumbency.

A tracheotomy was performed on all subjects, a tube inserted through the tracheal incision, and the mixture of inhalation gases and oxygen was reconnected to the endotracheal tube. The location of the midsternum was determined anatomically (as midpoint between the manubrium and the xyphoid). The midsternum was exposed by cauterizing the skin and the subcutaneous layers. A uniaxial accelerometer was attached to the sternum using bone screws. Catheter tip pressure transducers were inserted into the right femoral artery and vein and guided to the level of upper abdominal viscera. ECG leads (II) were permanently sutured to the limbs for monitor during the test. The swine was then rotated 180° to rest in a ventral recumbency. The thoracic spinous process transverse to the midsternum (T3 and T4) and that transverse to a location 5 cm below the tip of the xyphoid (T11 or T12) were exposed by cauterizing the skin and the subcutaneous layers. Two spinous clamps with mounted accelerometers and photographic targets were fastened to the exposed processes.

Particular adaptational aids were necessary for the quadruped to assure basal

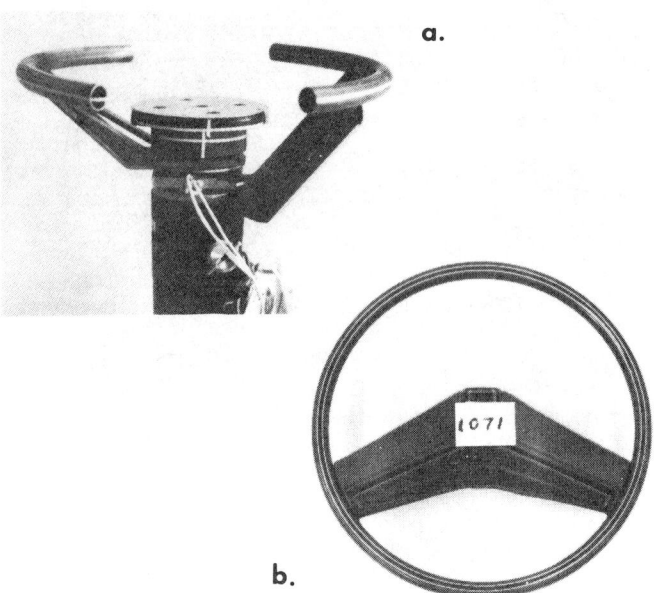

Fig. 6 Steering wheels used in the sled experiments. (a) Simulated wheel. (b) Two-spoke wheel.

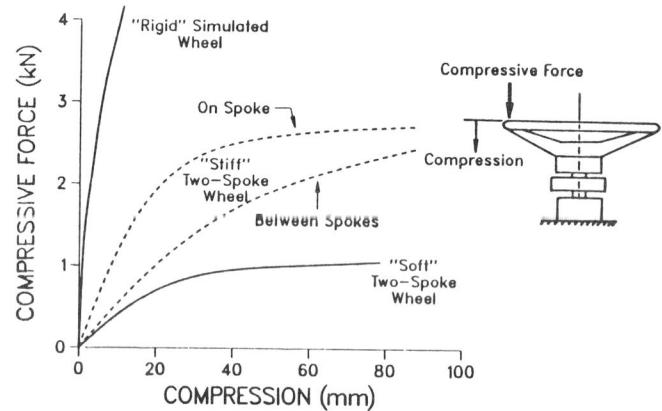

Fig. 7 Wheel quasistatic deformation characteristics for loading as shown in diagram.

physiologic functions in vertical suspension during the sled experiment. Before the suspension, an increase in blood volume was induced by intravenous infusion of 250 mL of isotonic lactated Ringer's solution to mitigate orthostatic hypotension (transient pooling of blood due to change in position). The animal was supported in a suspension suit with belts originating from four tethering points for attachment to the sled fixture (Fig. 5). The suit had adjustable abdominal supports which were securely tightened to minimize blood pooling in the pelvic girdle and the lower extremities. The suit was open at the steering wheel rim impact site. Since no surgical procedures were performed on the swine during the suspension, the concentration of halothane was reduced to maintain a level of 0.5%. With these provisions, the swine retained normal cardio-vascular physiologic function during vertical suspension.

Just before the onset of the test, the swine was disconnected from the inhalation gases and breathed room air for less than two minutes during the sled test. Immediately following the test, the swine was returned to a dorsal recumbency and inhalation gases were reconnected. The animal showed no signs of distress or sensation during or after the experiment. It was observed for 15 minutes, sacrificed by an overdose of sodium pentobarbital (>60 mg/Kg), and a truncal necropsy was performed immediately.

THE NECROPSY - The abdominal viscera were exposed by a midsagittal incision of the linea alba. Hemoperitoneum when present was noted and classified. Hemoperitoneum was considered moderate if peritoneal blood loss was less than 200 mL, hemorrhage stopped spontaneously and bleeding did not resume upon exposing the abdominal cavity to atmospheric pressure. Hemoperitoneum was considered severe if peritoneal blood loss was more than 200 mL and hemorrhage resumed as the abdominal cavity of the sacrificed animal was exposed to atmospheric pressure, indicating that hemorrhage initially stopped because peritoneal pressure equilibrated with central venous pressure. The liver, the spleen, the kidney, the stomach, and the intestines were then examined for lacerations or contusions. The number of independent tears was used as a measure of injury severity for each organ. An AIS score was assigned reflecting the overall severity of abdominal injury, the extent of concomitant hemorrhage, and possible prognosis if resuscitation were attempted.

The right and left diaphragms were incised from the abdominal cavity and possible pneumothorax or hemothorax were noted. The thoracic cavity was exposed by bisecting the left and right ribs and reflection of the sternum. Attention was paid not to interfere with any existing fractures, the number and location of which were noted. The lung, the major vessels and the pericardium were then examined for contusions or lacerations. The heart was excised from the chest. The epicardium and endocardium of all four chambers were examined for possible lacerations, contusions, and petechiae. All heart valves were similarly examined. To differentiate impact injury from possible artifacts resulting from the procedure, the necropsy was also performed on a sham operated swine which received identical treatments as the experimental swine including the vertical suspension, excluding the sled test.

RESULTS

INJURY - The impacts resulted in no cardiac arrhythmia among the test subjects. Only two animals from the "stiff"-wheel tests and the animal from the "rigid" wheel test died within the 15-minute observation period post impact. The immediate case of death was respiratory arrest, although they also received critical liver injuries. The other animals all breathed spontaneously following the experiments.

Gross necropsy showed that liver laceration was the only abdominal injury. Liver injury ranged from none to extensive laceration. The most frequently observed lacerations were tears of the Glisson's membrane and submembrane tissue (Fig. 8a). A less frequent but more critical injury was laceration of the central venous junction between lobes (Fig. 8b). Junctional lacerations always resulted in severe hemoperitoneum, an immediate potential threat to life.

The most severe thoracic injury was multiple rib fractures. None of the thoracic injury appeared life threatening. Pulmonary injury was restricted to isolated areas of contusion. The only cardiac injury observed were occasional petechiae on the endocardium. No tearing of valves or chordae tendineae were noted. No cases of hemothorax or pneumothorax were observed. The aortic, the pulmonary and the vena caval blood vessels received no injury.

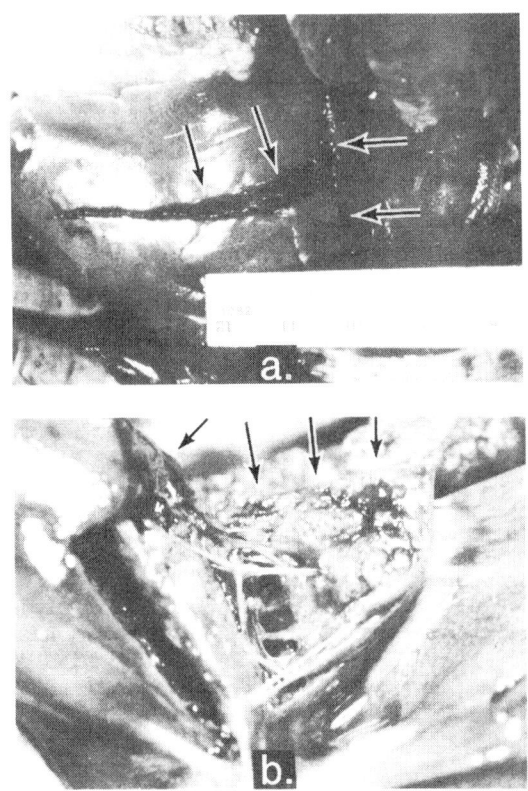

Fig. 8 Examples of liver injury from the "stiff"-wheel tests. (a) Laceration of the posterior surface of the right medial lobe. (b) Junctional laceration between adjacent lobes tearing the central venous junction.

Table 1 - Summary of test conditions and responses

Wheel Stiffness[1]	Column Angle	Spoke Position	Number Rib Fractures	Liver Laceration AIS	Liver Laceration Number	Abdominal Compression Maximum Percent[2]	Abdominal Compression Maximum V*C (m/s)[3]	Lower Spine Acceleration 3 ms (g)[4]
"Stiff"	20°	Vertical	12	5	10	42	1.7	41
			6	5	3	43	2.1	28
		Horizontal	8	5	5	36	1.6	43
			7	5	4	50	2.3	47
"Stiff"	30°	Vertical	7	5	10	41	2.0	--
			6	5	5	45	2.0	34
		Horizontal	10	5	7	41	1.5	55
			4	5	9	38	1.2	33
"Soft"	20°	Vertical	0	0	0	32	0.9	47
			6	0	0	34	1.0	43
		Horizontal	7	0	0	36	0.9	43
			6	0	0	33	0.8	46
"Soft"	30°	Vertical	10	4	1	33	0.9	44
			11	4	2	39	1.1	31
		Horizontal	1	0	0	36	0.7	59
			7	4	1	32	0.8	40
"Rigid"	30°		14	5	Extensive	50	2.4	32

[1] See Fig. 7.
[2] Compression normalized by subject thickness at lower rim contact point.
[3] Normalized compression multiplied by velocity of compression.
[4] Accelerometer located at T-11 or T-12.

Table 2 - Correlation of injury with steering assembly parameters. The mean amplitude is given for each level of the listed parameter variation.

Parameter	Rib Fracture Number per Subject	Liver Laceration AIS	Liver Laceration Number per Subject
Spoke position Vertical/Horizontal	7.25/6.25 p 0.57	3.75/3.38 p 0.45	3.88/3.25 p 0.53
Column angle 20°/30°	6.50/7.00 p 0.78	2.88/4.25 p 0.38	2.75/4.38 p 0.12
Wheel stiffness "Stiff"/"Soft"	7.50/6.00 p 0.40	5.63/1.50 p 0.0002	6.63/0.50 p 0.0001

Injury outcome as a function of steering wheel parameters is given in Table 1. Analysis of injury outcome as a function of steering wheel parameters is given in Table 2. Thoracic injury (number of rib fractures) was not influenced by column angle, spoke position, or rim deflection stiffness in these tests. Rib fractures ranged in number from 0 to 14.

Liver laceration was strongly influenced by the wheel deformation characteristic, a possible influence of column angle, but appears unaffected by spoke position. All eight animals in the "stiff"-wheel tests received critical to fatal liver injury, regardless of spoke position or column angle. The livers in five of the test animals were clearly irrepairable and likely fatal. Liver lacerations in these cases were extensive and involved all the major lobes. Liver laceration for the test with the "rigid" rim response of the simulated wheel was greatly increased compared with the worst case for the "stiff" version of the two-spoke steering wheel, and thus only one test was performed because of the severe outcome. By contrast, only three of eight animals in the "soft"-wheel tests received minor liver laceration. The other five animals sustained no abdominal injuries. The difference of liver injury between the "stiff"- and "soft"-wheel groups was obvious and statistically significant judged by the assigned AIS values. The difference was even greater based on the actual number of liver lacerations. Since hemoperitoneum resulted from the liver lacerations, there was also a parallel difference in the occurrence and the severity of hemoperitoneum between the "stiff"- and "soft"-wheel groups.

STEERING INTERACTION MECHANICS - The interaction mechanics can be viewed from laboratory (stationary) coordinates (Fig. 9), steering assembly coordinates (Fig. 10), or subject coordinates (Fig. 11). The sled was accelerated to test velocity before significant interaction of the rim with the abdomen, while the surrogate remained stationary. The rim would have compressed the abdomen at constant (test) velocity except for possible whole body motion of the surrogate, or motion of the rim relative to the sled by column compression or wheel deformation. However, the force generated by the rim compressing the abdomen was insufficient to produce significant whole body motion of the surrogate or column compression, which were initiated only by the greater forces associated with hub loading on the thorax. Hub contact occurred about 15 ms after abdominal contact. The only mechanism reducing abdominal compression response at test velocity before thoracic loading was wheel deformation. Since the "rigid" and "stiff" wheels exhibited relatively little wheel deformation, most of the sled displacement resulted in abdominal compression. The "soft" wheel exhibited relatively large deformation (Fig. 10) which reduced the velocity and extent of abdominal compression (Fig. 11).

CORRELATION BETWEEN INJURY AND MEASURED RESPONSES - Abdominal injury represented by AIS correlated significantly with the maximum "viscous" response $[V(t)*C(t)]max$, and adequately with maximum abdominal compression, $[C(t)]max$, (Table 3). There was no correla-

Table 3 - Correlation of AIS liver injury with response parameters

	Correlation Coefficient (R)	p-Value
3 ms Lower Spine Acceleration	0.46	0.0712
Maximum Abdominal Compression	0.62	0.0077
Maximum $[V(t)*C(t)]$	0.72	0.0012

*Probability that the value of the correlation coefficient (R) or greater will occur when in fact no correlation exists.

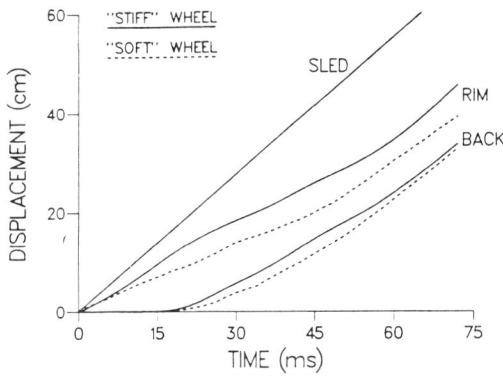

Fig. 9 Movement of the sled, the lower rim of the wheel, and the back of the surrogate in laboratory coordinates. Time zero is contact of the lower rim with the abdomen. Figures 9, 10 and 11 are from the same matched pair of tests having a "stiff" and a "soft" version of the two-spoke wheel.

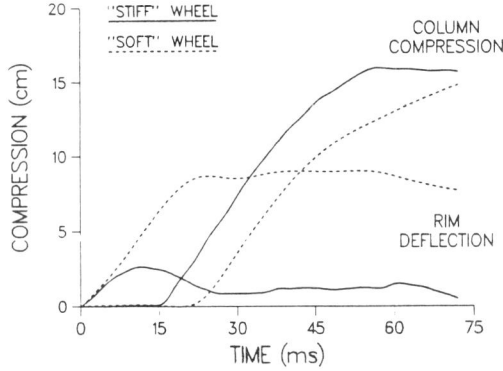

Fig. 10 Column compression and rim deflection (relative to wheel hub) measured in the direction of the column axis as a function of time from rim contact.

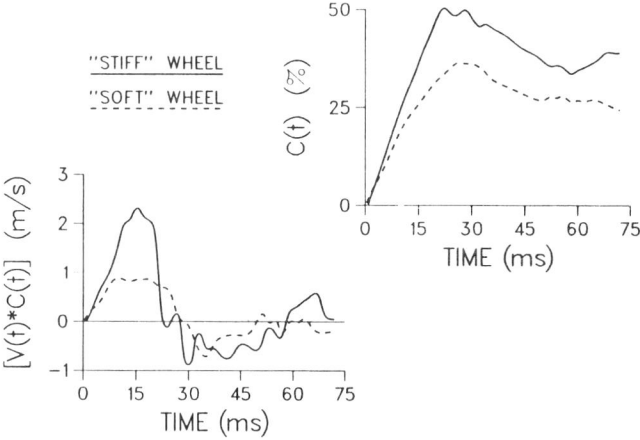

Fig. 11 Abdominal compression normalized by initial anterior-posterior thickness at contact location and the derived "viscous" response $[V(t)*C(t)]$ as a function of time from rim contact.

tion between abdominal injury and maximum upper or lower spinal acceleration (measured directly opposite to the impact site) nor with maximum sternal acceleration, or arterial or venous pressure. This suggests that dummy injury assessment for abdominal loading by the steering system should be based on measurement of the abdominal deformation as a function of time.

DISCUSSION

TEST ENVIRONMENT - A wide range of occupant alignments and impact severities and directions relative to the steering assembly occur in car crashes. Variations in vehicle design, vehicle crash kinematics, and vehicle crush all affect loading conditions for the occupant. Human factors such as occupant size, seating position, posture and reactions to an imminent crash provide additional variation. The response of the steering assembly strongly depends on impact severity and occupant alignment (5,6). The test environment in this study was chosen to focus on abdominal loading by the lower rim. The torso of the surrogate was upright with slight forward bowing before contact. This alignment of the surrogate to the steering assembly promotes interaction of the lower rim with the abdomen by delaying the contact between the hub and the thorax. Such an impact environment should be considered as one of various possibilities, depending on factors such as the knee impact with the vehicle interior. The test results were independent of the sled acceleration vs. time profiles because test velocity was reached prior to abdominal compression. The test severity provided a range of injury outcomes depending on the steering assembly parameters.

TEST SUBJECT - The 50-Kg swine was chosen for these experiments because we needed a physiological model which offered a good approximation of human function and size. At the midsternum and the impact site, the anterior-posterior dimensions of the experimental model were 27.2 ± 1.7 cm and 26.3 ± 1.5 cm, respectively. That compares favorably with similar dimensions of a 50th percentile male. The subject mass also approximated that of a 50th percentile anthropomorphic dummy interacting with the steering system. Slightly greater column compression occurred with the test subjects than for a seated Hybrid III dummy in a similar sled exposure, suggesting a slightly greater effective mass for the swine. The pelvic structure of the swine differs from that of the human and cannot be restrained similarly by a lap belt. The swine also lacks human-like knees which interact with the instrument panel and help to restrain the occupant in a crash. In a previous study where lap belts were used on swine (22), fatal abdominal injury resulted from belt loading. In the present study, we used an independent belt around each leg which restrained the lower torso with no abdominal loading. Together with the special adaptational support for the vertically suspended quadruped, the swine appears to be a good injury model for upper-abdominal loading by the rim under these controlled conditions. The swine was successfully used as an injury model for the torso in previous impact studies (12-16). One other study suggested that the swine was an unsuitable surrogate because of inconsistent hardware performance (22), a problem not encountered in our study.

INFLUENCE OF STEERING SYSTEM PARAMETERS - Among the steering wheel parameters, wheel stiffness had the greatest influence on the severity of abdominal injury. The spoke vertical configuration represents a stiffer contact interface than the spoke across configuration (Fig. 3) but no difference in injury was observed. The spoke vertical configuration of the "stiff" wheel had a greater abdominal contact area on impact, abdominal loading was distributed on the rim and the spoke, whereas it was concentrated on the rim in the spoke across configuration. Therefore, the effects of increased wheel stiffness and increased contact area may have compensated for each other in the spoke vertical configuration. The greater interaction force over a larger contact area resulted in no apparent difference in abdominal injury or kinematics. Spoke position did not affect the extent of wheel deformation, another indication of a compensating mechanism.

Column angle had no measurable influence on injury outcome for the "stiff" wheel -- all subjects had an AIS 5 liver injury. However, column angle appears to be a factor for the "soft" wheel tests -- at least on an AIS basis. AIS increases from 0 for no injury to 4 for any liver laceration but can be no greater than 5 for extensive liver laceration. Thus AIS is not a sensitive indicator of the extent of liver laceration. The number of liver lacerations does not suggest a strong correlation of injury with column angle. The loading severities represented by the "stiff" and "soft" wheels are near the injury extremes. Analysis of the influence of other factors might be more meaningful at an intermediate loading severity.

ABDOMINAL PROTECTION MECHANICS - The respective kinematics of the "stiff"- and "soft"-wheel tests explain the reduced abdominal compression and rates of compression and thus the reduced "viscous" response and injury by the "soft" wheel. There was no column compression and rearward displacement of the spine until after 15 ms of abdominal contact by the lower rim of the wheel. For that 15 ms, only the wheel or the abdomen could deform to account for the instantaneous sled displacement. Since the "soft" wheel deformed significantly more than the "stiff" wheel (Fig. 10) the instantaneous abdominal compression and velocity of compression (Fig. 11) were similarly reduced in the "soft"-wheel tests. Even the "stiff" wheel had appreciable deformation at this time; and an increase in wheel stiffness further exacerbates abdominal injury as exhibited by the "rigid" wheel test. We observed that the maximum "viscous" response occurred before column compression initiated, and hypothesize that liver injury is occurring before column compression. Thus abdominal protection must be provided by steering wheel characteristics.

In our test environment, the lower rim contacted the abdomen before the hub contacted the thorax. Column compression and significant whole body motions were associated with the greater force due to thoracic loading. A wheel with a deep dish would delay thoracic contact and might increase the potential for abdominal compression. Occupant alignment with the steering wheel at contact is an important parameter.

In our tests abdominal compression by the rim did not produce sufficient force to cause column compression. If column compression force is reduced to protect the abdomen from rim loading, the column would have a significantly lower energy absorbing capacity than it has today which would affect the higher severity collision protection of drivers well-aligned with the steering wheel. Severe frontal crashes require high energy absorption capacity which implies high column compression forces. Thus the wheel, not the column, is probably the steering system component best suited to limit compression of the abdomen. For our test situation and results, the data suggest that the rim and spoke should deform before sufficient force is developed to produce a high level of "viscous" response and abdominal compression. However, the test environment represents only one of many occupant interaction configurations. Thus, other loading conditions and body regions should be considered in a full analysis of occupant protection provided by the steering system.

ACKNOWLEDGMENTS

Many persons have contributed to the reported study. In particular the authors express appreciation to Donald Barker, Mary Foster, Richard Gasper, Gerald Horn, Edward Jedrzejczak, Joseph McCleary and Kathleen Smiler for their technical support and contributions.

REFERENCES

1. C. J. Kahane, "An evaluation of federal motor vehicle safety standards for passenger car steering assemblies," DOT HS-805 705, National Highway Traffic Safety Administration, Washington, DC, 1981.
2. A. C. Malliaris, R. Hitchcock, and J. Hedlund, "A search for priorities in crash protection," SAE Paper 820242, 1982.
3. A. C. Malliaris, R. Hitchcock, and M. Hansen, "Harm causation and ranking in car crashes," SAE Paper 850090, 1985.
4. S. Parks, "Relative risk of driver and right front passenger injury in frontal crashes," GMR-4802, August 3, 1984, Transportation Research Dept., General Motors Research Laboratories.
5. J. D. Horsch, K. R. Petersen, and D. C. Viano, "Laboratory study of factors influencing the performance of energy absorbing steering systems," SAE Paper 820475 (SP-507), 1982.
6. J. D. Horsch and C. C. Culver, "The role of steering wheel structure in the performance of energy absorbing steering systems," SAE Paper 831607, 1983.
7. J. D. Horsch and D. C. Viano, "Influence of the surrogate in laboratory evaluation of energy-absorbing steering systems, SAE Paper 841660, 1984.
8. J. W. Garrett and D. L. Hendricks, "Factors influencing the performance of energy absorbing steering columns in accidents," Fifth International Technical Conference on Experimental Safety Vehicles, 1974.
9. P. F. Gloyn and G. M. Mackay, "Impact performance of some designs of steering assembly in real accidents and under test conditions," Proceedings of 18th Stapp Car Crash Conference, SAE, 1974.
10. D. F. Huelke, "Steering assembly performance and driver injury severity in frontal crashes," SAE Paper 820474, 1982.
11. C. W. Gadd and L. M. Patrick, "System versus laboratory impact tests for estimating injury hazard," SAE Report 680053, 1968.
12. J. P. Verriest, A. Chapon, and R. Trauchesses, "Cinophotogrammetrical study of procine thoracic response to belt applied load in frontal impact -- Comparison between living and dead subjects," SAE Paper 811015, 1981.
13. D. C. Viano, C. K. Kroell, and C. Y. Warner, "Comparative thoracic impact response of living and sacrificed porcine siblings," SAE Paper 770930, 1977.

14. D. C. Viano and C. Y. Warner, "Thoracic impact response of live porcine subjects," SAE Paper 760823, 1976.
15. M. E. Pope, C. K. Kroell, D. C. Viano, C. Y. Warner, and S. D. Allen, "Postural influences on thoracic impact," SAE Paper 791028, 1979.
16. C. K. Kroell, M. E. Pope, D. C. Viano, C. Y. Warner, and S. D. Allen, "Interrelationship of velocity and chest compression in blunt thoracic impact," SAE Paper 811016, 1981.
17. D. C. Viano and V. K. Lau, "Role of impact velocity and chest compression in thoracic injury," Journal of Aviation, Space and Environmental Medicine, 54(1):16-21, January, 1983.
18. V. K. Lau and D. C. Viano, "Influence of impact velocity and chest compression on experimental pulmonary injury severity in an animal model," Journal of Trauma, 21(12), December, 1981.
19. D. C. Viano and I. V. Lau, "Thoracic impact: A viscous tolerance criteria," 1985 NHTSA Symposium on Experimental Safety Vehicles, Oxford, England, June 1985.
20. S. W. Rouhana, I. V. Lau, and S. A. Ridella, "Influence of velocity and forced compression on the severity of abdominal injury in blunt, nonpenetrating lateral impact," Journal of Trauma, 25(6), 1985.
21. V. K. Lau and D. C. Viano, "Influence of impact velocity on the severity of nonpenetrating hepatic injury," Journal of Trauma, 21(2):115-123, February, 1981.
22. R. G. Snyder, J. W. Young, and M. Q. Doyle, "Biomechanical evaluation of steering wheel design," SAE Paper 820478, 1982.
23. V. K. Lau and D. C. Viano, "An experimental study of hepatic injury from belt-restraint loading," Journal of Aviation, Space and Environmental Medicine, 52(10):611-617, October, 1981.

851737

Thoraco-Abdominal Response to Steering Wheel Impacts

Guy S. Nuscholtz, Patricia S. Kaiker, Donald F. Huelke, and Bryan R. Suggitt
TRI

ABSTRACT

Mechanisms of thoraco-abdominal trauma were investigated utilizing unembalmed, repressurized human cadavers subjected to frontal impact with a steering wheel assembly. The focus of this research program was on trauma to the soft-tissue organs surrounded by the thoracic cage, as well as on the kinematic response of the thoracic cage. The results are compared to other thoraco-abdominal research programs conducted at the University of Michigan Transportation Research Institute (UMTRI) during the last eight years.

INJURIES TO THE THORACO-ABDOMINAL ORGANS AND VESSELS follow head injuries as the second most frequent cause of death [29][1]. Of these, injuries to the spleen or liver and their vessels are especially significant.

One of the most common physiological responses to blunt abdominal impact is hypovolemic shock due to the laceration of blood vessels, and subsequent intraperitoneal bleeding [62]. A wide range of hepatic injuries have been clinically observed and defined. At one extreme are complex rupture injuries of the hepatic parenchyma and laceration of the hepatic and portal veins. These injuries are almost invariably associated with shock at the time of initial presentation and are generally fatal [45]. In contrast, some AIS 2-3 hepatic lacerations stop bleeding by the time of operation [1,62].

The extensive literature on abdominal trauma addresses many of the mechanical and physiological processes that take place during blunt impact to the thorax-abdomen, yet still leaves many questions unanswered [1-97]. Living human response to abdominal blunt impact has been modelled with both cadaver and animal surrogates [45,83].

In one study of hepatic injury in which cadaver livers were injected with barium to reproduce their vertura turgor and then dropped from varying heights, the results showed that 0.3 N-M of energy produced capsular tears and 2.8-3.4 N-M were needed to produce bursting injuries [45]. Apparently, turgidity in ex-vivo livers significantly influences injury [45]. Isolated, perfused ex-vivo non-human primate livers have been subjected to controlled blunt impact and the results compared to those produced by blunt upper and lower abdominal impact [85]. To produce an AIS 3 liver injury in an intact animal, 3.3 N-M of energy was needed, while only 1.4 N-M was needed to produce a similar injury in the directly exposed liver [85]. As might be expected, when impact was directed to the lower abdomen, much higher forces were necessary to create a liver injury similar in severity to that produced by upper abdominal impact [63]. Longitudinal lacerations of the liver were associated with liver displacement in both the medial-lateral (right-left) and inferior-superior directions [62] without severe thoracic compression. During impacts of 12 ms duration or less, the hepatic system was observed to act as a deformable structure with little response attributable to rigid body motion, and AIS-rated degree of injury was lower in unrepressurized postmortem subjects than in live, anesthetized animal subjects [62].

This paper reports the findings of a biomechanics laboratory research program which investigated the response of the thoraco-abdominal system to frontal impact. Mechanisms of hepatic trauma were investigated using 8

---

[1] Numbers in parentheses denote references at end of paper.

unembalmed, repressurized human cadavers[2], subjected to impacts by a steering wheel assembly. The results were compared to other thoraco-abdominal research programs conducted at UMTRI during the past eight years [62,63,74].

METHODOLOGY

The instrumented, repressurized stationary test subject was struck by a steering wheel assembly affixed to a 65 kg moving mass impactor at velocities up to 11 m/s. Six accelerometers affixed to the skull and eighteen accelerometers mounted on the thoracic skeletal system documented impact response. Vascular pressure in the descending aorta was measured. In addition, gross whole body motion was recorded through the use of high-speed photokinemetrics. String-pot transducers measured displacement at four points on the steering wheel rim and at one point on the test subject (at T12 thoracic vertebra). Injury/damage was assessed by gross autopsy.

The results are presented in the form of time-histories of the kinematic variables (accelerations, forces, velocities, displacements, pressures, auto- and cross correlations). Impact transfer functions are also presented in terms of mechanical impedance, as well as transfer functions between paired kinematic variables. Force deflection characteristics of the thorax-abdomen under different loading conditions are presented and the limitations of this type of data are discussed.

<u>Anatomical Considerations</u> - Important anatomical considerations pertinent to thoraco abdominal biomechanics research are discussed elsewhere [32]. A brief summary follows.

The torso, between the base of the neck and the hip joint area, includes the thorax above and the abdominal-pelvic region below. The abdomen and the pelvic cavities, although frequently described separately, are continuous from one to another, with bony landmarks used as reference points to separate the two.

Extending between the stomach and the liver is a very thin filamentous peritoneal layer, the gastro-hepatic ligament. At its lower free end this peritoneal sheet surrounds the blood vessels that pass to and from the liver, the associated autonomic nerves, and the common bile duct. This portion of the gastro-hepatic ligament actually attaches to the upper portion of the duodenum and is most properly termed the "hepato-duodenal" ligament. It extends from the hilum--the entranceway to the liver, to the posterior body wall at the right side of the vertebral column near where the duodenum is affixed against the posterior body wall.

The liver is a solid blood-filled organ which represents approximately 1/40th of the total body weight. It is located in the upper-right quadrant of the abdomen and is firmly attached to the underside of the diaphragm by very short reflections of the peritoneum covering the liver, the liver capsule. These thin peritoneal attachments are less than a centimeter long, adhering directly to the undersurface of the diaphragm. With the rise and fall of the right dome of the diaphragm during respiration, the liver moves in synchrony with breathing. Anteriorly, laterally, and posteriorly, the lower ribs cover a major portion of the liver.

The spleen is a very small blood-filled organ about the size of a fist, which lies against the posterior body wall on the diaphragm at the 9th, 10th and 11th rib level. It is

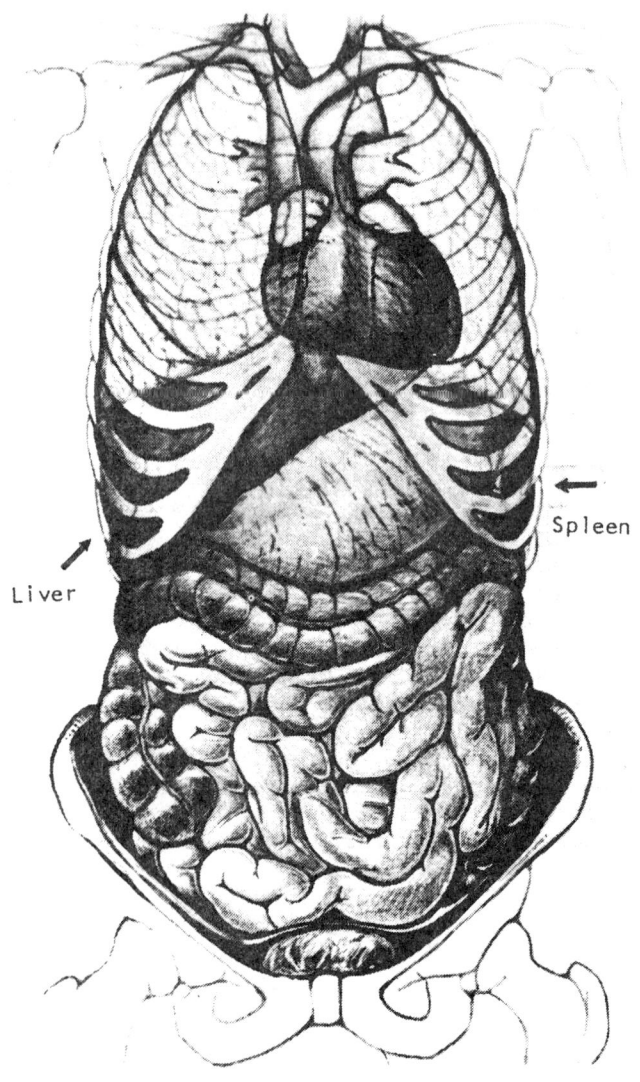

Figure 1. Position of Liver and Spleen and Associated Organs with Respect to Thoracic Cage

---

[2]The protocol for the use of cadavers in this study was approved by the University of Michigan Medical Center and followed guidelines established by the U.S. Public Health Service and recommended by the National Academy of Sciences, National Research Council.

basically free to move, as it possesses an encapsulation of peritoneum. All of its blood vessels enter and leave the spleen through the hilum, which is attached to the posterior body wall.

Both the liver and spleen are anatomically considered abdominal organs. However, from an anterior view, the liver is almost completely housed and protected by the lower ribs (see Figure 1). The spleen lies similarly housed in the lower left posterior rib area. Thus, functionally, in an impact event, the liver and the spleen react as thoracic soft-tissue organs protected by the rib cage rather than as abdominal organs. Not infrequently, impacts to the lower rib cage will cause the underlying liver to rupture. Similarly, impacts to the left side, especially the left lower posterior rib area, will rupture the spleen. A further detailed description of thoracic and abdominal anatomy and common injuries can be found in [31].

IMPACT METHODOLOGY

A test series using unembalmed, repressurized cadavers was conducted to investigate thoraco-abdominal impact response and kinematics secondary to steering wheel impact in the laboratory setting. The impactor, the UMTRI pneumatic impact device, accelerated a 65 kg free-traveling ballistic pendulum which was fitted with a steering wheel assembly. A load cell was affixed to the steering column to measure the axial steering wheel assembly force. In addition, string pot transducers mounted at four points on the steering wheel, at one point on the ballistic pendulum, and at one point on the twelfth thoracic vertebra of the test subject recorded displacements. The test subject was instrumented with 6 accelerometers rigidly affixed to the head and 18 accelerometers affixed to the thoracic skeleton. Tests were controlled by an electronic timing device and gross kinematic motion was documented on high-speed film. Induced injury/damage was assessed by gross autopsy.

<u>UMTRI Pneumatic Ballistic Pendulum Impact Device</u> - The impact device consisted of either a 25 or 65 kg ballistic pendulum mechanically coupled to the UMTRI pneumatic impact device (cannon) which was used as the energy source. The cannon consisted of an air reservoir and a ground and honed cylinder with a carefully fitted metal-alloy piston. The piston was connected to the ballistic pendulum with a nylon cable. The piston (Figure 2) was propelled by compressed air through the cylinder from the air

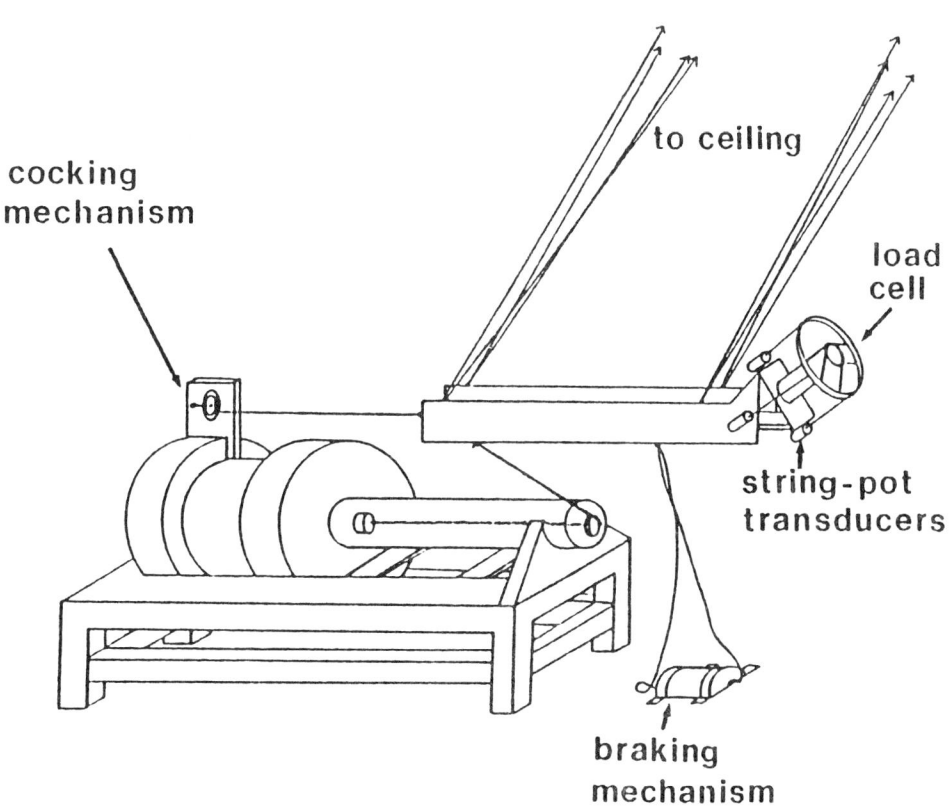

Figure 2. Pneumatic Ballistic Impact Device - test configuration

reservoir chamber, accelerating the ballistic pendulum to become a free-traveling impactor. The ballistic pendulum was fitted with an inertia-compensated load cell which was rigidly mounted to a steering wheel (Figure 3 A,B).

The steering wheel angle (defined as the angle formed between a vertical line and a line tangent to the top and bottom of the steering wheel) could be changed in 5° increments in a

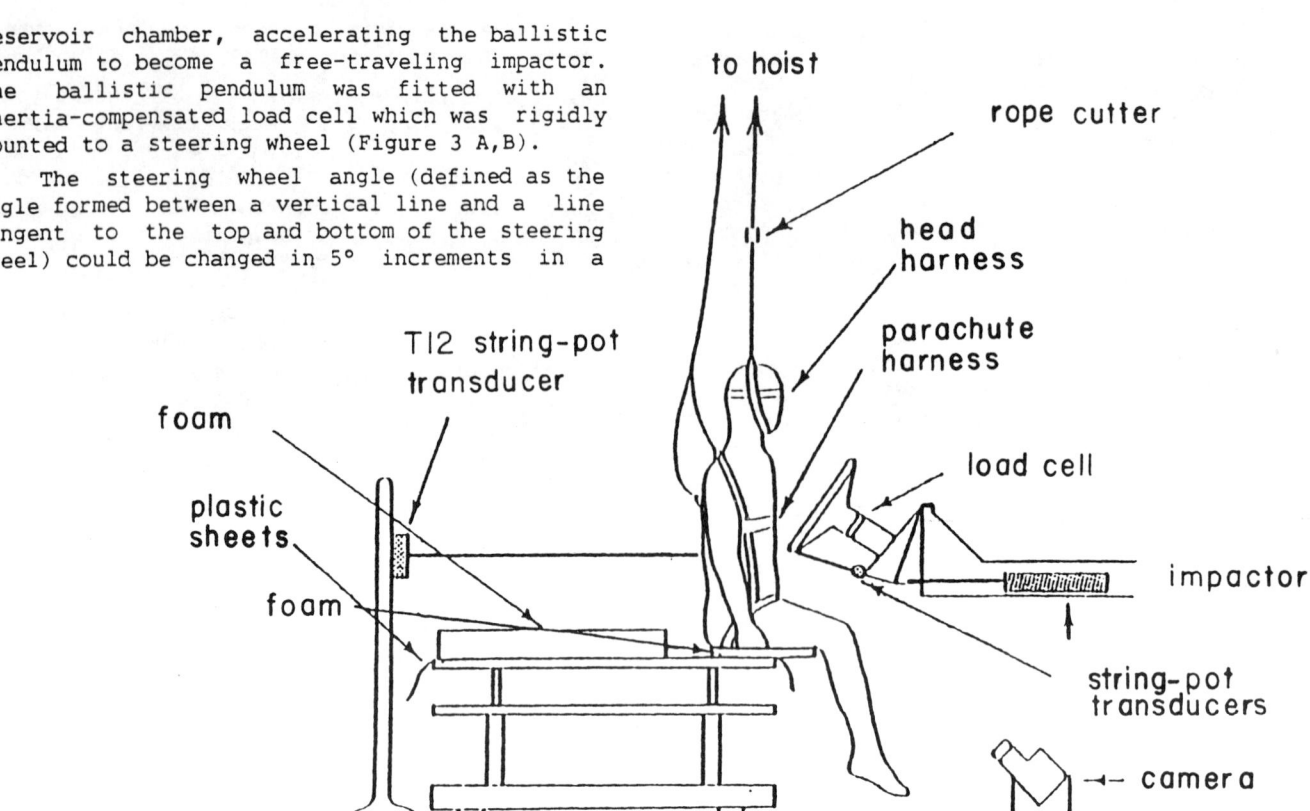

Figure 3A. Impact test setup

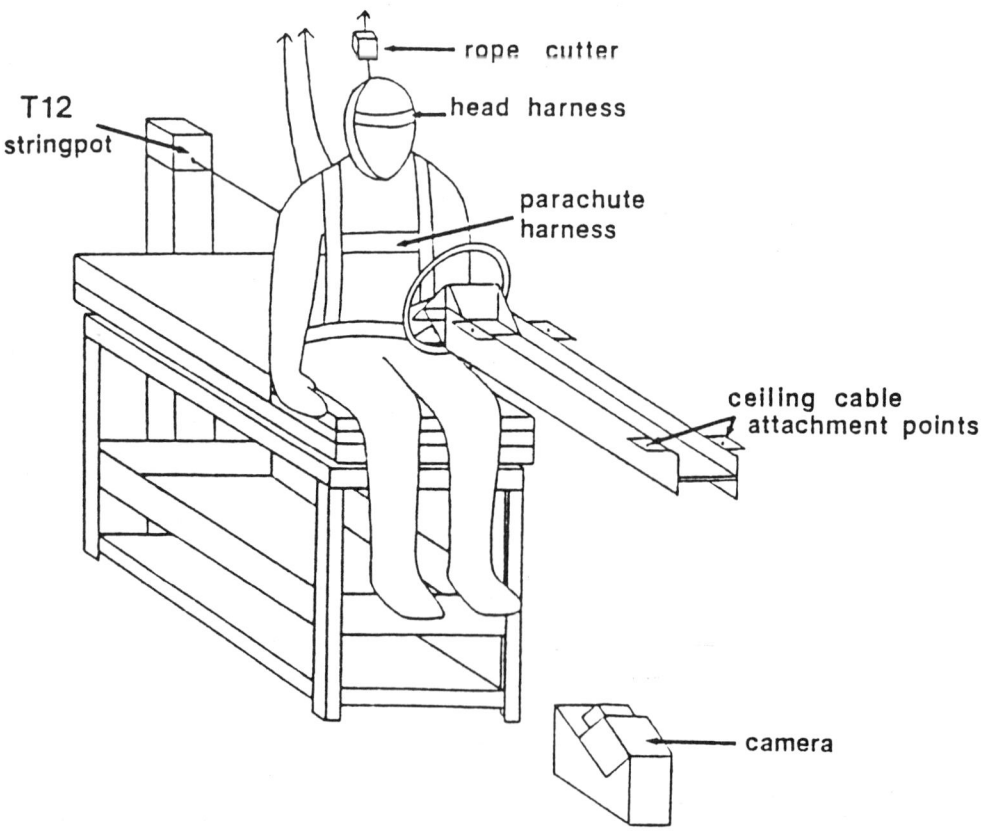

Figure 3B. Isometric view test setup

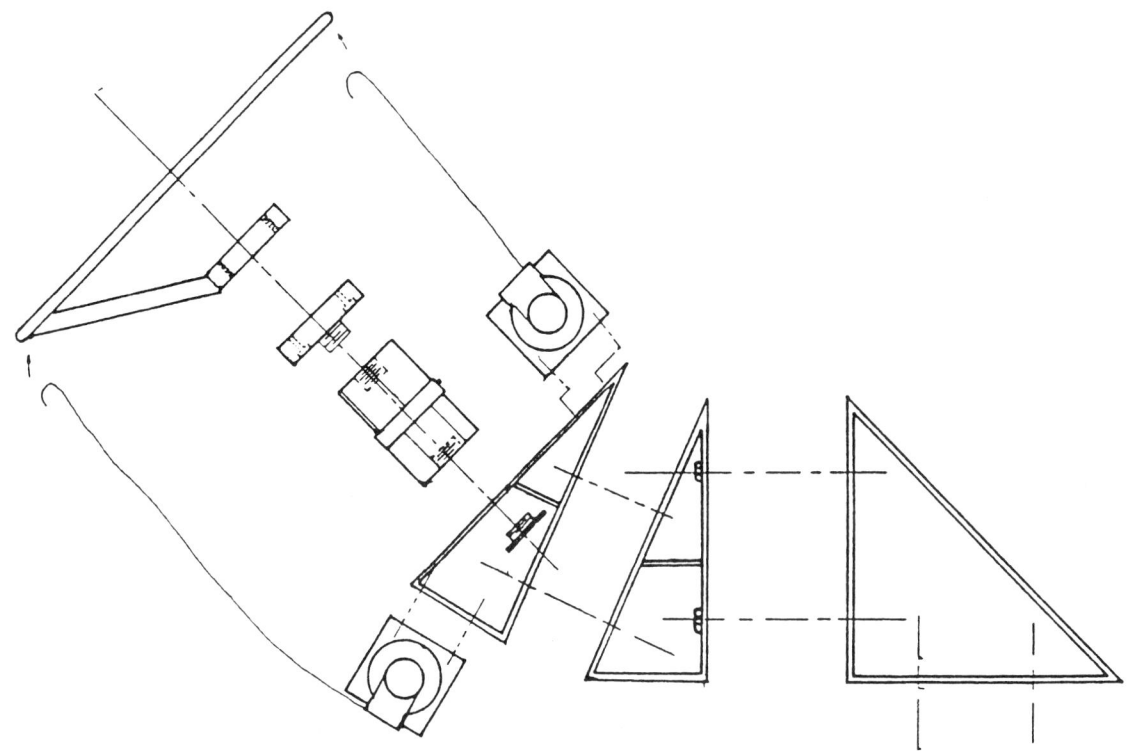

Figure 4. Steering Wheel Mounting System
Wedges of different sizes can be inserted to vary
steering wheel angle in 5 degree increments.

range of 0°-45°. Either a 1981 Chevrolet Citation or 1979 Ford Mustang steering wheel was used. (See Figure 4.)

Subjects

The unembalmed cadavers used in these tests were obtained from the University of Michigan Department of Anatomy and stored in coolers at 4° centigrade. The cadaver was X-rayed as part of the structural evaluation for possible pre-test damage and surgical implants. Anthropomorphic measurements were taken. The cadaver was then sanitarily and surgically prepared, dressed in a vinyl and cotton outfit, and fitted with head and parachute harnesses (Figure 3).

In the impact laboratory, accelerometers, pressure transducers and phototargets were attached. The subject was placed in a seated position on a mobile adjustable-height table covered with friction-reducing clear plastic sheets, and supported via a ceiling mounted rope cutter by the head and parachute harnesses. The lower aspect of the rim of the steering wheel was positioned for impact 11 cm below the sternum (substernale).

Vascular Repressurization

The subject's abdominal vascular system was repressurized just prior to impact. A Kulite pressure transducer guided through the carotid artery, and positioned in the descending aorta just below the diaphragm, monitored both the degree of initial pressurization and the change in the vascular system pressure during impact. The pressurizing fluid was introduced via the catheters through a channel in the center of the two occluding balloons. Both balloons were positioned in the aorta, one above the diaphragm, the other above the aortic termination.

Surgical insertion of the modified catheters followed three patterns depending on whether access through the femoral arteries was possible. Through an incision in the femoral artery, a catheter was guided up the arterial system, where the balloon occluded the aortic termination. Another catheter was guided through an incision in the common carotid artery into the descending aorta, occluding it slightly above the diaphragm. When the femoral arteries could not be used, due to plaque accumulation, either a double balloon catheter was used to occlude the aorta below the diaphragm and at the common iliac arteries, or two catheters, one in each common carotid artery were used to occlude these same locations. Critical to the study was that the liver be fluid-filled before impact [45]. This was done by pressurizing the area between the two occluding balloons above normal physiological pressure. One to two minutes before impact the pressure was pulsed between 100-200 mm Hg. Immediately prior to impact the pressure was dropped to 70 mm Hg. Although it was clear from inspection of the abdominal organs at autopsy that these organs had been profused with black ink, it was not clear how much of the turgor that might have been lost due to the post-mortem state returned.

Pulmonary Repressurization - A tracheotomy was performed to place in the trachea a tube which was connected to a compressed air reservoir, so that the pulmonary system could be pressurized to 15 mm Hg. An Endevco pressure transducer was inserted into the tracheal tube to measure the dynamic pulmonary pressure at initial pressurization and during the change in pressure throughout the impact. The trachea tube was fitted with a valve such that direct communication between the lungs and the outside air was possible just before impact.

Acceleration Measurement - Triaxial accelerometer clusters, affixed to the head and thoracic skeleton, documented the kinematic response of the subject. A pair of triaxial accelerometer clusters was attached to a mounting plate on the subject's head. The thoracic skeleton was instrumented with 18 accelerometers such that the triaxes were rigidly attached to the lateral flat portions of the right and left eighth ribs (R8R and R8L), the lower sternum, and the thoracic vertebrae T1 and T12. Single accelerometers were affixed to the upper sternum and to the left and right fourth ribs (Figure 5).

Surgical Instrumentation of Accelerometer Mounts - For the head mount, several metal self-tapping screws were threaded directly into the right parietal and occipital bones of the skull through small pilot holes. Dental acrylic was molded around the screws to serve as a medium for rigid attachment of the plate to the skull. Two triaxial accelerometer clusters were then attached to the plate.

Skin incisions exposed the attachment points on the upper and lower sternum. Small nails placed in the exposed sternum formed a mooring for the dental acrylic which was used as a securing medium for the accelerometer mounts. For rib mounts, incisions were made over the fourth and eighth ribs on each lateral side so that the flat part of the rib was exposed. To ensure rigidity, the mounts were fitted with pins and tied with wire to the flat surface of each exposed rib.

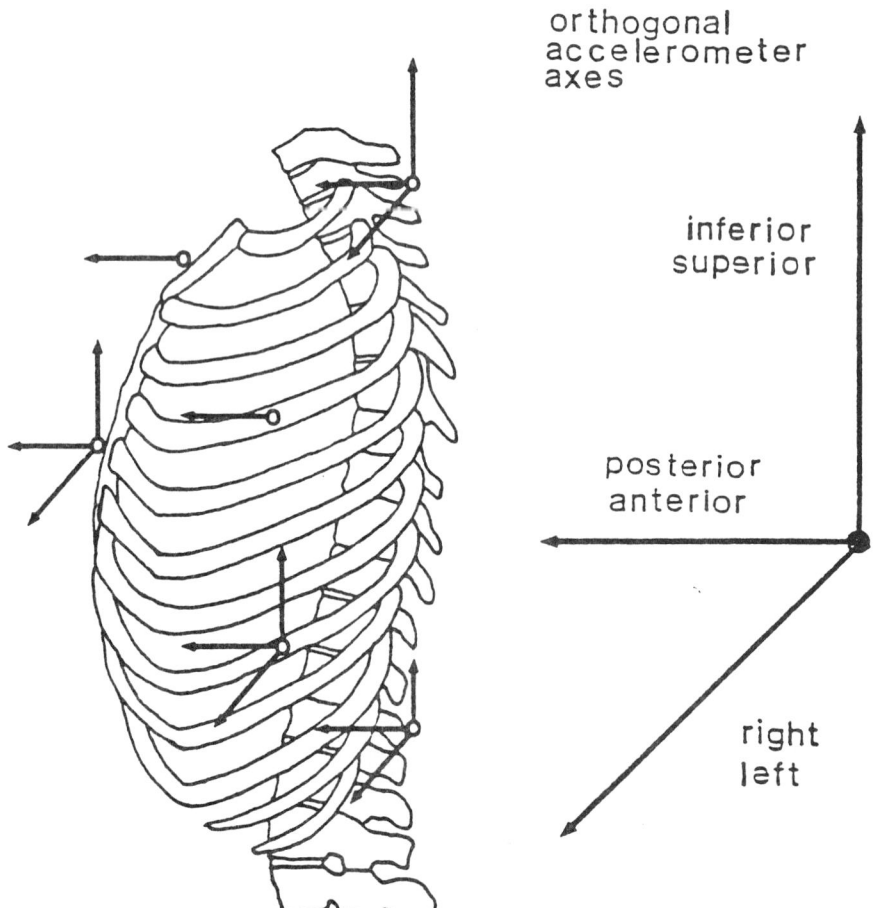

Figure 5. Location of thoracic accelerometers
Arrows represent the sensitive axis for the accelerometers for both uniaxes and triaxes.

For the T1 and T12 spinal mounts, deep incisions were made so that lateral supports for the accelerometer mounts were anchored on the lamina bilaterally. Acrylic was applied under and around the mounts to ensure rigidity.

METHOD OF ANALYSIS - The techniques used to analyze the results are outlined below. Additional information can be found in [62,63].

Frame Fields - As the thorax moves through space, any point on the thorax generates a path in space. In thorax injury research one is interested in the description of the path of instrumented points on the thorax and events which occur as these points move. A very effective tool for analyzing the motion of each point, as it moves along a curved path in space, is the concept of a moving frame. The path generated as the point travels through space is a function of time and velocity. A vector field is a function which assigns a uniquely defined vector to each point along a path. Thus, any collection of three mutually orthogonal unit vectors defined on a path is a frame field. Therefore, any vector defined on the path (for example, acceleration) may be resolved into three orthogonal components of any well-defined frame field, such as the laboratory or anatomical reference frames.

In biomechanics research, frame fields are defined based on anatomical reference frames. Other frame fields such as the Frenet-Serret frame or the Principal Direction Triad, which contain information about the motion embedded in the frame field, have also been used to describe motion resulting from impact.

Principal Direction - One method of determining the principal direction of motion and constructing the Principal Direction Triad is to determine the direction of the acceleration vector in the moving frame of the triaxial accelerometer cluster and then describe the transformation necessary to obtain a new moving frame that would have one of its axes in the principal direction. A single point in time at which the acceleration was a maximum is chosen to define the directional cosines for transforming from the triax frame to a new frame in such a way that the resultant acceleration vector (AR) and the "principal" unit vector (A1) are co-directional. This then was used to construct a new frame rigidly fixed to the triax, but differing from the original by an initial rotation. After completing the necessary transformation, a comparison between the magnitude of the principal direction and the resultant acceleration is performed.

Transfer Function Analysis - For blunt impacts in biomechanical systems using human surrogates, the relationship between a transducer time-history at a given point and the transducer time-history at another given point can be described in the frequency domain through the use of a transfer function. A fast Fourier transformation of simultaneously monitored time-histories from any two points in the system can be used to define a frequency response function relating the two points. In a case relating a force to a pressure, a transformation of the form:

$$X(iw) = F[F(t)]/F[P(t)]$$

can be obtained from the transformed quantities $F[F(t)]$ and $F[P(t)]$, the Fourier transforms of the impact force time-history and the pressure time-history, respectively where w is the given frequency and i implies the complex domain.

The transfer function is a complex-valued function which may be described by its magnitude and phase angle. A special form of the transfer function which relates impact force to the resulting velocity of a point is mechanical impedance, defined as:

$$Z(iw) = (w)F[F(t)]/F[A(t)]$$

for which w is the chosen frequency and $F[F(t)]$ and $F[A(t)]$ are Fourier transforms of the impact force and acceleration at the point of interest. Mechanical transfer impedance can also be defined as the ratio between simple harmonic driving force and the corresponding velocity at the point of interest [27].

Correlation Functions - To describe some of the fundamental properties of a time-history, such as acceleration or force, two types of statistical measures were used:
1. Auto-correlation Function. This measure is the correlation between two points on a time-history and is a measure of the dependence of the amplitude at time t_1.
2. Cross-correlation Function. This is a measure of how predictable, on the average, a signal (transducer time-history) at any particular moment in time is from a second signal at any other particular moment in time.

The auto-correlation function is formally defined as the average over the ensemble of the product of two amplitudes:

$$R_x(t_1,t_2) = \int_{-\infty}^{+\infty}\int_{-\infty}^{+\infty} x_1 \cdot x_2 \cdot P(x_1,x_2,t_1,t_2)\, dx_1 \cdot dx_2$$

where x_1, x_2 are the amplitudes of the time-history and $p(x_1,x_2,t_1,t_2)$ is the joint probability density. Normally the above definition cannot be used to generate an auto-correlation function directly. However, it can be shown that for a discrete time-history of a finite duration, a close approximation of the auto-correlation function can be obtained through the use of a Fourier transform [27].

In addition to auto-correlation, cross-correlation can be used to obtain useful information about the relationship between two different time-histories. For example, the cross-correlation between acceleration measurements at two different points of a material body may be determined for the purpose of studying the propagation of differential motion through the material body as well as load paths. Cross-correlation functions are not restricted to correlation of parameters with the same physical units; for example, one might determine the cross-correlation between the applied force and the acceleration response to that force. Similar to the auto-correlation function, the calculation of the cross-correlation of two signals begins by taking the Fourier transform of both time histories (Y_1, Y_2). The cross-spectral density is the complex-valued function (Y_1, Y_2). The cross-correlation is then the Fourier transform of the cross-spectral density [27].

Force Time-History Determination - In general the force-time histories were unimodal with a single maximum, smoothly rising, peaking and then falling. Force duration was determined using a boundary defining and least-squares straight-line fitting technique. This procedure began by determining the peak, or the first peak in the case of a bimodal waveform. Next, the left half of the pulse, defined from the point where the pulse started to rise to the time of peak, was least-squares fitted with a straight line. This rise line intersected the time axis at a point which was taken as the formal beginning of the pulse. A similar procedure was followed for the right half of this pulse, i.e., a least-squares straight line was fitted to the fall section of the pulse, which was defined from the peak to the point where the pulse minimum occurred. The point where this line intersected the time axis became the formal end of the pulse.

Force Deflection Measurement - String pot transducers were used to measure pendulum displacement, displacement of four points on the steering wheel rim located 90° apart, and displacement of a point on the subject's spine located at T12, which was opposite the lowest point on the steering wheel rim. The impactor force transducer assembly consisted of a piezoelectric load washer with a piezoelectric accelerometer mounted internally for inertial compensation. The uniaxial load cell was located on a rigid column directly behind the steering wheel hub. Deflection was obtained by appropriate addition of displacement signals obtained from the stringpot transducers, as well as from observed high-speed photokinematics. In several tests, the position of the steering wheel with respect to the test subject had the lower rim positioned just below the liver. This was accomplished through the use of pre-test in-place X-rays.

RESULTS

The data are presented in abbreviated form to show those trends which are felt to be representative of important factors in thoraco-abdominal impact response. Examples of raw transducer time-histories, auto- and cross-correlations, mechanical impedance, transfer functions and power spectrum are presented in the Appendix. In the accelerometer time-histories, the principal direction acceleration is A1, the secondary direction A2, and the tertiary A3.

Table 1 lists the Cadaver Steering Wheel Impact Injuries. Injuries that are classified as contusions are either extravasation of blood, repressurization fluid or a combination of both. Table 2 lists the Kinematic Test Summary. Table 3 lists velocities, pendulum mass and type of steering wheel.

DISCUSSION

The results presented in this paper on thoraco-abdominal impact response are from a research program conducted during the past two years. The mechanisms of injury associated with damage to the liver as well as the kinematic response of the thoracic cage and associated abdominal soft tissue were investigated using unembalmed repressurized cadavers subjected to steering wheel impacts. The data are presented in abbreviated form to show those trends that are felt to be representative of important factors in thoraco-abdominal impact response. Examples of the raw and processed data are presented in the Appendix. Comparisons are made between the results presented in this paper and the results of several other thoraco-abdominal research programs conducted at UMTRI over the last eight years [61-63].

The response of the thorax of a repressurized cadaver to direct loading from a steering wheel system was observed from: 1) the force obtained from a load cell placed directly behind the steering wheel hub, 2) accelerations obtained from the triaxial and uniaxal accelerometers fitted to the thoracic skeletal structure, 3) pressure transducers placed in the descending aorta and trachea, and 4) analysis of the high-speed photokinemetrics. The various accelerations were subsequently expressed as vectors and described in appropriate reference frames. While general trends were observed in a majority of the tests, the specific response was found to be dependent on: the impactor velocity, the impactor mass, the contact profile of the steering wheel with the thorax, as well as on the biovariablity of the population. In addition, the response of the thorax had certain characteristics in both the time and frequency domain that were similar to blunt impacts to the sternum using a flat impactor.

Table 1

CADAVER STEERING WHEEL IMPACT INJURIES

Test No.	Injuries
83E121C	Hemorrhage in diaphragm Contused spleen Hepatic vein torn 8 cm laceration at junction of major-minor lobes of liver 5 cm live tear in medial liver 1.3 cm tear in left liver Liver severed from its tethers
83E131C	Closed Fractured ribs R3L, R7L, R8L, R9L Hemorrhage left inferior pericardium Contusion in heart on right lateral side Contusion in tissue connecting esophagus-stomach Contused stomach Contused transverse colon 90% tear of disk between cervical vertebrae C6-C7 40% tear of disk between cervical vertebrae C5-C6 30% tear of disk between cervical vertebrae C4-C5 Partial tear of anterior longitudinal ligament at C5
84E142C	Closed fracture of the sternum Contusion stripes on diaphragm Hepatic vein torn Tear in liver Inferior tip of spleen torn Contused stomach Contused transverse colon
84E153C	Partial disconnection of right ribs at sternum R3R, R4R, R5R, - Mediastinal hematoma of pericardium Contused visceral surface of liver Contused transverse intestines
84E163C	Hemorrhage in fat over pericardium Contusion stripes on diaphragm Hemorrhage left kidney Ruptured, pulverized pancreas
84E173C	Closed fracture right rib R9R (twice) Fractured left ribs R8L (twice), R9L, R10L Massive hematoma in pericardium Petechial hemorrhage of diaphragm near aorta 10 cm tear in liver 4 cm tear of portal vein
84E181C	2 cm hematoma left inferior lung Severance of pericardium and diaphragm Ruptured pancreas Portal and hepatic veins torn Small laceration of liver at portal vein Contusion stripe on left kidney
85E193C	Partial tear of anterior longitudinal ligament at C7 Closed fracture of sternum at rib R5-R6 level Fractured ribs R5R (twice), R6R, R7R, R8R, R5L, R6L, R7L, R8L (twice) Contusion stripes on both lungs Small lacerations on superior surface of liver Partial tearing of portal and hepatic veins Capsular hemorrhage superior surface liver

Table 3
KINEMATIC TEST SUMMARY

Test No.	Force [N] (Time [ms])	Trachea Pressure [kPa] (Time [ms])	Aorta [kPa] (Time [ms])	A1:T1 [G] (Time [ms])	A1:T12 [G] (Time [ms])	A1:Ls [G] (Time [ms])	A1:R8R [G] (Time [ms])	A1:R8L [G] (Time [ms])	R4R [G] (Time [ms])	R4L [G] (Time [ms])
83E121-A	2000 (30)	2.1 (38)	N/A	24 (35)	19 (32)	11 (35)	16 (38)	9 (34)	3 66	N/A
83E121B	3000 (65)	4.1 (79)	N/A	29 (65)	N/A	69 (60)	42 (46)	17 (49)	23 (53)	N/A
83E121-C	10400 (11)	11 (37)	N/A	N/A	N/A	110 (26)	N/A	N/A	N/A	N/A
83E131-A	870 (87)	3.5 (75)	N/A	3 (81)	10 (109)	7 (22)	5 (57)	6 (49)	N/A	1 (44)
83E131-B	2700 (65)	6.2 (48)	N/A	14 (56)	9 (49)	27 (33)	22 (39)	47 (55)	8 (52)	7 (48)
83E131-C	4400 (51)	6.2 (48)	N/A	38 (59)	13 (71)	100 (43)	71 (40)	100 (45)	15 (56)	35 (50)
84E142-A	1800 (104)	7 (74)	11.7 (140)	6 (112)	4 (77)	6 (76)	6 (66)	6 (87)	2 (61)	1 (89)
84E142-B	3400 (68)	6.2 (64)	22 (94)	19 (105)	13 (62)	17 (45)	28 (56)	19 (49)	14 (43)	22 (72)
84E142-C	5700 (57)	14.5 (64)	102 (63)	46 (66)	30 (63)	78 (44)	48 (55)	56 (49)	31 (63)	21 (65)
84E153-A	850 (73)	2.1 (74)	79 (132)	5 (84)	5 (55)	11 (49)	7 (64)	10 (57)	3 (67)	2 (64)
84E153-B	2500 (67)	2.8 (64)	305 (64)	37 (75)	18 (69)	48 (61)	52 (61)	47 (65)	27 (66)	29 (65)
84E153-C	5400 (30)	4.1 (37)	320.6 (29)	37 (43)	16 (35)	96 (28)	70 (26)	66 (28)	14 (38)	32 (31)
84E163-A	1400 (102)	2.1 (85)	19.3 (95)	5 (98)	4 (84)	7 (76)	6 (90)	5 (77)	2 (81)	1 (80)
84E163-B	4000 (59)	.7 (85)	57.2 (87)	27 (65)	15 (56)	39 (42)	23 (52)	21 (56)	9 (48)	7 (42)
84E163-C	4900 (39)	.7 (27)	97.9 (55)	30 (40)	10 (49)	46 (30)	18 (33)	39 (30.31)	8 31	11 (36)
84E173-A	2300 (81)	10.3 (71)	N/A	9 (71)	8 (54)	N/A	N/A	N/A	N/A	N/A
84E173-B	4800 (60)	N/A	N/A	25 (55)	22 (61)	N/A	N/A	N/A	N/A	N/A
84E173-C	7400 (46)	6.9 (35)	N/A	53 (41)	32 (40)	N/A	N/A	N/A	N/A	N/A

Table 2

CADAVER STEERING WHEEL IMPACT

SUMMARY CONDITIONS

Test No.	Velocity m/s A	B	C	Steering Wheel	Pneumatic Ballistic Pendulum Mass
83E121	2.7	5	9.5	1981 C. CITATION	25 kg
83E131	2.7	5	12	1981 C. CITATION	25 kg
84E142	2.8	5.3	11.8	1981 C. CITATION	65 kg
84E153	2.7	5	11	1981 C. CITATION	65 kg
84E163	3	5	12	1979 F. MUSTANG	65 kg
84E173	2.7	4	7	1981 C. CITATION	65 kg
84E181	2.7	5.3	9.3	1981 C. CITATION	65 kg
85E193	3.6	4.4	11	1981 C. CITATION	65 kg

With the use of triaxial and uniaxal accelerometers attached to the thoracic skeletal structure, the response of the thorax was defined as a continuum of "events" characterized by the motion of the thorax as estimated by the accelerometers and the relationship of this motion to the steering wheel hub force. Examples of events which were used to characterize impact response for the force time-history were: the initiation of impact response, denoted by Q_1 (Figure 6 is an example); the positive maximum, denoted by Q_2; and the estimated end of impact, denoted by Q_3. In general, during an anterior-to-posterior direction steering wheel impact, the lower rim of the steering wheel contacted the abdomen at the Q_1 event. During the Q_1-Q_2 interval the steering wheel spokes interacted with the thoracic cage as the subject rotated forward. Finally, the hub of the steering wheel contacted the sternum close to the the Q_2 event, and the subject rotated far enough forward so that the chin protruded above the upper rim of the steering wheel, or the face contacted the rim. In general, the test subject stayed in this position for the remainder of the test. See Figure 7 for illustration of this motion.

Steering Wheel Force - The force time-histories were derived from the compensated force of the load cell positioned behind the steering wheel hub. The program consisted of three test types: low-, medium-, and high-velocity impacts to each of 8 unembalmed, repressurized cadavers. The

Table 3 (continued)

Test No.	Force [N] (Time [ms])	Trachea Pressure [kPa] (Time [ms])	Aorta [kPa] (Time [ms])	A1:T1 [G] (Time [ms])	A1:T12 [G] (Time [ms])	A1:Ls [G] (Time [ms])	A1::R8R [G] (Time [ms])	A1:R8L [G] (Time [ms])	R4R [G] (Time [ms])	R4L [G] (Time [ms])
84E181-A	2500 (80)	N/A	N/A	N/A	9 (41)	12 (42)	N/A	N/A	N/A	N/A
84E181-B	3800 (78)	N/A	N/A	N/A	21 (48)	23 (42)	N/A	N/A	N/A	N/A
84E181-C	5800 (45)	N/A	N/A	N/A	14 (41)	48 (31)	N/A	N/A	N/A	N/A
85E193-A	1300 (92)	N/A	N/A	8 (83)	3 (72)	8 (61)	N/A	N/A	N/A	N/A
85E193-B	1700 (71)	N/A	N/A	10 (74)	7 (63)	15 (38)	N/A	N/A	N/A	N/A
85E193-C	6200 (68)	N/A	N/A	35 (49)	11 (43)	77 (37)	N/A	N/A	N/A	N/A

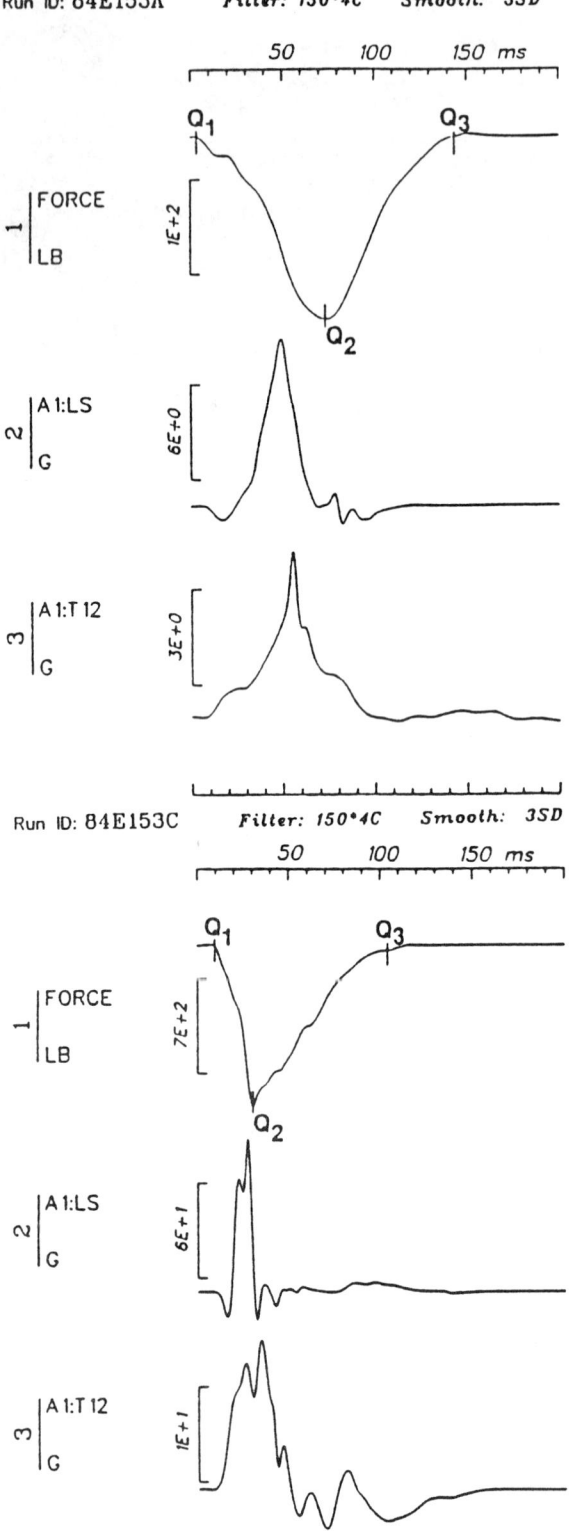
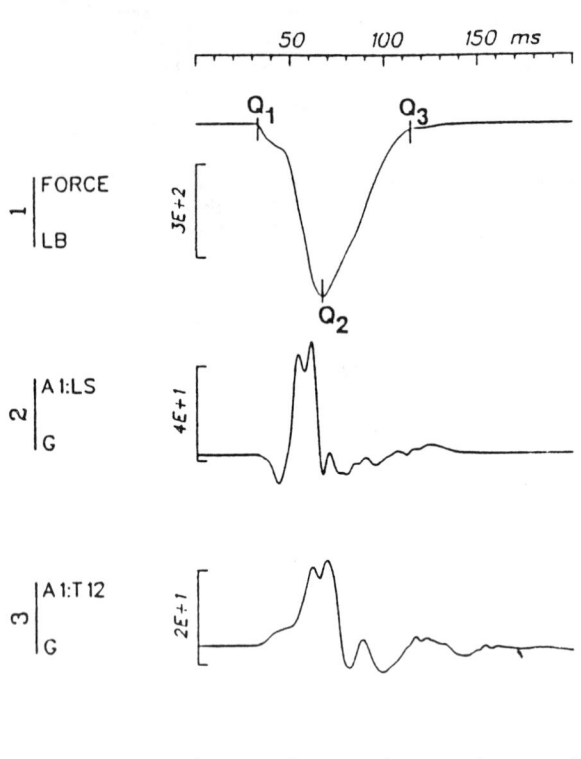

Figure 6. Graph of Force Time History Principal Direction of Acceleration for the sternum and spine.

low- and mid-velocity impacts were at non-injurious levels. The force time-histories were smooth, typically unimodal (only one significant local maximum) curves with occasional multimodal abberations (See examples given in the Appendix).

For the low-velocity impacts, the magnitude of the steering wheel hub force varied between 800 N and 2500 N, with an average value of 1600 N. In general, the Q_1-Q_2 interval was longer than the Q_2-Q_3 interval, indicating a greater rate of fall than rise. The Q_1-Q_2 interval was typically about 70 ms, with the Q_2-Q_3 interval about 50 ms. Exceptions to this general force time waveform came from the two low velocity tests in which a 25 kg impactor was used. In those cases, the Q_1-Q_2 interval and the Q_2-Q_3 interval were significantly different from the tests in which a 65 kg pendulum was used. This was consistent with observations based on the high-speed photokinemetrics. In these tests, the velocity of the pendulum during the Q_1-Q_3 interval decreased to a much greater degree than that of the 65 kg pendulum test. This phenomenon is believed to be a result of the interaction of the test subject with the pendulum in such a way that a significant percentage of the pendulum's energy was transferred to the test subject.

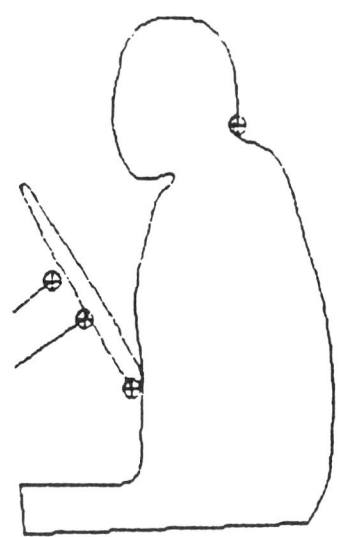 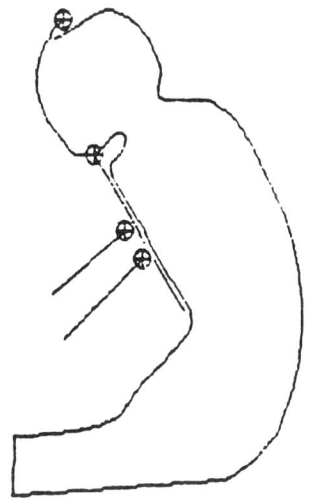

initial position   position at 50ms

Figure 7. Reconstruction of digitization of high-speed film for test 85E193-B.

For the mid-velocity impacts, the magnitude of the steering wheel hub force varied between 2500 N and 4500 N, with an average value of 3500 N. In general, the Q_1-Q_2 interval was the same as the Q_2-Q_3 interval, indicating a symmetric curve. The Q_1-Q_2 and Q_2-Q_3 intervals were about 50 ms each. Similar to the low-velocity impacts, the two tests in which the impact pendulum was of lower mass did not display a waveform similar to that of the higher mass pendulum.

For the high-velocity impacts, the magnitude of the steering wheel hub force varied between 4,500 N and 10,000 N, with an average value of 6200 N. In general, the Q_1-Q_2 interval was shorter than the Q_2-Q_3 interval, indicating a greater rate of rise than decline. The Q_1-Q_2 interval was about 30 ms, with the Q_2-Q_3 interval approximately 70 ms. Similar to the low- and mid-velocity impacts, the two tests in which the impact pendulum was of lower mass displayed a different waveform than that of higher mass pendulum impacts. The high-velocity steering wheel impact waveforms were most similar to other experiments which used a pendulum impactor with a flat surface striker [84].

Observations from the high-speed photokinemetrics, in conjunction with observations from the steering wheel hub force, indicated that for impactors using a moving pendulum, a difference existed between the flat surface impacts and the steering wheel impacts. In the steering wheel impacts the subject rotated forward (head toward the knees) in such a way that all the mass of the body trunk rested on the steering wheel (Figure 5). However, in the flat surface impacts, the impactor contacted the sternum and the subject rotated backwards (head and torso away from the knees) with a smaller portion of the body mass interacting with the pendulum. The increased effective mass of the test subject in a steering wheel impact as compared to a flat surface impact may indicate a necessity for using a heavier mass pendulum for steering wheel impacts than that used for flat surface impact to the sternum [62].

Acceleration Time-History - A comparison of the acceleration response of the thorax between the steering wheel impacts being reported here and flat surface impacts reported earlier [62] showed that steering wheel loading produced a more complex response from the thoracic skeletal structure. Differences in the waveform of the acceleration time-history, as well as the particulars of the impact conditions, limited the analysis to certain general characteristics of the response.

The gross overall motion of the thorax during steering wheel impact was, in general, three-dimensional. As the lower rim of the steering wheel penetrated the abdomen, the test subject started to rotate around the right-left axis. The thoracic cage was first deformed by the steering wheel rim near the lower ribs. Next, the thorax was deformed by the steering wheel spokes. Finally, the steering wheel hub contacted the sternum, compressing the midsection of the thorax (Figure 7). If the steering wheel deformed asymmetrically, the gross motion of the test subject moved out of the plane of the impact. Three-dimensional gross motion out of the plane impact was generally seen only in the high-velocity impacts.

In a general sense, the gross motion of the thorax in steering wheel impacts could be described for short time durations (less than 50 ms) using the principal direction acceleration triad. However, a one-dimensional acceleration description was not sufficient for description of the acceleration time-histories of several points on the thorax. This conclusion stems in part from comparison of the doubly integrated T12 acceleration as compared to the displacement obtained from film data and stringpots. After 50 ms, the acceleration time-history no longer was able to reliably predict the displacement. In addition, for triaxial accelerometers, in most cases, a secondary direction could not be found, so that no significant acceleration could be observed in the tertiary direction. In general, the response of the thorax in steering wheel impacts requires a three-dimensional description of the thoracic cage.

The results for blunt frontal thoracic impacts using a flat impactor reported [62] showed that: the magnitude of peak acceleration and the time at which the maxima occurred were found to be dependent upon the accelerometer location relative to the point of impact. The peak acceleration of a point nearest to the center of impact was typically three to four times greater in magnitude than a point furthest from impact. In addition, the relative phasing of the peak acceleration between the "sternum" and "spine" was sequential with the occurrence of the peak force.

In most tests reported here, the peak of the principal direction accelerations of the upper and lower sternum occurred prior to the peak force. The peak of the principal direction acceleration for those points further away from the center of impact--ribs R4R/R8R, R4L/R4R and thoracic vertebrae T1/T12--characteristically occurred after the peak force. The typical acceleration waveform of the sternum rose smoothly to peak acceleration, proceeded to a negative acceleration near peak force, and subsequently either became positive and returned to negative, or simply remained negative. On the other hand, the spinal acceleration response was more complex before peak acceleration. Either a multimodal waveform with several local maxima, or a delay between the initiation of impact and the most significant part of the acceleration response was observed. The spinal acceleration also lagged behind the peak force.

Unlike the flat surface sternal impact response reported [62], the steering wheel impact response being reported here shows that the propagation of this response as reflected in peak accelerations and the Q_2 event of the force time-history was impact velocity dependent for all triaxial accelerometer groups. For low-velocity steering wheel impacts (2.5-3 m/s), all acceleration maxima, in general, occurred before the Q_2 event of the force. In most cases, for mid-velocity steering wheel impacts, the maximum accelerations occurred before the Q_2 force event; however, occasionally, the maximum spine or sternal accelerations occurred after the Q_2 force event. For most high-velocity steering wheel impacts, the sternal accelerations occurred before the Q_2 force event, while the spinal acceleration maxima occurred after the Q_2 force event.

Differences in response existed between the magnitudes of the principal direction accelerations for the flat surface impacts [62] and for low- and mid- velocity steering wheel impacts. In the steering wheel impacts the principal direction magnitudes of sternal accelerations were 20-50 percent higher than those observed for the spinal accelerations. In contrast, the principal direction magnitudes of the high-velocity steering wheel impacts were 4-5 times as high as the spinal accelerations (similar to the flat surface impacts to the sternum [62]). The waveforms were significantly more complex for steering wheel impacts than for flat surface frontal impacts to the sternum [62], in terms of the number and magnitude of local maxima. This may have been the result of the complex interaction between the body trunk (which includes the thoracic cage and the abdominal area) and the steering wheel. In the abdominal impacts, different components of the steering wheel were able to contact the thoracic cage at different points in time, whereas the flat surface impactor [62] displayed a simpler contacting mechanism. In addition, both symmetric and asymmetric deformation of the steering wheel caused input loading of the thoracic cage that was not observed in the flat surface impacts to the sternum [62].

Auto- and Cross-Correlations - Due to the complex reponse pattern of the thoracic cage during a steering wheel impact, comparisons between its acceleration time-histories were made using auto- and cross-correlations. The three-dimensional motion in steering wheel impacts implied that comparisons should not be made beyond 50 ms lags. Peaks in the cross-correlation function correspond to the transmission lag between the two variables which were being correlated. For the steering wheel hub force and the principal direction acceleration variables, the physical path of energy transmission was not well determined. Therefore, the cross-correlation function gave an estimate of the average input transmission lag between the force time-history and the given accelerometer cluster.

The relative phasing of the maximum value of the cross-correlation function between the steering wheel hub force and the principal direction accelerations for the lower sternum, ribs R8R and R8L, and thoracic vertebrae T1 and T12 indicated that the force lagged all of the principal direction acceleration. The lags, in general, for the low velocity impacts were: for lower sternum, 20-25 ms; for ribs R8R and R8L, 20-25 ms; for thoracic vertebra T12, 15-25 ms; and for thoracic vertebra T1, 0-15 ms. The lags for mid-velocity impacts were: for lower sternum, 15-25 ms; for ribs R8R and R8L, 15-25 ms; for thoracic vertebra T12, 15-25 ms; and for thoracic vertebra T1, 0-15 ms. The lags for the high-velocity impacts were: for lower sternum, 5-15 ms; for ribs R8R and R8L, 5-15 ms; for thoracic vertebra T12, 0-10 ms; and for thoracic vertebra T1, 0-10 ms. In some of the tests, at all three impact velocities, the greatest lags were observed for the lower sternum, with intermediate lags for the ribs R8R and R8L, and the shortest lags for the spinal accelerations. However, this trend was not general enough to indicate a clear load path from the sternum to the spine. This observation is consistent with the concept that there was not one but several load paths occurring. In the blunt frontal sternum impacts with a flat surface impactor [62], the sternum was loaded first and then the rib and spinal accelerations resulted from the sternal motion. However, in the steering wheel impacts, the spine was initially loaded by the contact of the ribs with the spokes and lower rim of the steering wheel. Thus, in the steering wheel impacts, the loading of the sternum occurred after the initial load path had been established.

The maximum values of the auto-correlation functions (i.e., zero lag) of the principal direction accelerations from the triaxial groups were consistent with the maximum values of these accelerations when the raw accelerometer profiles were filtered at 150 Hz, 4th order. The maximum value of the auto-correlation function for the sternal acceleration for low- and mid-velocity impacts was 4-6 times higher than that of the maximum auto-correlation value for the spine at thoracic vertebra T12. For high velocity impacts, the maximum of the sternal auto-correlation function was 15-20 times the maximum of the spinal auto-correlation function.

Observations of the auto- and cross-correlation functions indicated that: 1) the most rapidly varying signal was the lower sternum, with ribs R8R and R8L acting intermediate, and the least varying signals were the spinal accelerations; 2) although ribs R8R and R8L showed the best correlations for low- and mid-velocity impacts, the high-velocity impacts did not indicate such parallel response for both sides of the thorax 3) at all test velocities, spinal accelerations showed the best correlations between principal direction acceleration and the force signal; 4) the high-velocity impacts were, to a greater extent, different from the low- and mid-velocity impacts than the low- and mid-velocity impacts were from each other; and 5) the varying load paths were most significant for the rib R8R and R8L triaxial accelerometer clusters.

Physically, these observations imply that the response of the thorax to steering wheel impact can be interpreted as the response of one deformable body (the thorax) in contact with another deformable body (the steering wheel). The waveform which was associated with the acceleration response of each point on the thorax was influenced by a number of load paths (originating from the steering wheel hub, the spokes, and the lower rim). The point in time at which each of these load paths became significant for a given steering wheel configuration depended on the impact velocity, the load paths, and the biovariability of the population.

Impact Response - Figures 8,9,10 represent the mechanical impedance transfer function for test 84E153 A,B,C. The results shown in these figures were generated from the principal direction triad of the sternum, R8R and T12 and steering wheel hub force and contain three traces per graph, one each for low-, mid-, and high-velocity impact. The transfer function includes the response of the steering wheel. The results presented here are considered representative of the general trends observed in a majority of the impacts.

The impact response of the thoraco-abdomen observed in the mechanical impedance data has the following characteristics similar to those of frontal thoracic impacts made with a flat surface impactor [62]: 1) local minima in impedance were observed for the uniaxial accelerometers and in all significant accelerations in the anatomical reference frames or the principal direction triad; 2) the magnitude of the lower sternum decreased from that at 15 Hz to the first local minimum; 3) a second local minimum was observed for some tests; 4) a greater value of mechanical impedance was observed from the level at 15 Hz up to the first local minimum for those instrumented points further from the center of impactor contact, with ribs R8R and R8L showing the most similar impedance values; 5) the impedance values for all significant accelerations increased as velocity increased, and 6) the first local minimum increased in frequency as impact velocity increased.

The impact response of the steering wheel reflected in the mechanical impedance data has the following characteristics which were different from those of the frontal flat surface thoracic impacts [62]: 1) the mechanical impedance values were higher in the steering wheel impacts in the low frequency range (below 15 Hz); 2) the low frequency components in the steering wheel data (those below 15 Hz) for a given impact velocity were characteristically the same for all principal directions; 3) the

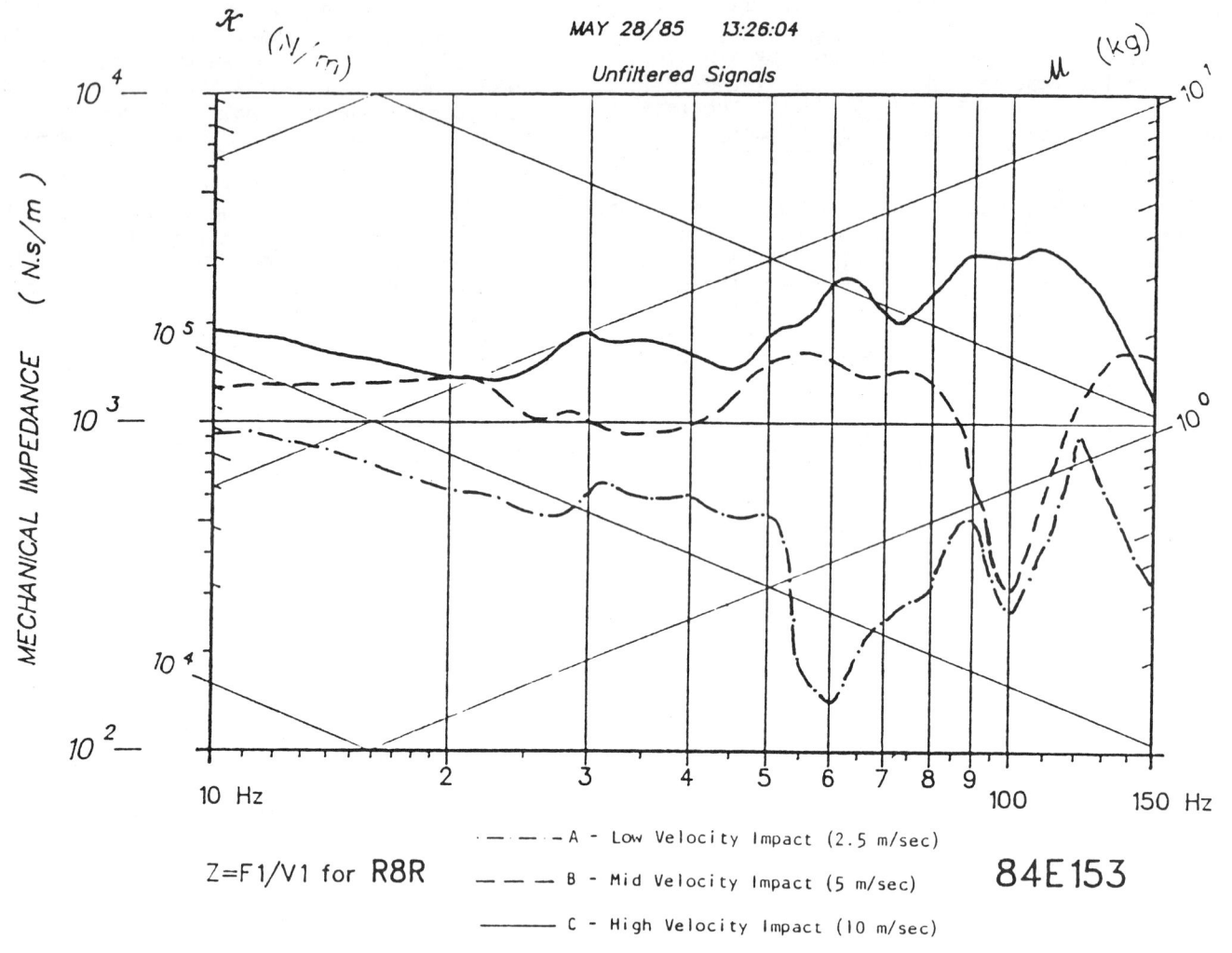

Figure 6. Mechanical impedance transfer function for 84E153 ABC

second local minimum for sternal impacts by the steering wheel generally occurred at a frequency 3 times higher than the first local minimum, while for frontal impacts with a flat surface impactor, the second local minimum occurred at a frequency 2 times higher than the first local minimum, 4) in general, the ribs R8R and R8L transfer function for the principal direction acceleration for steering wheel impacts differed from each other to a greater degree than those of the flat surface impacts, and 5) in the sternal impacts by a flat surface impactor [62], the first local minimum was clearly distinguishable in all mechanical impedance functions for any significant acceleration, while this was not always the case for the steering wheel impacts. The first local minimum of the mechanical impedance occurred in the 32-38 Hz range during the flat surface impacts to the sternum [62], while in the steering wheel impacts to the sternum of similar impact velocity, it occurred in the 20-25 Hz range.

The local minima observed in all tests were not necessarily related to resonances of the thoracic system due to free vibrations. During the force time-history, the steering wheel had a continually changing load surface as well as a continually changing load direction. In addition, the direction of the loading with respect to the test subject changed as the test subject rotated onto the steering wheel. In part, this may have caused the differences observed in the first local minima for the mechanical impedance for the different impact velocities. The complex loading conditions may have caused the differences in mechanical impedance profiles which were observed between the flat surface impacts and the steering wheel impacts.

The local minima (resonances) for the sternum were: for low-velocity impacts, 20-25 Hz; for mid-velocity impacts, 25-35 Hz; and for high-velocity impacts 30-45 Hz. Similar to the flat surface impacts reported [62], the decrease in the magnitude of the mechanical impedance up to the first local minimum for the lower sternum, provided spring values for steering wheel impacts; the value was 3×10^4 N/m for low-velocity impacts; 6×10^4 N/m for mid-velocity steering wheel impacts, and 9×10^4 N/m for high-velocity steering wheel impacts. Also similar to the flat surface frontal impacts [62], the magnitude of the mechanical impedance displayed spring-like characteristics, while the phase did not.

In many of the flat surface impact tests reported [62], the magnitude of the mechanical impedance for the T1 and T12 spine principal direction exhibited the behavior for a mass between 15-25 kg. In the steering wheel impacts, the magnitude of the mechanical impedance for the spine was closer to a damper of 1.5×10^3 N.s/m up to the first local minimum. However, similar to the spring-like behavior of the sternum, the phase of the transfer function was not damper-like. In addition, the complexity (larger number of maximum and minimum) of the mechanical impedance function was greater for the steering wheel impact than for the blunt sternum impacts [62].

The similarity in mechanical impedance magnitude between the sternal response of the steering wheel impacts and the flat surface impacts [62], is believed to be a result of the major loading of the steering wheel on the sternum from the steering wheel hub. The differences in the traces associated with the ribs (R8R and R8L) and the spine between the steering wheel impacts and the flat surface impacts [84], were a consequence of the numerous load paths to those anatomical structures.

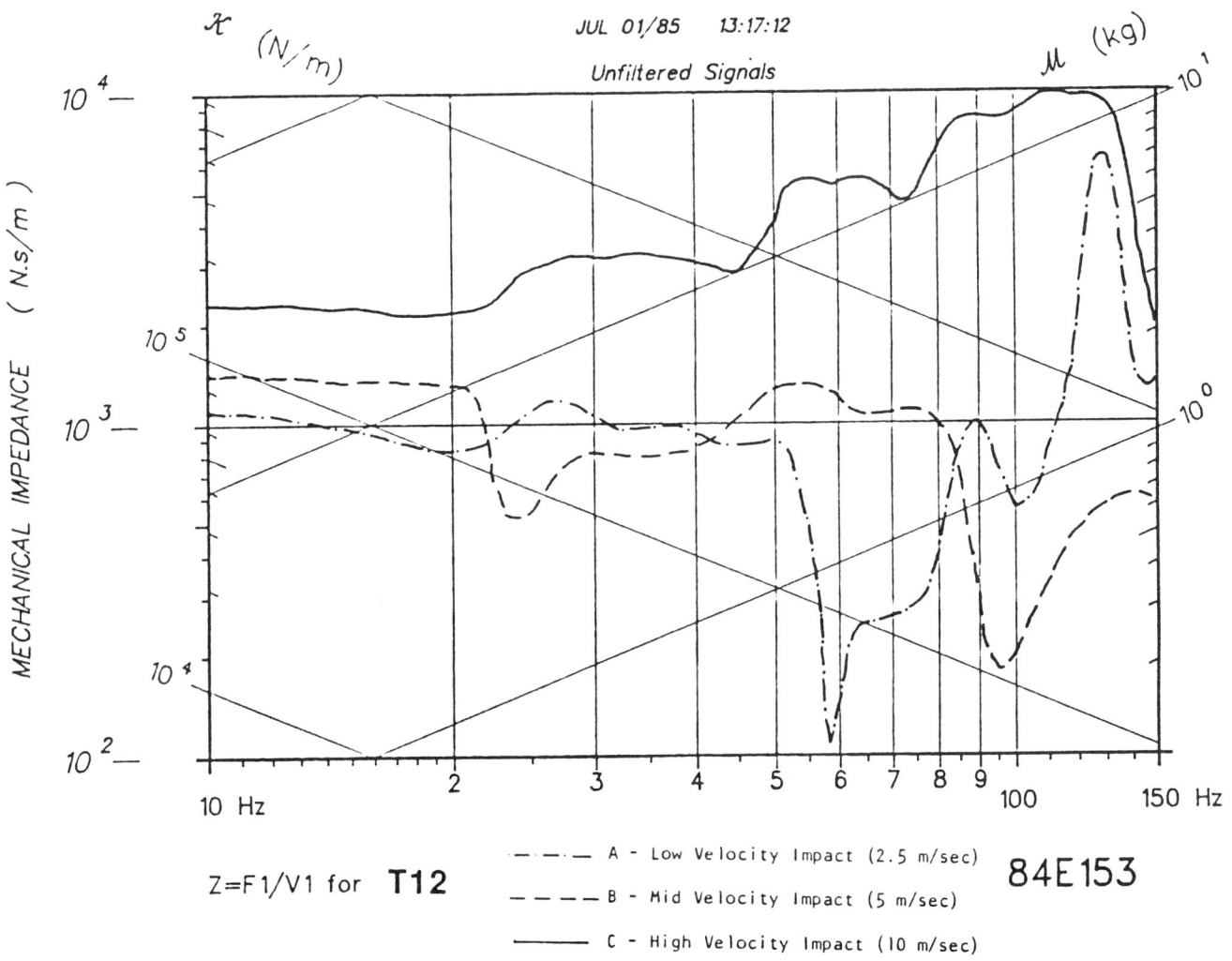

Figure 9. Mechanical impedance transfer function for 84E153 ABC

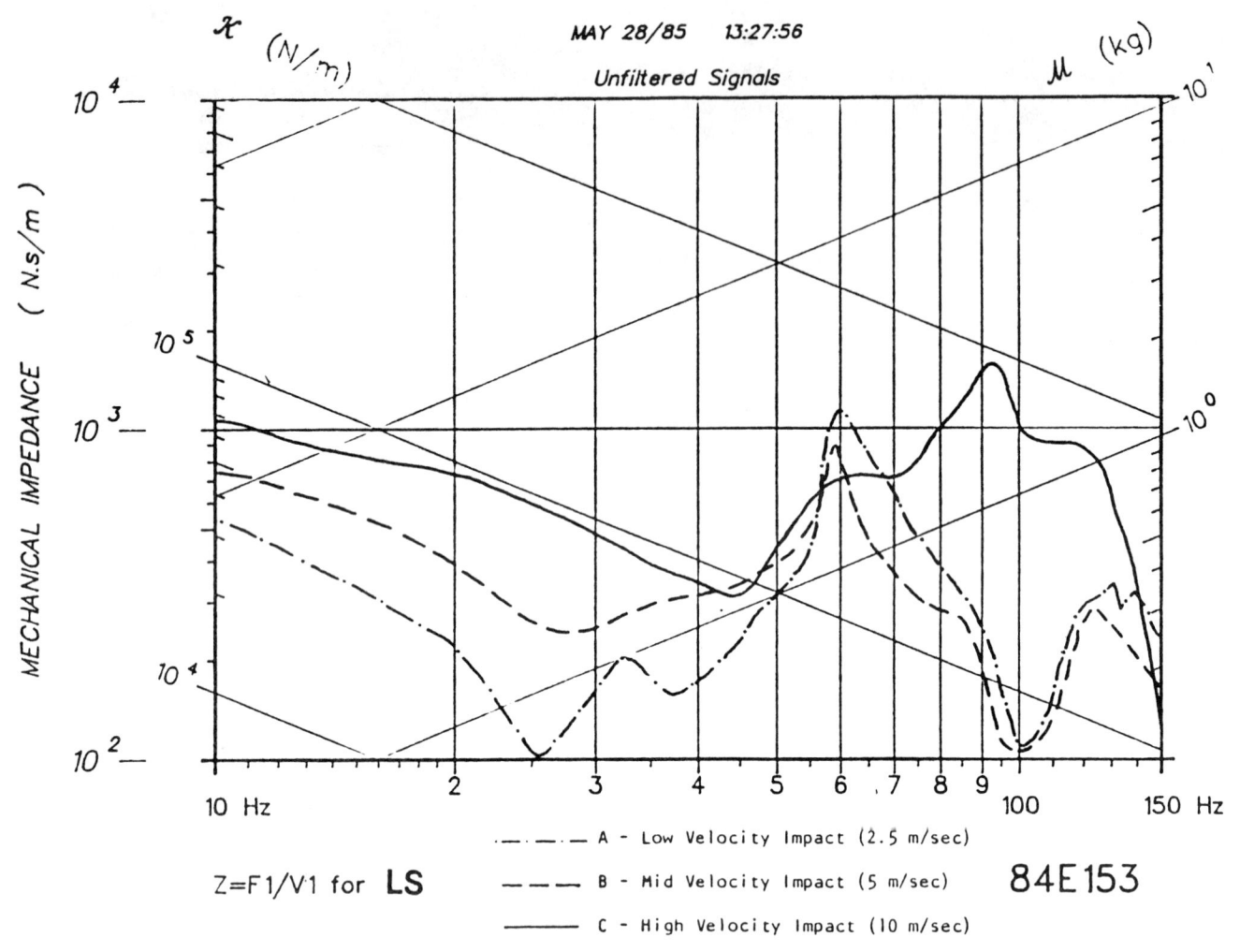

Figure 10. Mechanical impedance transfer function for 84E153 ABC

Transfer Functions - One of the goals of the present study was to quantitatively characterize the response of the thoracic skeletal structure by a transfer function between any two points on the thorax which possessed a significant component of acceleration. In this regard, transfer functions were generated between any given triaxial accelerometer package and any other given triax, resulting in several transfer functions for each point which could predict the corresponding response of every other point. When a transfer function was computed between two points such that the denominator was obtained from the accelerometer package of the sternum, the transfer function had the characteristics of a low-pass filter. Transfer functions which were generated further from the point of impact (R8R and R8L, T1 and T12) displayed an increasingly greater attenuation. In general, the transfer functions which were calculated from the significant acceleration components of the selected points on the thorax showed responses characterized by a general decrease in magnitude with increasing frequency and variations in phase at each different frequency. Although there was a general decrease in the magnitude of these transfer functions, the magnitude did not decrease to the same degree as for similar transfer functions generated when using a flat surface impactor. Therefore, if it is reasonable to assume that the thorax is a deformable structure, the response of the thorax is dependent upon the load path and upon the energy management of the thoraco-abdominal system (gross motion, differential motion, or dissipation).

For the low- and mid-velocity flat surface impacts, the transfer functions that were generated between the lower sternum and the thoracic vertebra T12 generally showed less attenuation than was observed for the same transfer functions in the low-velocity steering wheel impacts. Physically, this implies that the thoracic structure could have acted effectively stiffer as the impact velocity increased. A similar observation had been made previously [13,21] which suggested that the thorax stiffens under higher impact velocity.

In these tests, a complicated load path was obtained through the use of a steering wheel, and such effects as loading of a single rib may have occurred for short time durations. The increased complexity, as well as the larger variation in transfer functions generated in these tests compared to others [62], also indicated a much more complex loading path. Although there were clear similarities between the flat surface impacts [62] and the steering wheel impacts, the differences were significant enough to caution against using the results of flat surface impacts to predict the results in a steering wheel impact context.

Force Deflection Measurement

The force deflection measurements (the steering wheel hub force and the deflection associated with the lowest point on the rim and T12) recorded during the cadaver research program (these results are presented in the Appendix) may give useful information about the kinematic response of the abdomen which could be used to model the abdomen. However, the following problems exist:

1. The structural properties of the abdomen are mediated by bone, cartilage and soft tissue. The thoracic cage can form a protective structure for various aspects of the upper abdominal contents (liver, stomach, spleen, pancreas). The section of bone, cartilage, and soft tissue which interacts with the steering wheel during impact depends on the exact position of contact of the steering wheel. Therefore, to describe the force deflection characteristics so that they may be useful in understanding the response of the abdomen or contributing to the construction of an anthropomorphic test device (dummy), a series of force deflection curves, which depend on the position of impact, may be needed to characterize steering wheel impact.

2. The steering wheel undergoes permanent deformation. This activity may not be accurately reflected in the load cell's force time-history.

3. During the impact event, the soft tissue of the abdomen initially dominates external input to the steering wheel assembly. At some time during the impact event as the test subject rotates forward, the head, shoulders and upper thorax also make contact with the steering wheel, thus affecting the force time-history.

4. Loading of the steering wheel rim is not accurately represented under all conditions by the force measured at the center of the steering wheel.

5. The motion of the test subject is three-dimensional. This may lead to inaccuracies when using one-dimensional displacement transducers such as string pots.

The initial segment of the force deflection curve (up to 4 cm deflection) serves to represent the most usable portion of the curve. This is a result of the following:

1. In both dynamic and quasi-static testing, the force at the steering wheel rim was within 15 percent of that at the steering wheel center for up to 4 cm deflection of the lower aspect of the steering wheel rim.

2. Observations from the high-speed movies indicate that the abdomen is the only source of input to the steering wheel assembly during the first 4 cm of deflection. After that amount of deflection, the head, shoulders, and thorax make contact with the steering wheel, influencing the force time-history.

The most critical injuries to the region of the body trunk protected by the thoracic cage are thought to involve the internal soft tissue organs. In this regard, the liver and the spleen are important soft-tissue structures.

Mechanisms of Liver Injury - Two mechanisms of liver-spleen injury seemed to be operating in the steering wheel impacts. As the steering wheel lower rim contacted the abdomen, it penetrated below the thoracic cage. Shortly after contact, the spokes loaded the lower portion of the thoracic cage, compressing the liver. Next the steering wheel hub contacted the sternum, deforming the thoracic cage and further compressing the liver against the spine and posterior thoraco-abdominal wall. Finally, injury occurred when the liver was displaced beyond the range of motion that is normally permitted by the system's tethers, especially the hepatic and portal tethers, or when sufficient stresses developed from compression of the liver between the sternum and the posterior thoraco-abdominal wall so as to tear the liver at the lobular junction. Tearing of the hepatic portal vein and/or tearing of the interlobular junction of the liver seem to be reliably reproduced by careful positioning of the steering wheel with respect to the liver. This was accomplished through the use of in place X-rays. However, only a limited number of tests were conducted in which this procedure was used. More tests need to be performed before this conclusion can be generalized.

A second mechanism has been suggested by injuries which were not associated with tethered structures. These injuries were stellar and linear lacerations which occurred on the surface of the liver in the area closest to the thoraco-abdominal wall which was in contact with the steering wheel spokes and hub. Possibly, local stresses developed in the liver which were greater than the liver's stress tolerance, producing the observed injuries. If so, such stresses and injuries may be an impact velocity-sensitive phenomena.

CONCLUSIONS

1) Steering wheel impacts using a 25 kg pendulum produced significantly different results from that of a 65 kg pendulum, with regard to steering wheel hub force and thoracic cage acceleration. In a steering wheel impact using a low mass pendulum (25 kg), the amount of energy transferred to the test subject can significantly affect the velocity of the impactor during impact. Potentially, this could lead to greater variability in the impact response, as the test subject's mass would affect the impact response to a greater extent than the mass of a heavier pendulum (65 kg).

2) The liver and the spleen are soft-tissue organs which are partially protected by the thoracic cage. The responses of the bony structures of the thoracic cage are critical factors in the mechanism of injuries for these organs. Therefore, in view of their dynamic and injury responses, the liver and spleen should be considered thoracic organs rather than abdominal organs.

3) For frontal impacts using a steering wheel assembly, a single linear model seems inadequate to characterize thoracic impact response. In the interpretation of mechanical impedance (generated between selected points on the thoracic cage and steering wheel hub force) as well as transfer functions between two points on the thoracic cage, there seems to be a significant difference between low-velocity (non-damaging), mid velocity (non-damaging) and high-velocity (damaging) impact response.

4) The complex interaction of the steering wheel with the thoracic cage requires a three-dimensional description of impact response with regard to: 1) gross whole body motion, and 2) differential motion as determined by the acceleration response of selected points on the skeletal structure. The results obtained from accelerometers attached to the thoracic cage imply a complex thoracic response as well as multiple paths of energy transmission. When the body trunk is impacted by the steering wheel, load paths originate from the rim, the spokes, and the hub. The degree and point in time at which these load paths dominate the thoracic response is dependent upon the initial configuration of the steering wheel relative to the test subject, as well as upon the biovariability of the population.

5) Severe injuries, some of which involve the major arteries or veins in the organs protected by the thoracic cage, seem to be impact position dependent. Thoraco-abdominal impact tolerance levels based on deflection, velocity or a combination of both may be inappropriate for the events which occur in steering wheel impacts. Although velocity and deflection seem to be important parameters in determining thoraco-abdominal impact tolerance levels, severe injuries involving the major arteries or veins were observed to be impact position and initial test configuration dependent in the response programs reported here. Location of the liver with respect to the impact device is an important criteria that needs to be addressed in thoraco-abdominal impact.

ACKNOWLEDGEMENTS

The results presented in this paper were funded by the United States Department of Transportation, National Highway Traffic Safety Administration (Contract No. DTNH22-83-C-17019).

The authors wish to acknowledge the technical assistance of Bob Bennett, Nabih Alem, John Melvin, Paula Lux, Gail J. Muscott, Jean Brindamour, Zheng Lou, Steven Richter, Peter Schuetz, Wendy Gould, Shawn Cowper, Tim Jordan, Reza Salehi, Valerie Moses and Patrice Muscott. A special thank you goes to Jeff Marcus.

References

1. The Abbreviated Injury Scale (AIS), 1980 revision, American Association for Automotive Medicine, Morton Grove, IL.

2. Beckman, D.L. and Palmer, M.F. 1969. Response of the Primate Thorax to Experimental Impact. In: 13th Stapp Car Crash Conference Proceedings, pp. 270-281.

3. Beckman, D.L., Palmer, M.F. and Roberts, V.L. 1970. Thoracic Force-Deflection Studies in Living and Embalmed Primates. HSRI ASME 70-BHF-8.

4. Brinn, J. and Staffeld, S.E. 1972. The Effective Displacement Index--An Analysis Technique for Crash Impacts of Anthropometric Dummies. In: 15th Stapp Car Crash Conference Proceedings, pp. 817-824.

5. Brinn, J. and Staffeld, S.E. 1970. Evaluation of Impact Test Accelerations: A Damage Index for the Head and Torso. In: 14th Stapp Car Crash Conference Proceedings, pp. 188-202.

6. Burdi, A.R. 1970. Thoracic and Abdominal Anatomy. In: Huelke, D.F., ed., Human Anatomy, Impact Injuries, and Human Tolerances, SAE 700195, pp. 52-68.

7. Burow, K.H. 1972. Injuries of the Thorax and of the Lower Extremities to Forces Applied by Blunt Object. In: 15th Conference Proceedings American Assoc. for Automotive Medicine, pp. 122-150.

8. Burow, K. and Kramer, M. 1973. Experimental Investigations on the Type and Severity of Fractures in the Chest Cavity. [in German] International Conference on the Biokinetics of Impacts Proceedings, pp. 387-397.

9. Cheng, R., et al. 1982. Injuries to the Cervical Spine Caused by a Distributed Frontal Load to the Chest. 26th Stapp Car Crash Conference Proceedings, pp. 1-40.

10. Cotte, J.P. 1977. Semi-static Loading of Baboon Torsos. 3rd International Conference on Impact Trauma Proceedings, pp. 165-179.

11. Culver, R.H., et al., 1978. Evaluation of Intrathoracic Response Using High-speed Cineradiography. 6th New England Bioengineering Conference Proceedings, pp. 365-369.

12. Digges, K.H. 1983. Dynamic Response of the Human Thorax When Subjected to Frontal Impact. O.U.E.L. 1453/83. Oxford University (England), Dept. of Engineering Science.

13. Digges, K.H. 1983. Mathematical Model of the Human Thorax When Subjected to Frontal Impact During an Automobile Crash. O.U.E.L. 1454/83. Oxford University (England), Dept. of Engineering Science.

14. Eppinger, R.H. 1978. Prediction of Thoracic Injury Using Measurable Experimental Parameters. 6th International Technical Conference on Experimental Safety Vehicles, NHTSA, pp. 770-780.

15. Eppinger, R.H. and Chan, H.S. 1981. Thoracic Injury Prediction via Digital Convolution Theory. 25th Stapp Car Crash Conference Proceedings, pp. 369-393.

16. Fanyon, A., et al. 1978. Methods for Backing-up the Conclusions of Accident Reconstructions Carried Out with Instrumented Cadavers. Proceedings 3rd International Meeting on the Simulation and Reconstruction of Impacts in Collisions, pp. 220-233.

17. Fine, P.R., Kuhlemeier, K.V. and DeVivo, M.J. 1979. Residual Cardiovascular Damage Resulting from Nonpenetrating Steering Wheel Impact. Proceedings 23rd Conference American Assoc. for Automotive Medicine, pp. 28-42.

18. Frey, C.F., et al. 1973. A Fifteen-Year Experience with Automotive Hepatic Trauma. Journal of Trauma 13(11):1039-1049.

19. Frey, C.F. 1970. Injuries to the Thorax and Abdomen. In: Human Anatomy, Impact Injuries and Human Tolerances. SAE Paper No. 700195.

20. Gauthier, R.K. 1984. Thoracic Trauma. Emergency Medical Services 13(3):28, 30-35. May/June.

21. Gloyns, P.F., et al. 1979. Analysis of Additional Accident Data Relating to the Performance of Steering Systems Developed to Comply with Current Safety Regulations. Birmingham University (England), Dept. of Transportation and Environmental Planning.

22. Gloyns, P.F., et al. 1973. Field Investigations of the Injury Protection Offered by Some "Energy Absorbing" Steering Systems. International Conference on the Biokinetics of Impacts Proceedings, pp. 399-410.

23. Gloyns, P.F., Hayes, H.R.M. and Rattenbury, S.J. 1980. Protection of the Car Driver from Steering System Induced Injuries. In: Towards Safer Passenger Cars, London: Mechanical Engineering Publications, Ltd., pp. 23-30.

24. Got, C., et al. 1975. Morphological, Chemical and Physical Characteristics of the Ribs and Their Relationship to Induced Deflection of the Thorax. [in French] In: Cotte, J.P. and Presle, M.M., eds., Biomechanics of Serious Trauma, Bron: IRCOBI, pp. 220-228.

25. Granik, G. and Stein, I. 1973. Human Ribs: Static Testing as a Promising Medical Application. Journal of Biomechanics 6(3):237-240.

26. Gurdjian, E.S., et al. 1979. Impact Injury and Crash Protection, Springfield, IL: Charles C. Thomas.

27. Harris, C.M., and Crede, C.E. 1976. Shock and Vibration Handbook. New York, McGraw-Hill Book Company.

28. Hess, R.L., Weber, K. and Melvin, J.W. 1982. Review of Research on Thoracic Impact Tolerance and Injury Criteria Related to Occupant Protection. In: Occupant Crash Interaction with the Steering System, SAE 820474, pp. 93-119.

29. Hess, R.L., Weber, K. and Melvin, J.W. 1981. Review of Literature and Regulation Relating to Thoracic Impact Tolerance and Injury Criteria. UM-HSRI-81-38. Highway Safety Research Institute, Ann Arbor, MI.

30. Huelke, D.F. 1982. Steering Assembly Performance and Driver Injury Severity in Frontal Crashes. In: Occupant Crash Interaction with the Steering System, SAE 820474, pp. 1-30.

31. Huelke, D.F. 1976. The Anatomy of the Human Chest. In: The Human Thorax-Anatomy, Injury and Biomechanics, SAE P-67, pp. 1-9.

32. Huelke, D.F., Nusholtz, G.S., and Kaiker, P.S. 1985. Use of Quadruped Models in Thoraco-Abdominal Biomechanics Research. Submitted to: 29th Stapp Car Crash Conference Proceedings.

33. Kaleps, I. 1975. Thoracic Dynamics During Blunt Impact. In: Saczalski, K., et al., eds., Aircraft Crashworthiness, Charlottesville: University Press of Virginia, pp. 235-252.

34. Kallieris, D., et al. 1979. Thorax Acceleration Measures at the 6th Thoracic Vertebra in Connection to Thorax and Spinal Column Injury Degree. Proceedings 4th International IRCOBI Conference on the Biomechanics of Trauma, pp. 184-197.

35. Kalny, J. and Sezak, Z. 19?? Transport Fractures of the Sternum. [in Chechoslovakian] Acta Chirurgiae Orthopaedicae et Traumatologiae Chechoslovaca 42(5):459-466. Oct.

36. Kazarian, L.E., Hahn, J.W. and von Gierke, H.E. 1970. Biomechanics of the Vertebral Column and Internal Organ Response to Seated Spinal Impact in the Rhesus Monkey (Macaca mulatta). 14th Stapp Car Crash Conference Proceedings, pp. 121-143.

37. King, A.I. and Khalil, T.B. 1982. Crash Injury Studies. GMR-3904. Wayne State University, Detroit, MI.

38. Kramer, M. 1976. Injury Index in Accident--Simulated Trauma of Chest and Lower Leg. [in German] Unfallheilkunde 79(2): 61-69. Feb.

39. Kramer, M. and Heger, A. 1975. Severity Indices for Chest and Lower Leg Injuries. [in German] In: Cotte, J.P. and Presle, M.M., eds., Biomechanics of Serious Trauma, Bron: IRCOBI, pp. 229-239.

40. Kroell, C.K. 1976. Thoracic Response to Blunt Frontal Loading. In: The Human Thorax--Anatomy, Injury and Biomechanics, SAE P-67, pp. 49-77.

41. Kroell, C.K., et al. 1981. Interrelationship of Velocity and Chest Compression in Blunt Thoracic Impact to Swine. 25th Stapp Car Crash Conference Proceedings, pp. 549-579.

42. Liu, Y.K. 1968. The Human Body Under Time-Dependent Boundary Conditions. University of Michigan, Ann Arbor, Dept. of Engineering Mechanics. March.

44. Liu, Y.K. and Wickstrom, J.K. 1973. Estimation of the Inertial Property Distribution of the Human Torso from Segmented Cadaveric Data. In: Kenedi, R.M., ed., Perspectives in Biomedical Engineering, London: Macmillan Press, Ltd., pp. 203-213.

43. Martin, J.D., Jr., ed. 1969. Trauma to the Thorax and Abdomen. Emory University School of Medicine, Dept. of Surgery, Atlanta, GA.

45. Mays, E.T. 1966. Bursting Injuries of the Liver. Archives of Surgery 93(92)103.

46. Melvin, J.W., et al. 1973. Impact Injury Mechanisms in Abdominal Organs. 17th Stapp Car Crash Conference Proceedings, pp. 115-126.

47. Melvin, J.W., Robbins, D.H.; Stalnaker, R.L. and Eppinger, R.H. 1977. Prediction of Multidirectional Thoracic Impact Injuries. *3rd International Conference on Impact Trauma Proceedings*, pp. 281-285A.

48. Melvin, J.W. and Wineman, A.S. 1975. *Thoracic Model Improvements (Experimental Tissue Properties)*. HSRI UM-HSRI-BI-74-2-1/DOT/HS 801 557, UM-HSRI-BI-74-2-2/DOT/HS 801 558, and UM-HSRI-BI-74-2-3 DOT/HS 801 559.

49. Mertz, H.J. 1984. *A Procedure for Normalizing Impact Response Data*, SAE 840884.

50. Morris, J.M., Lucas, D.B. and Bresler, B. 1961. Role of the Trunk in Stability of the Spine. *Journal of Bone and Joint Surgery* 43-A(3):327-351. April.

51. Mulder, D.S. 1980. Chest Trauma - Current Concepts. *Canadian Journal of Surgery* 23(4).

52. Mulligan, G.W., et al. 1976. An Introduction to the Understanding of Blunt Chest Trauma. In: *The Human Thorax - Anatomy, Injury, and Biomechanics*. P-67, Warrendale, PA: Society of Automotive Engineers, October.

53. Nahum, A.M. 1973. Chest Trauma. In: *Biomechanics and Its Application to Automotive Design*, SAE, NY.

54. Nahum, A.M., et al. 1971. The Biomechanical Basis for Chest Impact Protection: I. Force-Deflection Characteristics of the Thorax. *Journal of Trauma* 11(10):874-882. Oct.

55. Nahum, A.M., et al. 1970. Deflection of the Human Thorax Under Sternal Impact. In: *1970 International Automobile Safety Conference Compendium*, SAE, pp. 797-807.

56. Nahum, A.M., Kroell, C.K. and Schneider, D.C. 1973. The Biomechanical Basis of Chest Impact Protection. II. Effects of Cardiovascular Pressurization. *Journal of Trauma* 13(5):443-459. May.

57. Nahum, A.M., Schneider, D.C. and Kroell, C.K. 1975. Cadaver Skeletal Response to Blunt Thoracic Impact. *19th Stapp Car Crash Conference Proceedings*, pp. 259-293.

58. Neathery, R.F. and Lobdell, T.E. 1973. Mechanical Simulation of Human Thorax Under Impact. *17th Stapp Car Crash Conference Proceedings*, pp. 451-466.

59. Newman, R.J. and Jones, I.S. 1984. A Prospective Study of 413 Consecutive Car Occupants with Chest Injuries. *Journal of Trauma* 24(2):129-135. Feb.

60. Nickerson, J.L. 1962. *International Body Movements Resulting from Externally Applied Sinusoidal Forces*. Chicago Medical School, IL. AMRL-TDR-62-81. July.

61. Nusholtz, G. 1977. Vascular and Respiratory Pressurization of the Thorax. *5th Annual Committee Reports and Technical Discussions International Workshop on Human Subjects for Biomechanical Research*, pp. 81-95.

62. Nusholtz, G.S., Melvin, J.W. and Lux, P. 1983. The Influence of Impact Energy and Direction on Thoracic Response. *27th Stapp Car Crash Conference Proceedings*, pp. 69-94.

63. Nusholtz, G.S., et al. 1980. Thoraco-abdominal Response and Injury. *24th Stapp Car Crash Conference Proceedings*, pp. 187-228.

64. Nusholtz, G.S., et al. 1985. Thoracic Response to Frontal Impact. Submitted to: *29th Stapp Car Crash Conference Proceedings*.

65. Patrick, L.M. 1981. Impact Force-deflection of the Human Thorax. *25th Stapp Car Crash Conference Proceedings*, pp. 471-496.

66. Plank, G.R. 1978. *Review of Chest Deflection Measurement Techniques and Transducers*. Final Report. Transportation Systems Center, Cambridge, MA.

67. Pope, M.E., et al. 1979. Postural Influences on Thoracic Impact. *23rd Stapp Car Crash Conference Proceedings*, pp. 765-795.

68. Raschke, K., Eckert, P. and Kohne, U. 1972. The Role of the Liver and Pancreas Injuries along with Multiple Injuries. [in German] *Monatsschrift fur Unfallheilkunde, Versicherungs-, Versogungs-und Verkehrsmedizin* 75(3):117-123.

69. Reddi, M.M., et al. 1975. Thoracic Impact Injury Mechanism. F-C3417/DOT/HS 801 710 and 711. Franklin Institute Research Laboratories, Philadelphia, PA.

70. Reddi, M.M. and Tsai, H.C. 1977. Computer Simulation of Human Thoracic Skeletal Response. F-C4216-1/DOT/HS 803 208, 209, 210. Franklin Institute Research Laboratories, Philadelphia, PA.

71. Roberts, S.B. 1975. Intrusion of the Sternum into the Thoracic Cavity During Frontal Chest Impact and Injury Potential. In: Saczalski, K., et al., eds., Aircraft Crashworthiness, Charlottesville: University Press of Virginia, pp. 253-271.

72. Roberts, V.L. 1967. Experimental Studies on Thoracic and Abdominal Injuries. In: Selzer, M.L., et al., eds., The Prevention of Highway Injury, Highway Safety Research Institute, Ann Arbor, MI, pp. 211-215.

73. Roberts, V.L. and Beckman, D.L. 1970. The Mechanisms of Chest Injuries. In: Gurdjian, E.S., et al., eds., Impact Injury and Crash Protection, Charles C. Thomas Publisher, pp. 86-100.

74. Robbins, D.H., Melvin, R.L., and Stalnaker, R.L. The Prediction of Thoracic Impact Injuries. 20th Stapp Car Crash Conference Proceedings. SAE Paper No. 760822.

75. Sacreste, J., et al. 1984. Evaluation of the Influence of Inter-Individual Differences on the Injury Level: Application to Accident Reconstructions with Cadavers. In: Benjamin, T.E.A., ed., Biomechanics of Impacts in Road Accidents, Luxembourg: Commission of the European Communities, pp. 246-269.

76. Sacreste, J., et al. 1979. Progress in the Interpretation of Cadaver Injuries. Proceedings 7th International Workshop on "Human Subjects for Biomechanical Research", pp. 209-211.

77. Sances, A., Jr., et al. 1984. Biodynamics of Vehicular Injuries. In: Peters, G.A. and Peters, B.J., eds., Automotive Engineering and Litigation, NY: Garland Law Publishing, pp. 449-550.

78. Schmidt, G. 1979. Rib-Cage Injuries Indicating the Direction and Strength of Impact. Forensic Science 13(2):103-110. March/April.

79. Schreck and R.M., Viano, D.C. 1973. Thoracic Impact: New Experimental Approaches Leading to Model Synthesis. 17th Stapp Car Crash Conference Proceedings, pp. 437-450.

80. Shatsky, S.A., et al. 1974. Traumatic Distortions of the Primate Head and Chest: Correlations of Biomechanical, Radiological and Pathological Data. 18th Stapp Car Crash Conference Proceedings, pp. 351-381. SAE Paper No. 741186.

81. Shatsky, S.A. 1973. Flash X-Ray Cinematography During Impact Injury. In: 17th Stapp Car Crash Conference Proceedings. SAE Paper No. 730978.

82. Society of Automotive Engineers. 1976. The Human Thorax--Anatomy, Injury, and Biomechanics, SAE P-67.

83. Stalnaker, R.L. and Mohan, D. 1974. Human Chest Impact Protection Criteria. 3rd International Conference on Occupant Protection Proceedings, pp. 384-393.

84. Strassman, G. 1947. Traumatic Rupture of the Aorta. American Heart Journal 33:508.

85. Terhune, K.W., Smist, T.E. and Hendricks, D.L. 1982. Steering Column Special Study Data Analysis. 6804-Y-1/DOT/HS 806 287. Calspan Field Services, Inc., Buffalo, NY.

86. Trollope, M.L., et al. 1973. The Mechanism of Blunt Injury in Abdominal Trauma. Journal of Trauma 13:962-970.

87. Verriest, J.P., Chapon, A. and Trauchessec, R. 1981. Cinephotogrammetrical Study of Porcine Thoracic Response to Belt Applied Load in Frontal Impact--Comparison between Living and Dead Subjects. 25th Stapp Car Crash Conference Proceedings, pp. 499-545.

88. Viano, D.C. 1978. Thoracic Injury Potential. Proceedings 3rd International Meeting on the Simulation and Reconstruction of Impacts in Collisions, pp. 142-156.

89. Viano, D.C., et al. 1988. Factors Influencing Biomechanical Response and Closed Chest Trauma in Experimental Thoracic Impacts. In: Huelke, D.F., ed., 22nd Proceedings American Assoc. for Automotive Medicine, pp. 67-82.

90. Viano, D.C., et al. 1978. Sensitivity of Porcine Thoracic Responses and Injuries to Various Frontal and a Lateral Impact Site. 22nd Stapp Car Crash Conference Proceedings, pp. 167-207.

91. Viano, D.C., Kroell, C.K. and Warner, C.Y. 1977. Comparative Thoracic Impact Response of Living and Sacrificed Porcine Siblings. 21st Stapp Car Crash Conference Proceedings, pp. 627-709.

92. Viano, D.C. and Haut, R.C. 1978. Factors Influencing Biomechanical Response and Closed Chest Trauma in Experimental Thoracic Impact. American Association for Automotive Medicine, Ann Arbor, MI, July.

93. Viano, D.C. and Lau, V.K. 1983. Role of Impact Velocity and Chest Compression in Thoracic Injury. Aviation, Space, and Environmental Medicine 54(1):16-21. Jan.

94. Viano, D.C. and Warner, C.Y. 1976. Thoracic Impact Response of Live Porcine Subjects. In: 20th Stapp Car Crash Conference Proceedings. SAE Paper No. 860823.

95. Walfishch, G., et al. 1982. Tolerance Limits and Mechanical Characteristics of the Human Thorax in Frontal and Side Impact Transposition of These Characteristics into Protection Criteria. Proceedings 7th International IRCOBI Conference on the Biomechanics of Impacts, pp. 122-139.

96. Walt, A.J. and Wilson, R.F. 1973. Blunt Abdominal Injuries: An Overview. In: Biomechanics and Its Application to Automotive Design, NY: SAE.

97. William, G., et al. 1976. An Introduction to the Understanding of Blunt Chest Trauma. In: The Human Thorax-- Anatomy, Injury, and Biomechanics, SAE P-67, pp. 11-36.

98. Wiott, J.F. 1975. The Radiologic Manifestations of Blunt Chest Trauma. American Medical Assoc. Journal 231(5):500-503. Feb.

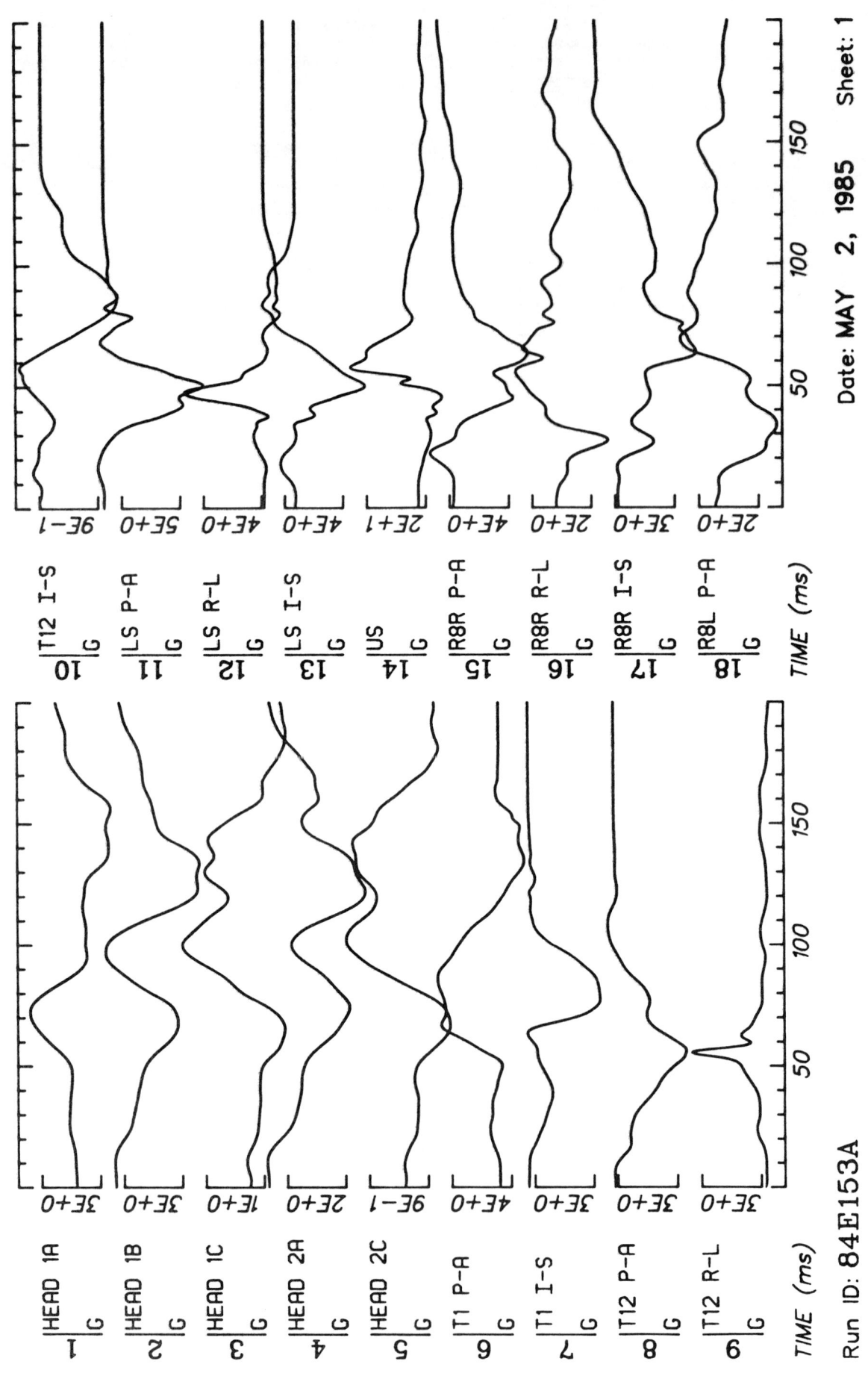

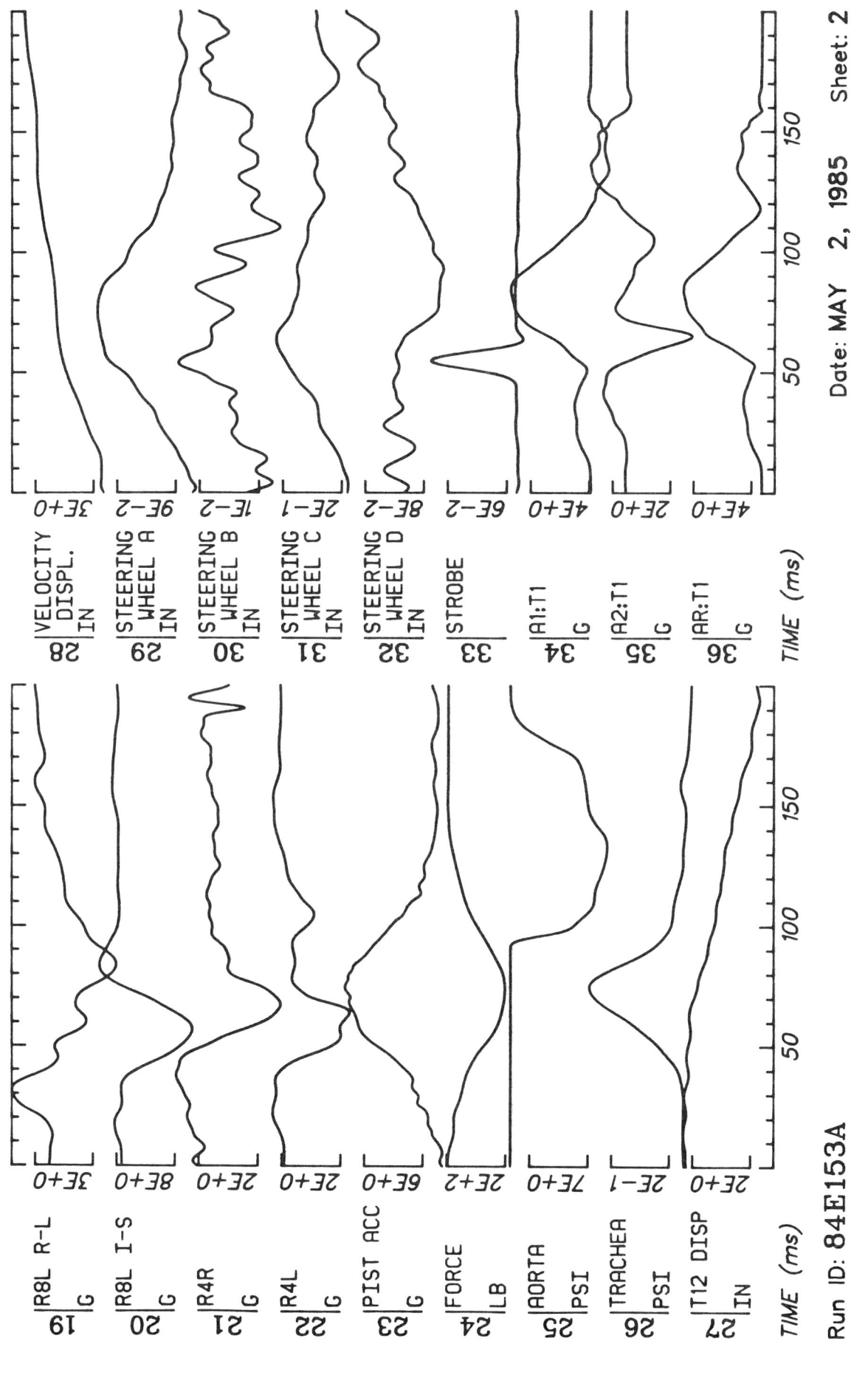

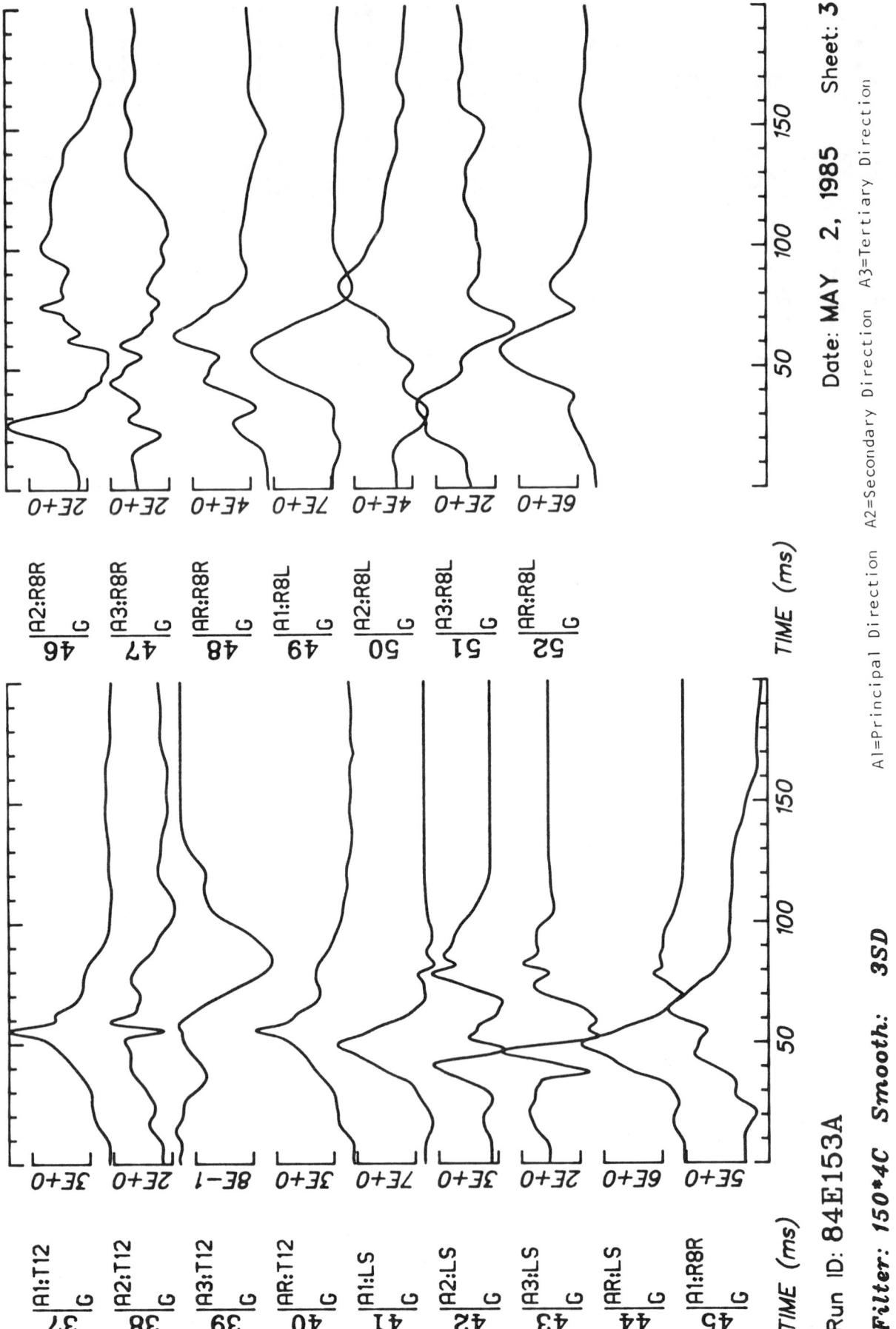

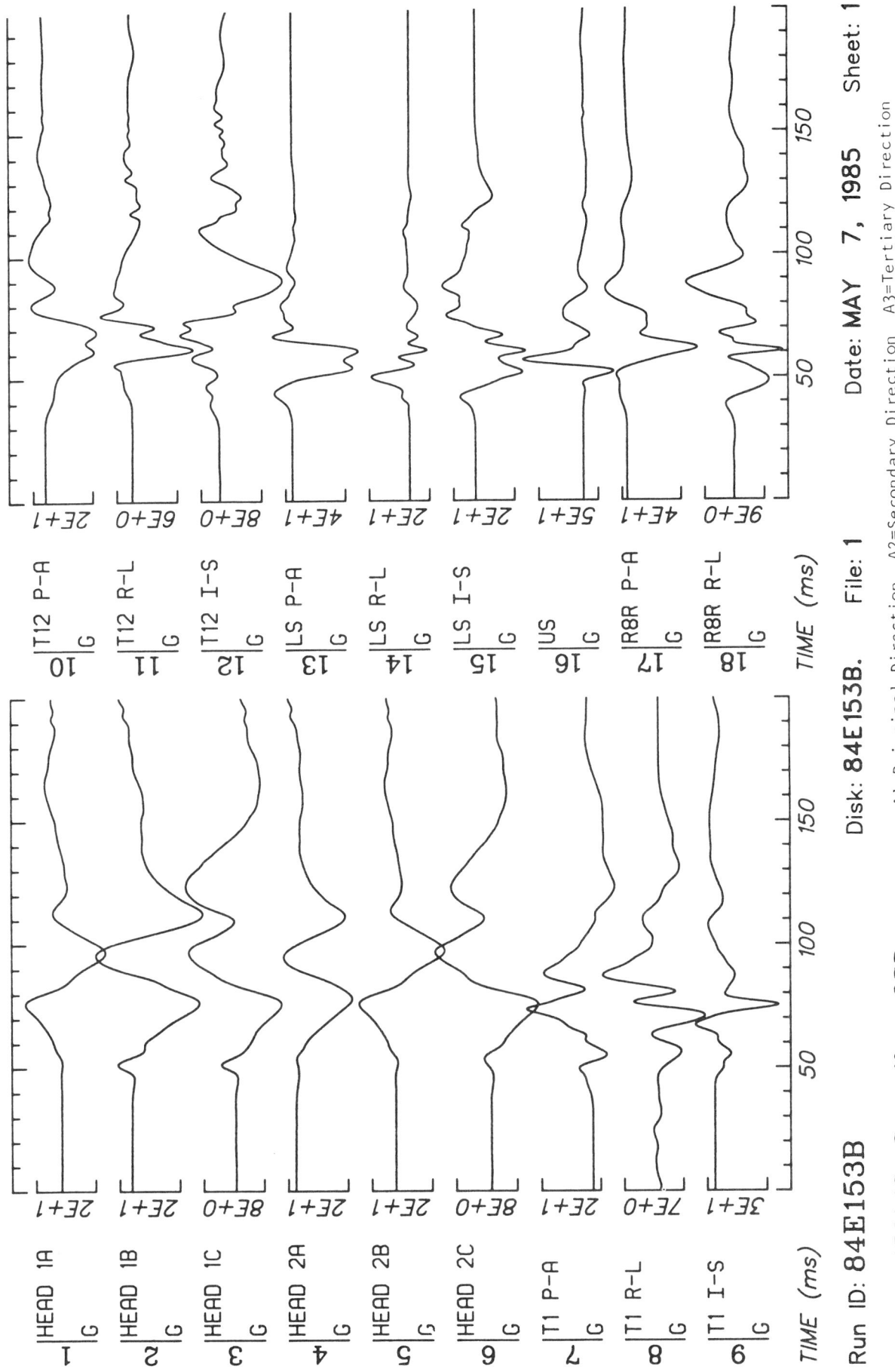

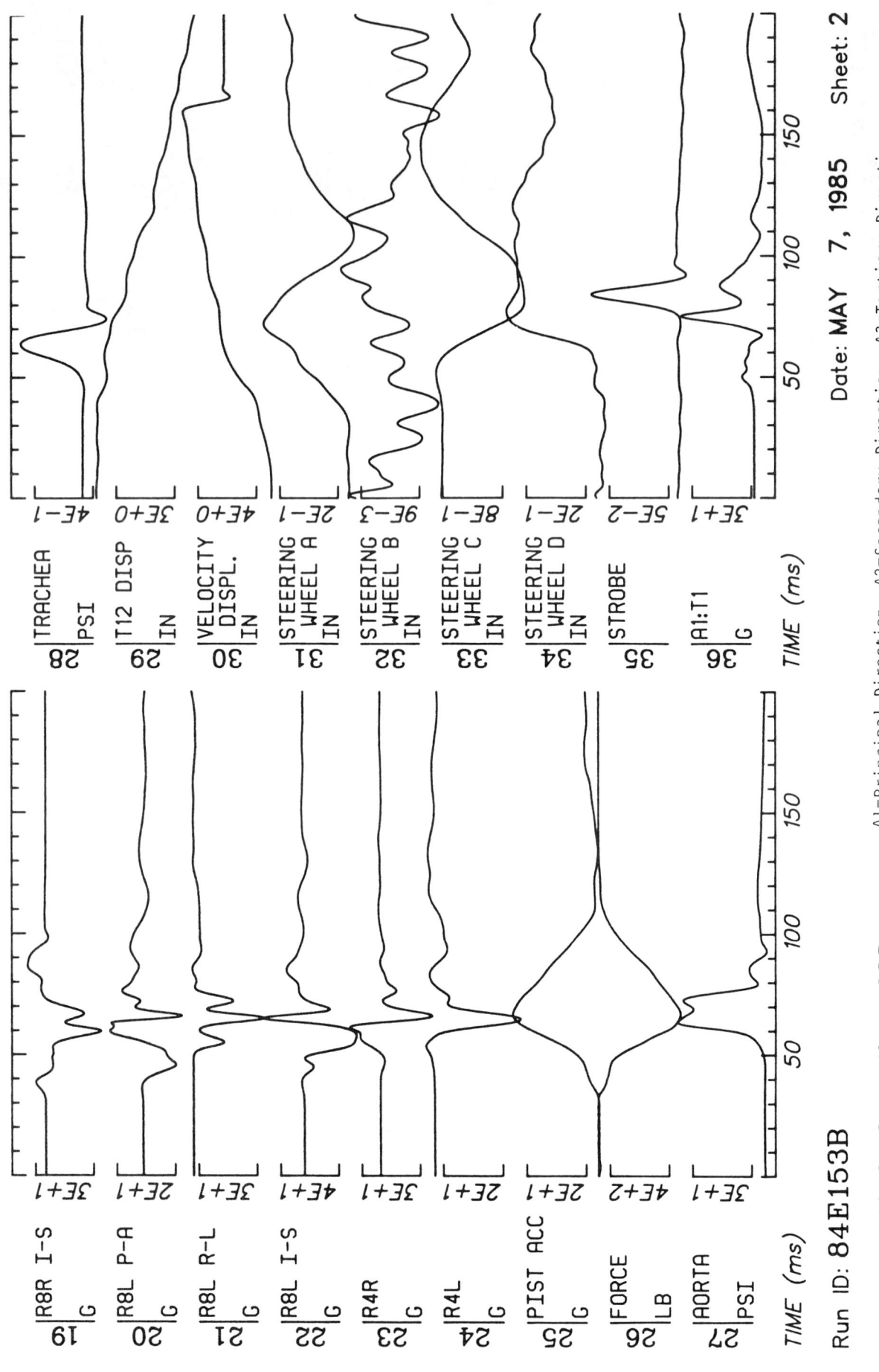

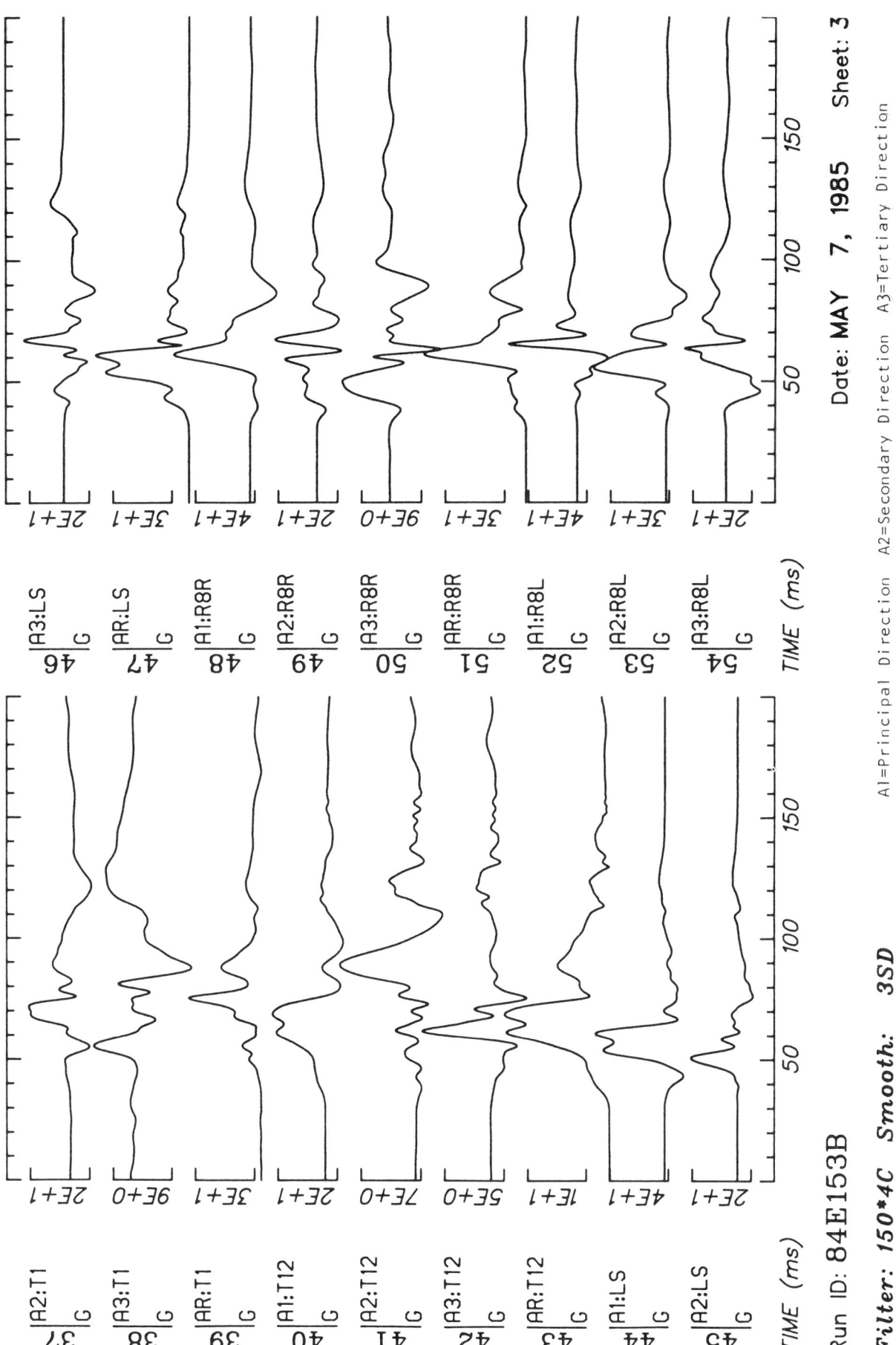

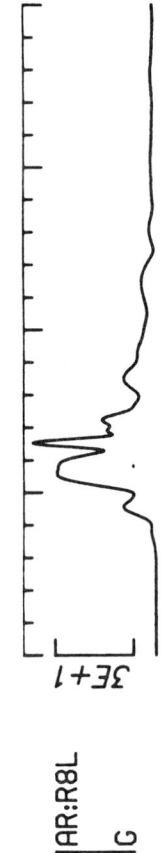

TIME (ms)

Run ID: **84E153B**

Filter: **150*4C** ***Smooth:*** **3SD**

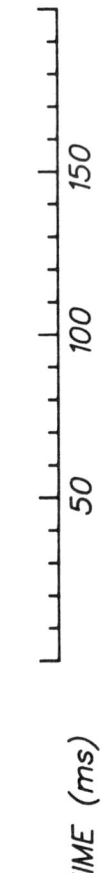

Date: **MAY 7, 1985** Sheet: **4**

A1=Principal Direction A2=Secondary Direction A3=Tertiary Direction

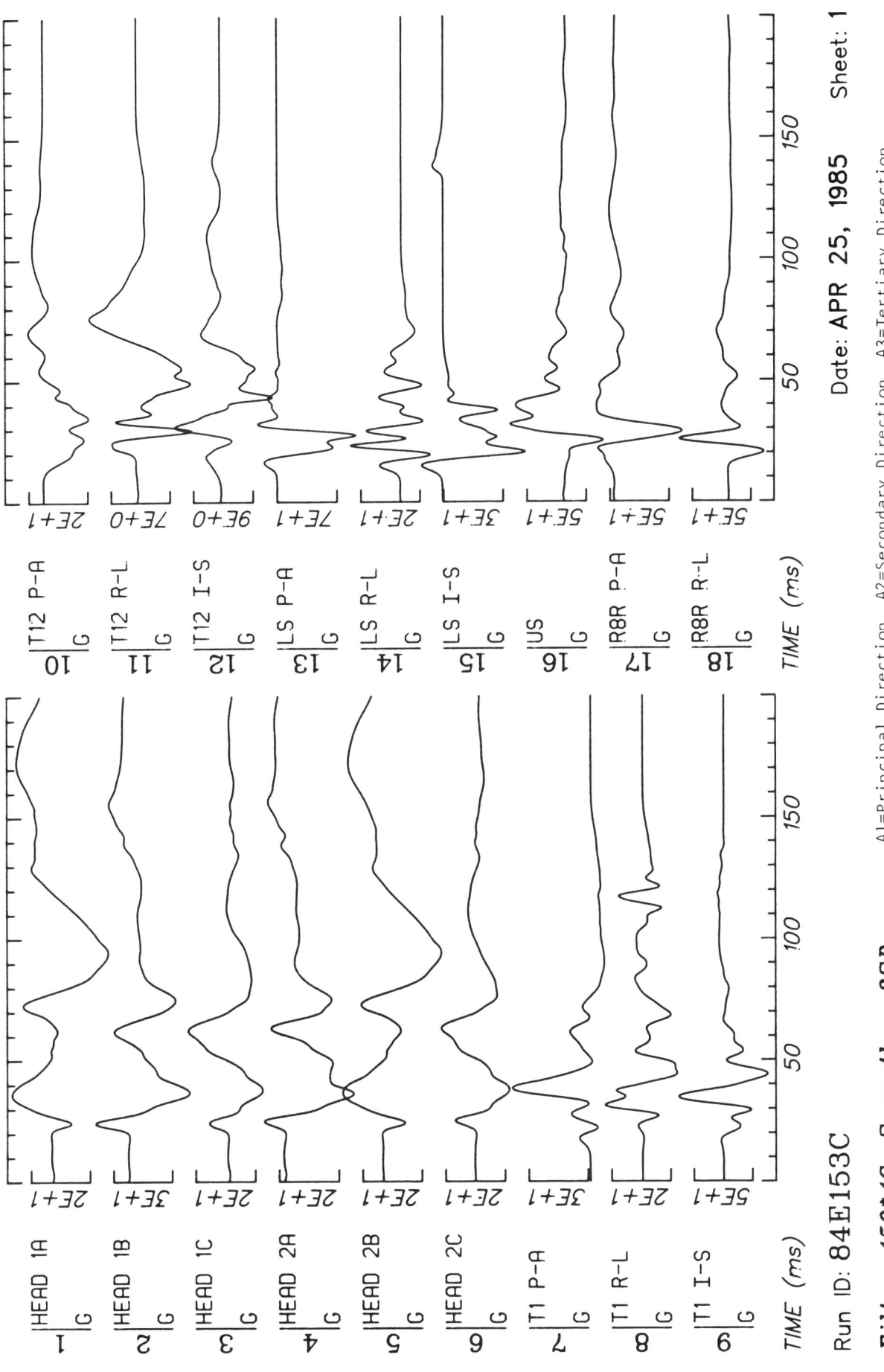

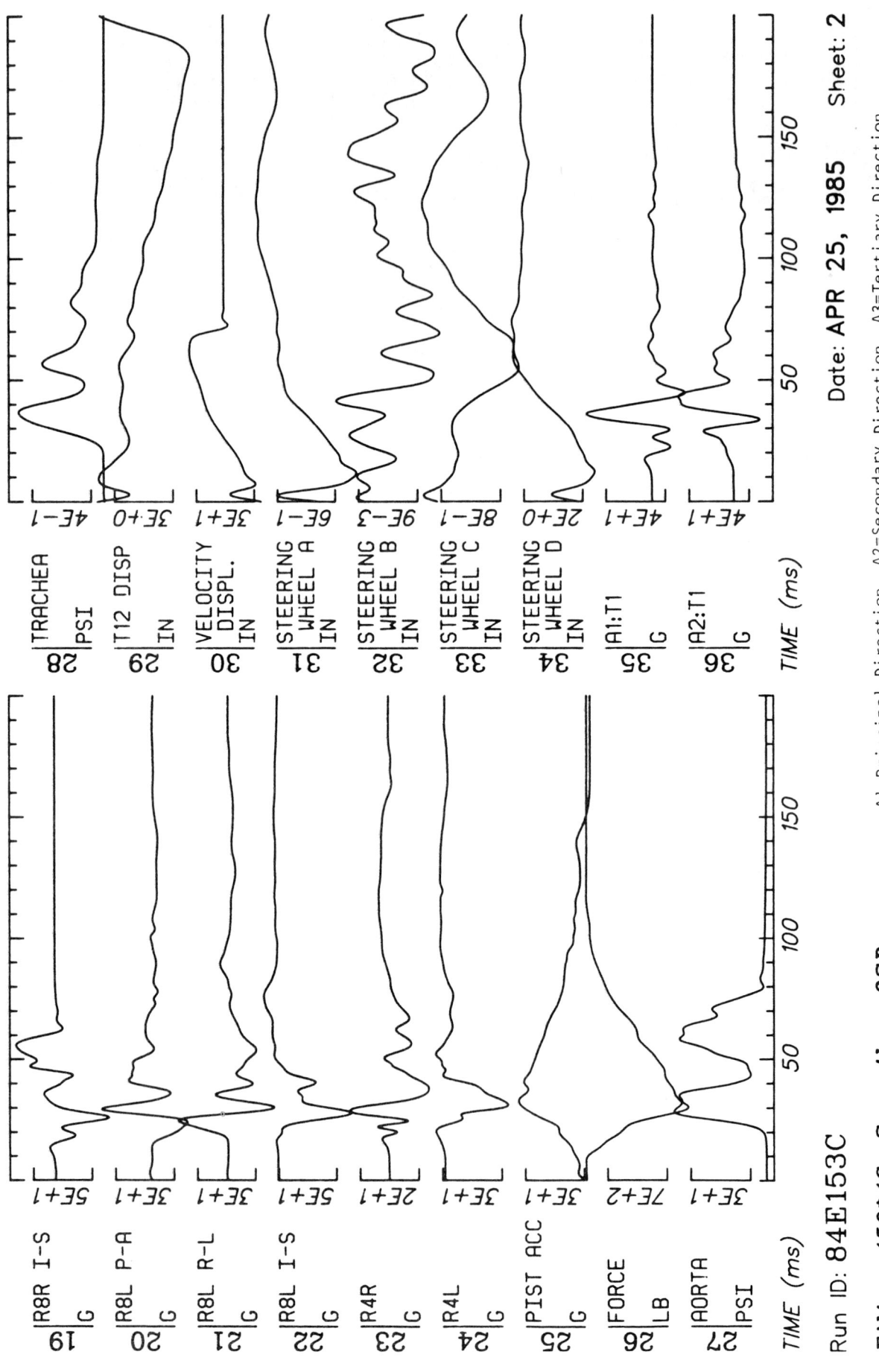

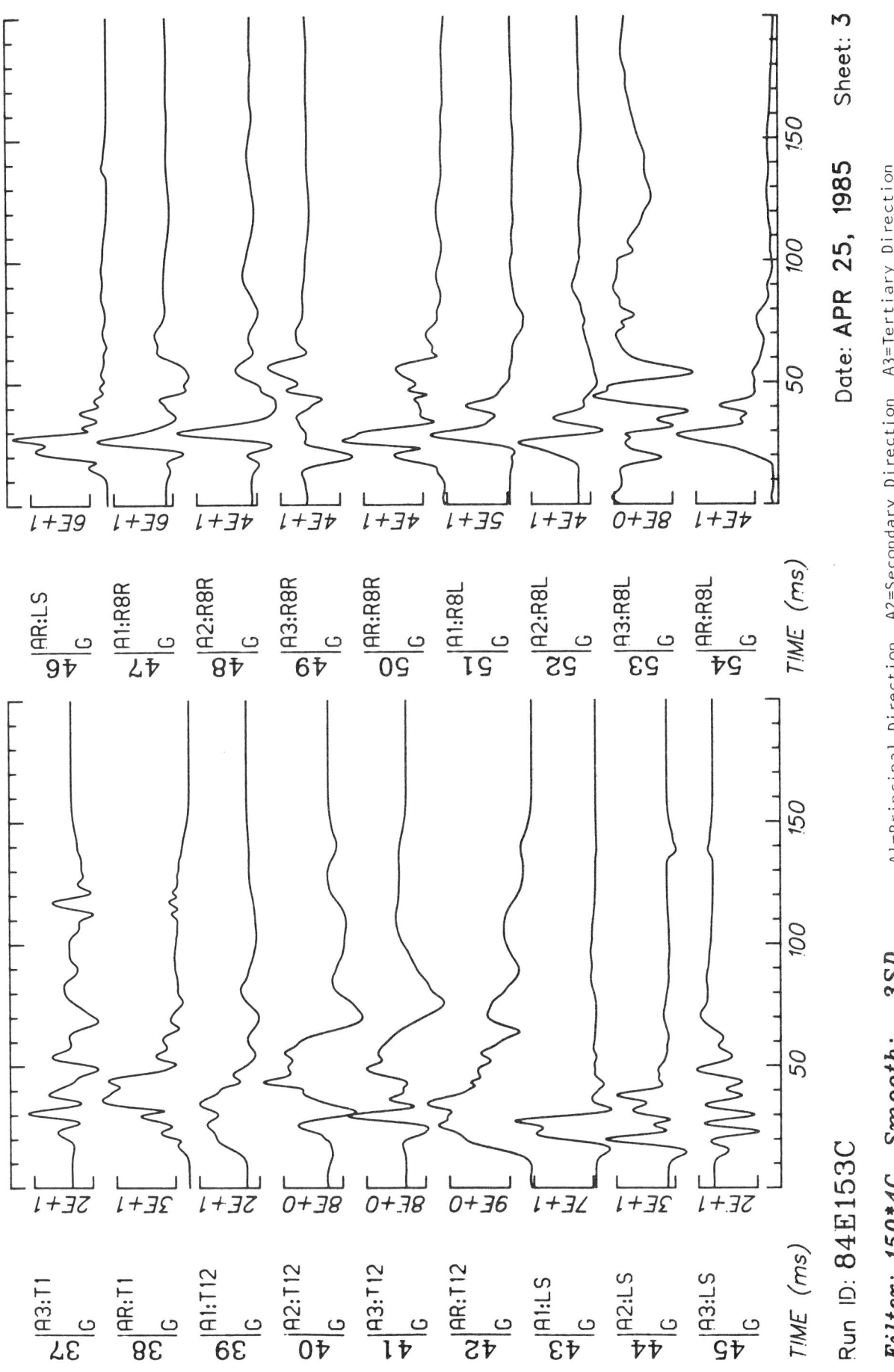

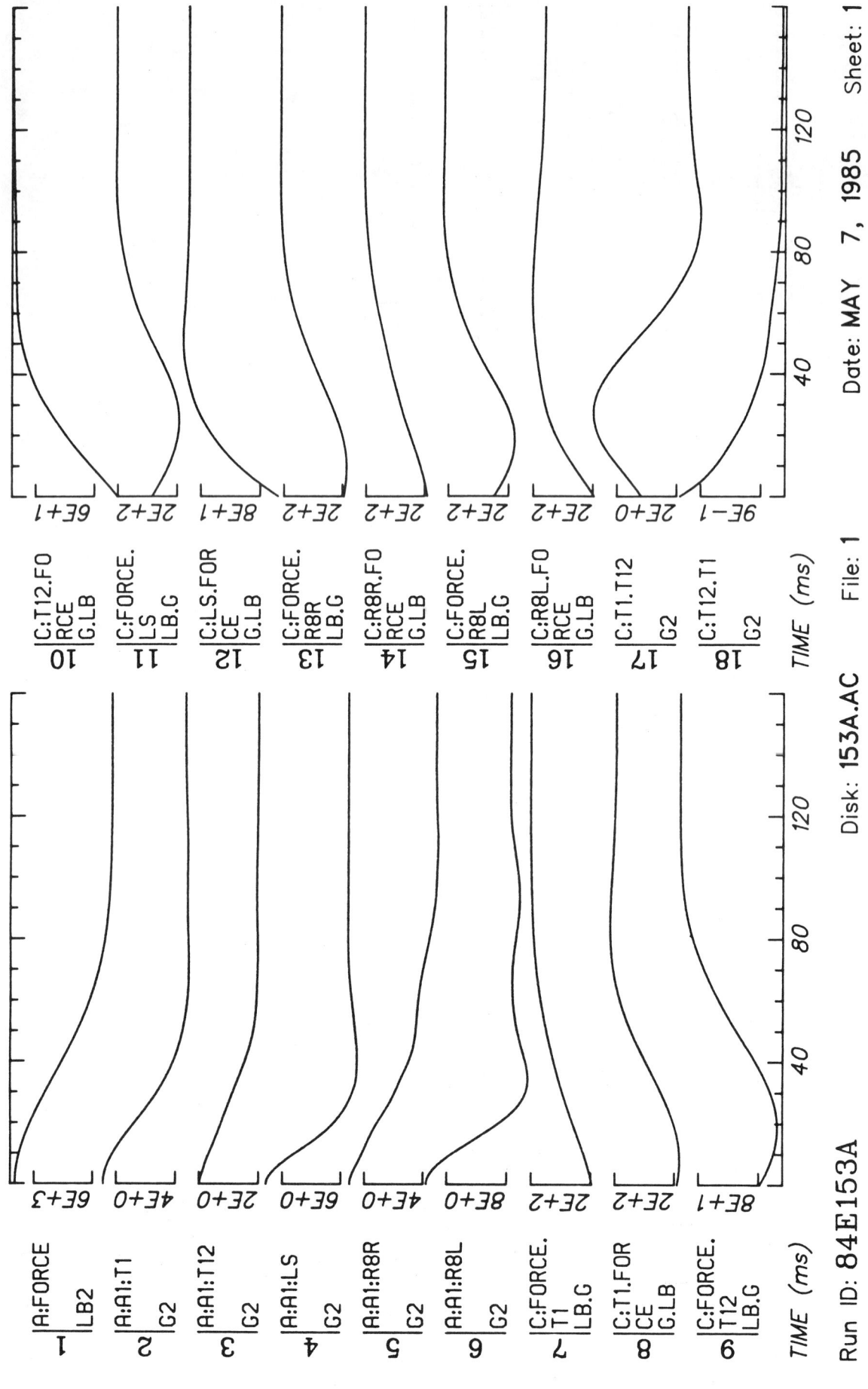

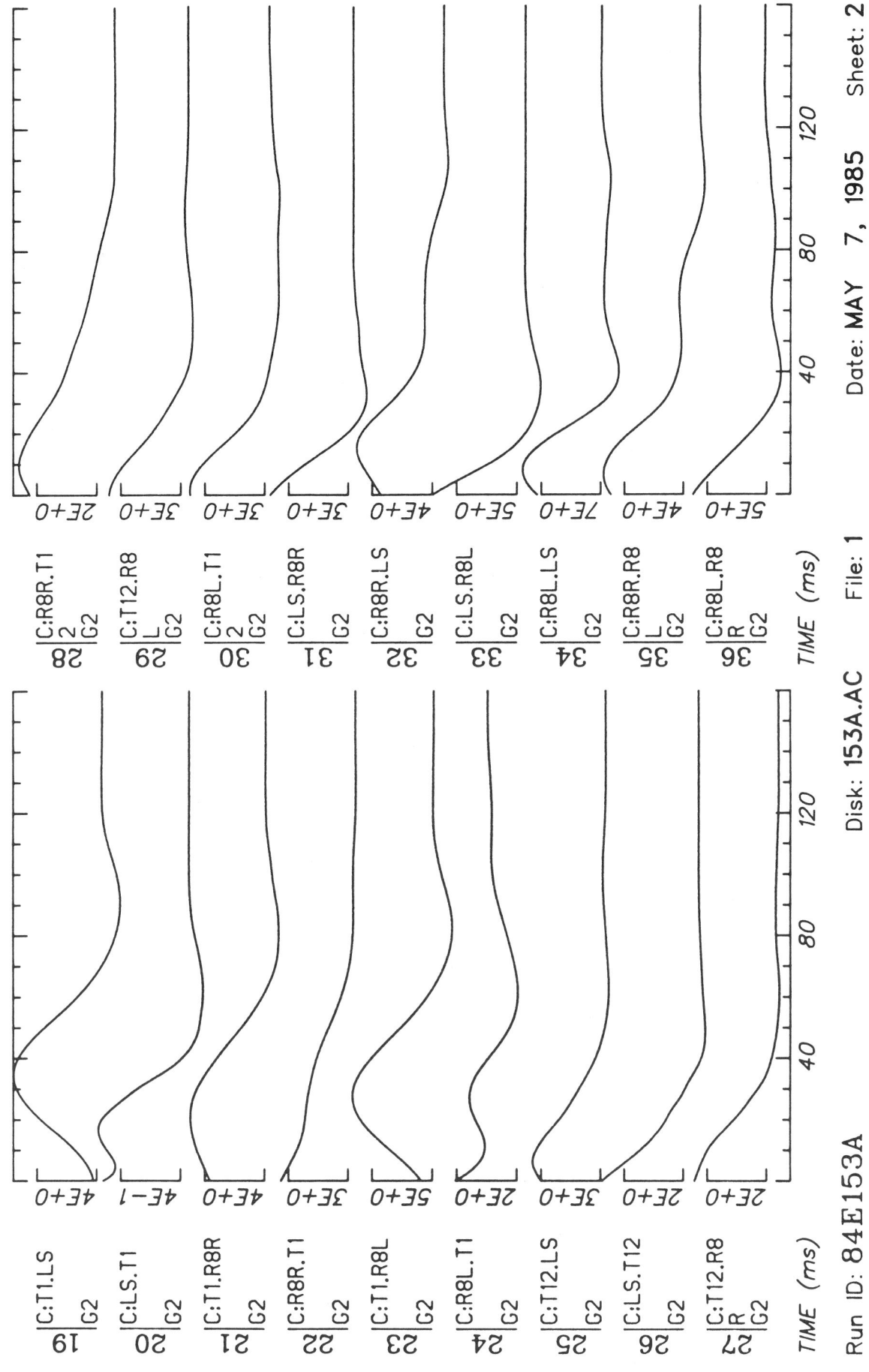

Auto- and Cross-correlations for Low-Velocity Steering Wheel Impacts for Principal Direction Acceleration and/or Force A=Auto C=Cross

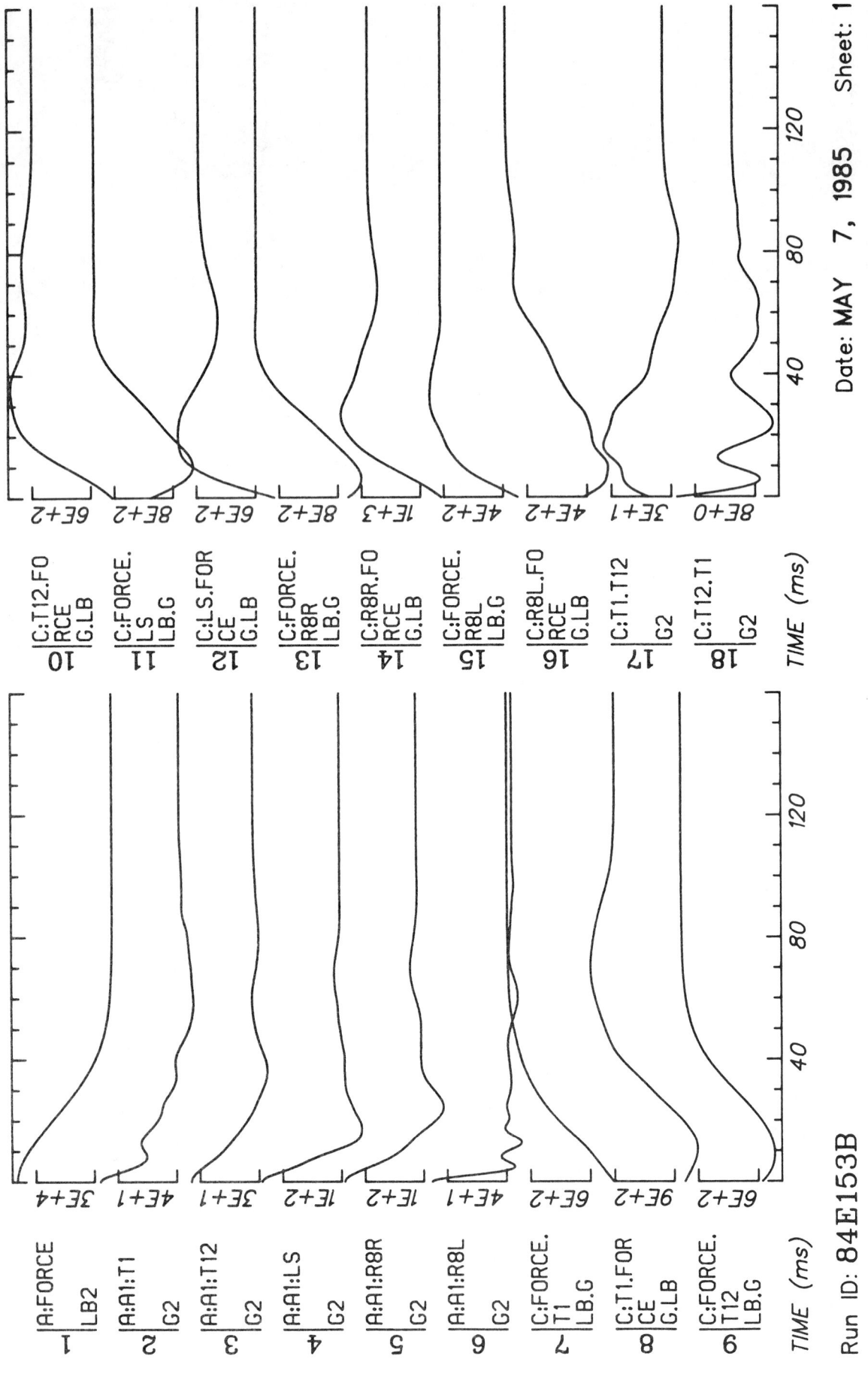

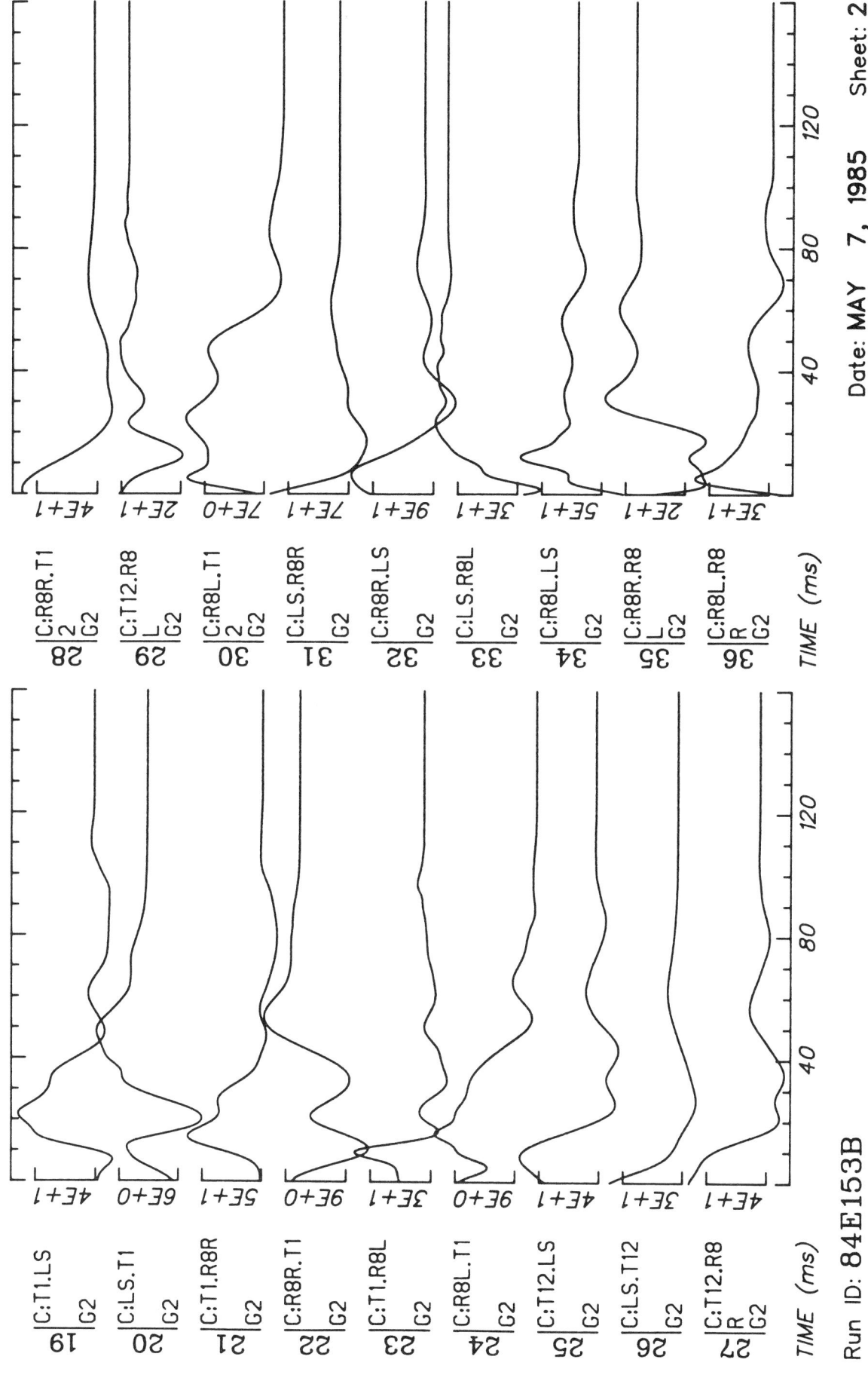

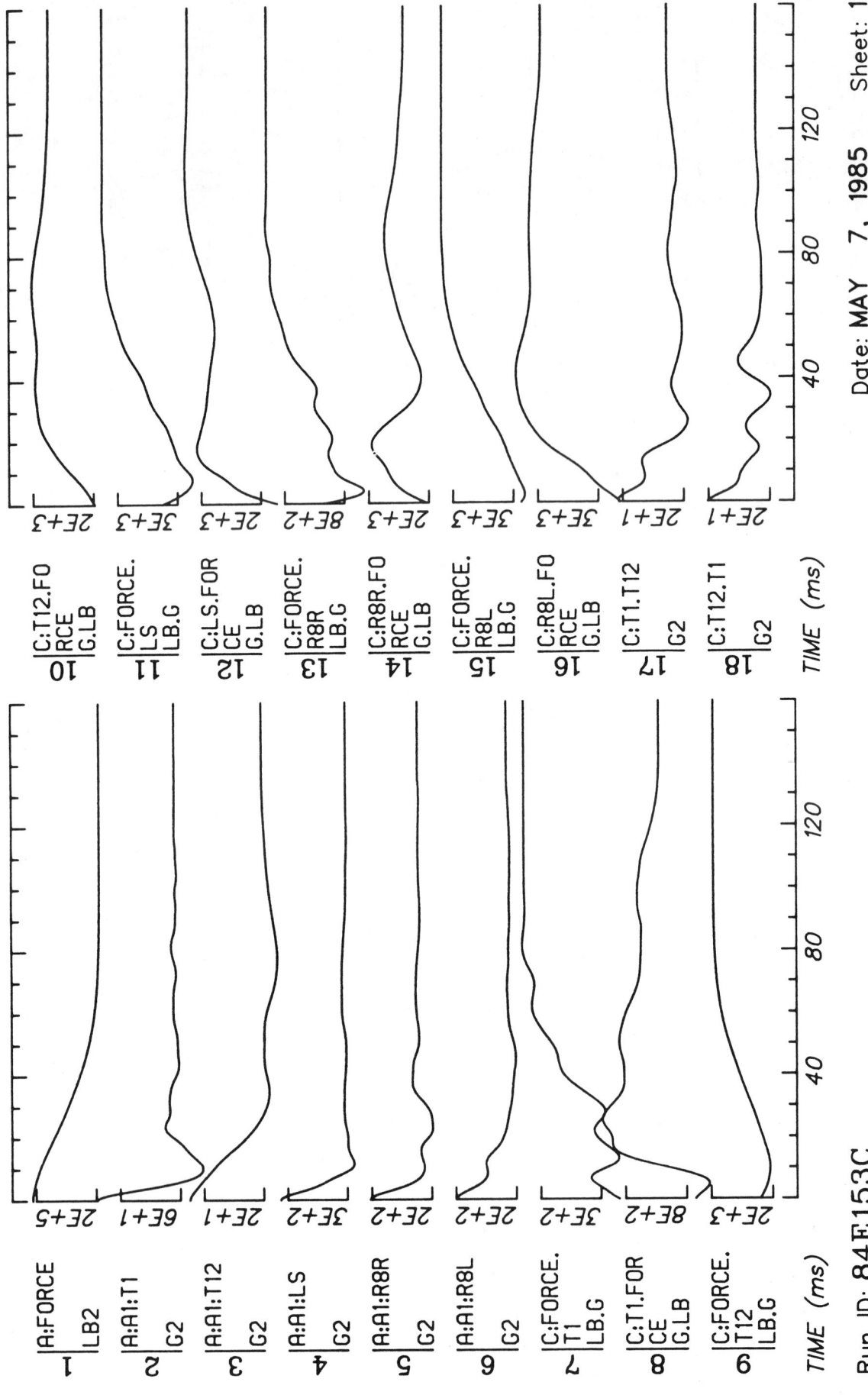

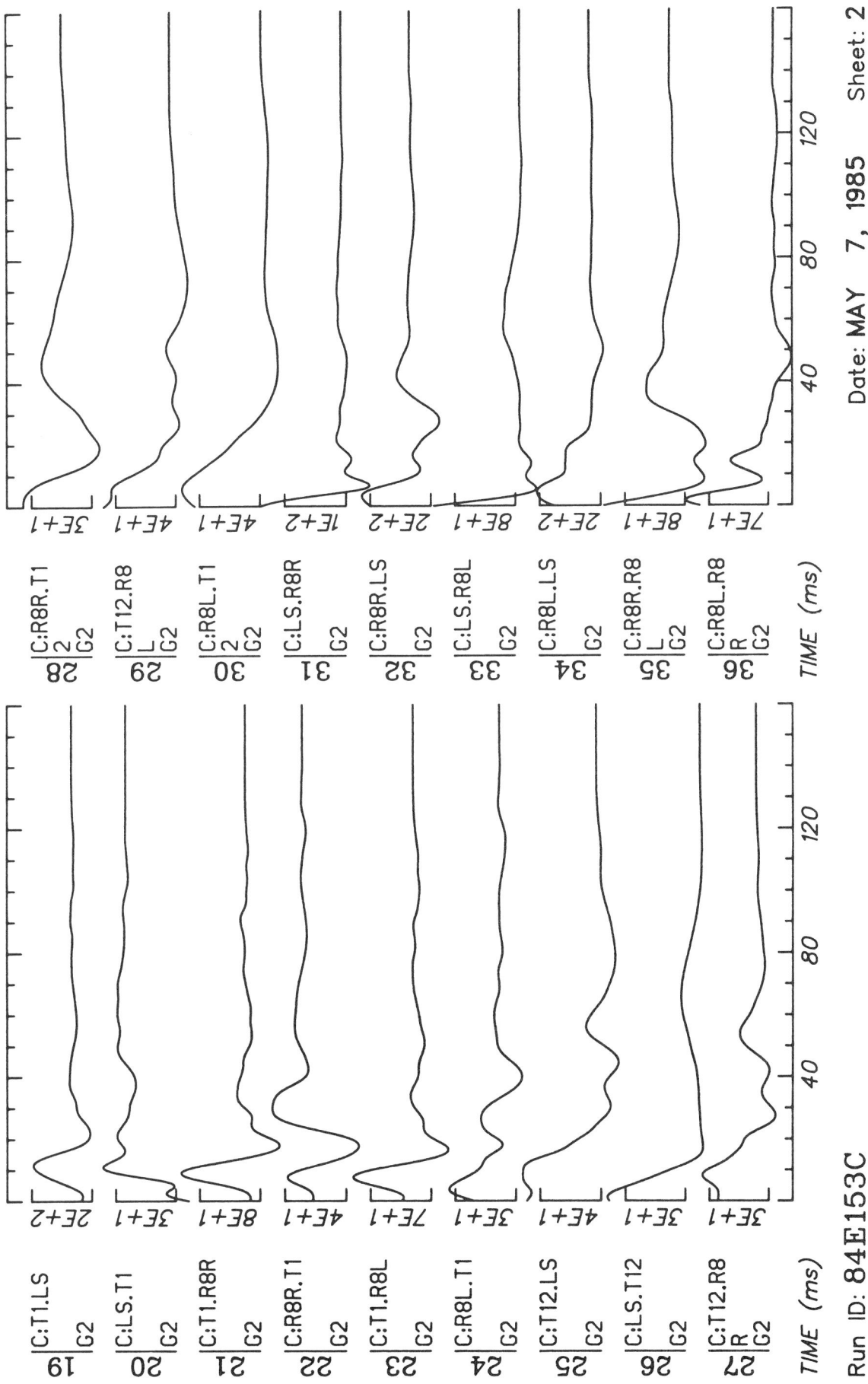

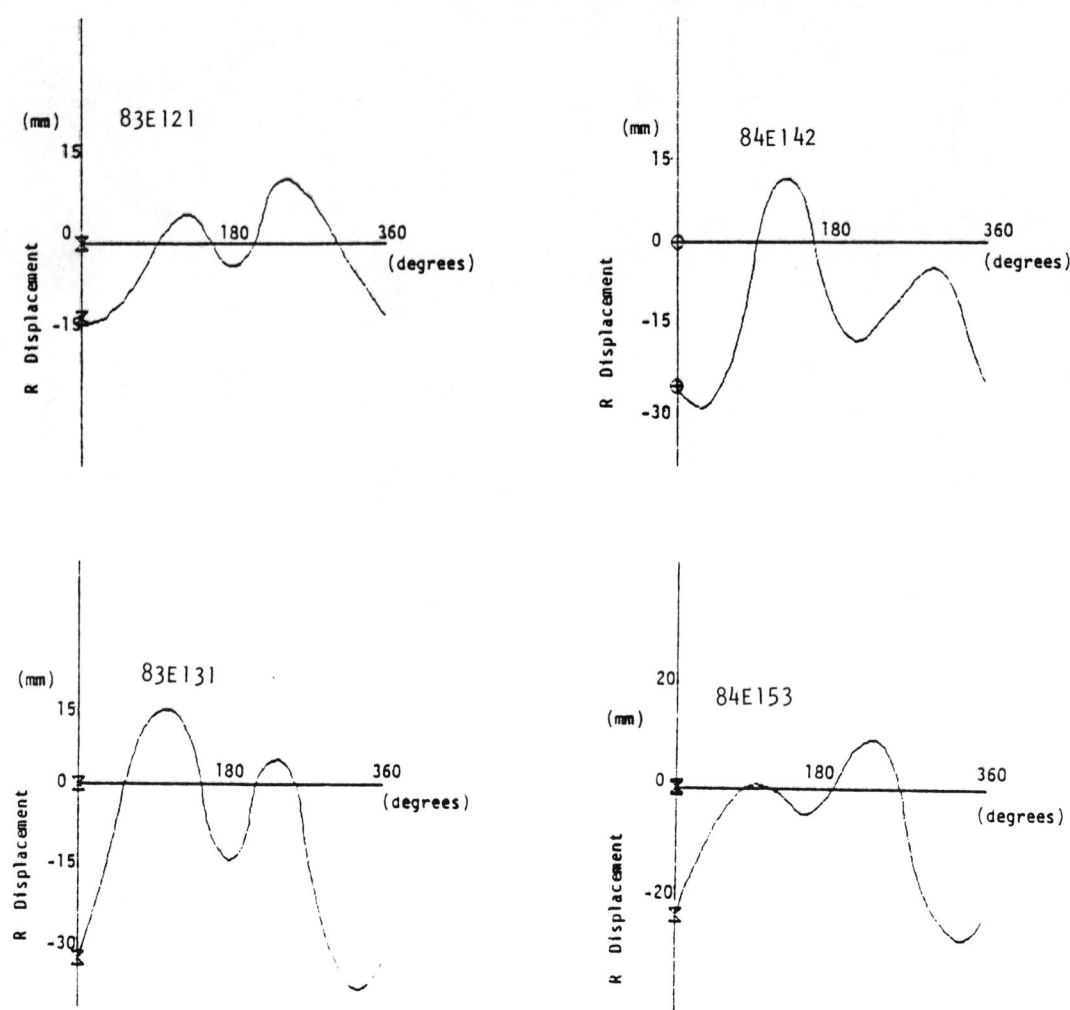

RADIAL DISPLACEMENT: STEERING WHEEL DEFORMATION

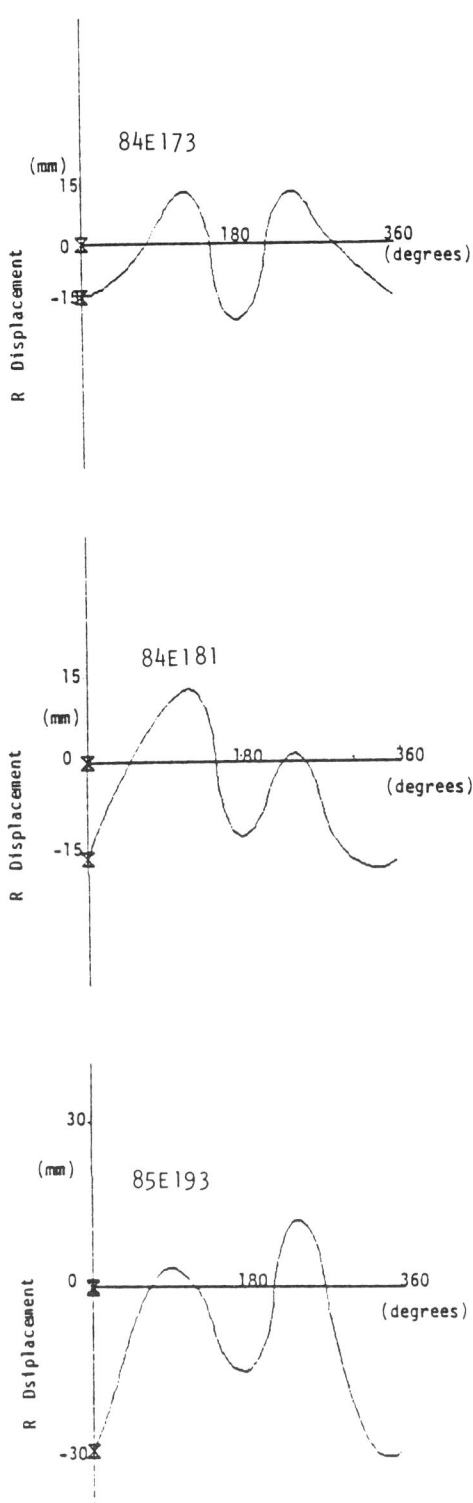

RADIAL DISPLACEMENT: STEERING WHEEL DEFORMATION

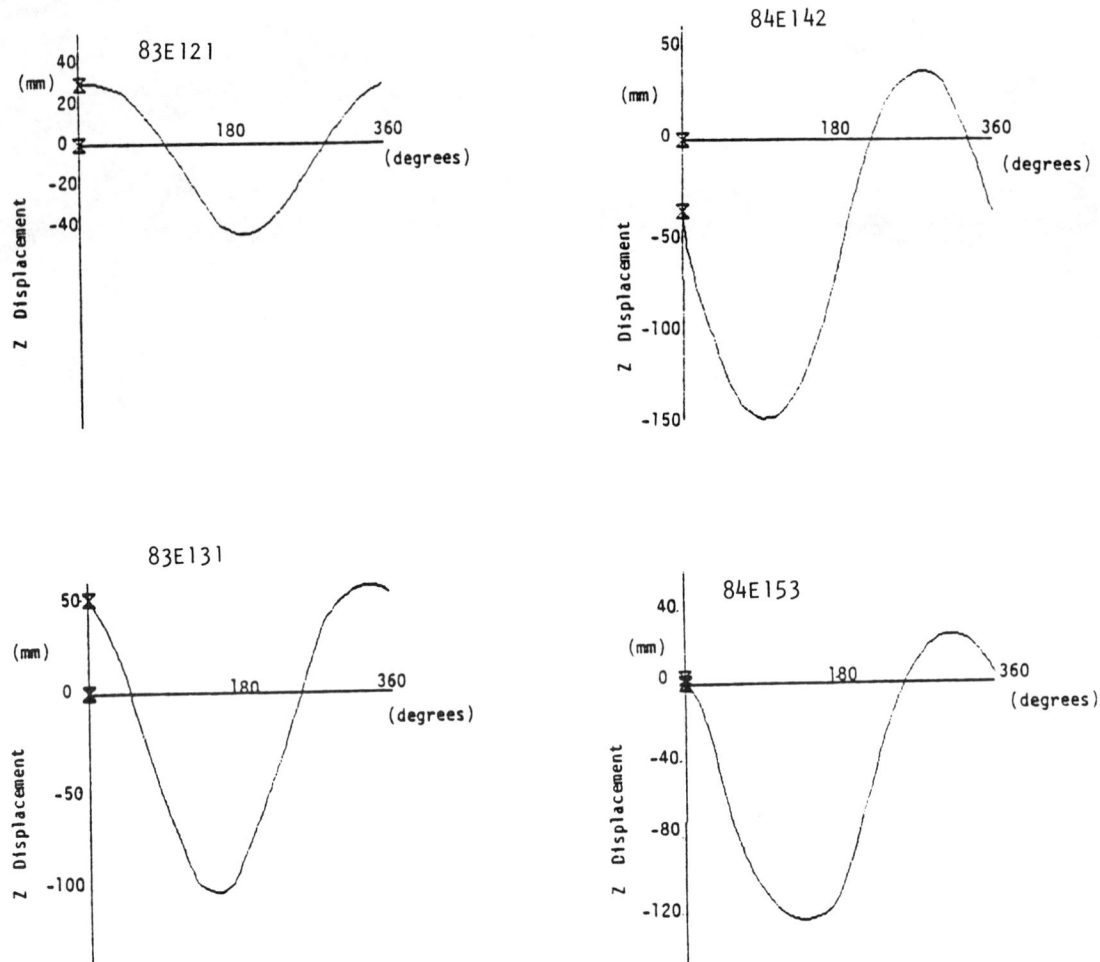

Z - AXIS DISPLACEMENT: STEERING WHEEL DEFORMATION

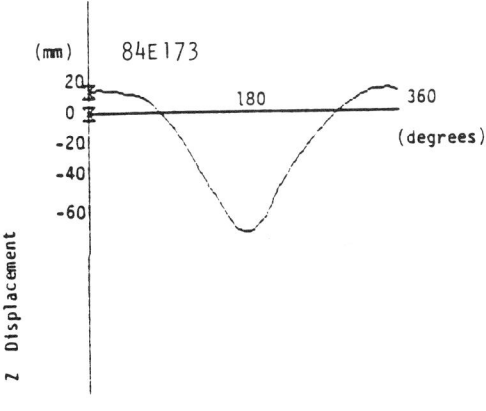
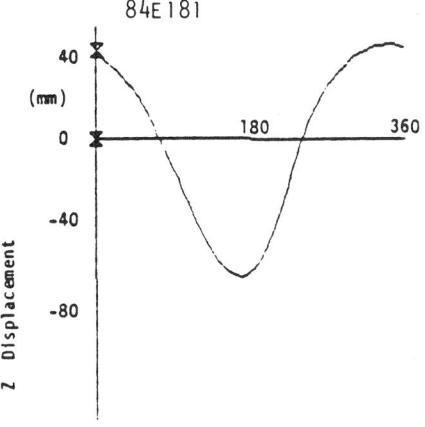
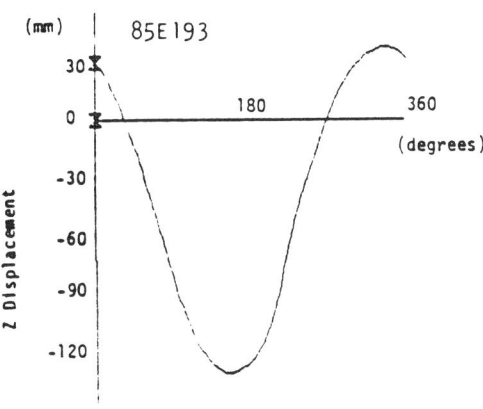

Z - AXIS DISPLACEMENT: STEERING WHEEL DEFORMATION

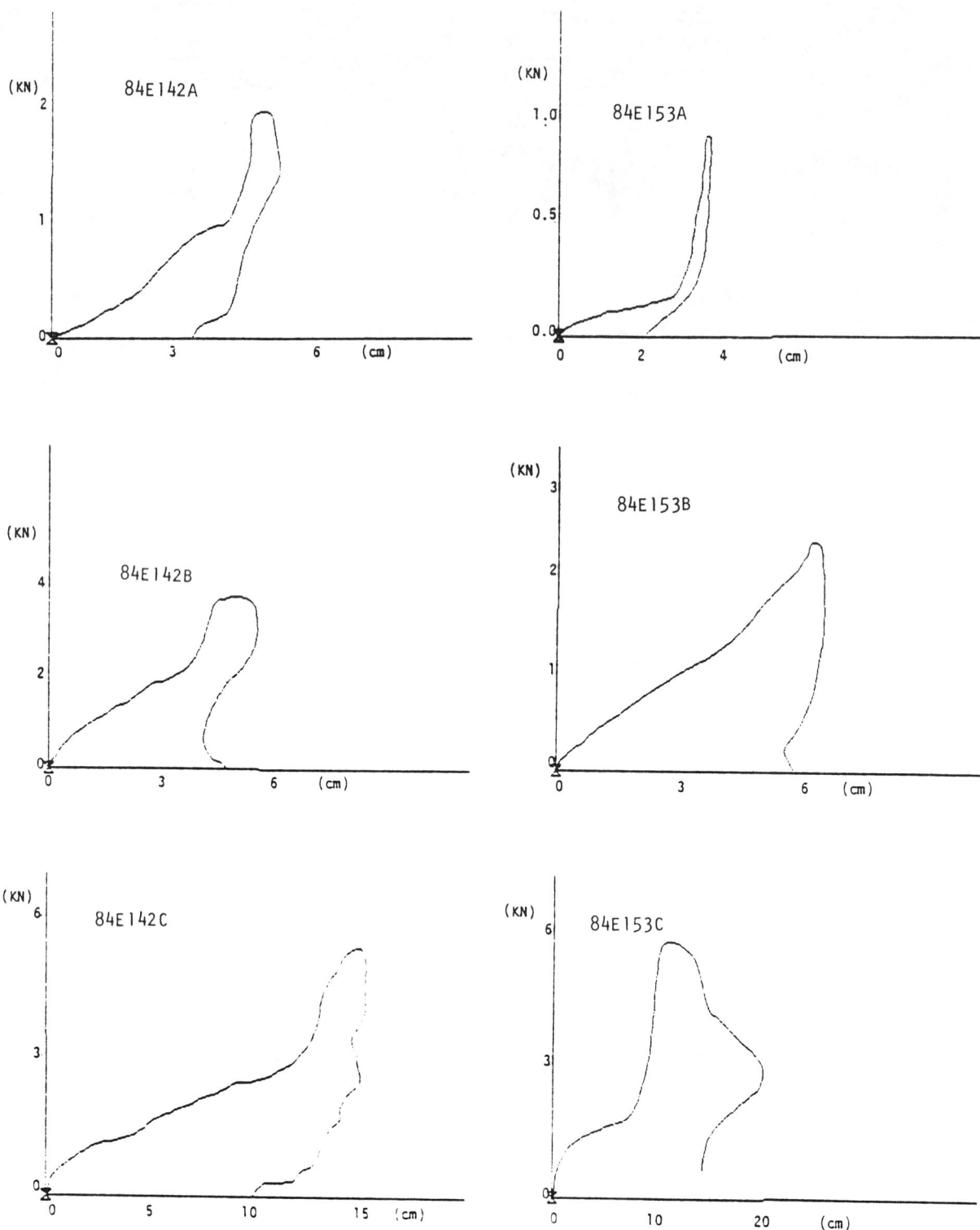

FORCE DEFLECTION: FORCE OBTAINED FROM STEERING WHEEL HUB, DEFLECTION OBTAINED FROM STRING POTS AND HIGH SPEED FILM ANALYSIS

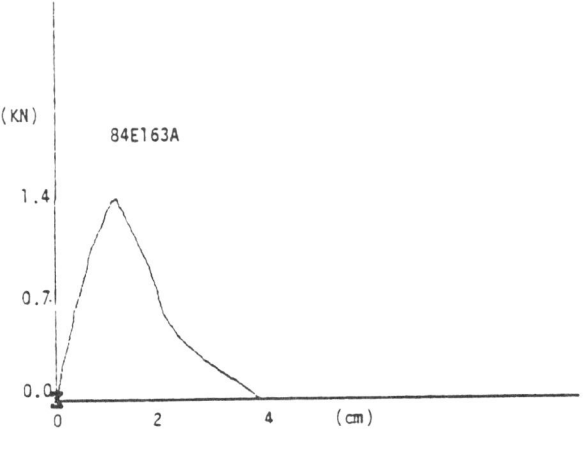
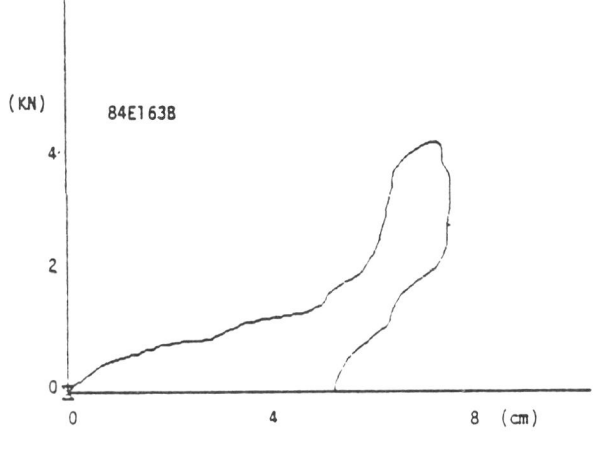
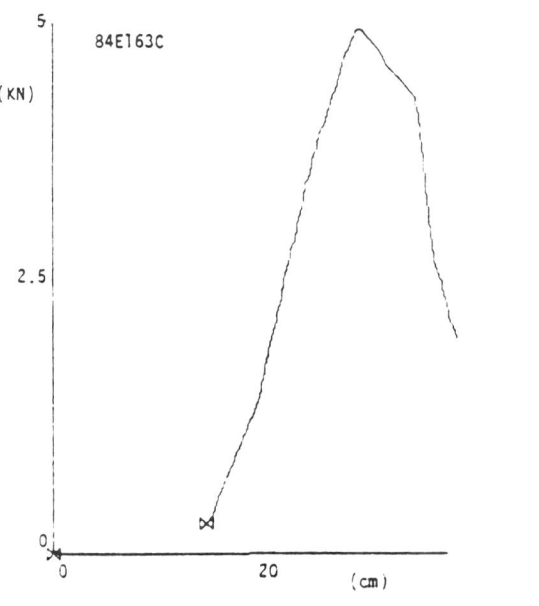

FORCE DEFLECTION: FORCE OBTAINED FROM STEERING WHEEL HUB, DEFLECTION OBTAINED FROM STRING POTS AND HIGH SPEED FILM ANALYSIS

872202

Interaction of Human Cadaver and Hybrid III Subjects with a Steering Assembly

Richard M. Morgan, Rolf H. Eppinger, and Jeffrey H. Marcus
U.S. DOT/NHTSA

Dennis C. Schneider, Alan M. Nahum, Joseph Awad, and David Dainty
Univ. of California at San Diego

Steve Forrest
MCR Technology

ABSTRACT   Nineteen sled impact tests were conducted simulating a frontal collision exposure for an unrestrained driver. The deceleration sled buck configuration utilized the passenger compartment of a late model compact passenger vehicle, a rigid driver's seat, and a custom fabricated energy-absorbing steering column and wheel assembly. Sled impact velocities ranged from 24.1 to 42.6 km/hr. The purpose of the study was to investigate the kinematic and kinetic interaction of the driver and the energy-absorbing steering assembly and their relationship to the thoracic/abdominal injuries produced.

The similarities and differences between human cadaver and anthropomorphic dummy subjects were quantified. A Hybrid III test subject subject developed (1) similar axial steering column forces to those produced by the cadaver subjects, (2) lower initial peak spinal acceleration than the cadaver subjects, and (3) larger steering wheel rim moments about the pitch axis than when the cadavers upper abdomen contacted the lower wheel rim. Calculations of the effective mass of the test subjects interacting with the column assembly also demonstrated similarity. The averages of the steering rim deformations suggest more rim deformation at the top and less deformation at the bottom for the cadaver relative to the Hybrid III. Maximum Abbreviated Injury Scale injuries sustained in the cadaver exposures ranged from 2 to 5. At the 42.6 km/hr test condition three out of seven cadavers sustained liver injuries. Energy calculations lead to the conclusion the cadaver thorax absorbed a greater proportion of the initial kinetic energy than did the Hybrid III thorax.

INTRODUCTION   Just over two decades ago, a component test with a body torso form was suggested as a means of introducing reasonable energy-absorbing elements into steering assemblies.[1]* Once energy-absorbing steering assemblies became common, it was found [2] "current energy-absorbing steering assemblies annually prevent 1300 fatalities and 23,000 nonfatal injuries requiring hospitalization." In spite of the propitious news about steering assemblies, Malliaris et al. found the steering assembly still accounted for 26.9 % of the total "harm" to restrained and unrestrained occupants. [3] A succession of papers [4,5,6,7] focused on "what to do next" by conducting sled tests with the torso form, the Part 572 dummy, the Hybrid III dummy, and porcine subjects. The present paper focuses on the unrestrained occupant/ steering assembly interaction by using cadavers and the Hybrid III dummy in sled tests.

TEST METHODOLOGY   The sled buck employed in the study was based on a Chevrolet Citation passenger compartment. Figure 1 illustrates the sled buck and the driver's position. The production steering column assembly was replaced with a generic energy-absorbing design based on the deformation of a steel tape in a roller assembly at the forward end of the column which provided a constant force versus column stroke characteristic shown in Figure 2 (the steel tape was moved about 2.54 cm through the rollers prior to the sled test to insure the mechanism was not stuck). The standard Citation column and the roller assembly column are shown in Figure 3. The stroking mass, or that mass lying between the occupant chest and the energy absorbing element, of the two designs are within 30 grams of each other. (The total mass of the production column is about 3.49 kg more than the generic design,i. e., the energy-absorbing steering assembly on the sled is matched to the stroking mass of the Citation steering column and not the total mass.) The production steering wheel, Figure 4, was modified to allow incorporation of instrumentation which permitted measurement of axial loads applied to the

---
* The number in brackets refers to references at the end of the paper.

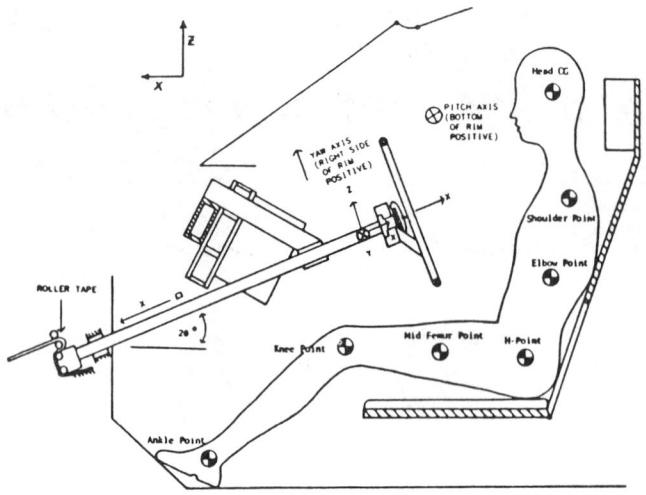

Figure 1 - Driver's Compartment Configuration

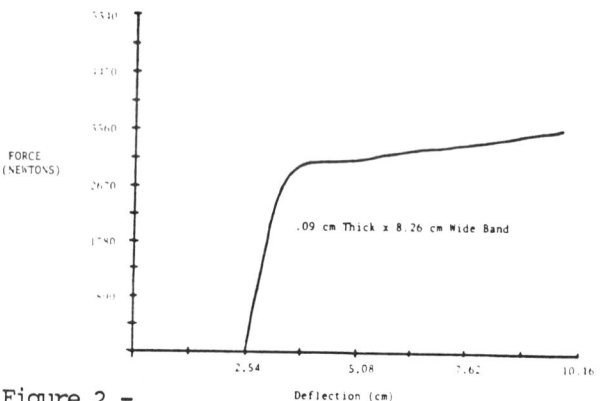

Figure 2 - Typical Steering Column Force/Deflection Characteristics under Axial Loading

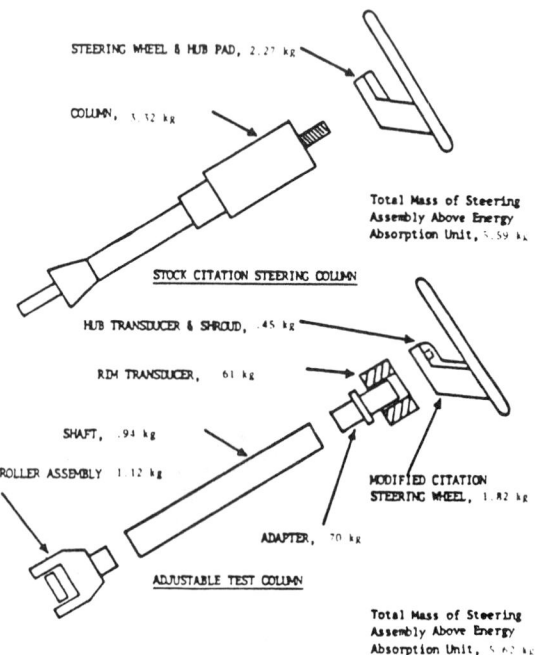

Figure 3 - Stock Citation versus Generic Steering Assembly

steering hub. Located between the wheel and column is a five axis transducer which measures (1) orthogonal forces along the column axis and perpendicular to it in a vertical and horizontal direction, and (2) moments applied to the steering wheel about the pitch and yaw axes. The direction and sign convention for the steering transducers are contained in Figure 1.

The production instrument panel was removed and occupant knee restraint was controlled by deformable blocks of semi-rigid polyurethane foam. A rigid seat back and cushion were adjusted longitudinally and vertically to accommodate stature changes of the cadaver subjects. The windshield was replaced following each sled exposure. The sled deceleration pulse utilized was a square wave, e. g., 7.5 G's magnitude and .114 seconds duration for a 24.1 km/hr sled test. All tests simulated a 12 o'clock frontal collision direction. A review of crash test data for the Citation vehicle indicated low levels of horizontal and vertical wheel movement for the velocity range of interest and therefore column intrusion was not simulated.

The instrumentation for the cadaver subjects included an array of 15 accelerometers placed around the thorax [8,9] as shown in Figure 5. A triaxial accelerometer was attached to the spinal column at the 4th thoracic vertebra. The thoracic accelerometer array secured to the Hybrid III included a triaxial accelerometer at the thoracic center of gravity location depicted in Figure 6. [10]

Chest deflection was measured directly on the Hybrid III dummy. Points on the dummy subject -- indicated by photographic targets placed around the body and on the buck -- were digitized. An algorithm was developed to determine the difference between the spinal marker and the sternal marker, or the chest deflection. In comparing the actual chest deflection in the dummy with the chest deflection determined by film analysis,

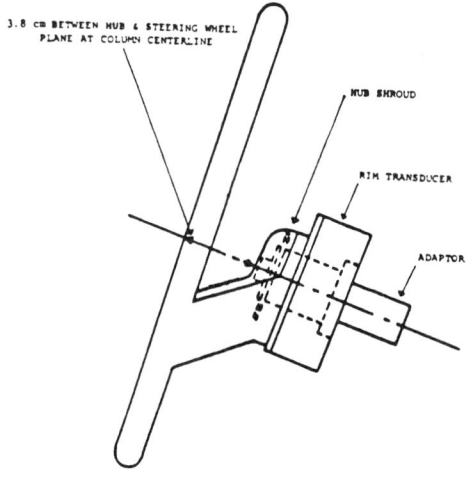

Figure 4 - Modified Citation Steering Wheel

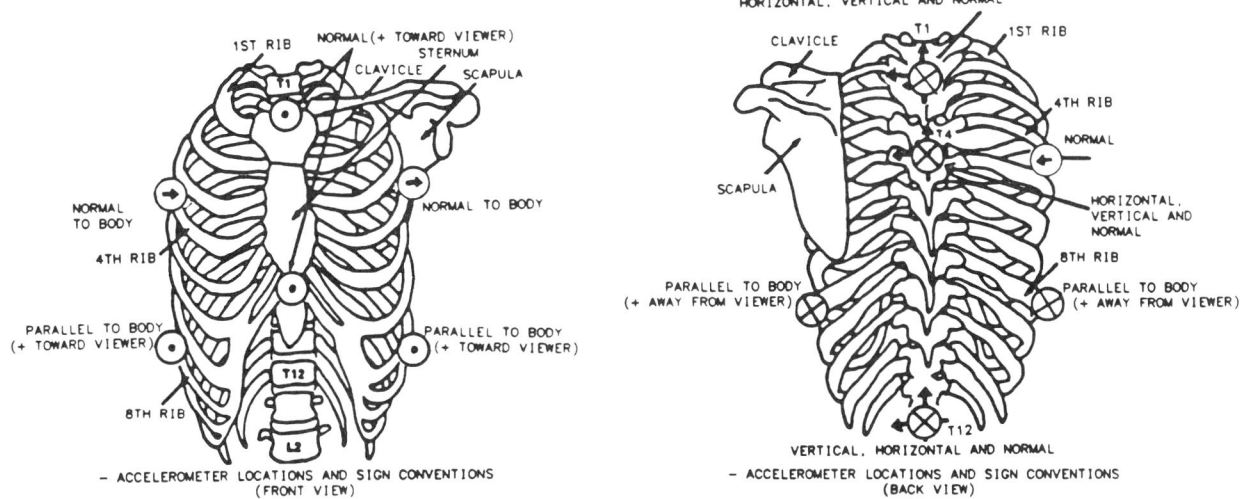

Figure 5 - Skeleton Accelerometer Locations

TEST NO	SLED INITIAL VELOCITY (km/h)	SLED CHANGE OF VELOCITY (km/h)	CONTACT RELATIVE VELOCITY (OCCUPANT TO STEERING ASSEMBLY) (km/h)	SUBJECT MASS (kg)	AGE (years)	SEX	MAXIMUM CHEST STROKE (cm)	MAXIMUM CHEST RESULTANT ACCELERATION (G's)	MAXIMUM LOWER STERNAL ACCELERATION (G'S)
HYBRID 3									
CI85015	25.4	27.4	19.0	74.4	NA	NA	3.7	17.6	73.3
CI85016	24.1	26.1	18.5	74.4	NA	NA	3.7	19.3	99.0
CI85013	34.1	40.5	24.9	74.4	NA	NA	6.0	24.1	92.7
CI85014	33.8	37.2	25.9	74.4	NA	NA	5.7	25.1	110.3
CI85017	42.6	47.5	26.5	74.4	NA	NA	7.7	44.2	88.2
CI85018	40.2	43.4	27.5	74.4	NA	NA	7.1	29.9	123.6
CI85019	40.1	43.0	27.5	74.4	NA	NA	7.1	33.7	129.9
CADAVERS									
CI85020	24.8	27.2	23.2	54.4	79	M	NA	52.9	55.4
CI85022	23.3	25.7	20.4	78.5	74	M	NA	38.0	41.0
CI85023	24.3	25.6	21.1	77.1	68	M	NA	27.8	79.0
CI85024	34.4	37.8	26.9	70.3	75	M	NA	46.8	77.4
CI86001	40.4	45.2	26.9	58.1	74	M	NA	59.3	170.3
CI86002	40.9	46.2	24.8	53.1	60	F	NA	62.9	67.9
CI86003	40.1	45.4	28.8	66.7	71	F	NA	59.4	61.9
CI86004	40.5	45.7	28.8	59.0	56	M	NA	75.3	77.6
CI86005	39.9	45.7	27.8	76.2	72	M	NA	65.8	155.8
CI86007	40.1	46.0	27.5	57.2	54	M	NA	65.7	233.4
CI86008	40.5	42.8	27.7	68.0	62	M	NA	56.5	212.9

* NA - NOT AVAILABLE OR NOT APPLICABLE

Table 1 - Summary of Frontal Impact Data (Non-Scaled Cadaver Data)

differences of up to 83% were observed. The film analysis technique was judged not accurate enough to be used for this paper. Future research will focus on determining an acceptable method of measuring chest deflection in the cadaver subjects.

A total of seven Hybrid III and twelve cadaver tests were conducted. The primary test variables are listed in Table 1. Pretest protocol was designed to produce test conditions as similar as practical between the cadaver and Hybrid III tests. The testing conditions were divided into three nominal sled velocities of 24, 34, and 40 km/hr. It should be noted that the early 24 km/hr cadaver subjects (test nos. CI85020, CI85021, and CI85022) were placed lower in the seat than their counterpart Hybrid III tests. A revised seating procedure was used for the later cadaver tests.

All curves used in this paper were filtered according to SAE Recommended Practice J211: chest acceleration is Channel Class 180, steering column force is Class 600, steering moment is Class 600, and steering column deflection is Class 180. The particular digital filter is a two pass, zero phase shift, second order Butterworth filter.

CADAVER/HYBRID III INTERACTION with STEERING ASSEMBLY An estimate of the "effective mass" of the occupant thorax which interacted with the steering wheel was obtained from an impulse - momentum calculation. The force versus time history of the steering column axial load was integrated and divided by the sled change-in-velocity to yield an effective mass value for the thorax. This was then normalized by the total mass of the subject. These data are listed in Table 2. The normalized effective mass for all subjects was found to be between 0.28 and 0.49 over the range of velocities studied.

The location of the steering wheel rim with respect to the chest shown in Figures 7 and 8 is based on photographic analysis of the high speed motion picture films. The rim appeared initially to contact the Hybrid III just below the "sixth" rib and -- because the horizontal steel 6th rib is rigidly attached to all the other ribs -- interacts with a fairly rigid chest structure. In contrast, the rim contacts the cadavers in the vicinity of the 8th through 10th ribs -- the upper abdomen -- and appears initially to load a more localized and softer region than with the Hybrid III.

Table 3 summarizes the dynamic steering column stroke for the Hybrid III and the cadavers. The dummy shows slightly greater -- say 1-inch -- column stroke. A word of caution about Table 3. The maximum allowable column stroke was set at 15.9 cm. Hybrid III tests CI85017 and CI85018 stroked the column all the way, or bottomed it. After the test series had been completed, an experimental problem was discovered which resulted in cadaver tests CI85024 and CI86003 bottoming at about 10.8 cm and cadaver tests CI86001 and CI86002 bottoming

TEST NO	SLED INITIAL VELOCITY (km/h)	∫Fdt (N-sec)	Effective * Subject Mass (∫Fdt/Delta V /Mass Subject)
HYBRID 3			
CI85015	25.4	189.0	0.33
CI85016	24.1	192.2	0.36
CI85013	34.1	252.2	0.30
CI85014	33.8	217.5	0.28
CI85017	42.6	329.6	0.34
CI85018	40.2	316.3	0.35
CI85019	40.1	252.6	0.28
CADAVERS			
CI85020	24.8	127.7	0.31
CI85022	23.3	168.1	0.30
CI85023	24.3	191.3	0.35
CI85024	34.4	277.6	0.38
CI86001	40.4	286.5	0.39
CI86002	40.9	331.8	0.49
CI86003	40.1	360.3	0.43
CI86004	40.5	255.3	0.34
CI86005	39.9	278.9	0.29
CI86007	40.1	278.4	0.36
CI86008	40.5	309.1	0.38

* - Using change-of-velocity of sled as delta v.

Table 2 -
Summary of Impulse Loading and Effective Mass
(Non-Scaled Cadaver Data)

INITIAL VELOCITY (km/h)	HYBRID III (cm)	CADAVER (cm)	CADAVER MASS (kg)	CADAVER TEST NO
24	4.6	1.2	54.4	CI85020
24	5.1	2.0	78.5	CI85022
24	4.6 *	2.3	77.1	CI85023
Average	4.7	1.8		
34	14.7	10.7	70.3	CI85024
40	15.7	13.7	58.1	CI86001
40	15.7	14.2	53.1	CI86002
40	15.6 *	14.2	66.7	CI86003
40		11.9	59.0	CI86004
40		12.2	76.2	CI86005
40		11.9	57.2	CI86007
40		11.9	68.0	CI86008
Average	15.7	12.9		

* - Data from an ancillary Hybrid III test conducted after main portion of testing was completed.

Table 3 -
Comparison of Dummy/Cadaver Dynamic Column Stroke
(Non-Scaled Cadaver Data)

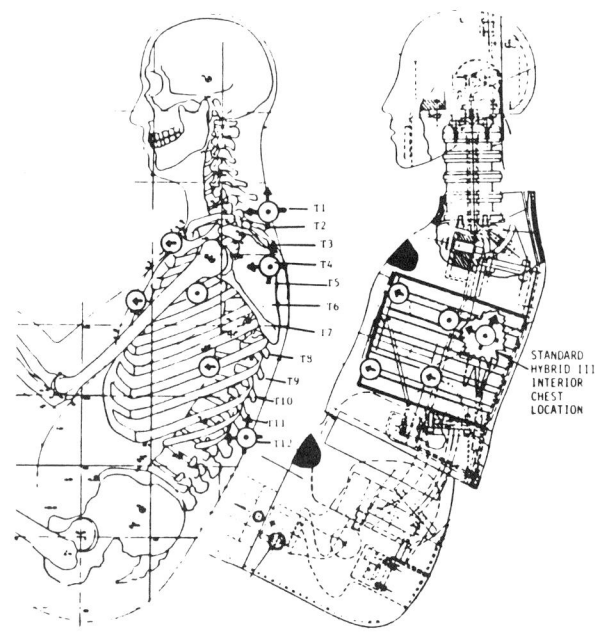

Figure 6 - Skeleton and Hybrid III Accelerometer Locations

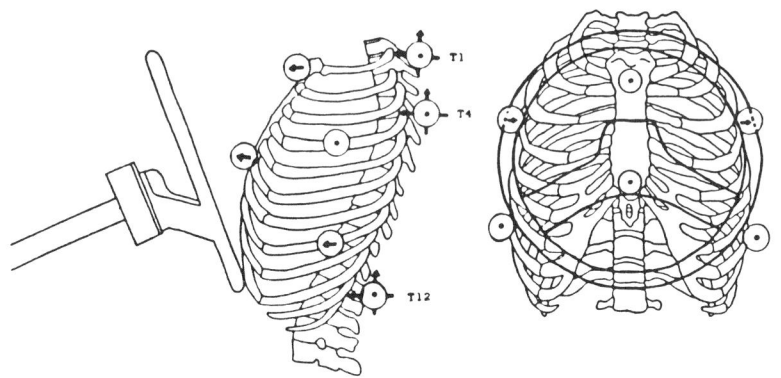

Figure 7 - Cadaver - Location of Steering Wheel with Respect to Chest

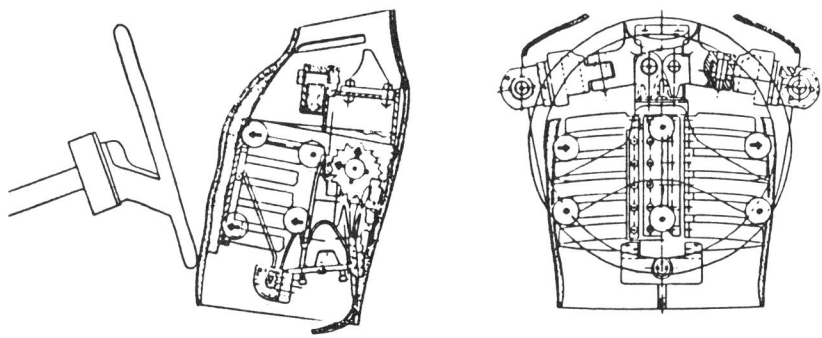

Figure 8 - Hybrid III - Location of Steering Wheel with Respect to Chest

at about 14.0 cm. Consequently, caution should be used in interpreting Table 3 for the higher test speeds. (The sources of the premature column bottoming have been identified; and a testing protocol developed to prevent its reoccurrence.)

Similarly to Reference 6, the Hybrid III in the 24 and 34km/hr tests recorded its maximum chest compression prior to a significant portion of the steering column stroke. For the 40km/hr tests however, the Hybrid III shows an initial chest compression before the column begins to stroke and -- see Figure 9 -- a rise to a maximum value after the column bottoms.

To quantify the amount of steering wheel rim deformation experienced during a test, pre- and post-test measurements were made according to the scheme shown in Figure 10. This figure divides the steering wheel rim into four segments represented by 3, 6, 9, and 12 o'clock positions. The steering wheel was placed on a flat surface both before and after the test and height measurements were taken from the plane of the steering wheel mounting surface to the o'clock position on the wheel rim. The differences between the pre- and post-test numbers are contained in Table 4. The source of the scatter in Table 4 has not been identified. There is no clear difference between cadavers and Hybrid III in pattern of lower rim and upper rim deformations. However, on the average,

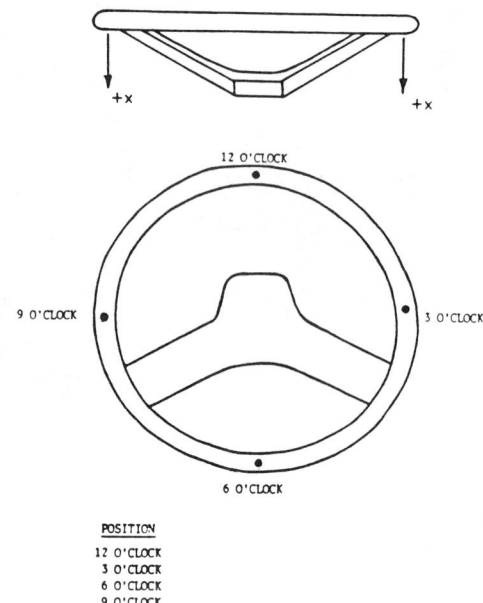

Figure 10 - Scheme for Determining Steering Wheel Deformation

INITIAL VELOCITY (km/h)	HYBRID III 12 O'CLOCK (cm)	HYBRID III 6 O'CLOCK (cm)	CADAVER 12 O'CLOCK (cm)	CADAVER 6 O'CLOCK (cm)
24	2.29	2.29	2.29	0.25
24	1.52	2.79	7.37	-1.02
24	1.91 *	3.18 *	3.56	0.00
Average -->	1.91	2.75	4.40	-0.25
34	3.81	2.29	4.57	0.51
40	1.02	4.57	6.10	2.79
40	-0.51	5.33	6.10	4.57
40	7.62 *	1.52 *	5.59	6.60
40			0.25	3.05
40			3.30	2.29
40			3.56	1.52
40			7.62	2.29
Average -->	2.71	3.81	4.64	3.30

* - Data from ancillary Hybrid III test conducted after main portion of testing was completed.

Table 4 - Summary of Steering Wheel Rim Deformation (Non-Scaled Cadaver Data)

there is more deformation at the 12 o'clock position and less at the 6 o'clock position for the cadavers relative to the Hybrid III. This observance supports the above kinematic observation; namely the stiffer Hybrid III more fully loads the lower rim causing a pattern of higher deformation at 6 o'clock, while the cadaver more heavily loads the top rim, leading to the higher 12 o'clock deformations.

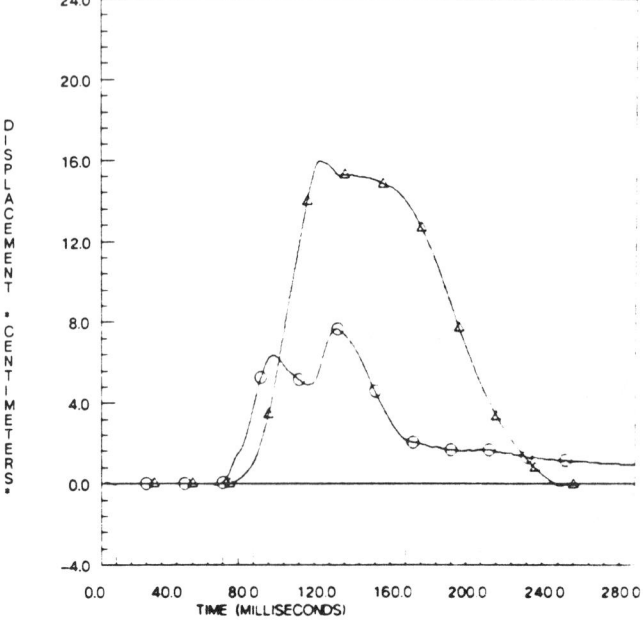

Figure 9 - Chest Displacement versus Column Stroke in Hybrid III

RESPONSE SCALING   The cadavers in Table 1 have different masses and dimensions relative to the Hybrid III. The responses of the cadavers should undergo modification following a set of compatible scaling laws prior to comparison with the Hybrid III. One set of model scaling laws has been used by some of the authors in the past. [11,12]

To review briefly, λ = the scaling constant, s = subscript for the scaled data which is suppose to mimic the Hybrid III, and i = subscript for i-th subject. If mass density (mass/volume) and modulus of elasticity are assumed constant, then the following relationships are true:

Velocity	$V_s = V_i$
Mass	$M_s = \lambda^3 M_i$
Acceleration	$A_s = \lambda^{-1/3} A_i$
Length	$L_s = \lambda^{1/3} L_i$
Time	$T_s = \lambda^{1/3} T_i$
Force	$F_s = \lambda^{2/3} F_i$
Moment	$M_s = \lambda\ M_i$

For example, for test no. CI85020, the value of λ would be $(165/120)^{1/3}$. This scaling algorithm does not alter the velocity, but it does modify most other parameters of interest, e. g., acceleration, time, force, etc. The cadaver responses of Figures 11 through 18 have been scaled according to the above scheme where the standard weight of the scaled model (the Hybrid III) is assumed to be 165 lbs. Figures 11 through 18 are discussed in the next section.

HYBRID III BIOFIDELITY   The biofidelity of an anthropomorphic test device can be defined as the extent to which the anthropomorphic test device mimics the dynamic response of a living human under a particular test condition. Frequently in impact testing, the assumption is made that a human cadaver will respond similarly to a living human. If true, then the extent to which an anthropomorphic test device's response replicates the response of cadavers is a measure of the dummy's biofidelity. In this study, the Hybrid III's biofidelity will be assessed by examining the extent to which it fits within the corridor of several response parameters.

For the three test velocities there exist both a Hybrid III dummy and one or more cadaver exposures. Using the scaling approach described above and then calculating cadaver plus and minus one standard deviation (or one sigma) curves, [13] the Hybrid III can be overlaid on the cadaver corridor for each test velocity (not possible in the case of the 34 km/hr test condition in which there was only one cadaver exposure). For example, the crosshatching in Figure 11 is the cadaver corridor for that test condition and is bounded by the plus and minus one standard deviation curves.

Figure 11 shows the force transmitted along the column (measured at the location labeled "rim transducer" in Figure 3) versus time for the 24km/hr test. The single line is the average of the Hybrid III while the crosshatched area is the cadaver corridor. The Hybrid III is within the corridor and reasonable given the fact the early 24km/hr sled tests were conducted with the cadaver seated a little low.

The Hybrid III is compared against the one cadaver tested at 34km/hr in Figure 12. The two are very similar. The cadaver trace does show a second peak which corresponds to the column prematurely bottoming due to an experimental problem. (The column bottoming previously discussed in the section CADAVER/HYBRID III INTERACTION with STEERING ASSEMBLY.)

The 40km/hr results are in Figure 13. The Hybrid III is within the cadaver corridor. Although averaging techniques have been used, the second peak -- which occurs when the column bottoms -- can be clearly seen.

The next comparison concerns spinal acceleration (see Figure 6). The cadavers had a triaxial accelerometer located at the fourth thoracic vertebra (T4). The Hybrid III's accelerometer was mounted at the standard center-of-gravity position. A plane parallel to the floor of the sled buck and passing through the T4 accelerometers of the cadaver would be slightly higher than a similar plane through the center-of-gravity accelerometer's of the Hybrid III, i. e., the cadaver's accelerometers are above the Hybrid III's. In retrospect, it might have been better to position the cadaver accelerometer cluster at the seventh thoracic vertebra. However, given the variability in (1) cadaver size and weight, (2) cadaver kinematics due to differences in size, and (3) positioning a flaccid cadaver to sit like a rigid dummy, the small difference of 5 to 7 cm in locating the accelerometer cluster along T4 to T7 is probably not important.

The resultant chest acceleration of the Hybrid III is compared with the cadaver corridor (chest resultant acceleration) for 24, 34, and 40km/hr in Figures 14, 15, and 16. Relative to cadavers, the Hybrid III produces lower peak spinal acceleration. As shown in Figures 7 and 8 and as previously discussed, the steering wheel rim initially loads all the Hybrid III's thorax while the rim initially reacts with the cadavers locally in the region of the 8th through 10th rib. In Figures 14 through 16, the Hybrid III exhibits an initially lower chest acceleration corresponding to a higher effective mass being coupled to the lower rim. Subsequently, the Hybrid III falls within the top of the cadaver corridor (in Figure 14 through 16, this phenomenon roughly begins after the curves pass the 16 G value on the vertical scale).

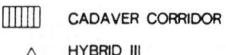
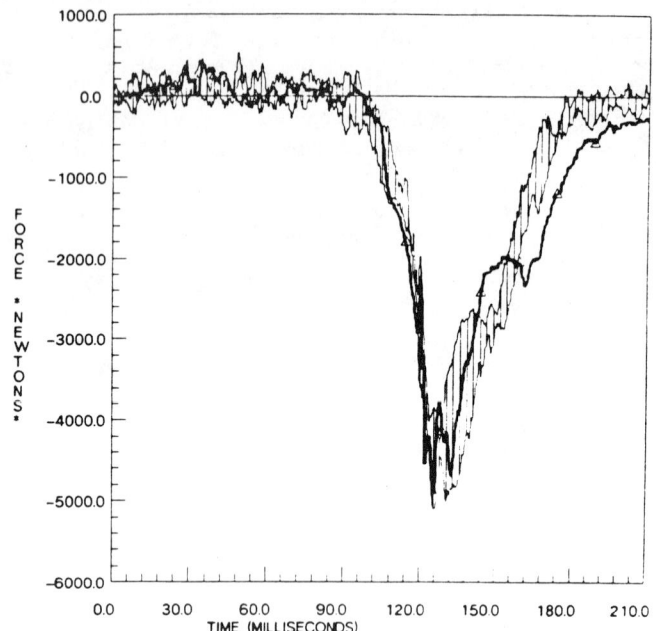

Figure 11 - Column Force - 24 km/hr Test
(Scaled Cadaver Data)

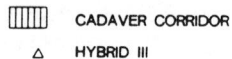
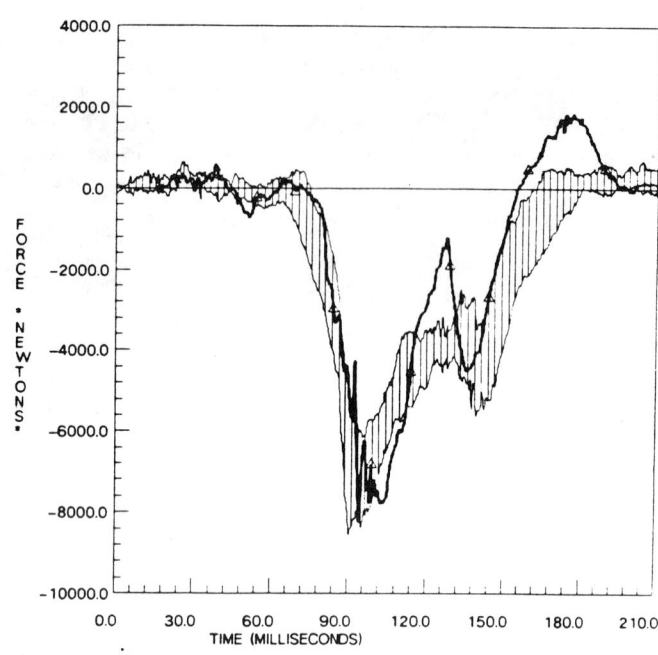

Figure 13 - Column Force - 40 km/hr Test
(Scaled Cadaver Data)

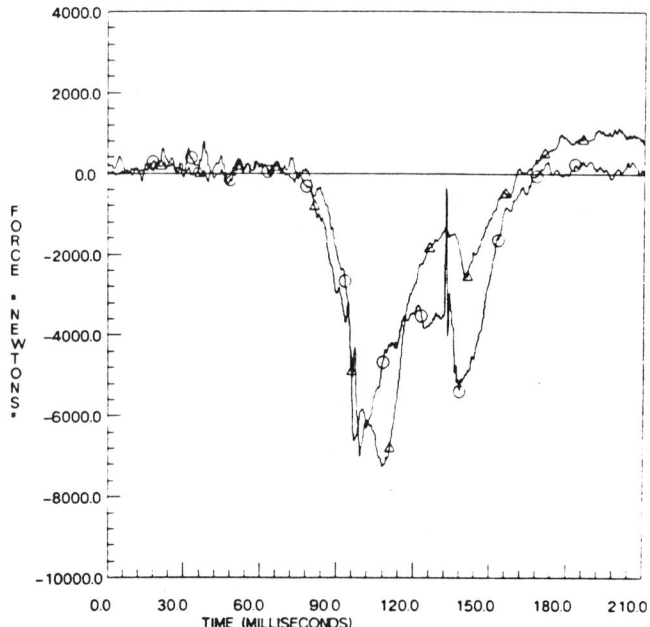

Figure 12 - Column Force - 34 km/hr Test
(Scaled Cadaver Data)

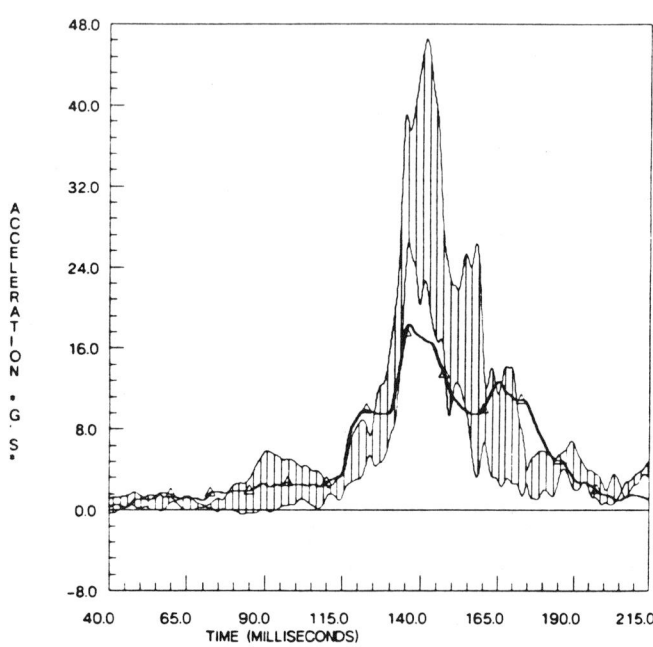

Figure 14 - Resultant Chest Acceleration
24 km/hr Test
(Scaled Cadaver Data)

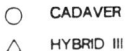
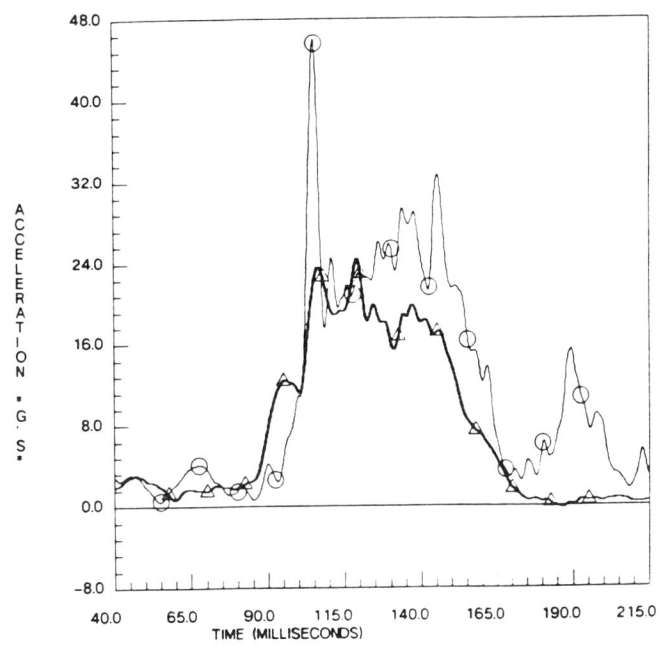

Figure 15 – Resultant Chest Acceleration
34 km/hr Test
(Scaled Cadaver Data)

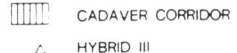
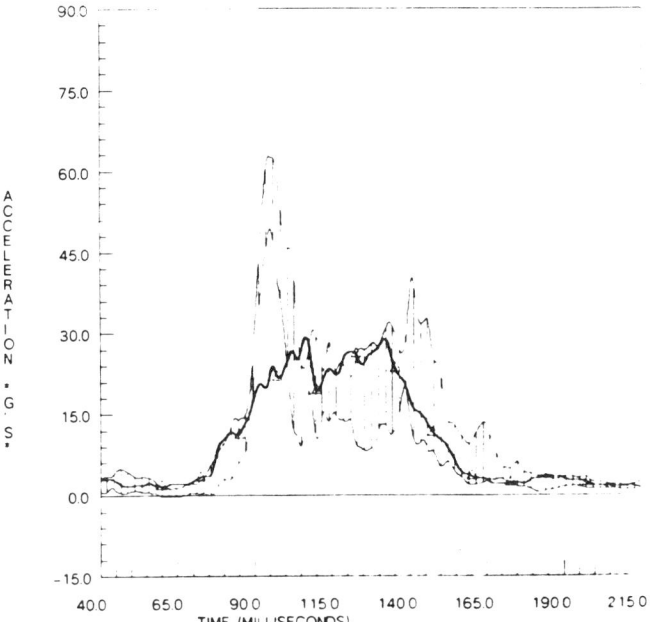

Figure 16 – Resultant Chest Acceleration
40 km/hr Test
(Scaled Cadaver Data)

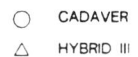
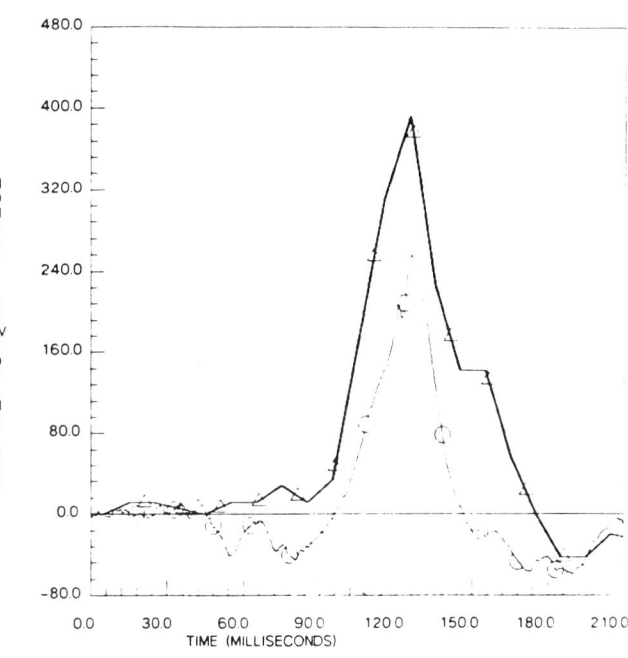

Figure 17 – Moment Curves – 24 km/hr Test
(Scaled Cadaver Data)

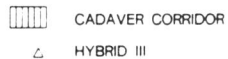
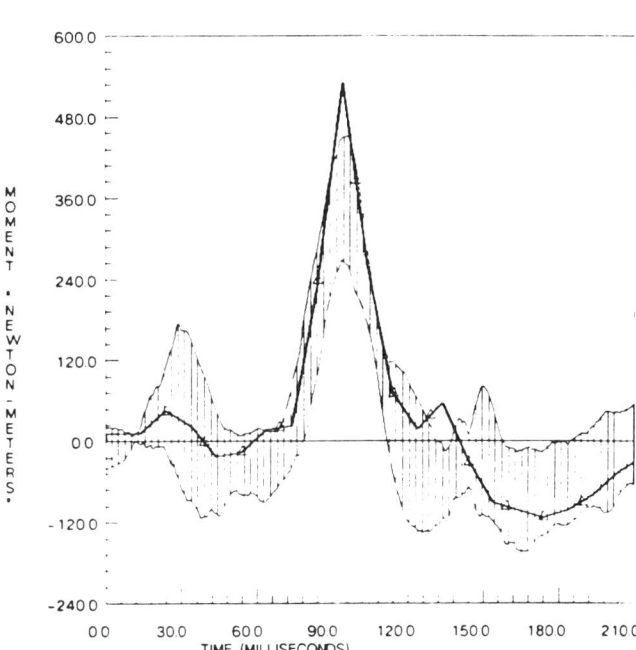

Figure 18 – Moment Curves – 40 km/hr Test
(Scaled Cadaver Data)

The rim transducer (see Figure 3) also measures pitch moment (y-axis). This channel was missing in some of the early tests preventing as complete a comparison as can be made for the force and acceleration data above. Figure 17 shows the pitch moment for one cadaver and the Hybrid III at 24km/hr. Figure 18 presents the dummy against the cadaver corridor for the 40km/hr condition. The Hybrid III response is slightly higher than the cadavers in this regard.

<u>ENERGY-ABSORBING CONSIDERATIONS</u> The human cadaver and the Hybrid III dummy interact with the energy-absorbing steering assembly. There is a certain amount of kinetic energy before the collision and -- assuming the change-of-velocity is used as the measure of velocity [14] -- no kinetic energy after the event. Where does the energy go and how fast does it go ? To determine the answer to this question, we need both column force and column stroke velocity.

The steering column displacement was measured against time in all sled tests. The differentiation of the column stroke has special interest with respect to the "rim-to-upper-abdomen" photographic analysis discussed earlier in the section <u>CADAVER/HYBRID III INTERACTION with STEERING ASSEMBLY</u>. If the more rigid lower ribs of the Hybrid III make first contact on the lower rim of the steering wheel, while the lower rim makes first contact with the softer upper abdomen of the cadavers, then the column stroke velocity would be higher for the Hybrid III than for the cadavers for identical collision severity. Figure 19 illustrates the column stroke velocity for a Hybrid III and a cadaver at the 40km/hr condition. Table 5 shows the column stroke velocity for all the sled tests. In each case, the Hybrid III column stroke velocity is higher than the cadaver column stroke velocity at the same sled velocity. This Table gives support to the supposition that the lower rim interacts differently with the lower ribs of the Hybrid III than it does with the upper abdomen of the cadavers.

The rate of energy absorption, power, in the steering column energy-absorption unit is

$$P(t)_{col} = F(t)_{hub} * \frac{dX_{col\ stroke}}{dt}$$

where

P = power

F = force along the column axis

$X_{col\ stroke}$ = column stroke

and

$\frac{d}{dt}$ = differentiation with respect to time.

In other words, the column power is calculated by multiplying the axial force by the column stroke velocity. The peak value of column power is recorded in Table 5. Again, the peak column power for the Hybrid III is higher than the cadaver for similar test conditions. Since the Hybrid III and cadaver column force is shown in Figures 11 through 13 to be similar, it follows the Hybrid III peak column power is larger because the Hybrid III column stroke velocity is higher.

Having calculated the power which is associated with the absorption of the energy in the steering column energy-absorption unit (which is denoted by column power), the next step is to calculate the larger power associated with the total motion of the steering column through space. This total power is the column force times the hub velocity. The hub velocity is

$$V_{hub} = [\Delta V - \int_{t_o}^{t} a_{sled}\ dt]\cos(\theta) + \frac{dX_{col\ stroke}}{dt}$$

where

ΔV = sled change-of-velocity

a_{sled} = sled acceleration

$\cos(\theta)$ = cosine of angle of steering column.

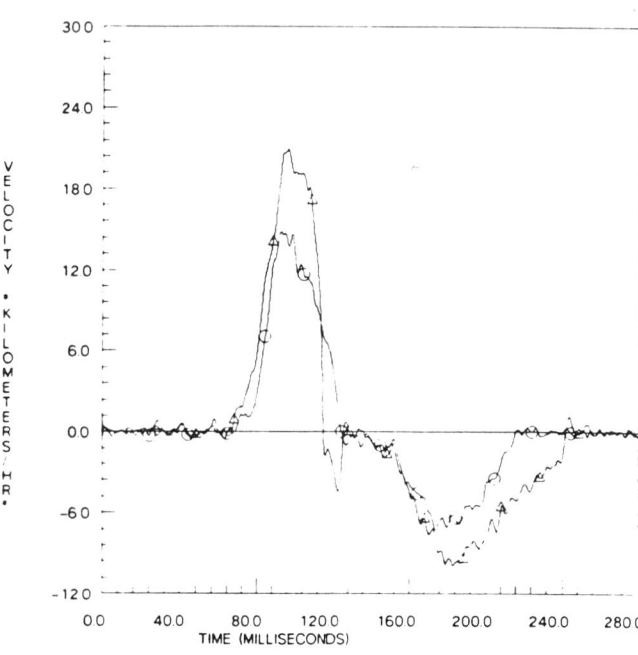

Figure 19 - Steering Assembly Velocity as Energy - Absorbing Device Strokes (Relative to Sled Buck)

TEST NO	SLED INIT VEL (km/h)	SLED DELTA VEL (km/h)	COLUMN VEL (km/h)	SUBJECT MASS (kgs)	PEAK COLUMN POWER (watts)	PEAK TOTAL POWER (watts)	INITIAL KINETIC ENERGY THORAX (joules)	MAX TRANSF ENERGY SLED-COLUMN COMPLEX (joules)	ENERGY TRANSF SLED-COLUMN COMPLEX (percent)	MAX COLUMN ABSORBED ENERGY (joules)	COLUMN ENERGY ABSORBED (percent)	ENERGY ABSORBED THORAX (joules)	FRACTION INITIAL KINETIC ENERGY ABSORBED THORAX (percent)
HYBRID 3													
CI85015	25.4	27.4	8.4	74.4	6551	9656	806	275	34	132	16	530	66
CI85016	24.1	26.1	14.0	74.4	8474	9181	731	244	33	161	22	487	67
				AVERAGE	7513	9418	769	260	34	146	19	509	66
CI85013	34.1	40.5	14.6	74.4	22421	27499	1770	743	42	412	23	1027	58
CI85014	33.8	37.2	15.8	74.4	21212	27658	1487	654	44	393	26	834	56
				AVERAGE	21817	27579	1629	698	43	402	25	930	57
CI85017	42.6	47.5	20.9	74.4	34696	53125	2426	1399	58	725	30	1026	42
CI85018	40.2	43.4	21.1	74.4	33432	44647	2032	1321	65	755	37	711	35
CI85019	40.1	43.0	20.1	74.4	35001	37401	1987	1100	55	746	38	887	45
				AVERAGE	34376	45058	2148	1273	59	742	35	875	41
CADAVERS													
CI85020	24.8	27.2	2.6	54.4	2644	4077	582	88	15	38	7	494	85
CI85022	23.3	25.7	9.5	76.5	4837	8240	753	160	21	69	9	593	79
CI85023	24.3	25.6	4.7	77.1	5855	8659	730	210	29	91	12	520	71
				AVERAGE	4446	6993	689	153	22	66	9	536	78
CI85024	34.4	37.8	12.9	70.3	15469	27987	1455	761	52	443	30	694	48
CI86001	40.4	45.2	15.6	58.1	20541	34857	1718	1054	61	601	35	664	39
CI86002	40.9	46.2	13.2	53.1	16573	34367	1638	1204	74	570	35	434	26
CI86003	40.1	45.4	12.2	66.7	15927	26683	1987	971	49	487	25	1016	51
CI86004	40.5	45.7	15.4	59.0	24220	40361	1782	887	50	500	28	895	50
CI86005	39.9	45.7	14.8	76.2	24487	39982	2303	980	43	536	23	1323	57
CI86007	40.1	46.0	13.5	57.2	18419	36287	1752	990	57	526	30	762	43
CI86008	40.5	42.8	14.6	68.0	24229	30675	1804	922	51	557	31	883	49
				AVERAGE	20614	34745	1855	1001	55	540	30	854	45

Table 5 — Summary of Energy Transferred and Absorbed by the Steering Assembly

In this paper the cosine term multiplier (.94) is neglected. The column force times the hub velocity gives the total power through the wheel. The peak total power is shown in Table 5. Integration of the column power and the total power give the energy absorbed by the column and the total energy out. For example, in test no. CI85015, the energy absorbed in the column is 132 joules and the total energy absorbed by the sled-column complex is 275 joules.

To determine the initial kinetic energy of the thoracic structure, the factor 0.37 -- a roughly average value taken from Table 2 -- is multiplied by one-half the subject mass times the change-in-velocity squared. In Table 5, the subject for CI85015 had an initial kinetic energy of about 806 joules (column called "INITIAL KINETIC ENERGY THORAX" in Table 5).

The ratio of energy transferred to the sled-column complex divided by the initial kinetic energy is calculated in the column called "ENERGY TRANSF SLED-COLUMN COMPLEX" in Table 5. For the 24, and 40km/hr tests, the Hybrid III transfers on the average a larger portion of the initial kinetic energy to the sled-column complex than does the cadaver.

Expressed another way, the amount of energy absorbed by the subject thorax is the difference in the initial kinetic energy and the energy absorbed by the sled-column complex. For example, in CI85015, roughly 530 joules of the original 806 joules is absorbed by the thorax. The energy absorbed by the thorax divided by the initial kinetic energy gives the fraction of the total initial energy absorbed by the occupant. This fraction is figured in the column called "FRACTION INITIAL KINETIC ENERGY ABSORBED THORAX" in Table 5. For the 24 and 40km/hr tests on the average, a greater proportion of the total initial energy is absorbed by the cadavers than by the Hybrid III.

CADAVER INJURY Following each sled run, the cadaver is removed from the sled buck and all the accelerometers are removed from their mounts. The subject is then returned to refrigerator storage. The time lapse between running the test and conducting the necropsy was no longer than three days and usually the following day. The injuries observed are recorded and special note is taken of the relationship of these to any external markings due to the impacting steering assembly.

Table 6 summarizes the hard thorax injuries for the twelve cadaver tests. The hard thorax injuries include not only the thoracic contents such as the heart, lungs, and ribs; but also the thoracic spinal column and the abdominal organs contained inside the rib cage such as the liver, kidneys, and spleen. At the 40km/hr test velocity, three of the seven cadavers had liver injury. Additional injury details are gathered in Table 7.

Figure 20 shows the the relative occurrence of an injury greater than or equal to a specific AIS level by test severity as measured by initial sled velocity.[15]

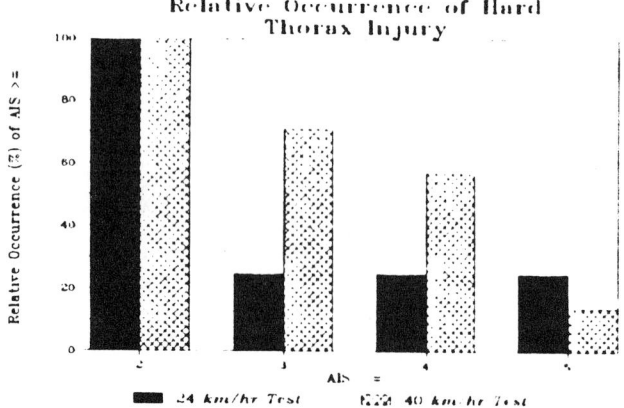

Figure 20 - Hard Thorax Injury

TEST NO	MAXIMUM AIS	INJURY DESCRIPTION OF HARD THORAX
		24 KILOMETERS/HOUR
CI85020	5	8MM INTERNAL LACERATION TO PULMONARY ARTERY. 20CM LIVER LACERATION.
CI85021	2	RIGHT RIBS 7, 8, 9, 10 FRACTURED 15CM LATERAL TO MID-LINE. LEFT RIBS 4,5,7,8,9 FRACTURED 10CM LATERAL TO MID-LINE.
CI85022	2	FRACTURES OF LEFT RIBS 4,5,6,7,8.
CI85023	2	LEFT RIBS 4,6,7,8 ARE FRACTURED IN MID-CLAVICULAR LINE. RIGHT RIBS 3,6,8,9,10 FRACTURED. SEPERATION OF RIGHT CLAVICLE AT STERNO-CLAVICULAR JOINT.
		34 KILOMETERS/HOUR
CI85024	2	LEFT RIBS 5, 6, 9, 10 FRACTURED LATERALLY. RIGHT RIBS 3, 5, 6 FRACTURED LATERALLY. LEFT AND RIGHT STERNO-CLAVICULAR SEPARATION.
		40 KILOMETERS/HOUR
CI86001	4	FLAIL CHEST - FRACTURE OF LEFT RIBS 3, 4, 5, 6, 7. FRACTURE OF RIGHT RIBS 4, 5, 6, 7, 8. FRACTURE OF LARYNGEAL PROMINENCE FOR 1CM. FRACTURE OF STERNUM.
CI86002	5	AVULSION OF BASEBALL-SIZE PORTION OF LEFT LOWER LIVER. SEVERAL LACERATIONS (DEEP) OVER ANTERIOR SURFACE OF LIVER. DISLOCATION OF RIGHT AND LEFT STERNO-CLAVICULAR JOINT. RIGHT RIBS 4, 5, 6, 7, 8 FRACTURED ANTERIORLY. LEFT RIBS 2, 3, 4, 5, 6, 7 FRACTURED ANTERIORLY.
CI86003	2	FRACTURES OF LEFT RIBS 4 AND 5. BILATERAL DISLOCATION OF STERNO-CLAVICULAR JOINT.
CI86004	4	3CM LACERATION OF LIVER DIRECTLY UNDER-LYING XIPHOID PROCESS. LEFT STERNO-CLAVICULAR PARTIAL SEPERATION. LEFT 8TH RIB FRACTURE.
CI86005	4	10CM POSTERIOR-INFERIOR, TRANSVERSE LIVER LACERATION. LEFT RIBS 3, 4, 5, 7, 8, 9 FRACTURED. TRANSVERSE FRACTURE OF STERNUM. LEFT STERNO-CLAVICULAR JOINT PARTIALLY SEPARATED.
CI86007	2	RIGHT RIBS 8, 9 FRACTURED. LEFT RIBS 5, 8, 9 FRACTURED. PARTIAL SEPARATION OF RIGHT STERNO-CLAVICULAR JOINT.
CI86008	3	PNEUMOTHORAX, MULTIPLE RIB FRACTURES. TRANSVERSE FRACTURE OF STERNUM.

Table 6 - Summary of Injuries

TEST NO	VELOCITY (km/hr)	*	REGION	DESCRIPTION
C185020	27.2	5	Chest	8mm internal laceration to pulmonary artery
		4	Abdomen	20cm liver laceration
		2	Back	Fracture of T-1 body
		2	Face	Dislocation of tempo manibular bilateral joint
		1	Chest	Fracture of 4th and 6th right ribs
		1	Chest	Fracture of 8th and 9th left ribs
C185021	27.0	2	Chest	Fracture of 7th, 8th, 9th, and 10 right ribs
		2	Chest	Fracture of 7th, 8th, and 9th left ribs
		1	Chest	Fracture of 5th left rib
		1	Chest	Fracture of 4th left rib
C185022	25.7	2	Chest	Fracture of 4th, 5th, 6th, 7th and 8th left ribs
		2	Face	Fracture of right mandible
		2	Face	Dislocation of right tempero mandibular joint
		2	Face	Laceration of vallecula inferior to the tongue
C185023	25.6	2	Neck	Fracture of hyoid bone left ramus
		2	Shoulder	Separation of right clavicle at sterno-clavicular joint
		1	Chest	Fracture of 4th, 6th, 7th, and 8th left ribs
		1	Chest	Fracture of 3rd, 6th, 8th, 9th and 10th right ribs
C185024	37.8	2	Shoulder	Left and right sterno-clavicular separation
		2	Chest	Lateral fracture of 5th, 8th, 9th, and 10th left ribs
		1	Chest	Lateral fracture of 3rd, 5th, and 6th right ribs
C186001	45.2	4	Neck	Fracture of laryngeal prominence for 1cm on midline
		4	Chest	Flail chest - Fracture of left ribs 3,4,5,6,7 and right ribs 4,5,6,7, and 8
		2	Chest	Fracture of sternum - 4cm superior to xiphoid
		1	Neck	Fracture of hyoid bone
		1	Face	Abrasion over right jaw
		1	Shoulder	Abrasion over right clavicle
C186002	46.2	5	Abdomen	Avulsion of baseball-size portion of left liver
		5	Abdomen	Several deep lacerations over liver
		2	Shoulder	Dislocation of left sterno-clavicular joint

* Abbreviated Injury Scale, 1980 Revision.

TEST NO	VELOCITY (km/hr)	*	REGION	DESCRIPTION
C186002 (Continued)		2	Shoulder	Dislocation of right sterno-clavicular joint
		2	Chest	Fracture of posterior sternum
		2	Chest	Anterior fracture of 4,5,6,7 and 8 right ribs
		2	Chest	Anterior fracture of 2,3,4,5,6 and 7 left ribs
		1	Face	Superficial abrasion over right zygomatic bone
C186003	45.4	2	Knee	Deep laceration of medial left knee
		2	Chest	Fracture of 4th and 5th right ribs
		2	Shoulder	Bilateral dislocation of sterno-clavicular joint
		1	Face	Laceration of lower lip and tongue
C186004	45.7	4	Abdomen	3cm laceration of liver
		2	Shoulder	Separation of left sterno-clavicular joint
		1	Chest	Fracture of 8th left rib
		1	Face	Multiple lacerations of forehead
C186005	45.7	4	Abdomen	10cm posterior-inferior transverse liver laceration
		2	Chest	Transverse fracture of sternum
		2	Chest	Fractures 3,4,5,7,8 and 9 left ribs
		2	Shoulder	Left sterno-clavicular joint partially separated
		1	Chest	Closed fracture of 5th rib
C186007	46.0	2	Head	Deep 6cm laceration over frontal scalp
		2	Shoulder	Separation of right sterno-clavicular joint
		2	Chest	Fracture of 8th and 9th right ribs
		2	Chest	Fracture of 8th and 9th left ribs
		1	Chest	Fracture of 5th left rib
C186008	42.8	3	Neck	Rupture/separation of disk @ anterior aspect C2&C3
		3	Neck	Rupture/separation of disk @ anterior aspect C5&C6
		3	Neck	Rupture/separation of disk @ anterior aspect C6&C7
		3	Chest	Open/displaced 4th left rib (pneumothorax)
		2	Chest	Closed fracture of right ribs 4-9
		2	Chest	Fractures of left ribs 4-10
		2	Chest	Transverse fracture of sternum
		1	Head	2cm laceration on forehead

* Abbreviated Injury Scale, 1980 Revision.

Table 7 - Detailed Summary of Injuries

Table 8 –
Application of Neathery et al. Equation
to this Data Set

CADAVER TEST NO	INITIAL SLED VELOCITY (km/hr)	NEATHERY et al. EQUATION AIS	EXPERIMENTALLY OBSERVED AIS
CI85020	24.3	1.0	5
CI85021	24.5	0.88	2
CI85022	23.3	0.95	2
CI85023	24.3	0.65	2
	AVERAGE	0.85	2.75
CI85024	34.4	2.44	2
	AVERAGE	2.44	2
CI86001	40.4	3.49	4
CI86002	40.9	3.05	5
CI86003	40.1	3.29	2
CI86004	40.5	2.92	4
CI86005	39.9	3.42	4
CI86007	40.1	2.86	2
CI86008	40.5	3.11	3
	AVERAGE	3.18	3.43

Table 9 –
Distribution of Injury by Body Region

TEST NO	NOMINAL INITIAL SLED VELOCITY (km/hr)	THORAX AIS *	ABDOMEN AIS *	NECK AIS *
CI85020		5	4	0
CI85022	24	2	0	0
CI85023		1	0	2
CI85024	34	2	0	0
CI86001		4	0	4
CI86002		2	5	0
CI86003		2	0	0
CI86004	40	1	4	0
CI86005		2	4	0
CI86007		2	0	0
CI86008		3	0	3

* – Abbreviated Injury Scale, 1980 revision

The development of an injury index based on this frontal impact experimental setup should wait until a larger cadaver base has been accumulated. One equation for the prediction of thoracic injury is based on a large cadaver data base. [16] Viano [17] observed that the thorax reaches it's maximum deflection limit at about the AIS 3 level at which point the chest bottoms. The Neathery equation is:

$$AIS = 17.4\, P/D + 0.0313\, Age - 5.15$$

where
  P = chest penetration,
  D = subject chest depth,
  Age = subject age.

Since the measurement of the cadaver chest penetration was not reliable, the average Hybrid III internally measured chest deflection will be used for each sled test condition. To use the Neathery equation, 1.27 cm was added to the chest deflection recorded by the Hybrid III. The 1.27 cm is added to account for skin thickness. The Hybrid III chest depth is about 23.6 cm. The only other variable is Age, for which each cadaver's age was substituted. The predicted results are shown in Table 8. For this limited number of cadaver tests, the Neathery equation predicts high for 24 km/hr but close for 34 and 40km/hr.

Does the distribution of injury by body part vary as test severity increases ? To answer this question, Table 9 was constructed from Table 7. Viewed in this way, most of the more significant injuries to the abdomen and the neck occur at the higher speeds while thoracic injuries remain relatively constant. There is a need for future research into these neck and abdominal injury mechanisms.

CONCLUSIONS

o In these experiments of unrestrained subjects into a steering assembly, the Hybrid III performed in a gross motion sense as the cadavers did. They showed similar "effective" mass based on impulse - momentum considerations. They exhibited similar steering column axis force-versus-time histories.

o Localized loading in the sixth rib region of the Hybrid III appeared to couple the steering wheel to a larger thoracic mass than is the case when the wheel contacts the upper abdomen region of the cadaver. The Hybrid III had lower initial peak spinal acceleration. The Hybrid III produced higher pitch moment (on the steering wheel) resulting from the abdomen contacting the lower steering wheel rim. The averages of the steering rim deformations suggested more rim deformation at the top and less deformation at the bottom for the cadaver relative to the Hybrid III. The column stroke velocity was higher for the Hybrid III.

o At 40km/hr initial sled velocity, three out of seven of the cadavers had liver injuries. Future research should focus on obtaining additional numbers of cadaver impacts so that the development of an injury index will have a statistically significant basis.

o For this experimental setup of the unrestrained occupant impacting the steering assembly, the Hybrid III exhibited a higher peak absorbed column power than did the cadaver. On the average for the 24 and 40km/hr sled tests, the cadaver thorax absorbed a greater proportion of the initial kinetic energy than did the Hybrid III thorax.

ACKNOWLEDGMENTS   The work upon which this paper is based was supported by Contract No. DTNH22-83-C-57019 with the Department of Transportation, National Highway Traffic Safety Administration.

DISCLAIMER   The views presented are those of the authors and are not necessarily those of the National Highway Traffic Safety Administration, U. S. Department of Transportation.

REFERENCES

1. Fredericks, R. H., "SAE Test Procedure for Steering Wheels," Ninth Stapp Car Crash Conference, October 1965.

2. Kahane, C. J., "Evaluation of Current Energy-Absorbing Steering Assemblies,"SAE Paper 820473, February 1982.

3. Malliaris, A. C., Hitchcock, R., and Hedlund, J., "A Search for Priorities in Crash Protection," SAE Paper No. 820242, February 1982.

4. Horsch, J. D., Petersen, K. R., and Viano, D. C., "Laboratory Study of Factors Influencing the Performance of Energy Absorbing Steering Systems," SAE Paper No. 820475, February 1982.

5. Horsch, J. D., and Culver, C. C., "The Role of Steering Wheel Structure in the Performance of Energy Absorbing Steering Systems," Twenty-Seventh Stapp Car Crash Conference, October 1983.

6. Horsch, J. D., and Viano, D. C., "Influence of the Surrogate in Laboratory Evaluation of Energy-Absorbing Steering System," Twenty-Eighth Stapp Car Crash Conference, November 1984.

7. Horsch, J. D., Lau, I. V., Viano, D. C., and Andrzejak, D. V., "Mechanism of Abdominal Injury by Steering Wheel Loading," Twenty-Ninth Stapp Car Crash Conference, October 1985.

8. Robbins, D. H., Melvin, J. W., and Stalnaker, R. L., "The Prediction of Thoracic Impact Injuries," Twentieth Stapp Car Crash Conference, October 1976.

9. Eppinger, R. H., Augustyn, K., Robbins, D. H., "Development of a Promising Universal Thoracic Trauma Prediction Methodology,"Twenty-Second Stapp Car Crash Conference, October 1978.

10. Haffner, Mark P., Personal Communication.

11. Eppinger, R. H., Marcus, J. M., and Morgan, R. M., "Development of Dummy and Injury Index for NHTSA's Thoracic Side Protection Research Program," SAE Paper No. 840885, May 1984.

12. Whittaker, E. T., A Treatise on the Analytical Dynamics of Particles and Rigid Bodies, Cambridge University Press, 1965, pg. 47.

13. Morgan, R. M., Marcus, J. H., and Eppinger, R. H., "Correlation of Side Impact Dummy/Cadaver Tests," Twenty-Fifth Stapp Car Crash Conference, September 1981.

14. Eppinger, R. H., and Marcus, J. H., "Production of Injury in Blunt Frontal Impact," Tenth International Technical Conference on Experimental Safety Vehicles, July 1985.

15. The Abbreviated Injury Scale, American Association for Automotive Medicine, Morton Grove, Illinois, 1980 Revision.

16. Neathery, R. F., Kroell, C. K., and Mertz, H. J., "Prediction of Thoracic Injury from Dummy Responses, Nineteenth Stapp Car Crash Conference, November 1975.

17. Viano, D. C., "Evaluation of Biomechanical Response and Potential Injury from Thoracic Impact," Aviation Space and Environmental Medicine, Vol. 49, No. 1, ASEMCG 49(1) 1-348, 1978.

892440

Assessing Submarining and Abdominal Injury Risk in the Hybrid III Family of Dummies

Stephen W. Rouhana, David C. Viano,
Edward A. Jedrzejczak, and Joseph D. McCleary
General Motors Research Labs.

ABSTRACT

This paper details the development of an abdominal injury assessment device for loading due to belt restraint submarining in the Hybrid III family of dummies. The design concept and criteria, response criteria, choice of injury criterion, and validation are explained. Conclusions of this work are:
1) Abdominal injury assessment for belt loading due to submarining is now possible in the Hybrid III family of dummies.
2) The abdomen developed has biofidelity in its force-deflection characteristics for belt loading, is capable of detecting the occurrence of submarining, and can be used to determine the probability of abdominal injury when submarining occurs.
3) Installation of the abdomen in the Hybrid III dummy does not change the dummy kinematics when submarining does not occur.
4) When submarining does occur, the dummy kinematics are very similar to baseline Hybrid III kinematics, except for torso angle. The change in torso angle is or may be a result of a more human-like compliance in the abdomen.

A SIGNIFICANT AMOUNT OF RESEARCH HAS BEEN DONE to assess the effectiveness of safety belts. Evans [1] applied a double pair comparison method to the 1975-86 FARS data and determined an overall effectiveness of (42 ± 3)% in fatality prevention with lap-shoulder belt use by front seated occupants. His more recent analysis [2] indicates that the highest level of driver fatality prevention by belt wearing is (82 ± 5)% in crashes where rollover is the first harmful event. Protection of the driver by lap-shoulder belt use is lowest in left-side impacts (27 ± 17)%.

There are essentially two components to occupant protection by safety belt use. One is anti-ejection protection and is primarily due to the lap portion of the belt system [3]. The other is mitigation of interior impact and is largely contributed by restraint of the upper body from the shoulder harness.

CONCEPT OF EFFECTIVE SAFETY BELT RESTRAINT - A principal design feature of lap-shoulder belts is to provide controlled loading and occupant restraint during a crash by routing safety belts over the bony structures of the pelvis, upper thorax, and shoulder. This takes advantage of a relatively high tolerance to impact forces for these regions of the skeleton and avoids concentrating load on the more compliant abdominal and lower thoracic regions. Control of occupant kinematics helps ensure maximum protection by belt restraints.

Adomeit [4-6] first espoused the fundamentals of effective belt restraint. The kinematic criteria, shown in Figure 1, help maintain the lap-portion of the belt low on the pelvis. This minimizes pelvic rotation and reduces the tendency for the lap belt to slide off the ilium and directly load the lower abdomen. Kinematic controls contribute to directing restraining forces onto the skeletal structures and away from more compliant body regions which are more vulnerable to critical injury.

Another component of effective restraint is to ensure that the biomechanical responses measured in crash testing, and related to assessment of occupant protection, consider human tolerance. While the Hybrid III dummy is considered to have biofidelity in its chest deflection response, and is considered to be a suitable tool for assessing injury risk by the Viscous and compression criteria [7-10], there is no injury assessment capability currently available for its abdominal region. In addition, the dynamic location of the belts is frequently obscured from direct photographic observation, especially in full-vehicle barrier crash testing. These situations complicate abdominal injury assessment.

HUMAN TOLERANCE - The human body has significant tolerance to impact loading as evidenced by survival in extremely severe motor vehicle crashes. In spite of the compliance of the chest and abdomen, these body regions are capable of tolerating impact force because of elastic and viscous resistance to body deformation. The pioneering work of Gadd and Patrick [11] demonstrated a tolerance to concentrated loading of the sternum of 3.3 kN (740 lb) and a tolerance of 8.0 kN (1800 lb) for distributed loading on the chest and shoulder. This research underscored the importance of the shoulder region as a load path for occupant restraint.

More recent studies have shown the importance of the Viscous response as a mechanism of impact injury of the abdomen and chest [9,10,12,13,14], and of compression [7,8] as a mechanism of crushing injury of the chest. Impact force is generally an inadequate predictor of abdominal injury [15]. However, Rouhana [13] demonstrated that the product of force and compression is a good predictor of abdominal injury. Following a limited series of experiments [16] on upper abdominal injury by a shoulder belt, Miller [17] recently determined injury tolerances of lower abdominal organs for direct lap belt loading. A Viscous tolerance of VC = 1.4 m/s and compression tolerance of C = 48% was determined for a threshold risk of 25% probability of critical abdominal injury (AIS 4+). Miller also confirmed the adequacy of the force and compression product in prediction of abdominal injury from direct belt loading. Sacco, et al [18] recently showed a 10.5% probability of death given an AIS 4+ abdominal injury by analysis of trauma patients in the Multiple Trauma Outcome Study (MTOS). This establishes the Viscous and compression tolerance for lap belt loading of the lower abdomen at approximately 2.6% probability of death (25% risk of 10.5% fatality outcome).

LIMITS OF CRASH PROTECTION - A recent analysis by Viano [19] brought together the results of several studies on crash protection. One was a crash investigation study and analysis which determined that approximately 50% of fatalities to unrestrained occupants are not preventable by the use of lap-shoulder belts or lap belt and air bag combination. This limit, in part, reflects the severity of many fatal crashes which involve extreme vehicle damage and forces on the passenger compartment, unusual crash configurations and causes of death, and unique situations associated with particular seating positions and crash dynamics. This implies that fatality risk depends on the particular occupant seating position with respect to the principal impact point. Rouhana and Foster [20] found a more than 19 to 1 increase, and Evans [21] found more than a 7 to 1 increase in fatality risk for a right-front passenger exposed to a right side (nearside) versus a left side (farside) impact in the NCSS and FARS data bases, respectively.

If the results of belt effectiveness and unpreventable deaths are compared, currently available lap-shoulder belt restraints provide a very high degree of effectiveness. There is approximately 7% additional safety potential achievable by the addition of interior safety features which supplement belt usage, such as air bags, restraint enhancements, and friendly interiors. However, the fact that lap-shoulder belts are only 42% effective in preventing fatalities underscores that absolute protection is not achievable by occupant restraints. Furthermore, it suggests that despite a significant overall net safety gain by restraint usage, injury and fatality will continue to occur to belt wearers even if belt restraints are supplemented by airbags.

BELT RELATED INJURIES - With the advent of lap belts in passenger cars in the late 1950's and early 60's, physicians started reporting new injury patterns for belt restrained victims. The typical pattern of facial and upper body injury to unrestrained occupants was replaced by belt related injury to abdominal organs and tissues [22-28]. These injuries led to the phrase "seat belt syndrome" [29-30] as the new injury patterns in motor vehicle crashes received attention due to concentrated forces on the lower abdominal region for lap belt wearers. In many cases improper belt wearing was identified as a cause of abdominal loading and injury [31]. The potential for improper use has continued with the advent of lap-shoulder belt systems, particularly placement of the shoulder harness under the arm [32] and wearing of the lap belt high on the abdomen with poor seating posture.

The most frequent belt related injuries are to the liver and spleen which are organs in the upper quadrant of the abdomen [33-35]. Injuries to lower abdominal tissues do occur [36,37] but at lower incidence suggesting a greater tolerance to abdominal compression. In some situations, upper abdominal injuries may be incorrectly assigned to the lap belt of the 3-point restraint system, when in fact the shoulder harness or steering wheel may have caused the injury. In very severe crashes, injuries may extend to the lumbar spine [38-39].

ABDOMINAL INJURY ASSESSMENT - With the introduction of lap-shoulder belts as standard equipment for front-seat occupants in the late 1960's, safety and design engineers saw the need to modify the test dummies and add new components to evaluate belt loading during crash testing. This work has continued as efforts have intensified to reduce the potential for belt-related injuries. There has also been continued progress in belt system design as injury mechanisms become better understood [40-45].

An indirect approach to abdominal injury assessment involved the insertion of load-measuring bolts at three levels in the ilium of the dummy pelvis to study the dynamics of lap belt loading and load transfer on the hip [46]. Later, the research group at Association Peugeot

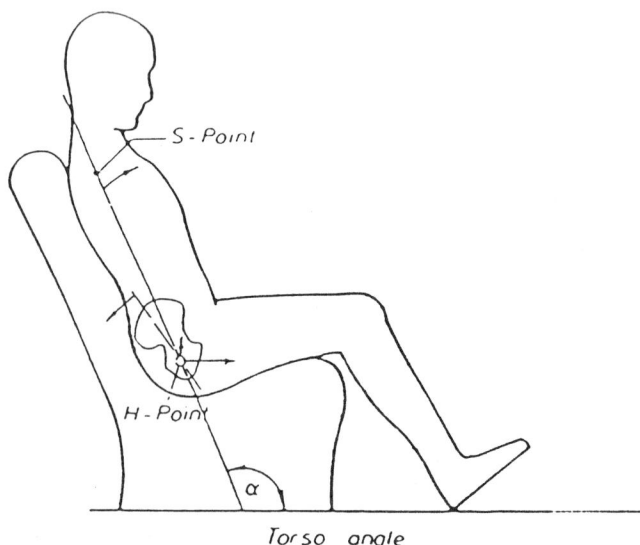

Figure 1. Adomeit's Motion Sequence Criteria
- H-point vertical disp. ≤ ±50 mm
- H-point horizontal disp. ≤ 250 mm
- Pelvic rotation < 30° CCW
- Torso axis ~90° at max. shoulder belt load

Renault [47,48] added a load cell above the ilium which could react to belt loading if the restraint slipped off (above) the pelvis. Research has also focused on improving the anthropometry of the dummy pelvic structure as more detailed information on the human seating posture became available. Melvin and Weber [49] developed a fluid filled, abdominal "intrusion sensor" for the Part 572 3 year old child dummy. While the abdomen could discriminate among various restraint systems, they noted that they did not attempt to make the response of abdomen biomechanically realistic. In fact, none of the early efforts included biofidelity in the dummy abdomen or injury assessment using a valid biomechanical response and injury criterion [50].

The importance of abdominal biofidelity and injury assessment has been discussed recently [51-53] as greater belt wearing has been achieved in the United States and passive belt systems are being introduced. Our development of an injury assessing abdomen for belt restraint loading involved matching the force-deflection properties of the human abdomen, and knowledge of the criteria upon which to estimate the risk of injury. Once a design was conceived and built, we conducted tests to ensure that the modified dummy and abdominal components functioned according to the design and development criteria.

The same basic design will be used in each member of the Hybrid III family of dummies. Values for the 50th percentile male used in the development phase have been scaled to the 5th percentile female dummy and other dummy sizes.

Early in the project we decided to develop a frangible abdomen (literally, "one that breaks readily or easily"; Webster) using plastic or foam, an approach which proved to be successful. The remainder of this paper details our design, development, and validation of an abdominal injury assessment insert for the Hybrid III family of dummies.

METHODS

DESIGN CONCEPT AND CRITERIA FOR THE ABDOMEN - The conceptual design for the injury assessing abdomen is a frangible insert that possesses biofidelity in belt restraint loading and minimizes changes to the Hybrid III dummy. The design concept involves the removal of the current "gut sack" and chest deflection potentiometer. Both of these components are situated in the abdominal region of the dummy in the location chosen for this abdominal injury transducer. The design includes a reaction surface for the frangible insert which is attached to the pelvis, rather than the rib cage, so that the orientation of the abdomen during belt loading remains fixed relative to the pelvis. The frangible insert design has biofidelity and the capability for measuring an abdominal injury criterion. The final design ensures that the amount and the characteristics of the rotation of the lumbar spine in the Hybrid III are preserved.

The design criteria for the frangible abdomen were grouped into two categories, viz., those that apply to the material chosen for the abdomen, and those that apply to the interface between the abdomen and the dummy

Material Criteria for the Abdominal Insert - The following criteria were developed and applied to the selection of the material used for injury assessment in the abdomen:
1) The force-deflection characteristics of the material must fall into established corridors.
2) When loading typical of submarining is encountered, the integrity of the material must not be compromised.
3) Restitution (or elastic spring-back) of the material does not occur, or if it does the amount of restitution is well characterized.
4) The material is easily machineable or moldable.
5) There is minimal variability between batches in production of this material.

Abdomen/Dummy Interface Criteria - The following criteria were developed for the attachment interface between the dummy and the abdomen:
1) There should be minimal modifications to Hybrid III family of dummies.
   a) Any mass and inertial changes should be well known so that reballasting of the dummies can be performed.
   b) There should be no effect on dummy posture.
   c) Performance of the dummy, as measured by dummy kinematics, should be unaffected when there is no submarining. Dummy kinematics may change when submarining occurs because the belt/dummy interaction will take place through the frangible abdomen which will be human-like and will differ in stiffness and crush performance from the existing Hybrid III abdomen.
2) Physical modifications to the dummy should not require major machining or installation procedures.
3) The frangible abdomen should be easy to install and remove after a test.

ABDOMINAL FORCE-DEFLECTION RESPONSE CRITERIA - Normalization of Force-Deflection Data for the Porcine Abdomen - While some data exists in the literature for the force-deflection properties of the abdomen most of it is for blunt loading with rigid objects Miller recently published the results of a series of experiments in which belt loading on the abdomen was examined [17]. We obtained the original data and normalized it to account for mass and antero-posterior dimensional differences between subjects. The normalization method used the equal stress/equal velocity scaling approach as suggested by Eppinger [54], Langhaar [55], and Mertz [56].

We chose to scale the force-deflection data, because it was necessary to preserve this characteristic in the design of the abdomen. Scaling was performed in a manner analogous to Mertz's scaling of force-time data, using a force scale factor, and a displacement scale factor. Because both time scales are identical, the time data did not have to be scaled. Scaling the force-deflection data in this manner is equivalent to scaling the force-time and displacement-time data separately, and then cross-plotting them.

The force and displacement are scaled according to equations (1) and (2).

(1) $\quad F_s = \lambda_f * F_i$

(2) $\quad D_s = \lambda_d * D_i$

where F_s = the normalized force (force on a standard subject),
F_i = the unnormalized force (force on the "ith" subject),
D_s = the normalized displacement,
D_i = the unnormalized displacement,
and λ_f, λ_d are determined by equations (3) and (4).

(3) $\quad \lambda_f = \sqrt{\dfrac{M_s L_s}{M_i L_i}}$

(4) $\quad \lambda_d = \sqrt{\dfrac{M_s L_i}{M_i L_s}}$

where M_s = the average mass of the porcine subjects tested
M_i = the mass of the ith subject
L_s = the average antero-posterior depth at the 4th Lumbar vertebrae
L_i = the A-P depth at L4 of the ith subject

Determination of Abdominal Force-Deflection Properties of Porcine Cadavers - The only force-deflection data available was from live anesthetized porcine and human cadaver subjects. Therefore, a small number of experiments was carried out to determine the force-deflection characteristics of the porcine cadaver for comparison with the data from the live anesthetized porcine subjects.

Fifteen experiments were performed on 7 Landrace-Yorkshire crossbred males* with an average mass of 46.1 ± 1.3 kg (101.4 ± 2.9 lbs). The subjects were preanesthetized by intramuscular injection of Acetylpromazine Maleate (0.37 mg/kg) and Ketamine HCl (33 mg/kg). They were then induced into deep surgical anesthesia by inhalation of Nitrous Oxide (50% for induction) and Methoxyflurane (3% for induction). Euthanasia was administered by overdose of anesthesia which was increased to lethal levels. Death was assured by examination of heart rate, respiration rate and volume, and neurological signs.

The protocol followed in these experiments simulated that used in human cadaver experiments such as those done by Kroell [7]. Within 6 hours after euthanasia, each subject was placed in a refrigerator where it remained at 2 °C until tested. Refrigeration times ranged from 2 to 8 days. The subjects were removed from the refrigerator at 6:00 AM on the day of the test, and allowed to warm at room temperature for approximately 8 hours. Rectal temperatures at the time of test ranged from 8 to 12 °C (47 to 54 °F).

Most subjects were utilized in more than one test in an attempt to obtain as much biomechanical information as possible. As seen in the matrix of experiments (Table 1), multiple experiments on a single subject were performed in order of increasing velocity. The primary focus of these experiments was a determination of force-deflection curves at velocities similar to those used by Miller. A determination of abdominal injury in the porcine cadavers was also made for comparison with the data from live anesthetized porcine subjects.

Each subject was placed in dorsal recumbency on a plexiglas V-block support which was bolted to the platen of a hydraulic, materials testing machine (MTS). The V-block was positioned such that impact would occur approximately at the level of the fourth lumbar vertebrae. The impacting object was the same 381 mm (15") length of 5.0 cm wide polyester safety belt used by Miller. The belt was attached to a yoke through two pivots (Figure 2), and the yoke was attached to the actuator piston of the MTS through an inertially compensated biaxial load cell (GSE 3182).

Prior to impact, the piston was lowered to the point where all belt slack was removed, but negligible preload was developed. The MTS piston was then cycled through a programmed displacement stroke and velocity. Total axial force developed, belt force at the pivot points (measured using strain gauges), and piston stroke were recorded on FM tape. Velocities ranged from 0.2 to 5.3 m/s, and piston stroke ranged from 118 to 126 mm (45 to 69 % of the antero-posterior dimension of the subject).

An abdominal necropsy was performed after last test on each subject, with abdominal injuries recorded and assessed using the Abbreviated Injury Scale (AIS-85) [57].

Extrapolation of Porcine Data and Human Cadaver Data to Corridors for Living Humans - Our desire was to determine the force-deflection characteristics of living humans. It was unknown whether force-deflection properties are independent of species (Porcine versus

---

* The rationale and experimental protocol for the use of an animal model in this program have been reviewed by the Research Laboratories' Animal Research Committee. The research follows procedures outlined in the Guide for the Care and Use of Laboratory Animals, U. S. Department of Health and Human Services, Public Health Service, National Institutes of Health NIH Publication 85-23, Revised 1985, and Public Health Service Policy on Humane Care and Use of Laboratory Animals by Awardee Institutions, NIH Guide for Grants and Contracts, Vol. 14, No. 8, June 25, 1985, and complies with the provisions of the Animal Welfare Act of 1966 (P.L. 89-544), as amended in 1970 (P.L. 91-579) and 1976 (P.L. 94-270), and the Food Security Act of 1985 (P.L. 99-158).

TABLE 1. Matrix of Porcine Cadaver Experiments

Expt #	Subject #	AP Dimen (mm)	Velocity (m/s)	Compression (mm)	(%)	AIS
1	1	207	.23	126		
2	1	"	.84	123		
3	1	"	5.3	118	57.1	5
4	2	242	NA	NA		
5	2	"	NA	NA		
6	3	268	.22	122		
7	3	"	5.2	120	44.6	4
8	3	"	5.0	119		
9	3	"	4.6	120		
10	4	181	.59	124		
11	4	"	.85	125	68.8	0
12	5	211	.86	125		
13	5	"	.88	125	59.2	3
14	6	199	.86	124	62.3	2
15	7	183	5.2	118	64.3	4

Human), or if the force-deflection properties of living subjects should be equivalent to those of cadaver subjects (assuming that tissue properties may change after death). Therefore, the force-deflection curves from porcine cadavers were compared to the curves from human cadavers, and to the curves obtained for living anesthetized porcine subjects. Any observed differences could then be used to extrapolate human cadaver force-deflection data to living human force-deflection data.

CHOICE OF ABDOMINAL INJURY CRITERION FOR BELT LOADING - Previous work has shown that the risk of abdominal injury can be predicted using a number of different criteria. The viscous criterion has been shown to apply to the abdomen by Rouhana [12], Viano and Lau [9,10], and Stalnaker [58] for rigid loading, and recently by Miller [17] for belt loading. In addition, Rouhana showed that the product of maximum force and maximum compression was a good indicator of the probability of abdominal injury for human cadavers. Miller [17] has shown that this criterion also worked well in live anesthetized porcine subjects. Miller also proposed that compression alone is a good indicator of abdominal injury in <u>belt</u> loading to the abdomen. Tolerance values for compression are presented in Figure 3 [17].

Verriest, et al. [59] have shown that belt loading is a low velocity phenomenon (Figure 3) which occurs at around 3 m/s. Given this low velocity loading, maximum compression is the injury criterion of choice for assessment of abdominal injury from belt restraint submarining.

DESIGN VALIDATION - The design of the frangible abdomen was validated in material tests and sled tests.

<u>Material Tests</u> - All material tests were performed on the hydraulic testing system (MTS) described above. The material tests were performed to assess:

a) Force-deflection of the design - Samples of the frangible abdomen were placed in a Hybrid III dummy pelvis which had been modified to accommodate a support structure for the abdomen. The same belt yoke and protocol that was used to determine the porcine force-deflection data was used to develop and assess the force-deflection data for the frangible abdomen samples. The abdomen was loaded by a standard belt in what is an anterior to posterior direction, *in situ*, in the dummy pelvis. The force-deflection of the final design could then be compared to the established corridors.

b) Repeatability of the force-deflection curves - Five samples were tested at 1 m/s and five at 6 m/s using the protocol described in a). Each force-deflection curve was compared to others generated at the same velocity.

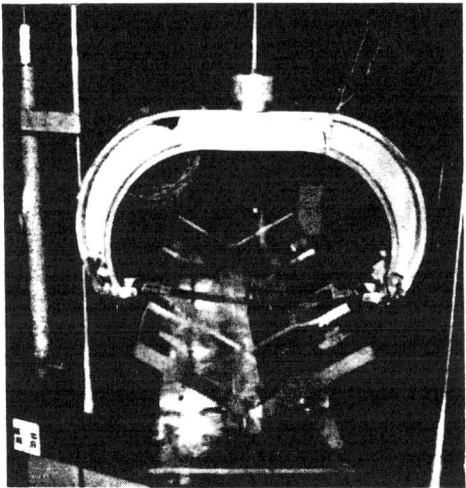

Figure 2. MTS impactor with yoke and belt used in live anesthetized and porcine cadaver experiments.

c) Rate dependence of the material chosen - Five samples were tested at 1 m/s and five at 6 m/s using the protocol described in a). The force-deflection curves generated at 1 m/s were then compared to those generated at 6 m/s.

d) Restitution of the material chosen - A small number of experiments were conducted during the development phase using a 51 x 127 mm (2 x 5 inch) rectangular aluminum impactor. Elliptical samples of the proposed material with a major axis of 279 mm (11.0") and a minor axis of 203 mm (8.0") were placed in a test fixture on the MTS platen. A programmed deformation-time history was then imposed on it. The restitution of the material chosen for the frangible abdomen could be determined by subtracting the amount of residual deformation of the material (measured after the test) from the amount of piston travel programmed. For example, if the programmed piston travel is 76 mm (3.0"), and the residual deformation is 70 mm (2.75"), then the restitution would be 6 mm (0.25").

e) Function and integrity of the material - The function of the material was assessed during the development phase by performing experiments as described in a), but varying the belt loading direction and amount of slack. The loading for all tests in this series was in an antero-posterior direction at a 30° angle to a transverse plane through the material, coupled with one of the following: no slack in the belt; 25 mm (1.0") of slack in the belt; or the initial position of the belt contact point either on an edge or in the center of the material. The structural integrity of the material was assessed post-loading. In addition, the "behavior" of the material (symmetric crush for symmetric load, etc.) was assessed.

f) Interaction between the rib cage and abdominal element - In sled or barrier tests in which submarining does not occur, a dummy can experience torso flexion (bending forward about the hip in which the front of the thorax (chest) moves toward the top of the knees). During torso flexion, the bottom of the rib cage interacts with any material in the area between the rib cage and the pelvis. Thus, if the kinematics of the dummy are to be preserved, the interaction of the bottom rib with the abdomen should be similar to current dummies.

To assess this interaction, MTS tests were performed using a simulated lower rib. This rib was made of a half steering wheel segment and was mounted to the hydraulic piston through the biaxial load cell described above. The force-deflection properties were recorded for the frangible abdomen, the abdomen from a Hybrid-III 5th percentile female, and both abdomens from a Hybrid III 50th percentile male (the abdomen with a clearance notch for the chest potentiometer arm, and the abdomen without the notch). Each abdomen was tested four times with vertical loading, and four times with the direction of loading at a 30° angle to the vertical (Figure 4). For each loading direction, 2 of the four tests were performed quasi-statically at .36 m/s and the other 2 were performed at 89 m/s.

Sled Tests - Sled tests were performed to assess the kinematics of the dummy and the function of the foam in actual use (indication of submarining, integrity after loading in a dummy, and ease of installation and handling.)

The sled tests were performed with a generic restraint system in a body buck on a Hyge Sled. The sled buck had a single bucket seat in the driver's position, and there was no instrument panel or steering system. The seat used in these tests was constructed of foam on a zig-zag spring suspension and sheet metal frame. The foam Indentation Load-Deflection characteristic was 240 N. The seat pan angle was 8° and the seat back angle was approximately 26° (not a reclining seat).

The dummy was in the driver's seat wearing a single retractor continuous loop lap/shoulder belt system with a cinchable latch plate. The retractor was on the shoulder portion of the belt system. Three types of tests were run which were classified by the intended degree of submarining:

a) no submarining - The lap portion of the belt system was positioned below the anterior superior iliac spines of the dummy pelvis and was cinched snug. The shoulder belt was pulled out of the retractor and allowed to retract until there was a "fistful" of slack in the belt (25-38 mm (1-1.5") of webbing). The retractor was locked before the test to avoid any changes in configuration.

b) incipient submarining - The lap portion of the belt system was positioned below the anterior superior iliac spines of the dummy pelvis and but was not cinched. Instead, the lap belt was left loose with 76 mm (3.0") of slack. The shoulder belt was "cinched" tight by pushing the back of the dummy into the seat back, retracting all shoulder belt slack, and locking the retractor

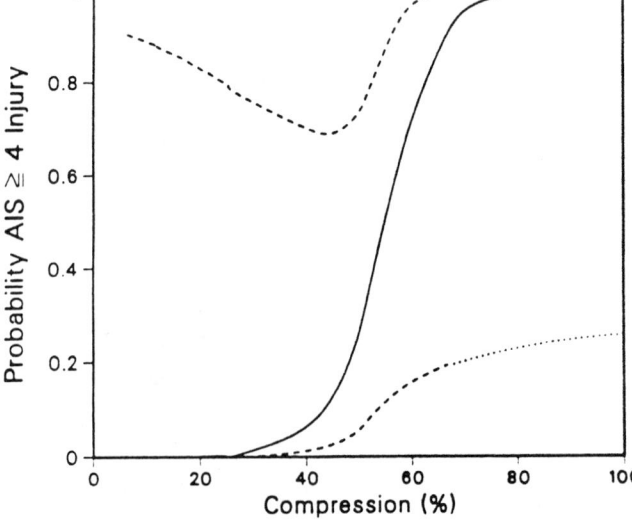

Figure 3. Probability of AIS ≥ 4 abdominal injury as a function of compression. (From logistic regression analysis of Miller data.)

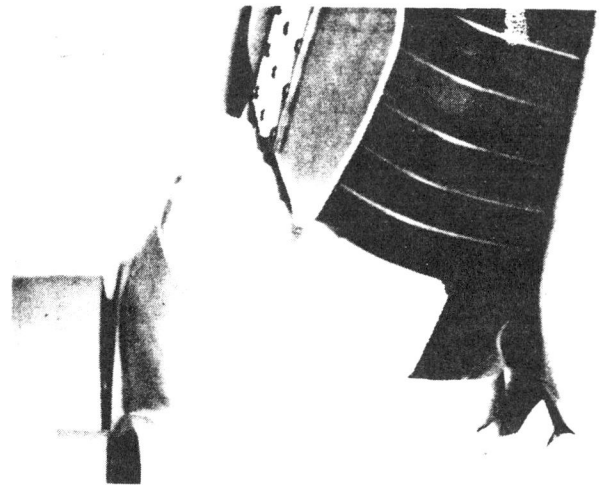

Figure 4a. Side view of Hybrid III showing position of rib cage relative to foam insert.

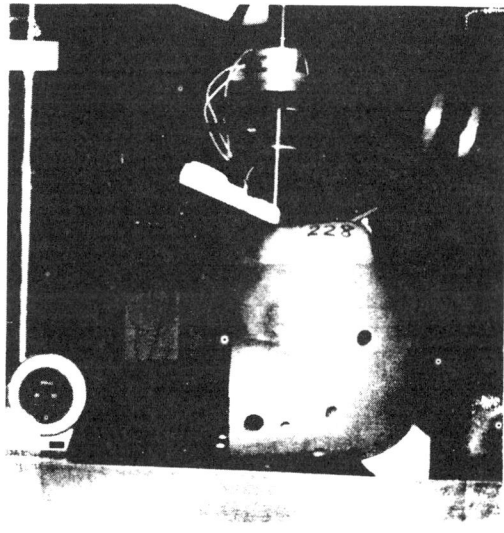

Figure 4b. Superior/inferior loading simulation.

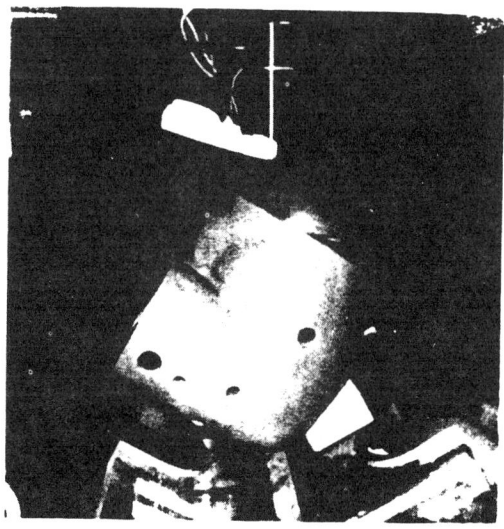

Figure 4c. Torso flexion loading simulation.

before releasing the dummy.

c) presubmarined - The lap portion of the belt system was positioned <u>above</u> the anterior superior iliac spines of the pelvis and lightly cinched without preloading the abdomen. The shoulder belt was also "cinched" into position by pushing the back of the dummy into the seat, retracting all slack, and locking the retractor before releasing the dummy.

All tests used a single 50th percentile male Hybrid III dummy. Shoulder belt loads were monitored using a GSE Belt Load Cell in a position midway between the guide loop and dummy shoulder. Inboard belt loads were also measured between the inboard anchor and the buckle. Sled parameters were set to provide a generic crash pulse with a 30 mph delta-v.

In all tests, high speed movies were taken with an onboard camera view from the driver's right side. The movies were used to compare baseline Hybrid III dummy kinematics to kinematics of the Hybrid III with the frangible abdomen. Dummy motion was assessed using Adomeit's kinematic criteria [4-6] and other criteria. Specifically, we monitored: the maximum excursion of the head in the x and y direction (by tracking the temporomandibular "joint" on the dummy with x forward/backward and y up/down); the angle of the neck at maximum head excursion (vertical was zero degrees, forward was increasing angle); the torso angle at maximum belt load (vertical was 90°, forward was decreasing angle); and the maximum excursion of the H-point in the x and y direction.

RESULTS

CONSTRUCTION OF DESIGN - The frangible abdomen is constructed of styrofoam floatation foam which is cut on a standard band saw. The shape of the foam after cutting is shown in Figures 5a-c. Since styrofoam floatation foam is extruded, the force-deflection properties may vary depending on the orientation of the sample within the billet. The frangible abdomen samples are machined as shown in Figure 6.

DESIGN CRITERIA - <u>Material for Frangible Abdomen</u> - Six materials were examined either physically on the MTS machine or by inspection of data provided by manufacturers. The materials included Betacore (a low density honeycomb composite), Dorvon, Ethafoam, Styrofoam floatation foam, a polyurethane foam, and a composite made of a fiber matrix embedded in a hardened resin. Styrofoam floatation foam was chosen for the frangible abdomen.

The shape of the frangible abdomen was designed to achieve a linearly increasing force (constant stiffness) which enabled Styrofoam to meet the first design criterion. The design allows the belt to penetrate into the frangible abdomen, where it is exposed to a linearly increasing area of foam with increasing compression (Figure 5c). With this geometry, the stiffness of the frangible abdomen (see Figures 16-18) is not significantly different from the porcine abdominal stiffness, at the .05 level of significance. The material and sled tests described below demonstrated that styrofoam also met design criteria 2-5.

<u>Abdomen/Dummy Interface Criteria</u> - The chest

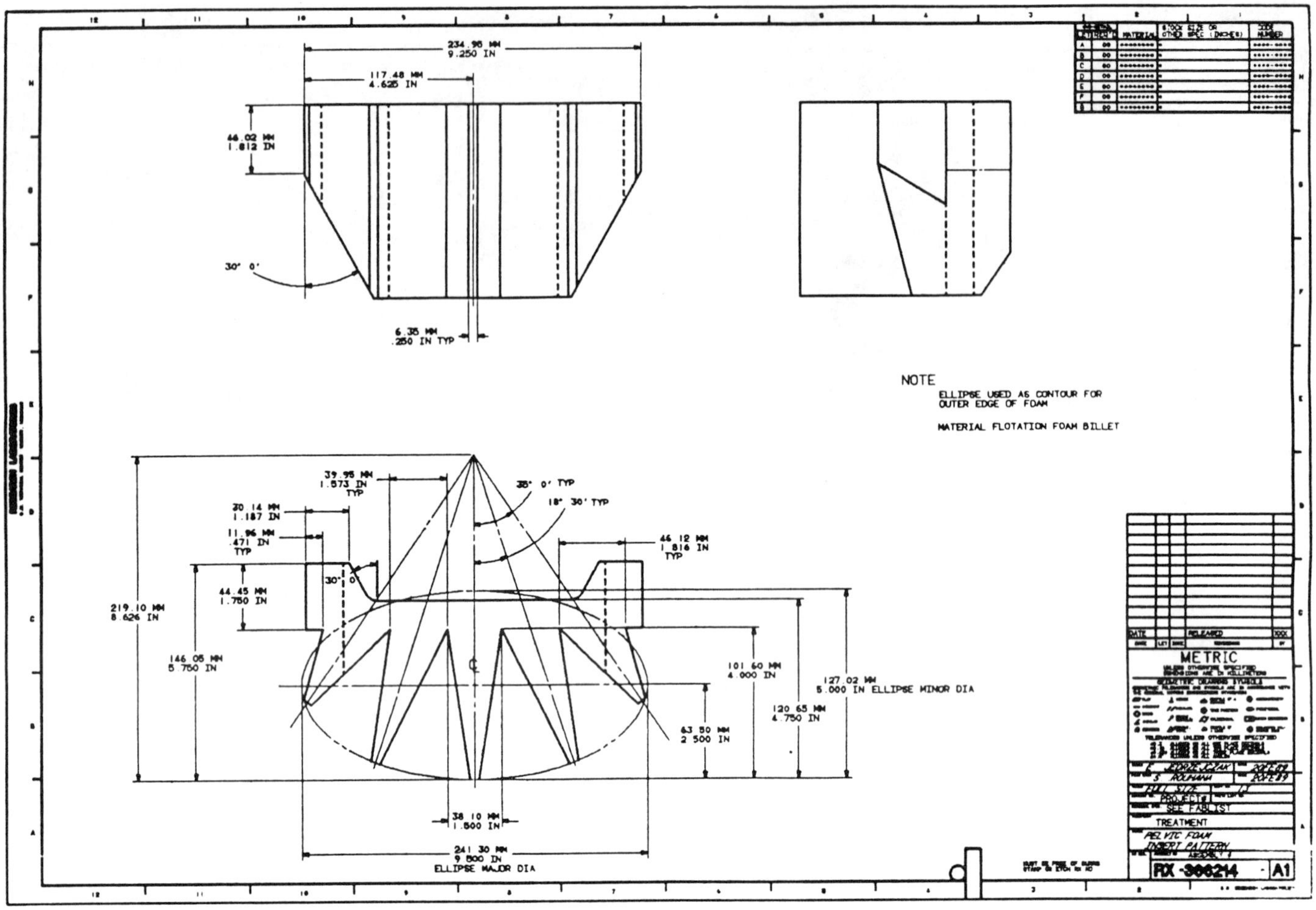

Figure 5a.

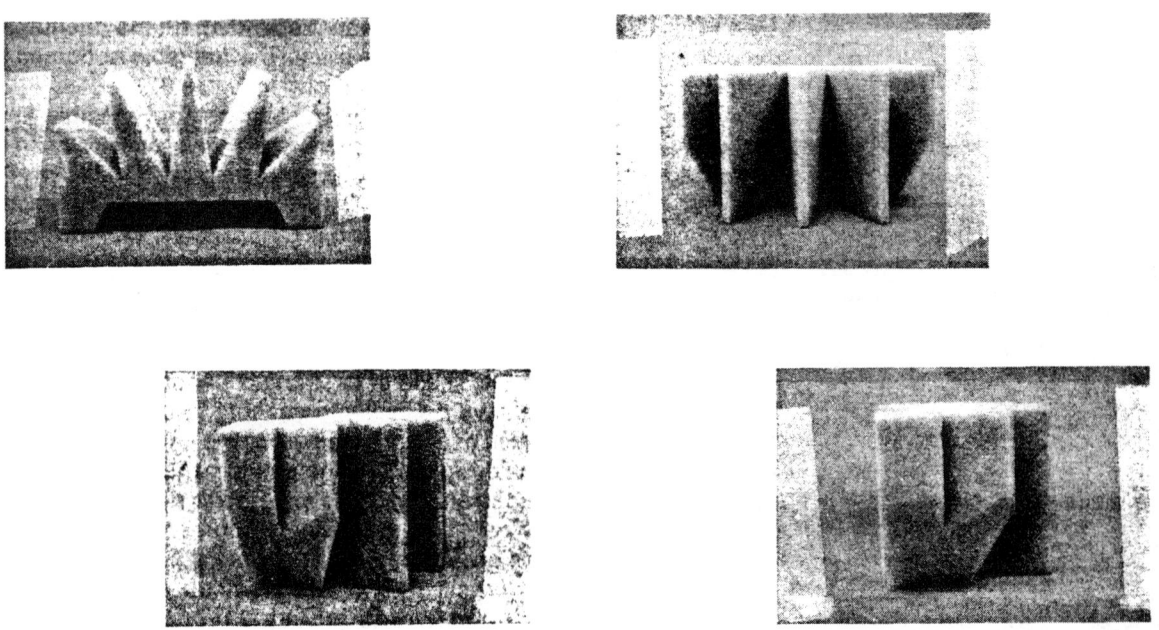

Figure 5b. Frangible abdomen foam insert.

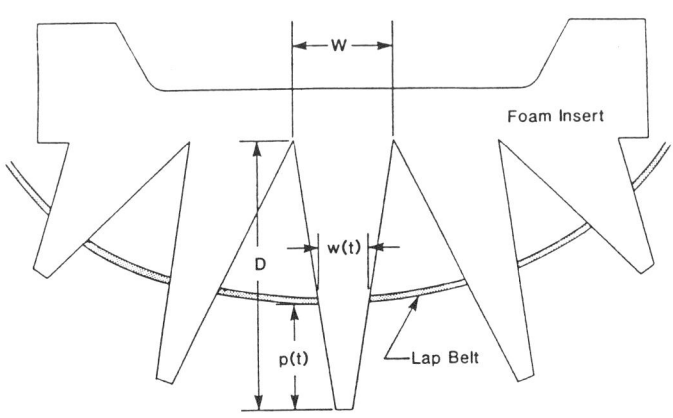

By similar triangles:

$$\frac{w(t)}{W} = \frac{p(t)}{D} \quad \text{so,} \quad w(t) = \frac{W}{D} p(t)$$

If the lap belt width is h, and if the area of foam exposed to the belt at any time is A, then A(t) = h w(t), or

$$A(t) = \frac{W h}{D} p(t) \quad \text{which is linear in } p(t).$$

Figure 5c. Geometric explanation for linearly increasing force-deflection.

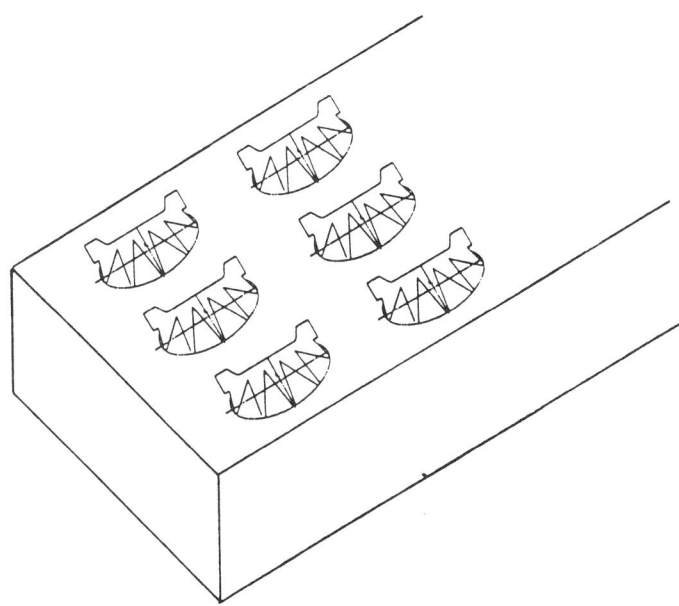

Figure 6. Location of foam sample within billet before cutting.

deflection measurement potentiometer had to be removed from the dummy for any practical design. The reason is apparent upon inspection of the Hybrid III with the standard abdomen removed (Figure 7). The chest potentiometer is in a location that is central to the abdomen, especially with the dummy in torso flexion. The chest deflection potentiometer is mounted on the anterior portion of the thoracic spine instrumentation adaptor (Hybrid III Drawing Number 78051-88). Its removal is accomplished by sawing off the front portion of the instrumentation adaptor (the part with the molded flexion stops) so that the remainder is flush with the front portion of the top of the lumbar spine. Removal of this piece, the chest deflection potentiometer, and arm, reduces the mass of the dummy by 0.845 kg. The part of the instrumentation adaptor that remains is used to mount the thoracic spine accelerometers.

A bracket shaped like a stirrup (henceforth, called "support bracket") served as a coupling between the abdomen and the pelvis of the dummy (Figure 8). The support bracket is constructed of welded and machined 6 mm (0.250") steel plate, which increases the height of the dummy by 6 mm. Another 6 mm (0.250") steel plate (henceforth called "reaction plate") is bolted to the support bracket and serves as a reaction surface for the foam insert (Figure 9). The design was accomplished by machining the lumbar spine mounting block (Figure 10).

The machined lumbar spine mounting block has a mass of 5.26 kg compared with the standard mounting block mass of 7.145 kg. The abdominal support bracket has a mass 2.63 kg. The standard abdomen mass is 0.656 kg, and the frangible abdomen insert mass is 0.062 kg. Then the net mass change of the Hybrid III dummy is a decrease of 0.694 kg.

Normalized Abdominal Force-Deflection Curves for Living Porcine Subjects - The zoometric data and test conditions from Miller's experiments, and the normalizing factors we determined are presented in Table 2. The force-deflection curves for the remaining tests are presented in Figures 11 and 12. Two separate graphs are given designated "higher velocity" and "lower velocity". The curves were separated because the higher velocity curves have a significantly greater stiffness than the lower velocity curves. Higher velocity curves were those above 5.8 m/s, and lower velocity curves were those below that velocity. Table 3 gives the average stiffness for the two different groups.

Abdominal Force-Deflection Curves for Porcine Cadavers - Force-deflection data from the porcine cadaver experiments is shown in Figures 13 and 14. Descriptions of the resulting injuries are given in Table 4, and comparison of stiffness with live anesthetized porcine data in Table 5.

Extrapolation of Porcine Data and Human Cadaver Data to Corridors for Living Humans - The force-deflection data from human cadaver experiments is shown Figure 15. Note that only low velocity data was used since this is the velocity range of belt loading [59].

DESIGN VALIDATION - Material Tests -
a) Force-deflection of final design - The force-deflection curves obtained from 5 tests of the frangible abdomen at 1 m/s are shown in

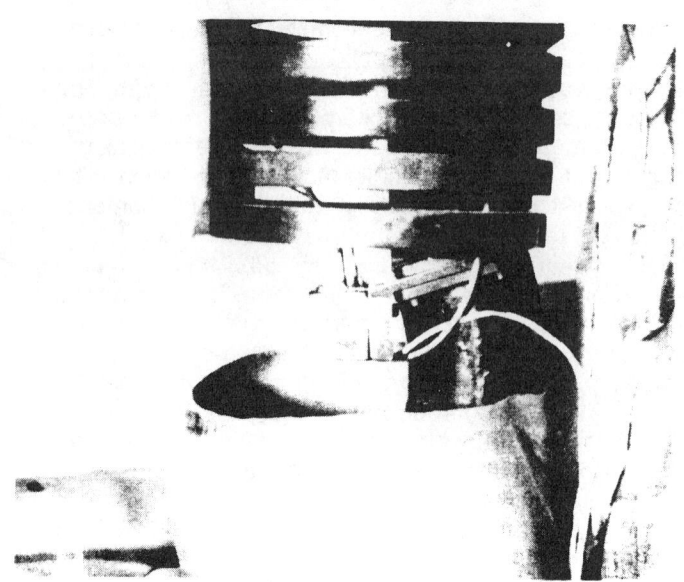

Figure 7a. Side view of Hybrid III dummy showing location of chest deflection potentiometer.

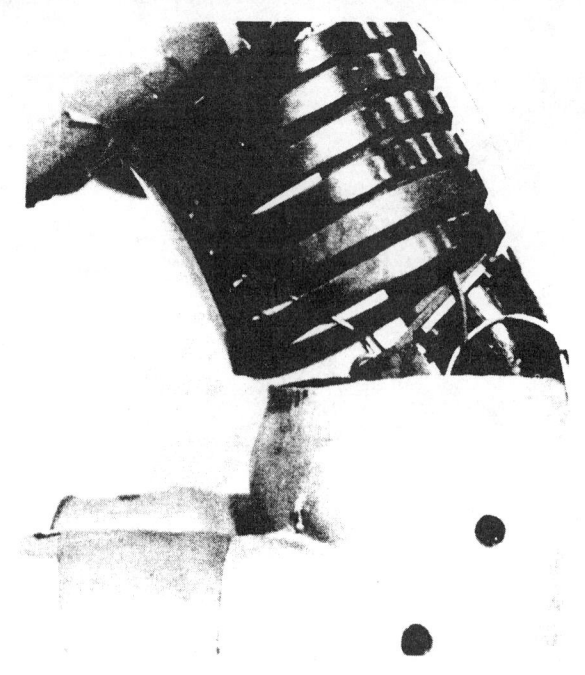

Figure 7b. Side view of Hybrid III dummy in torso flexion

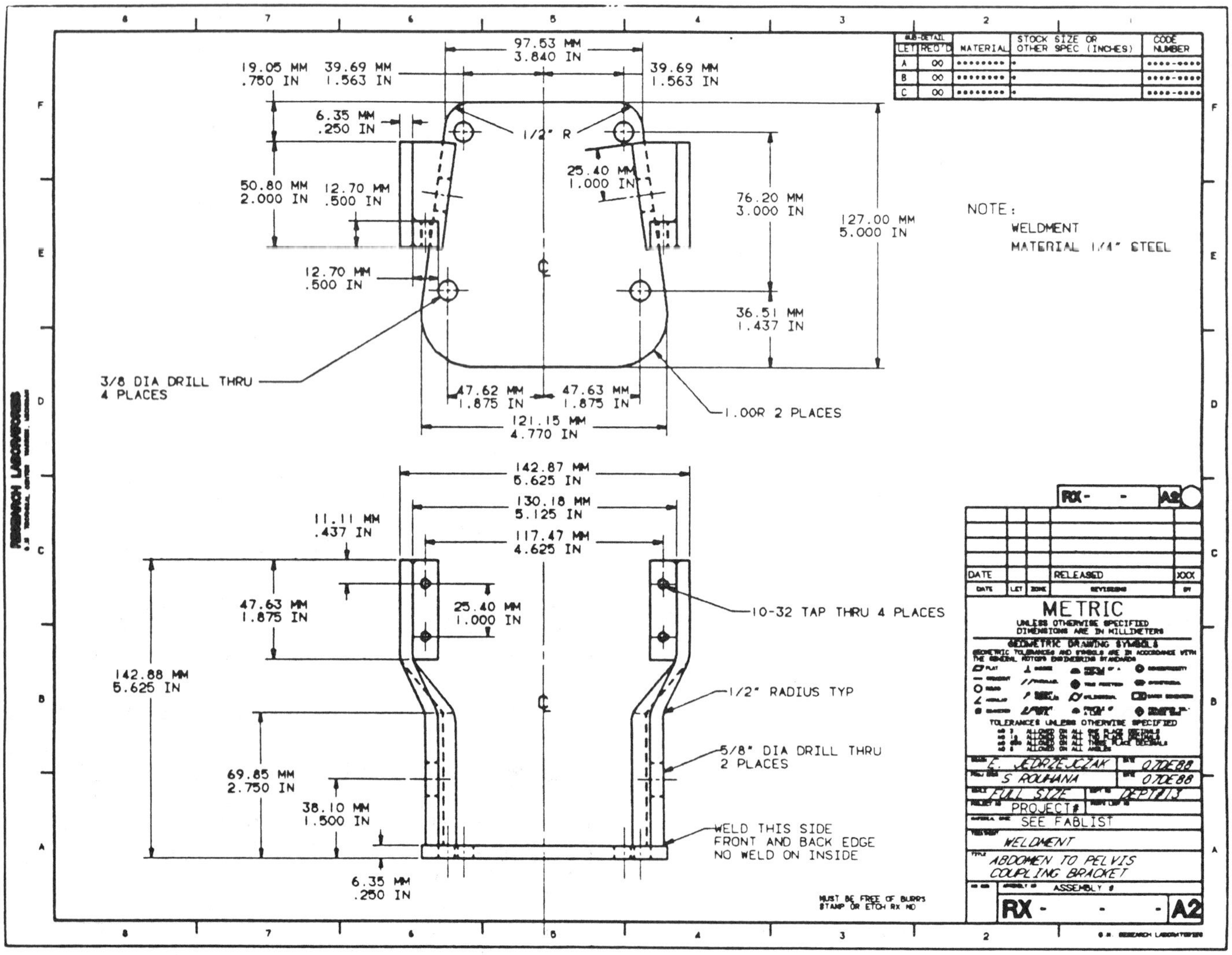

Figure 8.

Figure 9.

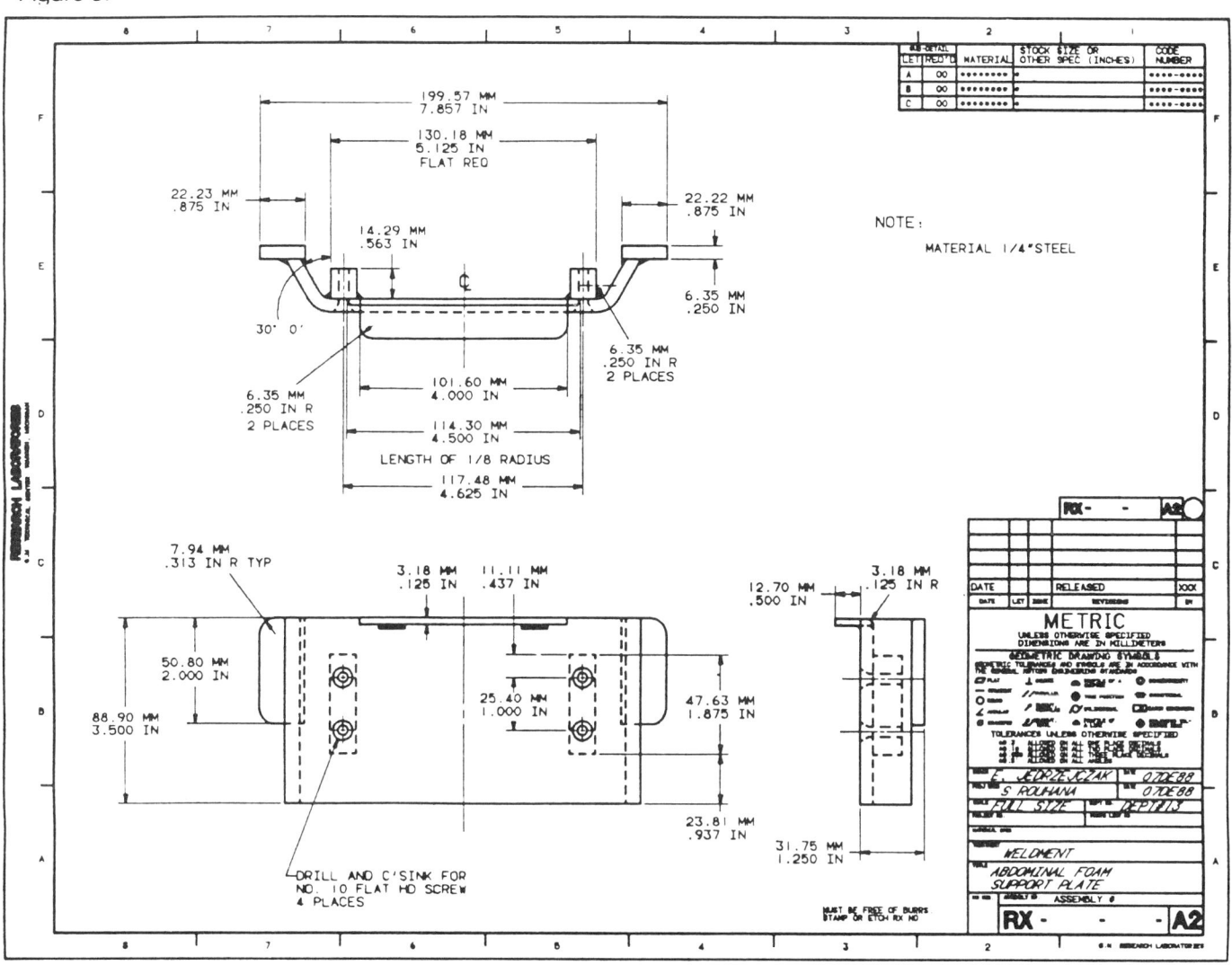

TABLE 2. Anesthetized Porcine Experiments

Expt. #	AP Diam (mm)	Mass (kg)	Normalizing Factors λf	λd	Impact Velocity (m/s)	Compression (mm)	(%)
2*	310	48.7	0.858	1.083	3.3	62	20
3	285	44.8	0.933	1.083	3.5	62	22
4	272	45.3	0.950	1.052	3.5	62	23
5	252	38.6	1.069	1.097	3.7	62	25
6	253	40.0	1.048	1.080	3.5	62	24
8	242	50.5	0.954	0.940	5.0	109	45
9	221	53.6	0.969	0.872	6.0	124	56
10	218	45.4	1.060	0.941	6.6	113	52
13	138	50.0	1.270	0.713	2.7	55	40
14	180	37.7	1.280	0.938	3.0	108	60
15	253	38.6	1.067	1.099	4.2	67	26
17	230	45.4	1.032	0.966	2.5	27	12
18	250	43.6	1.010	1.028	3.8	45	18
20	278	46.4	0.929	1.051	5.5	73	26
21	250	49.7	0.946	0.963	3.6	29	12
Avg	238 ± 45.6	45.3 ± 4.5	N = 15		{Low Velocity: N = 13} {High Velocity: N = 2}		

* For tests 1,7,11,12,16,19,22,23 data was missing or unusable.

Figure 10.

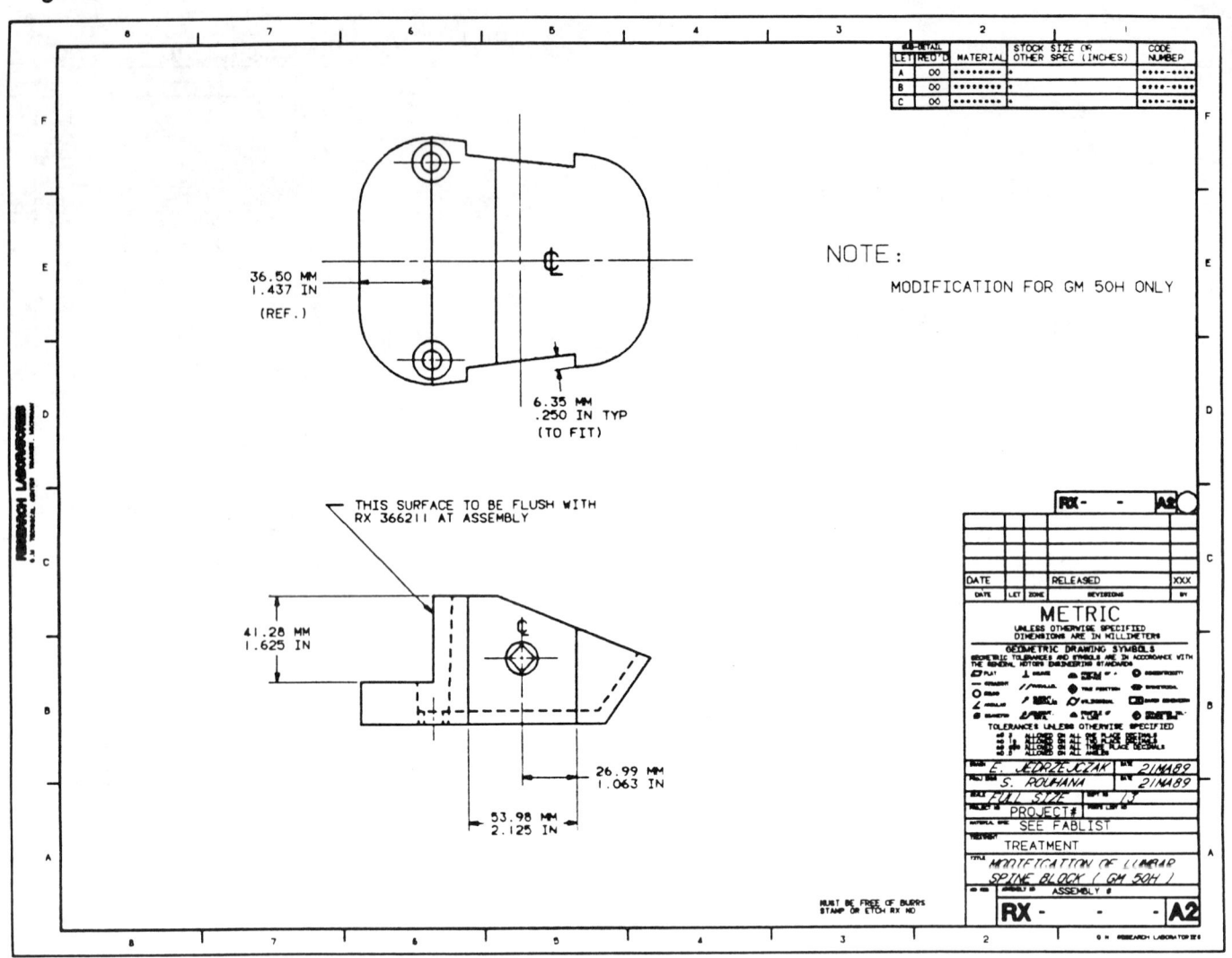

TABLE 3. Anesthetized Porcine Abdominal Stiffness

Experiment Series	N	Stiffness (N/mm)	Velocity (m/s)
Lower Velocity	13	23 ± 10	3.7 ± .84
Higher Velocity	2	63 ± 13	6.3 ± .42

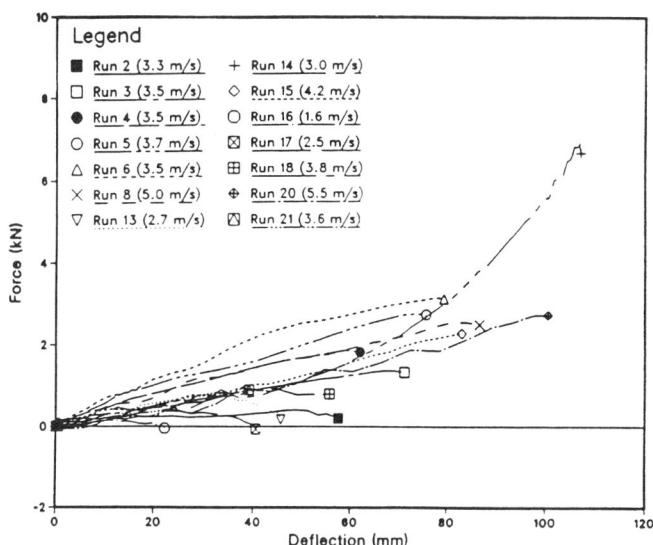

Figure 11. Force-deflection curves of live anesthetized porcine subjects in low velocity lap belt impacts.

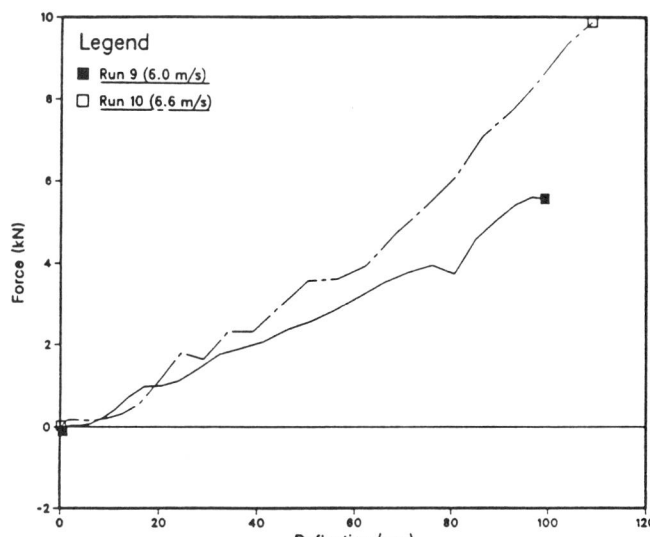

Figure 12. Force-deflection curves of live anesthetized porcine subjects in high velocity lap belt impacts.

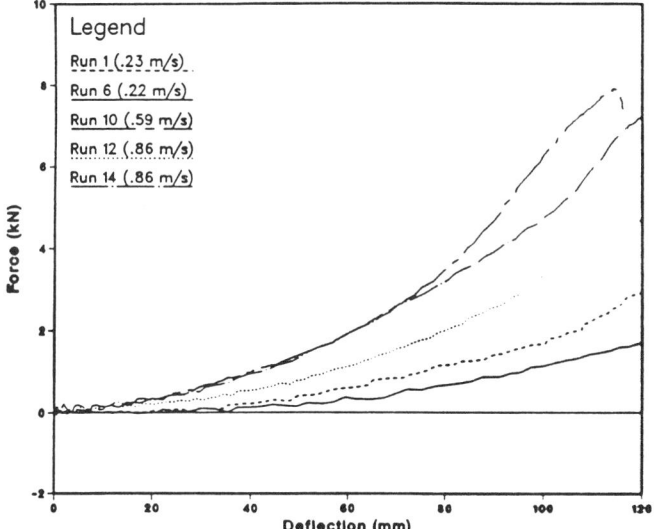

Figure 13. Normalized force-deflection curves for porcine cadaver subjects from low velocity lap belt impacts. (These are from the first impact to each subject.)

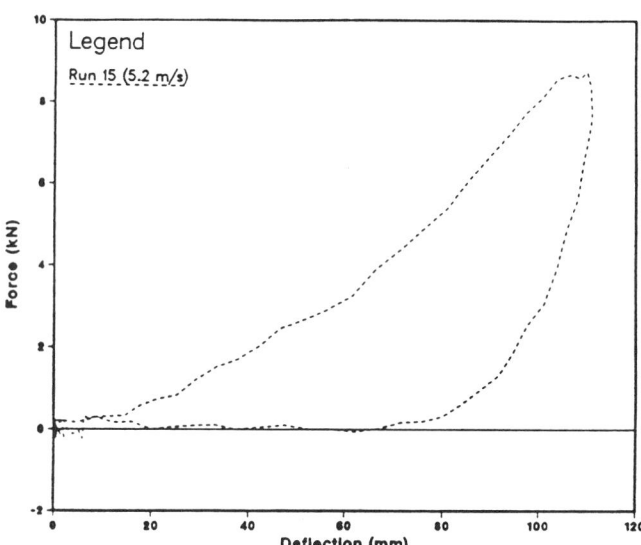

Figure 14. Normalized force-deflection curves for porcine cadaver subjects from high velocity lap belt impacts. (These are from the first impact to each subject.)

TABLE 4. Abdominal Injuries in Porcine Cadaver Experiments

Test	Injury Description	AIS
1	Large Intestine: Major Rupture	5
2	Large Intestine: Rupture with contam.	5
3	Large Intestine: Rupture	4
4	No Injury	0
5	Small Intestine: Rupture	3
6	Hemoperitoneum: Origin Unknown	2
7	Spiral Colon: Rupture	4

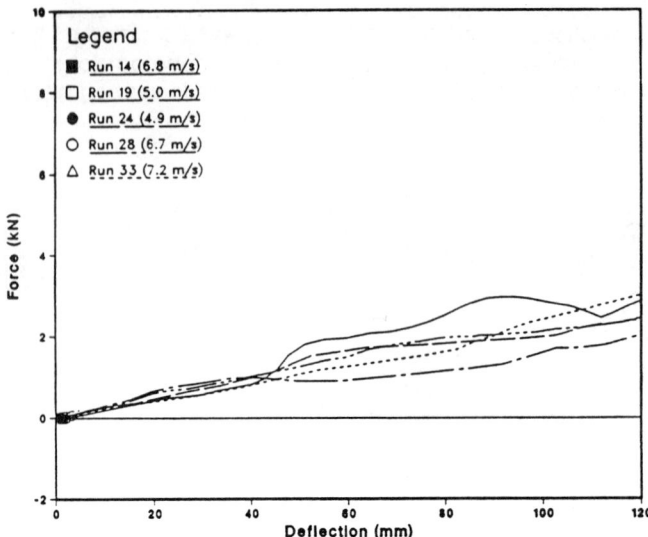

Figure 15. Force-deflection curves for human cadaver subjects, from Cavanaugh, et al.

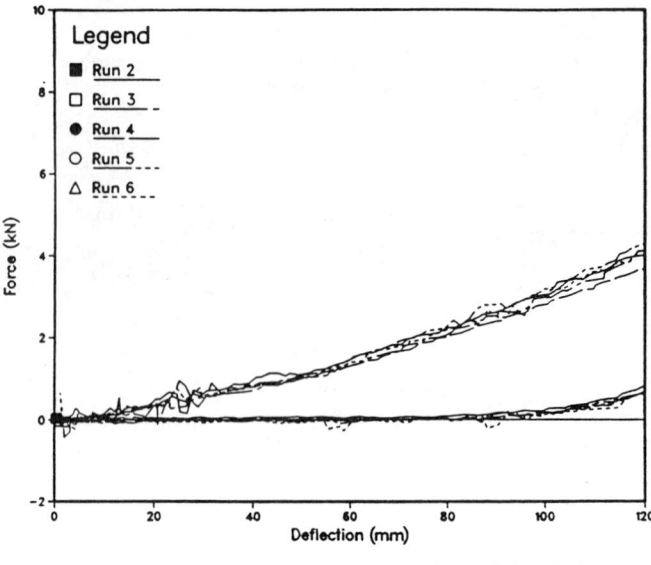

Figure 16. Force-deflection curves for frangible abdomen in 1 m/s lap belt impacts.

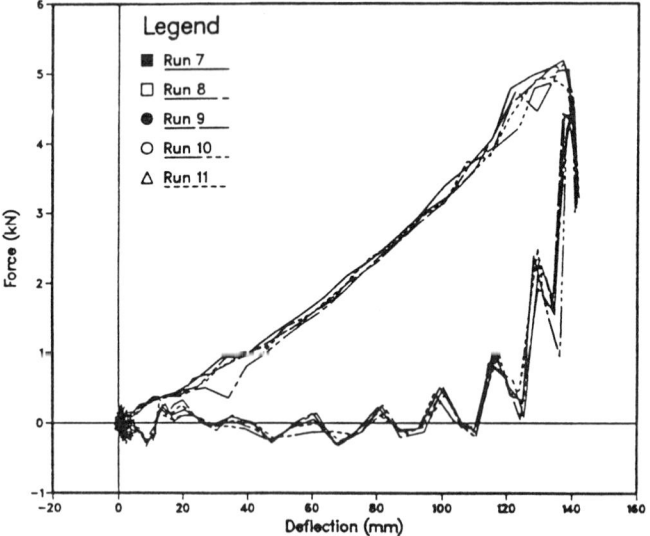

Figure 17. Force-deflection curves for frangible abdomen in 6 m/s lap belt impacts.

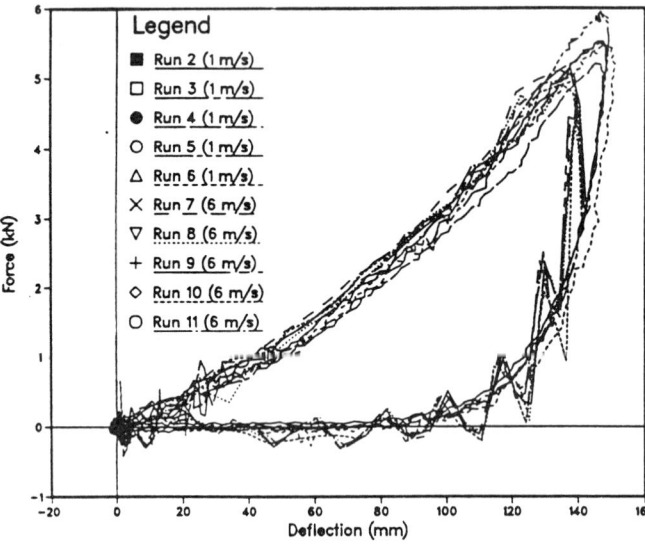

Figure 18. Overlay of 1 m/s and 6 m/s force-deflection curves for frangible abdomen.

TABLE 5. Stiffness of Porcine Cadavers
Low Velocity; First Test on Cadaver

Velocity (m/s)	Stiffness (N/mm)
0.23	12.8
0.22	27.8
0.59	28.4
0.86	22.0
0.86	59.2

Average Stiffness = 31 ± 9 N/mm (N=5)
Average Velocity = 0.55 ± .32 m/s

Figure 16.
b) Repeatability of the force-deflection curves - see a).
c) Rate dependence of the styrofoam - The force-deflection curves obtained from 5 tests of the frangible abdomen at 6 m/s are shown in Figure 17, and are overlaid on those of (a) in Figure 18.
d) Restitution of styrofoam - The tests performed with a rigid impactor indicated that the amount of restitution experienced when styrofoam is crushed 3.0" (76.2 mm) is between 0.16"-0.39" (4-10 mm).
e) Function and integrity of the styrofoam - Figure 19 shows a typical sample from the tests with angled impact and varying belt slack and position. In all cases the foam crush was very well behaved, and structural integrity of the undeformed foam was well maintained.
f) Interaction between the rib cage and the frangible abdomen - The stiffness of each abdominal element is given in Table 6.

Sled Tests - Figure 20a is a photograph of the foam sample used in the sled test in which there was no submarining, 20b-d are from the tests in which there was incipient submarining and 20e-f are from the tests in which the dummy was presubmarined.

When there was no submarining, the upper segment of the foam insert showed no deformation from the lap belt, and minor deformation from interaction with the rib cage. The lower segment of the foam insert showed some deformation because the foam protrudes forward of the anterior-superior iliac spines and is loaded by the belt as it hooks onto the pelvis. Such loads are insignificant when applied to the pelvis.

In the tests with incipient submarining, the deformation pattern occurs at a slightly superior (higher) location on the foam insert. In the first two tests the belt appeared to slip between the upper and lower segment of the foam insert. There is slight deformation to the insert in the first test, but, in the second test (Figure 20c) there is a clear indication that unilateral submarining was occurring on the right side of the dummy (left side of the photograph). A third test was run in which the upper and lower segments were glued together. Again there was some deformation to the foam, but the glue may have influenced the stiffness.

When the dummy was presubmarined, the degree of submarining was clearly manifested in the foam (Figures 20e-f). The submarining was unilateral (right side of the dummy, left side of the photograph) and extensive.

In all of the above tests the integrity of the foam was preserved, and it was easily removed after each test.

Figure 21 shows a comparison of the kinematics of the Baseline Hybrid III versus the Hybrid III with the frangible abdomen for tests in which submarining did not occur. Figure 22 shows the same comparison for tests in which submarining did occur. There were no sled tests run with the Baseline Hybrid III in the incipient submarining set up, so a comparison of those kinematics was not performed.

DISCUSSION

The final design of the frangible abdomen is a five-pointed, crown shaped piece of styrofoam. It has biofidelity in abdominal force-deflection properties which are very close to the established corridor. Installation of the frangible abdomen in the Hybrid III is easily accomplished by two people in less than a few minutes. Hanging the dummy by the cranial eyebolt helps open the abdominal cavity relative to the seated dummy. Then the foam is pushed into place by one person as the other person folds the abdominal skin down to expose the abdominal cavity.

The foam frangible abdomen satisfies the design objectives by providing an unambiguous indication of the occurrence of submarining, and by allowing an objective measure of the probability of abdominal injury from submarining.

FORCE-DEFLECTION PROPERTIES OF THE ABDOMINAL INSERT - The force-deflection data from each group of experiments was "self-normalized" using equal velocity/equal stress scaling. The purpose of the self-normalization was to account for mass and geometry

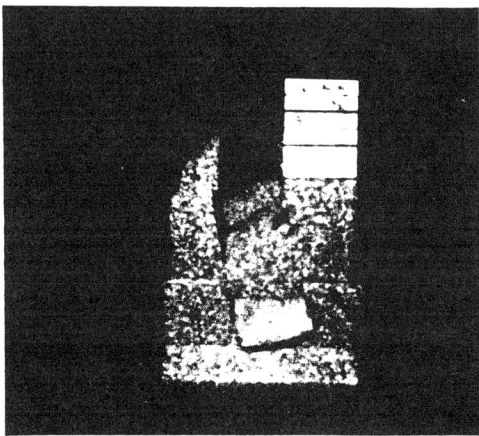

Figure 19. Crush of typical styrofoam sample in angled lap belt impact on MTS machine.

TABLE 6. Dummy Abdomen Stiffness Superior-Inferior Loading

Abdomen Type	Low Speed Stiffness (N/mm)	High Speed Stiffness (N/mm)
Hybrid III (old)	6.0	6.8
Hybrid III (new)	9.7	12.3
Frangible Abdomen	13.1	11.4
5th Female - HybIII	20.2	19.1

(a) No Submarining

(b) Incipient Submarining

(c) Incipient Submarining

(d) Incipient Submarining

(e) Pre-Submarined

(f) Pre-Submarined

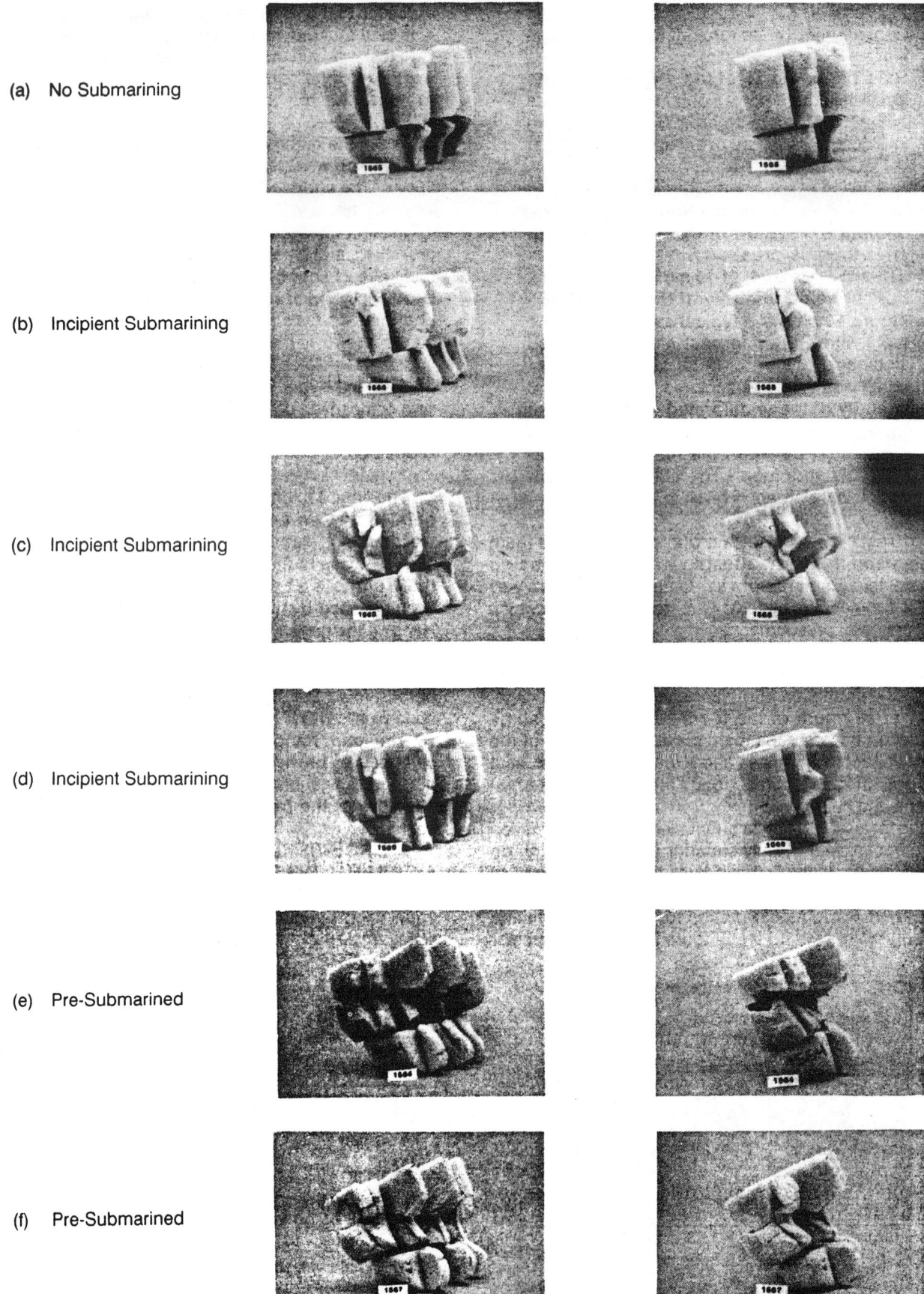

Figure 20. Crush pattern of frangible abdomen in various sled tests.

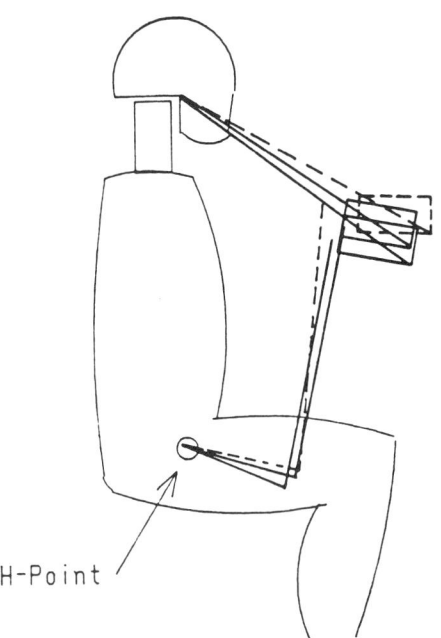

Figure 21. <u>Tests with no submarining.</u> Pictorial summary of kinematic analysis including maximum head excursion and neck angle, maximum H-point excursion and torso angle. (Dashed line represents one sled test with the frangible abdomen in the Hybrid III; solid lines represent two sled tests with the baseline Hybrid III.)

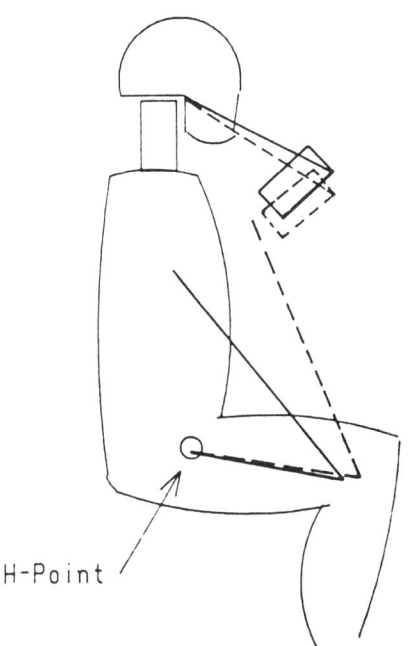

Figure 22. <u>Tests with submarining.</u> Pictorial summary of kinematic analysis including maximum head excursion and neck angle, maximum H-point excursion and torso angle. (Dashed line represents one sled test with the frangible abdomen in the Hybrid III; solid line represents one sled test with the baseline Hybrid III.)

differences between various subjects. While in principle normalization could make the data within each group of experiments fall onto a single curve, that rarely happens in practice. Instead a corridor is determined by the upper and lower bound of the curves.

As mentioned previously, several tests were performed on each porcine cadaver subject in an attempt to gain the most information possible from each test. However, the force-deflection data was not well behaved for the tests after the first on each subject. A likely explanation is that the cadaver tissues do not have the same restitution as the tissues of living subjects. These test were performed in rapid sequence without much time in between. It was noted during testing that the subjects did not return to their original shapes. Therefore, only the force-deflection data from the first test on each subject was used for this analysis.

The porcine cadaver data was also scaled to the Cavanaugh Human Cadaver data using equal velocity/equal stress scaling, and is shown in Figure 23. This scaling was mathematically equivalent to the normalization described in the previous paragraph, but allowed direct comparison between the human and porcine cadaver subjects. The use of equal velocity/equal stress scaling in this instance may not be appropriate, because the basic premise of geometric similitude may be violated. The amount by which the shape of the porcine subjects differs from that of human subjects determines the scaling error.

Stiffness was determined as the slope of the force-deflection curve (in units of N/mm), and these are shown in Table 7. The slopes were determined graphically, by visually fitting a straight line to the initial loading portion of each force-deflection curve. The mean and standard deviation of these stiffnesses for each group of experiments was determined, and the means between groups were compared using single factor Analysis of Variance (ANOVA). Specifically, we compared the stiffness between:

1) Self-Normalized Porcine Cadaver Data
2) Self-Normalized Live Anesthetized Cadaver Data
3) Self-Normalized Human Cadaver Data
4) Porcine Cadaver Data Scaled to Human Cadaver Data

At the .05 level of significance, there were no differences found: between the mean porcine cadaver stiffness and mean live anesthetized porcine stiffness; or between the mean porcine cadaver stiffness and mean human cadaver stiffness; or between mean scaled porcine cadaver stiffness and mean human cadaver stiffness.

Although the porcine stiffness data appears to be very similar the human cadaver stiffness data, they were not determined in the same manner. The porcine cadaver data was determined using standard safety belt material as the loading surface, but the human cadaver data was determined using a rigid bar as the loading surface. In addition, the human cadaver low velocity data was actually performed at a higher velocity range than these porcine experiments (Porcine low velocities were 1.6-5.5 m/s; Human low velocities were 4.9-7.2 m/s). While this may make the comparison less than ideal, there is no

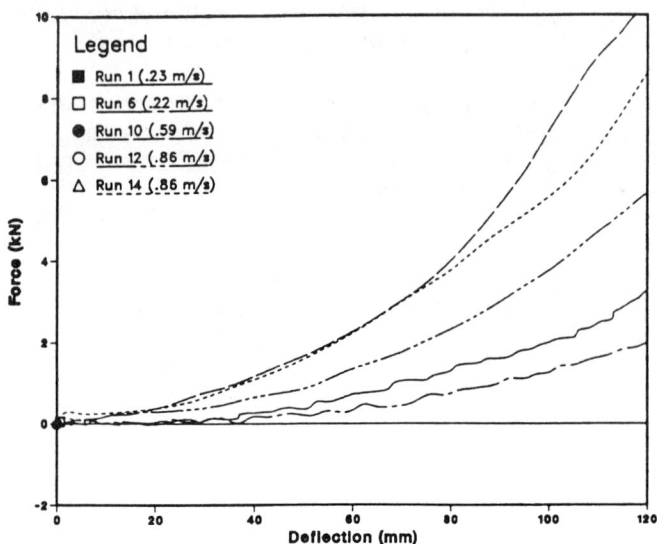

Figure 23. Force-deflection curves for porcine cadaver subjects normalized to human cadaver data.

other data available which gives the human cadaver stiffness with belt loading.

Given the above considerations, the target stiffness for the frangible abdomen was determined to be 23.0 N/mm.

The results from the MTS tests which were performed to assess interactions between the dummy ribs and abdomen are shown in Table 6. The frangible abdomen is stiffer in the superior/inferior direction than the old standard Hybrid III abdomen, about as stiff as the new Hybrid III abdomen with the notch for the chest deflection potentiometer arm, and less stiff than the Hybrid III 5th percentile female abdomen. With this relative stiffness, we do not expect unusual kinematics to result from interaction of the dummy ribs with the frangible abdomen.

REACTION SURFACE AND OTHER DUMMY MODIFICATIONS - Care was taken in the design of the support bracket and foam reaction plate to ensure that the ability of the dummy to flex forward, and sit "naturally" was maintained. A minimum clearance of 16 mm (0.625") between the flexible lumbar spine and the rigid reaction plate was designed after static dummy bending tests to ensure no contact during flexion. Sled tests with a prototype plate and bracket were performed which confirmed no interaction between the spine and plate.

TABLE 7. Stiffness Comparison

Anesthetized Porcine		Porcine Cadavers		Porcine Scaled to Human	
Test	Stiffness (N/mm)	Test	Stiffness (N/mm)	Test	Stiffness (N/mm)
2	8	1	25	1	26
3	19	6	21	6	19
4	30	10	41	10	52
5	37	12	26	12	28
6	40	14	41	14	52
8	29				
13	20				
14	21	Average (N = 5)		(N = 5)	
15	21	Stiffness: 31 ± 9 N/mm		35 ± 16 N/mm	
17	8	Velocity: .55 ± .32 m/s		.55 ± .32 m/s	
18	15				
20	25				
21	24				
		Human Cadaver Average Stiffness			
		From Cavanaugh (N = 5)			
Average (N = 13)					
Stiffness: 23 ± 10		Stiffness = 23 N/mm			
Velocity: 3.7 ± .84 m/s		Velocity = 6.1 ± 1.1 m/s			

As noted in the results, a height increase was introduced into the dummy by the support bracket. The support bracket raises the lumbar spine mounting block relative to the pelvis. This causes an offset between the H-point access hole and wrench socket which makes it difficult to set the H-point using standard tools. Since the lumbar spine mounting block must be machined for this design to work, a reasonable approach could be to incorporate the support bracket into the casting of the lumbar spine mounting block. This would eliminate both the 6 mm (0.250") height increase, and any difficulty setting the H-point.

With the addition of the support bracket, machining of the lumbar spine block, replacement of the standard abdomen, and removal of the chest deflection potentiometer, the net change in dummy mass is a decrease of .694 kg. This does not constitute a major modification to the Hybrid III since the dummy mass can be returned to its exact specified mass and inertia by addition of ballast material.

A important change with the frangible abdomen design is the removal of the chest deflection potentiometer. The ability to measure chest deflection and viscous response during impact at the same time as submarining injury potential is highly desirable. Use of high tension string potentiometers has recently been discussed as replacement technology for rotary chest potentiometer. The mounting locations under discussion are within the thoracic cavity, and as such would not interfere with the function of the frangible abdomen. If the rotary potentiometer is replaced with these advanced string potentiometers this concern would be alleviated.

Since these design changes have not been inspected by the NHTSA at this date, the Hybrid III dummy with the frangible abdomen cannot be used in certification tests. In addition, the force-deflection curves upon which the abdomen is based were generated using belt loading. They may also be applicable for impact with rigid objects, but further validation would be necessary. However, the reader is cautioned that impacts with rigid objects, such as those of unbelted occupants into steering wheels, may occur at higher velocities than belt loading. Then because of the rate sensitivity of the human abdomen, and the lack of rate sensitivity in the frangible abdomen, the stiffness of the frangible abdomen would have to be adjusted to a higher velocity stiffness to examine such phenomena.

DUMMY KINEMATICS WITH THE FRANGIBLE ABDOMEN - The kinematics of the dummy in tests without submarining appeared to be independent of whether or not the Frangible Abdomen was installed in the dummy. As can be seen in Figure 21, the head excursion, neck angle, torso angle, and H-point motion are all very similar in the baseline Hybrid III and the Hybrid III with the Frangible Abdomen installed.

When there was submarining, the head, neck, and H-point excursions were again independent of presence of the Frangible Abdomen (Figure 22). However, the torso angle was 16° greater in the Baseline Hybrid III, than in the Hybrid III with the frangible abdomen (129° vs 113°; where at 90° the dummy is sitting straight up, and at 180° it is lying flat on its back). A difference in torso angle during submarining might be expected when the frangible abdomen is in place because the reaction force of the lap belt in submarining acts directly upon the torso, probably via the lumbar spine. Based on the patterns left in the foam after the sled tests, one might speculate that with the frangible abdomen in place, a submarining belt will not have significant freedom to move in a superior/inferior direction because it becomes enveloped in the crushed foam. In contrast, in the baseline Hybrid III, the belt may compress the "gut sack" and possibly ride over the top of it to react directly against the lumbar spine. In the latter case, the moment arm on the torso is longer relative to the center of rotation (the H-point).

In the tests with submarining, the centerline of the belt within the frangible abdomen was 3" above the H-point, but a likely moment arm for a lap belt in the baseline tests would have been 6" above the H-point. If this postulate is correct, and if the forces on the torso in the baseline Hybrid III and the Hybrid III with the frangible abdomen are similar, then the difference in moment in these sled tests could have been near a factor of two. If so, the rotation will be greater in the case of the longer moment arm, viz. the Baseline Hybrid III.

POST-TEST CRUSH PATTERNS IN THE FRANGIBLE ABDOMEN - The frangible abdomen, as designed, functioned very well in bench test loading on the MTS and in sled tests. The foam crushed when loaded, but in a very well behaved manner. In particular, off-axis loading did not change the foam response, the crushed foam remained in one piece, it did not shatter or splinter, and was able to be removed without falling apart. The original design was limited to a two piece configuration as seen in Figures 20a-f because of the size of the billets available at that time. We now obtain billets twice as thick, which allow one piece construction (Figure 5a).

In the incipient submarining tests, the results were limited by the two piece design of the foam. While it was clear that submarining occurred, the exact amount of deformation of the foam was uncertain because part of the penetration of the belt into the abdomen occurred in between the two pieces of foam.

In the sled tests in which the dummy was presubmarined, and the tests in which no submarining took place, the ability of the foam to determine whether submarining had occurred was quite clear. Deformation to the foam above the location of the anterior-superior iliac spines indicated the occurrence of submarining.

INJURY ASSESSMENT WITH THE FRANGIBLE ABDOMEN - Because the force-deflection characteristics of the foam are known to match human force-deflection characteristics, the abdomen has biofidelity, and we can estimate the injury potential associated with the its deformation. For example, if the measured deformation of the abdomen after a test is 3.5" (89 mm), then when the elastic springback of the foam is accounted for, the maximum deformation during the test would be approximately 3.9" (99 mm) . A 50th percentile male has an abdominal depth of 8.1" (205 mm). The percent compression associated with 3.9" deformation is 48%. Using Figure 3 such belt loading would have a 25% probability of causing an AIS $>= 4$ abdominal injury. Thus, the frangible abdomen demonstrates the occurrence of submarining and the associated risk of injury.

The procedure for determining the probability of injury in a test with lap belt submarining is to remove the foam post-test and measure the maximum deformation of the middle three points. This deformation can be converted into a compression of the 50th percentile male abdomen by dividing by 206 mm (8.1"), and the probability of injury can be determined using Figure 3.

The frangible abdomen force-deflection characteristics were designed for low velocity loading (2-6 m/s). This is consistent with belt loading rates cited in the literature, but in higher velocity loading it could overestimate the probability of injury. Such an overestimate could occur because the stiffness of the human abdomen is rate sensitive. That is, at higher velocities, it takes more force to compress the human abdomen than at lower velocities. Therefore, if load from a higher velocity impact is applied to a dummy abdomen which is not rate sensitive and has been developed for a lower velocity impact, the loading will probably cause more deformation than it would have if the dummy abdomen was stiffer or rate sensitive. Thus, a dummy abdomen which is either stiffer, or one which is rate sensitive is desireable to study higher speed loading events that may take place (such as loading to the abdomen of an unbelted occupant).

Another consideration which indicates the need for a rate sensitive abdomen is that belt loading of an occupant in a vehicle has both loading and unloading phases. Near the end of the loading phase the rate of compression decreases, while the magnitude of the compression continues to increase, and the force may continue to increase. As the rate of compression decreases a rate sensitive abdomen would become less stiff, but a non rate sensitive abdomen would maintain a constant stiffness. Then the rate sensitive abdomen may compress more than the non rate sensitive abdomen. This indicates that the constant stiffness abdomen may underestimate the compression from actual belt loading.

HYBRID III FAMILY OF DUMMIES - Work continues in our laboratory to develop an abdomen that is rate sensitive, reusable, and gives a deformation time history. Concepts being explored include a fluid filled abdomen with advanced deflection sensors and a set of damped springs similar to Hybrid III ribs.

While this development was done with a 50th percentile male Hybrid III dummy, the same principles apply to other size dummies. At the time this project was started, the 5th percentile female dummy was in the process of being upgraded to Hybrid III status. Since no dummies were available we decided to work only on the 50th percentile dummy, and later scale the results down to the size of the 5th female. A foam reaction plate and support bracket have been designed for this dummy, and are shown in Figure 24. The lumbar spine block has been incorporated into the support bracket for simplicity. A need for submarining detection is not anticipated for the 95th percentile male dummy, but the principles and technology presented here apply as well.

The frangible abdomen has been transferred to the Safety Research and Development Laboratory at the Milford Proving Ground for use in sled and barrier testing. Biomedical Science will serve as the focal point for the results of these tests until a large enough data base has been developed to standardize the data analysis and procedures. Work is also proceeding on a version of frangible abdomen for the 5th percentile female Hybrid III dummy.

CONCLUSIONS

1) Abdominal injury assessment for belt loading due to submarining is now possible in the Hybrid III family of dummies.
2) The abdomen developed has biofidelity in its force-deflection characteristics for belt loading, is capable of detecting the occurrence of submarining, and can be used to determine the probability of abdominal injury when submarining occurs.
3) Installation of the abdomen in the Hybrid III dummy does not change the dummy kinematics when submarining does not occur.
4) When submarining does occur, the dummy kinematics are very similar to baseline Hybrid III kinematics, expect for torso angle. The change in torso angle is or may be a result of a more human-like compliance in the abdomen.

ACKNOWLEDGEMENTS

The authors acknowledge the contributions of many people that went into the successful execution of this project. In particular, we thank:
Dennis Andrzejak - for photographic work;
Joseph Balser - for technical discussions related to dummy development and use;
Howard Bender, Gerald Horn, Timothy Sorenson, Todd Townsend - for technical support;
Clyde Culver - for technical discussions;
Mary Foster - for computer support, assistance with figures, and paste-up of the final manuscript;
William Hering - for providing results of his own material tests on various foams;
John Horsh - for technical review;
Ahmed Kabir - for computer support;
John Melvin - for technical discussions, especially as

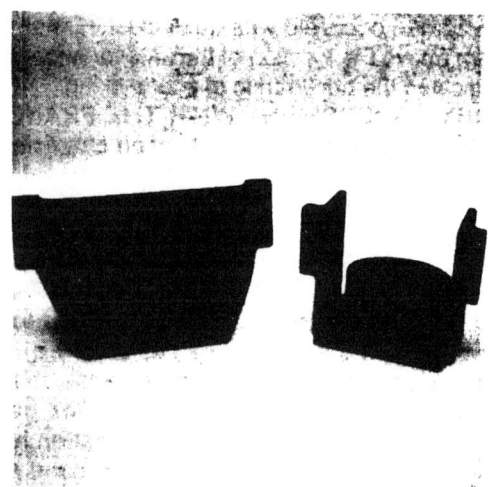

Figure 24. Support bracket and foam reaction plate for 5th percentile female Hybrid III dummy.

related to scaling and compression of a constant stiffness abdomen;

Mary Alice Miller - for providing raw force-deflection data from her initial porcine lap belt loading experiments;

Jeff Welch - for technical discussions related to foams.

REFERENCES

1. Evans, L., "Double Pair Comparison -- A New Method to Determine How Occupant Characteristics Affect Fatality Risk in Traffic Crashes." *Accid Anal & Prev* 18(3):217-227, 1986.

2. Evans, L., "Restraint Effectiveness, Occupant Ejection from Cars, and Fatality Reductions." General Motors Research Laboratories Report GMR-6398, September, 1988.

3. Evans, L., "Rear Seat Restraint System Effectiveness in Preventing Fatalities." *Accid Anal & Prev* 20(2):129-136, 1988.

4. Adomeit, D. and Heger, A., "Motion Sequence Criteria and Design Proposals for Restraint Devices in Order to Avoid Unfavorable Biomechanic Conditions and Submarining." In Proceedings of the 19th Stapp Car Crash Conference, SAE Technical Paper #751146, Warrendale, PA, 1975.

5. Adomeit, D., "Evaluation Methods for the Biomechanical Quality of Restraint Systems During Frontal Impact." In Proceedings of the 21st Stapp Car Crash Conference, SAE Technical Paper #770936, Warrendale, PA, 1977.

6. Adomeit, D., "Seat Design -- A Significant Factor for Safety Belt Effectiveness." In Proceedings of the 23rd Stapp Car Crash Conference, SAE Technical Paper #791004, Warrendale, PA, 1979.

7. Kroell, C.K., "Thoracic Response to Blunt Frontal Loading." In *The Human Thorax-Anatomy, Injury and Biomechanics,* SAE Publication P-67, pp.49-78, Warrendale, PA, 1976.

8. Neathery, R.F., Kroell, C.K., and Mertz, H.J., "Prediction of Thoracic Injury from Dummy Responses." In Proceedings of the 21st Stapp Car Crash Conference, SAE Technical Paper #751151, Warrendale, PA, 1975.

9. Viano, D.C. and Lau, I.V., "A Viscous Tolerance Criterion for Soft Tissue Injury Assessment." *J Biomech* 21(5):387-399, 1988.

10. Lau, I.V. and Viano, D.C., "The Viscous Criterion: Bases and Applications of an Injury Severity Index for Soft Tissue." SAE Transactions, vol. 95, 1986, P-189, In Proceedings of the 30th Stapp Car Crash Conference, pp. 123-142, SAE Technical Paper #861882, October, 1986.

11. Gadd, C.W. and Patrick, L.M., "Systems Versus Laboratory Impact Tests for Estimating Injury Hazard." SAE Technical Paper #680053, Society of Automotive Engineers, 1968.

12. Rouhana, S.W., Lau, I.V., and Ridella, S.A., "Influence of Velocity and Forced Compression on the Severity of Abdominal Injury in Blunt, Nonpenetrating Lateral Impact.", *J Trauma* 25(6):490-500, 1985.

13. Rouhana, S.W., "Abdominal Injury Prediction in Lateral Impact - An Analysis of the Biofidelity of the Euro-SID Abdomen.", In Proceedings of the 31st Stapp Car Crash Conference, pp.95-104, SAE Technical Paper #872203, Warrendale, PA, 1987.

14. Viano, D.C., "Cause and Control of Automotive Trauma." *Bulletin of the New York Academy of Medicine,* Second Series, 64(5):376-421, June, 1988.

15. Rouhana, S.W., Ridella, S.A., and Viano, D.C., "The Effect of Limiting Impact Force on Abdominal Injury: A Preliminary Study.", SAE Transactions, vol. 95, pp. 634-648, 1986, In Proceedings of the 30th Stapp Car Crash Conference, pp. 65-79, SAE Technical Paper #861879, Warrendale, PA, October, 1986.

16. Lau, V.K. and Viano, D.C., "An Experimental Study on Hepatic Injury from Belt Restraint Loading." *Avia Space Envir Med,* 52(10):611-617, October, 1981.

17. Miller, M.A., "The Biomechanical Response of the Lower Abdomen to Belt Restraint Loading." *J Trauma,* in press, 1989.

18. Sacco, W.J., Jameson, J.W., Copes, W.S. et al, "Progress Toward a New Injury Severity Characterization: Severity Profiles." In Computers in Biology and Medicine, December, 1988.

19. Viano, D.C., "Limits and Challenges of Crash Protection." *Accid Anal & Prev* 20(6):421-429, 1988.

20. Rouhana, S.W. and Foster, M.E., "Lateral Impact - An Analysis of the Statistics in the NCSS.", SAE Transactions, vol. 94, 1985, In Proceedings of the 29th Stapp Car Crash Conference, pp. 79-98, SAE Technical Paper #851727, Warrendale, PA, 1985.

21. Evans, L. and Frick, M., "Seating Position in Cars and Fatality Risk." General Motors Research Laboratories Report GMR-5911, July, 1987.

22. Kulowski, J. and Rost, W.B., "Intra-abdominal Injuries from Safety Belt in Auto Accident." *Arch Surg* 73:970-971, December, 1956.

23. Sube, J., Ziperman, H.H. and McIver, W.J., "Seat Belt Trauma to the Abdomen." *Amer J Surg* 3:346-350, March, 1967.

24. Porter, S.D. and Green, E.W., "Seat Belt Injuries." *Arch Surg* 96:242-246, February, 1968.

25. Mackay, G.M., "Abdominal Injuries to Restraint Front Seat Occupants in Frontal Collision." In <u>Proceedings of the American Association for Automotive Medicine</u>, pp. 146-148, 1982.

26. Ryan, P. and Ragazzon, R., "Abdominal Injuries in Survivors of Road Trauma Before and Since Seat-Belt Legislation in Victoria." *Aus N.Z. J Surg* 49(2):200-202, 1979.

27. Gallup, B.M., St-Laurent, A.M., Newman, J.A., "Abdominal Injuries to Restrained Front Seat Occupants in Frontal Collisions." In <u>Proceedings of the 26th Annual American Association for Automotive Medicine Conference</u>, Ottawa, Canada, October, 1982.

28. Dalmotas, D.J., "Mechanisms of Injury to Vehicle Occupants Restraints by Three Point Seat Belts." In <u>Proceedings of the 24th Stapp Car Crash Conference</u>, pp. 439-476, SAE Technical Paper #801311, Warrendale, PA, 1980.

29. Fish, J. and Wright, R.H., "The Seat Belt Syndrome -- Does it Exist?" *J Trauma*, 5:746-750, November, 1965.

30. Garrett, J.W. and Braunstein, P.W., "The Seat Belt Syndrome," *J Trauma*, 2:220-238, May, 1962.

31. Cocke, W.M. and Meyer, K.K., "Splenic Rupture Due to Improper Placement of Automobile Safety Belt," *JAMA*, 183:693, February, 1963.

32. States, J.D., Huelke, D.F., Dance, M., and Green, R.N., "Fatal Injuries Caused by Underarm Use of Shoulder Belts." *J Trauma,* 27(7):740-, 1987.

33. Trollope, M.L., Stalnaker, R.L., McElhaney, J.H., et al, "Mechanism of Injury in Blunt Abdominal Trauma." *J Trauma,* 13(11):962-970, 1973.

34. Huelke, D.F., Lawson, T.E., "Lower Torso Injuries and Automobile Seat Belts." Society of Automotive Engineers Technical Paper #760370, Warrendale, PA, 1978.

35. Dardik, H., Ibraham, M.I., "The Spectrum of Seat Belt Injuries." *Lawyer's Med J*, 6:50-75, 1977.

36. Williams, J.S., Lies, B.A., Hale, Jr., H.W., "The Automotive Safety Belt, in Saving a Life, May Produce Intra-Abdominal Injuries." *J Trauma*, 6:303, 1966.

37. Witte, C.L., "Mesentery and Bowel Injuries from Automotive Seat Belts." *Ann Surg*, 167:486, 1968.

38. Smith, W.S. and Kaufer, H., "Patterns and Mechanism of Lumbar Injuries Associated with Lap Safety Belt." *J Bone Joint Surg* 51-A, 239-254, 1969.

39. Dehner, J.S., "Seat Belt Injuries of the Spine and Abdomen," *Amer J Roentgen,* VIII:833-843, April, 1971.

40. Denis, R., Allard, M., Atlas, H. and Farkouh, E., "Changing Trends with Abdominal Injury in Seatbelt Wearers." *J Trauma,* 23(11):1007-1008, November, 1983.

41. Arajarvi, E., Santavirta, S. and Tolonen, J., "Abdominal Injuries Sustained in Severe Traffic Accidents by Seatbelt Wearers." *J Trauma*, 27(4):393-397, April, 1987.

42. Shanks, J.E. and Thompson, A.L., "Injury Mechanisms to Full Restrained Occupants." In <u>Proceedings of the 23rd Stapp Car Crash Conference</u>, SAE Technical Paper #791003, Warrendale, PA, 1979.

43. Dalmotas, D.J., "Mechanisms of Injury to Vehicle Occupants Restrained by Three-Point Seat Belts." In <u>Proceedings of the 24th Stapp Car Crash Conference</u>, SAE Technical Paper #801311, Warrendale, PA, 1980.

44. Society of Automotive Engineers, <u>Advances in Belt Restraint Systems: Design, Performance and Usage</u>, P-141, Society of Automotive Engineers, Warrendale, PA, 1984.

45. Society of Automotive Engineers, <u>Passenger Comfort, Convenience and Safety: Test Tools and Procedures</u>, P-174, Society of Automotive Engineers, Warrendale, PA, 1986.

46. Daniel, R.F., "Test Dummy Submarining Indicator System." United States Patent 3,841,163, October, 15, 1974.

47. Tarriere, C.H., "Proposal for a Protection Criterion as Regards Abdominal Internal Organs." In <u>Proceedings of the 17th American Association for Automotive Medicine Conference</u>, pp. 371-382, 1973.

48. Leung, Y.C., Tarriere, C., Fayon, A. et al, "A Comparison Between Part 572 Dummy and Human Subject in the Problem of Submarining." In <u>Proceedings of the 23rd Stapp Car Crash Conference</u>, pp. 677-720, SAE Technical Paper #791026, Warremdale, PA, 1979.

49. Melvin, J.W. and Weber, K., "Abdominal Intrusion Sensor for Evaluating Child Restraint Systems.", In Passenger Comfort, Convenience and Safety: Test Tools and Procedures, P-174, SAE Technical Paper #860370, Society of Automotive Engineers, Warrendale, PA, 1986.

50. DeJeammes, M., Biard, R., and Derrien, Y., "Factors Influencing the Estimation of Submarining on the Dummy." In Proceedings of the 25th Stapp Car Crash Conference, pp. 733-762, SAE Technical Paper #811021, Society of Automotive Engineers, Warrendale, PA, 1981.

51. Leung, Y.C., Tarriere, C., Lestrelin, D., et al. "Submarining Injuries of 3 Pt. Belted Occupants in Frontal Collisions - Description, Mechanisms and Protection." SAE Technical Paper #821158, pp. 173-205, Society of Automotive Engineers, Warrendale, PA, 1982.

52. Mooney, M.T. and Collins, J.A., "Abdominal Penetration Measurement Insert for the Hybrid III Dummy." SAE Technical Paper #860653, Society of Automotive Engineers, Warrendale, PA, 1986.

53. Biard, R., Cesari, D. and Derrien, Y., "Advisability and Reliability of Submarining Detection." In Restraint Technologies: Rear Seat Occupant Protection SP-691, pp. 27-38, SAE Technical Paper #870484, Society of Automotive Engineers, Warrendale, PA, 1987.

54. Eppinger, R.H., "Prediction of Thoracic Injury Using Measurable Experimental Parameters.", The 6th International Conference on Experimental Safety Vehicles, pp. 770-780, 1976.

55. Langhaar, H.L., Dimensional Analysis and Theory of Models, Wiley, New York, 1957.

56. Mertz, H.J., "A Procedure for Normalizing Impact Response Data.", SAE Technical Paper #840884, 1984.

57. American Association for Automotive Medicine, "The Abbreviated Injury Scale", 1985.

58. Stalnaker, R.L. and Ulman, M.S., "Abdominal Trauma - Review, Response, and Criteria.", In Proceedings of the 29th Stapp Car Crash Conference, pp. 1-16, SAE Technical Paper #851720, Warrendale, PA, 1985.

59. Verriest, J.P., Chapon, A., and Trauchessec, R., "Cinephotogrammetrical Study of Porcine Thoracic Response to Belt Applied Load in Frontal Impact - Comparison Between Living and Dead Subjects.", In Proceedings of the 25th Stapp Car Crash Conference, pp. 499-545, SAE Technical Paper #811015, Warrendale, PA, 1981.

896032

Experimental Investigation of Rear Seat Submarining

Thomas F. MacLaughlin, Lisa K. Sullivan
National Highway Traffic Safety Administration
Christopher S. O'Connor
Transportation Research Center of Ohio

Abstract

An experimental investigation was conducted to determine the effects of certain seating and restraint parameters on the tendency for an adult rear seat passenger to submarine (i.e., for the lap belt to ride over the pelvic iliac crests and penetrate the abdomen) in a 30 mph delta-v frontal collision. Four parameters were investigated: type of restraint (lap belt only or three-point belt), seat cushion stiffness, seat cushion height, and lap belt angle (within the range from 20 to 75 degrees, as specified in FMVSS 210, "Seat Belt Assembly Anchorages"). The experiments were done on the HYGE sled, using a Hybrid III dummy with a "submarining pelvis" which contains three load cells mounted on each iliac crest to indicate lap belt location. The test matrix was a fractional factorial design, which enabled determination of the statistical significance of the parameters on submarining tendency and other occupant responses. Lap belt angle was found to be a highly significant parameter—the shallower the angle, the greater the submarining tendency. The tendency to submarine also appeared to be greater for three-point belted occupants than for lap-only belted occupants, although lap belt forces were much less for three-point belts. Results indicated that only one injury (AIS 1) would have occurred out of six cases of submarining in three-point belts.

Introduction

United States FMVSS No. 210, "Seat Belt Assembly Anchorages", requires that the lap belt angle from the Seating Reference Point (SRP) to the anchorage fall within the range from 20° to 75° relative to the horizontal. Although front seat lap belt angles are typically close to 75°, rear seat installations in a number of cars, particularly small cars, have lap belt angles near 20°. Accident data indicate that, with the lap belt angle at or near 20°, there may be a possibility that rear seat occupants will slide under the lap belt (submarine), exposing themselves to abdominal injuries. Other parameters, such as seat cushion stiffness, the presence of a shoulder belt, etc., also may influence submarining tendency and other occupant responses.

We conducted a sled test program to determine (1) what parameters are significant in causing rear seat occupant submarining and (2) the effects of the more significant parameters on the occurrence of submarining and on other dummy responses. Prior to testing, we reviewed current literature to identify parameters which are believed to contribute to occupant submarining, and which are reproducible and repeatable in a controlled test situation. A listing (not necessarily all-inclusive) of parameters which appear to affect the tendency of the occupant to submarine is contained in table 1. Based on this review, the following factors were chosen for investigation: (1) type of restraint, (2) seat cushion stiffness, (3) seat cushion height, and (4) lap belt angle. These four factors were incorporated into a generic HYGE sled buck, allowing for the simulation of the rear occupant compartment of any vehicle. A series of 22 HYGE sled tests was then performed. For more details than are contained in this paper, the reader should see the project final report (1).*

Table 1. Parameters that affect submarining

A. Belt Parameters:
 1. Lap Only versus Lap/Shoulder Restraint
 2. Lap Belt Angle in Side View
 3. Lap Belt Angle in Top View
 4. Retractor Force
 5. Slack in the Lap Belt
 6. Slack in the Shoulder Harness
 7. Hysteresis in the Shoulder Harness Webbing
 8. Location of the Buckle
 9. Latch Plate Design
 10. Shoulder Belt Anchor Location
 11. Lap and Shoulder Belt Lengths

---

[1] Currently with the Ford Motor Company.

*Numbers in parentheses designate references at end of paper.

B. Seat Parameters:
1. Angle of the Seat Cushion
2. Stiffness of the Seat Cushion
3. Friction Coefficient between Occupant and Cushion
4. Angle of the Seat Back
5. Seat Height

C. Constraint Forces:
1. Restraint on Knees by Front Seat Back
2. Toe Board Restraint

D. Input Forces and Accelerations:
1. Time History of the Deceleration
2. Deceleration Magnitude

E. Occupant Parameters:
1. Amount of Clothing on the Occupant
2. Friction Coefficient between Occupant and Belt
3. Initial Position of the Occupant
4. Size of the Occupant
5. "Relative Bigness" of the Occupant (Weight divided by Height cubed)
6. Slope and Stiffness of the Abdomen
7. Locations of the Centers of Mass of the Body
8. Orientation of the Sartorius
9. Joint Stiffnesses and Damping Coefficients
10. Contraction of the Quadriceps Muscle

Test matrix design

The sled test matrix was designed to provide the most information possible about the statistical significance of the four factors in causing rear seat occupant submarining. The four factors and their levels were:

Table 1. Parameters that affect submarining

Factor	Level
type of restraint	lap belt only three-point belt
seat cushion stiffness	soft / hard — quantified in "Seat Cushion Stiffness Determination" and "Seat Height Determination"
seat height	low / high
lap belt angle (off horizontal)	20° 34° 47.5° 61° 75°

Three of the factors were tested at two levels; the fourth factor, lap belt angle, had five levels. The matrix is shown in figure 1, where conducted tests are designated by "X's". One repeat test was conducted to provide a basis for estimating experimental error, which was desirable to statistically analyze results.

This matrix is called a "half-factorial" or "half-replicate" because it calls for testing under only half the conditions present. The main features of factorial experimental designs are that (1) they allow the effects of independent variables on the dependent variable to be determined quan-

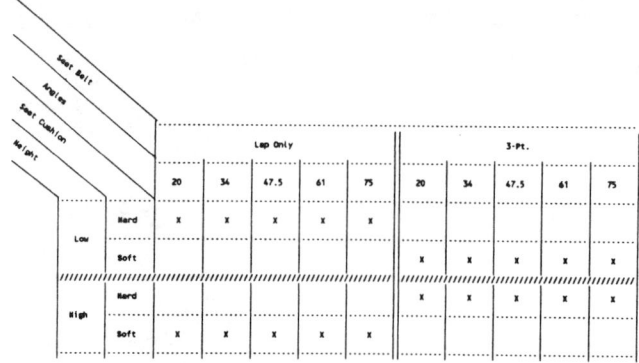

Figure 1. Sled test matrix.

titatively (statistically) and (2) they allow determination of interaction effects among independent variables. (For example, knowing the "first order", or "two-way", interaction effect between lap belt angle and seat cushion stiffness provides an answer to the question: Is the effect of lap belt angle on submarining different for soft seat cushions than for stiff?). In half-factorial designs, such as ours, some of the main effects and two-way interactions are confounded with higher-order interactions. It is assumed, because it is usually true, that any effect seen is due to the lower-order interaction; i.e., that higher-order interactions are negligible compared with main and two-way interaction effects.

Our primary interest was in the factor Belt Angle. Thus, we designed the sled test matrix to obtain statistical information about the four main effects and the two-way interactions involving the main effect Belt Angle (Belt Angle/Belt Type, Belt Angle/Seat Height and Belt Angle/Cushion Stiffness). Information about all other interactions was not discernable due to the confounding present.

For the statistical analyses (presented later in the paper), the null hypothesis was that the four main effects do not have an effect on the causation of occupant submarining or other responses of interest. The level of significance for rejecting that hypothesis was chosen to be 5% (5% is generally used in analyses of this type). Thus, if the "p-value" from the analysis was 5% or less, the risk of rejecting the null hypothesis when it was in fact true is minimal and we are confident in saying that the factor in question does have an effect on submarining. In addition, we felt that levels of significance in the 5% to approximately 15% range indicated "marginal" significance (i.e., we were unwilling to accept unconditionally the hypothesis that no effect existed, if the analysis indicated an 85% chance of an effect being present).

HYGE sled buck

We determined the values of several parameters in current vehicles to enable fabrication of a "generic" HYGE sled test buck. Nine parameters were selected which described the geometry of the rear passenger compartment (see figure 2). On the basis of 1986 sales figures and vehicle availability, we selected ten domestic and imported automobiles in different weight categories to determine average

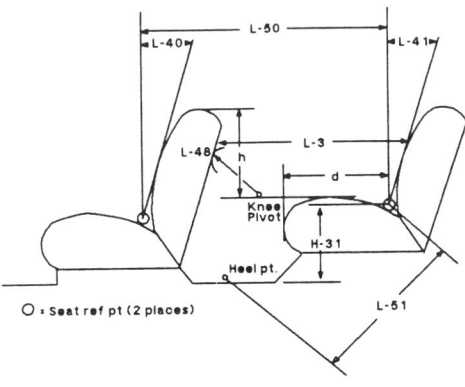

L-40 -- Front Seat Back Angle
L-3 -- Front of Rear Seat Back to Back of Front Seat Back
L-41 -- Rear Seat Back Angle
L-48 -- Rear Occupant Knee Pivot to Front Seat Back
L-50 -- Front Occupant H-Pt. to Rear Occupant H-Pt.
L-51 -- Rear Occupant H-Pt. to Heel pt. Distance
H-31 -- Rear Occupant H-Pt. to Heel pt. Vertical Distance
h -- Vertical Distance from Rear Occupant's H-Pt. to Top of Front Seat Back
d -- Depth of Rear Seat Cushion from Front Edge of Cushion to Occupant's H-Pt.

Figure 2. Passenger rear compartment geometry parameters.

values for the nine parameters. The vehicles were as follows:

Weight category	vehicle	1986 sales position:
1	1985 Ford Escort	#6 domestic
1	1984 Honda Accord	#3 imported
2	1985 Pontiac Grand Am	#4 domestic
2	1985 Pontiac Sunbird	#3 domestic
2	1983 Toyota Camry	#1 imported
3	1985 Chrysler New Yorker	#9 domestic
4	1985 Olds Ciera	#1 domestic
4	1986 Ford Taurus	#5 domestic
5	1983 Volvo GL	#8 imported
5	1986 Buick Electra	#11 domestic

The average values for the nine parameters are listed below:

Specification	average:
L–40	25.5°
L–3	26.76″
L–41	25.5°
L–48	2.23″
L–50	31.91″
L–51	35.94″
H–31	10.67″
h	17.97″
d	15.69″

The seat belt hardware consisted of the standard, automatic-locking type retractor generally used in the rear outboard seating positions. The original manufacturer's webbing was removed and replaced with a 5-bar webbing from one roll to minimize webbing differences. The same type of retractor was used for both the lap only and the three-point belts. The "D" ring chosen for the three-point belts was the locking type—over one half of the vehicles randomly surveyed had this type of "D" ring. Belt systems were replaced after each test to ensure integrity of each system. Load cells were used to record the inboard and outboard lap belt loads and the shoulder belt load, where applicable.

The Escort front bucket seat was chosen to represent the average front seat in overall height and seat back angle. Although not measured, its seat back stiffness appeared to be typical of most car seats; there was very little structure to resist rear occupant knee penetration. The Escort seat was replaced after each test to ensure an undamaged surface for the occupant to contact. The HYGE sled buck, in a pretest set-up, is shown in figure 3.

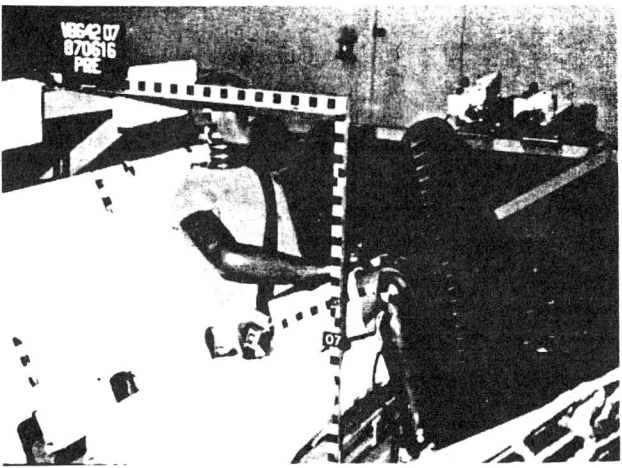

Figure 3. HYGE sled test set-up.

Seat cushion stiffness determination

The stiffness values for the seat cushions were determined to identify the "softest" and "hardest" seats from the 10 vehicles selected above. Each rear seat cushion was tested in two places: (1) at the center of the occupant seated position and (2) on the forward edge of the cushion. Figure 4 shows the forward position test set-up. The apparatus consisted of a hand-pumped hydraulic jack with a load cell and string potentiometer attached. The load was applied at a rate of approximately 1″ per minute through a universal swivel joint to an 8″ diameter plate. Force applied to the plate and

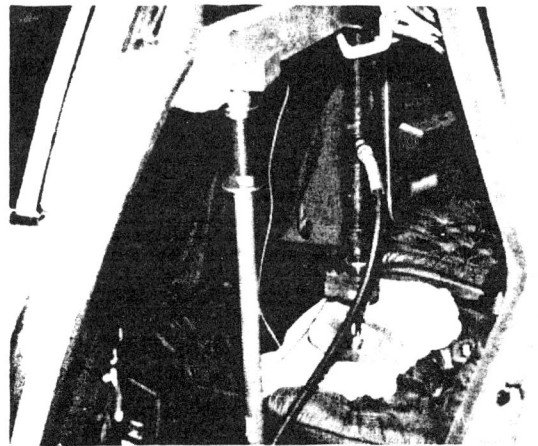

Figure 4. Cushion force-deflection test set-up (forward position).

vertical displacement of the plate into the cushion were measured.

Force versus deflection curves for all 10 vehicles are shown in figures 5 and 6. The Toyota Camry cushion was one of the stiffest, and the Buick Electra cushion was one of the softest; therefore, these two were selected for use in the sled test matrix.

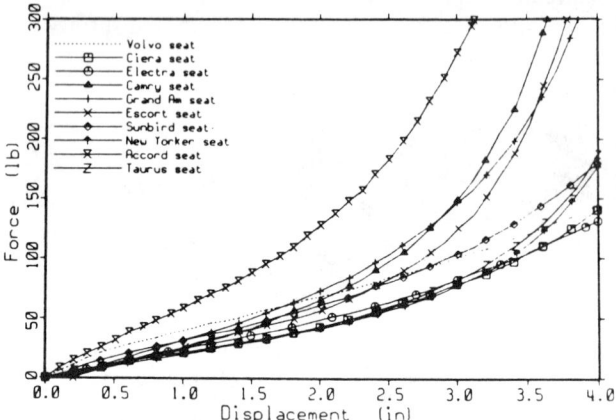

Figure 5. Seat stiffness at center (in loading).

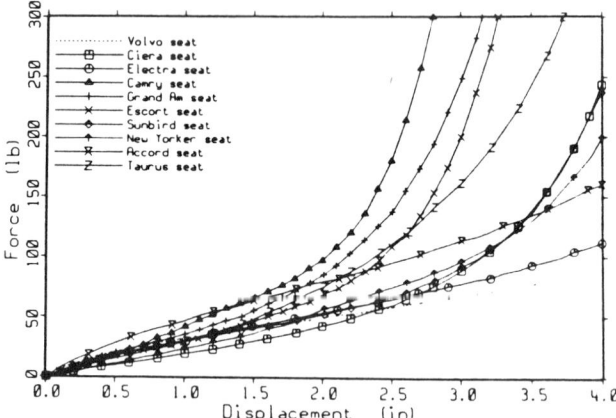

Figure 6. Seat stiffness at front (in loading).

Seat height determination

The vehicle rear seat height was measured as the vertical distance from the Seating Reference Point (SRP) to the occupant's resting heel position ("H-31" in figure 2). We obtained these values for a total of 31 vehicles (the 10 vehicles selected above plus a random sample of 21 vehicles). They were non-uniformly distributed; only 6.5% of the sample were in the 5.5"–9.5" range and 93.5% were in the 9.5"–13.5". The median range values for these two groups were 7.5" and 11.5", respectively. The final height values chosen were 8" and 12".

Crash pulse simulation

The sled tests were conducted at a test velocity of 30 mph using a half-sine pulse. The pulse duration was approximately 100 msec, resulting in peak sled accelerations of approximately 22 G's. This crash simulation pulse was based on similar pulses used for other occupant submarining studies performed by Adomeit (2, 3) and DeJeammes (4).

Hybrid III

The anthropomorphic test device used for the sled series was the Hybrid III 50th percentile male dummy. A simple procedure was developed for seating the dummy such that its seated posture in the rear seat would appear more natural than was obtained by using the standard FMVSS 208 seating procedure, developed primarily for front seating. First, a male human subject (approximately 50th percentile) was instructed to sit in a "normal and comfortable" position in a typical automobile rear seat. The dummy was then placed next to the subject, and its posture adjusted to simulate that of the human. This was repeated with three other human subjects. The procedure which resulted was to seat the dummy initially according to FMVSS 208, then move the pelvis forward enough to allow a space of about 2 inches between the rear seat back and the buttocks of the dummy.

Instrumentation for the Hybrid III consisted of:

- Triaxial accelerometer packages in the head, thorax and pelvis.
- Femur load cells and knee shear transducers in the legs.
- The "Submarining" pelvis, consisting of three load bolts distributed along the anterior surfaces of the right and left ilium.
- Denton six-axis upper neck load cell.
- Abdominal air bladder insert.

Filtering of the data consisted of SAE Class 1000 for the head accelerometer data, SAE Class 600 for neck forces and moments, pelvic load bolts and femur loads and SAE Class 180 for thorax and pelvic accelerometer data and knee shears. The abdominal bladder insert data and all of the seat belt loads were filtered using a SAE Class 60 filter.

Prior to this project, an air pressure abdominal bladder insert for the Hybrid III dummy (5) was developed for measuring the depth and rate of steering wheel penetration into the abdominal region. We used the bladder insert during this project in an attempt to (1) determine if and when submarining occurred, and (2) measure the amount of abdominal penetration caused by the belt when submarining occurs, hoping to determine the severity of the submarining. We found that, in its present form, the insert did not clearly indicate occurrence of submarining or penetration resulting from submarining, and would need more development work for this application. Therefore, it is not discussed further in this paper (see reference 1).

Sled test results

A summary of the test conditions and whether or not submarining occurred are contained in table 2. Test #843 was to have been a three-point test. However, the retractor failed to lock during the test making the test suspect for consideration in the matrix. Thus, the matrix contains 21 tests—20 of different conditions and 1 repeat test.

Of these 21 tests, full submarining occurred in 9 tests, "one-sided" submarining in 2 tests and submarining did not occur in 10 tests. In general, we were able to detect very

Table 2. Sled test conditions and results.

Test No.	Seat Belt Type	Seat Belt Angle	Seat Cushion	Seat Height	Submarining Occur ?	Time of Submarining
843	* Lap Only	20 Deg.	Soft	Low	yes	57 msec
844	Three-point	20 Deg.	Soft	Low	yes	47 msec
845	Three-point	75 Deg.	Soft	Low	yes	72 msec
#846	Lap Only	75 Deg.	Soft	High	no	NA
853	Lap Only	20 Deg.	Soft	High	yes	58 msec
891	Three-point	20 Deg.	Hard	High	yes	43 msec
892	Three-point	75 Deg.	Hard	High	no	NA
893	Lap Only	75 Deg.	Hard	Low	no	NA
#894	Lap Only	20 Deg.	Hard	Low	yes	43 msec
895	Three-point	47.5 Deg.	Hard	High	1/2 yes	75 msec
896	Three-point	47.5 Deg.	Soft	Low	yes	55 msec
897	Lap Only	47.5 Deg.	Hard	Low	no	NA
898	Lap Only	47.5 Deg.	Soft	High	no	NA
899	Three-point	47.5 Deg.	Hard	High	no	NA
904	Lap Only	34 Deg.	Soft	High	no	NA
905	Lap Only	34 Deg.	Hard	Low	yes	73 msec
906	Three-point	34 Deg.	Soft	Low	yes	47 msec
907	Three-point	34 Deg.	Hard	High	1/2 yes	57 msec
908	Lap Only	61 Deg.	Hard	Low	no	NA
909	Lap Only	61 Deg.	Soft	High	no	NA
910	Three-point	61 Deg.	Hard	High	no	NA
911	Three-point	61 Deg.	Soft	Low	yes	54 msec

* - #1 was to have been a three-point; retractor failed to lock.
\# - Lap Belt broke late in event (after 80 msec).

clearly the occurrence of submarining from the films, the lap belt force-time responses and the force-time responses of the load-measuring bolts on the pelvis (three located on each side).

In addition to noting whether submarining occurred or not, the following five elements were analyzed:

1. Tendency for rear seat occupant submarining.
2. Occupant head forward (X) velocity.
3. Occupant Head Injury Criterion (HIC).
4. Occupant peak chest acceleration.
5. Peak chest deflection for three-point belted occupants.

Tendency for rear seat occupant submarining

In addition to noting simply whether or not submarining occurred under certain conditions, we devised a rating method to indicate the "tendency" for submarining to occur. By "tendency", we mean (1) if submarining did not occur, how close it came to occurring and (2) if it did occur, whether it was on both sides, and how early it was in the crash event. As a measure of the near-occurrence of submarining, we determined the location of the lap belt on the pelvic iliac crests, as indicated by the pelvic load cell bolts. From our literature review, time of occurrence, and whether one- or two-sided, were seen to be important indicators of submarining tendency. The rating method, therefore, incorporated three factors: (1) how high on the pelvis belt loading occurred, (2) whether submarining, when it did occur, was one-sided or two-sided and (3) the time of initial indication of submarining.

The rating scheme consisted of six categories, which are listed below (although somewhat arbitrary, selection of the time intervals in categories 4–6 was based on the natural grouping that occurred in the experiments):

1. No submarining occurred; loads on pelvic lower load bolts *only*.
2. No submarining occurred; loads on pelvic lower and middle load bolts *only*.
3. One-sided submarining occurred.
4. Full (two-sided) submarining occurred; initial submarining in 70–79 msec.
5. Full (two-sided) submarining occurred; initial submarining in 50–59 msec.
6. Full (two-sided) submarining occurred; initial submarining in 40–49 msec.

In none of our tests did loading occur on the upper-most pelvic load cells without submarining occurring; nor did submarining initiate in the time frame of 60–69 msec in any of our tests.

Each of the 21 tests was rated according to the above scheme. The categorization results of the tendency for occupant submarining are shown in the matrix format in figure 7.

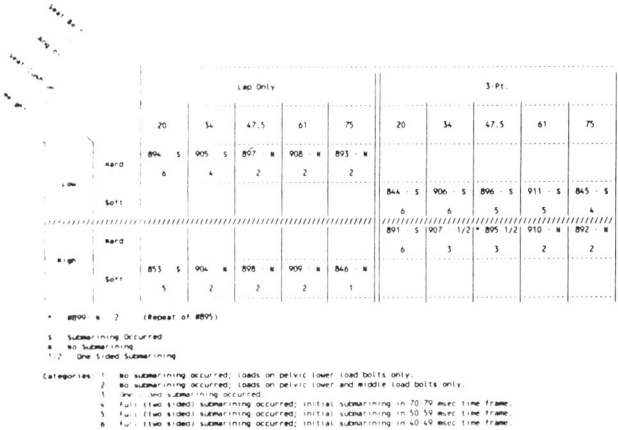

Figure 7. Tendency for submarining.

The categorization results were analyzed statistically to determine which of the four main factors and two-way interactions were significant. Figure 8 presents the four main effects of the test matrix. Each bar represents the average response for all tests conducted at the particular level (e.g., lap only) of the particular factor (e.g., Belt Type). Three of the factors have two levels each; one (Belt Angle) has five levels. If the difference between the average responses of different levels of a factor is "sufficiently large" compared with the response variances and the error estimate, then the statistical analysis will indicate that the main effect of that factor is "significant". Whether or not the main effect was found to be statistically significant is indicated beneath the effect, along with the p-value (as a percentage). Belt Angle, Belt Type and Seat Height all had highly significant effects on the tendency to submarine. (Significance levels were less than 1%). Cushion Stiffness had a marginal effect (10.77% significance level). No two-way interactions of main effects were significant (i.e., the effect a particular factor had on the submarining tendency was the same regardless of the level of other factors).

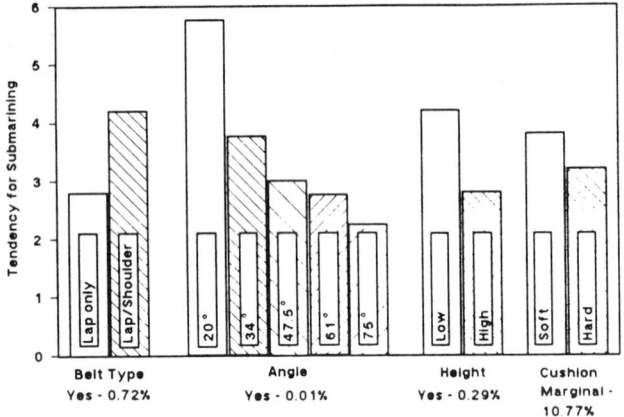

Figure 8. Tendency for rear seat occupant submarining.

The data indicating submarining tendency are presented in more detail in figures 9, 10, 11 and 12. Each point in figures 9, 10 and 11 represents an average of two tests (or three, when the repeatability test result was included), chosen to illustrate particular main and interaction effects.

In figure 9, lap-only and three-point belt results are plotted separately. It is clear that submarining tendency is different for the two restraint types (i.e., the Belt Type main effect is significant). Also, lap belt angle strongly affects submarining tendency for both restraint types, indicating the absence of a Belt Angle/Belt Type interaction effect.

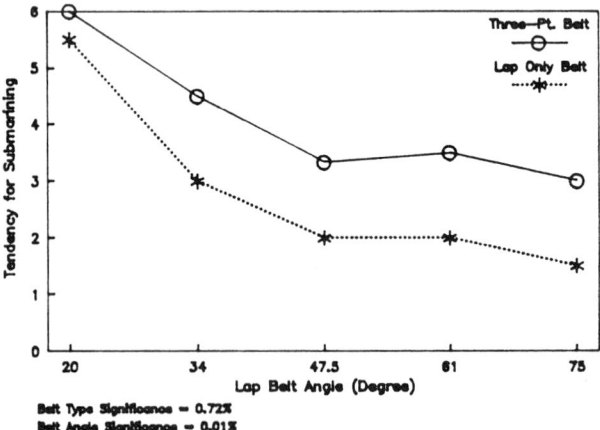

Figure 9. Tendency for submarining versus lap belt angle for belt type.

In figure 10, results are shown separately for the low and high seat heights. Submarining tendency differs for the two seat heights, but is strongly influenced by lap belt angle for both heights (similar to Belt Type results in figure 9).

Figure 11 suggests similar trends for the factor Cushion Stiffness. However, separation of the two curves is less

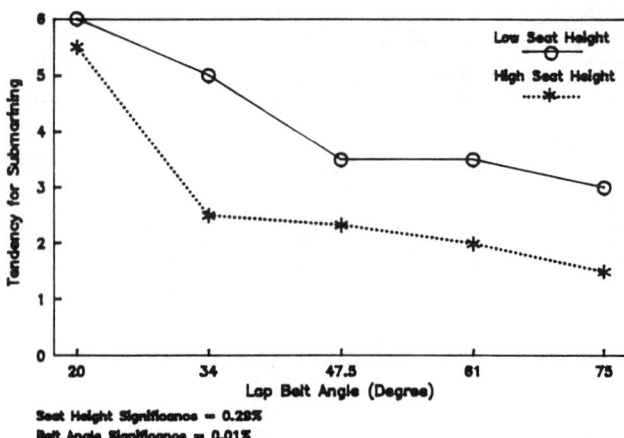

Figure 10. Tendency for submarining versus lap belt angle for seat height.

distinct, indicating marginal difference between the two cushion stiffnesses in the submarining tendency versus lap belt angle relationship (as was indicated in the statistical analysis).

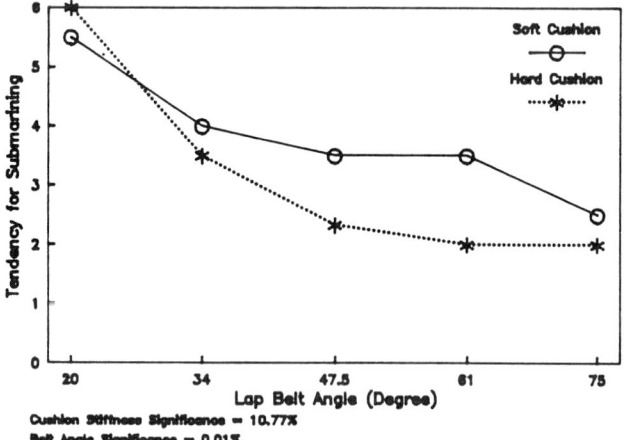

Figure 11. Tendency for submarining versus lap belt angle for cushion stiffness.

Figure 12 contains the results for each individual test. An interesting observation, which puts some degree of uncertainty on trends discussed thus far, is that three of the curves fall closely together, while the fourth is very different. One could conclude from this that the relationship between submarining tendency and lap belt angle is the same, regardless of type of restraint or seat cushion stiffness or seat height, except when the low seat is combined with the soft cushion. If this were true, it would indicate that the two-way interaction effect, Seat Height/Cushion Stiffness, is significant. This effect is confounded with the main effect of Belt Type, and, as previously stated, when confounding occurs, we have assumed that the observed effect is due to the lower-order interaction (i.e., the higher-order interaction effect is negligible). It is possible that this assumption is incorrect; however, we feel that is highly unlikely, since both logic and past experience indicate that submarining is more likely to occur in a three-point belt than in a lap-only belt. The only way to know for sure, however, would be to conduct more tests in the matrix.

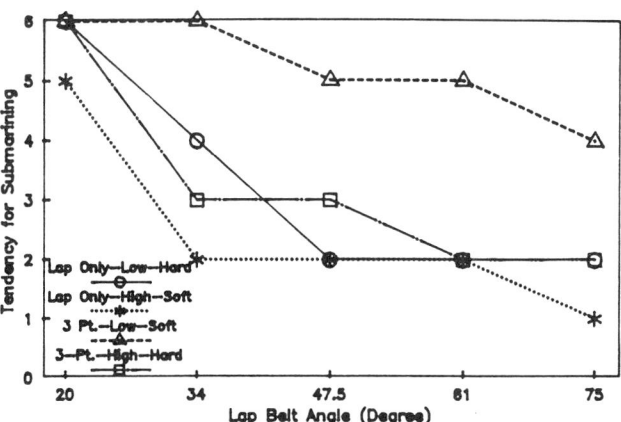

Figure 12. Tendency for submarining versus lap belt angle for belt type/seat height/cushion stiffness.

There is another issue which raises some uncertainty; the effect of seat height on submarining tendency, as observed in the sled tests, may have questionable validity. The Hybrid III dummy has a fixed angle between the lower spine and the upper legs. Therefore, when the dummy is placed in the lowered seat, the pelvis rotates with the upper leg, exaggerating the pelvic angle and predisposing the dummy to submarining more than is likely for the human. (The reader should bear in mind that the feet are constrained against moving forward by the front seat).

Occupant head forward (X) velocity

The occupant's head forward velocity was derived by film analysis—digitizing the 1" target at the head C.G. location and obtaining both longitudinal and vertical displacements of the C.G. The longitudinal head trajectory was differentiated to obtain the corresponding velocity.

Prior to testing, the occupant's head was located, on average, slightly over 20" behind the Escort front seat back. Therefore, 20" was considered the maximum distance the head could travel without impacting the front seat back. When the occupant was restrained by the three-point belt, maximum head excursion was less than 20". When restrained by the lap belt only, his head travelled at least 29". Thus, head impact was considered a possibility only for the lap-only belt system.

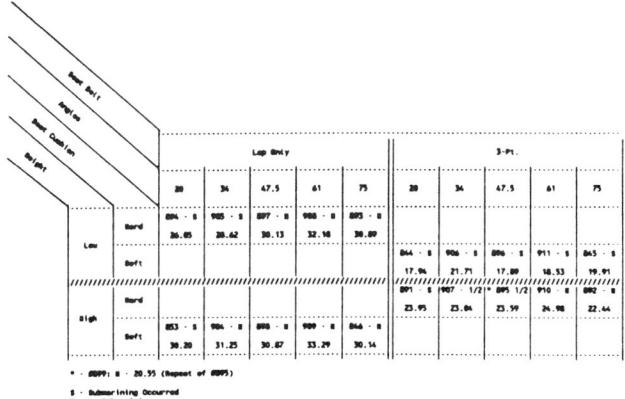

Figure 13. Head forward (X) velocity (mph).

In figure 13, longitudinal head velocities are presented in the matrix format. For the three-point belt, the velocities are maximum values, and range from 18 to 25 mph. For each lap belt only test, the longitudinal component of head velocity was determined at the point at which the head had travelled forward 20" (the rearmost point at which head impact might occur). These are the values which appear in figure 13 for the lap belt only; they ranged from 26 to over 33 mph, and, therefore, were considerably greater than maximum non-contact head velocities for the three-point belt restrained occupants.

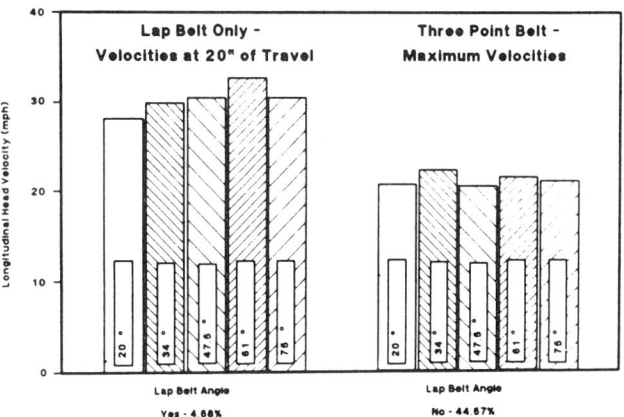

Figure 14. Effect of lap belt angle on head longitudinal velocity by restraint.

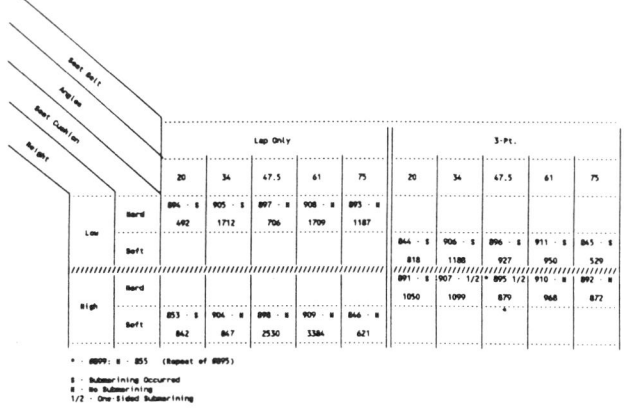

Figure 15. Head injury criterion (HIC).

Since our main concern in analyzing head motion was to determine potential contact velocities, we statistically analyzed head velocities separately for the lap-only and three-point belt restrained occupants. These results, shown in figure 14, indicate that Belt Angle has a small but significant affect on the head velocity of lap belt restrained occupants, at the point at which head impact may occur; but does not affect maximum head velocity of three-point belt restrained occupants. Also, this figure clearly shows that head velocities at 20" of excursion for the lap-only tests greatly exceed maximum head velocities for the three-point tests.

Head injury criterion (HIC)

The HIC was determined using the head C.G. resultant acceleration. Figure 15 contains the HIC values for the sled series.

The statistical analysis indicated that none of the four main effects or interactions appear to have a strong effect on the occupant's HIC value, which is shown by the bar charts in figure 16. However, the difference between the average lap-only and the three-point belt HIC's is substantial, and, at a 15.63% level of significance, is considered marginally significant. HIC values, separated by Belt Type and plotted against Belt Angle, are presented in figure 17. These curves, and the individual HIC values shown in figure 15, show that HIC was far more erratic for occupants restrained by the lap belt only. Observations of the films indicated the reason; head contact occurred in nine of the ten tests involving lap belt only, but did not occur in any of the eleven three-point belt tests. (Specifically, the head contacted either the front seat back or the dummy's knee in test 853, 893, 894, 897, 898, 904, 905, 908 and 909.

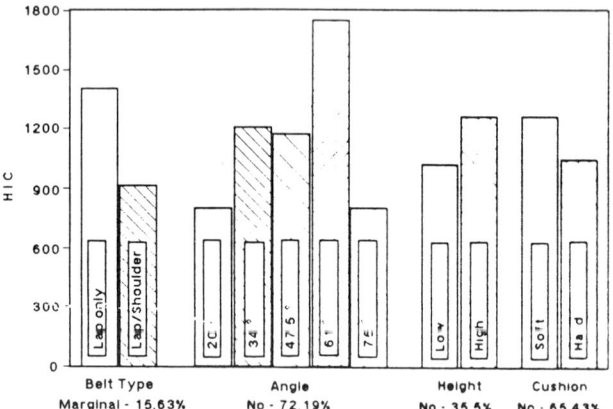

Figure 16. Head injury criteria for rear seat occupants.

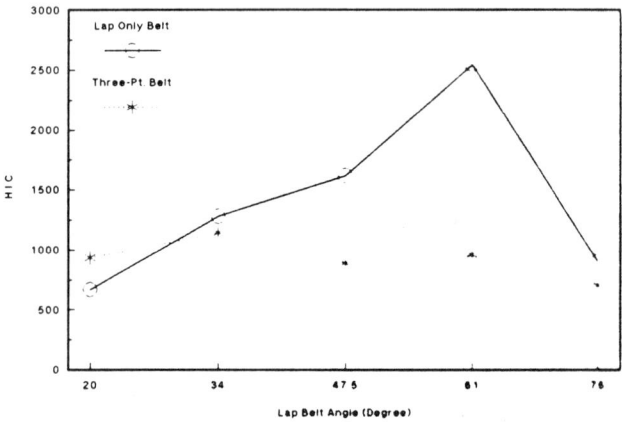

Figure 17. Head injury criterion (HIC) for rear seat occupants.

Occupant peak chest acceleration

The occupant's peak chest resultant accelerations are summarized in figure 18.

The statistical results are shown in figure 19. Cushion was the only main effect which was shown to be significant in effecting the chest acceleration, with a p-value of 2.5%. The remaining main effects and interactions were not significant.

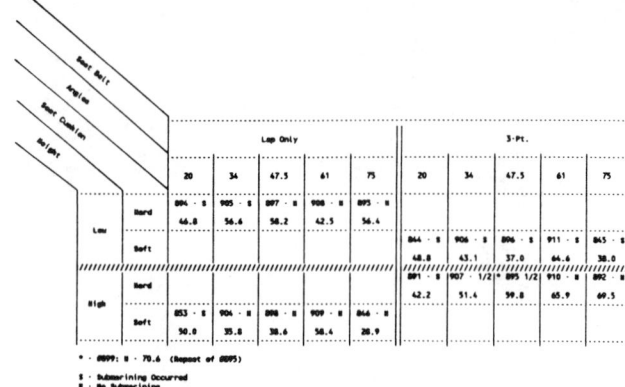

Figure 18. Peak chest resultant acceleration (G's).

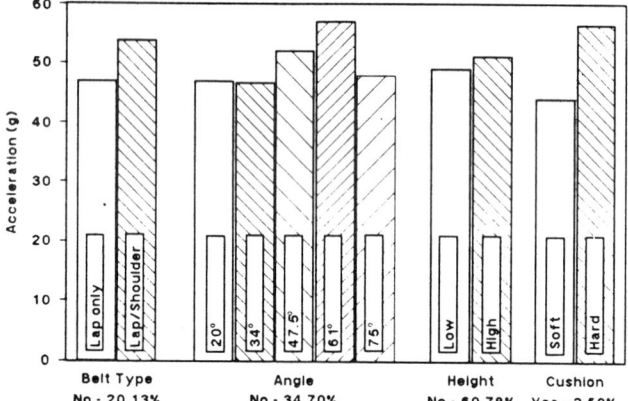

Figure 19. Peak chest acceleration for rear seat occupants.

Peak chest deflection for three-point belted occupants

The peak chest deflections are summarized in figure 20 for those tests where a three-point belt system was used. It is interesting that the two tests where submarining did not occur resulted in the least amount of chest deflection.

The statistical results are displayed in figure 21. Note that only 1 main effect is present in the statistical model—Belt Angle. It is significant, with a p-value of 1.11%. Seat Height

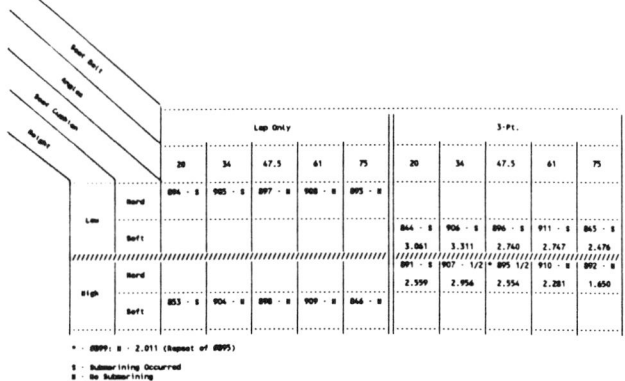

Figure 20. Peak chest deflection (inches) for three-point only.

and Cushion Stiffness are confounded, so the main effect due to either one cannot be discriminated without more testing. Interestingly, the confounded main effect is significant, with a p-value of 1.31%, indicating that one of the factors, or a combination of the factors (low seat and soft cushion versus high seat and hard cushion) is significant.

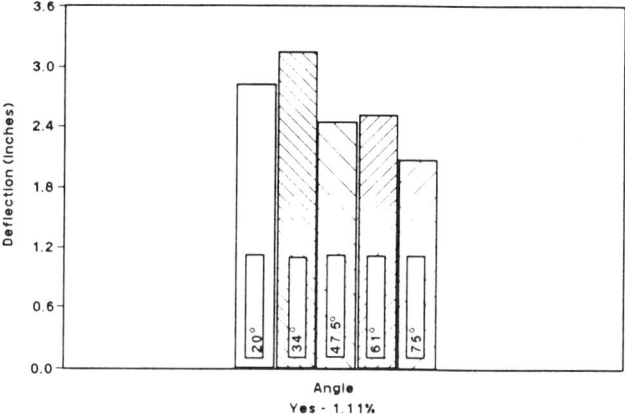

Figure 21. Chest deflection for lap/shoulder belted rear seat occupants.

Abdominal injury severity

Leung, et al., (6) conducted 10 sled tests, in which human cadavers were restrained by three-point belts, to develop an abdominal injury criterion associated with submarining. Nominal sled velocity was 30 mph and peak decelerations ranged from 21 to 30 g. Most of the cadavers were tested in a rear seat configuration. Upper and lower shoulder belt loads and inboard and outboard lap belt loads were recorded. Autopsies were performed.

They observed a relationship between post-submarining peak force on the lap belt (average of both sides), normalized with respect to the mass of the part 572 dummy, and abdominal injury severity. This relationship, reproduced from Reference 6 and shown in figure 22, represents an approximate injury criterion which can be applied to our three-point belt test results. The criterion should not be applied to tests involving lap belt only, because the lap belt would be expected to penetrate a different region of the abdomen, causing injury to different organs, and, therefore, a different overall injury severity for a given force, than would occur in a three-point belt system.

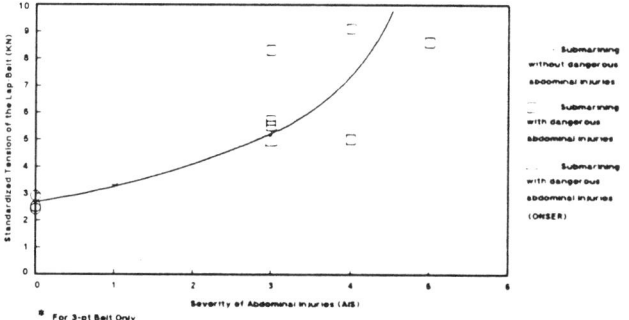

Figure 22. Relationship between the standardized tension of the lap-belt* (after submarining) and the abdomen AIS.

Lap belt forces (average of both sides) from all of our sled tests are shown in figure 23. For tests where submarining did not occur, values shown are maximum forces. For tests with submarining, values shown are the highest forces that were generated after submarining (full or half) occurred. No statistical analyses were performed on lap belt force because differences in injury consequences of high belt forces would be expected to greatly vary, depending on whether or not submarining occurs. As expected, maximum values (from tests with no submarining) were much higher for the lap-only belt (2000 to 3000 lbs or 8.9 km to 13.4 km) than for the three-point belt (approximately 1400 lbs or 6.2 km). Post-submarining belt forces for the lap-only belts having the shallowest angles (20° and 34°) were comparable in magnitude to peak forces that resulted in tests with no submarining. Maximum belt forces after full submarining in the three-point system ranged from 240 to 700 lbs (1.1 km to 3.1 km).

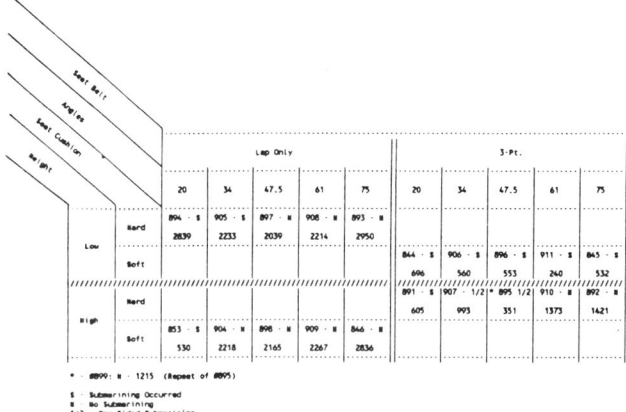

Figure 23. Peak lap belt forces (both sides averaged) (lbs).

For the three-point belt tests, injury severities (AIS levels) were obtained from the post-submarining lap belt forces, by means of the relationship in figure 22. These are presented in figure 24, and indicate that, although full submarining occurred in six out of the eleven tests, only one injury would have occurred and it would have been of minor severity (AIS 1). (Although not specifically stated in reference 6, it is assumed that the lap belt force/injury relationship of figure 22 applies only for full submarining).

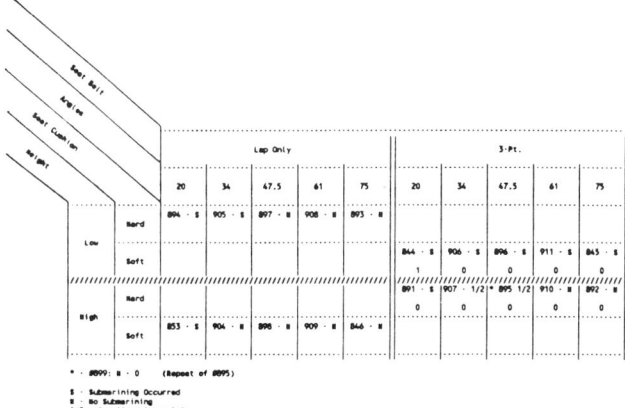

Figure 24. Injury severity (AIS) for three-point only.

Summary and Conclusions

Based upon the results of the sled test series, the following summary and conclusions are made about the occurrence of submarining for rear seat occupants:

1. The occurrence of submarining, in general, was very clearly detected by observing test films, force-time responses of the load cells mounted in the submarining pelvis and force-time responses of lap and shoulder belt load cells.

2. Of the four factors investigated in the test matrix, Lap Belt Angle has a statistically highly significant effect on the tendency for submarining to occur. Belt Type (lap belt only versus three-point belt) and Seat Height appear also to have a significant[2] effect on, and Cushion Stiffness appears to marginally affect, submarining tendency. (While the effect of Lap Belt Angle is clear, a small degree of uncertainty exists with regard to the effects of the other factors, because of the confounding inherent in half-factorial designs).

    a. The shallower the angle (off horizontal), the greater the tendency for submarining to occur. A lap belt angle of approximately 45° appears to be a transition, below which the tendency for submarining to occur increases rapidly with decreasing angle.

    b. The tendency to submarine appears to be greater for three-point belted occupants than for lap belt only occupants. This appears, from the films, to be due to the shoulder belt (1) pulling up on the lap belt and (2) preventing forward jackknifing motion of the upper torso.

    c. It appears that submarining tends to occur more frequently when the height between the occupant's H-Pt. and heel resting position is low (8") than when that height is relatively high (12"). The probable explanation for this is that with the lower height, the occupant's pelvis is rotated rearward more than at the higher height. However, the effect of seat height on submarining tendency is questionable, due to lack of leg articulation in the Hybrid III dummy, and the resulting uncertainty regarding the dummy properly duplicating the human pelvis orientation for low seating heights. We feel the dummy's pelvis probably was rotated more in the lower seat than a human's would be, exaggerating the pelvic angle and predisposing the dummy to submarining more than is likely for the human.

    d. Although statistical significance is marginal, submarining tendency appears to be greater for the softer seat cushion.

3. Forward head excursions and velocities were much greater for dummies in lap belts only than in three-point belts. Lap belt only restrained dummies had head velocities around 30 mph at a point representing the rearmost location of a front seat back; they appeared to be slightly higher for steeper lap belt angles. Head excursions of three-point belt restrained dummies were less than that which would cause head contact; maximum head velocities were approximately 21–22 mph.

4. HIC values were marginally higher, and more variable due to some head/front seat back contacts and head/knee contacts, for dummies in lap-only belts than in three-point belts. HIC's averaged approximately 1400 in the lap-only restraint, and 920 in three-point belts.

5. Peak chest acceleration values were significantly affected only by seat cushion stiffness, averaging just under 60 g's for the hard cushion and just under 45 g's for the soft cushion.

6. Peak chest deflections (three-point belt restrained dummies only) were significantly affected by lap belt angle, ranging from about 2.1 inches for the steepest angle to around 3 inches for the shallowest angles. The two tests where submarining did not occur resulted in the least amount of chest deflection.

7. Maximum post-submarining lap belt forces of 2839 and 2233 lbs occurred for the lap-only belts having the shallowest angles (20° and 34°, respectively).

8. Maximum lap belt forces after full submarining in the three-point belt system ranged from 240 to 700 lbs.

9. A useful, though approximate, injury criterion exists for evaluating severity of submarining for three-point belt restrained occupants only. Injury severity can be inferred from peak lap belt forces that occur after full (two-sided) submarining (6). Although full submarining occurred in six out of eleven tests involving three-point belts, only one injury (AIS 1) was indicated. No criterion appears to exist for determining submarining severity when only a lap belt is worn; therefore, no conclusions can be made regarding submarining injury severity in lap-only belted occupants.

Acknowledgments

The views and findings in this paper are those of the authors and do not necessarily represent the policy of the NHTSA.

The authors are grateful to Rodney Herriott, Doug Hayes, William Gwilliams, Claude Melton and Timothy Schock for their technical support in the fabrication of the test buck and processing of test data.

A special thanks goes to Susan Weiser for the preparation of the manuscript.

---

[2] Throughout the Summary and Conclusions, the term "significant" or "significance" is used to denote statistical significance.

References

(1) MacLaughlin, T.F., Sullivan, L.K., and O'Connor, C.S., "Rear Seat Submarining Investigation," DOT HS 807 347, National Technical Information Service, Springfield, VA 22161, May 1988.

(2) Adomeit, D. and Heger, A., "Motion Sequence Criteria and Design Proposals for Restraint Devices in Order to Avoid Unfavorable Biomechanic Conditions and Submarining", SAE Paper 751146.

(3) Adomeit, D., "Seat Design—A Significant Factor for Safety Belt Effectiveness", SAE Paper 791004.

(4) DeJeammes, M., et al, "Factors Influencing the Estimation of Submarining on the Dummy", SAE Paper 811021.

(5) Mooney, M.T. and Collins, J.A., "Abdominal Penetration Measurement Insert for the Hybrid III Dummy", SAE Paper No. 860653, SAE International Congress & Exposition, Detroit, Michigan, February 24–28, 1986.

(6) Leung, Y.C., et al, "Submarining Injuries of Three-Point Belted Occupants in Frontal Collisions—Description, Mechanisms and Protection", SAE Paper 821158.

902316

Steering Assembly Impacts Using Cadavers and Dummies

Paul C. Begeman, James M. Kopacz, and A. I. King
Wayne State University

ABSTRACT

Studies have shown that dummies can be used to study various issues relating to an unrestrained driver's interaction with the steering system in frontal crashes. However, current dummies have limitations in simulation of car occupants and to assess the spectrum of injury types and mechanisms. Human cadaver subjects were used to study abdominal injury and "severe" steering wheel deformation as part of an evaluation of energy absorbing steering systems.

A predominant factor influencing abdominal injury in these tests was the impact location of the lower rim, injury being associated with the rim aligned 50 mm below the xiphoid. The dummies developed approximately twice the impact force than the cadaver subjects in these severe tests with a noncompressible column, in part due to the chest of the dummies "bottoming" out on a rigid spine. Flexibility of the human spine resulted in the cadaver "inverting" the steering wheel rim below the hub in the most severe test with a noncompressible column. In contrast, the dummies did not invert the wheel rim inspite of much greater impact force. However, wheel deformations caused by the Hybrid III dummy were closer to those from the cadaver tests than wheel deformations caused by the Part 572 dummy.

ENERGY ABSORBING STEERING SYSTEMS have reduced injury associated with steering assembly contact [1]. Despite these reductions, the steering system remained the leading contact source of occupant injury and more than 25% of car occupant HARM was reported to be associated with steering assembly contact [2,3]. In viewing the incidence of injury associated with steering assembly contact, it is important to recognize that the presence of the steering system does not increase and might decrease the risk of injury for an unrestrained driver, based on the relative injury risks between drivers and right front passengers [4,5]. The steering assembly is frequently involved due to its high exposure rate -- most car occupants are drivers, generally in close proximity to the steering assembly.

A strategy to further improve the occupant protective function of the steering system for unrestrained drivers should be based on the understanding of occupant interaction with the steering system over the range of situations resulting in injury in actual car crashes. Analysis of car crash data suggests that injury is strongly influenced by belt restraint use, and occurs over a wide range of impact alignments and severities, with the head, face, thorax, and abdomen being the primary body regions to be considered [2,3,6].

The Hybrid III dummy is now accepted as more human-like and provides a wider range of injury assessment than other current frontal dummies or body forms for study of the protection provided by the steering system [7]. The Hybrid III has been compared with cadaveric subjects in impacts with steering systems [8], demonstrating general similarities of kinematics and steering assembly loading. However, some issues relating to driver impact protection cannot be directly addressed with current dummies, due to insufficient injury assessment or to non-human-like response under some impact conditions. The current study used cadaveric subjects to address two important issues relating to impact performance of the steering system: 1) abdominal injury; and 2) "severe" steering wheel deformation.

Abdominal injury is an important body region relating to the distribution of HARM associated with steering assembly contact for drivers not using the belt restraint, as shown in Figure 1. However, the current Part 572 and until recently Hybrid III dummies [12] have not provided abdominal injury assessment. Abdominal injury related to loading of the abdominal region by the lower rim of the steering wheel has been addressed by several methods. A previous study used an animal model [6]. The current study used cadaveric subjects.

Wheel deformation has been demonstrated as an important steering system response to impact in terms of force limiting, energy absorption, and change of load distribution [6,9,10]. Thoracic injury has been shown to be associated with steering wheel deformation [11], suggesting that deformation has decreased load distribution. However, most deformed wheels are not associated with injured occupants [10], suggesting that force limiting and energy absorption are also important characteristics. Large wheel deformations that have been observed in car crashes could not be duplicated in severe sled tests, using the Hybrid III or Part 572 dummies or the SAE J944 body block, limiting the usefulness of these dummies to fully address load deformation and force limiting associated with wheel deformation. One possibility was that the dummies are not human-like in terms of large wheel deformations. Cadaveric subjects were used to study this issue by comparing biomechanical responses and wheel deformations with those from tests with the Hybrid III and Part 572 dummies.

METHODOLOGY

The research consisted of a series of severe frontal tests on the WHAM III sled. The test severity was based on obtaining "severely" deformed steering wheels under direct thoracic impact conditions. Severe impacts were continued for study of abdominal injury resulting from impact by the lower wheel rim because abdominal injury was not found in the noncompressible (rigid) column tests. The fixture did not model a vehicle. It consisted of a hard seat and seat back (reclined 7 deg.), a rigid frame for support of the steering assembly, knee restraints consisting of 100 mm of styrofoam, and a padded head stop, as shown in Figure 2. The general configuration was based on previous studies [6,7,9,10]. The mid-sagittal plane of the subject was centered behind the steering column. The sled was accelerated to approximately 37 to 42 km/h and then stopped over a distance of 305 mm by a hydraulic snubber. By positioning the subjects approximately 380 mm from any potential impact surface, the sled had almost stopped before there was significant interaction of the test subject with the test environment. Thus the velocity of impact was nearly that of the sled. Although this eliminated "ride down", it improved analysis of the test responses.

Energy absorbing and rigid columns were used, mounted at either 15 deg. or 30 deg. from the horizontal. "Soft" and "stiff" two-spoke steering wheels were used, the "stiff" wheel being the same as the "stiff" wheel used with an animal model [6] (the "soft" wheels were not similar). Soft wheels were modified for inclusion of a hub load transducer.

Instrumentation included a triaxial load transducer located between the column and mounting structure, a triaxial load transducer was located on the top of the steering column to which the steering wheel was mounted, and a uniaxial load transducer was mounted in the hub of some wheels. Rim loads were calculated as the difference between the axial steering wheel load and the hub load. Triaxial accelerometers were used in the head and chest of dummies, and head and T1 accelerometer clusters on the cadavers. Photographic targets were attached to the spinous process of T1, T8, and T12 of cadavers. The vascular system of the cadavers was pressurized to approximately 100 mm Hg and a pressure transducer recorded aortic pressure during the tests. One on-board and two off-board high speed cameras recorded the kinematics.

Severe wheel deformation was studied using rigid columns with severe impact conditions (to generate "high" impact forces) and a "soft" wheel to minimize the test energy required to produce "severe" wheel deformation similar to that shown in Figure 3. The impact was aligned such that the upper steering wheel rim passed under the chin.

Abdominal injury was studied using energy absorbing columns and the "stiff" wheel which had produced liver injuries with an animal model [6]. The nominal test velocity was 42 km/hr. The severe impact conditions used to study wheel deformation were adopted for the abdominal injury study since no abdominal injuries were observed in the wheel deformation tests. Wheel stiffness, column angle, and other parameters were changed in an attempt to cause abdominal injury.

RESULTS

Test conditions and responses for the tests with the rigid column are provided in Table 1. Similar information for the tests with the energy absorbing column are provided in Table 2. Relevant cadaveric information and injury summary is provided in Table 3, bone strength data in Table 4. Bone strength (BCF) data are provided to further define the test subject [13]. BCF (bone condition factor) is an indicator of thoracic body resistance based on mineralization and mechanical tests of rib fragments from the test subjects. Subjects with better than average resistance will have a BCF < 0 and those less resistant than average will have a BCF > 0. The purpose of the BCF index is to help define a tolerance criterion for thoracic injury. No correlation of BCF with the number of fractures in these subjects or with AIS was apparent.

WHEEL DEFORMATION - A "severely" deformed wheel from a high-speed frontal car crash in which the investigator assigned a crushed chest to steering wheel contact is shown in Figure 3. In this instance, the rim has been displaced below the hub. Previous tests with dummies had not been successful in causing a similar wheel deformation. In the current study, a similar wheel deformation mode which displaced the rim aproximately 60 mm below the hub resulted for tests 9 and 10. Cadaveric subjects were used to impact a rigid column at 42 km/h. Tests at a lower severity, or with an energy absorbing column did not result in the rim being displaced below the hub. In no test with the dummy did the rim displace below the hub in spite of higher forces compared with tests using cadaveric subjects. Figure 4 shows a wheel from the rigid column tests at 42 km/h for the cadaver, the Hybrid III dummy, and the Part 572 dummy. Clearly the wheels were deformed the most in tests with the cadaver and the least with the Part 572 dummy.

The dummy chests bottomed out in tests at 37 and 42 km/h while the cadavers showed evidence of bottoming only in the 42 km/h test. Figures 5 and 6 show the column and hub loads for a dummy and cadaver tested at 37 km/h. The loads were considerably higher and of shorter duration for the dummies compared to those generated by the cadaver (note the inertial load on the force transducers due to sled deceleration). Figures 7 and 8 show the column and hub loads for the 42 km/h tests for the dummy and cadaver. The loads at 42 km/h were significantly greater than those at the 37 km/h test severity. The dummy imposed a much greater load on the steering assembly than did the cadavers.

Table 5 lists peak response amplitudes for the rigid column tests. Column and hub loads in tests with dummies were about twice those for tests with cadaver subjects. Load distribution between the rim and hub showed large differences among subjects. Fuji film (pressure sensitive film) indicated a much more uniform load distribution on the wheel for cadaver tests as compared with the dummy tests which demonstrated local spots of high contact pressure.

Table 6 summarizes the peak reponse amplitudes for the energy absorbing column tests. Column loads were significantly reduced as compared to rigid column loads. Peak column loads were generally associated with the "bottoming" out of the column as it reached the end of its stroke. The difference in column loads between cadaver and dummy subjects was not as significant as with the rigid column.

All but one cadaver sustained multiple rib fractures, some of which could result in a flail chest in a living subject. Some subjects had cervical or thoracic spine injuries in these severe exposures.

ABDOMINAL INJURY - No abdominal injuries were observed in the wheel deformation tests, with the "soft" wheel, either with or without a energy absorbing column. Energy absorbing columns were used for the study of abdominal injury. However, the severity of the sled exposure resulted in the column bottoming out in many of the tests. To emphasize lower rim loading of the abdominal region a "stiff" steering wheel and a 30 deg. column angle were selected. A more reclined back angle (increased from 7 deg. to 17 deg.) was also used to further emphasize lower rim loading. Two lower rim contact locations were tested, 50 mm below and approximately 100 mm below the xiphoid process.

Abdominal injuries consisting of a lacerated liver were observed in both tests with the lower rim 50 mm below the xiphoid. These tests used the "stiff" wheel. No abdominal injuries were found with the lower rim aligned 100 mm below the xiphoid. The liver injuries appear associated with lower rim alignment in these tests. A previous study has demonstrated that when the rim was aligned with the liver, abdominal injury is strongly associated with wheel stiffness (rim deformation force), and that injury had occurred by the time column compression was initiated [6].

CHEST COMPRESSION - Chest compressions were measured photographically by tracking a target on the steering column and targets on the spine of the subject at the level of T8. Chest data was then taken as the change in the resultant distance between a T8 and steering column target starting at the time of hub contact with the torso. Peak chest compression and the resulting calculated viscous criterion, V*C, are tabulated in Tables 5 and 6. Internal chest deflection, as measure by a chest potentiometer, of some of the dummy tests are also listed in Table 6. Some of the resulting force-deflection responses for the rigid column are plotted in Figure 15. The forces plotted are axial column loads normalized by multiplying by $(76/\text{body mass})^{2/3}$ and the deflections are normalized by multiplying by $(76/\text{body mass})^{1/3}$. The bottoming out of the Hybrid III chest (Test 11) at approximately 80 mm is clear. The two cadavers run at 37 km/h

(Tests 4 and 5) have chest compressions of approximately 90 mm while the two cadavers tested at 42 km/h (Tests 9 and 10) have compressions of more than 120 mm and show evidence of bottoming out forces. Because the steering wheel load is shared by the rib cage, shoulders, and abdomen, the force is not the force acting to compress the chest.

Results for the energy absorbing column tests show that there is less chest compression in cadavers for similar or higher velocity tests than in the rigid column tests, as well as lower peak column loads for both dummies and cadavers. The lower chest compressions may be due to a number of factors. Besides the energy absorbing column, tests with the stiff wheel would have provided a more distributed load on the thorax, and in the tests with the 30 degree column angle the subjects had considerable abdominal compression from the rim loading and a subsequent "lifting" of the torso. For the tests with the stiff wheel at 30 degrees it was not possible to generate force-deflection reponse for the chest. Force-deflection response of the chest for the tests with the 15 deg. column angle and soft wheel are shown in Figure 16. The lower column loads are not only due to the energy absorbing column, but because of the column compression more load went into the dash board also. Table 7 summarizes all the test results with injury parameters. The data is grouped and averaged for ease of comparisons. Cadaver chest injuries (ais) increased with chest compression as well as V*C. Chest acceleration did not appear to be a good injury predictor. Hybrid III matched cadaver chest compressions better with the energy absorbing column, while the Part 572 was consistently too low.

DISCUSSION

The biomechanical responses reported in this paper demonstrate that for very severe impacts with the steering assembly, current dummies have limitations in simulating human and/or cadaveric response. This study addressed two issues relating to assessment of occupant protection performance of steering systems: 1) Abdominal injuries and 2) "Severe" steering wheel deformation. Abdominal injuries were associated only with contact by the "stiff" wheel rim aligned with the liver. These tests demonstrate that abdominal injuries can be caused by steering assemblies and that the current dummies are not able to assess them. The deformation force of the steering wheel rim has been shown to strongly influence abdominal injury due to rim loading [6].

Wheel deformations are considerably different between cadavers and dummies for severe impacts with a "soft" wheel and a rigid column. The larger magnitude and shorter duration column loads seen with dummies are indicative of the chest bottoming out and of a relatively stiff system. In contrast the column loads in cadaver tests are of lower magnitude and longer duration suggesting a more compliant interaction. It is more compliant due to more flexibilty in the spine and shoulders, which is evident from viewing the kinematics recorded on film. Cadavers tend to wrap themselves around the steering wheel. Compliance is also in the chest itself. Evidence of this can be discerned by examining rim loads as a percentage of total column load. For a dummy impact, this is shown in Figure 9 as a function of time. The percentage is high at initial contact, followed by a sharp drop to a low value at the time of peak loading. As the subject rebounded, the hub unloaded first, and since the rim was not deformed past the hub, the rim load percentage is high at the end. Figure 10 shows the percentage rim loads for a cadaver test. They started out in the same manner but, since the rim was deformed past the hub it unloaded first and the percentage rim load dropped to zero and never recovered while the hub was still carrying load. From these two figures it can also be seen that the wheel contact time for the dummy was considerably shorter. Actual rim loads versus time are shown in Figures 11 and 12. The drop in the cadaver rim loads, shown in Figure 12, at approximately 190 ms could be due to rim "snap-through". The higher rim loads in the dummy run must be mostly distributed on the spokes near the hub since the rim did not "snap-through".

When energy absorbing columns are used measured responses of cadavers and dummies are similar, particularly for the Hybrid III. An example of column axial loads for Hybrid III and a cadaver are given in Figures 13 and 14. The first peak and plateau, after the sled inertia loading, is the force level of the column compressing. This is followed by the maximum peak when the column bottoms out. Responses are in general agreement with those reported by Morgan et al in similar testing with energy absorbing columns [8].

SUMMARY

This study indicates that dummies do not fully simulate unrestrained occupant interaction with the wheel in high severity impacts, particulary when the severity is great enough for the dummy chest to bottom out. The stiffer dummies do not distribute wheel loads as do cadavers, resulting in different wheel deformations.

As expected, reductions in peak column loads were seen with the use of energy absorbing columns. However, the severe test exposure resulted in the column bottoming out against a rigid frame. Liver injuries caused by contact of the steering wheel rim were associated with "stiff" wheels and alignment of the rim with the liver. Current dummies do not have the capability of assessing this and other abdominal injuries.

ACKNOWLEDGEMENTS

This research was sponsored by the Biomedical Science Department of General Motors Research Laboratories. The authors would like to thank Mr. John Horsch for his helpful contributions to the formulation of the study, analysis of the data and completion of this paper.

REFERENCES

1. Kahane, C.J.; "An Evaluation of Federal Motor Vehicle Safety Standards for Passenger Car Steering Assemblies"; DOT HS-805 705, National Highway Traffic Safety Administration, Washington, DC, 1981.

2. Malliaris, A.C., Hitchcock, R., and Hedlund, J.; "A Search for Priorities in Crash Protection"; SAE Paper 820242, 1982.

3. Malliaris, A.C., Hitchcock, R., and Hansen, M.; "Harm Causation and Ranking in Car Crashes"; SAE Paper 850090, 1985.

4. Parks, S.; "Relative Risk of Driver and Right Front Passenger Injury in Frontal Crashes"; GMR-4802, August 3, 1984, Transportation Research Department, General Motors Research Laboratories.

5. Evans, L. and Frick, M.C.; "Seating Position in Cars and Fatality Risk"; American Journal of Public Health, Vol. 78, pp. 1456-1458, 1988.

6. Horsch, J.D., Lau, I.V., Viano, D.C., and Andrzcjak, D.V.; "Mechanism of Abdominal Injury by Steering Wheel Loading"; SAE Paper 851724, 29th Stapp Car Crash Conference, 1985.

7. Horsch, J.D. and Viano, D.C.; "Infuence of the Surrogate in Laboratory Evaluation of Energy-Absorbing Steering Systems"; SAE Paper 841660, 1984.

8. Morgan, R.M., Marcus, J.H., Schneider, D.C., Awad, J., Eppinger, R.H., Dainty, D., Nahum, A,M., and Forrest, S.; "Interaction of Human Cadaver and Hybrid III Subjects with a Steering Assembly"; Thirty-First Stapp Car Crash Conference, November, 1987.

9. Horsch, J.D., Petersen, K.R., and Viano, D.C.; "Laboratory Study of Factors Influencing the Performance of Energy Absorbing Steering Systems"; SAE Paper 820475 (SP-507), 1982.

10. Horsch, J.D. and Culver, C.C.; "The Role of Steering Wheel Structure in the Performance of Energy Absorbing Steering Systems"; SAE Paper 831607, 1983.

11. Hess, R.J., Weber, K., and Melvin, J.W.; "Review of Research on Thoracic Impact Tolerances and Injury Criteria Related to Occupant Protection"; SAE Paper 820480, February, 1982.

12. Rouhana, S.W., Viano, D.C., Jedrzejczak, E.A., and McCleary, J.D.; "Assessing Submarining and Abdominal Injury Risk in the Hybrid III Family of Dummies"; SAE Paper 892440, 33rd Stapp Car Crash Conference, 1989.

13. Sacreste, J., Brun-Cassan, F., Fayon, A., Tarriere, C., Got, C., and Patel, A.; "Proposal for a Thorax Tolerance Level in Side Impacts Based on 62 Tests Performed with Cadavers Having Known Bone Condition"; SAE Paper 821157, 26th Stapp Car Crash Conference, 1982.

TABLE 1

Test Conditions for Rigid Column Tests

Test No.	Subject	Velocity km/h	Wheel Type	Spoke Posn	Column Angle	Seat Back Angle
3	Pt572	37.8	soft	hor	15	7
4	C238	37.9	soft	hor	15	7
5	C200	36.7	soft	hor	15	7
6	HybIII	39.8	soft	hor	15	7
7	HybIII	38.9	soft	ver	15	7
8	Pt572	42.2	soft	hor	15	7
9	C277	41.4	soft	hor	15	7
10	C274	42.2	soft	hor	15	7
11	HybIII	42.8	soft	ver	15	7

TABLE 2

Test conditions for Energy Absorbing Column Tests

Test No.	Subject	Velocity km/h	Wheel Type	Spoke Posn	Column Angle	Seat Back Angle
12	Pt572	40.2	soft	hor	15	7
13	Pt572	48.3	soft	ver	15	7
14	C353	45.1	soft	hor	15	7
15	C359	45.1	soft	hor	15	7
16	HybIII	45.3	soft	hor	15	7
17	HybIII	45.3	soft	hor	15	7
18	C395	41.2	stiff	ver	30	7
19	C406	42.6	stiff	ver	30	7
20	Pt572	42.0	stiff	ver	30	7
21	Pt572	42.2	stiff	ver	30	17
22	HybIII	41.5	stiff	ver	30	17
23	HybIII	42.3	stiff	ver	30	7
24	C462	40.1	stiff	ver	30	17
25	C463	42.2	stiff	ver	30	17
26*	C559	42.7	stiff	ver	30	17
27*	C611	41.5	stiff	ver	30	17

* Rim contact 50 mm below the xiphoid, rim contact approximately 100 mm below xiphoid in other tests.

TABLE 3a

Relevant Cadaveric Data

Run No.	Cad. No.	Age/Sex	Weight (kg)	Height (cm)	Chest depth (mm)	Cause of Death
4	238	59M	49	164	180	Methane gas
5	200	57M	64	171	210	Myocardial Infarction(MI)
9	277	66M	86	170	280	MI
10	274	57F	70	161	230	MI
14	353	59M	57	166	190	MI
15	359	67M	61	168	190	Pnuem.
18	395	57M	99	178	275	MI
19	406	64M	82	177	235	MI
24	462	17M	75	193	205	Carbon mon.
25	463	50M	98	176	265	Cirrh.
26	559	69M	86	176	255	Stroke
27	611	67F	57	165	200	MI

Table 3b

Cadaveric Injury Summary

Run No.	Cad. No.	Injuries	AIS
4	238	Fx ribs 3 thru 6, right	2
		Fx rib 6, left	1
		Dislocated A-O joint	5
		Fx C4, with cord damage	6
5	200	Fx ribs 2 thru 8, right	
		Fx ribs 2 thru 8, left	
		Flail chest	4
		Sep. C5-C6	3
9	277	Fx ribs 1 thru 7, right	
		Fx ribs 2 thru 8, left	
		Flail chest	4
10	274	Fx ribs 4 thru 9, right	
		Fx ribs 4,5,7 thru 9, left	
		Flail chest	4
		Fx T1, sep. T1-T2	4
14	353	Fx ribs 2 thru 7, right	
		Fx ribs 4 thru 7, left	
		Flail chest	4
		Fx C6	3
15	359	Fx ribs 2 thru 5,7,8, right	2
		Fx C6	3
18	395	Fx ribs 3,4,5,7,8,9, right	
		Fx ribs 4 thru 6,9, left	
		Flail chest	4
19	406	Fx rib 4, right	1
		Fx rib 8, left	1
		Sep. C5-C6	3
24	462	None	0
25	463	Fx ribs 2,3,4,6,7,8, right	
		Fx ribs 4,5,6, left	
		Flail chest	4
26	559	Fx ribs 2 thru 6, right	
		Fx ribs 2 thru 9, left	
		Flail chest	4
		Sep. C6-C7	3
		Sep. T6-T7	3
		Laceration of liver	4
		Laceration of spleen	4
27	611	Fx ribs 3 thru 10, right	
		Fx ribs 5 thru 8, left	
		Flail chest	4
		Fx femur, bilaterally	1
		Fx tibia, left	1
		Laceration of liver	4

TABLE 4

Cadaveric Bone Strength Data from Ribs

Cad. No.	Modulus GPa	Frac. Stress MPa	Ash Content %	BCF
200	10.96	118.6	31	-.335
238	9.93	71.7	19	.839
274	13.31	95.1	25	.558
277	7.93	120.0	29	.198
353	2.48	98.6	32	.023
359	1.31	20.0	41	.487
395	1.79	64.1	40	-.285
406	2.48	34.6	45	-.160
462	1.65	15.9	44	-.292
463	1.10	35.2	35	.341
559				
611	2.07	23.4	48	.500

TABLE 5
Peak Data Summary - Rigid Column

Run	3	4	5	6	7	8	9	10	11
Occ	Pt572	C238	C200	Hyb3	Hyb3	Pt572	C277	C274	Hyb3
Vel(km/h)	37.8	37.9	36.7	39.8	38.9	42.2	41.4	42.2	42.8
Colx(N)	17500	8500	7200	19250	21000	19000	13000	12500	29000
Coly(N)	-1130	1010	-1980	-2000	2100	3800	1500	1100	5600
Colz(N)	-2600	-2300	-1400	-3500	-3400	-5600	-2500	-4000	-10000
Hub(N)	8750	3550	2250	11500	14000	10700	7800	7500	24000
Rim(N)	8750	5000	5000	7800	7000	8300	5200	5000	5000
Rim(%)	50	59	69	40	60	44	40	40	17
Headx(G)	-117	-254	-124	-58	-72	-	-197	-131	-100
Heady(G)	4	27	41	29	-8	-	-23	29	5
Headz(G)	56	122	40	126	49	-	89	50	92
Headres(G)	126	276	127	138	83	-	203	141	122
HIC(S)	1048	6631	1226	1087	613	-	3196	1493	1204
Chestx(G)	-62	-73*	-61*	-73	-71	-	-30*	-60*	-88
Chesty(G)	-21	-37*	30*	4	-9	-	-	22*	25
Chestz(G)	25	103*	-*	21	31	-	55*	53*	54
Chestres(G)	66	106	61	74	76	-	57	67	106
GSI(S)	327	918*	171*	470	441	-	888*	392*	1142
CHDf(mm) (external)	60	98	94	100	88	-	128	124	93
V*C(M/S)	0.17	2.31	1.55	1.61	1.40	-	1.18	2.18	1.11
VasPr(KPA)	-	65	-	-	-	-	-	85+	-
WhDf(MM)**	17	51	33	39	43	19	114	109	51

* - Accelerations not at the same location as dummy (T1 vs T8)
\+ - Signal saturated
** - Measured as the average displacement of the rim at the spokes

TABLE 6
Peak Data Summary - Energy Absorbing Column

Run No.	Subj No.	Sled Vel km/h	Col Angle deg	Wheel Type/ Defmm	Back Angle deg	Max EA Crush mm	Col Load N	Chst Accel g	GSI S	Chest Dfl mm (ex)/in	V*C (ex) m/s
12	P572	40.2	15	Soft/8	7	Max	4400	125	1074	(58)	1.89
13	P572	48.3	15	Soft/14	7	Max	5700	160	1757	(67)	1.02
14	C353	45.1	15	Soft/25	7	Max	5500	97	1087	(85)	1.73
15	C359	45.1	15	Soft/57	7	Max	3000	132	1155	(100)	1.42
16	HIII	45.3	15	Soft/20	7	Max	·*	90	1406	(95)	1.45
17	HIII	45.3	15	Soft/34	7	Max	6500	71	511	(95)64	1.35
18	C395	41.2	30	Stiff	7	Max	4200	97	659	(60)	0.87
19	C406	42.6	30	Stiff	7	88	5000	57	447	(60)	0.69
20	P572	42.0	30	Stiff	7	Max	4500	73	277	(50)41	0.75
21	P572	42.2	30	Stiff	17	Max	5000	70	309	(50)50	0.68
22	HIII	41.5	30	Stiff	17	38	7200	108	331	(80)76	1.68
23	HIII	42.3	30	Stiff	7	83	6500	78	331	(77)75	1.17
24	C462	40.1	30	Stiff	17	Max	4500	99	500	(105)	1.06
25	C463	42.2	30	Stiff	17	57	#	53	247	(105)	1.14
26	C559	42.7	30	Stiff	17	95	-	52	329	(93)	1.52
27	C611	41.5	30	Stiff	17	89	6000	60	730	(55)	0.68

* = Data Lost   + = Analysis Incomplete
\# = Column Support Failure, no data
P572 = Part 572,   C = Cadaver,   HIII = Hybrid III
Column Angle wrt horizontal plane, Seat back Angle wrt vertical plane
Chest deflection external data from film analysis, internal data from chest potentiometer.
Maximum EA crush Max indicates full compression of column, nominally 100 mm but, with a range of 114 to 127 mm due to column support deformation.

Table 7
Summary Table

Rigid Column
(7 deg seat back, 15 deg col, soft wheel)

Test No.	Vel. kph	Cad/ Dum*	Rim Defl mm	Force Rim kN	Force Hub kN	Chest Defl(ex) mm	(ext) V*C m/s	Chest Accel g	Chest Injury ais
4,5	37	C	42	5.0	2.9	96	1.9	83	3
6,7	38	H	42	7.4	12.7	94	1.5	75	-
3	38	P	17	8.8	8.8	60	0.2	66	-
9,10	42	C	110	5.1	7.6	126	1.68	62	4
11	42	H	51	5.0	24.0	93	1.11	106	-

EA Column
(7 deg seat back, 15 deg col, soft wheel)

				Column load	Column disp				
14,15	45	C	41	4.2	max	92	1.57	103	3
16,17	45	H	27	6.5	max	95	1.40	82	-
13	48	P	14	5.7	max	67	1.02	151	-

(7 deg seat back, 30 deg col, stiff wheel)

18,19	42	C	-	4.6	88-max	60	0.78	76	2
23	42	H	-	6.5	83	77	1.17	84	-
20	42	P	-	4.5	max	50	0.75	60	-

(17 deg seat back, 30 deg col, stiff wheel)

24-27	42	C	-	5.2	90	90	1.10	68	3
22	42	H	-	7.2	38	80	1.68	84	-
21	42	P	-	5.0	max	50	0.68	55	-

* C=cadaver, H=Hybrid III, P=Part 572

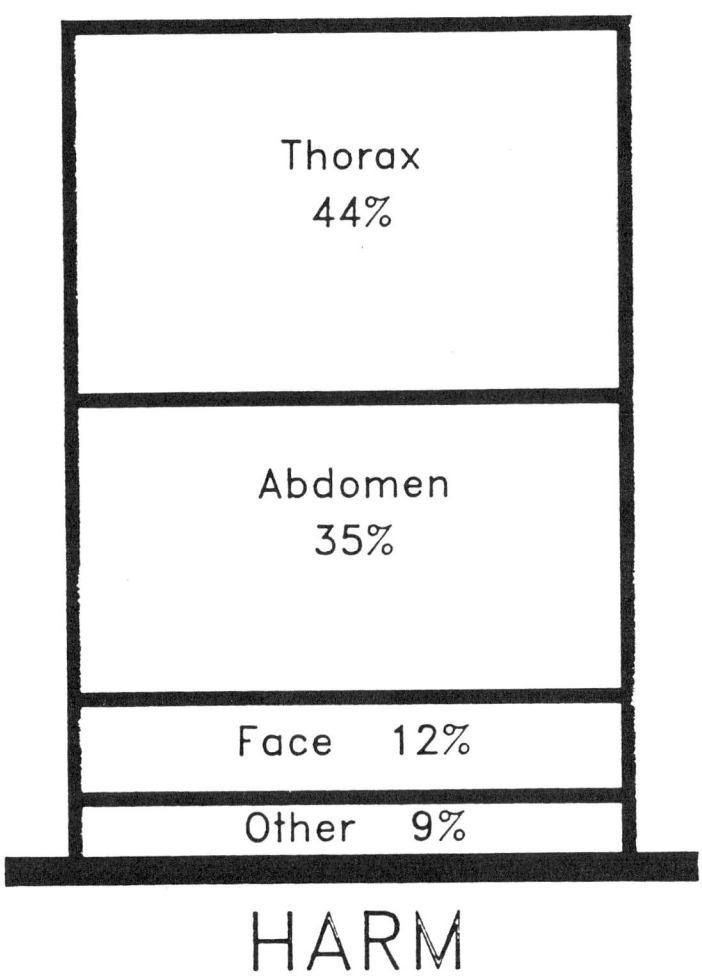

Figure 1. Distribution of HARM Associated with Steering Assembly Contact

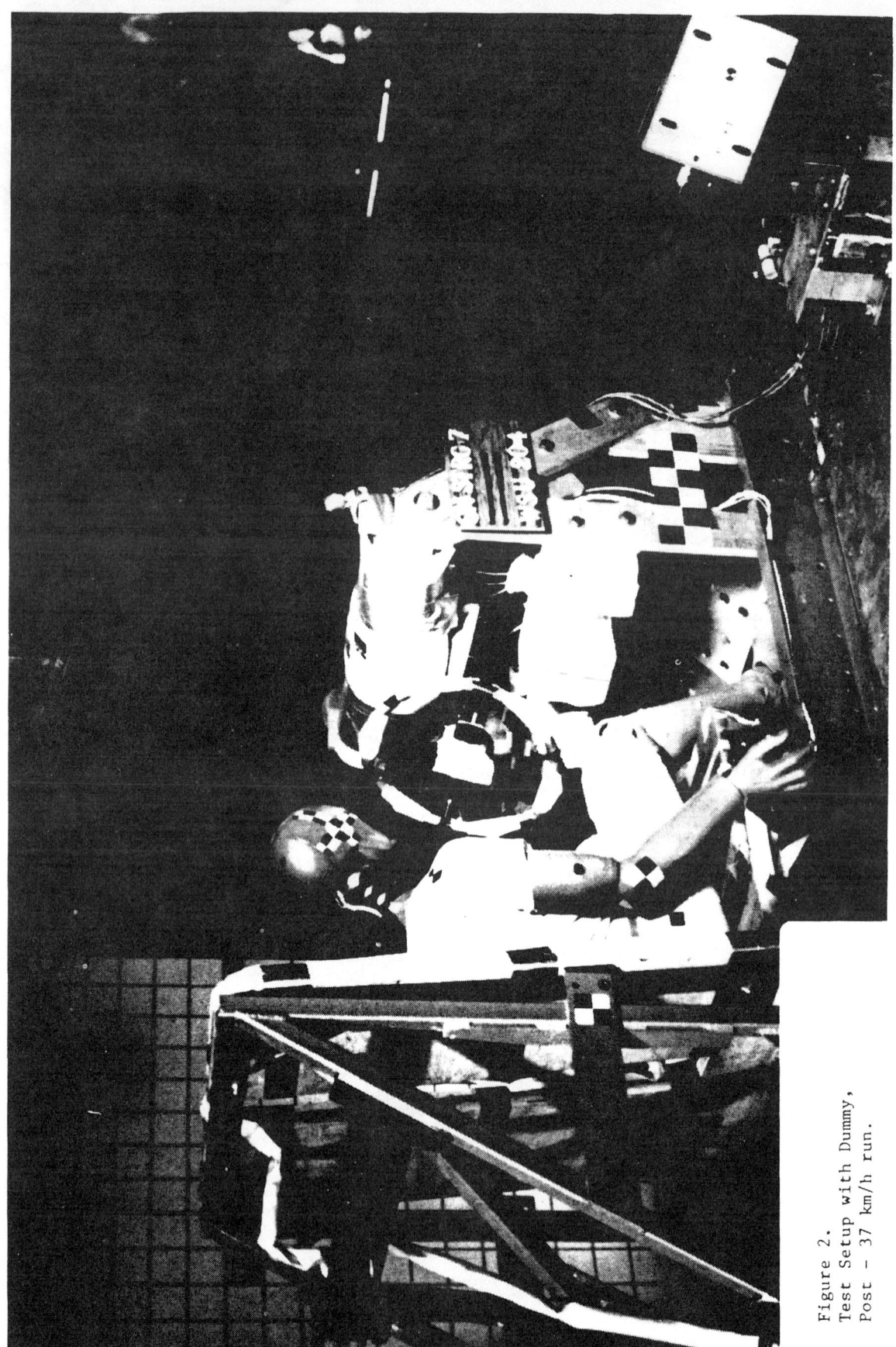

Figure 2. Test Setup with Dummy, Post - 37 km/h run.

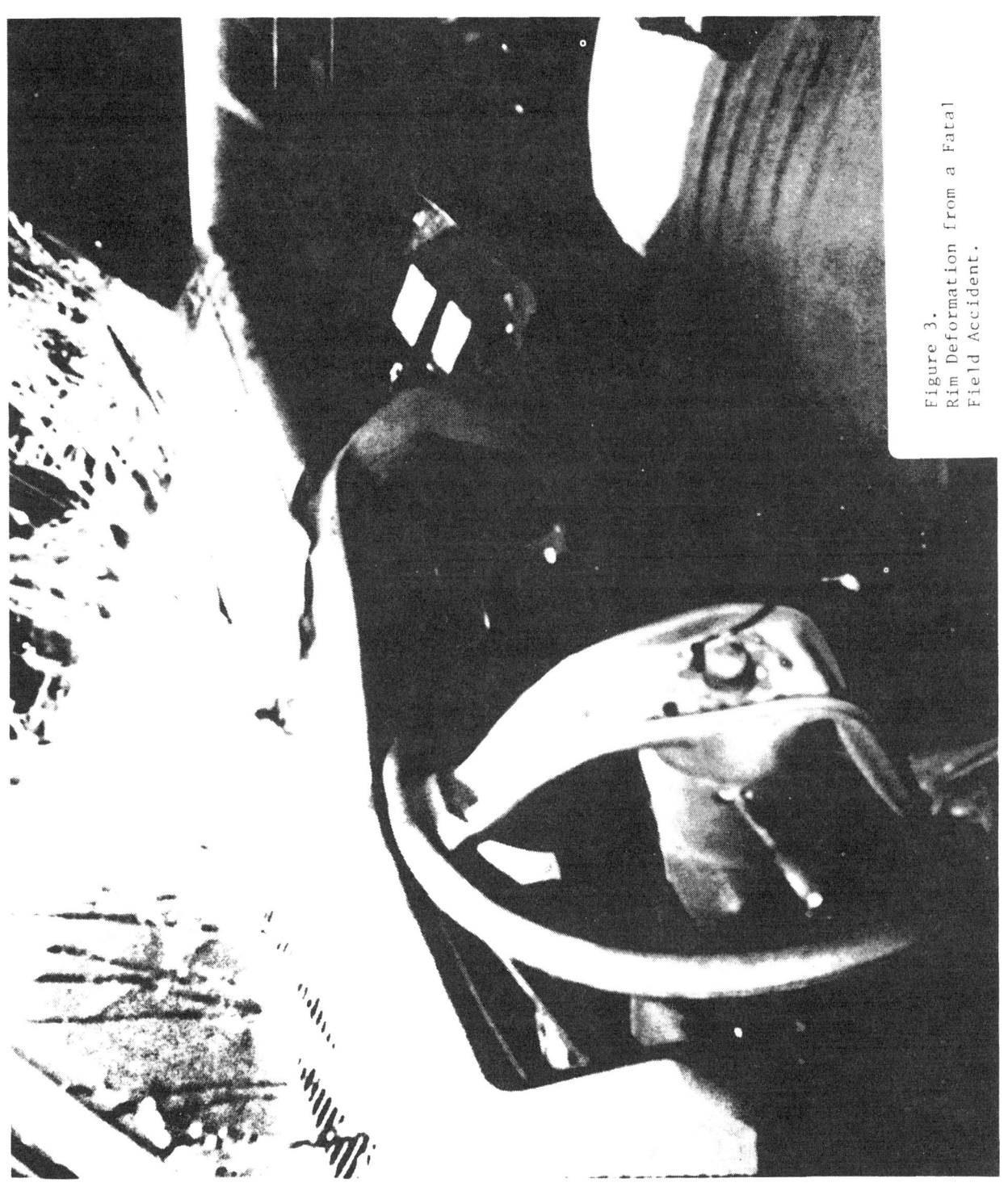

Figure 3. Rim Deformation from a Fatal Field Accident.

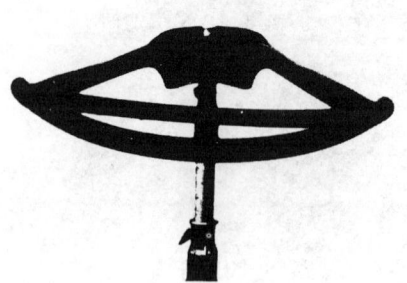

STRG8
Cadaver

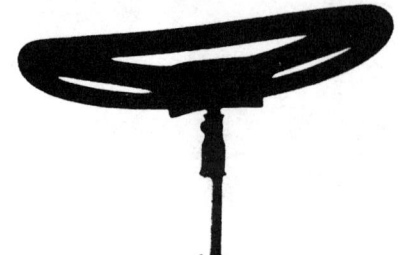

STRG9
Part 572

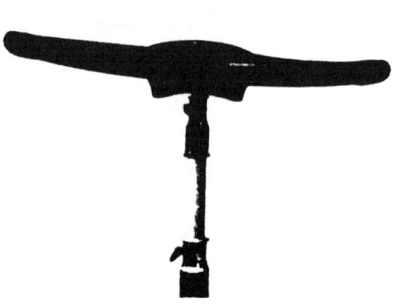

STRG11
Hybrid III

Figure 4.
Rim Deformations from Cadaver,
Hybrid III, and Part 572 Tests
at 42 km/h.

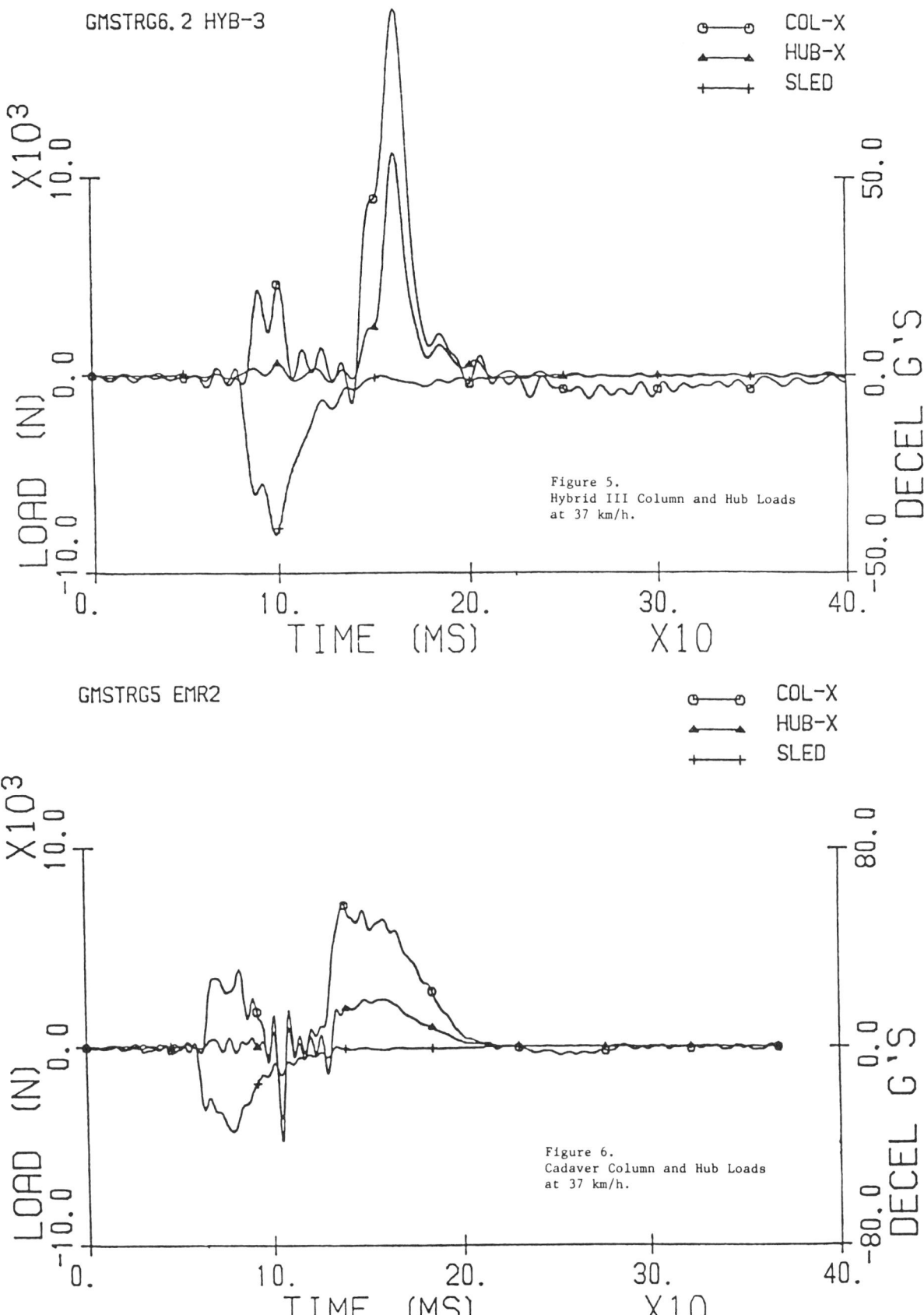

Figure 5. Hybrid III Column and Hub Loads at 37 km/h.

Figure 6. Cadaver Column and Hub Loads at 37 km/h.

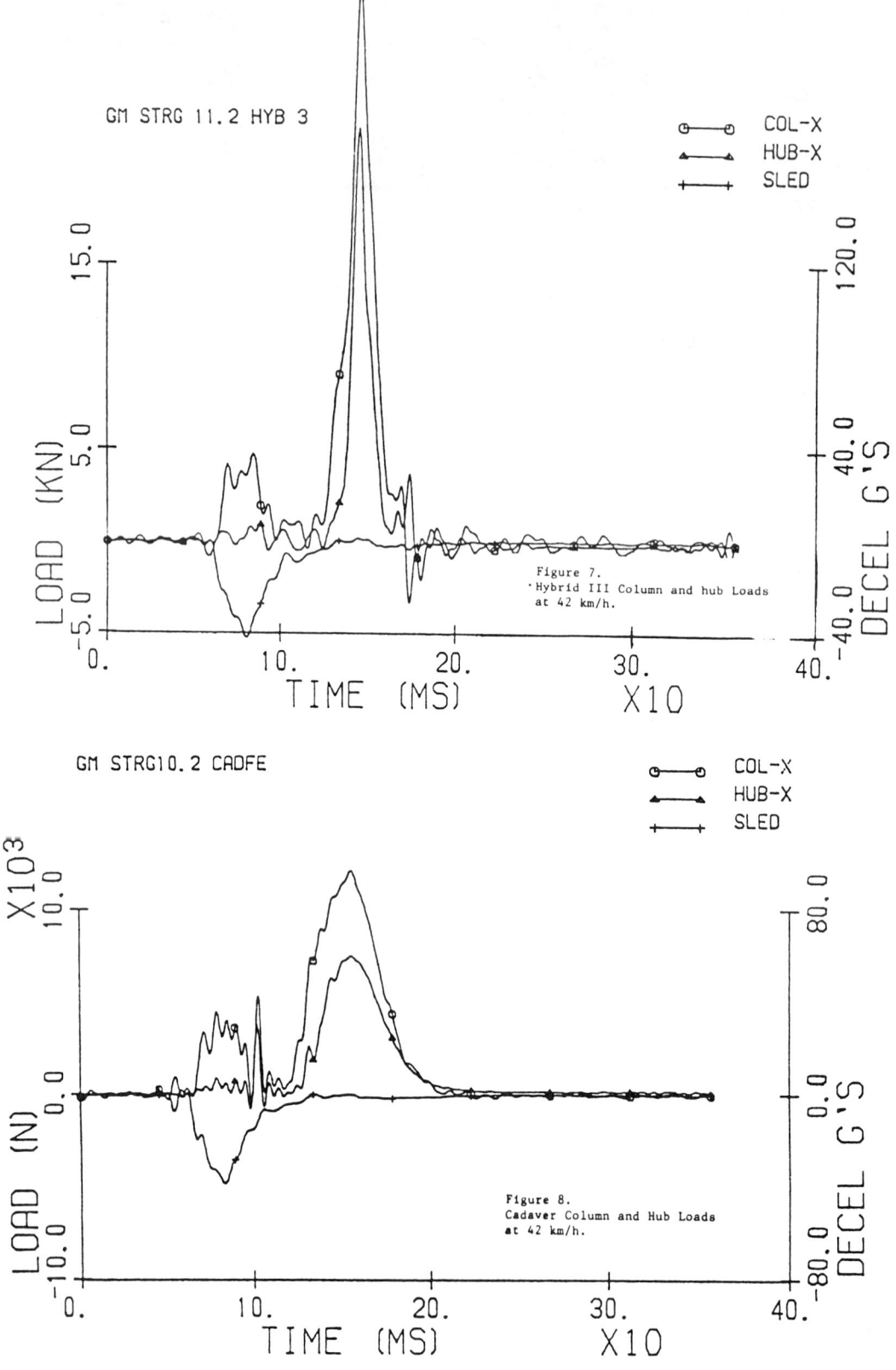

Figure 7. Hybrid III Column and hub Loads at 42 km/h.

Figure 8. Cadaver Column and Hub Loads at 42 km/h.

FIL 180 HZ FFT

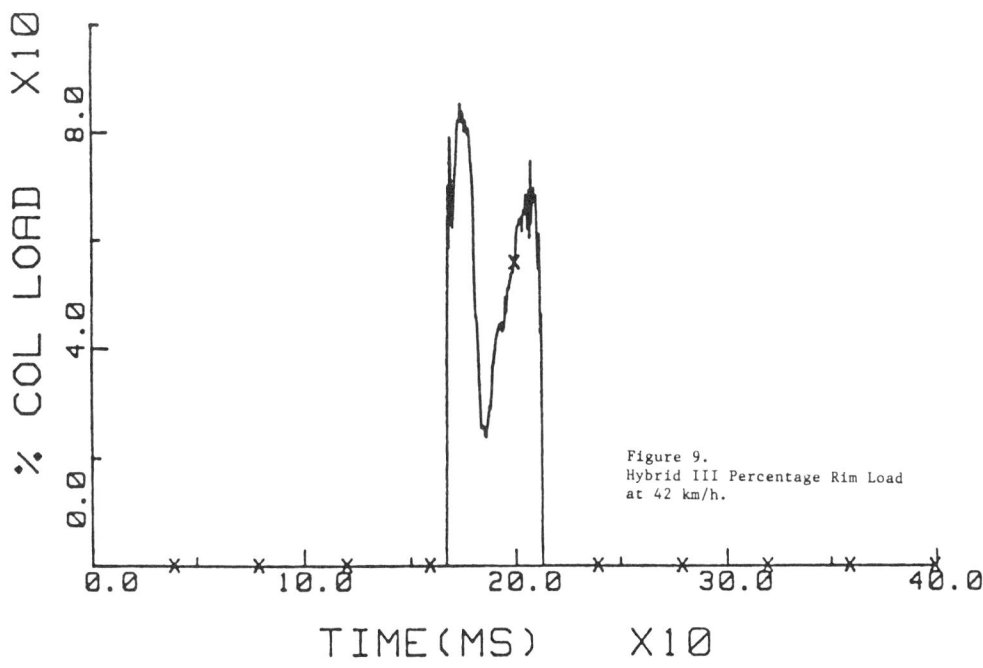

Figure 9.
Hybrid III Percentage Rim Load at 42 km/h.

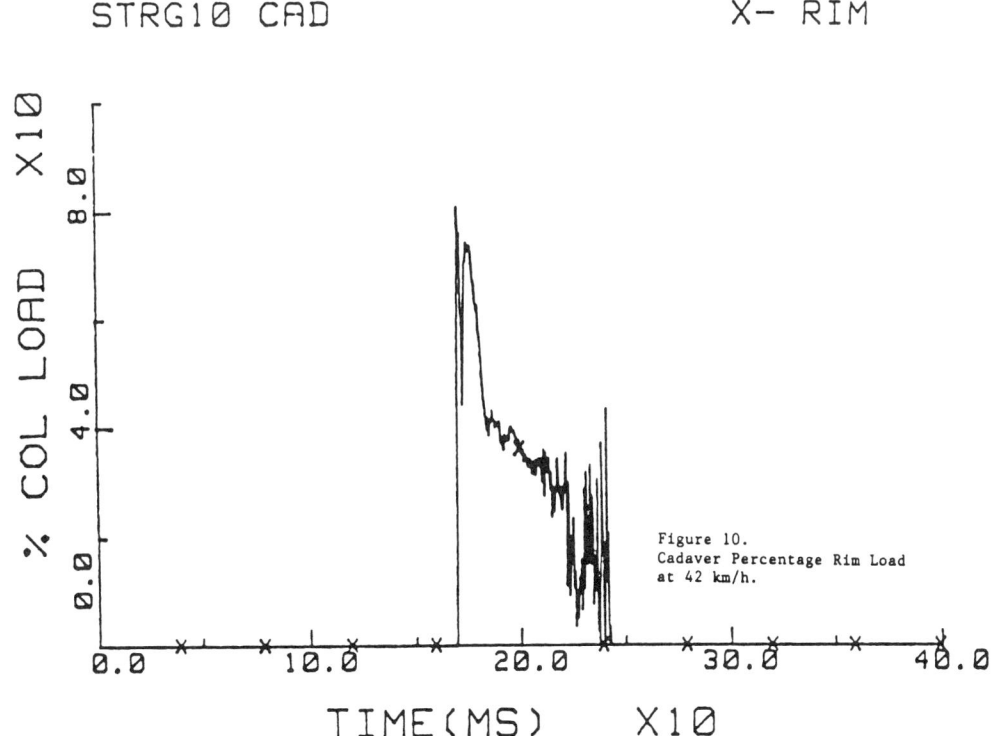

Figure 10.
Cadaver Percentage Rim Load at 42 km/h.

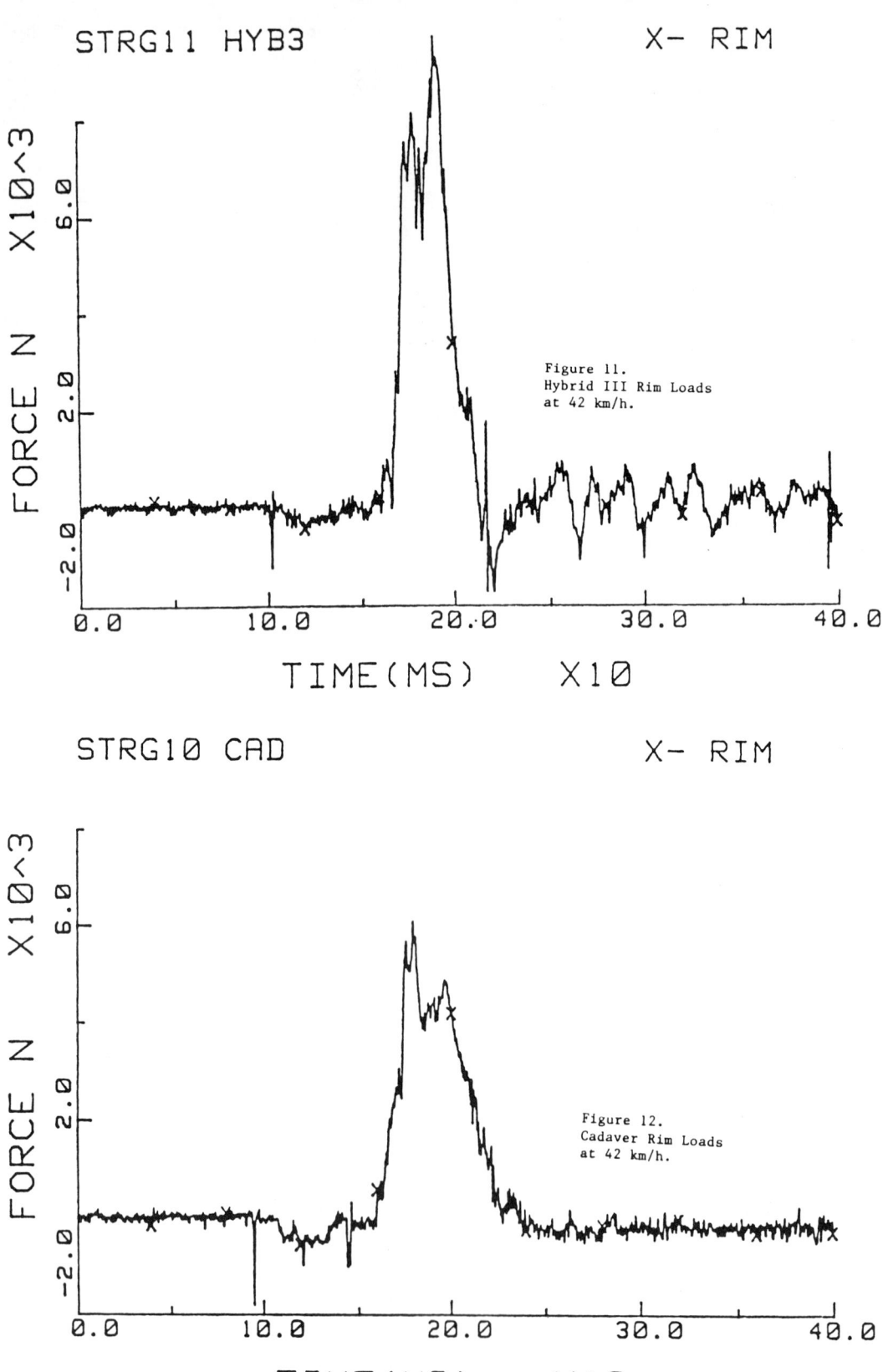

Figure 11. Hybrid III Rim Loads at 42 km/h.

Figure 12. Cadaver Rim Loads at 42 km/h.

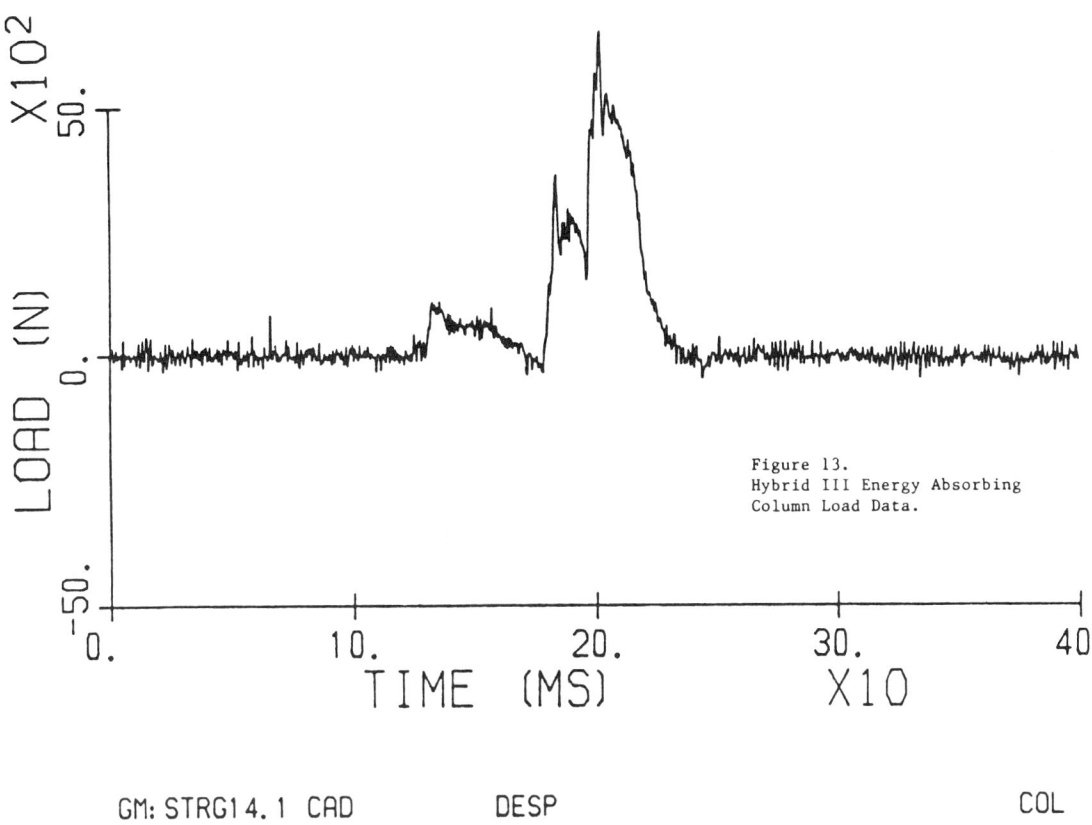

Figure 13.
Hybrid III Energy Absorbing Column Load Data.

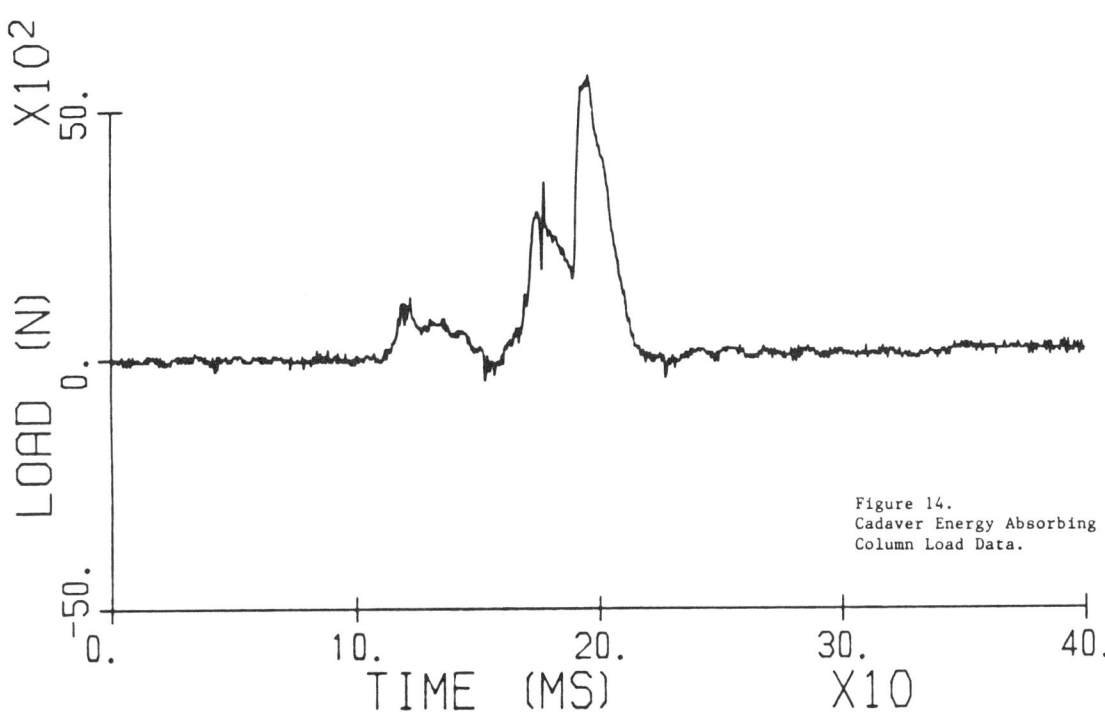

Figure 14.
Cadaver Energy Absorbing Column Load Data.

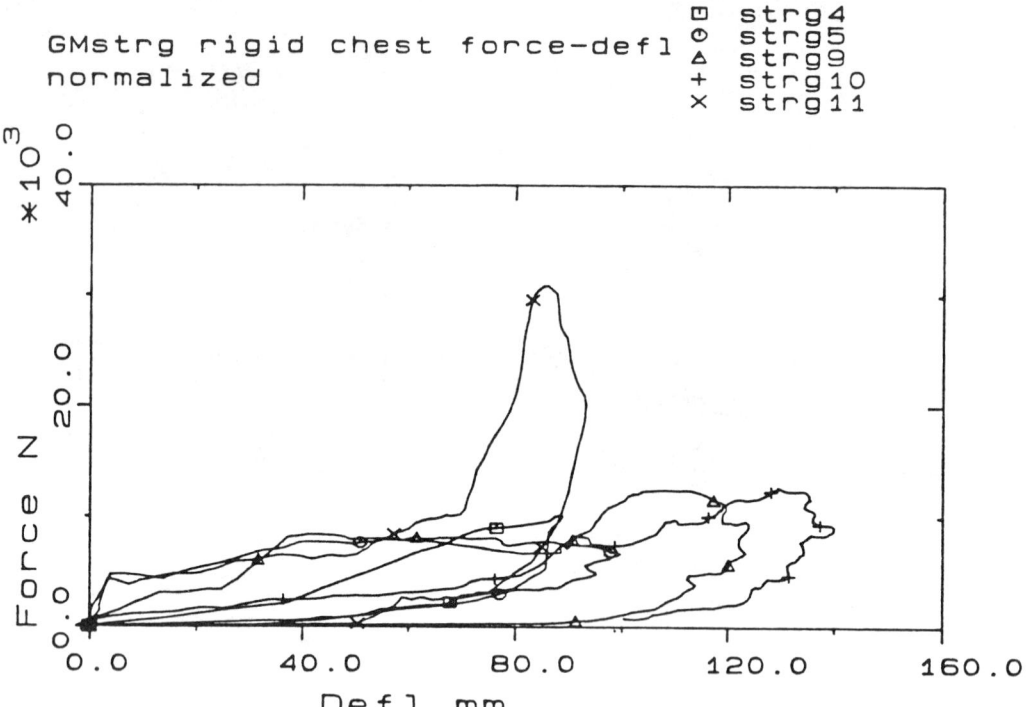

Figure 15. Rigid Column Wheel Force - Chest Deflections.

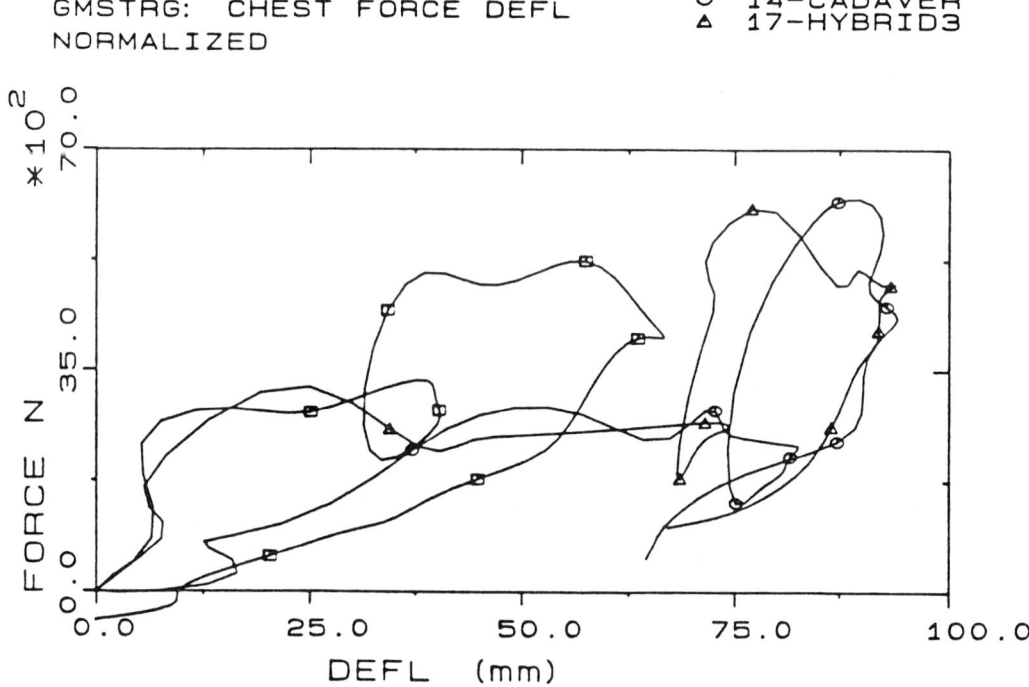

Figure 16. Energy Absorbing Column Wheel Force - Chest Deflection.

930639

Intraabdominal Injuries Associated with Lap-Shoulder Belt Usage

Donald F. Huelke
University of Michigan Transportation Research Institute and
University of Michigan Department of Anatomy & Cell Biology

G. Murray Mackay and Andrew Morris
University of Birmingham Accident Research Center

ABSTRACT

The "seat belt syndrome", first described in 1961, identified abdominal organ injuries related to the use of the lap belt. Many articles have further documented detailed descriptions of intraabdominal lap belt related trauma. Lumbar spine distractions were later added to this injury list. Lap belt injury literature not infrequently hypothecates that some, if not all, of these seat belt syndrome injuries would be prevented, eliminated, or at least significantly reduced in frequency by the use of lap-shoulder belts.

This report, based on data from crash investigations, documents lap-shoulder belt intraabdominal injuries occurring by belt loading alone, without significant intrusion and without significant dynamic flexing of the torso of the restrained front seat occupant.

INTRODUCTION

Abdominal injuries are not unknown in motor vehicle crashes, especially in the frontal type crash. The steering assembly, the rim, hub or spoke(s) are the primary impact site for the torso of the unrestrained driver in the frontal crash. For front seat passengers, abdominal injuries are mainly sustained by impact to the instrument panel in the frontal crash.

By the use of the lap-shoulder belt, some of the impact forces are absorbed by the shoulder portion of the belt, reducing abdominal/lap belt loading, thereby decreasing the number of intraabdominal injuries. Additionally the shoulder belt reduces driver torso/steering wheel contacts.

The seat belt syndrome, a term coined in 1961 by Garrett and Braunstein, generically describes injuries associated with the use of the lap belt [17]. Since then, injuries including lumbar fractures, or fracture-dislocations, abdominal wall injuries, as well as injuries to most all organs in the abdominal-pelvis cavity have been described (2,3,5,7,11,16,17,21-24,34,35,39,45,47,48,51,54,60,61).

Some researchers have presumed that by the use of the lap-shoulder belt these injuries would be prevented. Unfortunately, this is not true. Huelke found a 26% reduction of the more serious abdominal injuries in lap-shoulder belted front seat occupants who were in frontal crashes when compared to the unbelted [23] indicating that abdominal injuries still occur with lap-shoulder belt use.

MATERIALS AND METHODS

For this study a review of the medical-engineering literature on intraabdominal injuries to lap-shoulder belted occupants was conducted. Additionally, the National Accident Severity Study (NASS) file for years 1980-89 were reviewed. This file contains approximately 76,728 motor vehicle crashes and, in addition to the plethora of car crashes damage details, injury specifics and contact areas related to these injuries are available. Cases were reviewed from the field accident injury files at the University of Michigan where a motor vehicle injury causation study has been on-going since 1961. A similar study has been conducted at the University of Birmingham (England) and these files were also reviewed for case descriptions of lap-shoulder belted intraabdominal injuries. Only frontal collisions were selected where (at most) minimal intrusion due to crash forces was noted and where intraabdominal injuries of AIS 2 injury level or greater were identified (Table 1) [1].

Table 1

The AIS Scale

0	No Injury
1	Minor
2	Moderate
3	Serious
4	Severe
5	Critical
6	Maximum-virtually unsurvivable

LITERATURE REVIEW

Scattered throughout the medical and engineering literature are articles providing examples of the intraabdominal injury/lap-shoulder belt relationship. Banejee, in 1989, provided a good historical perspective on seat belt and injury patterns and noted that, because of the deceleration of the abdomen by the belt, there may be injuries to the abdominal wall musculature with associated hernia formation, as well as injuries to the various abdominal organs [9]. A decrease in severe injuries to the head, face and trunk has been reported in lap-shoulder belt wearers but with an increase in gastrointestinal injuries [4,15,57]. Ryan claims that this is due to improper wearing of the restraint [44].

Clyne and Ashbrooke reported a case of a 54-year old male wearing a lap and diagonal inertial seat belt [14]. Driving a approximately 30 mph he struck the back of a truck. After the crash he walked home. Later, at the hospital, it was noted that he had a small lower lip laceration, no thoracic or abdominal tenderness or bruising, but aortic bruising at the level of the renal arteries, with a small retroperitoneal hematoma causing distal aortic occlusion. Baker, et al, described a case of a 55-year old female, a lap-shoulder belted front seat passenger, involved in a head-on collision [8]. She sustained a rupture of the stomach, and a hematoma at the duodenojejunal flexure.

Green, et al., reported on the effectiveness of the three-point, i.e., lap-shoulder belt along with reports on intraabdominal lap-shoulder belt injuries [18]. In one of their cases a 1977 Toyota Corolla was involved in a frontal type collision with a 1975 Ford Pinto. The lap-shoulder belted driver sustained a nasal fracture and laceration. The lap-shoulder belted right front passenger, a 42-year old male (173 cm, 73 kg), sustained a laceration and perforation of the mid small bowel and a longitudinal tear in the mesentery, as well as a serosal tear of the cecum. Because the passenger had worn a bulky winter coat, it was postulated that the lap portion of the belt may have gotten out of position because of its looseness over the coat. In another of their cases, a 1981 Chevrolet Malibu Classic struck a tree at an estimated speed of 35 km/h. The 30-year old female right front passenger was fully restrained (174 cm, 67 kg). In addition to rib fractures, she sustained a ruptured spleen, laceration of the left lobe of the liver and a laceration of the inferior vena cava causing exanguination. All injuries were ascribed to restraint system loading. Through vehicle examination it was determined that there was a significant amount of slack in her belt system at the time of impact. They also reported on a front seat occupant with a severe lumbar spine fracture-dislocation. Loose shoulder belt and a misplaced lap portion of the restraint was reported as causing a splenic rupture [19].

Gallup, et al. in 1962, presented data on 314 fully restrained occupants of which 65 suffering an abdominal injury [16]. Of these, 25 were in frontal collisions with seven having the more severe injuries, and 17 having injuries to only the abdominal wall. Ruptures of the small bowel, sigmoid colon, spleen, cecum, jejunum and bladder were reported. The various cars involved were also described and included both domestic and foreign makes.

A front seat 46 year old female passenger sustained tears of the duodenum, anterior and posterior sides of the stomach and a hematoma of the ascending colon mescolon. Injuries were related to the 3-point seat belt [33].

Other authors have presented case examples or medical file reviews of lap-shoulder belted intraabdominal injuries primarily of the gastrointestinal tract (4,6,12,13,15,20,25,28,30,32,38,40-46,50, 52, 53, 55, 57, 58). In addition, Inappropriate (underarm) use of the lap-shoulder belt system aggravating injury severity has been reported [19,49].

UNIVERSITY OF MICHIGAN AND BIRMINGHAM STUDIES

In a review of the crash injury files at the University of Michigan and University of Birmingham, numerous cases were found of individuals who sustained intraabdominal injuries that could be related specifically to contact with the lap-shoulder belt. The extremely high speed motor vehicle crashes with significant interior crush and death of a lap-shoulder belted individual were not included, for it is difficult to separate the interior vehicle deformation from the lap-shoulder belt as the injury causation mechanism.

Listed below are examples which exemplify the issue at hand. In all of these it should be noted that the crashes include a variety of make, model, year of the cars. We did not find any specific car make or model which was more often related to intraabdominal injuries in this series.

Case 1

In a snowstorm, a 1976 Oldsmobile lost control and skidded sideways into oncoming traffic and was struck in a right rear of a 1982 Mercury Lynx (Fig.1). The lap-shoulder belted female driver (163 cm, 43 kg) of the Lynx had minor injuries of the face, knees, and fingers. Marked linear ecchymosis on the chest, flanks and lower abdominal outlined the 3-point belt placement. (UM-2151)

The female front right passenger (163 cm, 56 kg) slouched down just prior to impact. Injuries of the abdomen included a laceration to the right lobe of the liver, spleen and duodenal bulb, and a hematoma of the left adrenal gland. Abdominal wall ecchymosis, from the lap portion of the 3-point restraint, was noted above the umbilicus and below the rib cage.

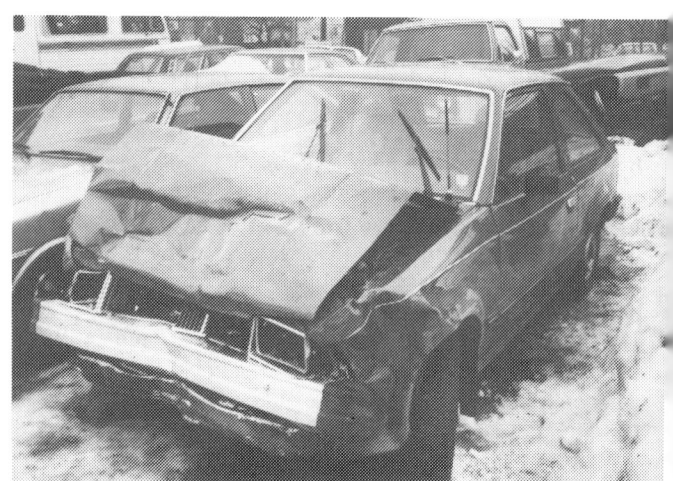

Figure 1

Case 2

On an expressway a 1984 Lincoln Continental struck a steel dumpster box that had fallen off the rear of a trash hauler (Fig. 2). The change in velocity was 48 km/h. The driver sustained minor injuries of the knuckles, eyelid, and a contusion band from the left clavicle diagonally to mid chest. A liver contusion was identified as shoulder belt induced injury. Lap belt markings (bilateral pelvic contusions) were also reported. (UM-2295)

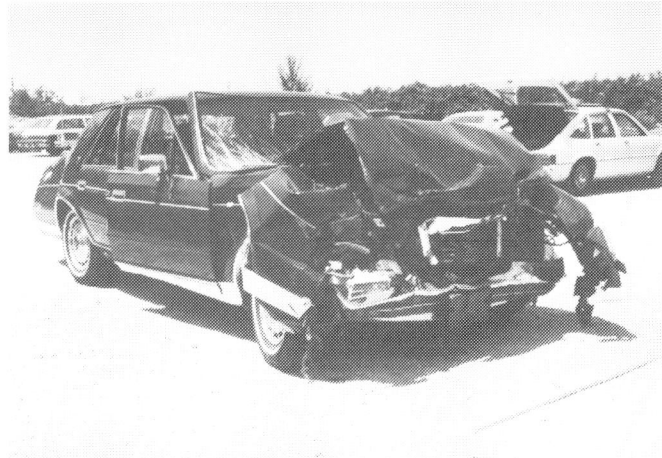

Figure 2

Case 3

In this intersection crash a 1984 Dodge Aries struck the right door area of a 1975 Corvette (Fig. 3). Both front seat occupants of the Dodge wore the lap-shoulder belts. The female driver (165 cm, 71 kg) sustained minor injuries of the head, shoulder and chest. The female passenger (75 years, 155 cm, 98 kg) sustained a tear of the ascending aorta, rupture of the left diaphragm, laceration of the spleen and a greater momentum, an abdominal aortic aneurysm and retroperitoneal hemorrhage. A contusion of the upper abdomen indicates an out-of-place lap portion of the 3-point restraint system. (UM-2375)

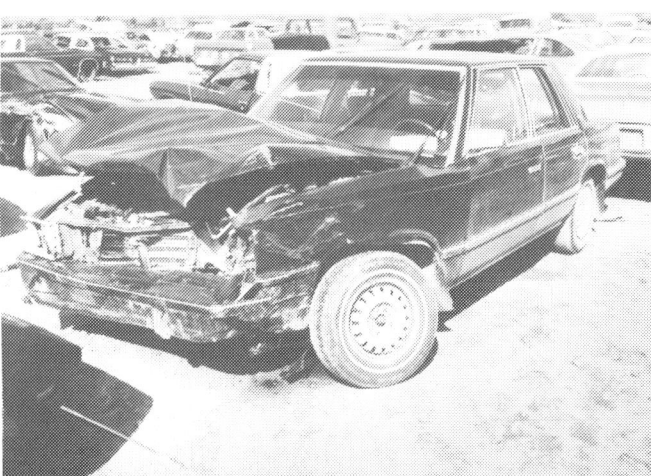

Figure 3

Case 4

A 1983 Plymouth slide into on-coming traffic striking a 1986 Mercury head-on (Fig. 4). Damage to the Plymouth was broadly distributed across the frontal area with heavier damage in the left front. The lap-shoulder belted male driver (188 cm, 82 kg) sustained but a minor leg laceration. The belted 45 year old belted female passenger (152 cm, 47 kg) had subcapsular hemorrhages of the liver and a lacerated spleen along with multiple rib fractures and a left hemothorax, all from belt loading. (UM-2764)

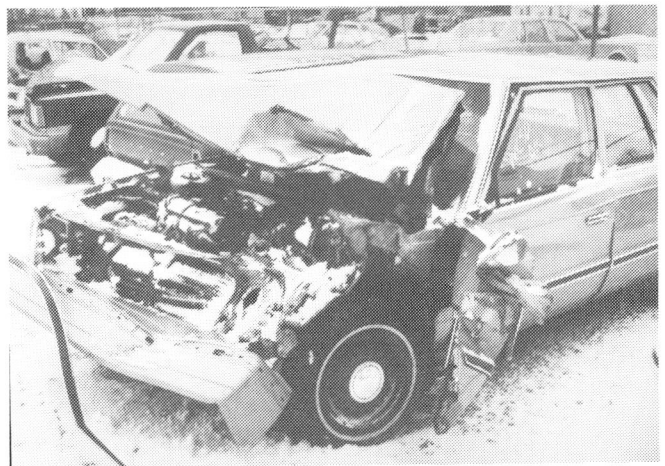

Figure 4

Case 5

A Citroen AX and a Ford Transit collided at a road junction (Fig. 5). A 62 year old male front seat occupant (168 cm, 70 kg) sustained a 5 cm tear in the lesser curve of the stomach, a tear in the mesentery of the small bowel and two cecal serosal tears all as a result of seat belt loading. (B7456)

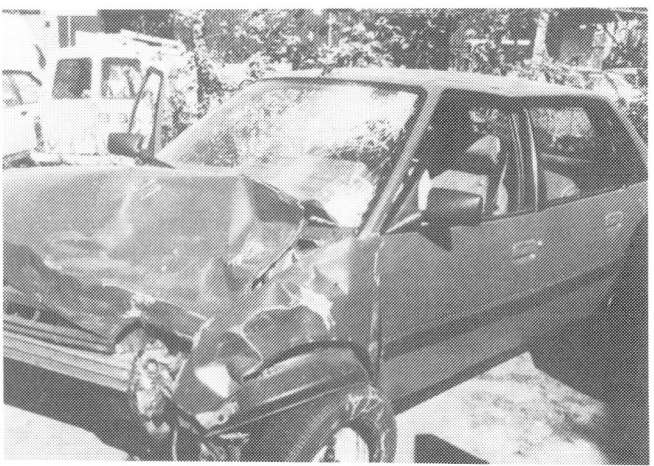

Figure 5

Case 6

A Toyota Corolla collided with an oncoming Metro (Fig. 6). The driver, a 59 year old male (168 cm, 74 kg), sustained fractures to the right femur and to the right ulna. Additionally he sustained a lacerated spleen, a lacerated colon and a complex liver laceration. All injuries are attributed to seat belt loading. (H5989)

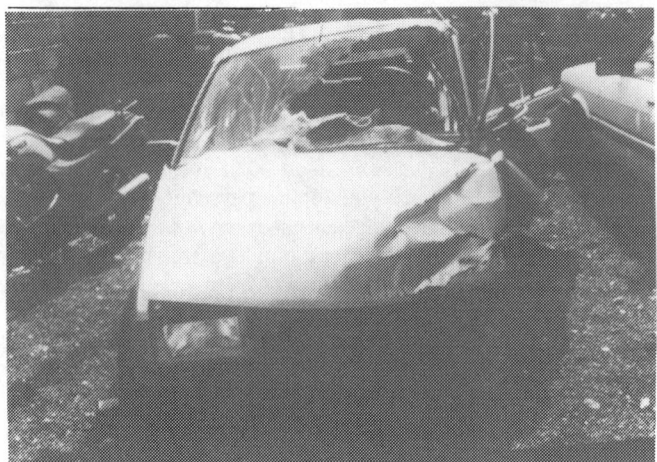

Figure 6

Case 7

This Austin Maxi collided head-on with an oncoming Austin Ambassador (Fig. 7). The ΔV was calculated to be 33 kph. The driver (height and weight unknown-described as 'obese' by the Coroner) was fatally injured but in addition to fracturing bones in the pelvis, arms legs and thorax, he also sustained a large tear in the mesentery attributed to seat belt loading. (B5001)

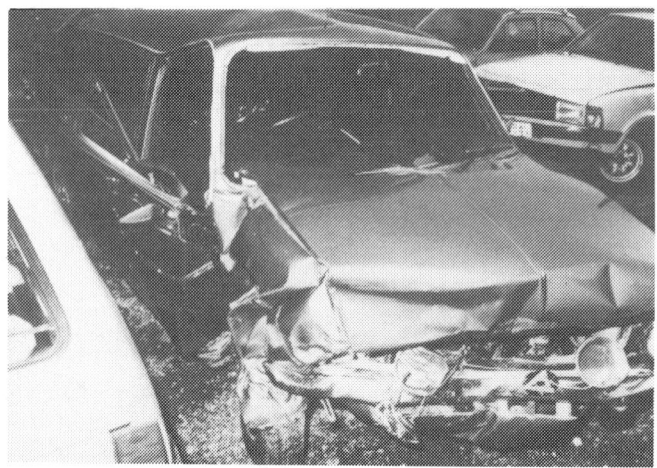

Figure 7

Case 8

A Lada struck an oncoming Escort which had spun out of control (Fig. 8). The male driver sustained only bruising but the 41 year old female front seat passenger (157 cm, 74 kg) sustained a stomach laceration in addition to other minor cuts and bruises. (B5250)

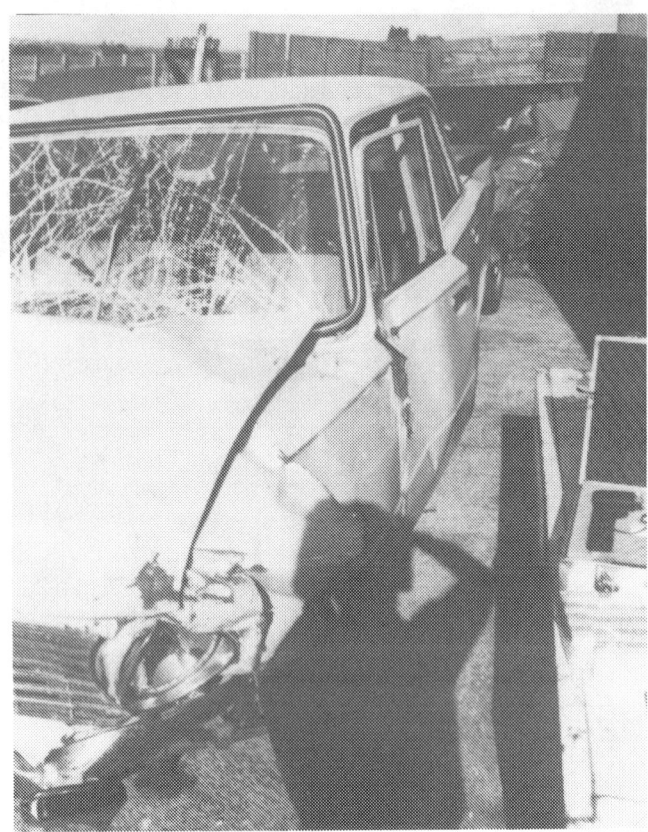

Figure 8

Case 9

A Nissan Micra spun out of control and collided with an oncoming Nissan Sunny on the opposite side of the road (Fig. 9). The front passenger sustained a fracture of the right tibia. The 20 year old female driver (175 cm, 60 kg) sustained only one injury-a jejunal trauma from the seat belt-which was operated upon. However, following the operation the wound developed complications and the patient died some 27 days after the accident from adult respiratory distress syndrome. (B7206)

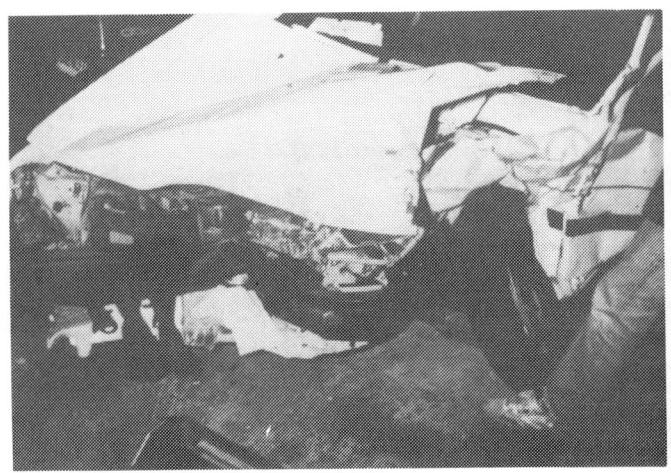

Figure 9

Case 10

The driver of a Triumph Dolomite lost control of his vehicle on a bend. The car struck a lamp post and then fell into a roadside ditch (Fig. 10). A 30 year old male occupant (unknown height and weight) sustained a perforation of the upper jejunum and a tear of the ascending colon without perforation. The injuries corresponded to the lap portion of the belt lying over the abdomen rather than the pelvic area. (B5484)

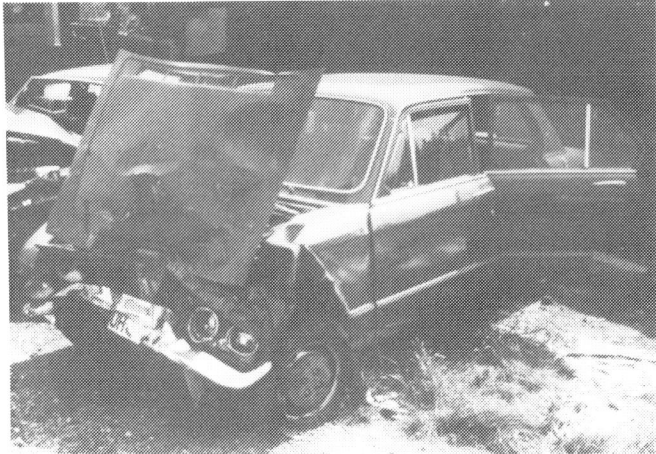

Figure 10

Case 11

A Mini collided head-on with an Alpha Romeo (Fig.11). The 39 year old female driver (unknown height and weight) sustained numerous lacerations, abrasions and bruising to various body regions. She also sustained a perforation of the small bowel and contusions to the cecum and right colon, all from the seat belt. (H6201)

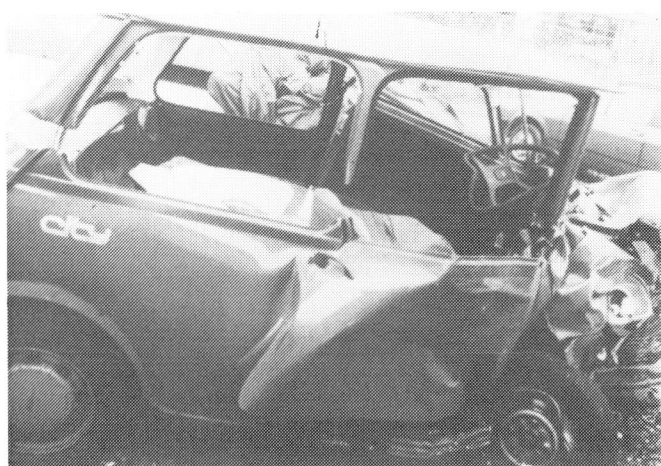

Figure 11

NASS DATA

The NASS file for years 1980-1989 were searched for lap-shoulder belted drivers, or front right passengers, who sustained a serious abdominal injury and were involved in frontal crashes (11-1 o'clock) crash direction. In this motor vehicle crash injury file there were 179 occupants identified with such injuries. Of these more serious intraabdominal injuries, 22% were reported to be due to the belt restraint system. Some of these occupants were fatally injured, but the cause of death was not necessarily due to the abdominal injuries.

Table 2 shows the increasing use of lap-shoulder belts in the NASS file, in frontal crashes. The noted increase in cases in the 1985-86 period is most probably due to the general increase in belt use in the United States, for the mandatory belt use laws were enacted at about that time.

NASS CASES

There are many cases in the NASS files where the injury source for abdominal injuries are listed as "belt restraint webbing". Some examples of these are presented below:

Case 1

A 1984 BMW 4-door sedan was involved in a frontal crash with another car with a change in velocity (ΔV) of 40 mph. The 48 year old female belted passenger (168 cm, 64 kg) sustained a laceration of the upper digestive tract. (In the NASS files specifics as to the exact intraabdominal injuries are sparse). (77 042C '89)

Case 2

A similar injury as in case No. 1, involved a 33 year old male front seat passenger (152 cm, 45 kg). A 1984 Subaru that was involved in a head-on crash, struck a 2-door coupe head-on at a ΔV of 15 mph. (72 122E '89)

Case 3

A 1988 Toyota pick-up truck collided with another car. The ΔV was 19 mph. The 17 year old female front seat passenger (170 cm, unknown kg) sustained a liver laceration. (80 100C '89)

Case 4

A 1989 Chevrolet Spectrum struck another car head-on. The 63 year old lap-shoulder belted female passenger (157 cm, 76 kg) was killed, sustaining, among other injuries, a liver laceration. The ΔV of the crash was 23 mph. (82 001A '89)

Many more NASS case documented significant injuries to the liver, kidneys, abdominal wall, a variety of arterial lacerations, as well as lacerations of all parts of the abdominal digestive tract and the urinary bladder--all from "belt restraining webbing" coded as the injury source (Table 3).

Table 2
NASS- '80-89
Frontal Crashes
Lap Shoulder Belted Passenger Car
Front Outboard Occupants
with Abdominal Injury of AIS 2 or Greater

Contacts	80-84	85	86	87	88	89	Total
Belt Restraint Webbing	3	2	6	5	16	9	41
Other*	3	13	19	10	48	46	139
Total Lap-shoulder belted occs. in file	1334	1164	1359	620	1195	970	6642

* Primarily steering wheel rim or hub, or (injury source) unknown. A few cases of side interior contact were identified.

MECHANISM OF INJURY

As the unrestrained driver moves forward and impacts the steering wheel in frontal crashes, or the front passenger impacts the instrument panel, so can the intraabdominal organs be disrupted due to forceful contact of the anterior abdominal wall with the webbing of a restraint system. Intraabdominal injuries, sustained by occupants wearing lap-shoulder belts occur for a variety of reasons. The lap portion of the 3-point belt restraint may be inappropriately positioned on the anterior abdominal wall prior to collision. Also there is a phenomena known as "submarining" where the individual moves forward and downward in the seat, thus changing the relationship of the lap portion of the belt and the anatomical anchor points--the anterior superior iliac spines--to an area higher on the abdominal wall. A shallow angle of the lap-portion of the restraint, combined with a too compliant seat, or a seat cushion with a low coefficient of friction, may play a role in the submarining event [27,30]. The shoulder portion of the restraint can directly load the liver, spleen or upper abdominal organs. The preflexed lumbar spine (sitting slumped) that allows pelvic rotation also can play a role in belt-to-pelvis displacement. Additionally, the shoulder portion of the belt may also "lift" the lap section of the restraint off of its proper pelvic location and onto the soft abdominal wall. Also heavy clothing may hinder proper belt placement [16].

Even with an appropriately positioned lap-shoulder belt, as indicated by belt markings on the chest and abdomen, the internal organs attempt to continue to move forward on vehicle deceleration. This inertial loading of the abdominal contents can cause injury even with the belt in the proper location [59]. Thus, there can be a tearing of the mesentery, or even of hollow viscera, due to the forward movement of these organs along with the bulging of the anterior abdominal wall. Increase in the intraabdominal pressure by the belt may be related to organ displacements as well as injuries due to direct organ-to-organ contact. Ryan and Ragazzon postulated that the lap portion of the system, when improperly worn, caused direct or shearing injury of the viscera, with diaphragmatic injuries, due to increased intraabdominal pressure [45].

Christophi, et al described three injury mechanisms of the jejunum and ileum, depending on the type of damage noted to the small bowel [13]. Their injury mechanism categories are deceleration, crush and transmitted forces ("blowout").

Compression impacts using rhesus monkey liver and kidneys in controlled laboratory studies (high speed testing machine with controlled ram velocity) were conducted by Melvin, et al [36]. The rate of loading was found to be an important factor, especially for liver injuries. The more serious liver injuries were produced at 45 psi. Kidneys failed at higher levels, probably due to the thicker renal capsule. Trollope, et al using squirrel, monkeys, rhesus monkeys and baboons, found a positive relationship between animal mass, duration of impact, the force and the surface area of the object impacted [56]. Liver injury biomechanics studies, i.e., impacts to steering wheels using swine surrogates, have been conducted by Lau, et al [29]. Injury occurred within the initial 15 ms of wheel contact, exceeding a combined velocity and compression sensitive tolerance limit. Anesthetized mongrel dogs were subjected to pendulum impacts. Flank impacts produced an increased incidence of hepatic and renal injuries. Only a small force was required to produce mesenteric injury [10]. Studies of the belt restraints in pregnant baboons have been documented by King, et al. [26]. In human cadaver impact studies, belt related intraabdominal injuries have also been noted [31]. Additional studies and a review of the literature has been presented by Mertz [37].

CONCLUSIONS

From our experience no redesign of contract areas in the occupant compartment will prevent or eliminate all injuries, although reduction in injury frequency and severity has been noted to almost all body areas by the use of restraints and redesign of the interior of the automobile.

Table 3
NASS Data-Frontal Crashes
Abdominal Lap-Shoulder Belt Injury Cases
Related to "Belt Restraint Webbing"

Vehicle	Occ.	Age/Sex	Vehicle	Occ.	Age/Sex
'89 Chevrolet Caprice	DR	33-M	'85 Pontiac T-1000	DR	35-M
'87 Ford Ranger PU	DR	34-M	'87 Nissan PU	FR	43-F
'87 Hyundai Excel	DR	22-F			
'86 Toyota Corolla	DR	37-F	'85 Pontiac J-2000	FR	22-M
'84 BMW	FR	48-F	'82 Oldsmobile Delta 88	DR	52-M
'76 Oldsmobile Cutlass	FR	14-M	'83 Chevrolet Chevette	FR	74-F
'84 Subaru	FR	33-F	'79 Ford Thunderbird	DR	20-F
'88 Toyota PU	FR	17-F	'85 Chevrolet Caprice	DR	47-F
'89 Chevrolet Spectrum	FR	63-F			
			'83 Pontiac 6000	DR	27-M
'82 Pontiac T-1000	FR	77-F	'87 Plymouth Caravelle	DR	19-F
'89 Chevrolet Cavalier	DR	32-M	'82 Chevrolet Malibu	FR	8-F
'87 Audi 4000	DR	53-F	'86 Honda Accord	DR	23-F
'84 Toyota Corolla	FR	17-M	'84 Buick LaSabre	FR	57-M
'87 Honda Civic	FR	14-M	'80 Mazda GLC	DR	30-M
'76 Ford Mustang PU	DR	58-M			
'80 Chevrolet Caprice	FR	88-F	'78 Cadillac Deville	DR	26-M
'84 Nissan 810	FR	12-F	'81 Plymouth Horizon	FR	61-F
'84 Chevrolet Blazer	FR	19-M			
'85 Dodge Lancer	DR	40-F	'80 Oldsmobile Cutlass	FR	30-F
'88 Mercury Cougar	DR	59-F			
'83 Plymouth Horizon	FR	19-F	'75 VW Rabbit	DR	17-M
'84 Dodge Colt	FR	23-F			
'79 VW Rabbit	DR	16-M	'79 Chevrolet Suburban	FR	38-F

Lap-shoulder belts reduce the frequency of the more serious injuries, especially in frontal car crashes. However, the 3-point restraints are related to intraabdominal injuries in some car crashes for a variety of reasons--positioning of the belt on the belly wall, submarining, or inertial loading of the organs. In addition the shoulder section can load the lower torso, cause rib fractures and associated trauma to the liver or other upper abdominal organs. Generally, these injuries are sustained in the higher speed crashes.

We strongly urge the proper use of the lap-shoulder belt by all car occupants. The cases documented here should not be considered a reason for non belt use. In our investigations we have noted a decrease in injury frequency and severity of crash injuries, directly related to belt use.

BIBLIOGRAPHY

1. American Association for Automotive Medicine, *The Abbreviated Injury Scale (AIS)-1990 Revision.* Des Plaines, IL 1990.

2. Anonymous, "Seat Belt Injuries", Br Med J, 3:4-5, 1968.

3. Appel, H, Vu-Han, V, Adomeit, D, "Misfunctions of Safety Belts Unavoidable and Avoidable Injuries", IRCOBI, pp. 27-40, Lyon, France, Sept., 1978.

4. Appleby, JP, Nagy, AG, "Abdominal Injuries Associated With the Use of Seatbelts", Am J Surg, 157: 457-458, 1989.

5. Arajarvi, E, Santavirta, S, Tolonen, J, "Abdominal Injuries Sustained in Severe Traffic Accidents by Seatbelt Wearers", J Trauma, 27:393-397, 1987.

6. Asbun, HJ, Irani, H, Roe, EJ, et al, "Intra-abdominal Seatbelt Injury", J Trauma, 30:189-193, 1990.

7. Backwinkel, KD, "Seat-Belt Injuries", Lawyers Med J, 5:397-405, 1970.

8. Baker, AR, Perry, EP, Fossard, D.P., "Traumatic Rupture of the Stomach Due to a Seat Belt", Injury, 17:47-48, 1986.

9. Banerjee, A, "Seat Belts and Injury Patterns: Evolution and Present Perspectives", Postgrad Med J, 65:199-204, 1989.

10. Baxter, CF, Williams, RD, "Blunt Abdominal Trauma", J Trauma, 1:241, 1961.

11. Bergqvist, D, Dahlgren, S, Hedelin, H, "Rupture of the Diaphragm in Patients Wearing Seatbelts", J Trauma, 18:781-783, 1978.

12. Buxton, B, "Rupture of the Duodenum Produced by a Safety Belt", Aust N Z J of Surg, 38:315-320, 1969.

13. Christophi, C, McDermott, FT, McVey, I, et al, "Seat Belt--Induced Trauma to the Small Bowel", World J Surg, 9:794-797, 1985.

14. Clyne, CAC, Ashbrooke, EA, "Seat-belt Aorta: Isolated Abdominal Aortic Injury Following Blunt Trauma", Br J Surg, 72:239, 1985.

15. Denis, R, Allard, M, Atlas, H, et al, "Changing Trends with Abdominal Injury in Seatbelt Wearers", J Trauma, 23:1007-1008, 1983.

16. Gallup, BM, St-Laurent, AM, Newman, JA, "Abdominal Injuries to Restrained Front Seat Occupants in Frontal Collisions", Proc. 26th Am Assn for Auto Med, pp 131-145, 1982.

17. Garrett, JW, Braunstein, PW, "The Seat Belt Syndrome", J Trauma, 2:220-238, 1961.

18. Green, RN, Nowak, ES, Thomas, LS, "Investigation of Injury Mechanisms Associated with Fully Restrained Passenger Vehicle Occupants in London, Ontario", Proc 21st Am Assn for Auto Med, pp 127-145, 1977.

19. Green, RN, German, A, Gorski, ZM, et al, "Improper Use of Occupant Restraints: Case Studies From Real-World Collisions", Proc 30th Am Assn for Auto Med, pp 423-438, 1986.

20. Hamilton, JB, "Seat-belt Injuries", Br Med J, 23:485-486, 1968.

21. Hudson, I, Kavanagh, TG, "Duodenal Transection and Vertebral Injury Occurring in Combination in a Patient Wearing a Seat Belt", Injury, 15:6-9, 1983.

22. Huelke, DF, Sherman, HW, Murphy, MJ, "Severe to Fatal Injuries to Lap-Shoulder Belted Car Occupants", SAE Int Auto Eng Cong and Expo, SAE #770149, 1977.

23. Huelke, D, "Death and Injuries Prevented by Lap-Shoulder Belt Usage in the United States", '70 Int Symposium on Seat Belts in Tokyo, Japan, pp. 159-162, 1979.

24. Jensen, AJ, Johnsen, T, "Fire Tilfaelde Af Sikkerhedsselelaesioner", Ugeskr Laeger, 139:1595-1596, 1977.

25. Johnstone, BR, Waxman, BP, "Transverse Disruption of the Abdominal Wall--A Tell-Tale Sign of Seat Belt Related Hollow Viscus Injury", N Z J Surg, 57:455-460, 1987.

26. King, AI, Crosby, WM, Stout LC, et al., "Effects of Lap Belt and Three-Point Restraints on Pregnant Baboons Subjected to Deceleration", Proc 15th Stapp Car Crash Conf, pp. 68-81,1971.

27. Kramer, F, "Abdominal and Pelvic Injuries of Vehicle Occupants Wearing Safety Belts Incurred in Frontal Collisions- Mechanism and Protection", Proc IRCOBI, pp 297-308, Berlin, Germany, 1991.

28. LeGay, D A, Petrie, DP, Alexander, DI, "Flexion-distraction Injuries of the Lumbar Spine and Associated Abdominal Trauma", J Trauma, 30:436-444, 1990.

29 Lau, IV, Horsch, JD, Viano, DC, et al, "Biomechanics of Liver Injury by Steering Wheel Loading", J Trauma, 27:225-235, 1987.

30 Leung, YC, Tarriere, C, Lestrelin, D, et al, "Submarining Injuries of 3 Pt. Belted Occupants in Frontal Collisions-- Description, Mechanisms and Protection", Proc 26th Stapp Car Crash Conf, pp 173-201, 1982.

31 Levine, RS, Patrick, LM, "Injury Assessment of Unembalmed Cadavers Using A Three Point Harness Restraint", Proc 19th Conf Am Assn for Auto Med, pp 80-92, 1975.

32 Ljungstom, K, "Skador Pa Bukvaggsmuskulatur Och Viscera Av Bilbalten", Lakartonngen, 75:1410-1412, 1978.

33 Lubbers, EJC, "Injury of the Duodenum Caused by a Fixed Three-Point Seatbelt", J Trauma, 17:960-963, 1977.

34 MacLeod, JH, & Nicholson, DM, "Seat-Belt Trauma to the Abdomen", Can J Surg, 12:202-206, 1969.

35 Mandelbaum, I, Enderle, FJ, "Seat Belt Injuries", J Indiana State Med Assoc, 63:340-342, 1970.

36 Melvin, J.W., Stalnaker, RL, Roberts, VL, et al, "Impact Injury Mechanisms in Abdominal Organs", Proc 17th Stapp Car Crash Conf, pp 115-126, 1973.

37 Mertz, HJ, Kroell, CK, "Tolerance of Thorax and Abdomen", Impact Injury and Crash Protection, pp 372-401, Charles C. Thomas, publisher, 1970.

38 Mills, PJ Hobbs, CA, "The Probability of Injury to Car Occupants in Frontal and Side Impacts", Proc 28th Stapp Car Crash Conf, pp 223-235, 1984.

39 Niederer, P, Walz, F Zollinger, U, "Adverse Effects of Seat Belts and Causes of Belt Failures in Severe Car Accidents in Switzerland During 1976", Proc 21st Stapp Car Crash Conf, pp 55-93, 1977.

40 Pedersen, S, Jansen, U, "Intestinal Lesions Caused by Incorrectly Placed Seat Belts", Acta Chir Scand 145:15-18, 1979.

41 Reid, AB, Letts, RM, Black, GB, "Pediatric Chance Fractures: Association With Intra-abdominal Injuries and Seatbelt Use", J Trauma, 30:384-391,1990.

42 Rouse, T, Collin, J, Daar, A, "Isolated Injury to the Intestine from Blunt Abdominal Injury", Injury, 16:131-133, 1984.

43 Rutledge, R, Thomason, M, Oller, D, et al, "The Spectrum of Abdominal Injuries Associated with the Use of Seat Belts", J Trauma, 31:820-826, 1991.

44 Ryan, GA, "The Performance of Seat Belts in Severe Crashes", Med J Aust 2:899-901, 1975.

45 Ryan, P, Ragazzon, R, "Abdominal Injuries in Survivors of Road Trauma Before and Since Seat Belt Legislation in Victoria", Aust N Z J Surg, 49:200-202, 1979.

46 Shennan, J, "Seat-Belt Injuries of the Left Colon", Br J Surg, 60:673-675, 1973.

47 Schneider, RC, Smith, WS, Grabb, WC, et al, "Lap Seat Belt Injuries; The Treatment of the Fortunate Survivor", Mich Med, 67:171-186, 1968.

48 Smith, WS, Kaufer, H, "Patterns and Mechanisms of Lumbar Injuries Associated with Lap Seat Belts", J Bone Jt Surg 51-A:239-254, 1969.

49 States, JD, Huelke, DF, Dance, M, et al, "Fatal Injuries Caused by Underarm Use of Shoulder Belts", J Trauma, 27: 740-745, 1987.

50 Stevenson, JH, "Severe Thoracic Intra-Abdominal and Vertebral Injury Occurring in Combination in a Patient Wearing a Seat Belt", Injury 10:321-323, 1979.

51 Sube, J, Ziperman, HH, McIver, WJ, "Seat Belt Trauma to the Abdomen", Am J Surg, 113:346-350, Mar. 1967.

52 Sund, C, "Sicherheitsgurt und Duodenalverletzung (Seat Belt & Duodenal Injury)", Mschr Unfallheilk, 76:528-530, 1973.

53 Tang, OT, Mir, A, Delamore, IW, "Unusual Presentation of Seat-Belt Syndrome", Br Med J, 4: 750, 1974.

54 Tolins, SH, "An Unusual Injury Due to the Seat Belt", J Trauma 4:397-399, 1964.

55 Trinca, GW Dooley, BJ, "The Effects of Seat Belt Legislation on Road Traffic Injuries", Aust N Z J Surg, 47:151-155, 1977.

56 Trollope, JL, Stalnaker, RL, McElhane, JH, et al, "The Mechanism of Injury in Blunt Abdominal Trauma", J Trauma 13:962-970, 1973.

57 Vellar, ID, Vellar, DJ, Mullany, CJ, "Rupture of the Bowel Due to Road Trauma", Med J Aust, i:694-696, 1976.

58 Wagner, AC, "Disruption of Abdominal Wall Musculature: Unusual Feature of Seat Belt Syndrome", Am J Roentgenol, 133:753-754, 1979.

59 Walfisch, G, Fayon, YC, Leung, C, et al, "Synthesis of Abdominal Injuries in Frontal Collisions with Belt-Wearing Cadavers Compared with Injuries Sustained by Real-Life Accident Victims", IVth IRCOBI, pp 151-159, 1979.

60 Walz, F, Niederer, P, Zollinger, U, et al., "Analysis of 115 Killed and 205 Severely Injured (OAIS≥ 2) Seat Belt Users", Proc 6th Int Assn Acc Traf Med, pp 393,406, 1977.

61 Williams, JS, "The Nature of Seat Belt Injuries", Proc 14th Stapp Car Crash Conf, pp. 43-65, 1970.

942205

Visocelastic Shear Responses of the Cadaver and Hybrid III Lumbar Spine

P. C. Begeman
Wayne State University

H. Visarius and L.-P. Nolte
Mueller Institute for Biomechanics

P. Prasad
Ford Motor Company

ABSTRACT

Due to the sparsity of cadaver lumbar shear stiffness data, tests on functional lumbar spinal units and a complete lumbar section (T12-L5) were done in both the anterior and posterior directions. Similar tests were performed on the Hybrid III lumbar spine for comparison.

Sixteen lumber motion segments were tested quasi-statically for their viscoelastic properties in a multi-directional (5-axis) spine machine. A hydraulic testing machine was used to carry out dynamic tests including cyclic tests at several rates of deformation (0.5 - 50 mm/sec) and relaxation tests (300 sec) to determine the associated viscoelastic properties in constrained and unconstrained modes. The specimens were then loaded to sufficient displacement to cause hard or soft tissue failures.

In the quasi-static tests the shear response was linear and the anterior stiffness (155 ± 90 N/mm) was found to be higher than posterior stiffness (104 ± 38 N/mm). In the relaxation tests the load decreased to approximately 60% of its peak value after 30 seconds. Moderate non-linearity was observed in cyclic loading with shear stiffness up to 750 N/mm, depending on the loading rate. Soft tissue only failures occurred in the unconstrained tests at 1290 N (0.5 mm/sec) and 1770 N (50 mm/sec) for anterior loading. Anterior constrained testing failures involved hard tissue at 2800 N and were not rate dependent. The Hybrid III spine elicited higher initial stiffness than cadaver specimens, but was comparable at shear loads greater than 500 N. It also had considerably greater hysteresis than cadaver specimens.

INTRODUCTION

During the last two decades a number of studies have dealt with the multi-directional *in vitro* stiffness of the cadaver lumbar spine. Initially focusing on the compressive and tensile axial behavior soon more advanced testing setups were developed to determine the three-dimensional rotational response of the spine. Although shear stiffness has been thought to be a principle requirement to maintain stability of the lumbar motion segment there are only a few studies on the spinal response in shear. Quasi-static *in vitro* data may be found in papers by Markolf (1972), Liu et al (1975), Panjabi et al (1977), Lin et al (1978), Berkson et al (1987), Edwards et al (1987), and McGlashen et al (1987). Only Liu et al (1975), analyzing vertebra-disc-vertebra units, isolated the shear stiffness from associated rotational stiffness by performing direct shear tests. Associated viscoelastic data on intervertebral discs from dynamic experiments are only available for rhesus monkey, Lantz et al (1980) and Kelley et al (1983). Moreover, there is no information in the literature on shear limit loads for motion segments at different rates of loading.

Advanced anthropometric test devices (ATD) are currently being used in crash testing and development. One of them, known as the Hybrid III dummy (Foster 1977), has instrumentation at the lumbosacral and thoracolumbar junctions to measure forces and moments developed at these locations during restraint systems testing. Whether restrained humans would also experience such loads in similar crash situations depends on the biofidelity of the lumbar spine used in the crash test dummy. The biofidelity of the lumbar spine in dummies has not been established, especially when subjected to shear loading.

The purpose of this study was (1) to test quasi-statically and dynamically cadaver lumbar spine motion segments in direct antero-posterior shear in order to determine the associated elastic and viscoelastic material properties, (2) to perform similar experiments on a Hybrid III dummy to evaluate the biofidelity of the lumbar spine, (3) to develop specifications for a biofidelic dummy lumbar spine, and (4) to determine the cadaver tolerance to direct shear by means of destructive testing.

MATERIALS AND METHODS

This study is based on sixteen lumbar functional spinal units (FSU, defined as two adjacent vertebrae and all interconnecting ligamentous soft tissues) obtained from donated human cadavers. The average age at the time of death was 51 ranging from 35 to 62 years. The distribution of the FSUs tested were as follows: one at the level L1-L2, one at L2-L3, 9 at L3-L4, and 5 at L4-L5. A specific FSU was used for one quasi-static test, one dynamic test, and one destructive test. These tests are explained below. In addition, one complete lumbar spine (T12-L5) was tested. The results reported here assume that the properties in shear at each level are approximately the same and are considered in total as properties of the lumbar spine. Within the population of the specimens, age, sex, and physical parameters (height and weight) and not considered.

The data are reported is relative to a clinical coordinate system in which the positive X-axis is in the lateral direction to the left, the positive Y-axis is in the superior direction and the positive Z-axis is in the anterior direction.

Anterior shear is defined as a force applied to an upper vertebrae in the anterior direction while a posterior force is applied to the lower vertebrae.

SPECIMEN PREPARATION - It was important for this study to exclude anatomic abnormalities and severe degenerative changes, in particular disc space narrowing and gross osteophyte formation by means of two planar radiographs. The spines were stored in plastic bags at -20° Celsius and gradually thawed to room temperature prior to testing. All musculature and extra soft tissue was then removed. Various bony parts of each vertebrae had to be reinforced with sheet metal screws before embedding in quick-setting epoxy blocks to provide a stable fixation during high load-level destructive testing as shown in Figure 1. Scaled radiographs were used to ensure the proper orientation of the specimens. The mid-disc planes were aligned in order to match with the horizontal plane of the clinical coordinate system, see e.g. Panjabi (1977). Alignment of the mid-disc plane was done by measuring the tilt angles of the disc relative to the inferior mount block and then adjusting the mounting fixture to compensate.

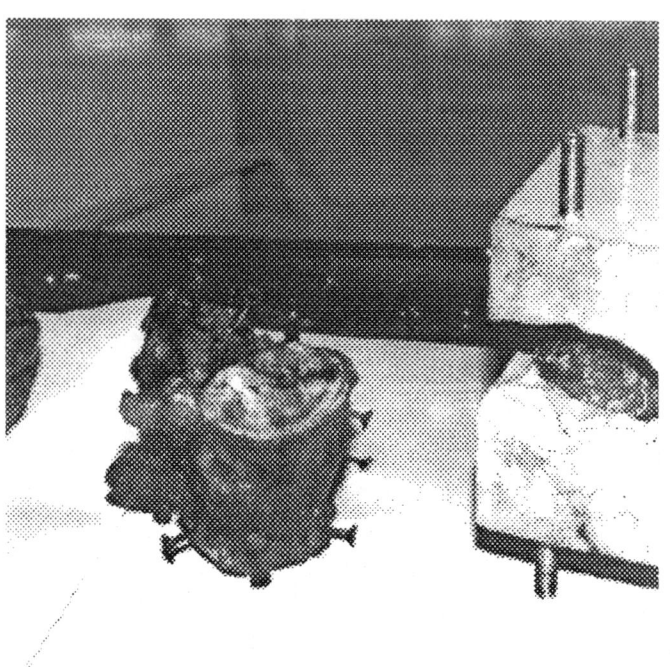

Figure 1: Specimen Preparation.

Each specimen was weighed before and after the molding of the upper vertebrae to allow for dead weight compensation of the molding blocks and fixturing during testing. A plexiglas marker carrier with three non-collinear marker points defined by light emitting diodes (LED) glued to it was rigidly fixed to the anterior surface of each epoxy block with sheet metal screws. The LED's were part of an OPTOTRAK displacement measuring system. A transformation between a local coordinate system located in the center of each upper vertebrae and any global system defined by the LEDs was established using two scaled planar radiographs of the spines. During an initial phase of specimen calibration this transformation was used to define the relative location of each marker point with respect to the center of shear for sagittal intervertebral motion. The lumbar spine of the studied anthropomorphic test device, the Hybrid III dummy, consists of a metal-rubber composite. Various adapter units, as shown in Figures 2 and 3, were designed for the proper fixation of the dummy spine to the testing setups.

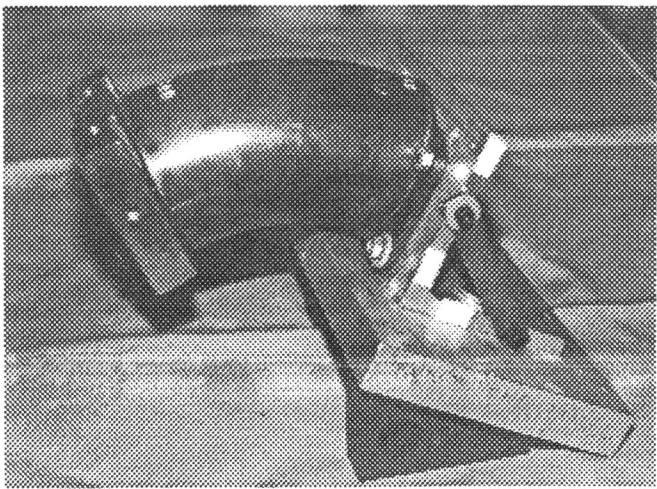

Figure 2: Total Hybrid III Lumbar Spine with Fixture.

NON-DESTRUCTIVE TESTING -
<u>Quasi-Static Loading</u> - For the quasi-static part of the non-destructive test series a multi-directional flexibility testing setup was used. This is a machine for precisely applying any of the six load components and is described in detail in Nowinski et al. (1993). Geometric and mass changes induced during the casting process of the specimens could be carefully compensated.

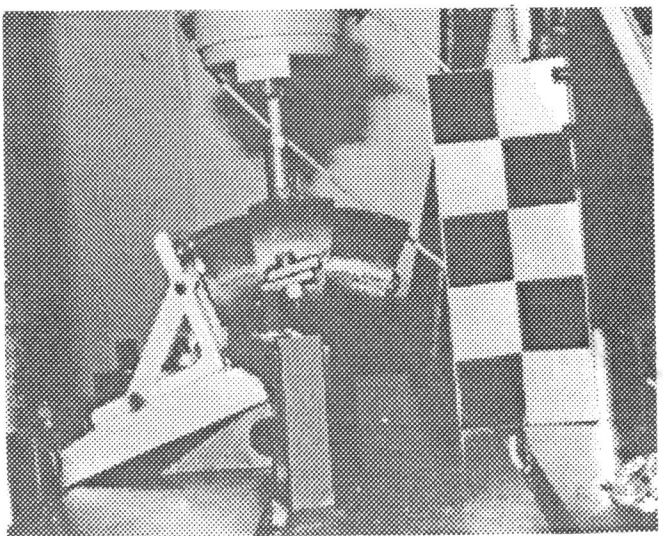

Figure 3: Hybrid III Lumbar Spine Segment Testing.

Before loading, the initial center of shear (COS) was determined experimentally by an iterative technique: The point of load application was manually altered until no rotation of the vertebral body could be measured (< 0.3 deg.) The COS was usually located within the intervertebral disk. Antero(+)-posterior(-) shear forces ($\pm FZ$) were then applied parallel to the mid-disc plane through the measured COS's via a top fixture which allowed for a variation of the point of loading in the vertical direction. Mechanically, this is the only way to isolate the antero-posterior shear stiffness from associated rotational and translational stiffness. Shear loads application at other points, i. e. above or below the COS would result in additional sagittal bending moments falsely implying a reduced or increased shear stiffness, respectively. Loading was applied under computer control using a system of pneumatic cylinders attached to the superior end of the FSU by cables and pulleys. Details are given in Nowinski et al. (1993). For a better characterization of the studied cadaveric material the following incremental moments were studied: flexion/extension ($\pm MX$), lateral bending ($\pm MZ$), and axial torque ($\pm MY$). Load magnitudes were chosen to be 150 N for the shear force and 15 Nm for each of the moments. Readings were taken 30 seconds after each load increment to account for creep effects. The rotational data allows these properties of the specimens to be compared to those of other investigators in order to "classify" these specimens.

For the single-level testing the total length of the Hybrid III dummy spine was subdivided into six levels, so that one-sixth of the lumbar spine would represent a FSU. This length (of the rubber spine) was approximately 40 mm. In this case the shear load was again applied parallel to the "mid-disc plane" defined at the lower one sixth of the arc-length of the composite column, orthogonal to the metal cables (see Figure 3).

For completeness comparative testing was performed on one complete lumbar spine specimen, T12-L5, and the entire lumbar spine of the dummy. In this case anterior and posterior shear forces ($\pm FZ$) were applied at the top of both lumbar spinal columns.

The motion of the upper vertebra was constraint-free, i.e. not affected by the load application. It was controlled by tracking the LEDs using an opto-electronic motion analysis system, OPTOTRAK 3D BAR (Northern Digital, Waterloo, Ontario, Canada).

Dynamic Loading - First, the information about the center of the shear gained in the quasi-static tests was transferred to the dynamic testing setup for proper adjustment of the point of load application. A custom-made loading-rig integrated into an INSTRON model 8500 material testing system (Instron Co, Canton, Massachusetts) allowed for constrained as well as constraint-free deformation of the spine specimen and the Hybrid III dummy (Figure 4). For constrained loading both ends of the spinal segment were rigidly attached to the testing machine, the inferior end to the bedplate and the superior end to the actuator, and hence the specimen was restrained from movement in every direction except the direction of applied loading. Constraint-free loading was realized by loading the superior end through a pair of mutually perpendicular linear bearings, and hence the superior end of the specimen was free to move in all directions.

The testing protocol for both the spine specimens and the Hybrid III dummy spine consisted of:

(a1) Anterior Relaxation Test
(a2) Posterior Relaxation Test
(b1) Anterior Cyclic Loading
(b2) Posterior Cyclic Loading

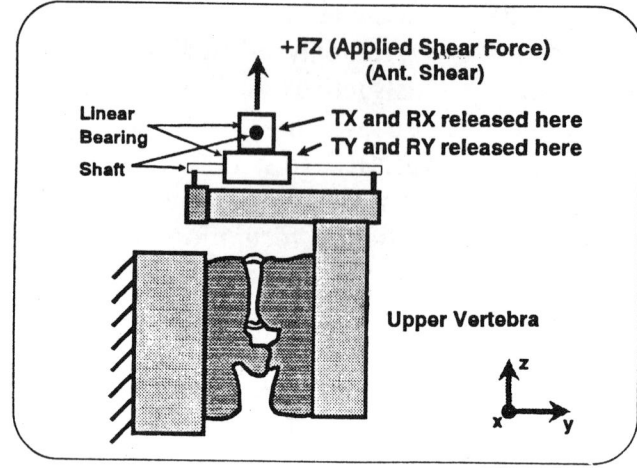

Figure 4: Constraint-free Dynamic Testing Setup.

The time period for the relaxation tests was chosen to be 300 sec with an initial displacement of 1.5 mm imposed with a linear ramp of 100 mm/sec to avoid significant initial relaxation. That is, for these tests, the specimen was displaced 1.5 mm in 15 ms and held at that displacement for 300 seconds while the force applied to the specimen is recorded. In the cyclic test series the specimens were tested at different loading rates: (a) 0.5 mm/sec, (b) 5 mm/sec, and (c) 50 mm/sec, again, with an amplitude of 1.5 mm. They were repetitively loaded for 10 cycles at a constant rate at each of the above mentioned rates, i.e. the displacement was a triangular waveform with an amplitude from zero to 1.5 mm.

DESTRUCTIVE TESTING - Cadaver spine specimens were loaded to sufficient displacements to cause hard or soft tissue failure in anterior direction only. Before testing, three stem type LED based markers were inserted into each vertebra using PMMA for fixation. By this method the motion of each vertebra could tracked and compared to the motion of the rigid epoxy blocks. Thus, failure of the fixation (detachment of the embedded vertebra from the epoxy) could be quantified, an important aspect at higher load levels. In order to provide a direct comparison to the resulting *in vitro* data the Hybrid III lumbar spine was tested in a single-level mode as outlined before. Spinal motion in destructive testing was not constrained. Two different loading rates, the slow 0.5 mm/sec and the fast rate 50 mm/sec were analyzed.

In a few destructive tests the pressure in the nucleus pulposus was measured by means of a miniature pressure transducer mounted in a hypodermic needle which was inserted into the disk.

RESULTS

For both the quasi-static and dynamic test series our molding technique has proven to be reliable. Only one specimen showed significant relative motion between the vertebra and the epoxy resin and was excluded from the data analysis. Pathology following the testing procedure did not indicate any further degenerative changes.

The resulting three-dimensional coordinates of all vertebral markers were further transformed to derive the associated three rigid body translations (TX, TY, TZ) and three rigid body rotations (RX, RY, RZ) by means of stereo-photogrammetric algorithms. For this purpose a rigid body attached coordinate system was defined in the center of shear. The software package Systat (Systat Inc., Evanston, Illinois, USA) was used for the statistical analysis.

NON-DESTRUCTIVE TESTING -
<u>Quasi-Static Loading</u> - First, comparative testing performed on one complete lumbar spine specimen T12-L5 and the composite dummy spine (which shall reflect the properties of T12-L5) was analyzed. The results for the translational motion at the top of both lumbar spinal columns in the direction of the applied force ±FZ are shown in Figure 5. It was very difficult to apply the force through the center of shear for the entire lumbar spine (especially in the *sequence* of the loading) with the result that the anterior shear test included a significant amount of flexion of the upper vertebrae (>12°) and the posterior shear test showed extension of the upper vertebrae (>7°). This might also explain the result that the anterior deformation was significantly larger than the posterior deformation in contrast to the expectation of higher anterior spinal stiffness set by the anatomic analysis. From the significant differences for the lumbar stiffness it can be easily seen that a muscle-free *in vitro* model cannot be used for the design and/or validation of the lumbar spine construct of an anthropomorphic test device. For this reason the multilevel test series was not extended further.

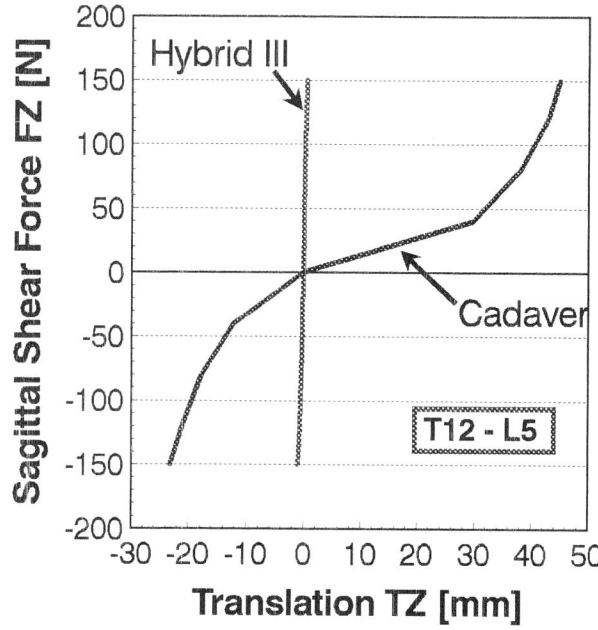

Figure 5: Comparative Multilevel Spine Shear Stiffness.

Twelve specimens were used for single-level tests. The initial center of shear was found to be located on the intersection of the sagittal and the mid-disc plane for the studied planar motion. This position did not change significantly during loading, in static as well as in dynamic mode, with measured sagittal rotations averaging 0.3°. In contradiction to the non-linear load-deformation relations obtained for the rotational motions, as depicted by the s-shaped curves in Figure 6, the antero-posterior translation was almost a linear function of the applied shear force in the quasi-static tests, implying a significant shear stiffness in the neutral, nonloaded position. Associated

Table 1: Shear stiffness in the quasi-static tests (N/mm)

Spec	1	2	3	4	5	6	7	8	9	10	11	12	Mean	SD
Ant	155	78	97	313	113	125	199	53	277	114	160	180	155	77
Post	104	98	140	108	124	110	136	54	37	129	95	113	104	31

Table 2: Comparison for shear test data

Author	Year	Force N	Displacement Ant/Post (mm)	Stiffness Ant/Post (N/mm)	Comments
Markolf*	1972	150	0.4/-	375/-	no post. elem.
Liu	1975	150	1.25/-	120/-	
Panjabi*	1976	150	3.2/1.2	47/125	
Lin*	1978	133	0.2-0.7/-	190-665/-	
Berkson*	1979	86	0.6/0.59	143/146	400 N preload
		145	0.85/1.21	171/120	400 N preload
Edwards*	1987			394/260	Var. preloads
McGlashen*	1987	160	2.05/2.21	78/72	
			4.26/3.54	38/45	no post. elem.
Janevic*	1991	160	1.35/1.03	119/155	
This Study	1994	150	0.97/1.44	155/104	Human FSU
This Study	1994	150	0.38/0.28	395/536	Hybrid III

*Specimen not loaded in the center of shear

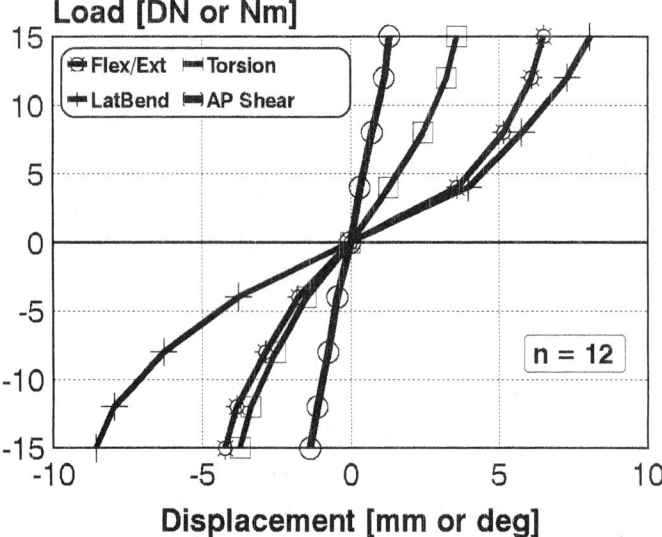

Figure 6: Average Quasi-static Response of Lumbar Functional Spinal Units.

average incremental load-deformation paths are shown in Figure 6.

Shear stiffness for all the specimens is given in Table 1. Analyzing differences in anterior and posterior direction it was found that the average anterior stiffness (155±90 N/mm) was higher than the average posterior stiffness (104±38 N/mm). Note also, that the standard deviation for the posterior stiffness is much smaller than for the anterior stiffness, identical to the findings of McGlashen (1987). A possible reason for this could be that in some of the specimens minor contact stresses in the facet joints could already be activated under the loads chosen, depending on the intersegmental stiffness and the geometry of the articular facets (Lin, 1978). Significant facet contact, indicated

Table 3: Relaxation force after 300 seconds (30 seconds) in % of the initial peak value.

SPEC	1	2	3	8	9	10	11	13	15	16	Mean
ANT	43 (60)	49 (63)	50 (63)	36 (42)	46 (52)	42 (62)	42 (64)	52 (62)	48 (60)	43 (57)	45 (4.5) 59 (6.4)
POST	54 (64)	47 (58)	57 (60)	53 (62)	53 (65)	51 (72)	43 (56)	49 (61)	45 (56)	40 (54)	49 (5.1) 61 (5.1)

by associated sagittal rotation +RX, was not observed in this test series. It was found that specimens with increased or decreased rotational stiffness did not in general show increased or decreased shear stiffness.

A comparison of the measured average *in vitro* shear stiffness with associated data from the single-level test of the Hybrid III dummy is given in Figure 7. The dummy spine had a significantly higher stiffness at lower load levels approaching more and more to the *in vitro* stiffness at higher load levels.

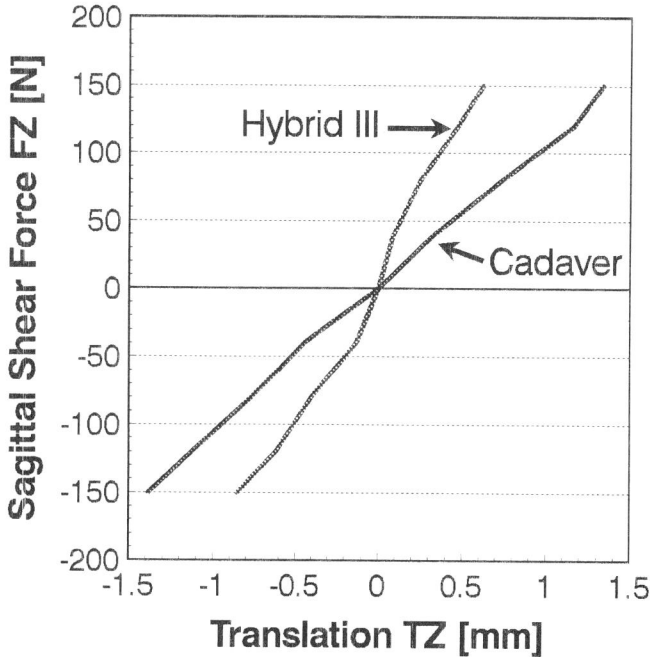

Figure 7: Quasi-static Single Level Response of the Hybrid III Compared to the Average Human Specimen.

Comparison of these data with results found in the literature is give in Table 2 (Publications are indicated by first author only). In many experiments the shear load was applied at the superior vertebra, leading to a combined loading situation (anterior shear and flexion, posterior shear and extension) as explained previously. This explains the higher deflections in anterior shear, which would be the result of flexion. Some authors removed the posterior elements prior to testing and thus altered the shear properties of their specimens (Lin et al, 1978, Asano et al, 1992). Adams and Hutton (1983) as well and Miller et al (1983) showed the importance of the apophyseal joints in general and for shear loads in particular. Markolf (1972) and McGlashen et al (1987) reported a linearity in the shear deformation and a significant initial static shear stiffness.

Dynamic Loading - Ten of the sixteen specimens were used in the relaxation and cyclic loading tests. In the relaxation tests a rapid load decrease to approximately 45 or 49% of the initial peak value was observed for the anterior and posterior directions, respectively (Figure 8. To further quantify the load decrease, the load at t=30 sec is also given in Table 3 (lower number in parentheses). It can be observed that the major share of the load decrease (to approximately 60% of the initial peak value) took part within the first 30 seconds after imposing a constant displacement of 1.5 mm.

Figure 8 also includes the anterior relaxation response of the Hybrid III lumbar spine. It can be assumed that the particular rubber content in the ATD is primarily responsible for the immediate force drop during the first ten seconds. At this time, the Hybrid III spine contains only 55% of its initial load peak, while the human specimen still holds approximately 75%. Especially in high speed tests, this might account for the large initial stiffness observed in the dummy tests. Furthermore, a larger amount of energy

Table 4: Peak loads (N) at 1.5 mm displacement

Rate	SPEC	1	2	3	8	9	10	11	12	13	15	16	Mean
0.5 mm/s	ANT	495	270	496	110	110	650	495	355	471	222	392	370 (166)
	POST	190	250	370	160	210	309	383	225	400	210	389	281 (86)
5.0 mm/s	ANT	530	310	520	125	115	710	561	428	482	261	460	409 (178)
	POST	210	260	420	175	255	319	394	246	419	245	425	306 (89)
50 mm/s	ANT	560	310	510	150	122	730	598	441	468	241	470	418 (183)
	POST	208	279	396	190	268	328	396	255	391	236	447	308 (83)

dissipation in a cyclic test as displayed by the hysteresis loop can be expected. However, the long term values (G(t=300 sec)) for the dummy spine are similar to the average human response (42% anterior, 48% posterior).

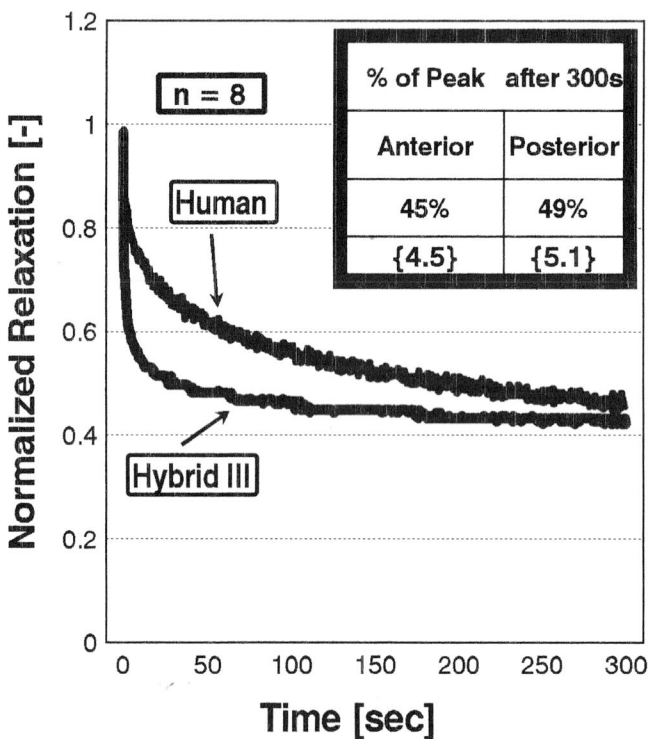

Fig. 8: A Typical Relaxation Test.

In cyclic loading the cadaveric spines showed a nonlinear behavior with load-displacement paths of sigmoid shape, as shown in Figures 9 and 10. The load-deflection curves followed the phase model as described by several authors (Rigby, 1959, Lanir, 1980, Sauren, 1983). After an initial linear phase of deformation a nonlinear transition phase was observed, beginning in the range of 0.4-1.5 mm translational motion. This indicates a redistribution in the load sharing between elastin and collagen fibers. Thus, the elastin, the transitional, and the collagen phase (Sauren, 1983) were observed. In order to compare the cyclic tests of the specimens the peak loads were reported for the anterior and posterior direction as well as for all loading rates in order to detect a possible loading rate dependency (Table 4).

It was observed that in most of the specimens the peak loads increased with the increase in loading rate (Figure 9). Peak loads in the anterior direction were found to be larger than in the posterior direction for all specimens. This finding coincides with the higher anterior stiffness found in the quasi-static tests. It is hypothesized that minor contact stresses in the facet joints can explain this phenomenon.

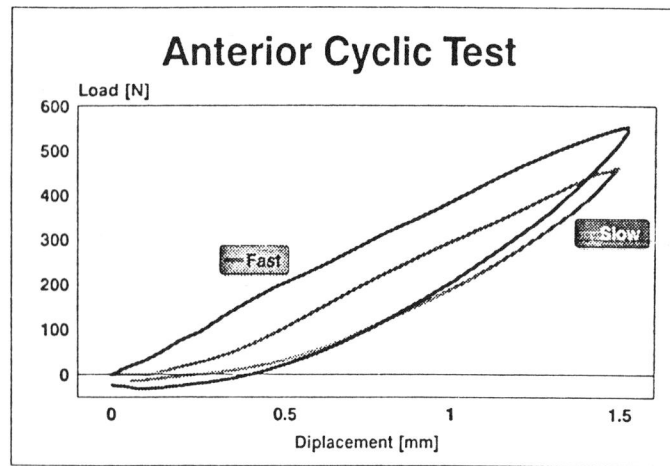

Fig. 9: Typical Cadaver FSU in an Anterior Cyclic Shear Test.

Table 5: Peak loads (N) at 1.5 mm displacement for the Hybrid III

Rate (mm/sec)	0.5	5	50
ANT	717	902	938
POST	785	922	938

Table 6: Hysteresis (% of total energy) for cadaver specimens (cycle 2(10))

Rate	SPEC	1	2	3	8	9	10	11	12	13	15	16	Mean (SD)
0.5 mm/s	ANT	34 (30)	31 (28)	27 (25)	28 (27)	21 (16)	33 (28)	30 (30)	38 (34)	36 (32)	27 (26)	44 (40)	32 (6.0) (29 (5.7))
	POST	23 (25)	18 (16)	25 (29)	26 (23)	26 (28)	24 (21)	41 (37)	23 (22)	20 (20)	23 (19)	31 (30)	25 (5.9) (24 (5.7))
5.0 mm/s	ANT	32 (28)	27 (25)	24 (22)	31 (29)	24 (23)	35 (26)	31 (31)	38 (35)	31 (28)	28 (26)	36 (34)	31 (4.4) (28 (3.9))
	POST	24 (25)	19 (17)	27 (28)	28 (25)	25 (23)	24 (20)	43 (38)	-	23 (20)	24 (21)	30 (29)	27 (6.1) (25 (5.7))
50 mm/s	ANT	48	42	42	57	42	37	-	50	49	50	53	47 (5.8)
	POST	55	46	49	63	45	41	56	36	35	37	48	47 (8.6)

Table 7: Hysteresis (% of total energy) for the Hybrid III (cycle 2 (10))

Rate (mm/sec)	0.5	5.0	50
ANT	37 (37)	42 (42)	59
POST	34 (34)	39 (42)	58

The peak loads for the Hybrid III in a single level test were higher than the corresponding loads for the cadaver FSUs. The data are shown in Table 5. The rate dependency of the peak loads is obvious. The dummy spinal segment also does not have a preferred direction of increased stiffness as it changes with loading rate.

In Figure 10 the response of a typical cadaver lumbar motion segment is compared with the dummy spine for one anterior loading cycle at the medium rate of deformation (5 mm/sec) and an amplitude of 1.5 mm. The dummy segment had a higher initial stiffness, reached a higher peak load, and showed more hysteresis, as could be expected from the larger force drop observed in the relaxation test.

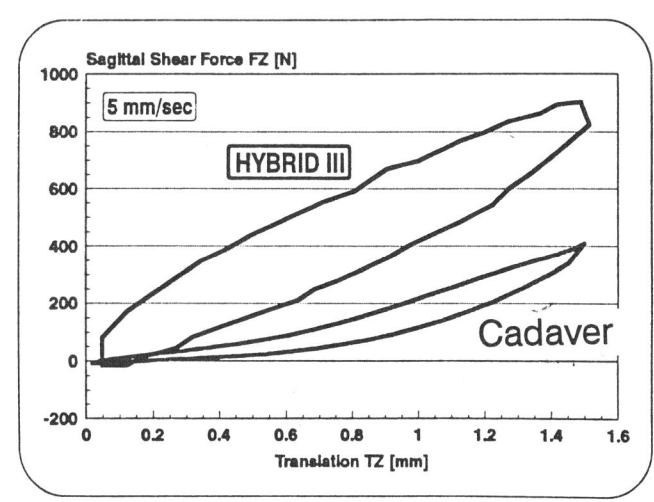

Figure 10: Comparative Loading Cycle for the Hybrid III Segment and a cadaver Single-level Specimen at 5 mm/sec Loading Rate.

Tables 6 and 7 show the percent of energy dissipated computed from the area of hysteresis loop for the cadaver specimen and the dummy, respectively. Especially at the highest loading rate the increase in energy dissipation is remarkable. The decrease of the hysteresis in the consecutive cycles of the human specimens was also noted by Liu et al (1975), Yahia et al (1993) and Viidik (1968).

DESTRUCTIVE TESTING - Anterior and posterior single-level tests on the Hybrid III dummy spine, as shown in Figure 3, were first carried out at higher load levels. Figures 11 and 12 show the rate-sensitive response of the single-level composite structure loaded to a displacement of ±4 mm. Note that the increase in intersegmental stiffness is more significant at higher rates of deformation. Due to the damping characteristics of the rubber-like material a high initial stiffness rate was observed. After this initial phase of approximately 1.5 mm the load-deflection curve is almost linear.

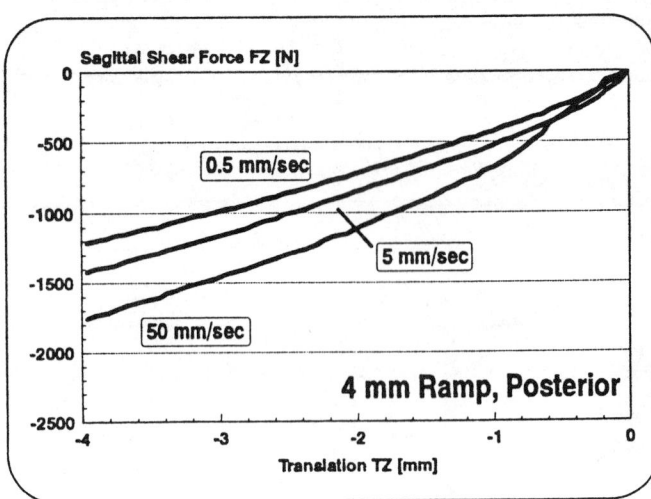

Figure 12: Response of the Hybrid III Lumbar Spine to Various Posterior Shear Loading Rates.

quasi-static tests, the dummy spine showed a larger initial stiffness while softening at higher loads. Note that the testing of the complete Hybrid III lumbar spine was performed with a deformation up to 10 mm and the tests of the single segments included deformations up to 4 mm. These limits were chosen in order to avoid permanent damage to the dummy spine.

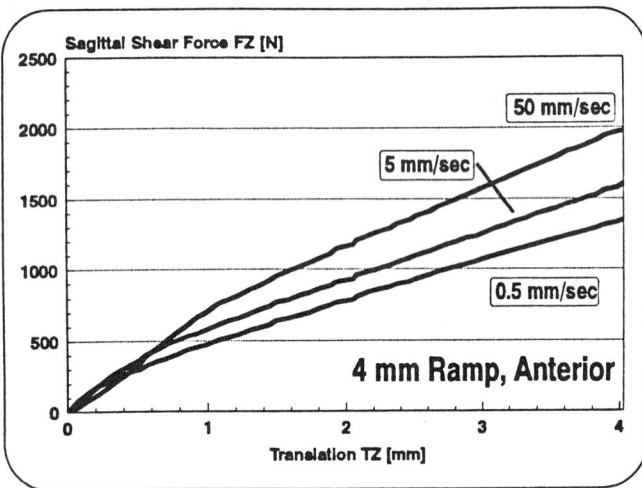

Figure 11: Response of the Hybrid III Lumbar Spine to Various Anterior Shear Loading Rates.

Destructive testing was conducted on thirteen out of the sixteen cadaveric specimens for four different test conditions. The four test conditions included constrained as well as unconstrained tests at slow (0.5 mm/sec) and fast (50 mm/sec) loading rates. Average results of the constrained and unconstrained tests are compared to the corresponding dummy data in Figures 13 and 14. As already seen in the

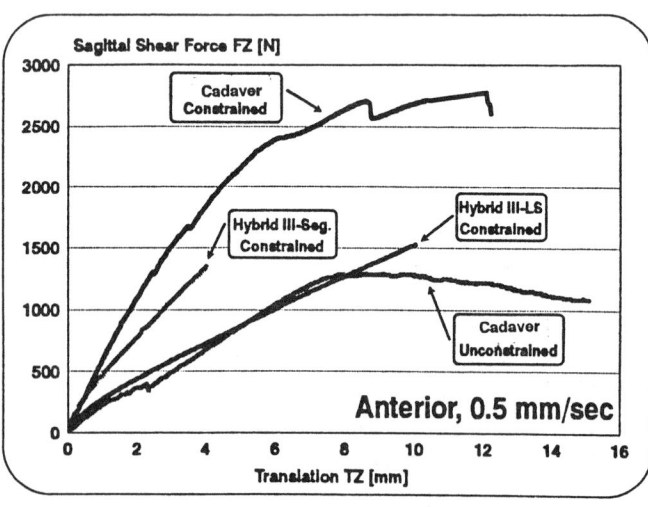

Figure 13: Comparison of Cadaver and Hybrid III Destructive Tests (0.5 mm/sec).

Table 8 summarizes the average failure loads and the corresponding translational (+TZ) and rotational (+RX) motions. The standard errors of the mean are given in parentheses. For completeness the translations

Table 8: Average failure loads and corresponding displacements

Rate (mm/s)	Cadaver Unconstrained			Cadaver Constrained			Hybrid III	
	FZ* (N)	TZ* (mm)	RX* (deg)	FZ* (N)	TZ* (mm)	RX* (deg)	TZ~ (mm)	RX (deg)
0.5	1292 (106)	8.48 (1.15)	14.5 (1.21)	2776 (390)	12.1 (0.68)	0	7.9	<2
50	1767 (460)	10.5 (0.33)	14.3 (1.9)	2894 (144)	10.7 (1.49)	0		

*Limit values, standard error in parentheses; ~For corresponding cadaver unconstrained load level

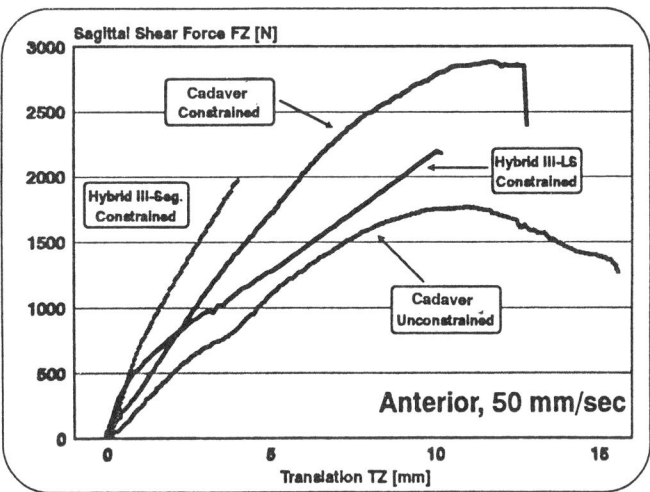

Figure 14: Comparison of Cadavaer and Hybrid III Destructive Tests (50 mm/sec).

and rotations of the dummy spine are given for equivalent load levels of the unconstrained human motion segment.

DISCUSSION

The complete cadaver lumbar spine was tested in shear as a comparison to the complete Hybrid III lumbar spine. The results showed that muscles and other torso tissues supply major rotational stiffness for the torso. In the ATD this torso stiffness is represented by the composite rubber lumbar spine. In addition shear response of the FSU for the ATD should be similar to the cadaver. It was not the purpose of this paper to compare the rotational properties of the two.

A comparison of data from the constrained and unconstrained tests shows that load response and peak loads attained were different. Constrained tests resulted in much higher loads than the unconstrained tests (Table 7). The performance of the Hybrid III segment is located in between the constrained and unconstrained test of the cadaver specimen for the low loading rate (Figure 13). However, its stiffness was higher than that of both average human specimens for the high loading rate (Figure 14). The load-deflection curve of the complete Hybrid III lumber spine matched quite well that of the average unconstrained human single-level specimen.

In the unconstrained tests on the human specimens, an analysis of the rigid body motion revealed that the motion was purely sagittal. A typical specimen response is shown in Figure 15. It can be seen that the sagittal rotation (RX) increased steadily while the other rigid body motions (RY, RZ) remain virtually unchanged.

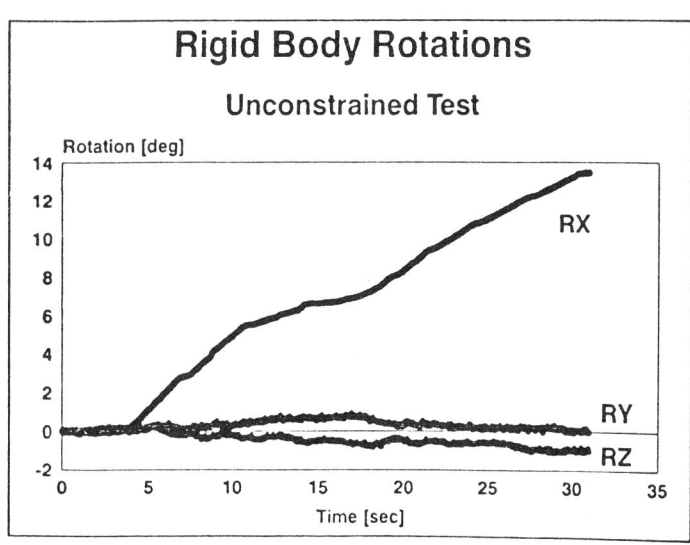

Figure 15: Rigid Body Rotations in an Unconstrained Test.

If this sagittal rigid body rotation is now investigated in comparison to the specimen force for the testing period, it can be observed that for a specific initial time range no sagittal rotation is present even though the loading has already started. It can be concluded that during this time period a pure translation takes place due to an initial, specimen-specific, gap between the facet joints (Figure 16). In the initial loading process the load-deflection curve had a concave shape, indicating soft tissue behavior with a low initial stiffness.

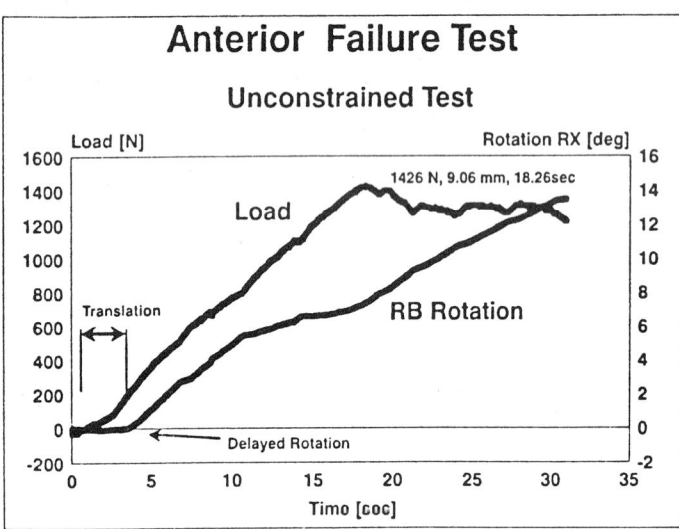

Figure 16: Failure Pattern in the Unconstrained Test.

After this translational phase the facet of the superior vertebra slipped over the inferior facet. This process left both facets intact and started a sagittal rotation which resulted in the complete failure of the posterior ligaments, termed a predominantly soft tissue failure. Pathologic examination revealed that tearing of the interspinous and supraspinous ligament as well as the ligamentum flavum were the predominant injuries. The facet capsules were torn while the bony structures remained intact and the anterior and posterior longitudinal ligaments were stretched. Injuries at the intervertebral disk included splitting and detachment from the bony end-plates.

The failure pattern in the constrained tests were different. As a sagittal rotation was prohibited, the superior vertebra was forced to move in a strictly translational fashion. This led to an audible breakage of the facet joints and a sudden increase in disk pressure, which will be denoted as hard tissue failure. Typical test results are given in Figure 17. This phenomenon supports the earlier findings by Yang and King (1984) that the load sharing was redistributed after failure of the facet joints. Note that the initial loading curve is convex shaped.

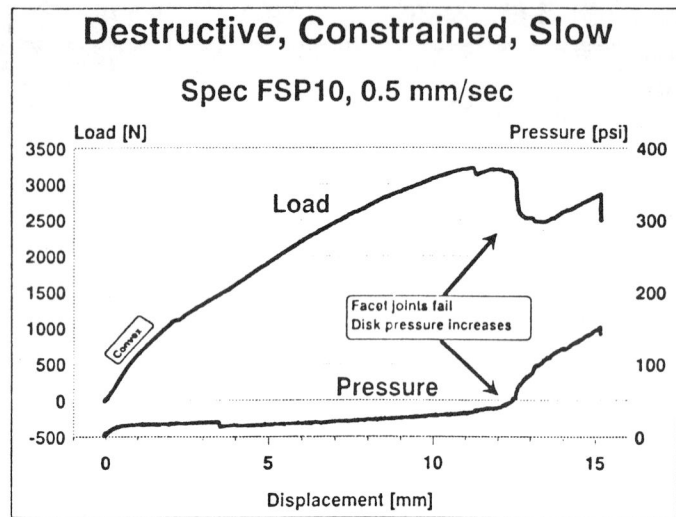

Figure 17: Constrained Destructive Test.

If the same test is repeated, it can be seen that the intervertebral disk is bearing the load without support from the facets, which fractured in the original test (Figure 18). The soft tissue loading curve is now concave and the disk pressure increases from the beginning of the test. The total failure load is now lower than in the original experiment.

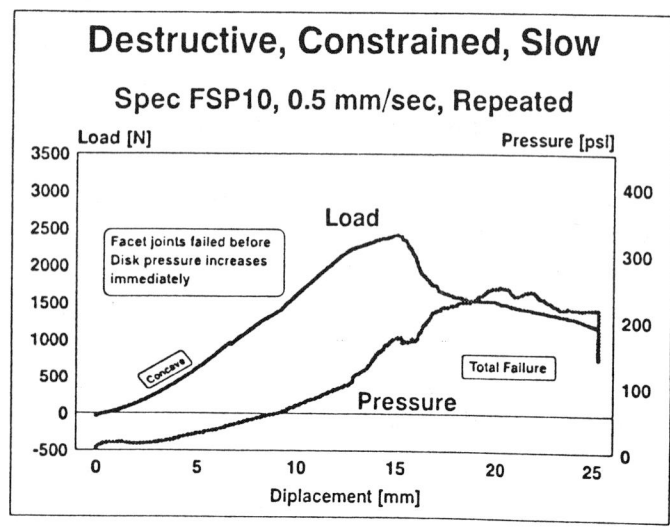

Figure 18: Repeated Constrained Destructive Test.

From the average failure loads it can be seen that soft tissue failure loads (unconstrained tests) were dependent on the loading rate, while hard tissue failure loads (constrained tests) were not. Under the assumption that the disk had none or only minor injuries from the preceding test, the average failure load of the disk alone (with facet joints already fractured and thus carrying no load) was found to be at 77% of the failure load of the original test. A facet failure occurred prior to a disk failure in all tests. These findings are comparable to those of Crowninshield and Pope (1976) and Lantz et al (1980). Adams and Hutton (1983) and Miller et al (1983) similarly reported high stresses occurring in the facet joints due to its load bearing role in shear.

From the displacement-load plots, such as Figure 7, it can be seen that there is no neutral zone in shear, i.e. stiffness is readily available even at low loads and displacements. Without this stiffness FSU's may be able to easily move in lateral and anterior/posterior directions relative to one another. This would make the spinal column a rather unstable structure. Shear stiffness plays a significant role in preventing or limiting these shearing motions and hence stabilizing the vertebral column.

CONCLUSIONS

The purpose of this investigation was to improve the current understanding of the behavior of the cadaver lumbar spine under shear loading. In order to achieve this goal, a quasi-static and a dynamic/destructive test setup were designed to conduct a comparative study of cadaver specimens and a dummy spine. Based on quasi-static and dynamic tests of isolated functional cadaver lumbar spine segments and the Hybrid III lumbar spine the following is concluded:

(1) An initial neutral zone, i. e. significant deformation at zero load level, was not observed in quasi-static shear tests. This is particularly relevant for cadaver specimens but, is true for Hybrid III also.

(2) For the cadaver specimens, the isolated quasi-static shear stiffness was substantially larger in the anterior direction (155 N/mm) than in the posterior direction (104 N/mm).

(3) The dynamic viscoelastic shear response of the cadaver data showed typical characteristics of soft tissue behavior in relaxation and rate dependencies. The stiffness increased more than 37% with increasing loading rates between 0.5 and 50 mm/sec.

(4) Hybrid III spine showed significantly greater initial stiffness than cadaver specimens, but had a comparable performance at shear loads greater than 500 N.

(5) Stiffness, peak loads, and hysteresis were found to be greater in anterior than in posterior direction for quasi-static as well as dynamic loading modes for cadaver specimens.

(6) Facet contact in the cadaver specimens could usually be noted at between 0.4 and 1.5 mm displacement from a change in stiffness and an increase in sagittal vertebral rotation.

(7) Cadaver anterior lumbar failure in shear started at 1200 N and depended on the loading rate as well as the test setup.

(8) The data support the hypothesis that the shear stiffness plays a major role in the stabilization of cadaver lumbar motion segments.

FUTURE WORK

Loading rate in automotive crashes may be 500 mm/sec or greater. Tests need to be done at higher loading rates. The effects of preload (primarily compression) need to be investigated for stiffness and failure loads. The results should be used to set up a nonlinear viscoelastic mathematical model.

ACKNOWLEDGEMENT

Support for this work came from the Ford Motor Company.

REFERENCES

1. Adams, MA, Hutton, WC; "The Mechanical Function of the Lumbar Apophyseal Joints", *Spine* 8(3), pp 327-330, 1983.

2. Berkson, MH, Nachemson, A, Schultz

A B; "Mechanical Properties of Human Lumbar Spine Motion Segments - Part II: Responses in Compression and Shear, Influence of Gross Morphology ", *J Biomech Eng*, 101, 1979 pp 53-57.

3. Crowninshield, RD, Pope, MH: "The Strength and Failure Characteristics of Rat Medial Collateral Ligaments", *J Trauma* 16(2), pp 99-105, 1976.

4. Edwards, WT, Hayes, WC, Posner, I, White, AA, and Mann, RW; "Variation of Lumbar Spine Stiffness With Load", *J Biomech Eng*, 109, 1987, pp 35-42.

5. Foster, JK, Kortge, JO, Wolanin, MJ; "Hybrid III - A Biomechanically-Based Crash Test Dummy", *Proc 21st Stapp Car Crash Conf*, SAE 770938, 1977, pp 973-1014.

6. Janevic, J, Ashton-Miller, JA, and Schultz, AB;, "Large Compressive Preloads Decrease Lumbar Motion Segment Flexibility", *J Orthop Res*, 9, 1991, pp 228-236.

7. Kelley, BS, Lafferty, JF, Bowman, DA, and Clark, PA ; "Rhesus Monkey Intervertebral Disk Viscoelastic Response to Shear Stress", *J Biomech Eng*, 105, 1983, pp 51-54.

8. Lanir, Y; "A Microstructure Model for the Rheology of Mammalian Tendon", *J Biomech Eng*, 102, pp 332-339, 1980.

9. Lantz, SA, Lafferty, JF, and Bowman, DA; "Response of the Intervertebral Disk of the Rhesus Monkey to P-A Shear Stress", *J Biomech Eng*, 102, 1980, pp 137-140.

10. Lin, HS, Liu, YK, and Adams, KH; "Mechanical Response of the Lumbar Intervertebral Joint under Physiological (Complex) Loading", *J Bone Joint Surg*, 60A, 1978, pp 41-55.

11. Liu, YK, Ray, G, and Hirsch, C; "The Resistance of the Lumbar Spine to Direct Shear", *Orthop Clin North Am*, 6, 1975, pp 33-49.

12. Markolf, KL; "Deformation of the Thoracolumbar Intervertebral Joints in Response to External Loads", *J Bone Joint Surg*, 54A, 1972, pp 511-533.

13. McGlashen, KM, Miller, JAA, Schultz, AB, and Andersson, GBJ; "Load Displacement Behavior of the Human Lumbo-sacral Joint," *J Orthop Res*, 5, 1987, pp 488-496.

14. Miller, JAA, Haderspeck, KA, Schultz, AB; "Posterior Element Loads in Lumbar Motion Segments", *Spine* 8(3), pp 331-337, 1983.

15. Nolte, LP, Visarius, H; "On the Viscoelastic Behavior of Biosoft Material", *ZAMM*, 73, pp 270-272, 1993.

16. Nowinski, GP, Visarius H, Nolte, LP, Herkowitz, HN; "A Biomechanical Comparison of Cervical Laminaplasty and Cervical Laminectomy", *Spine*, 18(14), pp 1995-2004, 1993.

17. Panjabi, MM, Krag, MH, and White, AA; "Effects of Preload on Load Displacement Curves of the Lumbar Spine," *Orthop Clin North Am*, 8, 1977, pp 181-192.

18. Rigby, BJ, Hirai, N, Spikes, JD, Eyring, H: "The Mechanical Properties of Rat Tail Tendon, *J Gen Phys* 43, 265-283, 1959.

19. Sauren, AASH, Rousseau, EPM; "A Concise Sensitivity Analysis of the Quasi Linear Viscoelastic Model Proposed by Fung", *J Biomech Eng*, 105, pp 92-95, 1983.

20. Viidik,A: "A Rheological Model for Uncalcified Parallel-Fibered Collagenous Tissue", *J Biomech* 1, pp 3-11, 1968.

21. Yahia, LH, Pigeon, P, DesRosiers; "Viscoelastic Properties of the Human Lumbodorsal Fascia", *J Biomed Eng*, 15, pp 425-429, 1993.

22. Yang, KH, King, AI; "Mechanism of Facet Load Transmission as a Hypothesis for Low Back Pain", *Spine* 9(6), pp 557-565, 1984.

942224

High Chest Accelerations in the Hybrid III Dummy Due to Interference in the Hip Joint

Edward Abramoski, Kris Warmann, Jim Feustel, Sripathi Nilkar, and N. J. Nagrant
Ford Motor Company

ABSTRACT

The design of the Hybrid III dummy's hip joint limits the allowable relative rotation between the dummy's lower torso and femur assembly. This limited motion is thought to cause abnormally high chest accelerations in some front barrier crash tests.

This paper describes static testing and computer modeling to quantify the hip joint range of motion and its effect on dummy chest accelerations. To verify model results, a series of HYGE sled tests were completed using modified hip joints.

INTRODUCTION

Interference in the Hybrid II dummy's hip joint was reported in 1982 by Taheda, et al of Honda [1]. They reported that when the dummy's upper leg impacts the rigid pelvis structure, a substantial shock is produced which causes unusual spikes in chest accelerations.

Similar abnormal chest accelerations in some tests using Hybrid III dummies led to the study of possible interference in the dummy's hip joint. This interference was believed to restrict the relative rotation between the dummy's femurs and lower torso resulting in forces being applied through the lumbar spine to the upper torso. To study this, a series of static tests was conducted to investigate the angle at which this interference occurs. Once the maximum angle of the hip joint was quantified, the crash victim simulation code MADYMO was used to study the effect this would have on dummy responses. Since modeling showed that a hard limit in the hip joint's upward rotation affected chest accelerations, a modification to the Hybrid III dummy's femur casting was developed. This modification was evaluated in a series of HYGE sled tests.

JOINT TESTING AND MODELING

JOINT STIFFNESS TESTING - The pelvis and upper legs of two Hybrid III dummies were tested. The pelvis was held rigidly at the lumbar spine attachment with the upper leg oriented to simulate the dummy in its design seating position. With the femur joint constrained such that no rotation could occur along its axis, a bar attached to the leg was manually loaded to rotate the leg to a maximum condition. A load cell on the end measured the applied force, and the relative angle was measured between the upper leg and pelvis so that a joint stiffness could be calculated. The initial setup is shown in Figures 1-3. The test was conducted for the left and right legs on both dummies with plan view angles of 0, +7 (inward), and -7 (outward) degrees. Each test was repeated three times.

Major differences were found between the left and right sides of each dummy, and also between the two dummies for the right sides in the +7 degree inward position. The difference in the left and right sides was attributed to the asymmetrical design of the pelvis casting. Examination of the right hip femur joint assemblies showed indentations around the retaining rings, Figure 4, and that the castings appeared bent where they attach to the ball joint. This was confirmed by dimensional analysis. The deformation of the joint indicates that the joint had bottomed out during at least some crash tests with forces substantial enough to bend the castings. The results for both dummies are shown in Figures 5 through 8.

RANGE OF MOTION TESTS - A second series of tests was done with the hip joints from the previous tests, a random set of hip joints (taken from inventory but appearing not to have been used), and a new set mounted to a pelvis casting with the foam skin removed. The relative pelvis / upper leg angle when metal to metal contact occurred was recorded using the same fixture as above. The tests were conducted for inward(+) / outward(-) upper leg angles of +35 to -65 degrees.

The results, shown in Figures 9 and 10, indicate that the difference in range of rotation between the right and left leg for a new hip joint is about 21 degrees. They also show that the available rotation angle for the right hip can vary by as much as 22 degrees due to permanent deformation from dynamic testing whereas the left hip shows very little degradation. In addition, moving either leg inward 10 degrees from nominal results in over a 10 degree reduction in allowable hip joint rotation.

MADYMO MODELING - MADYMO [2] occupant models were used to study the effect that reduced upward hip rotation would have on dummy responses. A passenger side model and driver side model were chosen that simulate 31 mph barrier tests in which the hip joint was suspected of bottoming out. Both models are unbelted with MADYMO finite element airbags.

The models were each run using the base function defining the upper leg upward rotational stiffness found in the MADYMO dummy database and a revised function with a 28 degree maximum angle to simulate the right joint interference condition. Model results are shown in Table 1 below..

Model Description	HIC	Resultant Chest G's (3ms)
Passenger side model:		
base joint function	301	36.2
revised joint function	302	48.8
difference:	+1	+12.6
Driver side model:		
base joint function	479	55.2
revised joint function	465	59.9
difference:	-14	+4.7

Table 1: MADYMO model results.

The 28 degree limit for hip joint rotation affected chest acceleration in both models. The passenger side increased 12 G's, and the driver side close to 5 G's. The lower increase for the driver can be explained by the lower relative angle between the lower torso and femur achieved due to the steering column mounted airbag restraint on the upper torso. The models indicate that a hard bottoming out at 28 degrees will show up in both longitudinal and vertical chest accelerations. Also, the vertical pelvis acceleration and lumbar spine shear load increase when the hip joint bottoms out, showing that these channels may be useful indicators of whether interference is actually occurring in a particular test.

HYGE SLED TESTING

HIP JOINT MODIFICATION - The next task was to develop a modification to the Hybrid III dummy hip joint that would better simulate a human. This meant eliminating the possibility for metal-to-metal contact in either hip joint. The revised femur casting is shown in Figure 11, with the changes outlined below:

1) Replace the neck of the femur casting by a 0.5" diameter steel rod.

2) Remove an 80 degree wedge from the reinforcement on the retaining ring to eliminate interference with the neck.

3) Replace the retaining ring cap head screw that is situated within the removed wedge with a flat head screw.

4) Remove a portion from the top of the femur casting to reduce the femur / ilium interaction.

These revisions resulted in a range of motion of approximately 52 degrees for both the right and left hip joints.[*]

HYGE SLED TESTING - The modified femurs were then tested with a series of HYGE sled tests. These tests simulated a 31 mph, 90 degree, frontal impact of a mid-sized four door sedan with a passenger side airbag. The only occupant was an unbelted Hybrid III dummy sitting in the front passenger seat. The dummy was instrumented with head, chest, and pelvis accelerometers as well as neck, femur, and lumbar spine load cells. Four sled tests were conducted where the only variable tested was the modification to the Hybrid III dummy hip joint. The first test was a baseline test with an unmodified dummy. The next two tests were conducted with the same dummy fitted with the modified hip joints. Finally, the last test was a second baseline test using the same dummy refitted with the original hip joints.

The results from each set of two tests were averaged and summarized in Table 2. It is clear from these results that the femur modification has a significant effect on dummy response. The vertical chest acceleration alone was reduced by 57%. The results also show a 28% reduction in the longitudinal chest acceleration. The improvements seen in the vertical and longitudinal chest accelerations translate into a 26% reduction in the 3ms clipped resultant chest acceleration. Since any forces generated in the hip would have to be transmitted to the chest via the lumbar spine, this data is also summarized in Table 2. The lumbar shear and moment were reduced by 33% and 37% respectively. The largest change in spine data was seen in the lumbar spine axial load which was reduced by 46%.

The data was further analyzed in an attempt to understand how the interference in the hip joint affects the dummy's chest response. Figures 12a and 12b show the pelvis vertical acceleration from the two tests using the unmodified Hybrid III dummy. Both tests show large spikes occurring at approximately 77 ms. These spikes are characteristic of accelerometer ringing seen in cases of metal-to-metal contact

---

[*] A subsequent study by a subgroup of the SAE Human Biomechanics and Simulation Standards Committee has recommended that a biofidelic range of motion starting from the supine position would be a maximum rotation of 135 degrees of the knee about the hip joint with some progressive resistance being encountered starting at 122 degrees. An angle of 83 degrees must be subtracted from this recommendation (yielding 39/52 degrees respectively for the soft/hard stop) to compare to the angles discussed in this report due to a 7 degree offset in the hip-knee angle below the pelvic reference plane (Figure 1).

Data channel	Unmodified Dummy Test Avg.	Modified Dummy Test Avg.
Chest Vert. Accel.	65.6 G's	28.3 G's
Chest Long. Accel.	69.6 G's	50.5 G's
Chest Res. Accel. (3ms)	74.0 G's	55.0 G's
Lumbar Shear	2021 lbs.	1358 lbs.
Lumbar Moment	3270 in-lbs.	2069 in-lbs.
Lumbar Axial	1584 lbs.	861 lbs.

Table 2: HYGE sled series results.

such as occurs with the hip joint interference suspected in this dummy. Comparing these two tests to the two tests using the modified Hybrid III dummy (figures 13a and 13b), it is clear that the modification has eliminated the metal-to-metal contact since no spikes appear in the pelvis accelerometer. Figures 14 and 15 show overlays of the lumbar spine shear and moment obtained in the four tests. The negative sense of the shear force indicates that the upper torso is attempting to slide forward relative to the pelvis and the pelvis is applying a restraining force on the lumbar spine attempting to stop this motion. The positive moment indicates that the pelvis is applying a moment to the lumbar spine that resists the forward rotation of the upper torso. Both the lumbar shear and moment show sharp spikes occurring slightly after the ringing is seen in the vertical pelvis acceleration. It can be inferred that the spikes are generated when pelvis rotation is suddenly stopped by interference in the hip joint. These two forces act to resist forward movement of the dummy's chest and create a significant negative longitudinal acceleration in the chest.

Figure 16 shows an overlay of the lumbar spine axial load obtained in the four tests. The positive sense of this force indicates that there is a tensile force between the dummy's pelvis and lumbar spine. This tensile force is a result of the rotation of the upper torso about the pelvis. When the rotation of the pelvis is suddenly stopped by the hip joint interference, the tension in the spine rapidly increases. In the tests using the unmodified dummy, this spike occurs in the axial force at the same time as the spikes in the lumbar shear and moment. This force acts to pull the dummy's upper torso downward and creates a significant positive spike in the vertical chest acceleration.

Figures 17-19 show overlays of the vertical, longitudinal and resultant chest accelerations obtained in the four tests. These figures illustrate the significant effect that the hip joint interference has on dummy response. Using the modified Hybrid III dummy, the vertical chest acceleration was reduced from over 65 G's to approximately 28 G's. The longitudinal acceleration is also significantly affected. Longitudinal accelerations are reduced from almost 70 G's to approximately 50 G's. When the resultant is calculated the 3ms CUMDUR is reduced from 74 G's to 55 G's.

CONCLUSIONS

The test results show that the maximum rotation angle of the femur relative to the pelvis before hip joint interference occurs in a new Hybrid III dummy is approximately 28 degrees for the right hip and approximately 49 degrees for the left hip. The results also show that this angle can decrease significantly if the leg is rotated in towards the center of the dummy. As a Hybrid III dummy is used in various crash tests, the maximum rotation angle between the pelvis and femur can change substantially due to deformation of the hip joint casting. This self-modifying nature of the hip joint causes a significant concern about the objectivity of any test results obtained using the Hybrid III dummy. Similar test conditions can create drastically different results simply due to the occurrence or non-occurrence of interference in the hip joint.

MADYMO modeling and HYGE sled testing clearly demonstrate that interference in the dummy's hip joint significantly increase not only the dummy's vertical chest acceleration but also the longitudinal acceleration. Increases of almost 20 G's in the clipped resultant chest acceleration have been caused by this interference. Both modeling and testing show that the pelvis and chest vertical acceleration and lumbar spine shear and axial forces, and moment are good indicators of hip joint interference.

RECOMMENDATIONS

It is recommended that the Hybrid III dummy be modified to allow for greater relative rotation between the upper legs and the pelvis to better simulate a human range of motion. This is particularly important for the right side which is restricted more than the left due to the asymmetrical geometry of the pelvis casting. The amount of rotation allowed should be based on the maximum range of motion for a human hip joint.

To evaluate whether hip joint interference occurs in tests using the current Hybrid III design it is recommended that the lumbar spine forces and the pelvis and chest vertical acceleration traces be examined.

ACKNOWLEDGEMENTS

The authors would like to thank G. Nowak of Ford Motor Company for his contributions in obtaining the static joint test data and R. Daniel and C. O'Connor, also of Ford Motor Company, for their assistance.

REFERENCES

1. Takeda, H. and Kobayashi, S., "Optimizing Knee Restraint Characteristics for Improved Air Bag System Performance of a Small Car", 9th International Technical Conference on Experimental Safety Vehicles, November 1982, Paper 826027.

2. MADYMO User's Manuals, Version 5.0, TNO Road Vehicles Research Institute, the Netherlands.

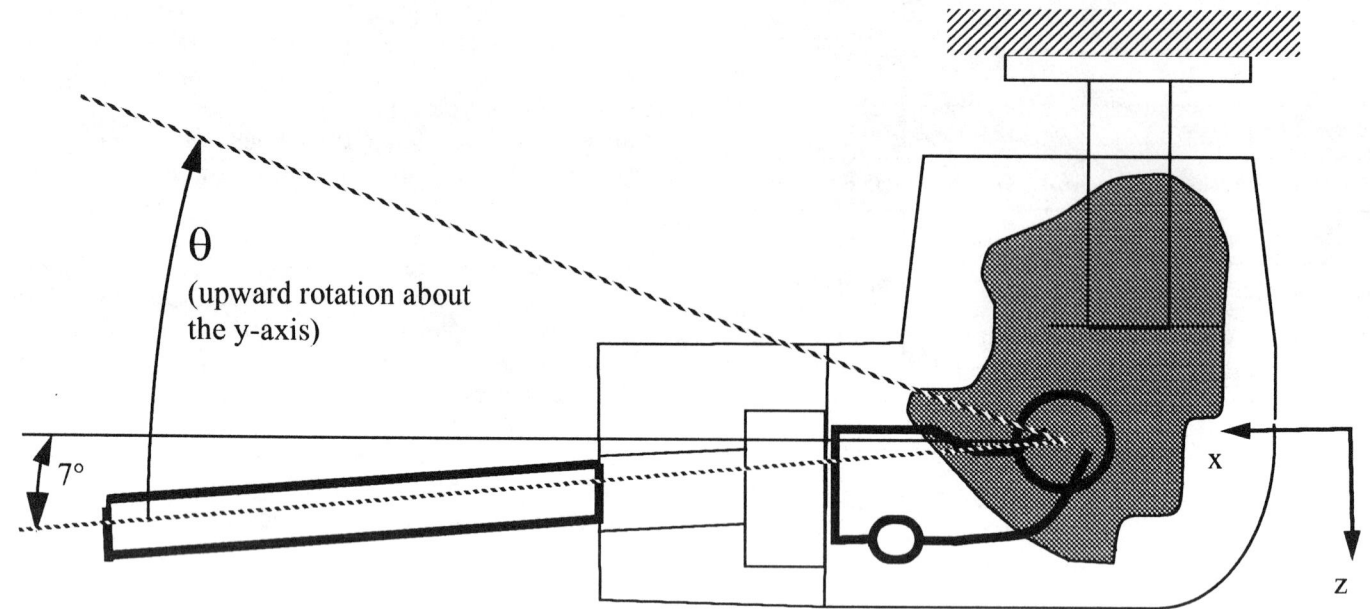

Figure 1: Side view of hip joint stiffness test setup.

Note: The bar on the end of the femur joint was constrained so that the joint could not rotate about the x-axis. Also, for the second series of tests only a pelvis casting and the femur castings were used (there was no foam skin on the pelvis).

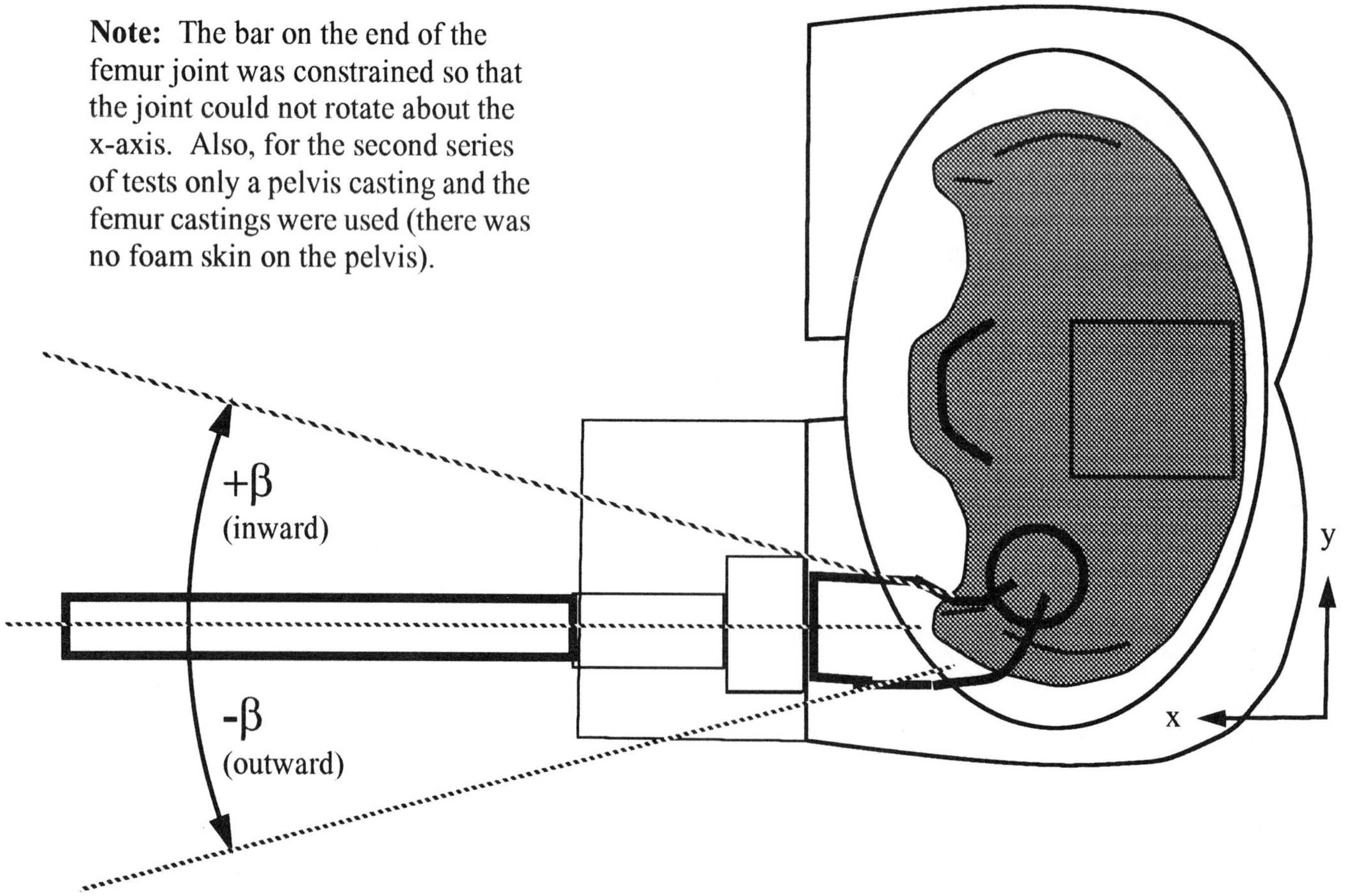

Figure 2: Top view of hip joint stiffness test setup.

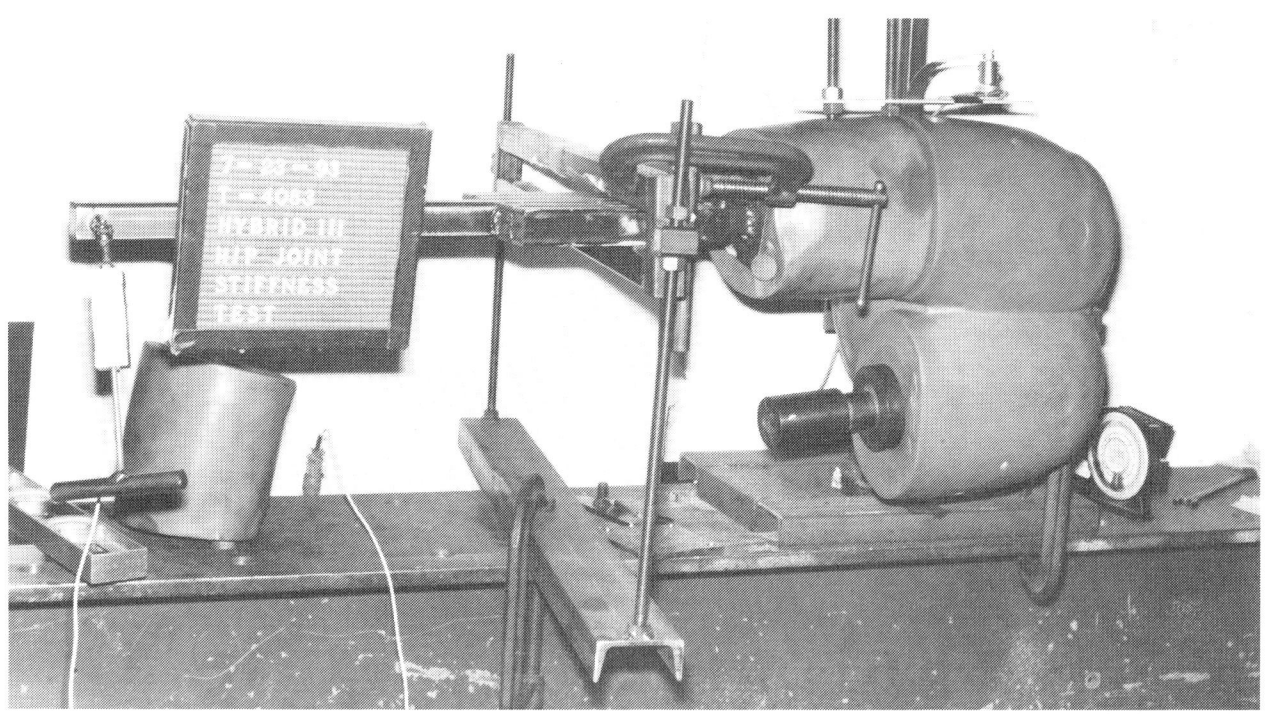

Figure 3: Hip joint test fixture.

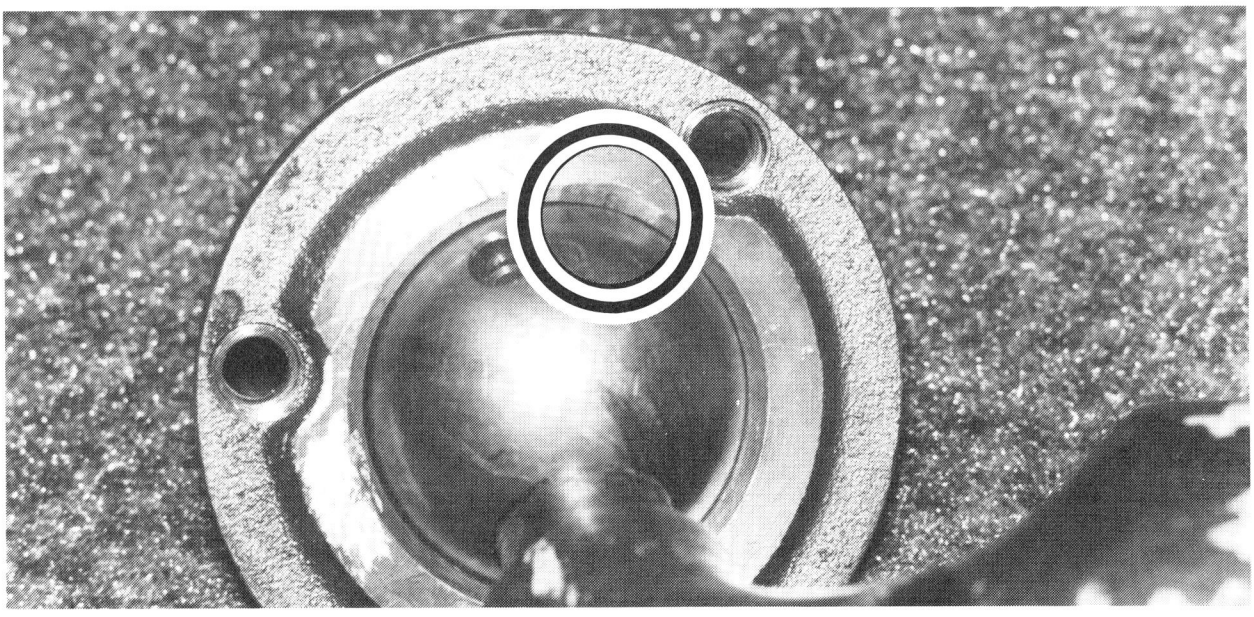

Figure 4: Indentations caused by the bottoming out of the femur casting against the retaining ring.

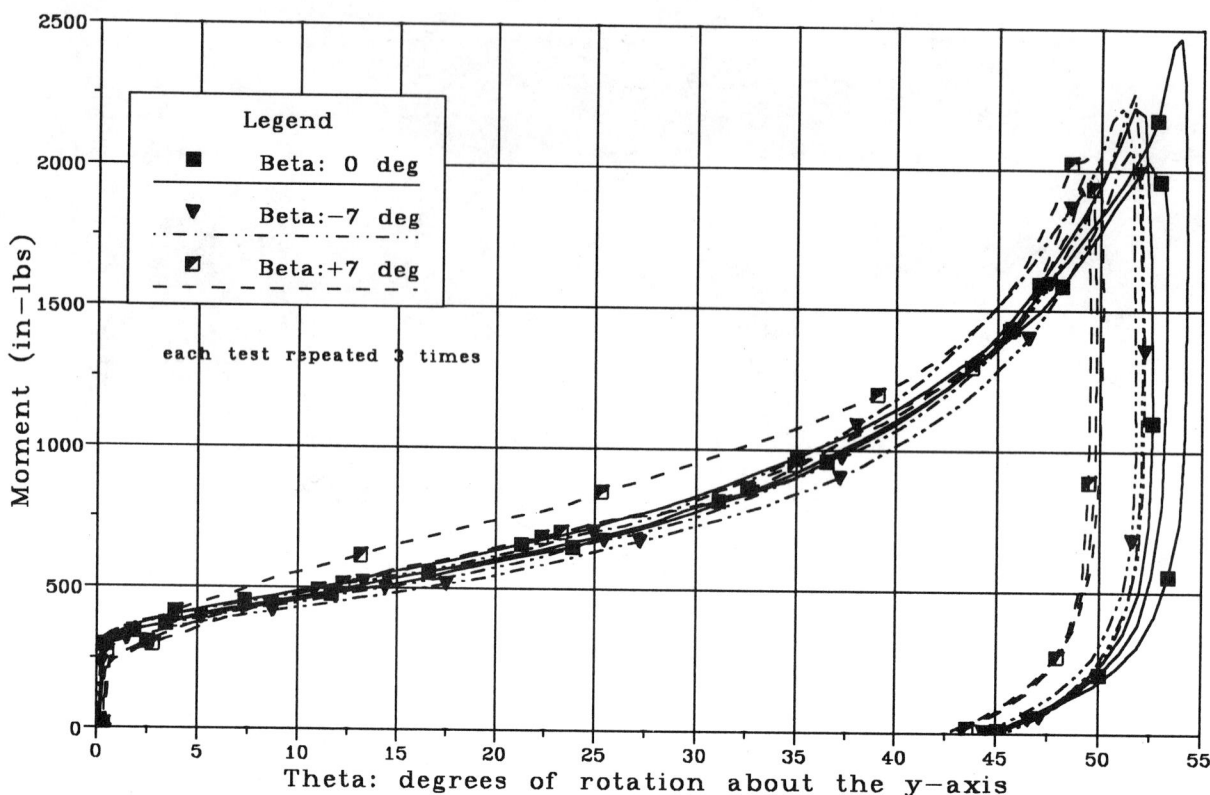

Figure 5: Left hip joint stiffness for dummy #1.

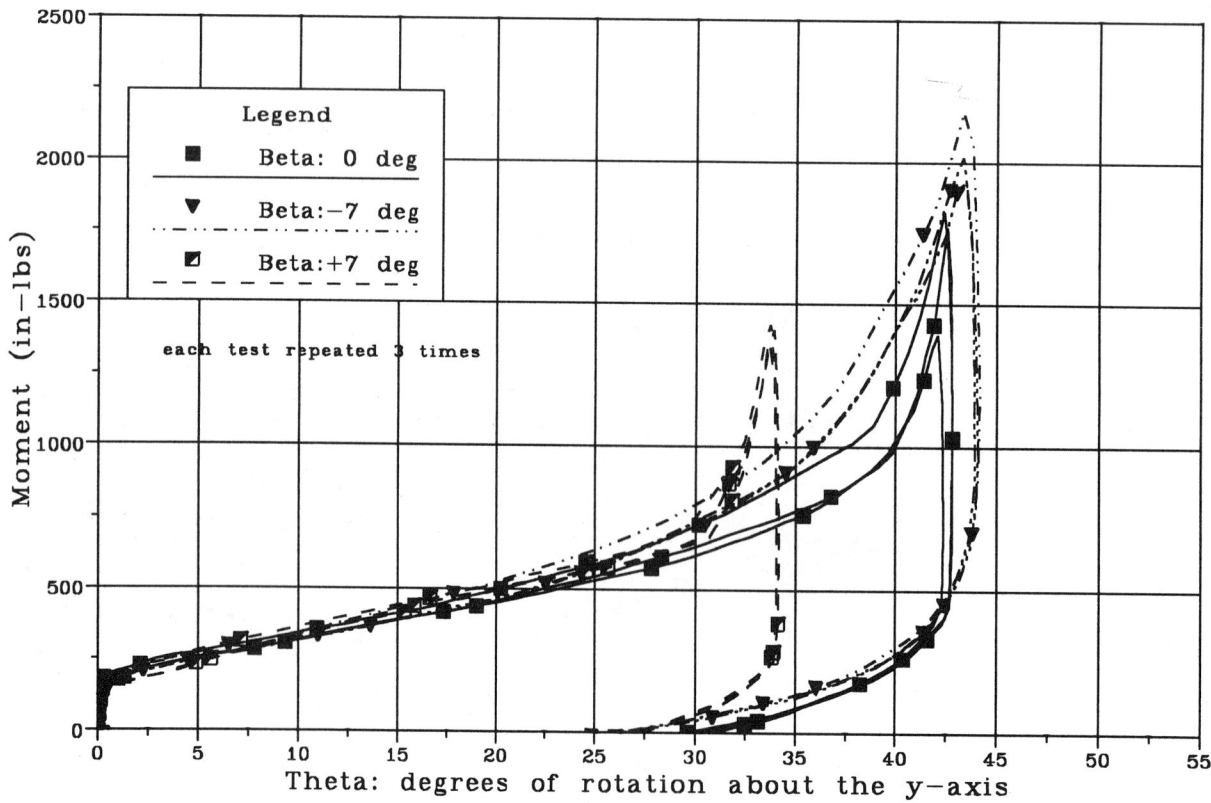

Figure 6: Right hip joint stiffness for dummy #1.

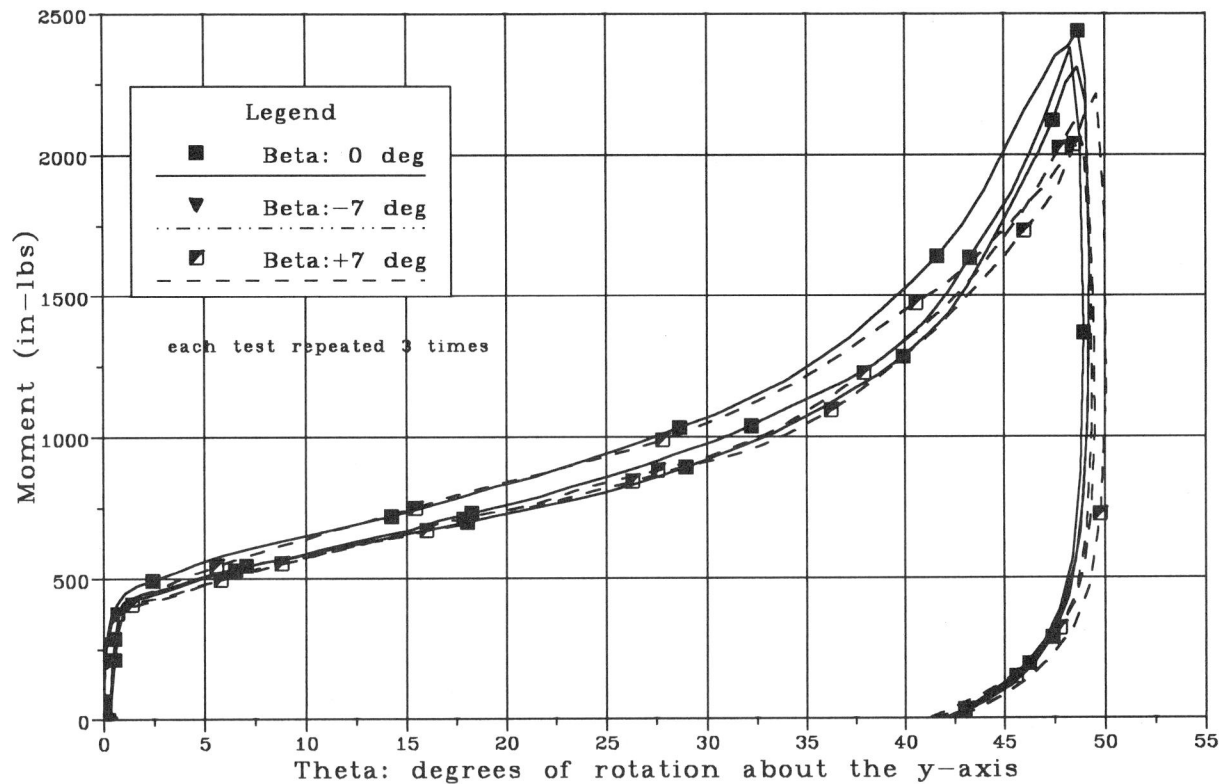

Figure 7: Left hip joint stiffness for dummy #2.

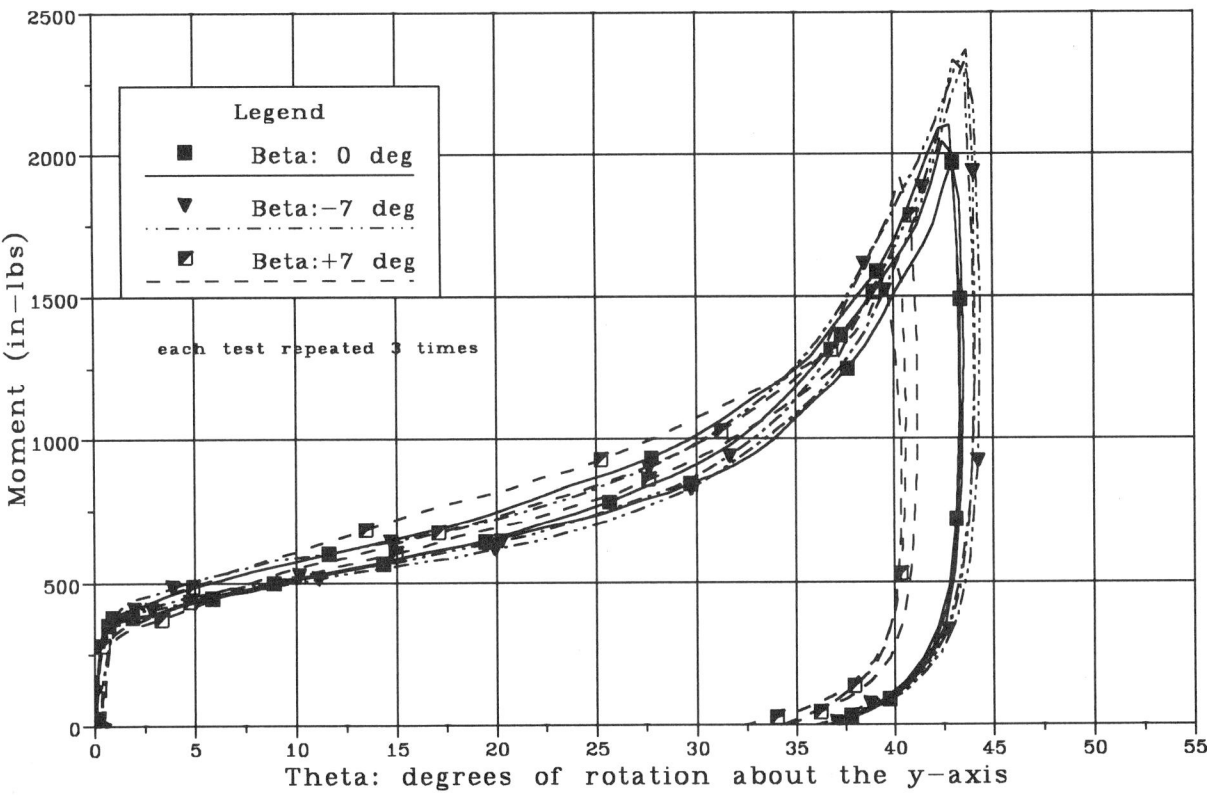

Figure 8: Right hip joint stiffness for dummy #2.

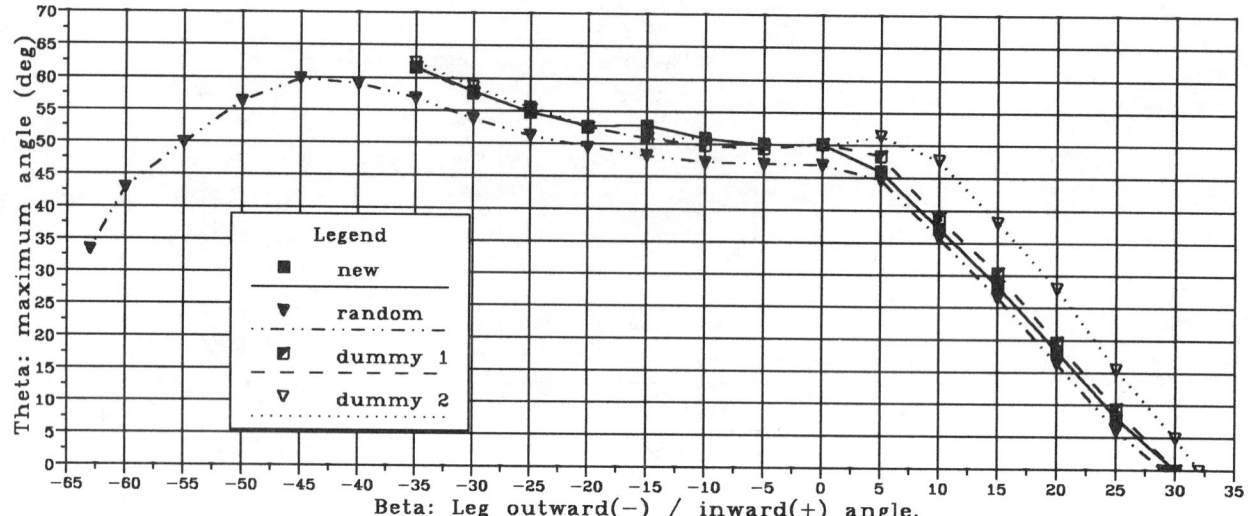
Figure 9: Left hip joint maximum rotation.

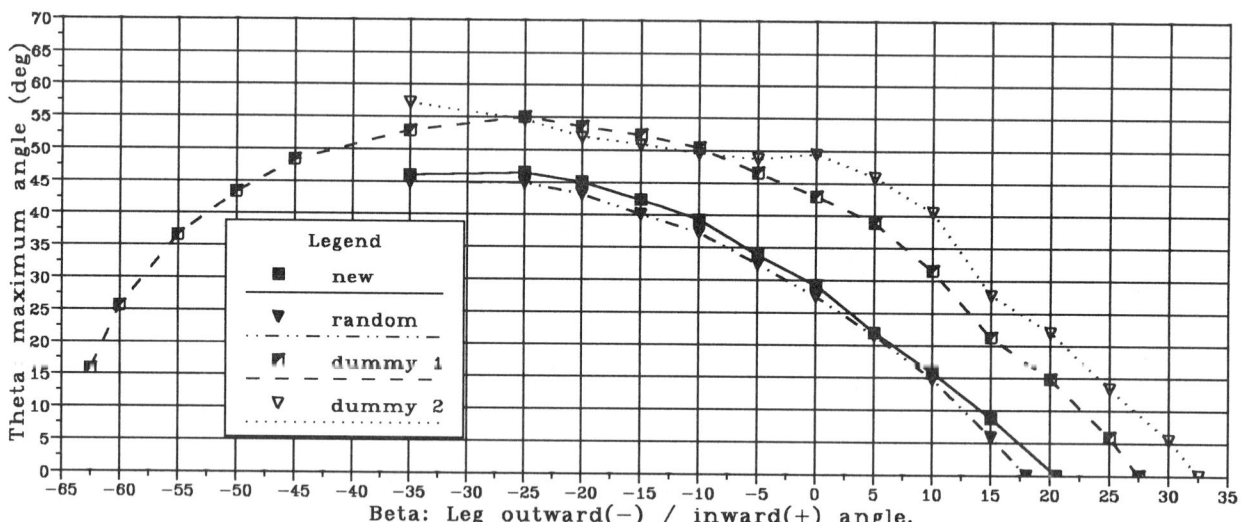
Figure 10: Right hip joint maximum rotation.

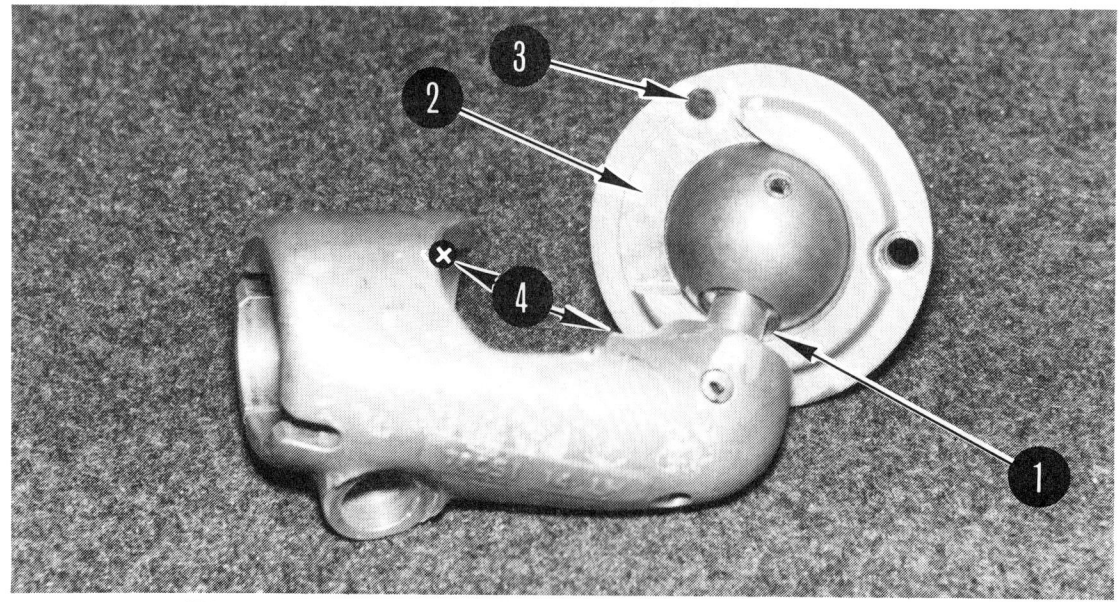
Figure 11: Modified femur casting.

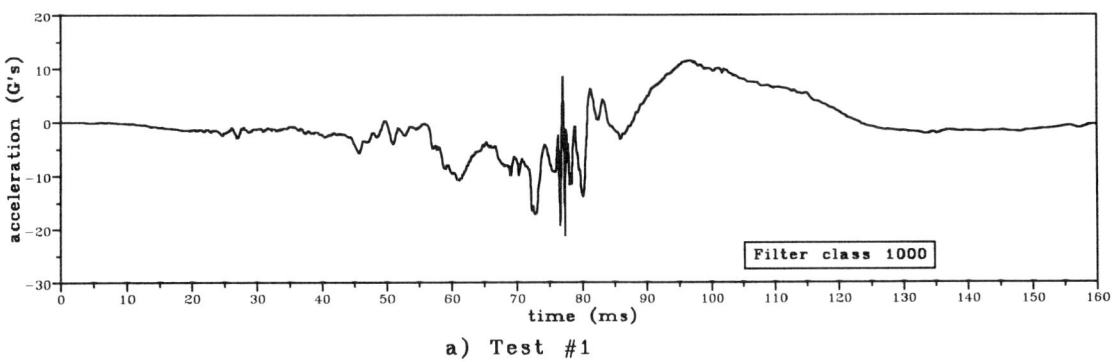

a) Test #1

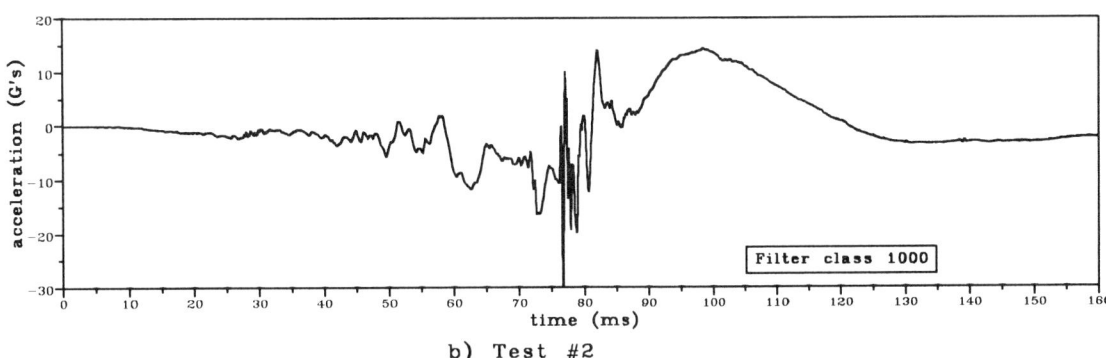

b) Test #2

Figure 12: Pelvis Vertical Acceleration (Unmodified dummy)

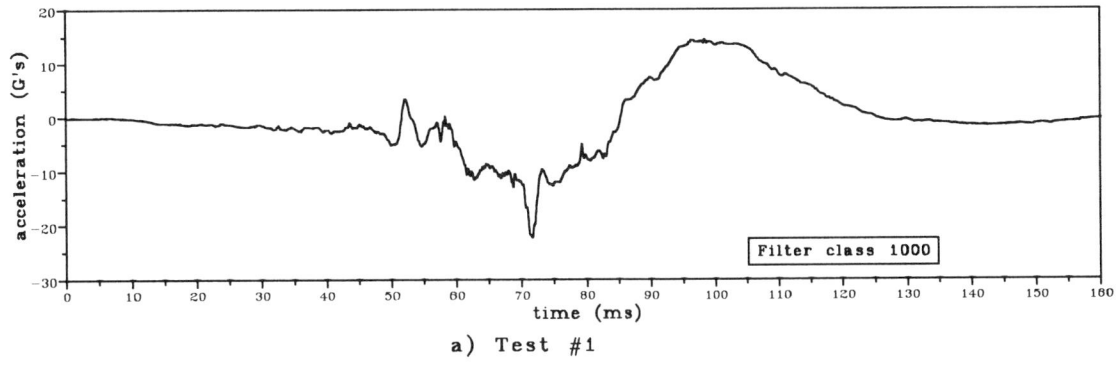

a) Test #1

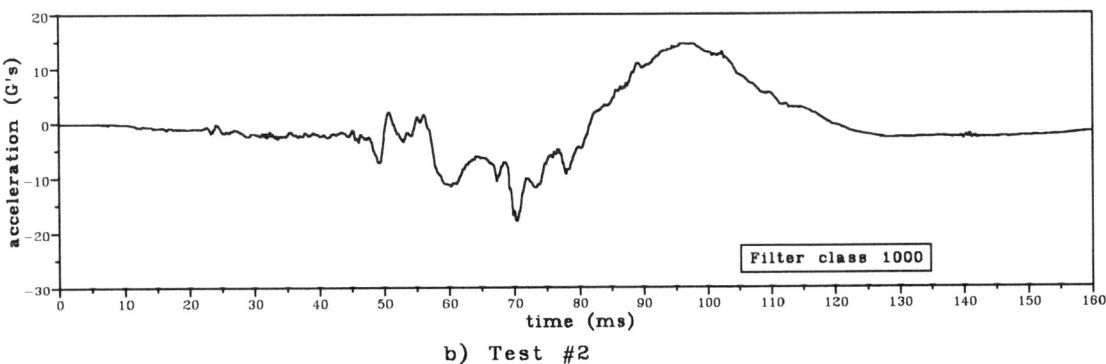

b) Test #2

Figure 13: Pelvis Vertical Acceleration (Modified dummy)

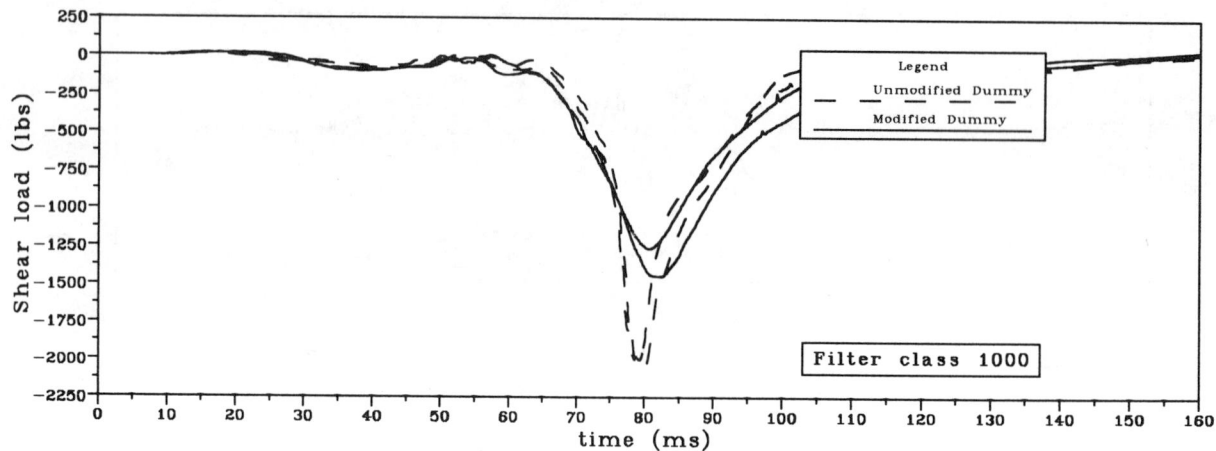

Figure 14: Lumbar spine shear load

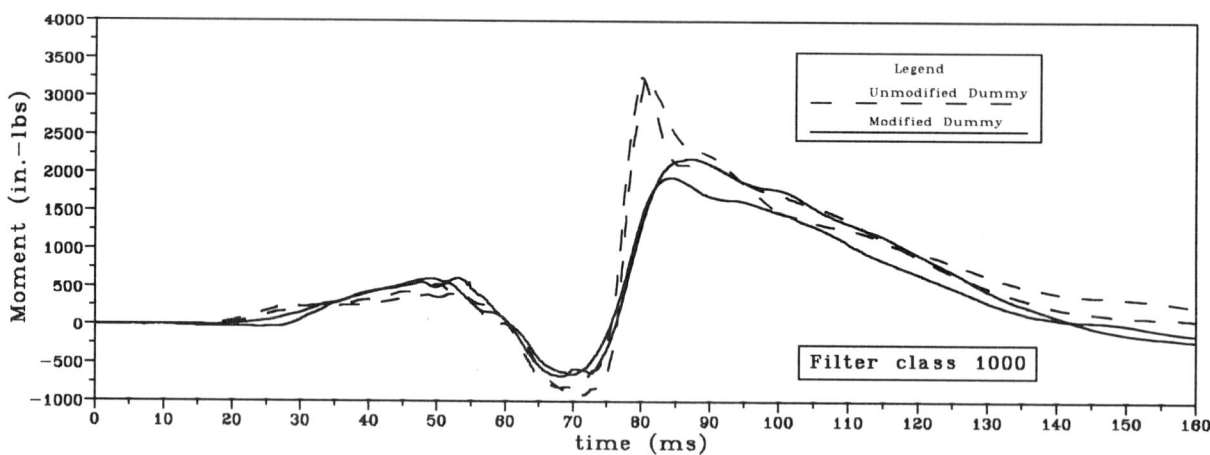

Figure 15: Lumbar spine moment

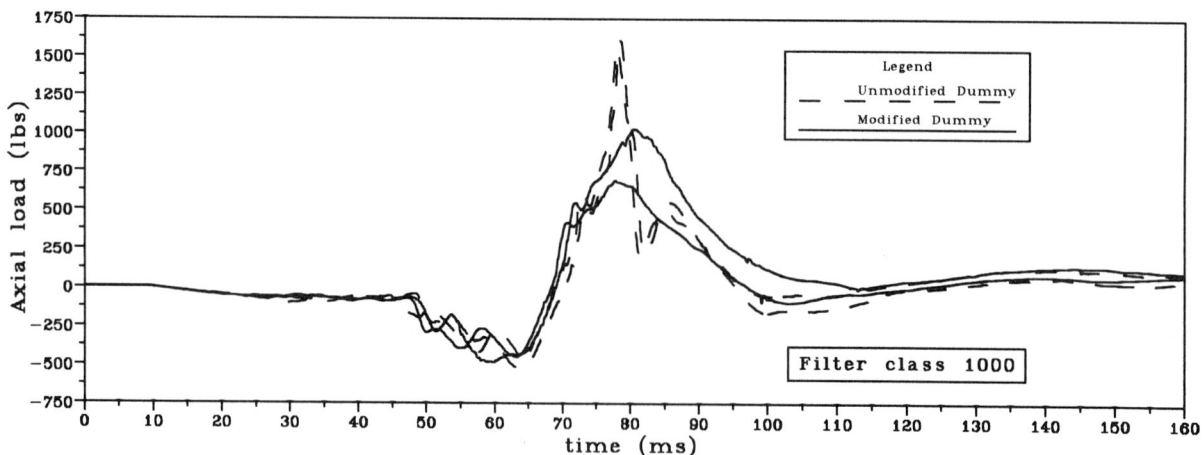

Figure 16: Lumbar spine axial load

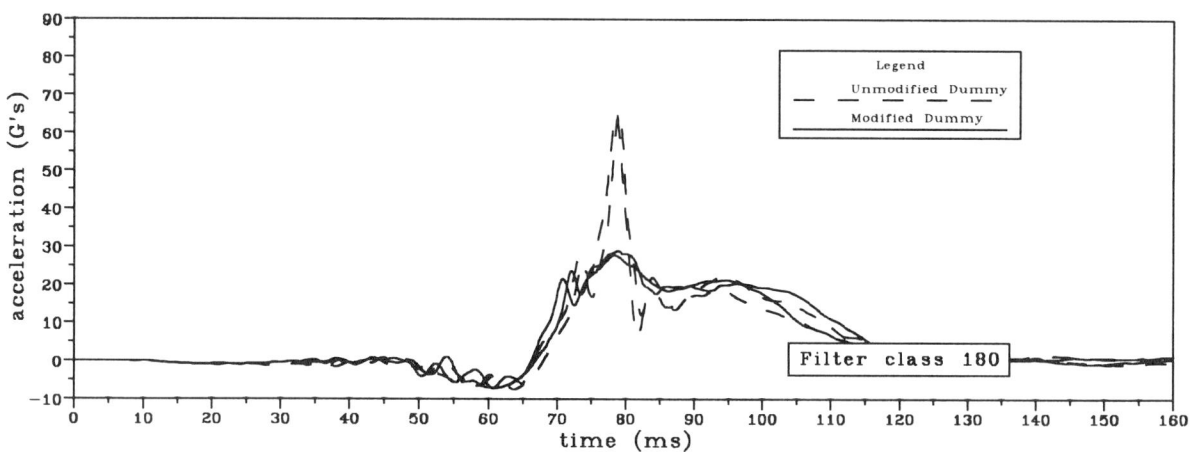

Figure 17: Chest vertical acceleration

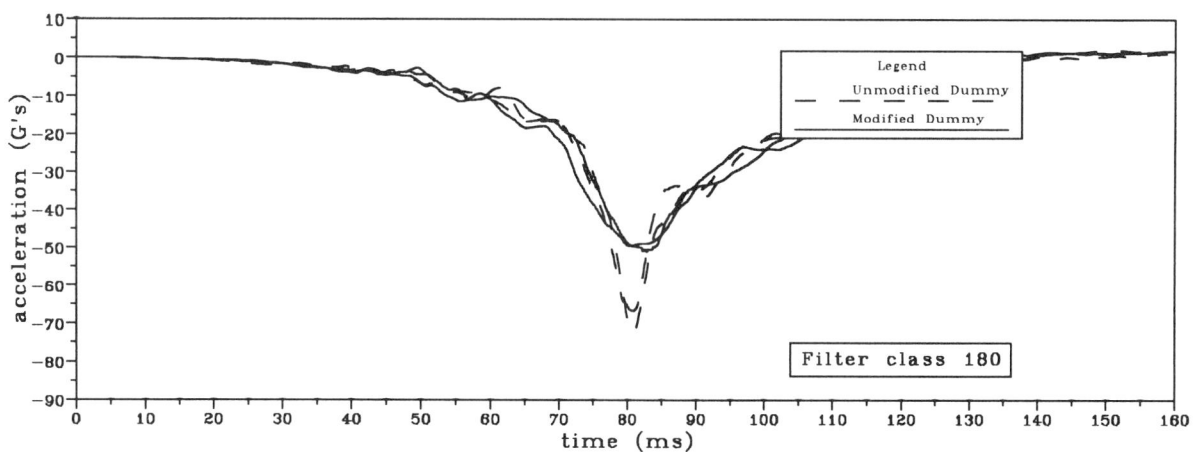

Figure 18: Chest longitudinal acceleration

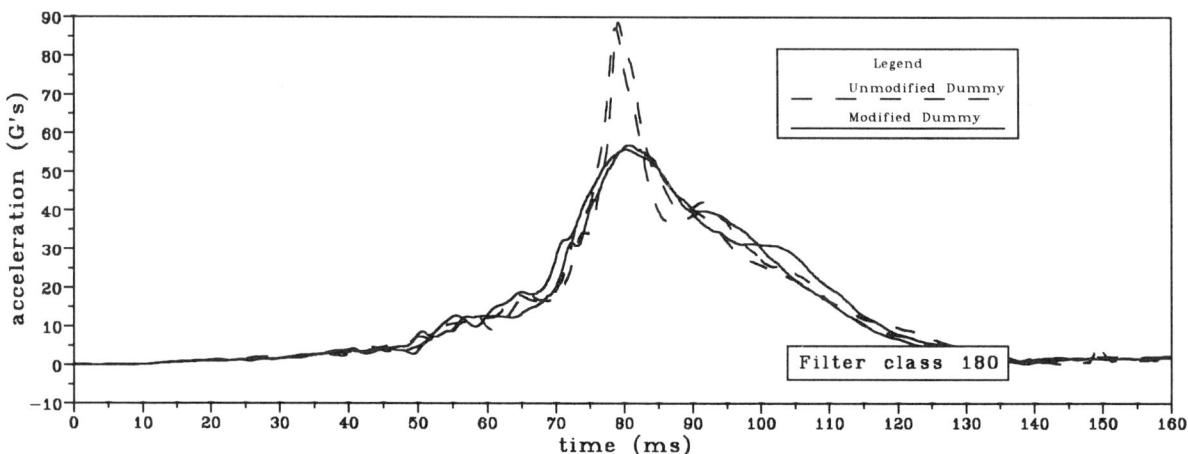

Figure 19: Chest resultant acceleration

Section 3:
Biomechanics, Impact Response and Trauma Assessed with Volunteers, Cadavers, Animal, and Mechanical Surrogates in Lateral Impacts

680773

The Pathology and Pathogenesis of Injuries Caused by Lateral Impact Accidents

John D. States and David J. States
School of Medicine, University of Rochester

Abstract

Forty-eight lateral impact accidents were studied correlating vehicle damage and occupant injury. Side-swipe accidents produced serious injury only when the occupant's elbow was protruding through a window or when the occupant space of the vehicle was seriously compromised. Intersection impacts and drifting impacts, particularly when the impact was caused by a vehicle approaching from the opposite direction, caused the most serious injuries. Fractures of the acetabulum with intrapelvic protrusion of the hip and fractures of the pubic rami are characteristic of lateral impact accidents. The door was the most common injury-producing structure of the vehicle. Deep wrap-around seat designs and stronger doors, door frames, and chassis structures are necessary to reduce occupant space penetration and to absorb impact energy in lateral impact accidents.

LITTLE ATTENTION has been directed to the problem of side or lateral impact accidents. The present study is an attempt to determine injury patterns in lateral impact accidents and to suggest design changes which will reduce or prevent these injuries.

National Safety Council data for 1966 revealed that 37% of urban and 23% of rural accidents were intersection collisions with lateral impact (1).[1] Ryan, of the Harvard School of Public Health reported that 46.7% of a group of urban traffic accidents in Adelaide, Austrailia, were lateral impacts (2).

In 1956 the first Liberty Mutual Safety Car, designed by Crandall, was introduced (3). Features protecting the occupants from lateral impact were wrap-around and lateral bumpers, roll bars incorporated in the front and rear door posts, heavily constructed and bolted doors, and a special seat design. Many of these features were incorporated in the Liberty Mutual Survival Car II, a modified production car developed in 1960. In particular, the seat design was further developed. Severy

---

[1]Numbers in parentheses designate References at end of paper.

tested this seat and concluded that it was the most important single design feature for the protection of an occupant in a side impact accident.

Severy, of UCLA, has provided extensive experimental data on the collision performance of vehicles in lateral impact accidents by conducting carefully instrumented and photographed crash tests (4). His studies, begun in 1949, have revealed many of the problems of production car designs in lateral impact accidents. His studies clearly demonstrated the phenomenon of overriding of the floor pan and frame rails by the impacting vehicle.

The New York State Safety Car was developed with a thick door of a metal honeycomb, designed to absorb impact. Frame roll bar bulkheads were used to prevent inward collapse of the passenger compartment.

Stock car racers found that lateral impact protection is necessary for competition vehicles. The National Association of Stock Car Automobile Racers (NASCAR) requires roll cages with heavily constructed side bars for lateral impact protection. (See Fig. 1.)

The American automobile industry has recognized the problem of lateral impact accidents. On March 12, 1968, the New York Times carried an article announcing structural changes for full-sized General Motors cars beginning with the 1969 models (5). Door frames, chassis frames, and floors will be reinforced, and a cross bar will be placed in the doors to prevent penetration.

Source of Data

The data and case studies to be presented have been drawn from a case series begun in 1959. The authors, both orthopedic surgeons, have examined the cars in which their patients were injured. In most instances, the accident scene and the other accident vehicles were examined as well. The four most comprehensively studied cases were contributed by the Research Accident Investigation Team of the University

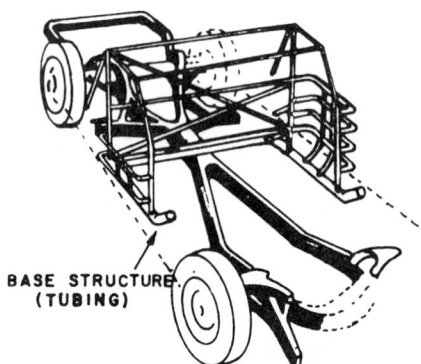

Fig. 1—Roll cage design required in NASCAR (stock car) racing

of Rochester School of Medicine. The R.A.I. Team is supported by contract funds from the Department of Transportation, Washington, D. C.

Case Selection

Case contact was made in two Rochester hospital emergency departments and in the authors' offices. For an accident to be included in the series, at least one occupant in an accident vehicle had to be injured.

Accident Classification

Lateral impact accidents are defined as those in which a vehicle was struck primarily on the side. Although damage to other surfaces may have occurred with the primary impact or other subsequent impacts, the initial and primary impact was to the side structures (the fenders,

Table 1—Injury Severity Categories[a]

Points	Category
0	No injury
1	Minor injury a. Contusion, abrasion, superficial laceration b. Trauma to head without fracture or loss of consciousness c. Teeth loosened or fractured d. Mild whiplash, resolved in 1 month e. Sprains f. Simple fractures and dislocations of nose or digits, chip fractures about ankles or wrists
2	Moderate injury a. Deep or disfiguring lacerations without dangerous hemorrhage b. Whiplash requiring more than 1 month to resolve c. Compound fractures of nose or digits d. Simple fractures of upper extremities, foot, patella (one fracture only) e. One or two rib fractures
3	Moderately severe injury a. Skull fracture without unconsciousness b. Concussion with unconsciousness up to 30 minutes c. Loss of eye d. Fracture of femur, tibia, acetabulum, pelvis, spine, facial bones (except nose) without dangerous hemorrhage e. More than one fracture (except digits and nose) f. More than two rib fractures
4	Life-threatening injuries a. Depressed skull fracture b. Intracranial or spinal cord injury c. Concussion with loss of consciousness for more than 30 minutes d. Neck injury with fracture or dislocation or neurological injury e. Rupture of internal organ f. Crush injuries of extremities g. Injuries causing cardiorespiratory distress h. Dangerous hemorrhage or shock due to fractures or extensive soft tissue injury
5	Fatal injury (death within 72 hr)

[a]From A.M. Nahum, et al. with modification.

wheels, doors, and door frames). Rollover accidents were included only when a rollover followed a side impact.

Lateral impact accidents were grouped according to the direction of impact and the objects struck. Cases were classified as intersection, side-swipe, fixed-object, and drifting accidents.

Intersection accidents are defined as those in which vehicles approached each other at an angle of 30-150 deg.

Side-swipe accidents were separated from this group. In these accidents, the vehicles were going in nearly the same or nearly the opposite directions and only minor changes in direction occurred after impact. Vehicle damage often extended over a large area, but involved only easily deformed sheet metal structures.

Drifting accidents are defined as those in which one vehicle was out of control and was slipping sideways on its tires. Drifting is a term used in racing to denote sliding sideways. In racing, it is intentionally produced, either with the rear wheels or with all four wheels, to stabilize a vehicle cornering at high speed.

In accident situations, drifting commonly occurs on straight or nearly straight sections of highway. Adhesion between the tire and the pavement is unusually and unexpectedly decreased. Rain, snow, and ice are the common causes of reduced adhesion leading to drifting accidents.

Fixed-object accidents are those in which the vehicles drifted or spun into an immovable roadside object: that is, trees, guard rails, lamp and sign posts, and bridge abutments. They are distinctive from collisions with other vehicles because fixed objects do not override the frame or floor of the vehicle.

Cases were also grouped by point of principle impact: that is, the occupant space, front fender, hood and wheel, or the rear fender, trunk, and wheel.

Injury and Damage Scaling

Arbitrary patient injury and vehicle damage scaling techniques were used to permit comparison of accidents. The injury scale was adopted from Nahum and Siegel Injury Scale, but with an added unit, "moderately severe." Numbers were assigned to the scale—zero denoted no injury, five denoted a fatal injury. The added unit of "moderately severe" permitted identification for scaling purposes of simple fractures and severe spine sprains without fracture. (See Table 1.)

The Cornell Accident Crash Injury Research Accident Severity Rating Scale was used for vehicle damage (Fig. 2). Points were similarly assigned, ranging from zero to five. Zero denoted no damage, and five denoted extremely severe damage. A nomogram supplied by ACIR was used in making these vehicle damage estimates.

Presentation of Data

The authors have studied a total of 204 cases since 1959. Forty-eight of these were lateral impact accidents. Utilizing the damage severity rating (DSR), damage from lateral impact accidents was 3.46. The DSR for the entire series of 204 cases is 3.22. The average injury rating (IR) for lateral impact accidents was 2.83. The average IR for the entire series was 2.44. (See Table 2.)

Table 2—DSR and IR Ratings

Category	Number	Damage Severity Rating (DSR)	Injury Rating (IR)
Accident Vehicles	204	3.22	2.44
Laterally Impacted Vehicles	48	3.46	—
Occupants in Laterally Impacted Vehicles	74		2.53

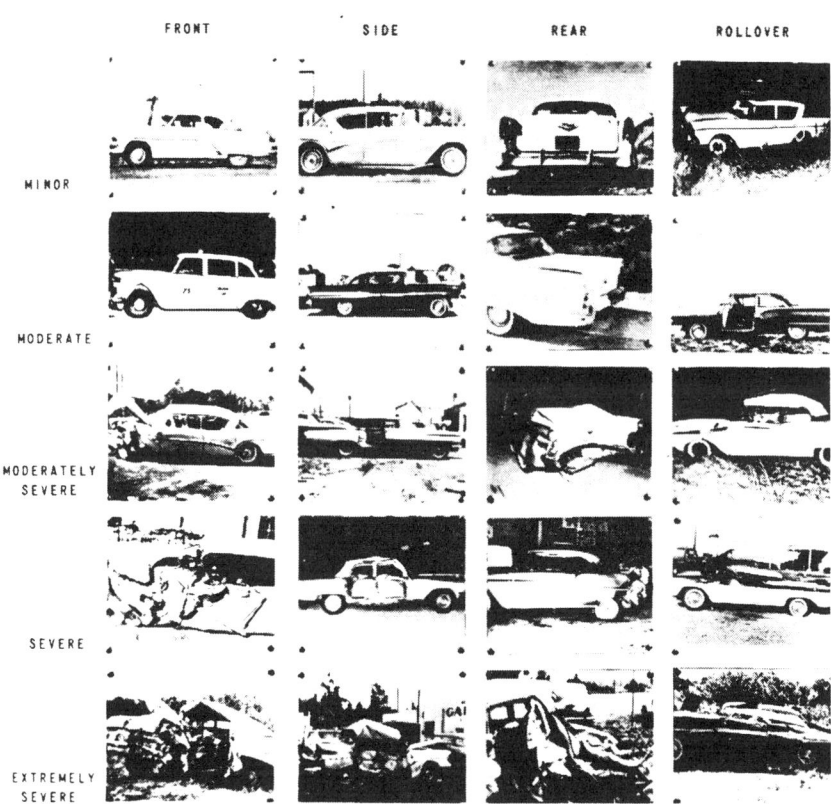

Fig. 2—Damage Severity Rating Scale (DSR), Automobile Crash Injury Research, Cornell Aeronautical Laboratory

Types of Accidents

Grouping the cars according to accident type revealed that intersection-type accidents were somewhat more common. The DSR and IR revealed that fixed-object and drifting accidents were more violent and that collision damage and injuries were more severe, particularly in the drifting type impact (Table 3). The reasons for this became evident when individual cases were examined. These cases will be presented in the Discussion Section.

Accident cases were also grouped by point of impact (Table 4). An obvious judgment is confirmed by these data in that impacts on the occupant compartment are much more injury-producing than impacts on the front or rear of the vehicle.

Model Years

There is a spread of 14 years of model years in the accident vehicle study (Table 5). In 1968, attention was directed to late model cars; but

Table 3—Accident Type and Injury and Damage Severity Ratings

Accident Type	No. of Cases	DSR	IR
Intersection Collision (angular impact by another vehicle)	19	3.3	2.0
Fixed Object	10	2.6	2.6
Drifting into Oncoming Car:	7	4.7	3.8
Side-swipe Accident	12	2.4	2.2

Table 4—Area of Impact

Area	No. of Cases	Injury Rating All Occupants	Injury Rating Occupant on Impact Side
Front Fender and Hood	14	1.9	2.8
Occupant Compartment	31	3.3	3.6
Rear Fender and Trunk	3	1.7	2.5

Table 5—Model Year of Vehicle

Year	No. of Cases	IR	DSR	Ejections	Seat Belts in Use
1955-1960	10	3.3	3.3	1	
1961	2	2.5	3.5		
1962	6	2.6	4.0	1	
1963	4	2.7	3.5		
1964	4	2.4	2.7		1
1965	6	1.7	3.3	1	2
1966	4	2.0	2.5		1
1967	11	2.5	3.8	1	1
1968	1	2.0	4.0		2
Totals or Average	48	2.53	3.46	4	7

in the past accident cases were studied regardless of vehicle age.

While the numbers are statistically insignificant, there is no evident pattern of change in the DSR. In contrast, there is a suggested downward trend in the IR, which may be due to improved interior safety designs introduced with 1966 model cars.

Seat Belts

Only 7 occupants out of a total of 74 were wearing seat belts at the time of their accidents. The usage rate is low, but this may be explained by the fact that most of the accidents occurred in suburban areas where frequent short trips are taken. The IR for occupants wearing belts was 1.9 and the DSR for their vehicles was 3.4. The IR for unrestrained occupants was 2.7 and the DSR 3.45. The DSR is a measure of the violence of the accident and is nearly equal for the two groups. The restrained occupants were significantly safer.

There were no shoulder harnesses in use in this series.

Injury Patterns

Head injuries were most common and were caused by contact with structures on the impacted side of the vehicle. The severity of head injuries ranged from bruises and lacerations to fatal skull and facial fractures. Upper extremity injuries were the next most frequent, but only

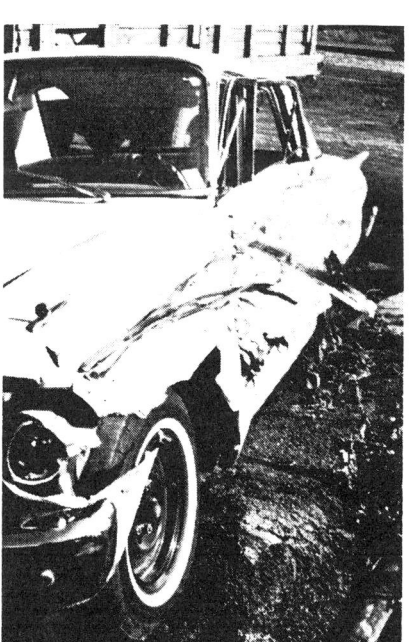

Fig. 3—Case study 1, driver's left arm was traumatically amputated (he was driving with his arm protruding from window)

one was life-threatening (IR, grade 4). The following case study is an example:

Case Study 1—A 39-year-old man, driving with his left elbow out of the door window of a 1963 Comet 4-door sedan, was sideswiped by an oncoming car on a country road. His left arm was amputated traumatically below the shoulder. He also sustained a concussion and a severe contusion of the left hip. (See Fig 3.)

Among other injury patterns which were nearly as frequent were head and upper-extremity injuries. These injuries were more serious and were often life-threatening. Multiple rib fractures were present in 15 patients. Nine patients had hemo or pneumothorax. The chest injuries were the most common life-threatening injuries in the series. Pelvic fractures occurred in 10 cases, but only when the vehicle was impacted on the occupant space. Pubic rami were fractured on the opposite side as frequently as on the impacted side. Fractures of the acetabulum always occurred on the impacted side. In three cases, the femoral head was driven through the acetabulum into the pelvis. (See Table 6.)

Life threatening injuries of the lower extremities (excluding hip and pelvic injuries) did not occur in this series. Most injuries were simple fractures or soft tissue injuries, most commonly in the knee region. The

Table 6—Area of Injury versus Impact Area

Injury	Front	Occupant Space	Rear
Head Injury			
Impact side	6	15	
Opposite side	1	1	
Neck	4		1
Upper Extremity			
Impact Side	4	17	
Opposite side			
Chest			
Impact side	1	12	
Opposite side	1	6	
Hemo- or pneumothorax	1	8	
Rib fractures	1	14	
Abdomen Contusions	2	6	
Ruptured visci	2	1	
Lumbar Spine	3	2	
Pelvis			
Pubic rami			
Impact side		5	
Opposite side		5	
Fractured acetabulum			
Impact side		6	
Opposite side		0	
Intrapelvic protrusion			
Impact side		3	
Opposite side		0	
Lower Extremity			
Impact side	3	10	
Opposite side	1	1	

Note: Ejected Occupants not included.

knee appears to be unusually vulnerable to injury because of its dependence on ligamentous and muscular structures for stability.

Ejected occupants were not included because the exact causes of their injuries could not be determined. It was assumed that in most instances injury occurred after ejection and was caused by contact with structures external to the vehicle.

Structures Causing Injury

Head injuries were caused by nearly all structures in the occupant area. Lacerations were usually caused by window glass but none were

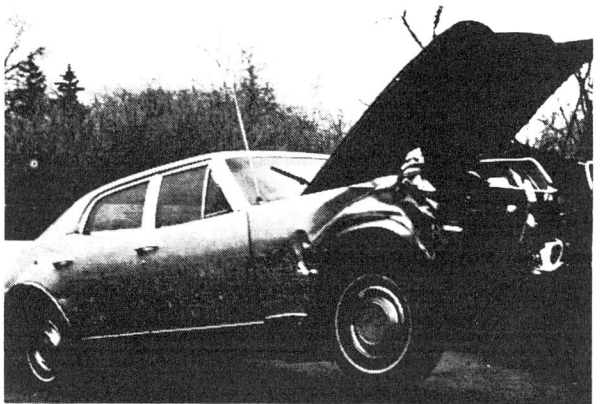

Fig. 4A—Case study 2, 1968 Oldsmobile side-swiped panel truck during overtaking maneuver, ran off the road, and struck clump of trees

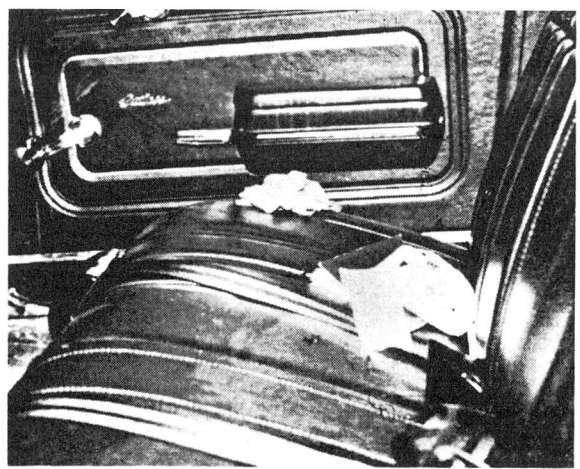

Fig. 4B—Case study 2, driver was thrown against right door, his head impacted window control. He was wearing loosely applied lap belt but slipped partially out of belt

severe. All of the vehicles were fitted with tempered side window glass.

The door was the single structure most commonly causing injury. All parts of the body were susceptible to injury from the door. Door controls were implicated in two cases. The following case illustrates an unusual injury mechanism producing an apical scalp laceraion from a window control:

Case Study 2—A 30-year-old man, driving a 1968 Oldsmobile Cutlass and wearing a lap belt, was thrown hard to the right when he side-swiped a panel truck he was overtaking. His head hit the window control on the right-hand door. He admitted that his belt was loosely applied. (See Figs. 4A-4C.)

Pelvic injuries were caused by direct contact with the door. In most instances, the role of the arm rest could not be determined. Collapsible arm rests in the 1967 and 1968 models may have reduced injury by absorbing impact energy. Pelvic fractures occurred only in occupants next to the impacted side of the car. Contact of the door with the occupant's greater trochanter transmitted the impacting force to the pelvis, resulting in fractures. Fracture of the acetabulum with intrapelvic protrusion of the femoral head and fractures of the pubic rami required the highest forces and occurred only when the occupant was next to the point of maximum deformation of the vehicle. (See Table 7.)

Case Study 3—A 20-year-old young man sustained a left, intrapelvic fracture-dislocation of his hip when his 1962 Corvette drifted into a telephone pole. He had skidded on an ice covered highway. The telephone pole penetrated the vehicle 20 in. (See Figs. 5A and 5B.)

Discussion and Conclusions

The ultimate objective of this study is the reduction of accident injury through vehicle design.

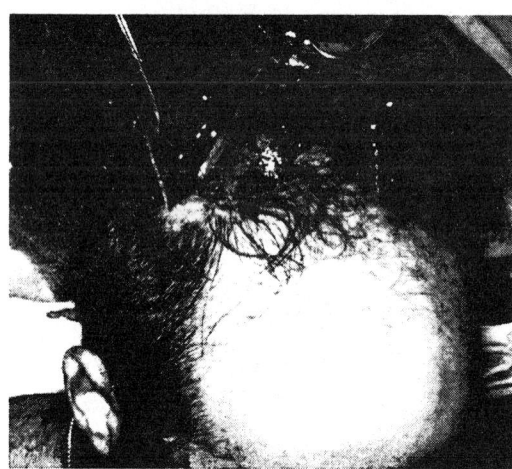

Fig. 4C—Case study, driver received deep scalp laceration because of contact with window control

Seat belts are the single most effective safety device. They are effective in lateral impact accidents because ejection is prevented and the occupant is held in place inside the car. In case study 2 the lap belt would almost certainly have prevented injury had it been applied snugly.

The only situation in which the lap belts do not function well is a direct impact on the occupant space with an occupant seated adjacent to the impacted area. This occurred in three instances (see case study 8). Injury was caused by direct impact, giving the belts no opportunity to protect the occupant. Two patients sustained lumbo-sacral spine strains while wearing lap belts. These injuries are grade 1 (minor injuries) and are attributed to the use of lap belts. However, the occupants would have sustained more serious injuries had they been unrestrained.

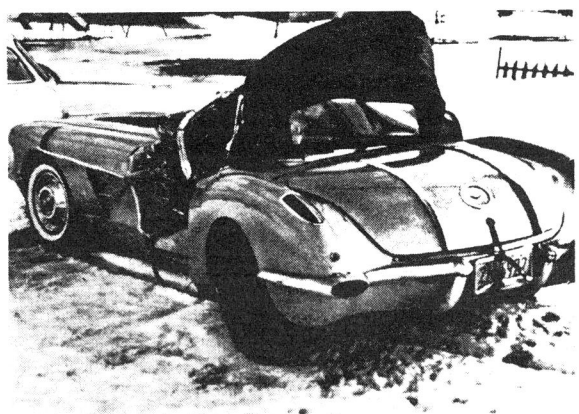

Fig. 5A—Case study 3, 1962 Corvette drifted into telephone pole impacting on left door

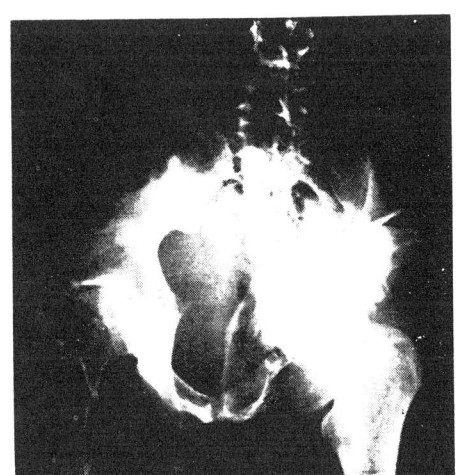

Fig. 5B—Case study 3, driver sustained an intrapelvic dislocation, dislocation of hip and fracture of acetabulum (characteristic injury of lateral impact accidents)

Seat design is an obvious means of occupant protection. The Liberty Mutual seat, as tested by Severy, protects the occupant from injury because of its unusual structural integrity and its high back and sides.

Competition car builders and drivers recognized the advantages of deep bucket seats with lateral support which hold the driver in position to maintain control of the vehicle (Fig. 6). Such a seat also prevents the occupant from striking objects on either side of the seat. NASCAR requires such seats and most other sophisticated racing vehicles use deep bucket seats.

Head protection can be achieved by seat design, particularly in lateral impact accidents. A high back with a wrap-around design affords

Table 7—Parts of Vehicle and Objects Causing Injury

Parts of Vehicle	Head	Neck	Chest	Upper Extremities	Abdomen	LS Spine	Pelvis	Lower Extremities
Impacting Object	4			6				1
Door, Front	5	1	11	12	6	1	10	7
Arm rest	1						1	4
Door controls	1							1
Rear Quarter Panel			1					1
Door Glass	11							
A Pillar	3							
B Pillar			1		1			
Header	1							
Dash	2			4				2
Windshield	6							
Steering Wheel and Column	2		3	1				
Lap Belt					2			

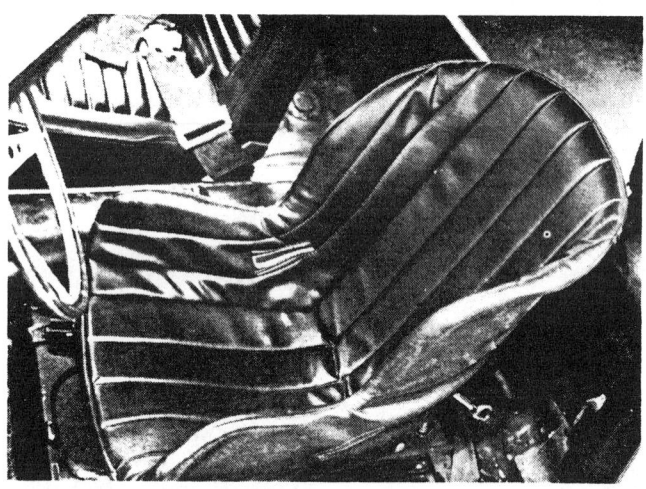

Fig. 6—Custom-made deep bucket seat used in sports car and stock car racing

protection from side and rear impacts. Such a seat is more acceptable for the driving public than crash helmets.

Door and door frame design is the area where the most can be achieved with lowest cost and least risk of consumer rejection. At present, doors are sheet metal structures which collapse with little energy absorption. Protrusion of the impacting object readily occurs and is productive of frequent and serious injuries.

Case Study 4—A 38-year-old woman sustained a fracture of her left tibia and fibula when the 1963 Buick sedan she was driving was struck on the left front door (Fig. 7). The A and B pillars remained in-

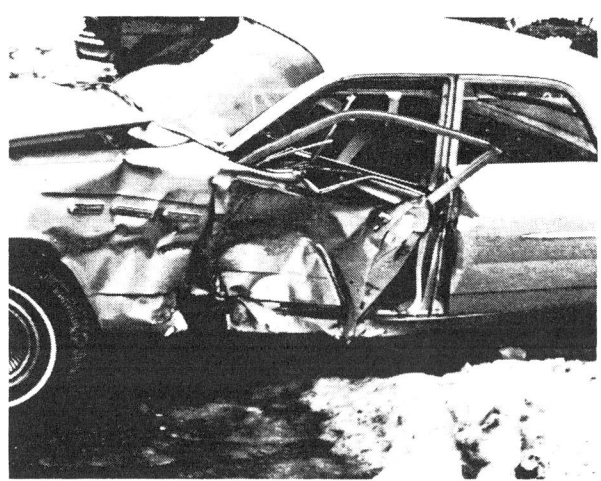

Fig. 7—Case study 4, 38-year-old woman sustained fractures of left tibia and fibula because of direct contact with the left front door. Impacting vehicle penetrated 12 in.

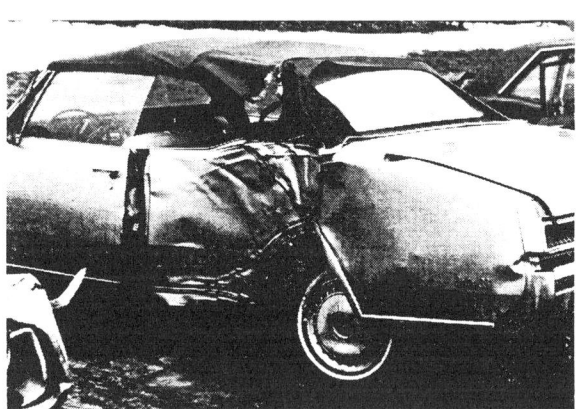

Fig. 8A—Case study 5. Three teenage boys received only minor to moderately severe injuries when 1968 Oldsmobile drifted into tree

tact, but the door permitted 12 in. penetration of the impacting vehicle and produced the left lower extremity fracture by direct contact. A more rigid and energy-absorbing door structure might have reduced or prevented injury.

Chassis frame structure must be coordinated with door design. The introduction of peripheral frames, beginning in 1965, has been a major improvement. Collision with poles and trees have demonstrated the effectiveness of this design in preventing intrusions into the occupant space.

Case Study 5—Three teen-age boys were riding in the front seat of a 1967 Oldsmobile Delta convertible. The driver lost control, overtaking another car. The Oldsmobile drifted into a large maple tree, contacting it just behind the rear left door opening. The frame was contacted, but very little penetration of the occupant space occurred (Figs 8A and 8B). None of the boys received life-threatening injuries.

The driver received a mild concussion because his head hit the windshield and the middle seat occupant received a fractured mandible and left clavicle as a result of contact with the steering wheel. The right seat occupant was uninjured. Seat belts were not in use.

In this case study the frame was hit at a point where it is cross braced and where penetration resistance is high. When the frame is struck in an unbraced section, collapse occurs as is demonstrated in case study 6.

Case Study 6—A 48-year-old man ran off a curve in a four-lane urban street and drifted into a large pine tree striking the tree with the right side of his 1966 Pontiac Le Mans 4-door sedan. He was wearing a seat belt and sustained superficial lacerations of his face and a fracture of the right seventh rib. The tree intruded into the occupant space 22

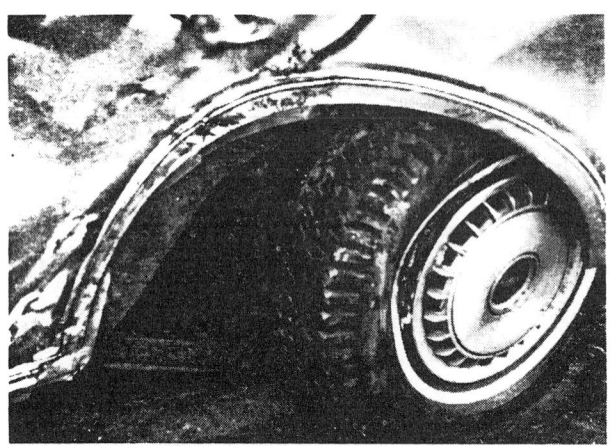

Fig. 6B—Case study 5, tree hit car just in front of rear axle where frame is cross-braced, limiting penetration of occupant space

598

in. in spite of the perimeter frame construction of the vehicle (Figs 9A and 9B).

Some unit body frame vehicles are particularly vulnerable in side impact accidents. The following is an example of a much higher speed accident in which the driver was killed:

Case Study 7—A 1967 Mustang, which is of a unit body construction and without a frame, drifted into a tree, killing the driver. The tree

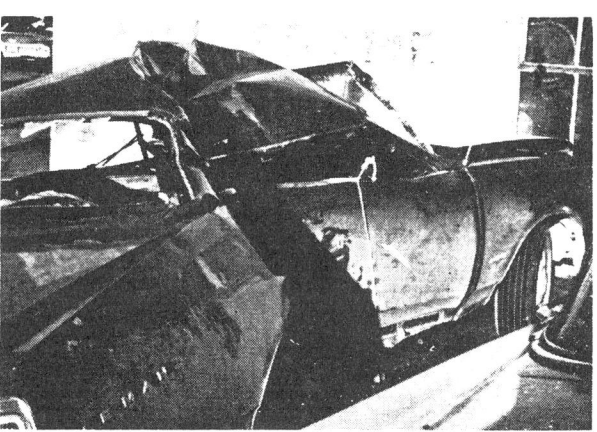

Fig. 9A—Case study 6, 1966 Pontiac drifted into large tree. Driver was wearing lap belt and received only moderate injuries in spite of compromised occupant space

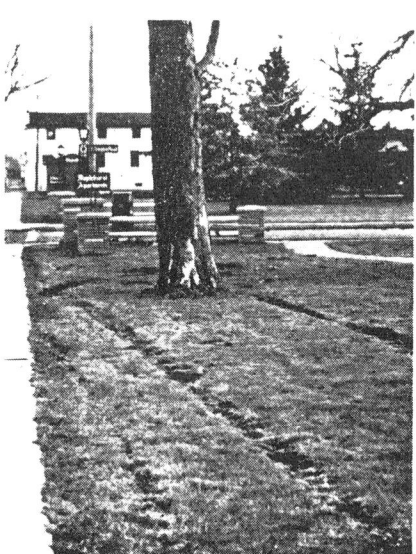

Fig. 9B—Case study 6, car drifted 155 ft before impacting tree

hit and penetrated the left door. The occupant space was penetrated 21 in. and the floor pan was torn open by the tree. It is believed that the occupant's head hit the tree directly. The estimated speed of impact was 45 mph. Death would almost certainly have occurred regardless of vehicle structure, but heavier lateral body or frame structures would have reduced intrusion of the tree into the occupant space. (See Figs. 10A-10C.)

Perimeter frame members or the lateral floor pan reinforcements

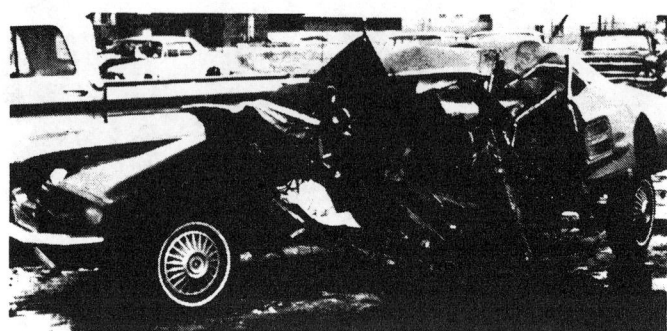

Fig. 10A—Case study 7, 1967 Mustang drifted into tree. Driver sustained fatal head and trunk injuries

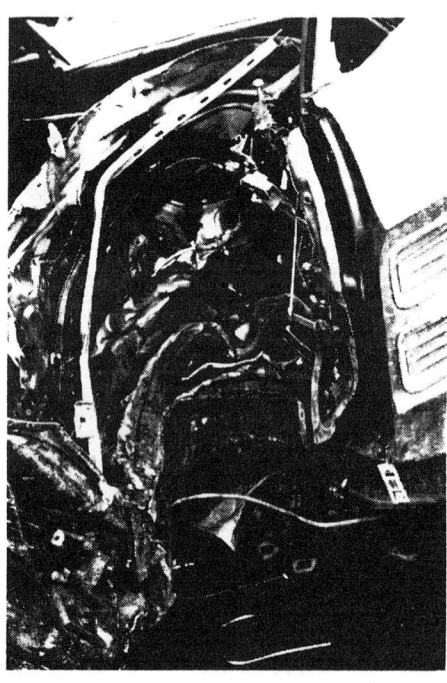

Fig. 10B—Case study 7. Tree hit car on left door and penetrated 21 in.

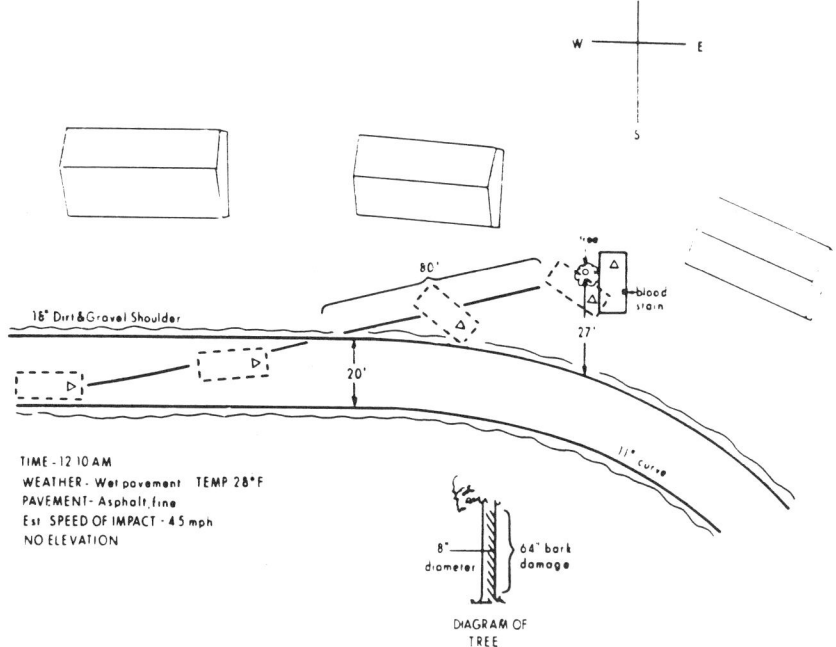

Fig. 10C—Case study 7, car ran off outside of unbanked turn and drifted over frozen ground before impacting tree

of a unitized body should be of sufficient strength to minimize penetration. In turn this will transmit forces to the entire car body which will permit the interior vehicle padding and the occupant restraint systems to function, protecting the occupant.

Door pillar (B pillar) construction and anchorage is essential to prevent penetration of impacting vehicles which override the frame and floor pan of struck vehicles. Hard top models are particularly vulnerable, in spite of heavy B pillars riveted to the floor and frame. Such pillars are tipped over because there is no roof support. This produces tension and shear stress on the floor attachments of the B pillar.

Case Study 8—A 38-year-old man driving a 1967 Buick Wildcat hardtop sustained a hemo-pneumothorax and multiple rib fractures when he was struck on the left door by a 1967 Ford Country Squire station wagon. He ran through a rural intersection, which was controlled by a stop sign which had been removed and thrown into a field by some pranksters. The Ford approached him at a 90 deg angle from the left, hitting his car on the left door and B pillar. The B pillar was tipped over, pulling out its floor attachments. (See Figs. 11A-11C.)

B pillar anchorages in sedans of conventional construction may shear off at the floor level, in spite of their roof anchorage.

Case Study 9—A 1967 Chevrolet Belaire 4-door sedan ran off

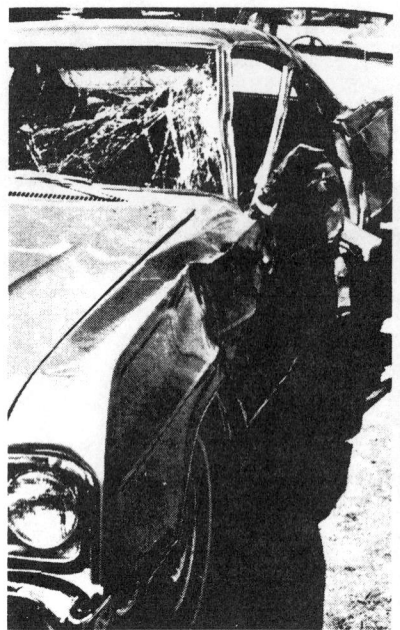

Fig. 11A—Case study 8, 1967 Buick Wildcat was impacted on left door by 1967 Ford Country Squire station wagon. Driver sustained life-threatening chest injuries.

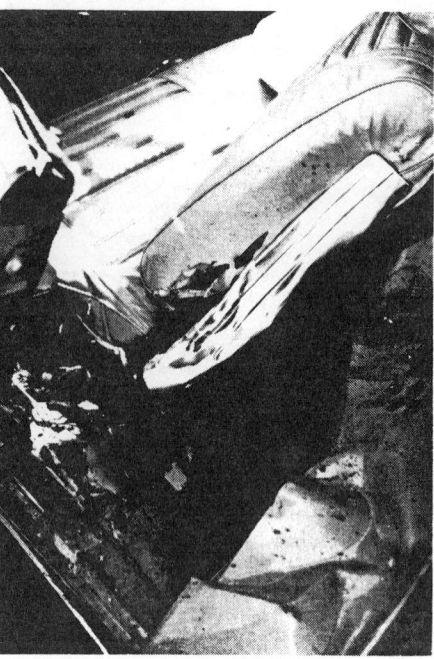

Fig. 11B—Case study 8, B pillar was pulled out of floor and front seat back partially collapsed

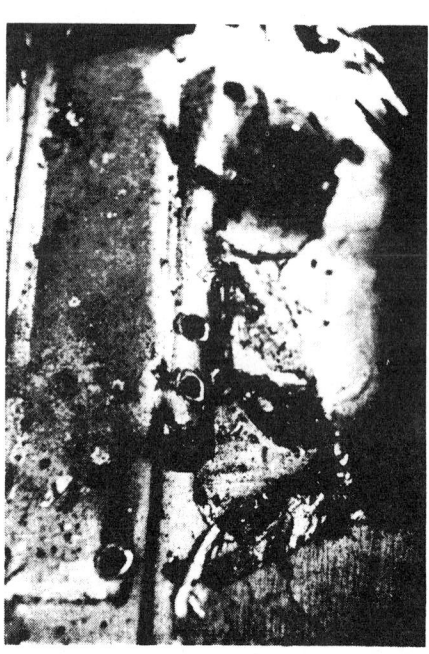

Fig. 11C—Case study 8, close-up view of B pillar anchorage to floor pan

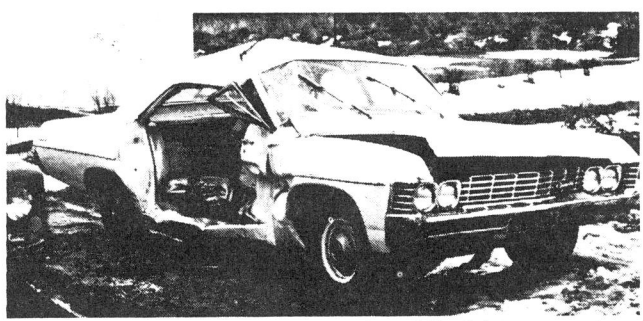

Fig. 12A—Case study 9, 1967 Chevrolet sedan drifted into oncoming 1966 Ford Fairlane station wagon. Seven-month-old infant in front seat sustained fatal head injuries and her mother sustained multiple fractures of pelvis when back of seat was hit by B pillar and impacting vehicle

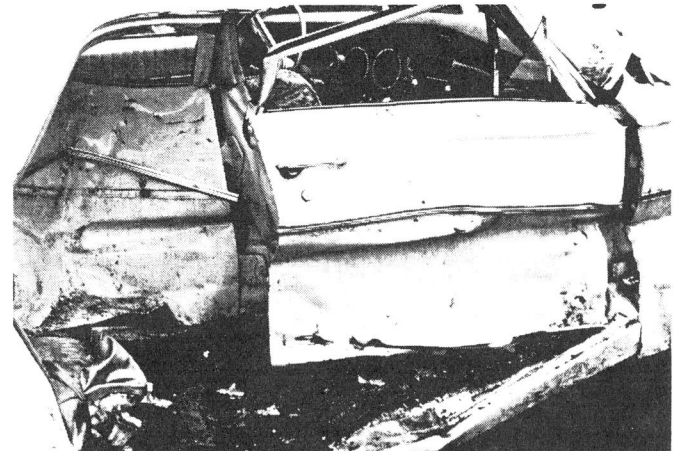

Fig. 12B—Case study 9, car was impacted on both right-hand doors

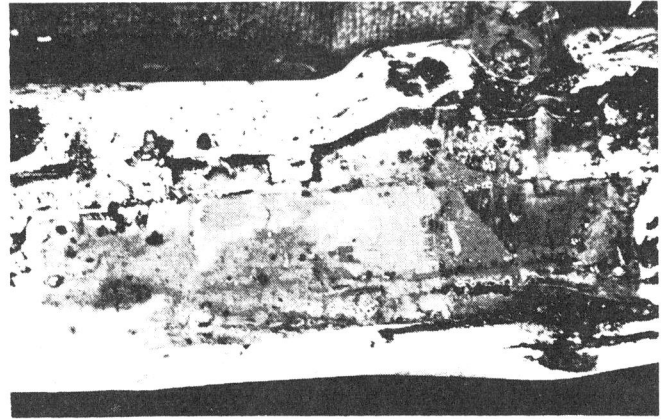

Fig. 12C—Case study 9, close-up of B pillar floor anchorage which was sheared off

766064

Biomechanics, Pedestrian Impact, and Dummies

J. W. Melvin, D. H. Robbins, and R. L. Stalnaker
University of Michigan

ABSTRACT

This paper presents results from a project studying the side impact response of anthropomorphic test devices and human cadavers.

Using a baseline test configuration of a flat rigid wall for initial tests and a contoured, padded surface to simulate a vehicle side interior configuration for subsequent tests, a series of experiments was performed with:

- Unembalmed human cadavers with head, thorax, and pelvis accelerometer instrumentation
- Part 572 test device with head, thorax, and pelvis triaxial accelerometer instrumentation
- Transport and Road Research Laboratory (TRRL) side impact test device with head, thorax, and pelvis triaxial accelerometers as well as shoulder, rib, and pelvis load cells

Comparisons of both the kinematic responses and the accelerometer data of the three types of test subjects are made. In addition, a discussion of the injuries produced in the cadaver tests with respect to test device interpretation is included with emphasis on the development of improved test response specifications.

INTRODUCTION

The subject of side impact injury protection in automobile crashes has received relatively little emphasis when compared to the research conducted on frontal impact protection. This is mainly due to the high priority of protecting vehicle occupants in frontal type crashes. As this goal is approached, attention has been shifted to consideration of the side impact problem. Protection of vehicle occupants sitting on the near side of a vehicle subjected to a side impact presents several difficulties, the major ones being:

- Minimal crush distance to attenuate and control the forces of the crash
- Penetration of the occupant compartment space
- Partial ejection of the occupant through the side windows—thereby allowing interaction with outside objects
- Difficulty of adequate lateral restraint of the occupant by conventional restraint systems.

The sequence of events that happen to a near side occupant in a side impact depend somewhat on the seating position relative to the point of impact and upon the geometry of the impacting structure. In the case of an unrestrained occupant seated near the point of impact, the initial acceleration of the vehicle due to the crash is not transmitted to the occupant—instead the vehicle undergoes a velocity change while the unrestrained occupant continues at the velocity he had in that direction at the start of the crash.

Eventually, the side structure of the vehicle (which may be moving toward the occupant due to intrusion) and the occupant meet in a second impact with a relative velocity which depends upon the crash velocity and the rate of intrusion. The forces generated by the impact of the occupant with the side structure depend on their relative velocity and the mechanical properties of both the occupant and the side structure. In many side impacts, the window glazing shatters upon the initial impact and is gone by the time the occupant reaches the side structure of the vehicle. This leads to additional concentration of the occupant impact loads into the thorax since the glazing no longer can serve as a load-bearing surface on the upper portions of the body. The shape of the interior surfaces of the side structure also influences the load distribution developed when the occupant's body impacts the side structure.

The protection of occupants in side impacts depends primarily upon controlling the magnitude and distribution of impact forces applied to the occupant's body as the vehicle side structure and the occupant collide. The design of the side structure interior surfaces to achieve this goal depends on a knowledge of the biomechanical characteristics of the human body under lateral impact—particularly of the shoulder, thorax, and pelvis—and the development of test devices based on such knowledge.

MATERIALS AND METHODS

The test subjects used in this study were unembalmed human cadavers, a Part 572 anthropometric test device, and a prototype side impact test device developed by Transport and Road Research Laboratory (TRRL).

Cadaver Test Subjects

The unembalmed human cadavers were stored under refrigeration (5° C) except when being surgically prepared and were allowed to reach room temperature (25° C) prior to testing. Testing took place typically 5 to 7 days post mortem, and the effects of rigor mortis were past at the time of testing. Instrumentation surgically attached to the cadavers included the following:

- An externally mounted array of uniaxial Endevco 2264-2000 piezo-resistive accelerometers on the right side of the head oriented one each in the anterior-posterior (A-P), superior-inferior (S-I) and left-right (L-R) directions
- An array of 10 uniaxial Endevco 2264-2000 accelerometers mounted on the thorax in a manner described in detail by Robbins, et al. [1], consisting of biaxial arrays on the first thoracic vertebra (T1) (A-P and S-I) and the twelfth vertebra (T12) (A-P and L-R) as well as various uniaxial mounts on individual ribs and the sternum
- An externally mounted triaxial array of uniaxial Endevco 2764-2000 accelerometers in the A-P, S-I and L-R directions on the rear of the pelvis in the mid-sagittal plane

All accelerometers were attached in a rigid manner to the bony structures indicated. In addition to the accelerometers, pressure transducers (Kulite miniature piezo-resistive units) were inserted into the trachea and aortic arch to measure airway and vascular system pressures. The vascular system of the cadavers was fluid-filled and the lungs were air-filled; both were pressurized to physiological levels prior to testing. The cadaver test subject data are listed in table 1 for the

Table 1. Cadaver test subject data

Test No.	Age (yrs)	Sex	Stature (cm)	Weight (kg)
003	60	M	181	102.1
009	75	F	156	44.1
010	84	M	162	87.8
011	69	M	170	74.9
029	67	M	167	62.5
039	72	M	187	73.9
042	58	F	178	64.5

seven cadavers used in this study. The cadavers were clothed in vinyl exercise suits to minimize moisture loss and then suited in cotton thermal underwear to provide an appropriate outer surface for testing.

Part 572 Test Subject

The Part 572 anthropometric test device used in the study was instrumented with triaxial arrays of uniaxial Endevco 2264-2000 accelerometers mounted internally in the required head, thorax, and pelvic locations. The dummy was suited in the same type of cotton thermal underwear as the cadavers.

TRRL Test Subject

The TRRL side impact test device was instrumented with triaxial arrays of uniaxial Endevco 2264-2000 accelerometers in the head, thorax, and pelvis in the same manner as the Part 572 dummy. In addition, this test device features load cells built into various of the side structures of the dummy. The load cells are contained in the shoulder, the four individual ribs which comprise the thorax, the iliac crest, and the hip. The details of this design can be found in the paper of Harris [2]. A notable feature of the device is the absence of arms—the shoulder load cells take their place. This dummy was also suited in cotton thermal underwear for the tests.

Test Methods

All tests in this study were performed at the Highway Safety Research Institute (HSRI) Impact Sled Facility. The sled is a deceleration sled which operates on the rebound principle. Since the tests were to simulate an unrestrained vehicle occupant in a side impact, the test technique utilized a test fixture consisting of a rigid bench seat mounted in a side impact configuration on the sled with a rigid wall structure representing the side of the vehicle at the left end of the seat. The test subject was placed a predetermined distance from the impact surface such that the subject was free to translate along the seat during the sled deceleration and impact the surface only after the sled deceleration had terminated. This technique produced an impact situation in which the test subject and the impact surface came together at the desired relative impact velocity while allowing the test subject decelerations to be determined solely by the interaction between the subject and the impact surface rather than the sled deceleration profile. Three test relative velocities were used—25, 33, and 43 km/h—designated low, medium, and high velocities, respectively. In addition, a special low velocity (16 km/h) test was performed on the TRRL dummy only.

The impact surface configurations consisted of a flat rigid wall and a contoured energy-absorbing structure. The flat wall buck configuration (shown in fig. 1) was constructed of one-inch plywood backed by

Figure 1. Test set up configuration for rigid wall impact tests.

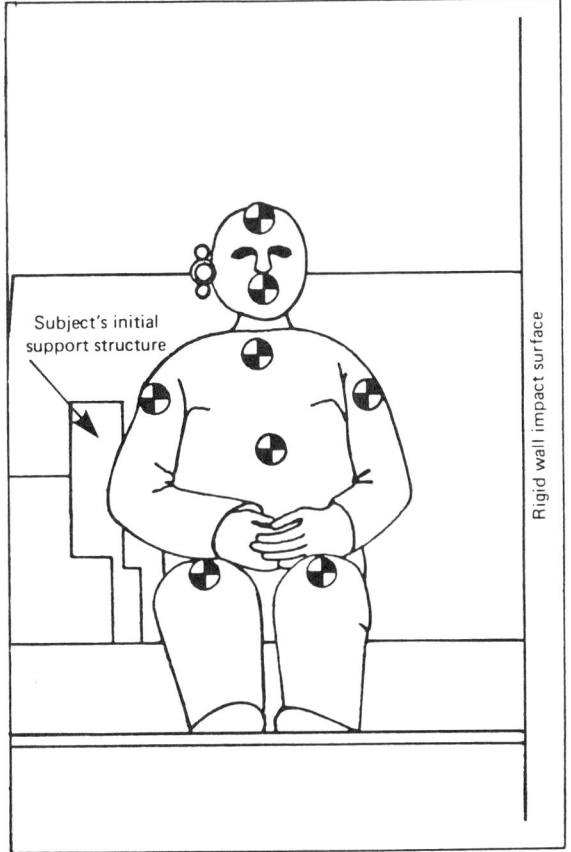

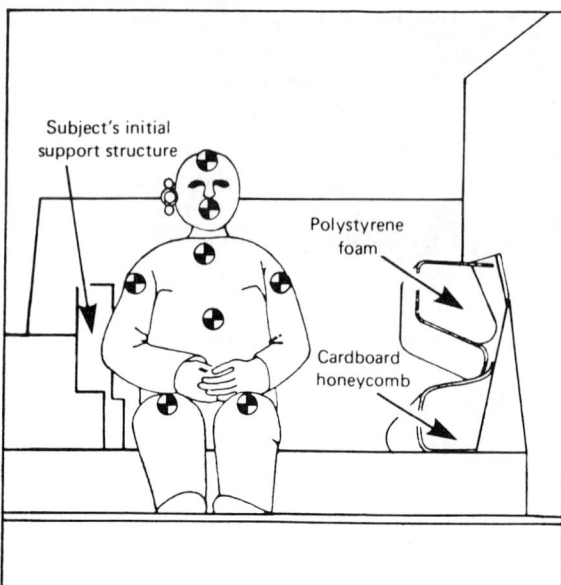

Figure 2. Test set up configuration for energy absorbing contoured side structure tests.

a steel beam reinforcing structure tied to the sled. The energy-absorbing structure (shown in fig. 2) consisted of thorax and pelvis bolsters developed in the NHTSA RSV program. The thorax bolster was constructed of 15 cm of polystyrene foam drilled with lateral holes to adjust crush strength and covered with 1.3 cm of Ensolite energy-absorbing vinyl foam. The pelvis bolster was constructed of 15-cm thick Hexcell cardboard honeycomb also covered with Ensolite. The bolsters were attached to the rigid wall surface of the buck, as shown in figure 2.

Lateral and overhead view high speed movies were taken of every test at 1 000 pictures/second.

TEST RESULTS

The results of the test program are presented in the following sections—first in terms of general kinematics and then followed by tabular summaries of transducer response and cadaver injury rating. The transducer signals were filtered according to SAE J211a specifications: head accelerations - Channel Class 1000; thorax and pelvis accelerations - Channel Class 180; and load cells - Channel Class 600.

Test Subject Kinematics

During the phase of the test when the test subject is sliding towards the impact surface, all three types of test subjects behaved similarly and exhibited uniform translation of the body with no relative motion of body parts. As soon as impact with the side structure begins, each type of test subject starts to exhibit individual impact behavior unique to the structural characteristics of the subject. The differences were most marked in the rigid wall impact tests. In the case of the Part 572 dummy, the side of the torso contacts the wall and then deforms slightly due to the low compliance of the dummy internal structure. This is quite pronounced in the shoulder region where the shoulder linkage transmits the forces directly to the base of the neck and thereby starts the head to rotate toward the wall. The resulting lateral flexion of the neck rotates the head almost horizontally, but the shoulder structure does not let the head fully contact the wall—it barely grazes it at the higher test velocities. With the TRRL dummy, the lack of arms allows the head to be much closer to the wall and thus the head contacts the wall more directly, although only after lateral neck flexion on the order of 30 to 45 degrees occurs.

The cadaver subjects exhibited a completely different head-neck response in the rigid wall tests. The shoulder linkage of the cadaver displaced laterally with little apparent resistance and the head-neck system does not undergo appreciable lateral flexion. The result is that the head strikes the wall in an upright position and the loads are carried by the lower parietal and temporal bone regions.

For the case of the padded structure impacts, the differences in head-neck response diminished somewhat due to the spacing of the torso impact surface away from the wall. The highly compliant cadaver shoulder structure still reduces the lateral neck flexion and allows head contact with the wall but the contact is more onto the parietal bone region. It should be noted that the shoulder bones were not broken or dislocated in any of the tests.

The general motions of the rest of the body below the shoulders were similar in all three types of test subjects. The pelvis region tended to rebound first followed by the thoracic region—leading to a marked tendency of the subject to rotate out of the seat in a counterclockwise manner.

Head Impact Response

The results of the head accelerometer peak readings are summarized in table 2. The lower acceleration values of the Part 572 dummy in all the tests are attributable to the lack of lateral shoulder compliance and its effect on head kinematics as discussed above. The lack of arms on the TRRL dummy allowed head impacts more like those produced with the cadavers to take place. Direct comparison of the A-P and S-I values between cadaver and dummies is questionable due to the external mounting of the accelerometers on the cadaver head. In those cases where skull fracture took place, it can be expected that high peak values may occur in various directions depending on fracture patterns.

Thorax Impact Response

The results of the thorax accelerometer peak readings are summarized in table 3. Due to the different accelerometer placement on the cadaver thorax, a direct comparison of transducers is not possible. The A-P and S-I values were taken from the biaxial accelerometer pair mounted on the first thoracic vertebra (T1) while the L-R values were taken from a uniaxial accelerometer mounted on the fourth rib on the right-hand side of the body (opposite the impacted side). Comparison of the L-R peaks in the rigid impacts shows that the values produced in the cadaver thorax were generally comparable to those obtained in the Part 572 dummy, while the TRRL dummy gave lower values. It is of interest to note that in the low velocity rigid test, the suggested tolerance

Table 2. Head peak accelerations (g)

a. Rigid wall impact tests										
	Low velocity			Medium velocity				High velocity		
Subject	CAD	572	TRRL	CAD	CAD	572	572	TRRL	CAD	572
Test No.	–	012	016	010	011	013	014	017	009	015
A-P	–	6	38	57	125	14	23	25	309	47
S-I	–	50	53	174	138	83	85	157	415	135
L-R	–	64	135	293	179	82	41	197	468	104

b. Padded side structure tests										
	Low velocity			Medium velocity			High velocity		
Subject	CAD	572	TRRL	CAD	572	TRRL	CAD	572	TRRL	
Test No.	029	028	045	039	043	030	042	044	046	
A-P	–	3	5	38	5	–	27	22	38	
S-I	–	17	36	278	38	–	233	72	183	
L-R	–	12	17	137	28	–	103	49	767	

Table 3. Thorax peak accelerations (g)

a. Rigid wall impact tests

	Low velocity			Medium velocity					High velocity	
Subject	CAD	572	TRRL	CAD	CAD	572	572	TRRL	CAD	572
Test No.	003	012	016	010	011	013	014	017	009	015
A-P	73	15	5	56	95	17	18	42	100	40
S-I	196	18	16	107	81	35	22	42	96	84
L-R	82	61	42	120	149	139	147	89	150	162

b. Padded side structure tests

	Low velocity			Medium velocity			High velocity		
Subject	CAD	572	TRRL	CAD	572	TRRL	CAD	572	TRRL
Test No.	029	028	045	039	043	030	042	044	046
A-P	14	5	5	25	4	11	44	14	13
S-I	24	8	5	37	12	7	51	24	26
L-R	56	28	37	19	102	40	175	145	88

Table 4. Pelvis peak accelerations (g)

a. Rigid wall impact tests

	Low velocity			Medium velocity					High velocity	
Subject	CAD	572	TRRL	CAD	CAD	572	572	TRRL	CAD	572
Test No.	003	012	016	010	011	013	014	017	009	015
A-P	22	10	3	41	—	21	24	28	54	42
S-I	65	14	93	63	70	63	47	96	47	61
L-R	53	60	49	70	149	286	278	147	279	379

b. Padded side structure tests

	Low velocity			Medium velocity			High velocity		
Subject	CAD	572	TRRL	CAD	572	TRRL	CAD	572	TRRL
Test No.	029	028	045	039	043	030	042	044	046
A-P	42	3	4	7	7	—	35	9	23
S-I	20	5	6	19	15	—	43	35	43
L-R	78	28	34	39	44	—	106	121	74

level of FMVSS 208 was exceeded by the cadaver and the Part 572 dummy and closely approached by the TRRL dummy, while in the padded low velocity test, only the cadaver exceeded the 45 g level.

Pelvis Impact Response

The results of the pelvis accelerometer peak readings are summarized in table 4. The external placement of the accelerometers on the cadaver pelvis is most likely the cause of the large differences which appear in the A-P and S-I values when comparing the cadaver values to the dummy values. The L-R values are, for the most part, quite comparable in both the rigid wall and padded structure tests. The exception to this is the low velocity padded test.

TRRL Dummy Load Cell Response

The peak readings of the various load cells of the TRRL dummy are listed in table 5.

Table 5. TRRL dummy peak load cell values (kN)

a. Rigid wall impact tests			
Test No.	109[a]	016	017
Left shoulder	9.79	19.06	–
Left rib 1	0.36	0.70	1.91
Left rib 2	0.52	1.04	2.18
Left rib 3	0.28	0.44	1.05
Left rib 4	0.37	0.65	0.77
Left iliac	16.69	–	–
Left hip	1.17	5.22	4.70

b. Padded side structure tests			
Test No.	030	044	046
Left shoulder	0.32	0.16	1.01
Left rib 1	3.10	2.09	4.49
Left rib 2	2.99	1.98	3.02
Left rib 3	1.84	0.47	2.41
Left rib 4	0.32	0.32	0.18
Left iliac	1.28	–	–
Left hip	10.07	2.71	10.85

[a]Special low speed (16 km/h) test.

The missing data in the table are due to either malfunctioning transducers or overload conditions. In the rigid wall tests, some ringing of the rib load cells was noted. The padding configuration in the energy-absorbing side structure tests was such that the shoulder load cell did not come into full contact with the padding, thereby producing low readings. The special low speed (16 km/h) test was necessary due to load cell overload in the rigid wall tests at the medium velocity level.

Cadaver Injury Ratings

The injuries sustained by the cadavers in the various rigid wall impact tests are listed in table 6 along with the assessments of the Abbreviated Injury Scale (AIS) ratings of the injuries. The moderate injuries sustained in the 25-km/h impact escalate sharply at the 33-km/h level indicating that in rigid wall impacts the AIS 3 level is most likely reached in the 28 to 30 km/h velocity range. The severity of the injuries at the 43-km/h level point out the serious need to manage the occupant kinetic energy in impacts at velocities considerably lower than those associated with frontal crashes.

The results of the injuries sustained in the padded structure tests are given in table 7. Although the severity of the injuries was reduced at the high velocity in comparison to the rigid wall test, the padded structure did not change the injury level of the thorax at the medium velocity and actually raised it slightly in the low velocity test. The padded structure did help to reduce head injuries in the low and medium test velocities even though the head hit the wall in the medium velocity test.

Some insight into the factors affecting injury production in the padded side structures can be gained by examining the resulting deformation patterns in the energy-absorbing materials used in the structures. The Part 572 dummy consistently produced larger penetrations of the thorax padding and in the medium- and high-velocity tests most likely bottomed the foam out (that is, completely penetrated it)—yet the deformations were more localized. This

Table 6. Cadaver injury summary—rigid wall impact tests

Test No.	Body part	Injuries	AIS rating
003 25 km/h	Thorax	Left side—minor rib fracture directly under fourth rib accelerometer mount	2
010 33 km/h	Head	Superficial bruising of brain at the base of the frontal lobe	4/5
	Thorax	Left side-fractures of ribs 1-8 in front and 3 and 4 in rear Right side—fractures of ribs 1-5 in front	4
011 33 km/h	Head	Depressed fracture of the left side of the skull, free blood in the cavity right side: subarachnoid hemorrhage left side: frontal lobe hemorrhage	5
	Thorax	Left side—fractures of ribs 2, 3, 4, 5, 6, 7, and 9 Right side—fractures of ribs 2-6 Spinal dislocation between C4/C5	4
	Abdomen	Liver—small tear on surface Spleen—crushed	4
009 43 km/h	Head	Left side—massive depressed skull fractures and extensive hemorrhaging in scalp, muscle, and dura mater	6
	Neck	Cervical spine fractures at C1 and dislocation between C2/C3	6
	Thorax	Left side—15 rib fractures in front and 11 rib fractures in rear Right side—13 rib fractures in front and 2 rib fractures in rear 7 cm tear of left lung with free blood 2 cm tear of pulmonary artery	6
	Abdomen	Crushed left kidney	5
	Pelvis	Left side iliac crest crushed severely with soft tissue damage	5

was due to the rigidity of the arm structure which penetrated the foam at load levels lower than the more distributed loading on the side of the cadaver thorax. In fact, the TRRL dummy with no arms produced thorax padding similar to those of the cadavers.

An additional feature was noted in the deformations of the pelvis honeycomb padding. The cadaver tests tended to produce crushing distributed along the honeycomb in contrast to the more localized crushing associated with the pelvis and knees of the dummies. This behavior may be due to the more concentrated masses of the dummy pelvis and knee structures as opposed to the more evenly distributed soft tissue masses of the cadavers.

Table 7. Cadaver injury summary—padded side structure tests

Test No.	Body part	Injuries	AIS rating
029 25 km/h	Thorax	Left side—4 rib fractures	3
039 33 km/h	Thorax	Left side—11 rib fractures, very slight surface hemorrhage on heart	4
042 43 km/h	Head	Left side—massive depressed skull fracture with fractures extending to the right side. Extensive hemorrhage over the right temporal and parietal lobes of the brain	5
	Thorax	Left side—12 rib fractures. Mid-shaft fracture of left humerus	4

SUMMARY AND CONCLUSIONS

A series of comparative side impact tests using unembalmed human cadavers, a Part 572 test device and the TRRL side impact test device has been presented in brief. The results of the program indicate the following:

- Significant differences in head-neck kinematics exist in the side impact behaviors of the three types of test subjects—the lack of lateral compliance of the shoulder structure in dummies contributes to this effect.
- The peak responses of the thorax accelerometers were similar in the three types of test subjects, but the resulting injuries in the limited cadaver test sample did not correlate well with suggested tolerance levels for lateral acceleration.
- The peak responses of the pelvis accelerometers were similar for the three types of test subjects.
- The differences between dummy and cadavers in lateral compliance of the shoulder and arm structures and in the distribution of masses in the lower body must be considered in the design of energy-absorbing side impact structures.

ACKNOWLEDGMENTS

This work was supported under NHTSA Contract No. DOT-HS-4-00921. The results and conclusions presented are those of the authors and do not represent statements and policy of the United States Government. The authors would like to acknowledge the diligent work of HSRI staff including J. Benson, J. Lehman, G. Nusholtz, T. Tann, and the impact sled laboratory staff in accomplishing this work.

REFERENCES

1. Robbins, D. H., Melvin, J. W., and Stalnaker, R. L. "The prediction of thoracic impact injuries." Proceedings of the 20th Stapp Car Crash Conference, Society of Automotive Engineers, Inc., Warrendale, Pennsylvania, SAE Paper No. 760822. 1976.
2. Harris, J. "The design and use of the TRRL side impact dummy." Proceedings of the 20th Stapp Car Crash Conference, Society of Automotive Engineers, Inc., Warrendale, Pennsylvania, SAE Paper No. 760802. 1976.

796033
Synthesis of Human Tolerances Obtained from Lateral Impact Simulations

C. Tarrière, G. Walfisch, A. Fayon, and J. P. Rosey
Laboratoire de Physiologie et de Biomécanique de l'Association Peugeot-Renault

C. Got and A. Patel
IRO/IRBA—Hôpital Raymond Poincaré

A. Delmas
Laboratoire d'Anatomie de l'Unité d'Enseignement et de Recherches Biomédicales des Saints Pères

ABSTRACT

The desirable protection criteria on dummies have to be defined from the best estimate of human tolerances. In lateral collisions, the state of knowledge stayed a long time less advanced than in frontal collisions. Research on fresh cadavers has been carried on for several years to fill this gap; a synthesis of recent results is presented.

Relating to the head, sufficient data has been collected in the cases of impacts simulating realistic conditions of ΔV and shock duration. Likewise, for the neck in the absence of head impact, for the thorax, and the pelvis, numerous experiments were conducted, which are used to define human tolerances.

The state of the transposition to dummies is evoked.

INTRODUCTION

The protection of occupants of a private car that is struck from the side is a complex and difficult problem. It is complex because a large number of parameters intervene, and difficult because very little volume is available for providing protection. The requisite conditions for finding proper solutions include a thorough knowledge of human tolerances to side impacts and the availability of dummies whose behavior and responses are correlated with the kinematics and potential injuries of accident victims. The matter dealt with in this report is a synthesis of the data that have essentially been gathered from biomechanical experiments on the cadavers of individuals who had willed their bodies to science.

This research was conducted under contracts with French Administration. The findings and views expressed here are those of the authors.

Tolerances of the Head to Side Impacts

Data concerning the tolerance of the head to impacts in the temporoparietal area, which are of likely occurrence in side impact collisions, were collected under the heading of research devoted to investigation of helmets for riders of two-wheeled vehicles. Some results are already published[5].

It should be noted that the speed variation sustained by the head in most of the corresponding experiments was on the order of 30 kilometers per hour, and that impact time-length, determined by the shock-absorbing material used, was such that tolerance estimates were compiled under impact-violence conditions pertinent to the case of a laterally-struck victim.

Testing procedure consisted of releasing cadavers into free falls, said cadavers being fresh, unembalmed and perfused, as shown in Figure 1 where the head hits a rigid and plane surface.

The subject lies in a metal cradle. His head, with or without a helmet, protrudes beyond the cradle. The unit is allowed to fall freely. The head is maintained in alignment with the trunk until impact.

The cradle containing the body comes to rest against a thick mattress. The head undergoes a relative movement in relation to the thorax.

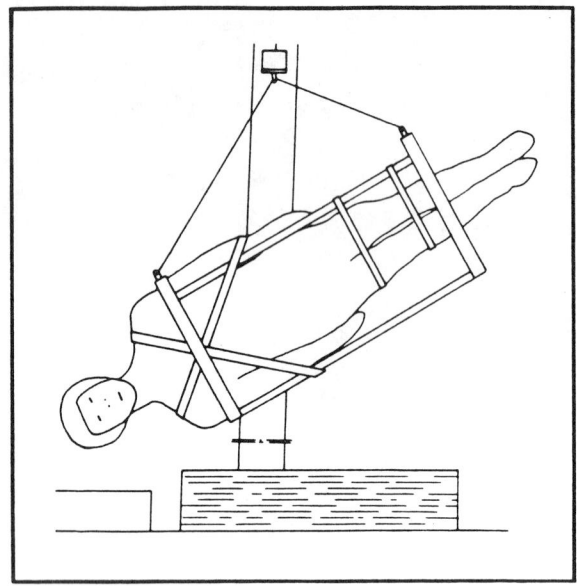

Figure 1. Free fall conditions for head impact tolerance experiments.

Each test is accompanied by anthropometric measurements, acceleration measurements and measurements of the percussion force, and a pressurization of the encephalon described below.

The impact is recorded on films.

Three accelerometers are attached to light alloy plates screwed into the subject's skull. On the basis of the acceleration measurements performed on the periphery of the skull, it is possible to compute the acceleration at the center of gravity of the head. A method of solution was used similar to that of Stalnaker, Alem[6].

Satisfactory results were achieved when nine correct $\gamma(t)$ pulses were available.

When it was not possible to use this method, an estimate of $\gamma(t)$ at C.G. was made according to the accelerometers closest to the C.G.

In order to detect the cerebral lesions, a perfusion of the encephalon was performed on each subject. The injected liquid is made of water, India ink (as a marker) and formaldehyde.

Vascular damage is hence marked by black extravasations around the ruptures, similar in appearance to hemorrhages observed in live persons.

The best estimate of the corresponding AIS value is made accordingly.

More details are published in Reference 5.

Observing the head kinematics during these tests and taking into account the estimates of head tolerance to angular accelerations, one may conclude that the observed injuries are linked to linear accelerations. Most of these injuries are lesions at brain stem level.

Figure 2 shows, for each subject, the estimate of AIS value versus the computed HIC.

This a priori does not reveal any relationship between two parameters. This is not surprising: in an identical injury-causing process, tolerance is a function of numerous parameters related to the subject; besides, the AIS is not a proportionate continuous scale.

Serious injuries (AIS $\geq$ 3) may appear in extremely low HIC values when the subject's brain is a poor state of conservation, but this result is not meaningful. The lowest HIC associated with serious injuries is this of No. 99, which is 1400.

Conversely, it is possible to obtain high HIC values without injuries. It should be noted that we found no serious injuries except when the accelerations maintained during three milliseconds at the most were more than 130 g.

It was finally found that during these lateral skull impacts, there is but slight likelihood of the occurrence of a serious injury for a value of HIC $\leq$ 1500.

A few characteristic tests were reproduced with Part 572 dummies for purposes of comparing the HIC values yielded by cadavers with those yielded by dummies at identical impact velocities. For the high HICs, we approached the limits of the helmets' shock-absorption capacities, and we found values in the same range. (For moderate violence, this did not apply, and the ATD values were then lower) (fig. 3). This confirms the absence of any constant relation between the accelerations measured on a dummy and those measured on a human subject: the relation is variable and depends on test conditions.

Although it is allowable to use a HIC 1500-type limit in the temporoparietal impact against a Part 572-type head, the fact must not be overlooked that this correspondence was approximately verified in the case of im-

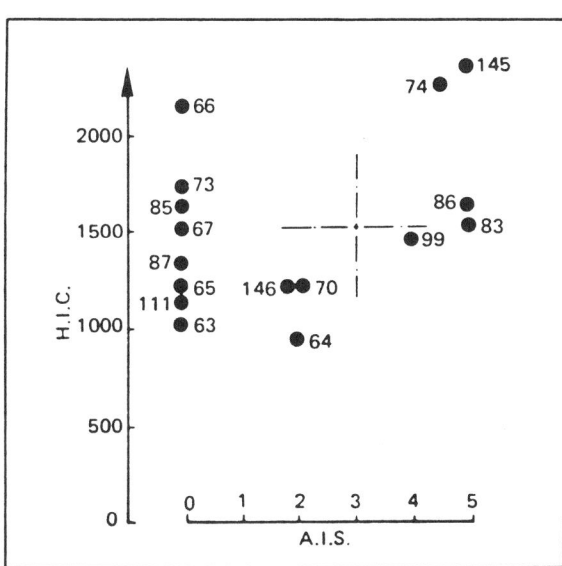

Figure 2. Relation between calculated HIC and AIS.

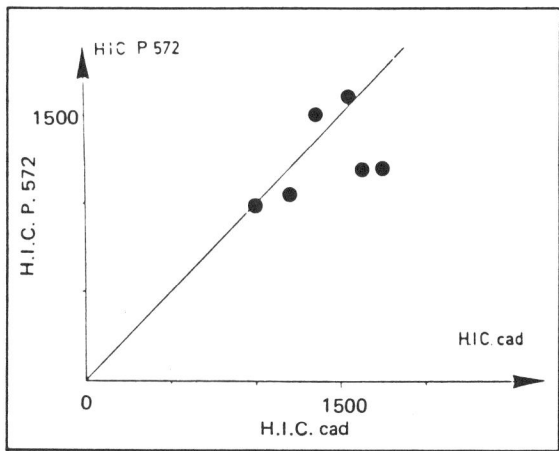

Figure 3. Comparison between the "Part 572" HIC and the cadaver HIC for same free fall tests with helmet.

pacts occurring at identical impact velocities for dummies and human subjects.

No positive conclusion will be possible concerning the validity of the protection provided in car-to-car side collisions unless the dummy's behavior yields a head impact velocity close to that of a human head, which is not the case when the shoulder acts as a brace and when the chest deflects insufficiently.

In addition, HIC 1500 can be used in the case of impacts carried out with a separate head, not using the complete dummy.

Tolerances of the Thorax to Side Impacts

Methodology

For the main part, collected data come from the results of the free-falls of human subjects. These strike rigid surfaces or surfaces covered with shock-absorbing materials side-on at the thorax and pelvis. These tests were reproduced with Part 572 dummies. Consequently, a contribution will be made to knowledge of human tolerance to lateral impacts, the desirable characteristics of a dummy for side-on impact and for protection paddings.

The subject or dummy is hung and then released in order to drop freely against the side, in the position shown in Figure 4. The side struck varies for reasons related to the experimental conditions.

The configurations used for the tests are on Figure 5.

Two positions for the arms were used.

The types of surfaces struck were rigid planes, hitting the shoulder or not, or pairs of shock-absorbing material blocks, one for the thorax and the other one for the pelvis (see fig. 5).

All the subjects were equipped with triaxial accelerometers. Among them, one accelerometer was screwed to the fourth dorsal vertebra, a second was also screwed to the sacrum in the median sagittal plane, 90 mm below the iliac crests.

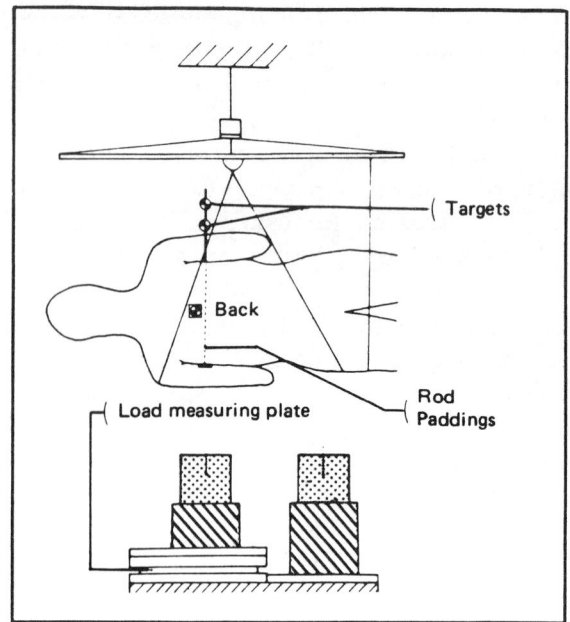

Figure 4. Lateral drop test conditions.

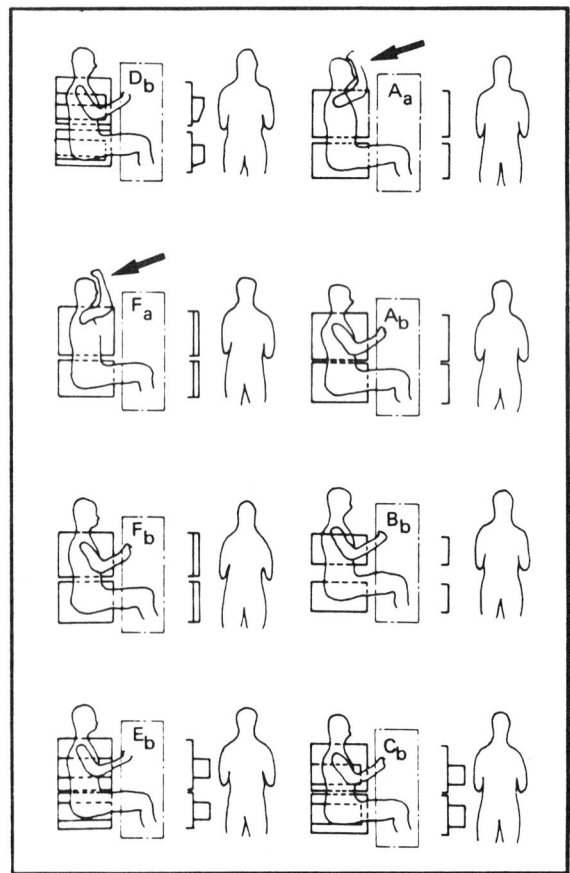

Figure 5. Test configurations.

618

The accelerometers and measuring channels meet the requirements of SAE J 211 b, F_H = 180 Hz.

Deflection of the thorax was measured by using films (a cylindrical rod was used inserted crosswise through the thorax).

A load measuring plate using Kistler cells was beneath the surface struck by the thorax. The load measured approaches that applied to the top of the trunk, in view of the small mass of the shock-absorbing material. The frequency F_H in this measurement is 180 Hz.

After the test, an autopsy was carried out on each subject.

Knowledge of the strength of their skeleton enables the results to be interpreted more finely. With this in view, undamaged parts of the ribs were sampled after the test and subjected to bending and shear mechanical tests as described in Reference 5. Likewise, the calcination of a fragment of rib made it possible to determine the percentage by weight of mineral salts in the bone. The overall results show that exceptional subjects the skeletal strength of which is too great or too small, would bias the results.

In order to eliminate these subjects from the analysis, subjects are illustrated in Figure 6 as a function of two parameters of mineralization of ribs, C/M and C/L.

C/M corresponds to the mass of ash obtained by calcination of a fragment of rib compared with the mass of the same fragment when fresh; this gives a good approximation of the percentage of the weight of mineral salts contained in the rib.

C/L corresponds to the weight of ash contained in 1 cm of length of rib; the values of C/L illustrated in the Figure 6 are average values obtained from several positions of samples; the same applies to C/M.

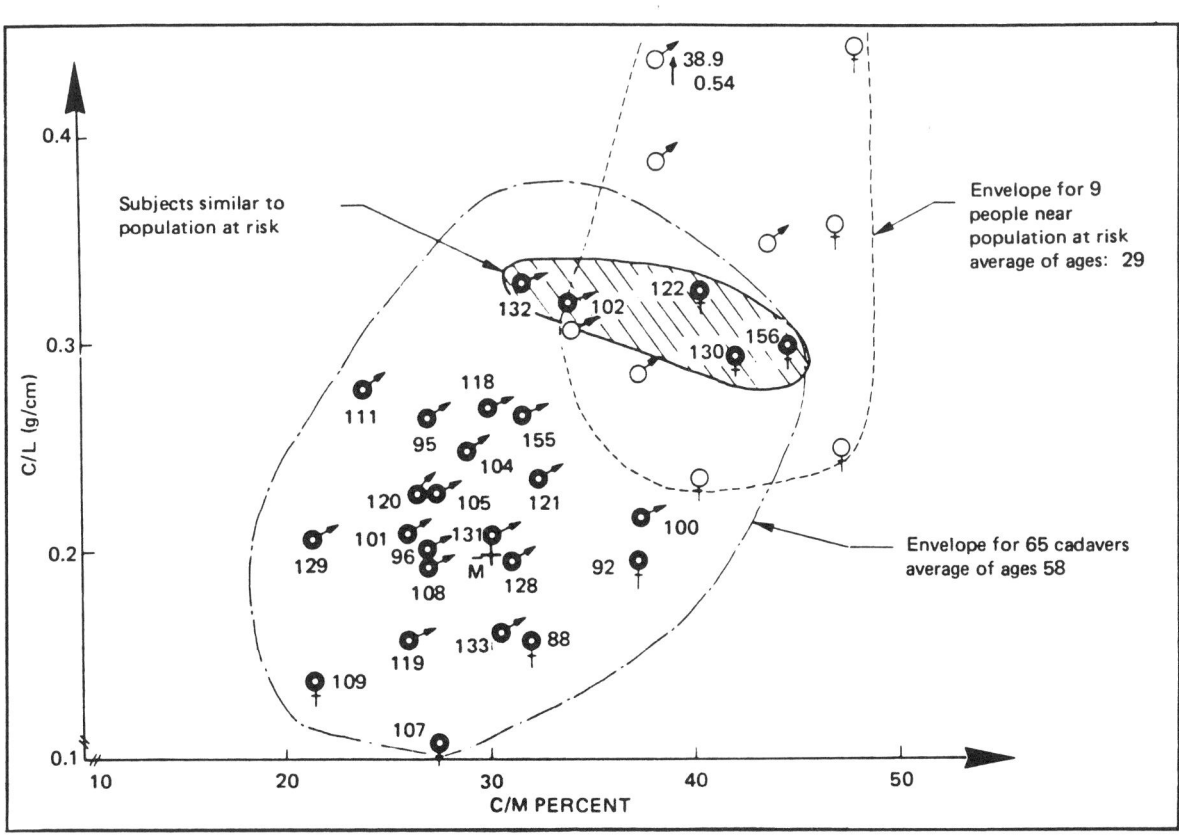

Figure 6. Rib mineralization of subjects (weight of mineral salts per unit of mass and per unit of length)

In order to assess the differences of mineralization between the subjects on which experiments were carried out and those of people actually exposed to the risk, fragments of rib were taken from cadavers autopsied after a sudden death without any previous illness (suicides, accidents, etc.) These subjects also are represented in the plane (C/M, C/L). As a comparison, it may be seen that subject 130, for example, may be considered as equivalent to people exposed to the risk of accident while it is reasonable to eliminate subject 109 from an analysis which relates to the mechanical characteristics of the thorax.

A rough ranking of the subjects is obtained by using C/L and C/M. But it is not sufficient to get an accurate hierarchy in any case. Some studies are dealing with this matter[7].

In the following, one will admit that the subjects No 122, 130, 132 and 156 are very similar to people exposed to the risk; subject No 102 does not enter this group because of his age.

Anthropometric data of the subjects are given in Table 1.

General Remarks Concerning the Injuries Found

The injuries that were found under the laboratory impact conditions were essentially rib

Table 1. Anthropometric data on subjects.

Test	Age	Sex	Weight (Kg)	THORAX (cm) Breadth	Depth	Circumference	Rib Mineralization C/M %	C/L (g/cm)
104	70	M	59	27	20	88.6	29.0	0.248
105	47	M	54	27	20	84.5	27.5	0.227
109	68	F	49	27	21	89.0	21.5	0.137
11	52	M	53	28	21	86.4	24.0	0.274
155	42	M	69	29	20	91.6	31.9	0.264
156	25	F	57	27	17	78.7	44.7	0.296
118	46	M	49	28	20	81.5	30.0	0.269
119	52	M	41	25	20	76.4	26.0	0.158
92	69	F	–	25	19	72.5	–	–
100	34	M	56	28	18	88.3	37.5	0.214
101	41	M	52	26	20	91,0	26,0	0.209
88	71	F	–	20	17	86.2	32.0	0.159
95	55	M	–	28	23	80.0	–	–
96	53	M	–	30	20	94.5	–	–
102	69	M	53	27	21	96.6	34.0	0.318
107	55	F	42	26	17	96.1	27.5	0.109
108	64	M	50	27	19	77.6	27.0	0.195
120	51	M	70	30	23	96.6	26.5	0.228
121	57	M	75	32	23	96.1	32.5	0.232
122	42	F	45	26	16	77.6	40.5	0.333
128	47	M	50	28	20	84.0	31.1	0.196
129	57	M	44	27	21	87.5	21.3	0.205
130	45	F	62	25	20	79.0	42.2	0.292
131	47	M	45	29	21	90.5	30.2	0.207
132	38	M	44	27	20	86.0	31.9	0.319
133	67	M	61	28	23	95.0	30.6	0.153

fractures. The number of fractures sustained can be an injury level indicator, and we endeavored to successively correlate the number of fractures occurring in the human subjects with the force applied to the chest, and also with the relative deflection of the chest as well as with thoracic acceleration.

When the injuries correspond to AIS ≤ 3, the fractures occurred on the impacted part of the chest. When they are more severe (AIS = 4 and more), what had occurred most frequently was a flail chest on the impacted side and rib fractures on the anterior or middle arches of the other part of the chest, which occasionally caused another flail chest in the plastron; in this case the AIS was 5.

In addition to the rib fractures, we found only one sternal fracture and one collarbone break in one subject, who had sustained a fall from a height of 3 meters. The shoulder was involved in the impact.

In no case did we find the occurrence of any intra-thoracic visceral lesion in the course of our testing.

The full set of results are given in Table 2. This table pertains to measurements performed on the subjects, and in no way presumes the conclusions yielded by the tests on dummies. In other words, the findings concern human tolerance and do not concern protection criteria.

Maximum Distributed Force Applied to the Chest

We endeavored to use the force applied to the chest as an injury level indicator. Figure 7 shows the findings.

The values of the forces applied to the chest were normalized, i.e. the measured values were corrected so as to most closely approximate the values that would have been found if the subject had weighed 75 kg.

The following formula (Eppinger[8]) was used:

$$\text{Normalized F} = \text{Measured F} \times \left(\frac{75}{\text{actual weight}}\right)^{2/3}$$

Seventy-five kg is a weight close to that of the 50th percentile male dummy.

Tests may be distributed in several groups. However, two groups of findings emerge:
- those yielded by tests on bare surfaces or on surface covered with overly-stiff paddings,
- those yielded by tests with the use of redesigned interior features that were more deformable and better adapted to thoracic tolerance.

For these latter subjects, a distributed normalized force close to 1,000 daN corresponds to a number of fractures inferior to equal to 8. This number of fractures constitutes the threshold above which injuries are in most cases considered to be intolerable. The reason is that a "flail chest" may theoretically appear if this number of fractures is exceeded. Practically, flail chests appear when the number of fractures is much higher.

The cross-hatched portion of Figure 7 represents subjects exposed to identical testing conditions; among them, we singled out those subjects whose bone condition could probably be that of accident victims and whose tolerance appeared to be higher. Unfortunately, they are not numerous.

Whatever the parameters used for evaluating human tolerances, the experimental findings reported on here will supply only an underestimation of these tolerances whenever it was impossible to assemble a sufficient number of suitable subjects.

The following table lists the findings, classified by AIS ratings:

A.I.S.	Nb of subjects	Average age	Measured daN F			Normalized daN F		
			Mini.	Maxi.	Average	Mini.	Maxi.	Average
0	4	45	240	700	437	330	780	550
1 + 2	1	25			–			–
3	9	49	460	1020	809	580	1356	993
4 + 5	12	59	590	1240	868	600	1250	900

Table 2. Thoracic results of subjects drop tests.

Test N°	Drop height (m)	Configuration	Acceleration (g) γR max.	γR 3 ms	S.I.	Force (daN) Measured	Normalized	Deflection ½ thorax δmm	δ%	Thorax δmm	δ%	Padding deformation (mm)	Injuries N. of rib fractures	AIS
\multicolumn{15}{c}{1° — Subjects with deflection measurement}
104	1	Aa	62	55	187	590	690	52	38	81	30		14	4
105	1	Aa	56	50	189	700	870	66	48	86	32		13	3
109	1	Ab	34	29	62	—	—	36	26	48	17,5		15	4
111	1	Ab	47	43	126	460	580	30	22	42	15		5	3
155	1	Ab	48	40	110	700	740	17	12	29	10		0	0
156	1	Ab	73	55	276	—	—	30	22	50	18,5		1	1
118	0,5	Bb	34	29	45	550	730	18	12	26	11		0	0
119	0,5	Bb	27	26	33	240	360	43	34	44	18		0	0
120	2	Cb	40	32	100	890	930	79	52	104	35		13	3
121	2	Cb	42	37	114	1,020	1,020	44	28	66	20	67	4	3
122	2	Cb	44	40	147	560	780	28	22	44	17	59	0	0
128	2	Db	68	60	280	810	1,061	56	40	90	32	17	8	3
129	2	Db	83	65	371	680	970	27	18	70	25	32	6	3
130	2	Db	62	50	210	840	954	38	30	70	28	20	4	3
131	2	Db	62	50	120	740	1,040	27	18	62	21	27	8	3
132	2	Db	74	50	300	950	1,356	40	30	75	28	27	7	3
133	2	Db	64	55	200	1,000	1,147	—	—	—	—	—	17	4
\multicolumn{15}{c}{2° — Subjects without deflection measurement}
92	2	Fa	69	59	324	1,090	—	—	—	—	—	—	18	4
100	2	Fb	54	51	209	630	770	—	—	—	—	—	12	4
101	2	Fb	42	38	131	800	1,020	—	—	—	—	—	20	5
88	3	Fb	84	65	436	950	—	—	—	—	—	—	18	4
95	3	Fa	83	74	410	1,240	—	—	—	—	—	—	12	4
96	3	Fa	128	90	688	1,160	—	—	—	—	—	—	21	4
102	3	Eb	82	60	345	870	1,100	—	—	—	—	—	23	5
107	3	Eb	75	70	392	640	940	—	—	—	—	—	15	4
108	3	Eb	70	62	335	840	1,100	—	—	—	—	—	25	5

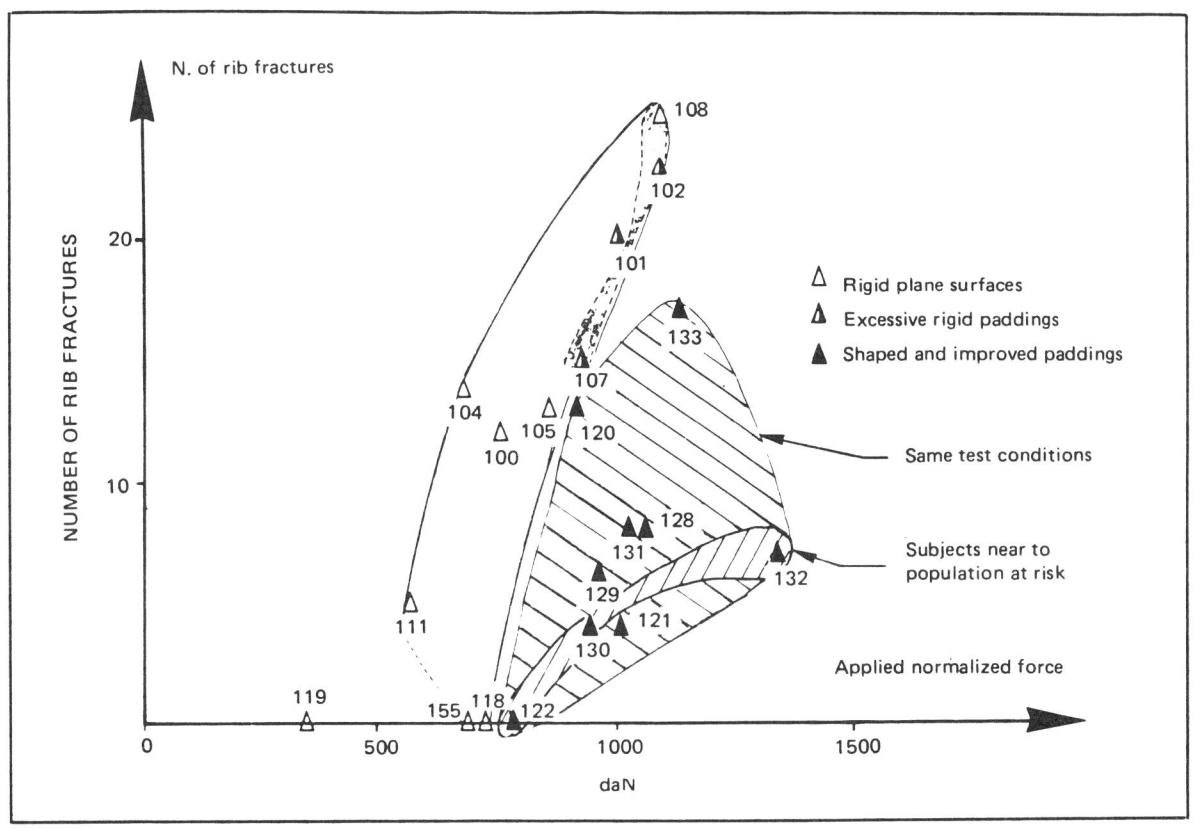

Figure 7. Relation between the normalized force applied to the thorax and the number of rib fractures.

The maximum measured force corresponding to an AIS = 0 is 700 daN (740 normalized daN).

The maximum measured force corresponding to an AIS = 3 is 1020 daN for a subject weighing 75 kg (121) and incurring four fractures, hence representing a case corresponding to only slight severity in the range covered by the AIS = 3 level.

Tolerance of Chest to Relative Deflection

It should be noted that this deflection was obtained by deformation of the chest over a relatively wide surface area, and that it is not comparable to a penetration.

Whole Chest. The relative deflection of the whole chest here is the ratio between the deformation of the chest measured on the films—definitely at the mesosternal level—and chest width at the same level prior to testing.

For the 16 subjects whose chest deflection was measured, this deflection appears to be a reliable injury level indicator (fig. 8) whatever the test conditions.

The following table lists the findings classified by AIS ratings, whatever the test conditions. When the shoulder is also directly hit, it seems that the relative deflection is lower for the same injury level.

As a conclusion concerning relative deflection of the whole chest, we can note as the maximum tolerable value, with reference to the cadaver, a relative deflection of approximately 30% of the chest width; this corresponds to a chest injury level that is con-

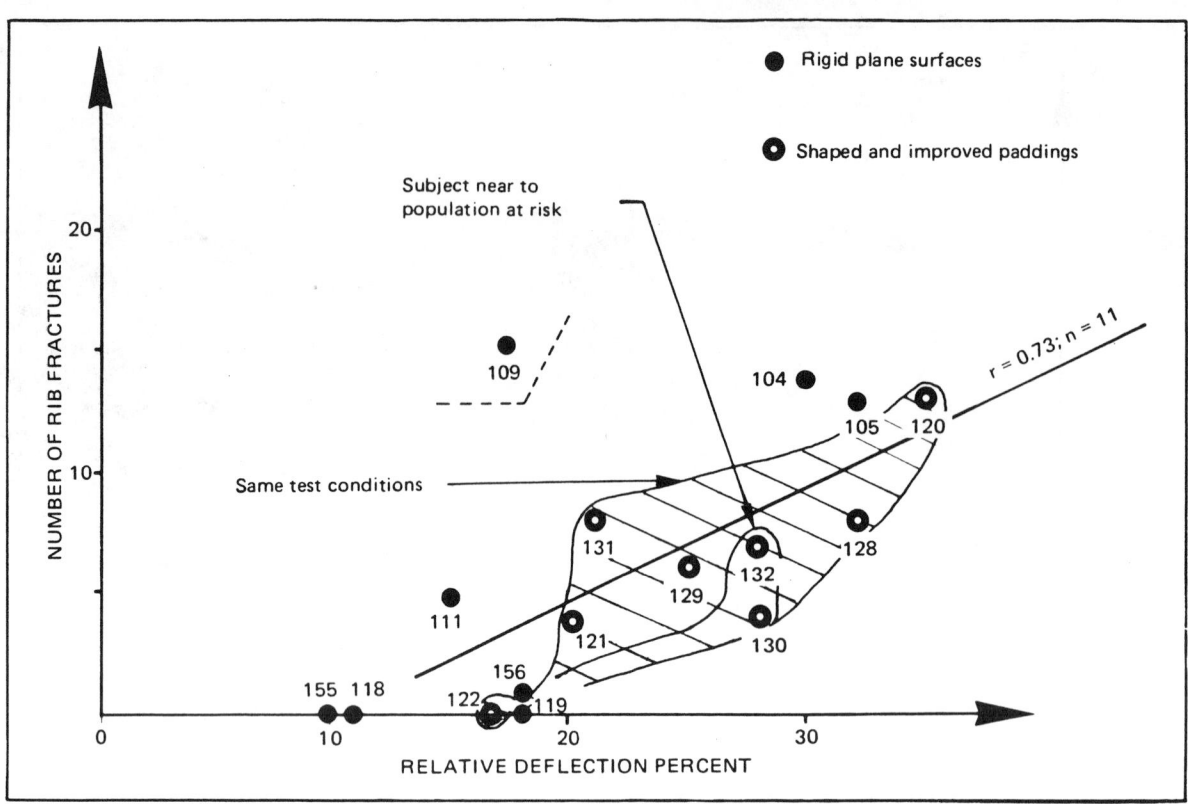

Figure 8. Relation between the relative deflection of the thorax and the number of rib fractures.

sistently less than, or equal to, 3 on the AIS scale.

Half Chest. We also investigated the deflection of the impacted half chest. As seems logical, this is the part of the chest that was the most extensively deflected; it was also the site of the greatest number of fractures sustained.

The findings (fig. 9) are more scattered than for deflection of the whole chest. However, it seems that an approximately 35% relative deflection of the impacted half chest is the maximum tolerable, if we refer to AIS ≤ 3 for human subjects.

In addition, the investigations enabled definition of the force/deflection dynamic characteristics of the impacted half chest. The corresponding data were used for the modification of a Part 572, designed to make it suitable for side impact (see references 9 and 10).

A.I.S.	No. of Subjects	Average Age	Relative Deflection of the Thorax (%)	Relative Deflection of the Half-Thorax (%)
0	4	45	10 to 18	12 to 34
1 + 2	1	25	18.5	22
3	9	49	15 to 35	18 to 52
4	1	70	38	30

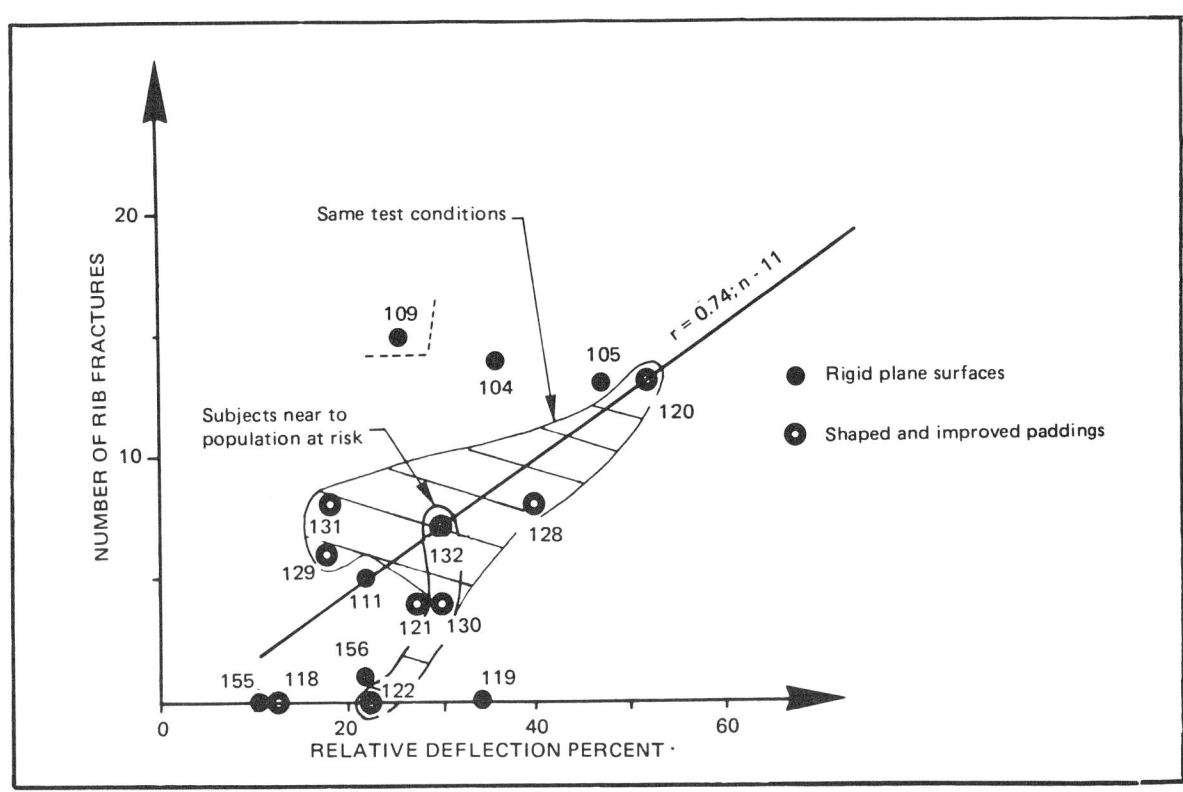

Figure 9. Relation between the relative deflection of the half thorax and the number of rib fractures.

Tolerance to Acceleration

Figure 10 shows that there is no close relation between the number of fractures sustained and the maximum resultant acceleration applied during 3 ms, measured on the subjects' fourth thoracic vertebra.

This does not mean that no conclusion can be reached on the basis of acceleration measurements (see references 11 and 12) concerning both tolerances and protection criteria.

It will further be noted that maximum acceleration is influenced by the subject's size characteristics, and that no correction was used similar to the one used for the applied force.[8] Some studies are dealing with this matter.[7]

The table below lists the findings. With the exception of subject No 101, rather weak, we found no occurrence of flail chest (AIS = 4) for γ(3ms) lower than 50 g in the subject.

Corresponding to an AIS = 3, the mean of the maximum accelerations applied during 3 ms was 49 g (nine subjects). The maximum and minimum recorded deviate from the mean by approximately 30%, with two of the

A.I.S.	No. of Subjects	Average Age	Resultant maximum Acceleration			Resultant Maximum Acceleration (at 3 ms)		
			mini.	maxi.	average	mini.	maxi.	average
0	4	45	27	48	38	26	40	34
1 + 2	1	25			73			55
3	9	49	40	83	60	32	65	49
4 + 5	11	59	42	84	70	38	74	60

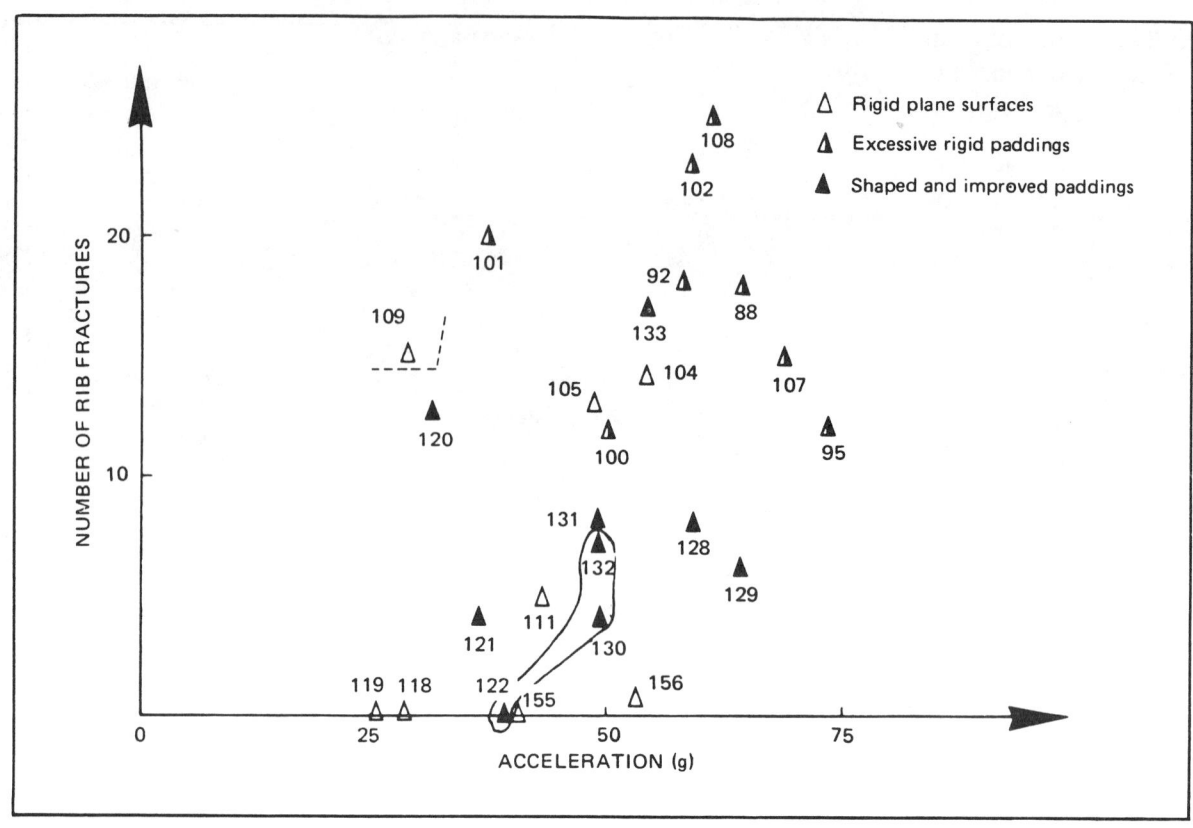

Figure 10. Relation between the thoracic acceleration at 3 sm measured at T 4 and the number of rib fractures.

nine subjects being exposed to $\gamma(3\ ms)$ respectively, equal to 60 and 65 g.

These nine subjects had a bone condition intermediate between that of the test subjects and that of the cadavers of individuals who had died sudden deaths, whose bone condition was considered to closely resemble that of the population exposed to risks.

Chest Protection Criteria

In the light of the tolerances whose levels have just been described, it is impossible to define a fully satisfactory protection criterion, for reasons not essentially related to the biomechanical data but primarily related to the dummies that were available. It is, however, possible to formulate provisional recommendations:

- Analysis of the force applied to the chest shows that padding pressed close against the side of the torso at a height of at least 14 cm—the height of the test materials—has to become crushed before a force of 1,000 daN is achieved; 800 daN would provide a better margin for the less robust segment of the population.

- Analysis of the deflection fails to yield a criterion that would be usable with the dummies currently available on the market. The findings could be transposed to the experimental APR dummy that is in the process of being developed as shown in references 9 and 10. The difference between the behavior of the presently existing dummies and that of the human body during a side collision is known and has been reported on (see references 2 and 14). Because of the difference between the transverse rigidity of the dummy and that of the human body, the distribution of the deflections and of the dissipation of energy between the chest and the padding is quite different depending on whether a dummy or a human being is involved.

As concerns acceleration, the present state of the findings, whether for the use of maximum acceleration in T4 or for tests with dummies, does not make it possible to define a protection criterion correlated with the injuries of individuals exposed to risk.

However, it will be possible to establish chest protection criteria once a sufficiently anthropo-dynamic dummy has been developed and can be tested via experiments yielding data linked to recognized injury levels for human beings.

Tolerances of the Pelvis (Table 3—Figure 11)

After subject No 109 is eliminated on account of the weakness of his skeleton, 4 cases of pelvis fractures remain among the 26 tested subjects. The corresponding AIS values are 2 when the fracture involves no displacement; the AIS level reaches 3 when a displacement occurs; such is the case of two subjects.

No abdominal lesion was observed. However, no perfusion had been made on subjects after No. 120 (the formaldehyde might have partially fixed the viscera). The maximum accelerations at 3 ms level sustained during the corresponding tests reached 74 g.

As regards fractures, the fracture without displacement (AIS 2) which occurred at the

Table 3. Pelvic results of subjects' drop tests (test configurations are illustrated in Tables 2, 3 and 4).

Test No	Drop Height (m)	Configuration	Age	Sex	Impacted Side	Weight (kg)	$\gamma.R$ Max.	$\gamma.R$ 3ms	AIS	Injuries
104	1	Aa	70	M	R	59	55	40	0	
105	1	Aa	47	M	R	54	153	66	0	
109	1	Ab	68	F	R	49	90	70	3	F. little displacement, R. ischio and ilio-pubic branches
111	1	Ab	52	M	R	53	89	47	0	
155	1	Ab	42	M	L	69	75	57	0	
156	1	Ab	25	F	L	57	69	55	0	
118	0.5	Bb	46	M	L	49	62	33	0	
119	0.5	Bb	52	M	L	41	34	30	0	
92	2	Fa	69	F	L	–	82	50	2	F. R + L ischio and ilio-pubic branches
100	2	Fb	34	M	R	56	44	38	0	
101	2	Fb	41	M	R	52	110	77	0	
88	3	Fb	71	F	L	–	65	60	0	
95	3	Fa	55	M	L	–	120	105	3	F. little displacement L. ischi pubic branch
96	3	Fa	53	M	L	–	135	90	0	
102	3	Eb	69	M	R	53	62	57	3	F. R. ilio-pubic branch, F. R. iliac wing F. + displacement R. cotyle
107	3	Eb	55	F	R	42	77	66	2	F. ischio and ilio-public branches
108	3	Eb	64	M	R	50	74	53	0	
120	2	Cb	51	M	L	70	37	30	0	
121	2	Cb	57	M	L	75	32	31	0	
122	2	Cb	42	F	L	45	34	34	0	
128	2	Db	47	M	L	50	48	40	0	
129	2	Db	57	M	L	44	48	34	0	
130	2	Db	45	F	L	62	–	–	0	
131	2	Db	47	M	L	45	50	45	0	
132	2	Db	38	M	L	44	60	47	0	
133	2	Db	67	M	2	61	84	74	0	

F = Fracture, R = Right, L = Left

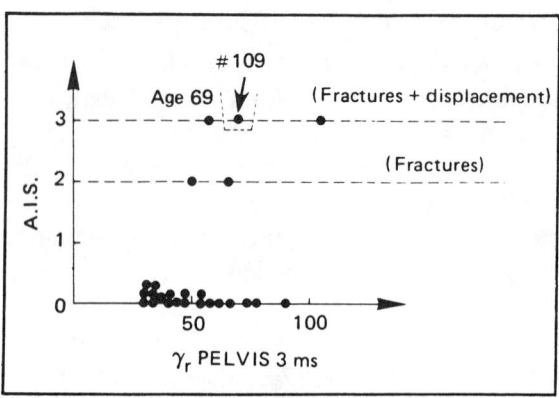

Figure 11. Relation between the AIS and the pelvic acceleration (at 3 ms).

lowest acceleration value is the fact of a 69 year old female subject at 50 g/3 ms of maximal acceleration. On the contrary, the highest acceleration level without a fracture was measured on a 53 year old man, at 90 g/3 ms.

Fractures with displacement occurred for a height of fall of 3 m, which gives a speed variation of about 35 kph (a little more than the impact speed).

The chronological order of tests was such that the subjects considered to be near the true-life accident victims sustained, for their main part, only moderate impacts at pelvis level.

When compared to the real-life accident conditions, test conditions are such that neither intrusion nor penetration occur. In padded impacts, the $\gamma(t)$ pulse of the pelvis has a smooth shape and a level near the maximum is sustained during a rather long duration. One could also observe from some tests carried out with dummies that the maxima of accelerations on dummies are likely to be a littler higher than on subjects (see references 9 and 10).

Due to the absence of noticeable human pelvis deformation during the impact, the "Part 572" pelvis does not raise the same problems as the thorax does. On the basis of these results and some others already published, 80 to 90 g/3 ms to the pelvis seem to be a conservative level of human tolerance for victims, generally younger than the subjects; the best protection criterion which may be associated to this tolerance level has not to ensure that no injury occurs in car crashes of low severities; the criterion has better to ensure an acceptable injury distribution in car crashes of higher severities. The injury distribution and the accident severities have to be defined by accidentological studies, so as to give finally a higher protective benefit for the whole population at risk. Therefore, for a protection criterion on a dummy such as "Part 572" one, a level comprised between 90 and 100 g/3 ms could be contemplated.

Neck Tolerance in Side Impact

The matter is the tolerance of the neck in the case of the imposed lateral flexion which is obtained when the side wall stops the thorax and that no head impact occurs.

With the experimental conditions, no cervical lesions were observed; lateral flexion attained 60° and the resulting acceleration of the head did never overpass 60 g. One has to observe that the thorax is already stopped when the acceleration reaches its maximum. It seems that there is no need for a neck protection criterion in the range of these impact severities.

CONCLUSIONS

This report dealt primarily with the findings of free-fall tests performed on cadavers over the past few years, and up to the present time for the most recent findings.

We were able to specify the human tolerance levels for most of the body parts what are frequently affected in actual car-to-car side collisions occurring on the highways. The findings are closely related to the particular conditions of each individual experiment and each individual subject; the emphasis was on reducing the causes of scatter. In any event, the figures set forth in this report enjoy maximum reliability in cases involving impact against prepared surfaces involving subjects closely resembling the population exposed to risk.

Another important point is the necessity for having a dummy whole behavior closely resembles that of the human being, so as to be able to transform the tolerance levels into protection criteria that will be closely correlated with the injury levels of real-life accident victims. Several research teams are currently devoting their efforts to defining a satisfactory dummy.

REFERENCES

1. R. L. Stalnaker, J. H. MacElhaney, R. G. Snyder, V. L. Roberts: "Door Crashworthiness Criteria", Paper 710 864, proceedings of 15th Stapp Car Crash Conference, SAE.
2. J. W. Melvin, D. H. Robbins, R. L. Stalnaker: "Side Impact Response and Injury", Proceedings of the 6th ESV Conference, Washington, Oct. 1976.
3. R. L. Stalnaker, V. L. Roberts, J. H. MacElhaney: "Side Impact Tolerance to Blunt Trauma", Paper 730 979, Proceedings of 17th Stapp Car Crash Conference, SAE.
4. A. Fayon, C. Tarriere, G. Walfisch, C. Got, A. Patel: "Contribution to Defining the Human Tolerance to Perpendicular Side Impact", Proceedings of the 3rd International Conference on Impact Trauma, Berlin, Sept. 1977, IRCOBI Secretariate, 109 ave. Salvador Allende, 69500 Bron, France.
5. C. Got, A. Patel, A. Fayon, C. Tarrière, G. Walfisch: "Results of Experimental Head Impacts on Cadavers: the Various Data Obtained and their Relations to Some Measured Physical Parameters", Proceedings of 22nd Stapp Car Crash Conference, SAE Paper 780 887.
6. R. L. Stalnaker, J. W. Melvin, G. S. Nusholtz, N. M. Alem, J. B. Benson: "Head Impact Response", Proceedings of 21st Stapp Car Crash Conference, SAE Paper 770 921.
7. J. Sacreste, A. Fayon, C. Tarriere, C. Got, A. Patel: "Theoretical and Experimental Study of Rib Fractures in Frontal and Lateral Impacts Based on Tests with Instrumented Cadavers", to be published in Proceedings of 4th International Conference on the Biomechanics of Trauma, Gothenburg, Sept. 1979, IRCOBI.
8. R. H. Eppinger: "Prediction of Thoracic Injuries Using Measurable Experimental Cadavers", Proceedings of 6th ESV Conference, Washington, U.S.A., Oct. 1976.
9. R. L. Stalnaker, C. Tarrière, A. Fayon, G. Walfisch, M. Balthazard, J. Masset, C. Got, A. Patel: "Modification of Part 572 Dummy for Lateral Impact According to Biomechanical Data", proposed paper to the 23rd Stapp Car Crash Conference, Oct. 1979.
10. A. Fayon, Y.C. Leung, R. L. Stalnaker, G. Walfisch, M. Balthazard, C. Tarriere: "Presentation of a Frontal and Side Impact Dummy Defined from Human Data and Realized from a "Part 572" Basis", Proceedings of 7th ESV Conference, Paris, June 1979.
11. D. H. Robbins, J. W. Melvin, R. L. Stalnaker: "The Prediction of Thoracic Impact Injuries", Proceedings of 20th Stapp Car Crash Conference, SAE Paper 760 822.
12. R. H. Eppinger, K. Augustyn, D. H. Robbins: "Development of a Promising Universal Thoracic Trauma Prediction Methodology", Proceedings of 22nd Stapp Car Crash Conference, SAE Paper 780 891.
13. D. Cesari, B. Friedel, Heger, G. M. Mackay, C. Tarrière, R. Weissner: "Preliminary Report About the Work of the Joint Biomechanical Research Project (KOB)", Proceedings of 7th ESV Conference, Paris, June 1979.
14. G. Walfisch, A. Fayon, C. Tarrière, C. Got, A. Patel: "Travaux Effectués pour Disposer d'un Mannequin et de Critères Convenables pour Améliorer la Protection en Choc Latéral", in "Ingénieurs de l'Automobile", March 1979.

801305

Thoraco—Abdominal Response and Injury

G. S. Nusholtz and J. W. Melvin, G. Mueller,
J. R. MacKenzie, and R. Burney
University of Michigan

LATERAL THORACO-ABDOMINAL IMPACT BIOMECHANIC studies using human cadavers (1,2,3,4) and animals (3,5,6,7) as surrogates of the human have been concerned with the many processes (both mechanical and physiological) that can take place as a result of blunt impact. These processes are of interest for a variety of reasons, ranging from developing an understanding of the fundamental nature of the interactions resulting from blunt impact and quantitatively determining the probabilities associated with resulting injury, to applying the data for the reduction of those probabilities.

One of the most common physiological responses to blunt abdominal impact is hypovolemic shock due to the laceration of blood vessels, and subsequent intraperitoneal bleeding; while a common biochemical response is disruption of cells resulting in the escape of pre-formed enzymes into the blood stream and/or the peritoneal cavity.

As clinical experience with thoraco-abdominal trauma has increased, a wide range of hepatic injuries have been observed and defined. At one extreme are complex bursting injuries of the hepatic parenchyma and laceration of the hepatic and portal veins. These injuries are almost invariably associated with shock at the time of initial presentation and were fatal in 22 out of 24 cases (90%) in one series (4).

In contrast, it has long been appreciated that many grade 1 or 2 (8) (AIS 2-3 (9)) hepatic lacerations will have stopped bleeding by the time of operation. It has recently been suggested (10) that, if identified non-operatively, some mild to moderate liver injuries might be safely observed thus avoiding the morbidity, disability, and expense associated with operation and post-operatic recovery. As of yet, no reliable method has been developed to assess the probability of continuation or cessation of the hemorrhage or the anatomic severity of liver injuries by non-invasive methods or by a safe, minimally invasive technique.

Mechanisms of traumatic hepatic injury have been studied previously. Cadaver livers have been injected with barium to reproduce their vertura turgor and then dropped from varying heights (4). It was found that .3 N-M of energy produced capsular tears: a 2.8 to 3.4 N-M were

_____ Abstract _____

This study[1] investigates the response of human cadavers, and live anesthetized and post-mortem primates and canines[2], to blunt lateral thoraco-abdominal impact. There were 12 primates: 5 post-mortem and 7 live anesthetized; 10 canines; 1 post-mortem and 9 live anesthetized; and 3 human cadavers.

A 10 kg free-flying mass was used to administer the impact in the right to left direction. To produce the varying degrees of injury, factors including velocity, padding of the impactor surface, location of impact site, and impactor excursion were adjusted. The injuries were evaluated by gross autopsy, and in the case of live subjects, current clinical methods such as sequential peritoneal lavage and biochemical assays were also employed. Mechanical measurements included force time history, intraortic pressure, and high-speed cineradiography to define gross organ motion.

---

[1] The protocol for the use of cadavers in this study was reviewed by the Committee to Review Grants for Clinical Research and Investigation Involving Human Beings of the University of Michigan Medical Center and follows guidelines established by the U.S. Public Health Service and recommended by the National Academy of Science/National Research Council.

[2] Animals cared for and handled according to AALAC guidelines.

needed to produce bursting injuries. Another test subjected isolated, perfused ex-vivo primate liver to controlled blunt impact and compared the injuries produced to those produced by blunt upper and lower abdominal impact (5). It was found that 3.3 N-M of energy was needed to produce a grade 2+(AIS 3) injury in an intact animal while only about 1.4 N-M was needed to produce a similar injury in the directly exposed liver. When the force of impact was held constant in these experiments, the liver injuries produced correlated with contact area, duration of impact, and the mass of the animal. As might be expected, it was also shown that much higher forces were necessary to create a liver injury similar in severity to that produced by upper abdominal impact when impact was made in the lower abdomen.

This paper discusses techniques used at the Highway Safety Research Institute (HSRI) for conducting blunt lateral thoraco-abdominal impacts with human cadavers, primates, and canines. Through the use of the high-speed cineradiograph (11) utilizing human cadavers and primates, organ motion descriptors have been developed. Employing current clinical methods, techniques have been developed to assess the rate of hemorrhage in the live model. Injuries are described by means of gross autopsy and in the case of primates and canines, sequential peritoneal lavage and biochemical assays.

EXPERIMENTAL METHODS

IMPACT TESTING - The impact tests were conducted with the HSRI pneumatic impact device. The details of the operation of this device have been reported previously (12). The device consists of an air reservoir which is connected to a honed steel cylinder. A driver piston is propelled down the cylinder by the pressurized air in the reservoir. The driver piston contacts a striker piston which is fitted with a piezoelectric accelerometer (Kistler 904A) and a piezoelectric load washer (Kistler 805A) to allow the determination of acceleration compensated contact loads applied to the test subject. The mass, velocity, and stroke of the striker piston can be controlled to provide the desired impact conditions for a particular test. The velocity of the impactor is measured by timing the pulses from a magnetic probe which senses the motion of targets on the impactor at 1.3 cm intervals.

AORTIC PRESSURE MEASUREMENT - Aortic pressures were obtained from the descending aorta at a point just inferior to where the aorta passes through the diaphragm. A Kulite model MCP-055-5f catheter tip pressure transducer was inserted through the right femoral artery. The location of the tip of the presssure transducer was checked by x-ray before the impact.

X-RAY CINERADIOGRAPH - Cineradiographs were taken from impact events at 1000 frames per second. The HSRI high-speed cineradiographic system (11) consists of a Photosonics 1B high-speed, 16-mm motion-picture camera which views a 2-inch diameter output phosphor of a high-gain, four stage, magnetically focused image intensifier tube, gated on and off synchronously with shutter pulses from the motion-picture camera. A lens optically couples the input photocathode of the image intensifier tube to x-ray images produced on a fluorescent screen by a smoothed direct-current x-ray generator. Smoothing of the full-wave rectified x-ray output is accomplished by placing a pair of high-voltage capacitors in parallel with the x-ray tube. A 22 cm diameter circular field was viewed in these experiments.

SEQUENTIAL PERITONEAL LAVAGE - The live anesthetized subject was placed in a supine position on a table in the Anatomy Room. A small midline incision was made between the umbilicus and the pubic bone and a trocath peritoneal dialysis catheter and stylet were introduced into the peritoneal cavity. The stylet was then removed and the distal tip of the catheter was advanced below the right lateral lobe of the liver. A 15 mg/kg body weight solution of normal saline or Ringer's lactate was infused into the peritoneal cavity. The animal was then rocked gently back and forth to insure complete mixing of the instilled fluid with the unclotted elements of the blood which had extravasated into the cavity from the wound created by the trauma. This mixture of saline and unclotted blood was then siphoned from the cavity into a collecting vessel and the fluid was examined for red blood cell (RBC) count and serum enzymes. Simultaneously, the peripheral blood was collected and similarly analyzed. The serum enzyme samples were centrifuged and chilled at 4^0 C until later biochemical analysis. This procedure was performed at 30, 90, 150, and 210 minutes.

The amount of unclotted blood which was free to mix with the instilled saline and which had been extravasated from the lacerated liver between the time intervals 0-30 minutes; 30-90 minutes; 90-150 minutes, and 150-210 minutes was calculated by the following formula:

$$B_i = \frac{Lc_{i-1} \times R_i - S_i \times Lc_i - R_i \times Lc_i}{Lc_i - Sc_i}$$

Where:

B_i - volume of blood lost to abdomen during a specified time interval.

Lc_i - lavage blood count at a specific sampling time.

Sc_i - serum blood count at a specific sampling time.

R_i - remaining fluid volume in abdomen at a specified sampling time.

S - fluid input during lavage.

It is recognized that this formula will most likely underestimate the actual amount of blood that has escaped from the blood stream into the peritoneal cavity since the RBC that are entrapped in the clotted blood will not be estimated by this method. However, few RBC are entrapped in blood clots after the first instillation of fluid into the peritoneum due to dilutional effects, therefore, B_i approaches the actual value of lost blood after the first instillation of saline.

After the sampling time, a laparotomy was performed to determine if the liver had stopped bleeding.

SEQUENTIAL BIOCHEMISTRY - Biochemical assays were performed for both the lavage fluid and serum. The lavage fluid was obtained from the sequential peritoneal lavage. The fluid was then mixed with EDTA. The arterial blood samples were taken from a catheter inserted into the femoral artery. The samples were centrifuged and chilled at 4°c until analysis.

The two assays discussed in this paper will be GOT (glutamic oxalacetic transaminase) and GPT (glutamic pyruvic transaminase). GOT levels of the serum are elevated in patients with hepatobiliary disease, cardiovascular disease, muscle disease, and some miscellaneous conditions. GPT levels are elevated in the serum of patients with hepatic disease. In other conditions elevations are negligible unless there is hepatic involvement (13).

TEST SUBJECT PREPARATION

HUMAN CADAVERS - The cadavers used in these experiments were obtained from the University of Michigan Anatomy Department in an unembalmed condition. Following transfer to the HSRI, the cadavers were stored in coolers at 4°c until further use. After being prepared in the HSRI Anatomy Room, the cadavers were transferred to the X-ray Room, where surgical preparation took place. A 6-8 cm incision was made over the right jugular vein, lateral to the larynx. A double balloon modified no. 20 Foley catheter was used to instill barium contrast media into the hepatic veins in a retrograde manner and was inserted through the jugular vein into the inferior vena cava. The catheter was positioned so that the perforations in the fluid passage used for contrast media insertion were at the point in the vena cava where the hepatic vein empties into it (Figure 1). The balloon above and below the perforations prevented the escape of the media into the vena cava.

The two balloons were inflated and used as markers to position the catheter using x-ray methods. One balloon was placed just above the diaphragm; the other 10 cm below it. The cadaver was then transferred to the Impact Laboratory where it was positioned in the test apparatus shown in Figure 2.

The cadaver was placed in a partially suspended position with its right side towards the impactor, so that the line of impact was in the mid-sagittal plane in the right to left direction. Positioning was obtained by a chair that was designed and constructed for the cadavers that could be adapted to the varying subjects and test conditions. In addition, two moveable overhead arms facilitated suspension of the cadaver. The cadaver was held in place with filament tape which grips the body under the arms and upper torso, suspending the torso from the overhead arms. The alignment was such that the impact went through the approximated center of gravity of the liver.

PRIMATES - Twelve primate subjects were used in these experiments: eleven macaca mulatta and one macaca assamensis. These were obtained by the HSRI from the University of Michigan Unit for Laboratory Animal Medicine (ULAM). Prior to use at the HSRI, the primate subjects had been used in one or more pharmacological research projects at the University of Michigan Medical Center.

Live anesthetized macacas were used in the first four and the three final experiments. The impacts of the fifth through the ninth macacas were conducted on post-mortem subjects. Upon termination they were stored in a cooler at 4°c for 48 hours before testing. The protocol for post-mortem primates was less complex than for that of the live primates, which is outlined below.

The primate was initially anesthetized by an intramuscular injection of ketamine. The animal was then catheterized for subsequent venous injection of sodium pentobarbitol at a dosage of 25 mg/kg body weight to maintain the anesthesia. An airway was established and then biometric measurements were taken. Next, a pressure transducer was surgically introduced into the right femoral artery and advanced into the descending aorta. An additional cannula was inserted through the left femoral artery and into the descending aorta for the purpose of taking blood samples.

The positions of the two catheters were checked by x-ray and then the primate was transported to the Impact Laboratory and positioned in a manner similar to that of the cadavers (Figure 2). Following the positioning of the animal in the test apparatus, a Polaroid photograph of the subject was taken through the cineradiographic system to check transducer positioning and x-ray contrast. Once the positioning and x-ray controls were set, the distance from the x-ray source and the distance from the midline of the primate were measured relative to the cineradiographic screen. The still camera was replaced by the high-speed movie camera and the impact test was conducted.

After impact, the primate was moved to the Autopsy Room and monitored for up to four hours (or until the primate expired). During this monitoring period, on tests 79A255, 79A257, and

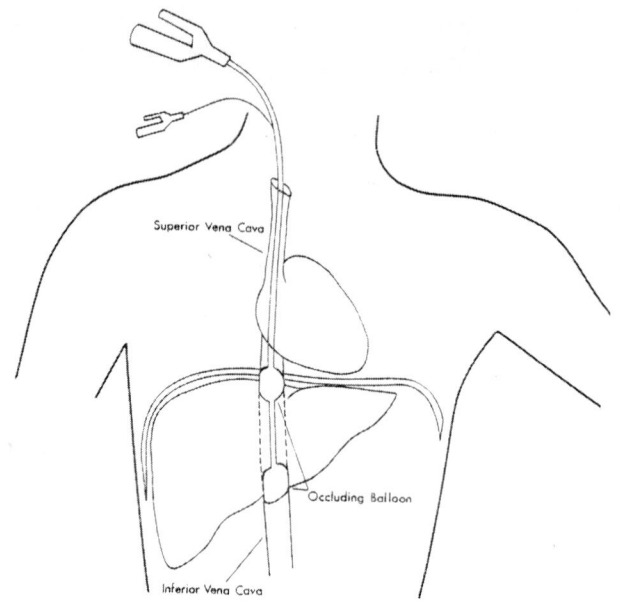

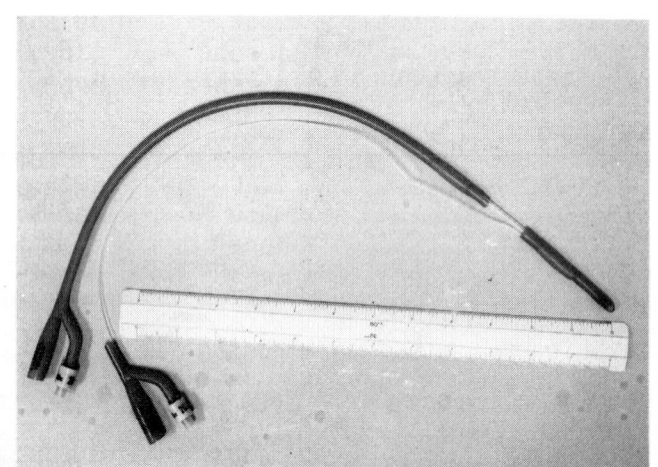

Fig. 1 - Catheter location

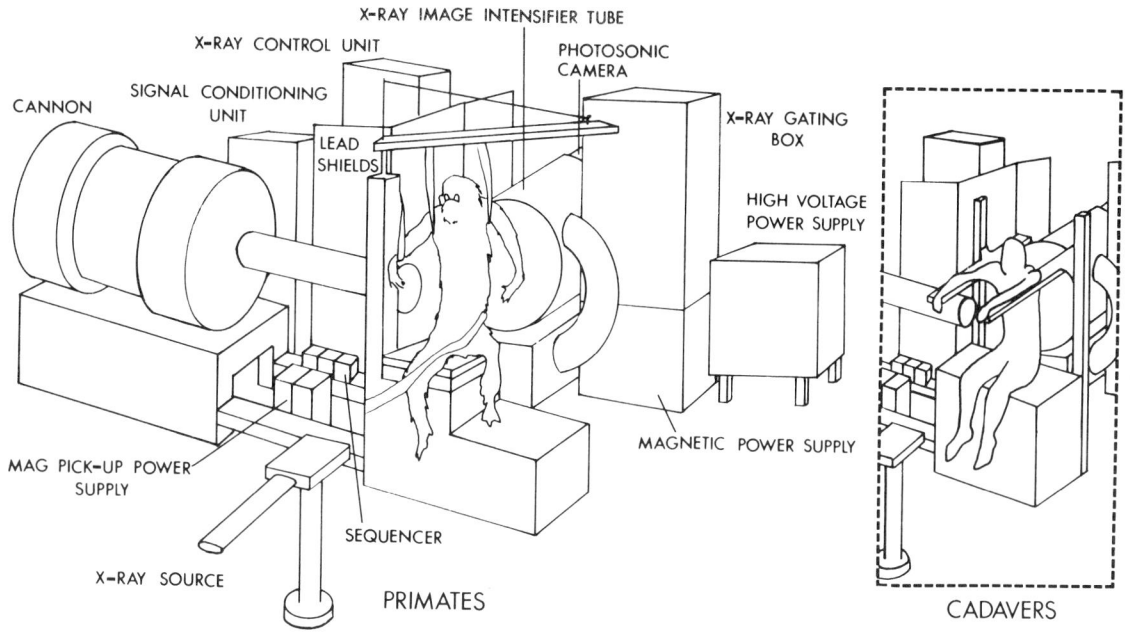

Fig. 2 - Test setups for cadavers and primates

79A259, sequential biochemistry and peritoneal lavage were performed. The primate was then euthanized by a 5 ml dose of Uthol (concentrated, unpure, sodium pentobarbital) injected via the hind leg catheter. A bilateral pneumothorax was performed to ensure termination. A thoracic and abdominal autopsy was then performed. The organs of each respective location were examined in situ for evidence of injury. All injuries were recorded and photographed.

In the test series with post-mortem primates, the ninth test subject (79A254) was tested with its vascular system pressurized in a manner similar to the techniques used with cadavers (14). A balloon-tipped catheter was inserted through the left common carotid into the descending aorta and inflated to occlude the superior vessels. The left femoral artery was cannulated and connected to a reservoir of normal saline. A Kulite pressure transducer was inserted into the right femoral artery and advanced to the level of the hepatic arteries and ligated securely.

CANINES - The subjects used in these experiments were live "chronic" mongrel canines weighing 13 to 33 kilograms. They were obtained from ULAM and housed there until the day of the test.

Each day the experiments involved one or two canines who were transported from ULAM to the HSRI. Prior to arrival, the canine was anesthetized by sodium pentobarbital injected through a catheter into the cephalic vein at a dosage of 30 mg/kg, to effect. The subject was then transported to HSRI where it was surgically prepared for aortic pressure measurement and blood sampling in a manner similar to the previously described primate preparation.

The canine was then transported to the Impact Laboratory and positioned in the following manner. A frame was designed and constructed for positioning of the canine to support either its natural quadrupedal posture or a posture which required a rotation from the horizontal to vertical position. This frame was also adaptable to the varying subjects and test positions.

The site of impact was determined in the following manner: a pre-test lateral x-ray of the canine was taken. From this x-ray, the position of the liver with respect to the ribs was obtained. The position of the liver can then be determined by palpation.

The thoraco-abdominal region was impacted. After the test, the subject was removed from the Impact Lab and transported to the Anatomy Room. A four hour monitoring period ensued in which biochemical assays and serial peritoneal lavage were performed. The canine was then euthanized by an I.V. injection of 5 cc Uthol and a bilateral pneumothorax was performed to ensure termination. The animal was then autopsied for injury determination.

PHOTOGRAMMETRIC ANALYSIS OF ORGAN MOTION DESCRIPTORS

Analytical photogrammetry is widely used in

biomechanics to describe the geometry of anatomical structures and their motion in the laboratory reference frame (15,16). The object space coordinates of points of interest can usually be obtained once the coordinates of well-defined points in an image space and the calibration translation and rotations are specified. The points in image space are normally obtained with cameras or radiographic equipment and preserved on film.

The motion of an anatomical structure in object space is generally obtained by measuring the time history of the position of a photographic target with a well-defined position and orientation relative to a predefined anatomical landmark. This motion is generally associated with rigid body motion, such as motion of the head with defined descriptors of translations and rotations (position, velocity, acceleration). Once these descriptors are obtained, they can then be used to characterize the dynamic response of the subject under study and assist, in some cases, in the understanding of injury mechanisms.

The cineradiograph system allows non-invasive viewing of internal anatomical structure *in vivo*. In the case of a rigid structure such as bones, the radiopaque targets can be placed on or near anatomical landmarks and motion can be similary described to that of standard photometric techniques. Problems arise when soft tissue is to be analyzed and rigid body dynamics no longer offer a good approximation.

Several methods could be suggested to produce analytical information describing soft tissue motion. In this paper, the descriptors chosen are based upon the shadows of objects associated with anatomical structures in a two-dimensional image space produced by a point source of x-rays. The descriptors are at most two-dimensional and do not take into account rotations and translations which move objects in and out of a plane of gross whole body motion. In addition, changes in the x-ray cross section of objects can lead to changes in the descriptors which do not have a direct relation to rigid body motion. Three descriptors were used for the cadavers, while four such descriptors were employed for the primates.

HUMAN MOTION DESCRIPTOR - Liver motion visualization was made possible by the use of radiopaque dye injection. The liver was the only organ observed in the cadaver due to its relative size. The descriptor utilizes a point defined by the intersection of two lines. The intersection is taken as the crossing of a radiopaque vein and a line perpendicular to the impactor (Figure 3). The excitation of this point is determined either by the instant in time at which this intersection of the veins becomes obscured by increased x-ray absorption or when motion of this intersection can be seen in the direction of the motion of the impactor. In test 79A225, with the vena cava visible, an additional descriptor was defined as the motion of the center of the visible segment. The third descriptor was the diaphragm motion described below for the primates.

HEART MOTION DESCRIPTOR - The position descriptor chosen for the heart is based upon an approximating ellipse which fits its image (Figure 4). The descriptor is then reduced to a point by only considering the intersection of the major and minor axes. This point, once obtained, defines an absolute position in the laboratory reference frame Y,Z(R-L, I-S) axis. As the point moves in space travels along a curve defined by its position as a function of time. This curve can then be used to obtain a velocity for this point. The curve generated by the heart descriptor is a function of the inputs to the heart and is partially related to its gross whole body motion. Changes in the curve can also be produced by other factors such as compression or distortion of the heart.

SPINE DESCRIPTOR - The descriptor for the spine is one dimensional with the z-coodinate fixed and determined before impact. This descriptor is obtained by choosing a point on the shadow of the spine half way between the shadow of the diaphragm and the shadow of the heart. This section of the spine is not always visible, but it is assumed that the image generated by the spine, which shows up as a curve with some thickness, is relatively smooth and that the point of interest be located by interpolation or, in some cases, extrapolation (Figure 4). In addition, the time derivative of this descriptor can also be obtained.

NEAR SIDE IMPACT DEFLECTION - The near body side deflection is not directly related to the impactor stroke. It is the difference, in the direction of the impactor motion, between the spine descriptor and the radiopaque density associated with the thoraco-abdominal wall (Figure 4). This does not take into account the response of the left half of the body. Total deflection, defined as the difference in distance between the right thoraco-abdominal wall and the left thoraco-abdominal wall, does not necessarily relate to the difference between the spine and either thoraco-abdominal wall. Large deflection as indicated by the descriptor could happen with a lesser amount of total deflections occurring.

DIAPHRAGM - The descriptor associated with the abdomen is the angle of a secant line that intersects the boundary of the radiopaque difference between the thorax and the abdominal cavity and spans the center third of this boundary (Figure 4). Once impact is initiated, the x-ray cross-section changes. Contact and the resulting dislocation of the thoraco-abdominal wall will then produce changes in the diaphragm position descriptor. These changes can be expressed by an angle and an angular velocity.

RESULTS

The tables and graphs presented here represent the data found to be most pertinent in discussing the test results. For a more

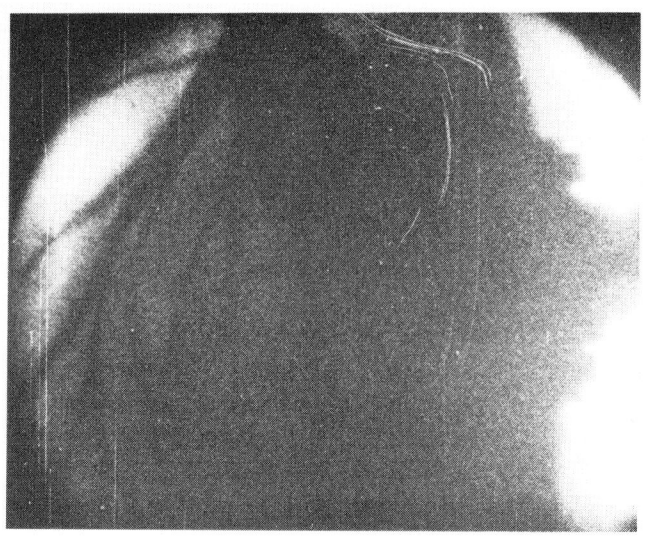
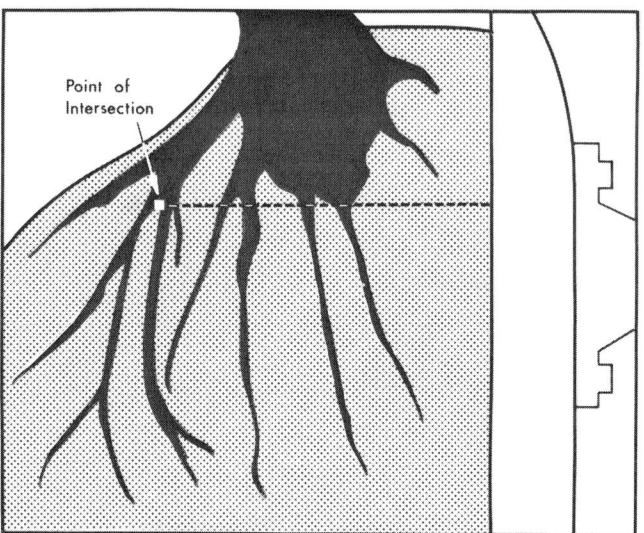

Fig. 3 - X-ray cineradiograph reconstruction and definition of human motion descriptor

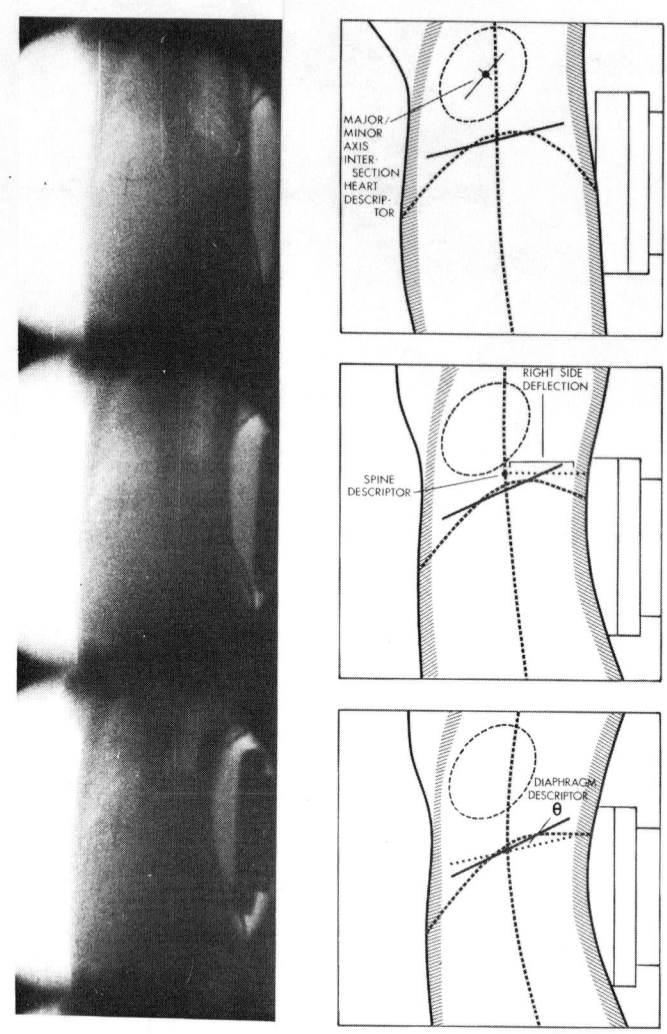

Fig. 4 - X-ray CRG reconstruction and definition of primate motion descriptors

Table 1

INITIAL CONDITIONS TEST SUMMARY

Primates

Test No.	78A231	78A233	78A235	78A237	78A240	78A242	79A250	79A252	79A254	79A255	79A257	79A259
Velocity (m/sec)	10.5	--	13.1	12.3	12.5	12.3	13.3	13.3	14.5	8.5	11.4	13.3
Piston Excursion (cm)	5.1	6.4	5.1	5.1	5.1	5.1	5.1	5.1	5.1	5.1	5.1	3.8
Surface Padding of a 10 cm Diameter Rigid Impactor (cm) (Ensolite)	2.5	NONE	NONE	NONE	2.5	NONE	2.5	2.5	2.5	2.5	NONE	2.5
Site of Impact (Distance from Diaphragm Spine Intersection) (cm)	2	--	1.5	1	2	--	--	-1	2	1.5	1	1

Canines

Test No.	79C001	79C002	79C003	79C004	80C005	80C006	80C007	80C008	80C009	80C010
Velocity (m/sec)	10.6	10.3	10.2	10.1	9.4	9.79	10.6	10.0	11.4	12.3
Piston Excursion (cm)	6.4	6.4	6.4	6.4	6.4	6.4	6.4	6.4	6.4	6.4
Surface Padding of a 15 cm Diameter Rigid Impactor (cm)	NONE	NONE	NONE	NONE	NONE	NONE	NONE	NONE	NONE	NONE
Site of Impact (Rib Number)	7	6	9	6	6	7	9	8	5	6

complete presentation, see (17). A summary of the initial test conditions are given in Table 1. The time histories of force filtered at SAE Channel Class 1000 are shown in Figures 5,6,7,8, and 9. A summary of the autopsy results can be found in Tables 2 and 3. Biochemistry and lavage results can be found in Table 4.

In order to define the pulse duration for force time history, a standard procedure was adopted which determines the beginning and end of the pulse. The left half of the pulse, defined from the point where the pulse starts to rise to the time of peak, is least squares fitted with a straight line. This rise line intersects the time-axis at a point which is taken as the formal beginning of the pulse. A similar procedure is followed for the right half of the pulse, i.e., a least-squares straight line is fitted to the fall section of the pulse which is defined from a point that initiates a rapid rate of decline, to the point where the first pulse minimum occurs. The formal end of the pulse is defined then as the point where the fall line intersects the time axis.

A summary of the test results is given for the cadavers and primates in Table 5 and for the canines in Table 6 which includes peak force, force duration, momentum and energy transferred, and the greatest positive and negative aortic pressures. Also in Table 5, the confidence intervals for comparison of post-mortem and live primates of these variables can be found.

The momentum transferred was determined by the integration of the force trace with respect to time. The energy transferred was defined by squaring the momentum transferred and dividing it by twice the mass of the impactor piston.

The biochemical assays, GOT and GPT, were evaluated by the Department of Pathology of University Hospital, The University of Michigan Medical Center. The total GOT and GPT were calculated using blood volume estimations of the test subject and calculating the total amount in the lavage by use of lavage biochemistry.

A summary of organ motion descriptors taken from the cineradiographs for the heart, spinal cord, and soft abdominal tissue is given in Table 7. Synchronization of the descriptors and force time histories was performed by the use of the gating circuit recorded on magnetic tape.

DISCUSSION

POST-MORTEM VS. LIVE MONKEYS - The time history of the applied force indicates that during the first 10 ms after contact, the impactor continues forward without a substantial loss of energy. This is arrived at by comparing the energy transferred to the available energy. In most cases, the force that is applied reaches a plateau and continues at that level until the impactor is arrested. During this interval, momentum and energy are being transferred to the subject (Tables 5 and 6). In general, a greater

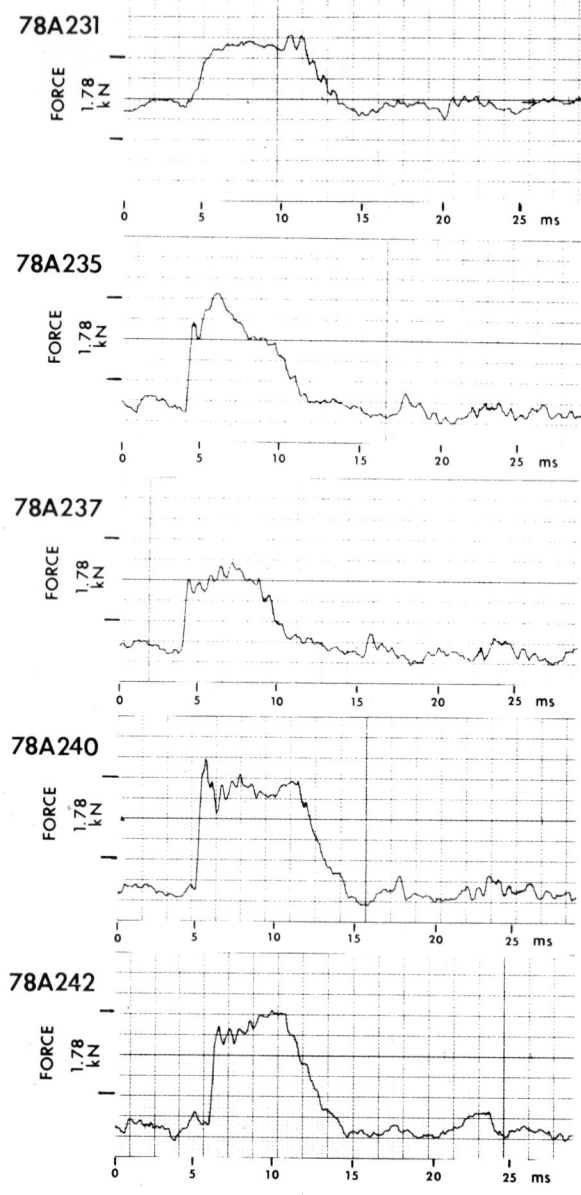

Fig. 5 - Primates force-time histories

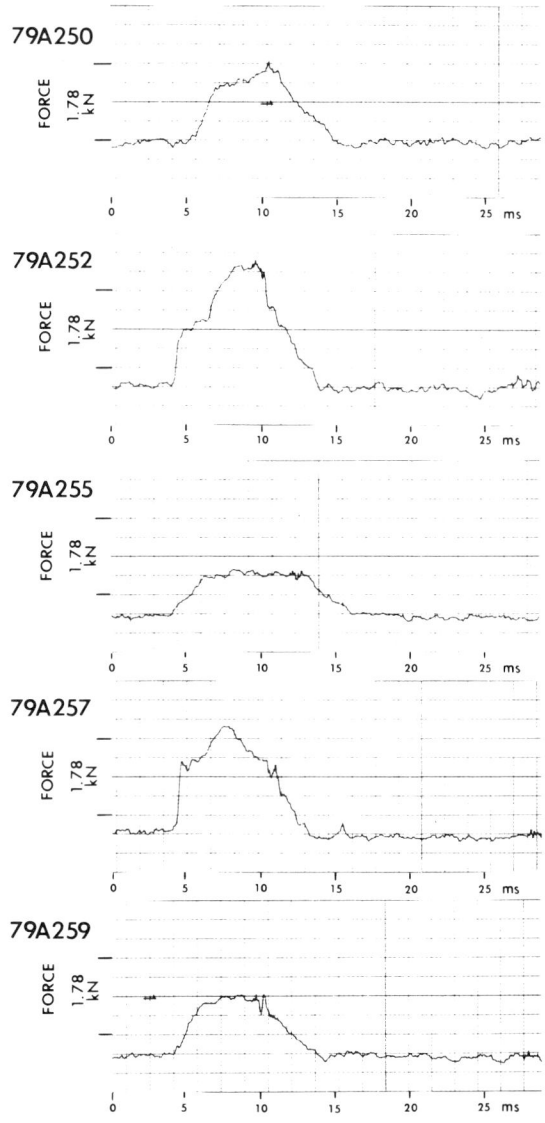

Fig. 6 - Primates force-time histories

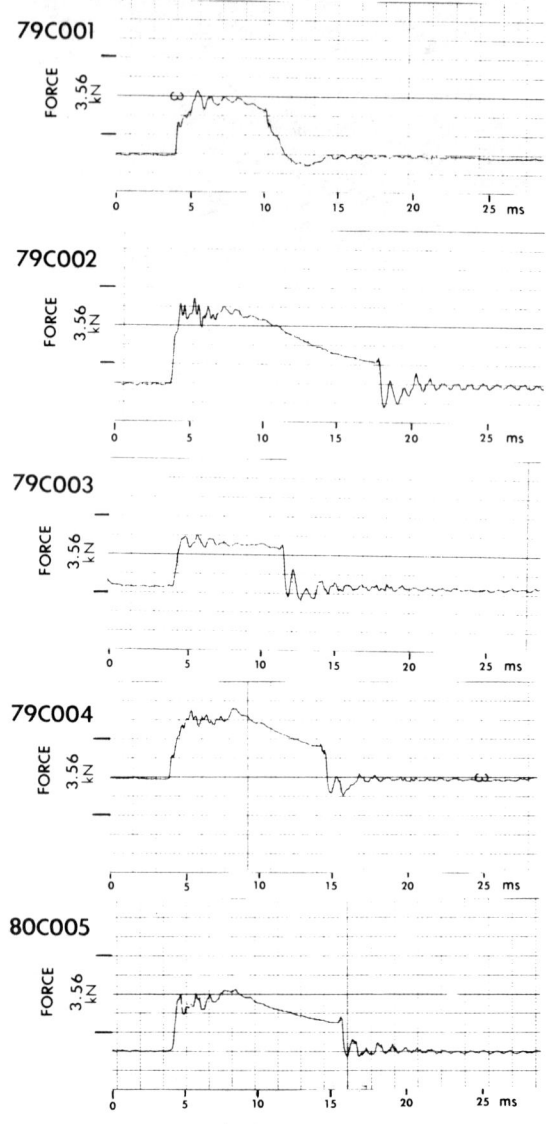

Fig. 7 - Canines force-time histories

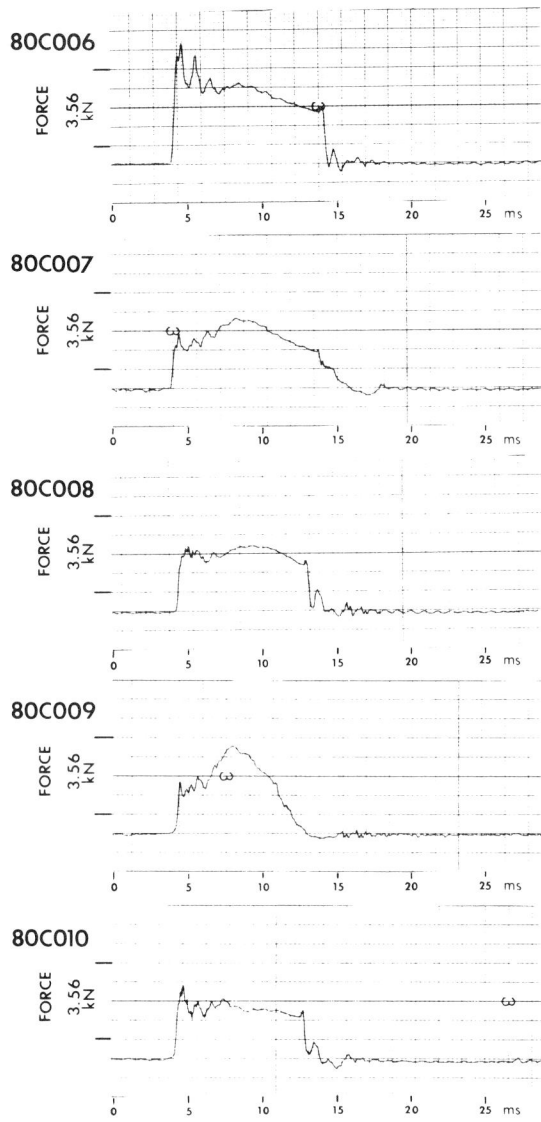

Fig. 8 - Canines force-time histories

Table 2

AUTOPSY SUMMARY

(Primates)

Test No.	Liver - Right Central Lobe	Liver - Right Lateral Lobe	Liver - Left Central Lobe	Liver - Left Lateral Lobe	Kidney - Right Side	Kidney - Left Side	Others	AIS Overall	AIS Liver	Grade
78A231	petechia hemorrhage				sub-capsular hematoma		petechia hemorrhage in left lower lobe of lung	3	2	1
78A233	1) longitudinal rupture 2) stellar rupture	longitudinal rupture			longitudinal rupture	sub-capsular hematoma completely surrounding the kidney longitudinal rupture	1) contusion at 8th right intercostal space 2) contusion on the right lung 3) hematoma - pancreas 4) hematoma - bladder	5	5	4
78A235	stellar rupture	longitudinal rupture	longitudinal rupture		1) surface tears in the capsule 2) tear in the renal vein		1) contusion - duodenum 2) contusion - stomach 3) contustion - right lung	5	5	4
78A237		longitudinal rupture					1) ribs 6,7,8,9 fracture near spine 2) mediastinal hematoma near the superior arteries 3) surface bruise over stomach	4	4	3
78A240*		longitudinal rupture	longitudinal rupture			longitudinal rupture	1) hematoma - pancreas 2) pneumothorax	3	3	2
78A242*	longitudinal rupture			bruise				3	3	2

*indicates post-mortem subject.

Table 2

AUTOPSY SUMMARY (cont'd.)

Primates

Test No.	Liver - Right Central Lobe	Liver - Right Lateral Lobe	Liver - Left Central Lobe	Liver - Left Lateral Lobe	Kidney - Right Side	Kidney - Left Side	Others	AIS Overall	AIS Liver	Grade
79A250*		rupture-G2		rupture-G1	1) petechiae hemorrhage 2) rupture		1) peritoneal attachments appear avulsed 2) fracture of left #7 rib 3) hematoma-pancreas, extending up hepato-duodenal ligament	3	3	2
79A252*	rupture-G2 Laceration of hematoma - G5	laceration-G2 both right and	rupture-G2 left hepatic vein with		laceration			5	5	5
79A254*					hematoma		hematoma on the inferior vena cava	3	0	0
79A255	laceration	laceration			subcapsular hematoma		hematoma - pancreas	4	4	3
79A257	laceration	1) laceration 2) hemorrhage	contusion	contusion			1) hemorrhage around right ribs #7 - #12 2) fracture of right ribs #8, 9, and 10 near spine	5	5	4
79A259	laceration			hemorrhage			1) hemorrhage on the fundus of gall bladder 2) hematoma - head of pancreas 3) small contusion - transverse colon 4) diaphragmatic hemorrhage near vena cava	3	3	2

*indicates post-mortem subject.

Table 3
AUTOPSY SUMMARY
(Canines)

Test No.	Liver: Left Center Lobe	Liver: Left Lateral Lobe	Liver: Right Center Lobe	Liver: Right Lateral Lobe	Liver: Quadrate Lobe	Liver: Caudate Lobe	Kidney: Left Side	Kidney: Right Side	Others	Degree of Injury: AIS Overall	Degree of Injury: AIS Liver	Degree of Injury: Grade
79C001			longitudinal rupture	stellar rupture and longitudinal rupture						4	4	3
79C002	stellar rupture	stellar rupture w/ hematoma	stellar rupture	longitudinal rupture w/ hematoma		stellar rupture				6	6	5
79C003		longitudinal rupture	stellar rupture	1) stellar rupture 2) subcapsular hematoma	stellar rupture					3	3	2
79C004	longitudinal rupture	longitudinal rupture w/ hematoma		longitudinal rupture		longitudinal rupture		longitudinal rupture w/ subcapsular hematoma		3	3	2
79C005	longitudinal rupture		1) longitudinal rupture 2) stellar rupture	longitudinal rupture w/ hematoma		stellar rupture			1) gall bladder -avulsion 2) right chest cavity-15 cc hematoma 3) right lung contusion	4	4	3
80C006	longitudinal rupture		longitudinal and stellar ruptures	1) stellar rupture 2) longitudinal and stellar ruptures						5	5	4

Table 3
Autopsy Summary (cont'd.)
(Canines)

Test No.	Liver: Left Center Lobe	Liver: Left Lateral Lobe	Liver: Right Center Lobe	Liver: Right Lateral Lobe	Liver: Quadrate Lobe	Liver: Caudate Lobe	Kidney: Left Side	Kidney: Right Side	Others	Degree of Injury: AIS Overall	Degree of Injury: AIS Liver	Degree of Injury: Grade
80C007	longitudinal rupture	longitudinal rupture and contusion	stellar rupture	stellar rupture		longitudinal and stellar rupture			gall bladder -avulsion	4	4	3
80C008				stellar rupture w/ subcapsular hematoma						3	3	2
80C009	Laceration		1) subcapsular hematoma 2) stellar & longitudinal ruptures	longitudinal rupture					gall bladder -avulsion	3	3	2
80C010				stellar rupture w/ subcapsular hematoma		stellar rupture			gall bladder -avulsion	4	4	3

Table 4

SERIAL BIOCHEMISTRY AND LAVAGE SUMMARY

Test No.	GOT SERUM IU/L				GOT LAVAGE IU/L				TOTAL GOT IU/KG				GPT SERUM IU/L				GPT LAVAGE IU/L				TOTAL GPT IU/KG				TOTAL UNCLOTTED BLOOD RELEASED ML/KG			
	*.5	1.5	2.5	3.5	.5	1.5	2.5	3.5	.5	1.5	2.5	3.5	.5	1.5	2.5	3.5	.5	1.5	2.5	3.5	.5	1.5	2.5	3.5	.5	1.5	2.5	3.5
79C001	1290	1616	1766	1806	705	407	269	116	114	25.5	12.5	3.6	1280	1675	1945	2050	728	419	276	109	113.6	31	21.7	28.1	3.9	1.6	0	0
79C003	781	865	861	848	1186	752	420	271	64.7	28.6	0	0	802	955	1038	1033	1238	765	424	264	80.5	17.2	9.4	4.8	7.0	0.7	0	0
79C004	1356	1862	1724	1684	2100	1800	1850	1500	130	35.5	20.5	6.3	613	933	904	959	1000	820	860	720	67.5	27.1	11.8	9.8	5.3	1.1	1.8	0.9
80C006	530	710	670	554	3190	2050	1390	870	145	9.4	0	0	730	810	1110	580	4290	2900	2100	1380	153.8	47.1	26.7	0	8.5	4.8	4.0	1.7
80C008	76	78	76	88	322	148	82	66	11.3	1.0	0.1	1.6	100	102	124	142	556	236	118	86	14.6	3.4	1.9	2.1	2.5	0.8	0	0
80C009	5420	6500	6200	7400	904	300	220	178	442	86.9	0	95.7	5120	6080	6000	7080	796	180	100	146	412	76	0	86.3	2.0	0.3	0.2	0.1

*Time in hours

Pre-test values GOT (Serum IU/L)		Pre-test values GPT (Serum IU/L)	
79C001	44	79C001	50
79C003	31	79C003	27
79C004	26	79C004	21
79C006	30	79C006	53
79C008	18	79C008	36
79C009	76	79C009	150

Table 5

IMPACT TEST SUMMARY

	Human Cadavers				Primates - Live							Primates - Post-Mortem							Single Tail T-test
	77A217	77A225	77A226	mean	78A231	78A235	78A237	79A255	79A257	79A259	mean	78A240	78A242	79A250	79A252	79A254	mean	Live vs. Post-Mortem
Duration (ms)	7.5	10.2	7.42	8.37	9.69	8.75	8.76	12.0	8.75	9.38	9.54	10.0	8.75	9.38	9.38	10.0	9.50	--
Peak Force (kN)	4.8	4.5	3.2	4.17	1.6	2.5	1.9	1.3	2.5	1.6	1.9	2.7	2.5	1.8	2.8	2.3	2.42	--
Momentum Transferred (N-S)	22.2	29.5	49.6	33.8	9.73	11.1	8.34	9.73	12.5	7.89	9.88	16.7	13.9	10.2	13.9	14.6	13.9	.99
Available Momentum (N-S)	97.5	94.5	128	107	105	131	123	85	114	133	115	125	123	133	133	145	132	.90
Energy Transferred (N-M)	24.7	43.5	123	63.7	4.73	6.18	3.48	4.73	7.8	3.11	5.01	13.9	9.66	5.23	9.66	10.7	9.83	.99
Available Energy (N-M)	475	446	819	580	552	855	756	360	653	888	677	781	756	888	888	1050	873	.90
Peak Aortic Pressure								+576/-58	+245/-14						+2130/-691			

Table 6

IMPACT TEST SUMMARY

(Canines)

Test No.	Peak Force (N)	Duration (msec)	Momentum Transferred (N-S)	Available Momentum (N-S)	Available Energy (N-M)	Energy Transferred (N-M)
79C001	2800	7.92	12.4	106	562	7.81
79C002	3560	14.	38.9	103	527	75.6
79C003	2220	7.8	18.1	102	516	16.3
79C004	3230	10.9	23.6	101	505	27.9
80C005	3110	12.5	27.4	94	441	37.6
80C006	5780	10.1	43.7	98	479	95.6
80C007	3340	12	26.4	106	557	34.8
80C008	2890	10.1	24.3	100	503	29.5
80C009	4090	8.75	19.8	114	650	19.6
80C010	3030	10.3	20.9	123	615	21.7
Mean	3440	10	25.6	105	536	36.6

Table 7

Descriptor Test Summary

Test Number	Percent Compression	Heart Velocity (Y) (ms)	Heart Velocity (Z) (ms)	Peak Velocity Resultant (m/sec)	Angular Velocity Diaphragm (rd/s) peak positive	Angular Velocity Diaphragm (rd/s) peak negative
78A231	36	7.1	1.1	7.2	31.2	-79.7
78A233	59	6.4	2.7	6.9	137.9	-115.2
78A235	80	7.4	1.5	7.5	136.8	-171.3
78A237	66	4.4	5.9	7.4	46.4	-122.2
78A240	95	7.7	2.6	8.1	90.1	-102.2
78A252	87	9.7	4.1	10.5	195	-183.3
78A254	59	6.6	5.4	8.5	70.1	-126.2
78A255	55	4.6	1.7	4.9	116.2	-127.9
78A257	69	7.9	1.5	7.9	145.3	-128.9
78A259	69	7.2	3.0	7.8	115.2	-478.9

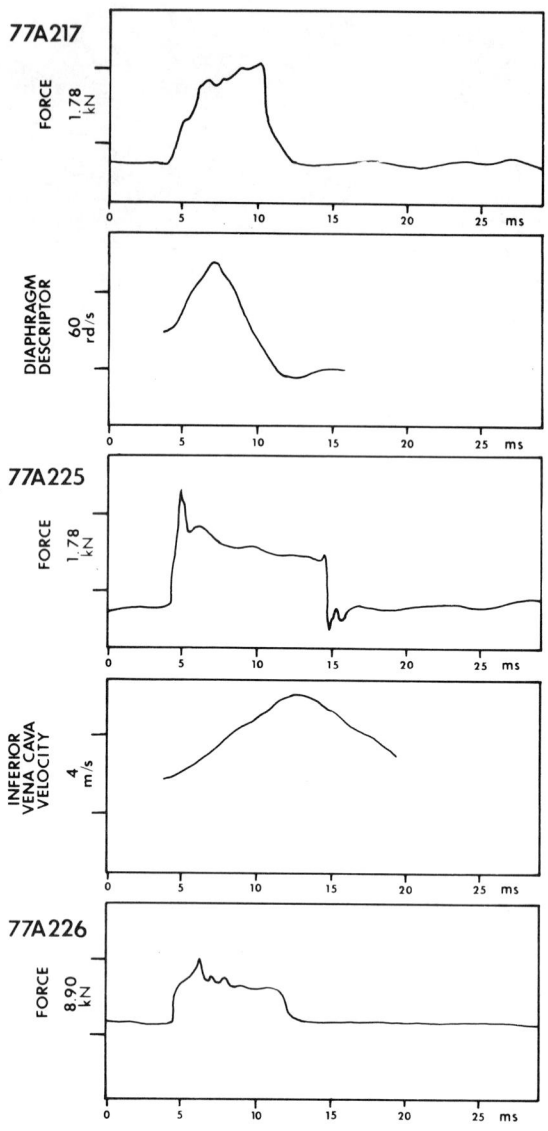

Fig. 9 - Human force-time histories and descriptors

percentage of available energy is transferred to the cadavers and canines, than to the primates.

A comparison of the average input characteristics taken from the force time history for the post-mortem and live groups of primates, shows noticeable differences between two variables (Table 5), momentum transferred and energy transferred, as indicated by a single tail t-test. A less noticeable difference occurs between the available energy and available momentum. An observation that seems pertinent to the variation in energy and momentum transferred is that the post-mortem subjects are in a more severe impact environment than that of the live subjects and that normalized energy transferred should be compared. When this is accomplished, there is a signficant reduction in the differences in the means indicating that the energy absorption response of the live primates is similar to that of the post-mortem. This method of comparison only takes into account the total energy transferred and not the response of the subject. Figures 10,11,12, and 13 show a composite of the responses of the primates as interpreted by the x-ray descriptors. From these results, no significant differences were seen between the post-mortem subjects and the live subjects. However, this response is only indicative of gross motion and the figures only transmit the idea of a general trend. To generalize these results, more tests would be needed. In addition, consideration must be given to the narrow range of velocity, padding, and stroke used in these tests. Therefore, this does not necessarily imply that in general, the energy transferred or the response for the live subjects during blunt impact is similar to that of the post-mortem subjects. The results utilized in the following comparison are that

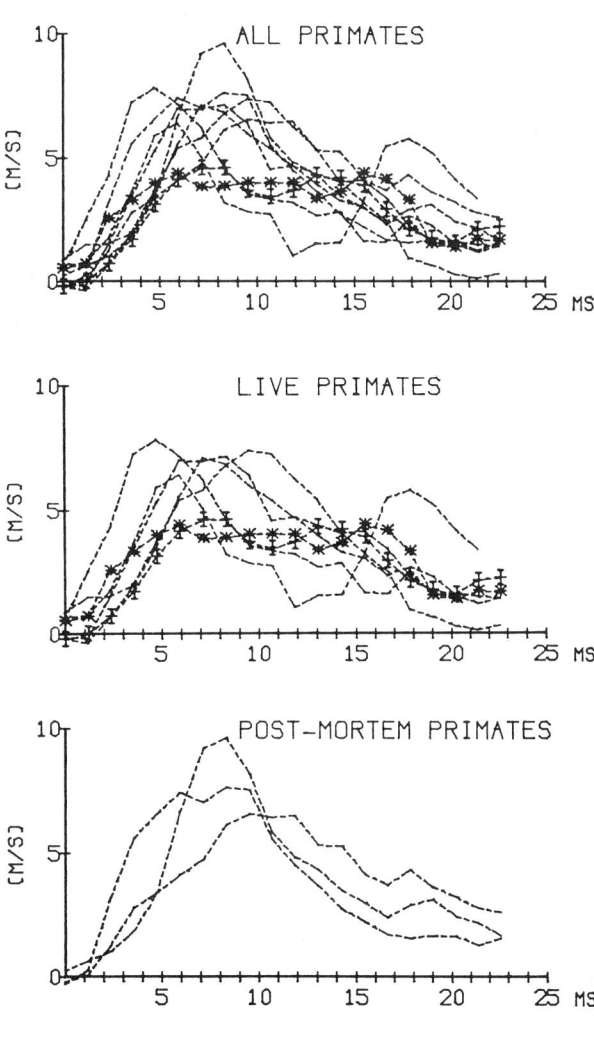

Fig. 10 - Primate descriptors

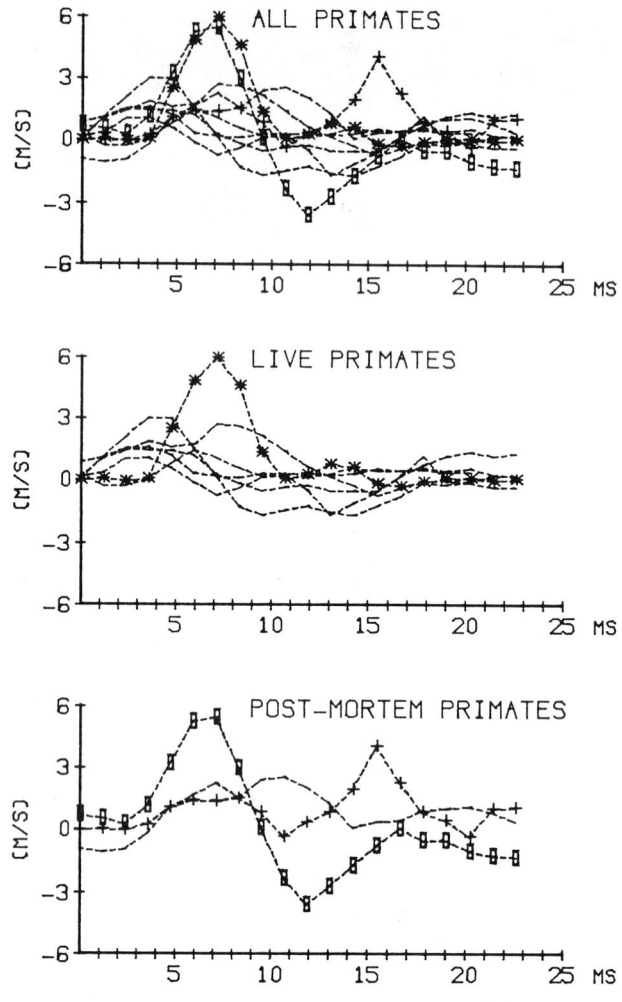

Fig. 11 - Primate descriptors

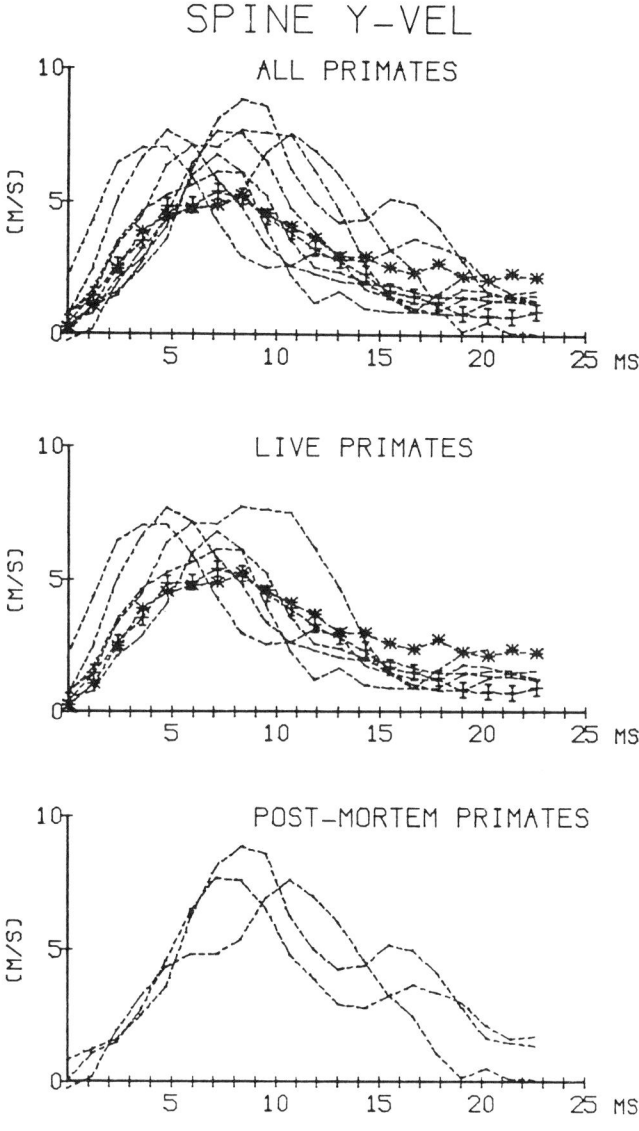

Fig. 12 - Primate descriptors

DIAPHRAGM ANG-VEL

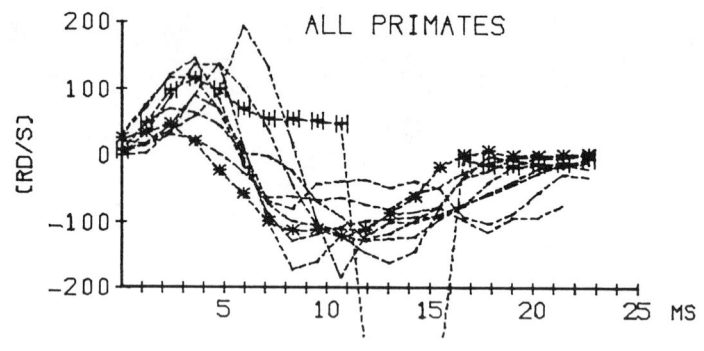

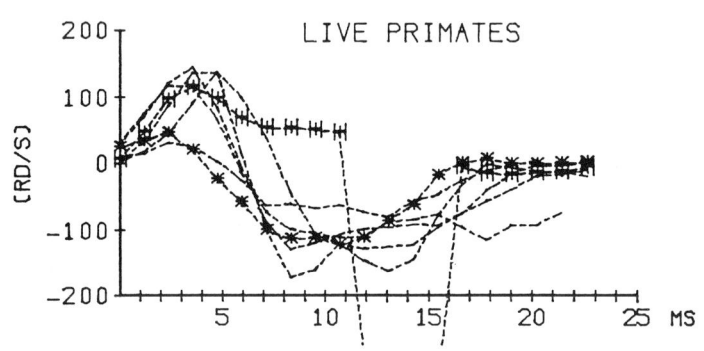

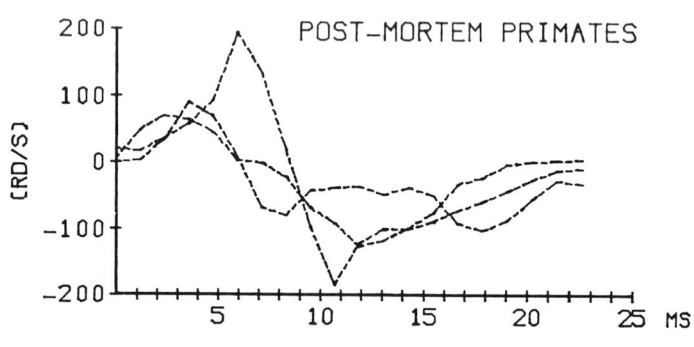

Fig. 13 - Primate descriptors

the impact environment of the post-mortem group was equal to or more severe than that of the live.

On the basis of overall AIS, the live primate injuries were more severe. In all but one of the live groups, there was an AIS of more than 4. In contrast, only one post-mortem subject obtained an AIS greater than 3 and that subject had an hepatic vein tear possibly due to the high location of the impactor. A possible explanation for the difference between the two groups could be the lack of pressurization in most of the post-mortem subjects. It has previously been found that turgidity in ex-vivo livers influences significantly the injury potential (4). One question not addressed is whether or not a more severe impact environment than that used for the post-mortem subjects in these tests can produce similar injury patterns to that of the live subjects. The trend seems to indicate that if it were possible, the impact environment would have to be made substantially more severe.

HUMAN CADAVER X-RAY CINERADIOGRAPH - The use of various descriptors based on radiopaque density and associated with an anatomical structure has proven to be a useful tool in the analysis of thoraco-abdominal response for human cadavers. There was no useful information obtained from the cineradiograph for test 77A226, and therefore, that test was not analyzed in that manner.

In these initial studies of right lateral blunt impacts, barium sulfate was used to quantitatively obtain information about the effect of such impacts on the hepatic system. The use of radiopaque dye injection made the venous tree visible during various phases of impact. The three test force time histories and responses as derived from the cineradiographs are summarized in Figure 9.

To obtain information from test 77A227, a variety of observations were made. Pre-impact radiographs clearly show sections of the right-hand hepatic venous system as well as a 10 cm section of the inferior vena cava. Excitation of the section of the liver within 2 cm of the most right-hand side started within 1 ms after the initiation of impact.

At 2 ms after impact, excitation at 3.5 cm from the right-hand side of the visible object space began and the vena cava started moving to the left. At 4 ms the hepatic right-hand tree had disappeared and reappeared after 8 ms indicating that the x-ray path thickness of the material bodies in close proximity to the venous tree had increased enough to obscure it during this interval.

One interpretation of this result is that the liver had increased its contact area with the thoraco-abdominal wall, thereby increasing its thickness in the posterior to anterior direction, while decreasing its right-to-left length. The thoraco-abdominal wall returns to the pre-impact condition following impact with a resulting decrease in the posterior-to-anterior liver thickness during this interval.

The vena cava was visible throughout the impact and displayed no significant rotation or translation. Its velocity is presented in Figure 12, and shows that there was an increase in velocity for the first 2/3 of the impact with subsequent decline after that.

The pre-impact radiographs for test 77A217 showed that, in this experiment, the radiopaque dye had located itself in the left-hand hepatic tree. If the response of the liver in this test was to be similar to that in test 77A225 then the excitation of event markers now on the left-hand side, should occur much later in the impact event. The first excitation at 9.8 cm, began at 6 ms, with motion at 13 cm following at 8 ms and motion at 16 cm following at approximately 9 ms, which confirms the estimated motion. In this test, the diaphragm descriptor was determined and is graphed in Figure 9. The descriptor velocity starts with a positive motion upon impact. This is associated with the thoraco-abdominal wall projecting into the thoraco-abdominal cavity and the boundary between the radiopacity and radiotransparency moving in the Z-direction (I-S) on the right side. This is similar to the results obtained from the excitation of event markers in which the liver is initially deformed from its initial configuration. The implication from the behavior of this descriptor is that some of the deformation is in the I-S direction and that the descriptor velocity then gives an estimate of the rate of deformation. There were no injuries produced in test 76A217 and 76A225. In test 76A226 longitudinal lacerations were present on the visceral surface of the right lateral lobe.

PRIMATE X-RAY CINERADIOGRAPHS - In tests 78A242 and 79A250, no attempt was made to obtain analytic data due to the poor quality of the x-ray cineradiograph. Test 79A259 (indicated in Figure 13 as I, had stomach bubbles that were positioned in such a way to cause the abdominal descriptor to differ vastly from the rest, 10 ms after initiation of impact. Test 79A240 also showed bubbles in the stomach, but it was judged that the usefulness of the abdominal motion descriptor was not hampered. In test 79A237 the majority of the heart had moved out of the range of the x-ray cineradiograph for the last 10 ms of sampling.

SPINE DESCRIPTOR - The data for the spine descriptor velocity are collectively presented in Figure 12 and give a general idea concerning its time history. In most cases, the peak velocity was reached after the majority of the momentum had been transferred. Test 79A237 and test 79A255 shown as * and # respectively in the accompanying graphs, have velocities less than that of the others. In test 79A255, the available energy is less than that of the other live tests. In test 79A237, ribs 7, 8, and 9 fractured near the spine, possibly limiting the load-transferring ability of the thorax.

HEART DESCRIPTOR - In general, the heart descriptor for the x-direction generates peak velocities from 6 to 9 m/s as shown in Table 7. The dynamic response of the heart as indicated by the velocities of the heart descriptor is judged to be controlled generally by direct contact of the heart with another material body. Such bodies include the thoraco-abdominal wall, the lung tissue trapped between the heart and the thoraco-abdominal wall, or the diaphragm. One such example is test 79A252. It was seen that no radiotransparent area existed between the heart and the thoraco-abdominal wall. Shortly following this, the heart flattened and then moved away from the contact. The heart then slowed down possibly due to the resistance of lung tissue. In test 79A237 and test 79A254 larger than normal Z-velocities were observed. In test 79A237, shown as a * in Figure 11, the heart moved up by contact with the abdominal wall, sliding up and over the indentation caused by the impactor. In test 79A254, shown as a I in Figure 11, the impactor was low enough such that the indentation was primarily in the abdomen. This caused the diaphragm to be displaced upward, contacting the heart and forcing it in the Z-direction. In test 79A252, shown as a +, the Z-velocity did not reach a peak until late in the impact, possibly due to the high location of the impactor and the resulting large distortion of the heart.

PRIMATE INJURIES AND DESCRIPTORS - Injuries to the hepatic system, obtained under the above described impact conditions, were principally longitudinal or stellar ruptures. Commonly, these were seen on the right central lateral lobes. Tests 78A235, 78A240, and 78A252 had longitudinal or stellar ruptures to the left central or lateral lobes and were at a distance from the impactor. In these tests, normalized compression (defined as the difference between the initial and minimum value of the near side deflection divided by the initial value) was 80% or greater. One possible explanation of these injury locations is that, due to the differential motion, the right central and lateral lobe are displaced or distorted to an extent that would allow greater interaction of the left central and lateral lobes with other material bodies. Of interest in this regard, are tests 79A257 and 79A259 which had the next highest compressions (69%). Contusions were located on the left central and lateral lobes.

The descriptor associated with the abdomen and the hepatic system is the diaphragm angle and its related derivative, angular velocity. This angular velocity is related to the rate of uplifting of the abdominal material and this would be related to the rate of deformation of the material bodies and thus, could be related to injury production. Figure 13 and Table 7 contain pertinent information regarding this concept. For the post-mortem state, although the test sample is small, there is no specific contraindication in the trend of increasing injury with increasing peak angular velocity. However, for the live state, there is one notable exception. In test 79A237, as noted previously, the ribs were fractured near the spine. This injury may have retarded the energy from being transferred to the spine resulting in reduced displacement of the opposing side of the rib cage. This, in turn, reduced the relative motion between the left side rib cage and the soft tissue.

Test 79A257 was initially evaluated as an AIS of 4 with a liver grade of 3. Consideration was then given to the profuse unclotted loss (9.6 ml/kg body weight during the first 1/2 hour with the animal expiring 1 1/2 hours after impact, probably due to shock) as an indication of injury severity. Utilizing this result, the liver grade was upgraded to a 5. Test 79A255 lost .6 ml/kg body weight in the first 1/2 hour, which was considerably less than test 79A257. The evaluation from gross autopsy had indicated that both tests should have had an equal level of injury, yet clearly test 79A257 was life-threatening and survival was questionable while test 79A255 was less severe. From these results, it is evident that the magnitude of internal bleeding can only be inferred by gross autopsy but not predicted.

SEQUENTIAL PERITONEAL LAVAGE AND BIOCHEMICAL ANALYSIS - The results of the serial peritoneal lavage and blood chemistry portions of this study are preliminary in nature and focus primarily upon the measurement of the release of unclotted blood into the peritoneal cavity of the canine test subjects. It was found that serial peritoneal lavage may be a useful technique for predicting when bleeding will cease. Tests 79C004 and 80C006 were the only tests in which the subject was still bleeding at the time of post-sample laparotomy. Both subjects displayed a significantly greater amount of unclotted blood entering the peritoneal cavity at that time (3.5 hr.) than the other subjects. No absolute statement can be made with respect to the efficacy of sequential peritoneal lavage as a method to chart the escape of unclotted blood from the site of injury into the peritoneal cavity due to the small sample size however.

The experimental results indicate that the magnitudes of the liver injury ratings obtained at autopsy do not correlate well, in this small series, with the ability of the liver to stop bleeding within the time frame of the experiments. Therefore, the rate of appearance of RBC from unclotted blood in the peritoneal cavity, due to liver injury, may be a functional characteristic which is as important in determining the necessity for operation as it is for determining the presence of the liver injury itself.

One method commonly used to define hepatic injuries clinically, is to measure certain biochemical assays. The two chosen to be presented in this report are GOT and GPT. In the tests presented here, the largest rate of release of GOT and GPT occurred in the first 1/2 hour. Elevated levls of GOT and GPT were found in both the serum and the peritoneal cavity. An interesting observation is that the GOT and GPT concentrations in the lavage fluid can be greater than the GOT and GPT concentrations in the serum. This may be due to the possibility that GOT and GPT, when released by bursting hepatocytes, can be flushed into the abdomen if there is a sufficient flow rate at the time of enzyme release.

CONCLUSIONS

Many features of the data presented in this paper are felt to be indicative of important factors in thoraco-abdominal impact. More work is necessary before findings can be generalized. The following specific conclusions can be drawn.

1. The x-ray cineradiograph has shown to be an invaluable tool in the understanding of thoraco-abdominal impacts. Quantitative motion determination of internal anatomical structures can be obtained in vivo with non-invasive techniques.

2. The response of the heart, during the time of contact in blunt lateral thoraco-abdominal impacts is affected by interactions with other material bodies. Direct contact with the diaphragm, thoraco-abdominal wall, and lung tissue can have an affect on the response of the heart.

3. During impacts of 12 ms or less, the hepatic system acts as a deformable structure with little response attributed to rigid body motion.

4. The degree of resulting injury, as interpreted by the AIS rating, was lower in the unpressurized post-mortem subjects than that of the live subjects.

5. Evaluation of abdominal injury severity by gross autopsy needs to be re-examined, critical factors such as hemorrhaging are only inferred and not directly interpreted.

6. Elevated levels of the enzymes GOT and GPT occur in both the circulatory system and the peritoneal cavity within one half hour following blunt abdominal impact trauma.

ACKNOWLEDGEMENTS

This work was conducted under the sponsorship of the Motor Vehicle Manufacturers Association. The authors would like to acknowledge the contributions of Jeffrey B. Axelrod, Jean S. Brindamour, Su-Hua Chen, Donna M. Head, Garry L. Holstein, and Valerie A. Moses in the performance of this work.

REFERENCES

1. J.W. Melvin, "Biomechanics of Lateral Thoracic Injury." The Human Thorax--Anatomy, Injury, and Biomechanics, Dearborn, Michigan, pp. 79-84, October 20, 1976.

2. D.H. Robbins, J.W. Melvin, and R.L. Stalnaker, "The Prediction of Thoracic Impact Injuries." Paper No. 760822, Proceedings of the Twentieth Stapp Car Crash Conference, Warrendale, Pa.: Society of Automotive Engineers, Inc., 1976.

3. R.L. Stalnaker, V.L. Roberts, and J. McElhaney, "Side Impact Tolerance to Blunt Trauma." Paper No. 730969, Proceedings of the Seventeenth Stapp Car Crash Conference, Warrendale, Pa: Society of Automotive Engineers, Inc., 1973.

4. E.T. Mays, "Bursting Injuries of the Liver." Archives of Surgery, 93:92:103, 1966.

5. M.L. Trollope, R.L. Stalnaker, J.H. McElhaney, and C.F. Frey, "The Mechanism of Injury in Blunt Abdominal Trauma." Journal of Trauma 13:962-970.

6. J.W. Melvin, R.L. Stalnaker, V.L. Roberts, and M.L. Trollope, "Impact Injury Mechanism in Abdominal Organs." SAE Paper No. 730968, Proceedings of the Seventeenth Stapp Car Crash Conference, Warrendale, Pa: Society of Automotive Engineers, Inc., 1973.

7. D.C. Viano, C.Y. Warner, K. Hoopes, C. Mortenson, R. White, and C.G. Artinian, "Sensitivity of Porcine Thoracic Responses and Injuries to Various Frontal and a Lateral Impact Site." Paper No. 780890, Proceedings of the Twenty-Second Stapp Car Crash Conference, Warrendale, Pa: Society of Automotive Engineers, Inc., 1978.

8. C.F. Frey, F. Trollope, W. Hampster, and R. Snyder, "A 15 Year Experience with Automotive Hepatic Trauma." Journal of Trauma, 13:1039-1049.

9. The Abbreviated Injury Scale, 1976 Revision, American Association for Automotive Medicine. Copyright 1976, Morton Grove, Illinois 60053.

10. R.P. Fischer, R.A. O'Farrell, and J.F. Perry, "The Value of Peritoneal Drains in the Treatment of Liver Injuries". Journal of Trauma, 18:393-398, 1978.

11. M. Bender, J.W. Melvin, and R.L. Stalnaker, "A High-Speed Cineradiograph Technique for Biomechanical Impact." Paper No. 760824, Proceedings of the Twentieth Stapp Car Conference, Warrendale, Pa: Society of Automotive Engineers, Inc., 1976.

12. G.S. Nusholtz, J.W. Melvin, and N.M. Alem, "Head Impact Response Comparisons of Human Surrogates," Paper No. 791020, Proceedings of the Twenty-Third Stapp Car Crash Conference, Warrendale, Pa: Society of Automotive Engineers, Inc., 1979.

13. I. Davidson and J.B. Henry, Clinical Diagnosis. Fourteenth Edition. W.B. Saunders Company, Philadelphia, Pa., 1962, p. 721.

14. G.S. Nusholtz, "Vascular and Respiratory Pressurization of the Thorax," International Workshop on Human Subjects for Biomechanical Research, Fifth Annual Meeting, Committee Reports and Technical Discussions, October 18, 1977, New Orleans, pp. 81-95.

15. Y.I. Abdel-Aziz and H.M. Karara, "Photogrammetric Potentials of Non-Metric Cameras," Report No. UILU-ENG-74-2002 on a study sponsored by National Science Foundation, University of Illinois, Urbana,

11, March 1974.

16. N.M. Alem, J.W. Melvin, and G.L. Holstein, "Biomechanics Applications of Direct Linear Transformation in Close-Range Photogrammetry." <u>Proceedings of the Sixth New England Bioengineering Conference</u>, New York: Pergamon Press, 1978.

17. G.S. Nusholtz, "Thoraco-Abdominal Response and Injury." Final report for Motor Vehicle Manufacturers Association of the United States, Inc., In Preparation.

801306
Evaluation of Pelvic Fracture Tolerance in Side Impact

Dominique Césari, Michelle Ramet, and Pierre-Yves Clair
Organisme National De Sécurité Routière

PELVIC GIRDLE FRACTURES are not very frequent (about 6% of all lesions) if every type of impact is considered. Nevertheless, this percentage rises to 10-14% if only nearside occupants in lateral impacts are considered. While restraint devices have a good efficiency mainly in frontal impact, few improvements have been effected up to now for reducing lateral impact severity.

A bibliographic survey points out that the frequency of side impacts account for between 15% and 28% of traffic accidents (1-2)*. In our investigation, side impacts represent 18.5% of traffic accidents. These accidents produce many injuries. As a matter of fact, WOLF (2) establishes that 15% of traffic accidents are lateral impacts and that they account for 22% of those injured. Besides, they are more severe than others and the death rate is higher than that of traffic accidents as a whole.

When comparing the distribution of injuries between injured occupants in lateral impact and injured occupants in all types of impacts, it can be noticed that the lesions to the pelvic and the abdominal content are more frequent in lateral impact, rising from 7.1% to 11.9% in our investigation (3). On the other hand, severity is linked to the occupant's seating place: as a matter of fact, the nearside occupant is generally the most severely injured, which confirms the importance of intrusion.

The experimental study of injury mechanisms in lateral impact (4-5) shows that for nearside occupants the lateral impact severity comes firstly from the intrusion of the impacted side panel and secondly from the shock of the occupant against the deformed panel.

So, to ensure a better protection in lateral impact, the panel intrusion has to be reduced and also the shock of the occupant against the vehicle inner door has to be absorbed. The first proposal (to reduce the intrusion) depends upon the vehicle design, whereas the second one (shock absorption)

---
*Numbers in parentheses designate references at end of paper.

ABSTRACT

Pelvic fracture is a typical lesion sustained by the occupant of a vehicle involved in a lateral impact collision who is seated on the impact side. If this fracture is generally not severe by itself, it is nevertheless often associated with severe abdominal lesions.

Study of injury mechanisms in lateral impact collisions shows that there are two ways of ensuring a better protection of the occupant in this type of accident: first by preventing intrusion so that the contact velocity "occupant/inner door" is decreased, secondly by absorbing the shock of the occupant against the inner door, especially at pelvis and thorax levels.

It is necessary to have a good knowledge of human tolerance to fracture of the considered body segment in order to determine the mechanical properties of the padding material.

The aim of this study is to determine the tolerance of the human pelvis. This study takes into account results of 36 impact tests against the pelvis of 10 cadavers and proposes injury criteria values to characterize the risk of pelvic fracture.

needs a good knowledge of human tolerance to this type of impact.

Thorax and pelvis are the two main body segments likely to come into contact with the inner panel.

This study deals with pelvic tolerance to lateral impact: in fact, pelvic fractures are not very severe from the vital point of view, but they are often accompanied with abdominal lesions in lateral impact, more especially at high speeds (6).

Besides, it can be noticed that pelvic lesions in lateral impact affect mainly os pubis rami, sacro-iliac joint and wings of ilium (7) whereas acetabulum injuries (dashboard injuries) are more frequent in frontal impact.

All these facts led us to carry out this study of pelvic tolerance in lateral impact in order to determine the properties of a padding material designed to protect the pelvis.

ANATOMICAL RECALL

The pelvis is formed by the sacrum and the two os innominata which are attached to the sacrum posteriorly by the sacro-iliac joint and are joined to each other anteriorly at the pubic symphysis. Each hip bone has 3 components: the ilium, the ischium and the pubis. The ilium is fan like and splays upward while the os pubis in front and the ischium behind form the lower part of the pelvic cavity and enclose an oval aperture: the obturator foramen. The banks of the foramen are the descending (ischiopubic) and ascending rami of os pubis. These three parts contribute to form the acetabulum, which constitutes, with the head of the femur a ball-and-socket joint. The large part of ilium forms the prominence of the hip and is called iliac wing.

Pelvic lesions seem to be a mechanism occuring by direct impact on the iliac crest or on the greater trochanter. Impact forces, working transversally on the pelvis's lateral part, bring closer the 2 parts of the pelvic girdle: there is then either a pubis symphysis disjunction, or a sacro-iliac disjunction or a posterior fracture of the iliac wing. But the compression works through the head of femur then there are the classical fractures of the ascending and descending rami of os pubis. The fractures of the acetabulum are not frequent although the compressive force works at the level of head of femur.

TEST METHODOLOGY

All the tests were performed using a device especially designed to reproduce impacts similar to those observed in real accidents. The procedure we used has been described in a previous paper (8) but it is briefly described below.

The device consists of a fixed frame and a mobile impactor, horizontally guided in order to hit a human subject seated on a rigid seat locked with the frame end. The mobile part is propelled by rubber extensible springs and the system is tightened through a small trolley guided on the same axis as the impactor and attached to a steel cable. It is possible to pull on the cable through a winch and then to move the trolley and the impactor back by tightening the rubber extensible springs. A bolt located between the trolley and the impactor releases the impactor which is then accelerated by the rubber extensible springs and hits the human subjects (Fig. 1).

The impactor mass is 17.3 kg and the impacting system is the portion of a sphere ($r = 600$ mm, $R = 175$ mm). Analysis of car-to-car side impact tests shows that the impacted door is deformed before hitting occupant. The deformations make the door stiffer, and the actual cars do not ensure a good protection in side impact, especially they have no padding material on the inner side. For these reasons we decided to use a rigid impactor in these tests. The impact force and impact acceleration are measured on the mobile system through transducers.

All the tests were performed with fresh human cadavers. They were incised along the iliac crest to expose the internal face of the wing of ilium. Three strain gauges were applied on this internal face: 2 below the iliac crest and 1 behind the acetabulum. These gauges were plastic sheathed, which made their fitting simpler. Then, the incision was sutured. A fourth gauge was placed on the same side on the upper face of the ascending ramus of os pubis as indicated on Fig. 2. Then, the cadaver was dressed up, weighed, measured and placed on the seat. The seat was adjusted in height and depth so that the impactor was centered on the greater trochanter tuberosity.

The seat used gave the cadaver a posture identical to that of a car driver. The subject was unbelted and without lateral support.

Several tests are performed with the same cadaver, until a pelvic fracture is produced. Therefore an X-ray picture is taken after each test to verify whether is produced a fracture or not. An X-ray picture is also taken before the tests to verify that there was no previous fracture or important osseous decalcification.

We decided to perform tests with unbelted subjects, because the analysis of car-to-car collisions shows that the safety belt is generally not solicited in lateral impact, at least not during the main phase of the impact.

36 impact tests on pelvis were performed for this study, using 10 cadavers (5 males, 5 females). The main results of these tests are shown in Tables 1 and 2. The various recordings made during a test are given in the appendix.

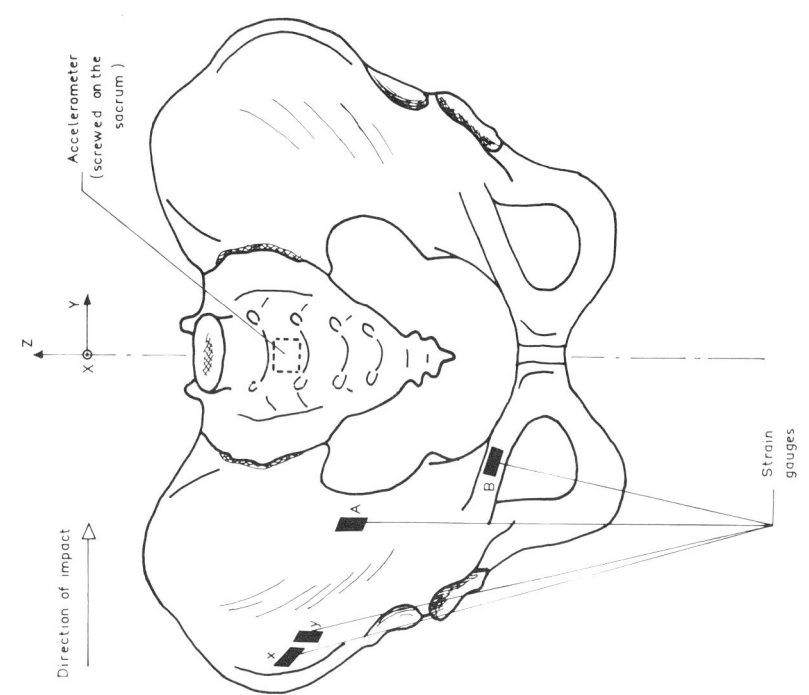

Fig. 2 - Locations of strain gauges on the pelvis of cadavers (impacted side)

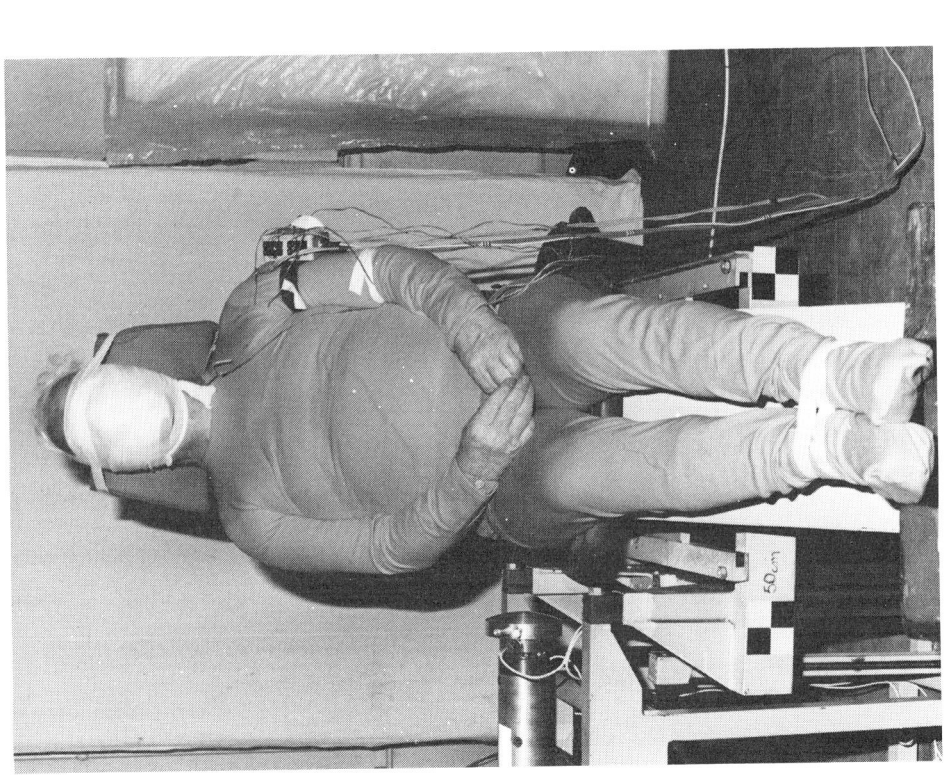

Fig. 1 - View of the cadaver seated and of the impactor

Table 1 - Test results (cadavers A to F)

Test	Sex	Age	Height cm	Weight kg	Speed m/s	Force N	3 ms accel. g	Impulse N.s.	AIS	LESIONS
A1	F	70	167	58	5.83	4170		63	0	
A2					7.22	5800		122	0	
A3					8.33	6960		163	0	
A4					11.39	11140		209	3	fract. of right os pubis rami, sacro iliac disjunction non complete fracture of sacrum
B1	F	84	154	70	5.83	5100		71	0	
B2					8.33	6260		131	2	fract. of the anterior superior iliac spine
B3					9.72	8120		161	3	fract. of right ischio pubic ramus, fract. of femoral neck and collapse of the femoral head
C1	M	69	173	78	7.11	5620		113	0	
C2					8.89	10120		136	0	
C3					10.94	10120		162	2	fract. of the right iliac wing
C4					13.19	13780		232	2	fract. of right femoral shaft
D1	F	63	160	52	6.94	4410	34	88	0	
D2					8.56	5240	45	115	0	
D3					9.92	4530	23	131	3	fract. of right os pubis rami, fract. of right femoral neck, sacro iliac disjunction
E1	F	72	156	60	7.00	5520	45	88	0	
E2					8.64	5520	34	112	3	fract. of right os pubis rami, sacro iliac disjunction
F1	F	59	152	55	7.86	5790	33	89	0	
F2					8.64	3860	24	90	0	
F3					9.72	5520	24	111	0	

Table 2 - Test results (cadavers H to K)

Test	Sex	Age	Height cm	Weight kg	Speed m/s	Force N	3 ms accel. g	Impulse N.s.	AIS	LESIONS
H1	M	69	175	86	7.08	6920	27	82	0	
H2					8.39	10760	42	99	0	
H3					9.61	11040	40	128	0	
H4					10.61	12690	-	140	0	
H5					11.67	9930	-	171	2	right femoral fracture
I1	M	63	181	63	7.08	10210	39	77	0	
I2					8.41	11040	49	97	0	
I3					9.86	11590	49	115	0	
I4					11.05	12690	35	139	0	
I5					12.52	13240	80	157	0	
I6					13.72	11040	36	174	2	fracture of the right iliac wing
J1	M	75	177	63	7.08	7730	34	79	0	
J2					8.50	6070	30	124	0	
J3					9.89	8270	62	131	3	fract. of right os pubis rami, pubis symphysis disjunction
K1	M	75	171	55	6.94	5520	34	73	0	
K2					8.55	7170	35	85	0	
K3					9.81	8280	40	102	0	

RESULTS

The impact is characterized by various physical parameters. They are mainly: impact velocity (or shock kinetic energy), maximum sustained force, impulse and pelvic acceleration.

ADMISSIBLE IMPACT VELOCITY - Fig. 3 shows the maximum admissible speed according to age. For each subject, the determined speed value is the average between the test speed provoking a fracture and the highest test speed without fracture. For both subjects that sustained no fracture (subjects F and K), the limit value is the speed value of the last test plus 2.5 km/h (which is half of the speed variation between 2 tests i.e. 5 km/h). We consider that the following test which would have been performed at a speed superior of 5 km/h would have then induced a lesion. These two subjects were not tested at higher velocities because the external examination made by a medical doctor revealed a pelvic fracture, and the X-ray pictures were not immediately processed. Unfortunately for these two subjects only, the autopsy and the X-ray pictures show that there was no bone fractures. These two subjects are more resistant than the average of the cadavers used for this study, so if we do not consider the results of these two cadavers we get lower values of human tolerance, whereas we are sure that they were able to sustain the last test that we performed on them.

In Fig. 3, we tried to establish a linear correlation between the various subjects. It can be noted that the admissible speed decreases according to the age, which is quite normal because the osseous resistance decreases according to the age. Female subjects have generally an inferior osseous resistance, but this resistance does not decrease much with age. On the contrary, male subjects have an osseous resistance which decreases very quickly with age. The literature is not unanimous in this field but it seems that the bone resistance falls after the age of 40, and that the bone resistance of female is weaker than the bone resistance of male (9).

The speed values of admissible speed are approximatively the same than those measured in car-to-car impacts: in car-to-car impact, it seems that pelvic fractures occur from a 35 to 40 km/h panel speed. Indeed in actual accidents pelvic fractures occur at an impact speed over 50 km/h (10) which corresponds to a door velocity change equal to 35/40 km/h (5). Nevertheless, it is difficult to measure the impact speed between the occupant and the inner panel during a car test. Moreover, the relationship between impact speed and severity is good only for a precise stiffness value of the impacting element. As a matter of fact, if the impacting element offers better padding properties, the human subject may "sustain" an impact at a higher speed. For all these practical reasons, it is advisable to link severity with a measurable parameter, especially on a dummy. This parameter may be either the impact force or a parameter deriving from

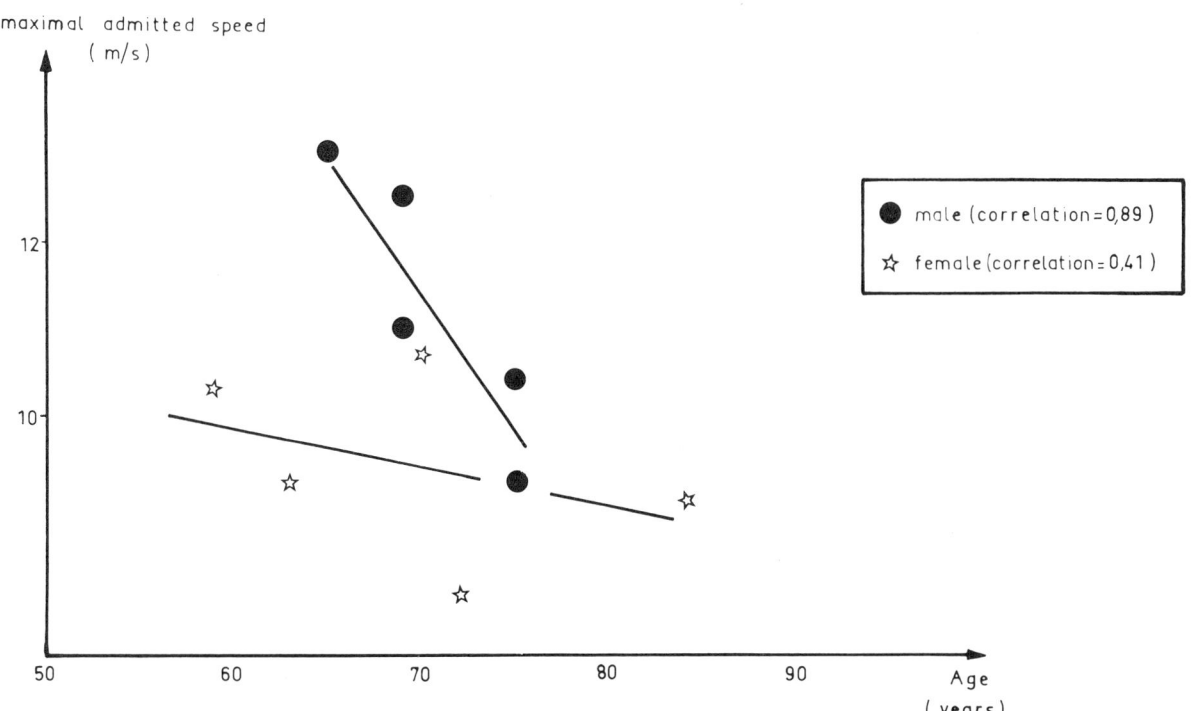

Fig. 3 - Maximum tolerable impact speed as a function of age and sex

the force, or the acceleration induced by the impact.

ADMISSIBLE IMPACT FORCE - The impact force has been measured during all the tests. Fig. 4 shows the maximum admissible force according to the test speed for the 10 subjects. The considered force value is that of the tests performed at the highest speed without provoking a fracture. It can be noticed that there is a quite good correlation between the speed and the impact force.

The maximum impact force recorded during fracture producing test was not always higher than the maximum load of the preceding test. When there was a fracture the force time record was often characterized by two peaks on the trace, but not always.

Figure 5 shows the impact force value of the test performed at the highest speed, without provoking any fracture and according to the age. There is a good relationship between the age and force for male subject, the permissible force decreasing quickly according to the age. However, for female subjects, age makes practically no difference to the admissible force in the considered age group. These differences have the same reasons as established in the analysis of the admissible speed. It can be noticed in Fig. 4 that the admissible force sustained by the pelvis is always superior to 5000 N. All female subjects have an admissible impact speed between 5000 and 7000 N, whereas male subjects have an admissible force varying from 7000 to 13000 N.

VALUE OF THE ADMISSIBLE IMPULSE - If only the maximum value of the admissible force is considered, the duration of loading is not taken into account. Nevertheless, given the viscoelastic properties of the human body, it would be advisable that the parameter linked with the tolerance takes into account the duration of loading. The impulse is a parameter linked with the impact which depends on the applied force and its duration. Its definition is:

$$\pi = \int_0^T F dt$$

Fig. 6 shows the impulse value according to the impact speed in 6 tests performed with subject n° 1. There is a very good correlation between these two parameters. This subject has been chosen because it was used to perform the greatest number of tests. This good correlation means also that the impulse value is also well linked with the kinetic energy of the impactor.

Fig. 7 indicates the relationship between the admissible impulse and the subject's age. With the admissible impact force, so the impulse decreases according to the age for male subjects, whereas the age seems to have little effect upon the impulse value for female subjects. For the 10 tested subjects, the admissible impulse varies between 90 and 170 N.s., but the admissible value is inferior to 100 N.s. for only one subject, the average value is therefore 129 N.s.

ADMISSIBLE ACCELERATION - The pelvic acceleration has been measured from subject D onwards i.e. for 7 subjects out of the 10. However, the pelvic acceleration value could not be measured in the last two tests performed with subject H because of a recording breakdown.

Results of the analysed tests given in Table 1 show that there is generally not a good correlation between the impact speed and the pelvic acceleration. Fig. 8 indicates the pelvic AIS value depending on the acceleration. This graph indicates for each subject both the acceleration value recorded during the most violent test without fracture and if a fracture occured, the acceleration value recorded during the fracture producing test. To compare the results of tests with and without fracture of the same subject references are indicated on this figure. It is noticeable that, except for one cadaver, the maximum acceleration recorded during a fracture producing test is always lower than the value recorded during the non fracture producing precedent test. Values recorded during tests with fracture are generally inferior to those proposed in a previous study (11).

DISCUSSION

COMPARISON OF INDUCED LESIONS - In real accident studies, the fractures of pelvic girdle in lateral impact, concern especially the ascending and decending rami of os pubis and the iliac wing often associated with sacro-iliac disjunction or pubic symphysis disjunction, bilateral fractures are not rare. Incomplete fractures of the sacrum are often observed. The fractures of the pelvic girdle are frequently associated with femoral fractures. During our tests, the lesions noted are the same type but never bilateral. These experimental tests did not produce bilateral fractures because we control the kinetic energy of the impactor, and we do not perform a more severe test as soon as a fracture occurs. In 4 cases we observe fractures of right ascending and descending rami of os pubis, i.e. on the impacted side. In one case the ischio pubic rami only is broken. The iliac wing is broken in 2 cases and associated in one case with femoral fracture. The disjunctions of the sacro-iliac joint are associated with rami of os pubis fractures in 4 cases. Only one pubic symphysis disjunction was observed. The upper part of the femur is broken in 3 cases. We can establish a good similitude between the lesions observed in real accident and in dynamic tests. We notice that, in spite of a localized impact on the trochanter major, we cannot induce any acetabulum fracture. Similarly in real accident, this type of lesion is not found whereas it is particularly frequent in frontal impact (dashboard injuries).

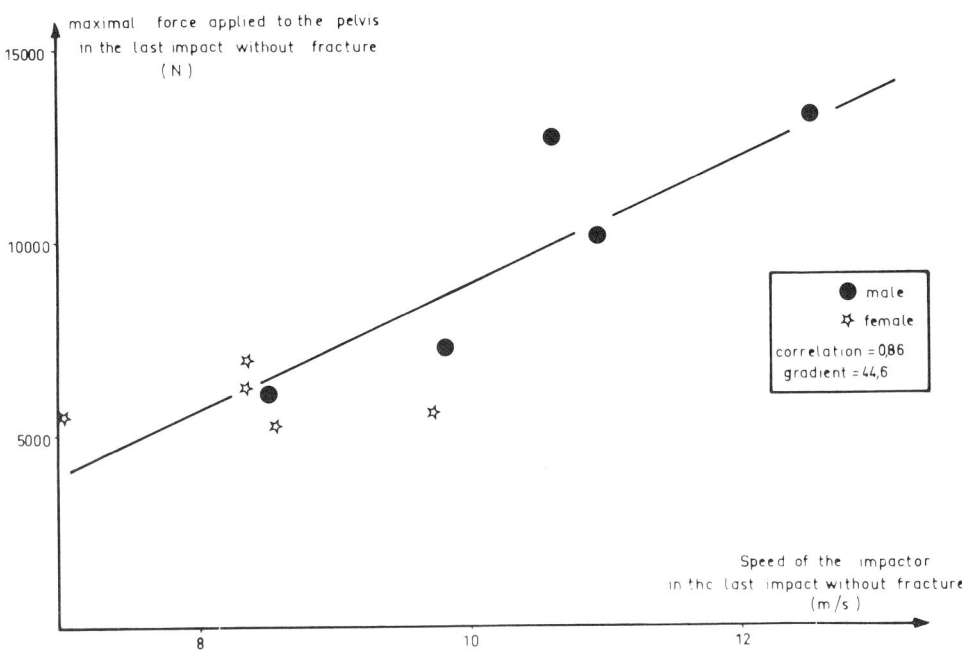

Fig. 4 - Relation between impact force and impact speed for the most severe test without fracture of each cadaver

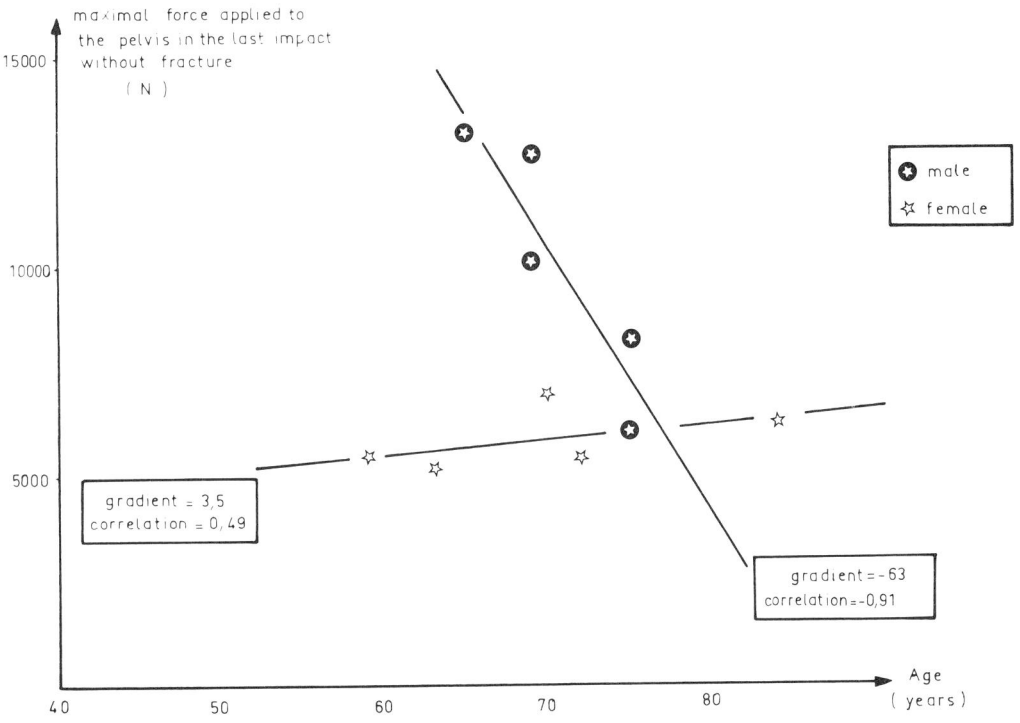

Fig. 5 - Maximum tolerable impact force, as a function of age and sex

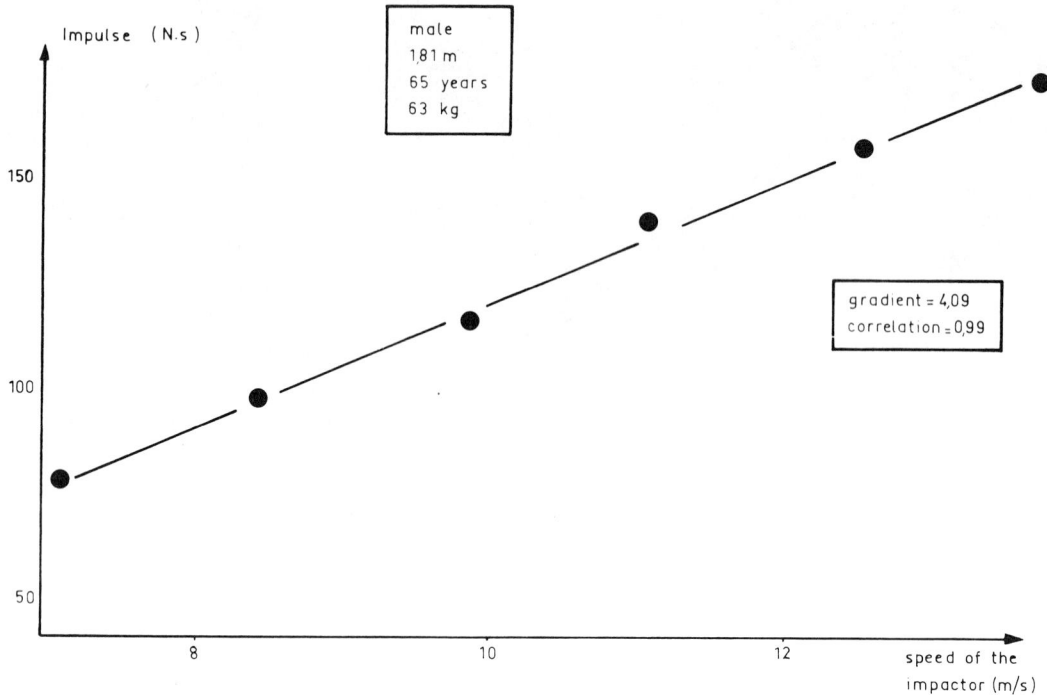

Fig. 6 - Relation between impulse and impact speed for the 6 tests of cadaver I

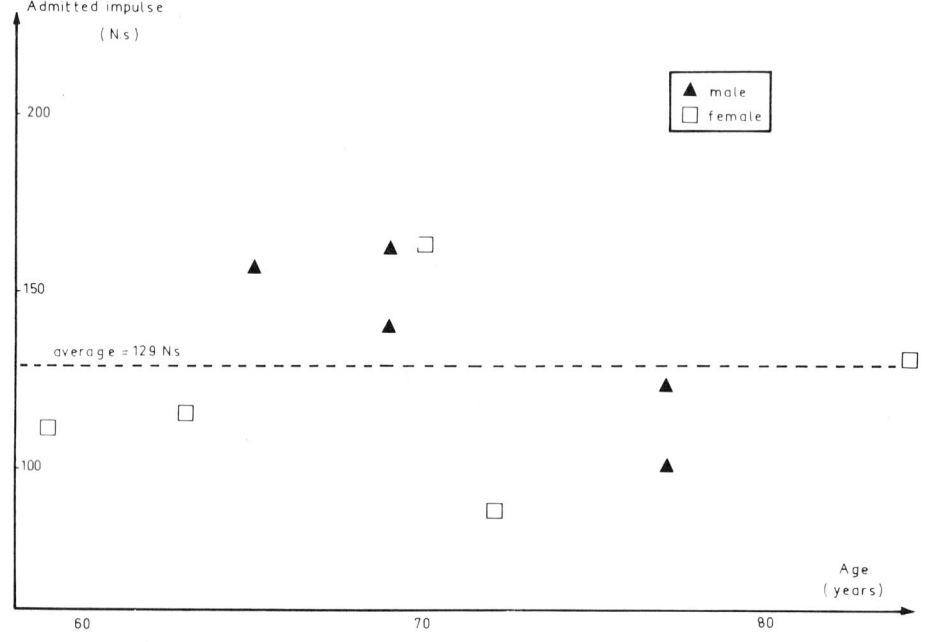

Fig. 7 - Maximum tolerable impulse as a function of age and sex

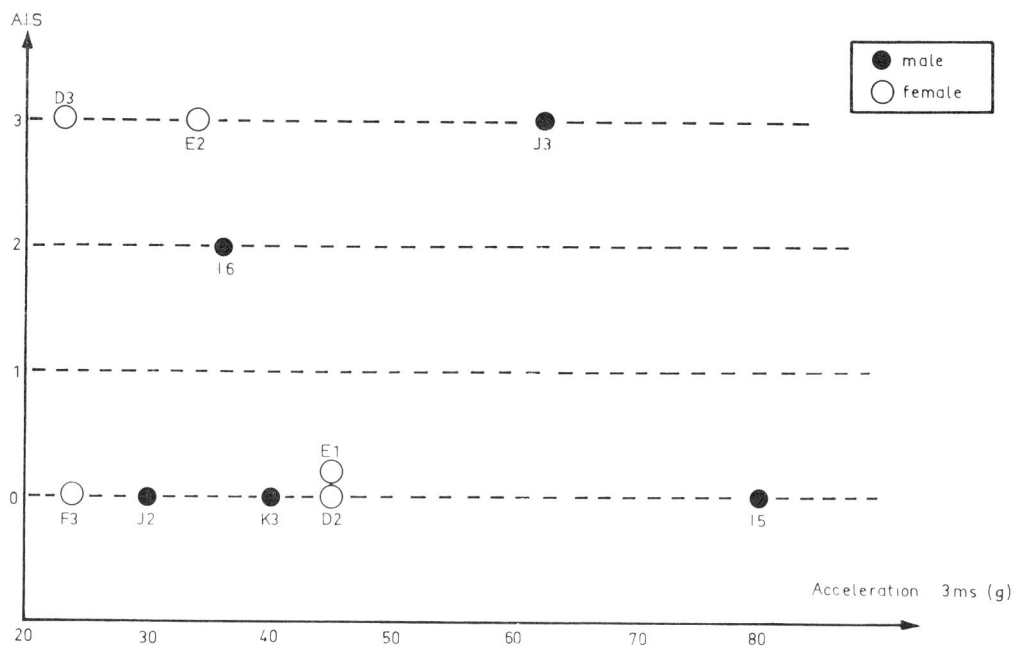

Fig. 8 - Relation between AIS and 3 ms pelvis acceleration

COMPARISON OF SUSTAINED IMPACTS - To establish the validity of the results obtained in this study, it is interesting to compare the impact sustained by the pelvis in this study with the impact sustained by a cadaver pelvis in a car-to-car impact. The only measure recorded both in this study and in car-to-car impact reconstructions is the transversal acceleration of the pelvis. The impactor acceleration may be associated with the door acceleration during the impact in a car-to-car crash, the impact point being located near the area struck by the pelvis.

Fig. 9 shows pelvis acceleration curves according to time, in a test performed with the impactor and in a car test; both tests are carried out under similar conditions with regards to the speed (impactor speed and door speed). Indeed the door velocity change is approximately equal to 75% of the impact speed, i.e. for this test 10.4 m/s. These curves have a similar shape, especially in the area where the acceleration is high. Differences are seen at the beginning of the impact. In particular, in the car test, the beginning of the pelvis acceleration is slower than that of the test with impactor. As a matter of fact, at the beginning of the impact, the cadaver deforms the door front face, whereas in the test with the impactor, it is not possible for the impacting element to sustain a deformation. This difference at the beginning of the impact does not call the use of the impactor into question: during the main impact phase, the acceleration curves of the cadaver pelvis obtained by performing both tests (with impactor and with car) are similar, especially concerning the acceleration slope and the maximal acceleration magnitude.

VALUES OF PELVIC TOLERANCE TO FRACTURE - The analyses of the results obtained by performing 36 tests during this study shows that the pelvic tolerance is not the same for males as it is for females and depends on the subjects age. Concerning the force, this tolerance would be about 5000 N and concerning the impulse, it would be 100 N.s. Some subjects, especially among the males, have a higher tolerance to fracture. If the selected tolerance value is higher than the one above mentioned, it would mean that old people, and especially women above 60, are not protected. Furthermore, in French traffic accidents, one out of eight killed or severely injured traffic accident victims is more than 65 years old and the traffic death rate is the highest at this age (12). Concerning the speed, the tolerance value established in this study indicates that the occupant seated on the impact side must be able to sustain an impact between two vehicles of same mass, the impacting vehicle speed being about 45 km/h. As a matter of fact, given the present vehicle design, experimental studies show that the contact speed between the occupant and the inner door is about 0.75 time the impact speed in a lateral impact involving two vehicles of same mass. Given the admissible speed limit is about 34 km/h, it corresponds for the panel speed to a car-to-car impact at 45.3 km/h performed with two vehicles of same mass. On the contrary, if intrusion could

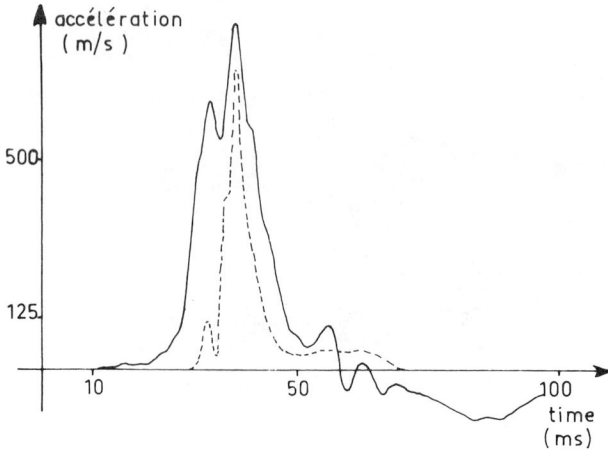

Fig. 9 - Pelvic acceleration in car-to-car test in comparison with pelvic acceleration in impacting machine test

be avoided the contact speed between occupant and inner door would be about half the impact speed in a lateral collision of two cars of same mass. So, the nearside occupant could sustain at the pelvis level a lateral impact at more than 65 km/h (both vehicles having the same mass).

CONCLUSION

Results of 36 transversal impact tests against the pelvis of 10 cadavers show that the fracture tolerance decreases according to the age and that female subjects have a lower tolerance than males.

Concerning the impact speed, the maximum limit value is between 30 and 35 km/h. It is better to choose, as pelvis injury criterion, the maximal impact force, or a parameter derived from the force such as the impulse, rather than the acceleration which has a bad correlation with the speed.

If the chosen tolerance value is that of the group of people having the lowest resistance, the pelvis tolerance limit is about 5000 N or 100 N.s. It could be possible to choose the most adequate injury criterion between force and impulse by performing additional tests during which the shock of the impactor against the pelvis is absorbed, and tests conducted with energy absorbing materials placed between the impactor and the cadaver should be complementary to this study.

ACKNOWLEDGMENTS

This work was sponsored by the French Ministry of Transportation, Direction des Routes et de la Circulation Routière and EEC, for which we are grateful.

REFERENCES

1. G.M. Mackay, "Causes and effects of road accidents", Department of Transportation and Environmental Planning, University of Birmingham, vol. 3, 1969.

2. R.A. Wolf, "Causes of impact injury in automobile accidents", National Academy of Science, 1962.

3. D. Césari, M. Ramet, "Influence of intrusion in side impact", 6th E.S.V. Conf., Washington, 1976, 1-19.

4. A.J. Padgaonkar, P. Prasad, "Simulation of side impact using the CAL 3D occupant simulation model", 23rd Stapp Car Crash Conf., 1979, 133-158.

5. D. Césari, M. Ramet, D. Herry-Martin, "Injury mechanisms in side impact", 22nd Stapp Car Crash Conf., 1978, 429-448.

6. F. Hartemann, J. Y. Foret-Bruno,

C. Thomas, C. Tarrière, C. Got, A. Patel, "Influence of mass ratio and structural compatibility on the severity sustained by the near side occupants in car-to-car side collisions", 23rd Stapp Car Crash Conf., 1979, 233-260.

7. N. Dejeammes, "Fractures du bassin au cours des chocs latéraux automobiles", Thèse Lyon 1978.

8. M. Ramet, D. Césari, "Experimental study of pelvis tolerance in lateral impact", 4th International IRCOBI Conf., Göteborg, 1979.

9. R. M. Kenedy, "Advances in biomedical engineering", Academic Press London and New York, 1971.

10. F. Hartemann, J. Y. Foret-Bruno, C. Thomas, C. Tarrière, "Compatibility of masses and structures in car-to-car lateral collisions", 7th E.S.V. Conf., Paris, 1979, 622-629.

11. A. Fayon, C. Tarrière, G. Walfish, "Contribution to defining the human tolerance to perpendicular side impact", 3rd International Conf. on impact trauma, IRCOBI, Berlin, 1977, 297-309.

12. "Accidents corporels de la circulation routière en France", SETRA, Ministère des Transports, 1977.

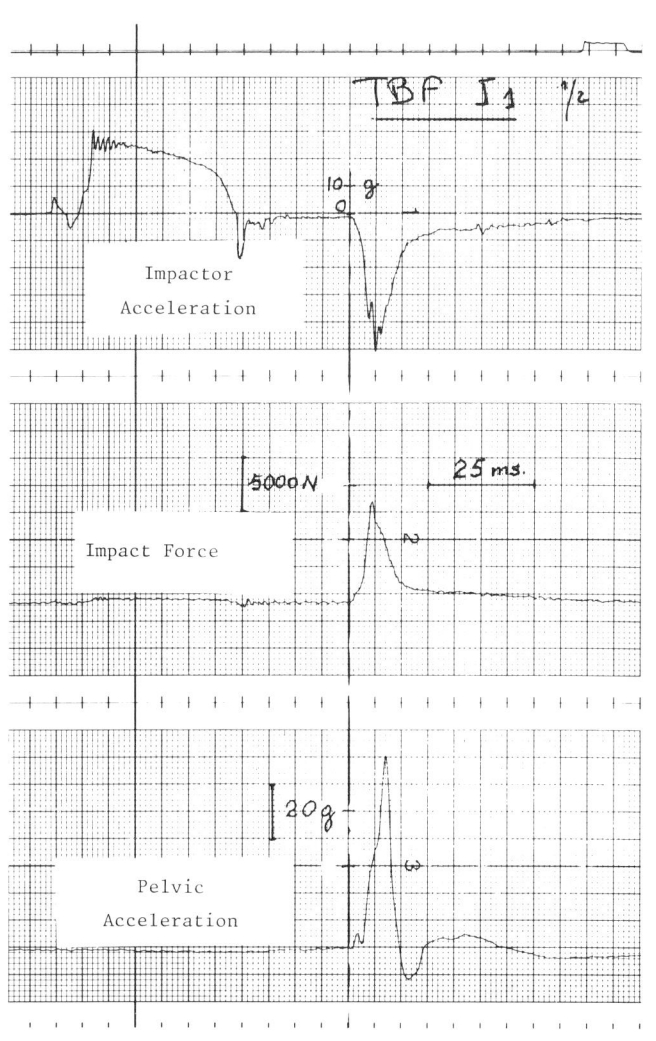

Fig. A1 - Acceleration and force traces

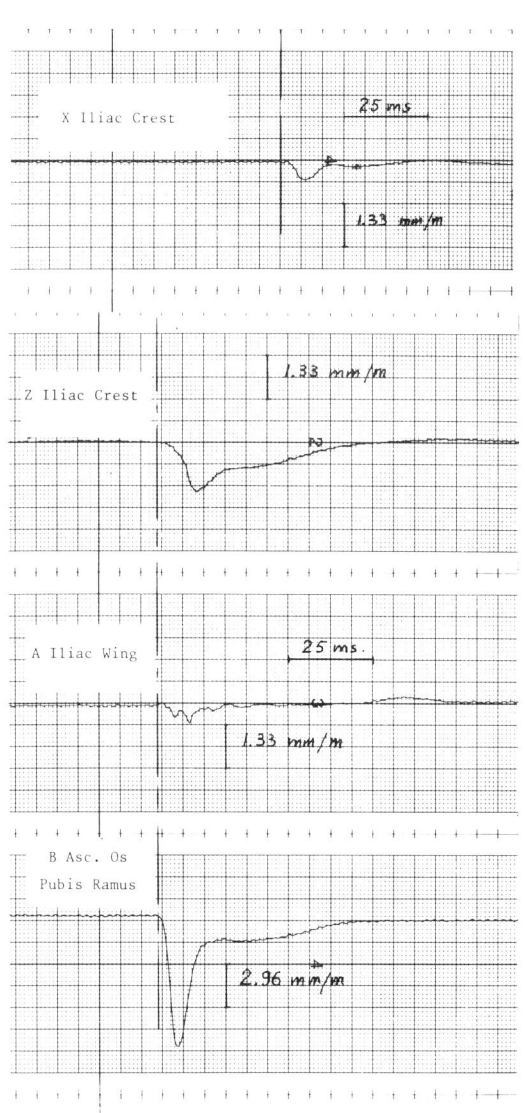

Fig. A2 - Strain gauges traces

811019

Development of a Dummy Abdomen Capable of Injury Detection in Side Impacts

J. Maltha and R. L. Stalnaker
Research Institute for Road Vehicles

Abstract

A prototype of an abdomen for injury detection in side impacts is developed. This design can in principle be built into existing side-impact dummies. Necessary biomechanical data was obtained from free-fall studies with cadavers simulating impacts with intruding doors.

The design consists of a structure with built-in tolerance limits and injury detection is obtained by a single channel go/no-go signal; thus complicated continuous force and penetration measurements are avoided. The abdomen has a rigid penetration stop at the critical tolerance level. This stop is covered by a composite material giving stiffness characteristics identical to the human abdomen. Coded contact switches activated by springs when a critical load is exceeded are mounted between this material and the rigid stop.

The abdomen is presented in detail together with the results of impact tests. The materials for the abdomen were selected with assistance of a computer aided design study described in this paper.

The interfacing with some existing dummies and a possible extension to frontal abdomen injury detection is discussed.

---

[*]Dr. R.L. Stalnaker is now working at the Southwest Research Institute, San Antonio, Texas.

THE CURRENT RESEARCH and coming regulations for assessment of the protection provided to car occupants in side-impacts need specially developed lateral crash dummies, which are capable of injury detection for the most endangered areas of the human body. In the beginning of side-impact test work the traditional dummies developed for frontal collisions, especially the Part 572, were used. It soon appeared, especially when these tests were compared with identical tests with cadavers, that these dummies were not representative, because of lack in biofidelity with respect to kinematical as well as to dynamical response (1), (2), (3), (4) and (5)*. A number of laboratories then started the development of specially designed lateral dummies, which were in some cases modifications of the Part 572 (2) and (3). The unrealistic behaviour of the Part 572 dummy in side-impacts was primarily caused by the high rigidity of the shoulder joint and of the chest structure, which caused an unrealistic motion of head and neck as a side effect. This and the fact that chest injuries were most frequently observed in real accidents made the laboratories concentrate on redesign of the chest and shoulder structures and protection criteria were established from cadaver testing. Work is in progress now to develop protection criteria for the head, neck and pelvis regions, and dummies are now being designed to predict also these types of injuries.

From studies by Hartemann (6), Walfish (7) and Stalnaker (8) it was recognized that the severity and occurrence of abdominal injuries in side-impacts, which were caused by an intruding door, ranks for nearside occupants about equal to head and thoracic injuries, which indicates the need of protection of the abdominal area. Biomechanical studies were done to find injury mechanisms and tolerance values (4) and (7). A study which especially focussed on the problem of an intruding armrest was carried out by Walfish (7) and resulted in a preliminary protection criterion giving the design base for the abdomen in this study.

The work presented here is a design description together with test results of a prototype of a dummy abdomen capable of detection of injuries, which can in principle be built into existing side-impact dummies. As the design is primarily developed to be used in regulations testing, and therefore should be simple and easy in use, it is based on a structure with built-in tolerance limits. The injury detection is then obtained from a single channel go/no-go signal, which avoids complicated continuous force and penetration or acceleration measurements.

---

*Numbers in parentheses designate References at end of Paper.

PROTECTION CRITERION

The starting point for the design work is the protection criterion developed from cadaver experiments, which is reported by Walfish (7) and Stalnaker (8). These experiments were specially performed to obtain the criterion for abdominal injury detection in dummies and was based on the next premises:
1. This criterion should only be used in addition to the side-impact criteria already developed for thorax and pelvis.
2. Only first-order injuries resulting from direct penetration of an intruding door or from other car structures will be considered.
3. The criterion is based on the worst cases, which are right-side liver injuries.
4. The criterion is associated with an AIS 3 value.

The lower-most part of the abdomen is effectively protected by the pelvic girdle while the upper-most part is partially protected by the lower ribs. For this reason the criterion focusses on penetration into the area from the sixth rib to the top of the ilium, which corresponds to the spacing of about 12 cm between last rib and top of pelvis moulding of the Part 572 dummy.

For a car occupant the object most likely to penetrate the abdomen in $90° \pm 20°$ side-impacts is the armrest or a reinforcement beam of an intruding door. This was simulated in the cadaver tests by free falls from a drop-height of 2 meters (corresponding to 22.6 km/h or 14.1 mph) with the side of the abdomen hitting a rigid simulated armrest with a width of 7 cm (fig. 1).

From these tests, forces and penetrations on the armrest were measured and normalized to match the 50 percentile male according to Eppinger's formula (9). For these test conditions it was found that an AIS = 3 corresponds to the following tolerance values:
1. 4500 N force on the simulated armrest.
2. 28% relative penetration of the half abdomen (39 mm for a 50 percentile dummy).

Based on the same cadaver tests a force penetration corridor is defined to enable the design of a dummy abdomen, which gives a correct dynamical response when it is loaded under the tolerable limits (fig. 2).

DESIGN PRINCIPLE

The design requirements were to construct an abdomen that would allow an easy interfacing with existing side-impact dummy prototypes and would have an easy-to-use and

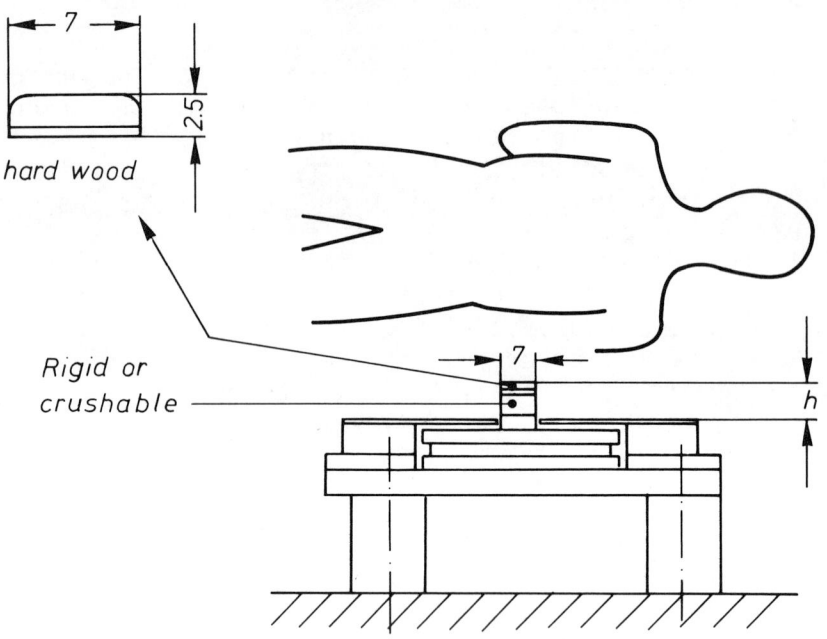

Fig. 1 - Lateral cadaver drop test set-up

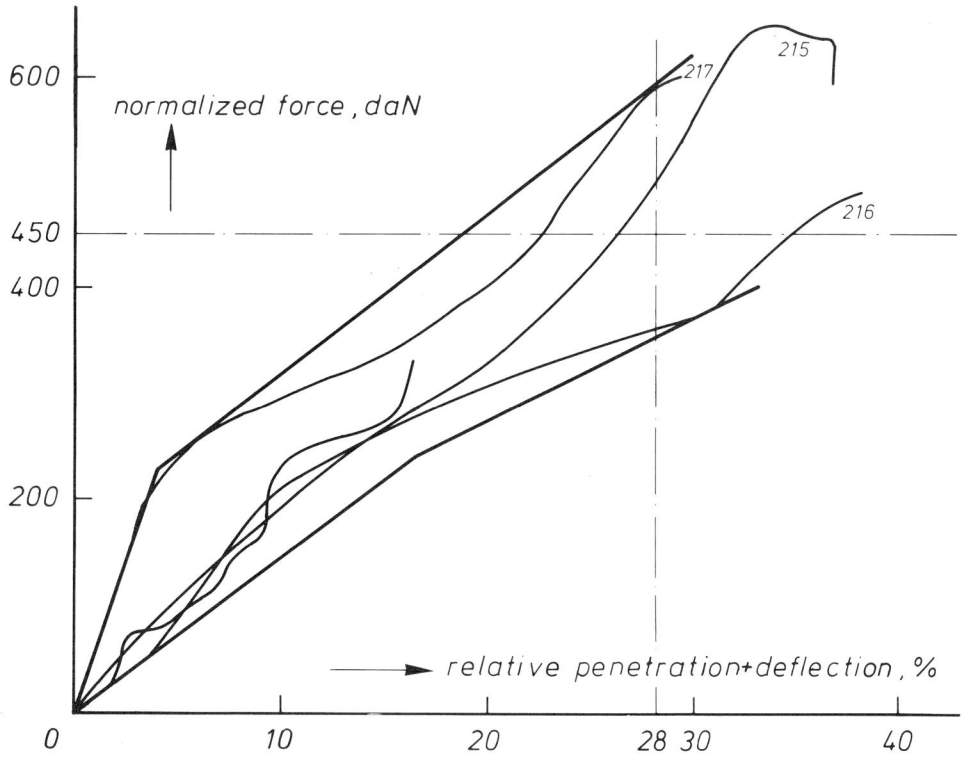

Fig. 2 - Force-relative penetration corridor

an easy-to-maintain measurement system for use in normally equipped test houses set up for regulations testing. Because repeated use of the dummy was required, devices with parts that would be permanently deformed or destructed were not considered.

The structure principally exists of a rigid light metal drum mounted firmly to the thorax-lumbar spine connection and which provides a solid base for a physical stop at the penetration limit. This drum is covered by a composite material giving a dynamical stiffness identical to that of the human abdomen under these conditions. A number of steel leaf springs are placed on the sides of the drum, which are activated through the compressed material and trigger a contact switch when load and penetration limits are exceeded (fig. 3).

In order to make the construction suitable for other than purely lateral impact directions three switches are attached at each side of the rigid drum to obtain injury detection for $90° \pm 30°$ impacts. Because of the low informational content of each separate on/off switch, the signals could be combined and used in one measuring channel only. Each switch is coded by a unique binary voltage, which is distinguishable in the single channel output signal in order to maintain all information obtained by opening or closing of each individual switch. More detail is given in the separate chapter about switches.

The design principle shows some basic limitations, which are thought to be acceptable for regulations testing:
1. Left and right sides give symmetrical response, which was based on the worst case; viz. right side liver injuries.
2. The dynamical response of the whole dummy under the impact loading is biomechanically correct until the maximum load and penetration for injury are reached; then the correct dynamical response is disturbed by the rigid penetration stop and the dummy kinematics may be affected.

MATERIAL SELECTION USING COMPUTER AIDED DESIGN

PROBLEM ANALYSIS - The first choices for abdominal material were urethane and rubber closed-cell foams because of their expected resemblance to abdominal tissue, and a number of dynamical impact tests were performed. Impacting body and impact velocity were identical to those of the cadaver testing and the impacted structure was a simulated half abdomen with the penetration stop allowing a 6 cm thick layer of foam to form an outside contour identical to those of the Part 572 dummy. The thickness of 6 cm was estimated from the maximum allowed penetration of 39 mm plus 21 mm for "bottoming" of the compressed foam (fig. 4).

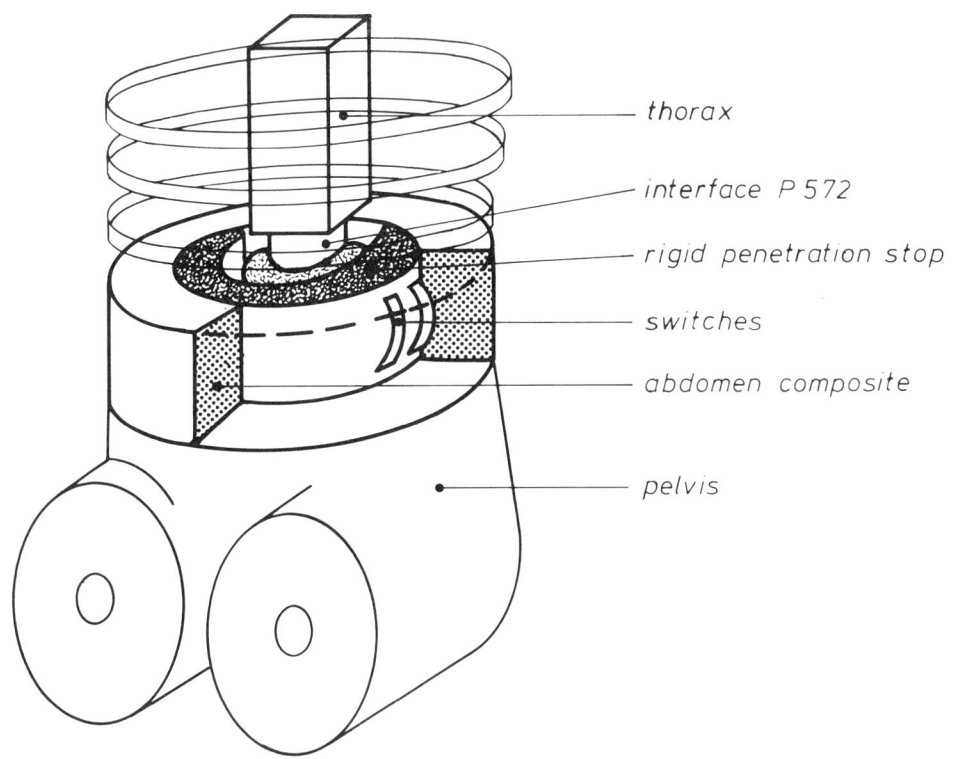

Fig. 3 - Design principle

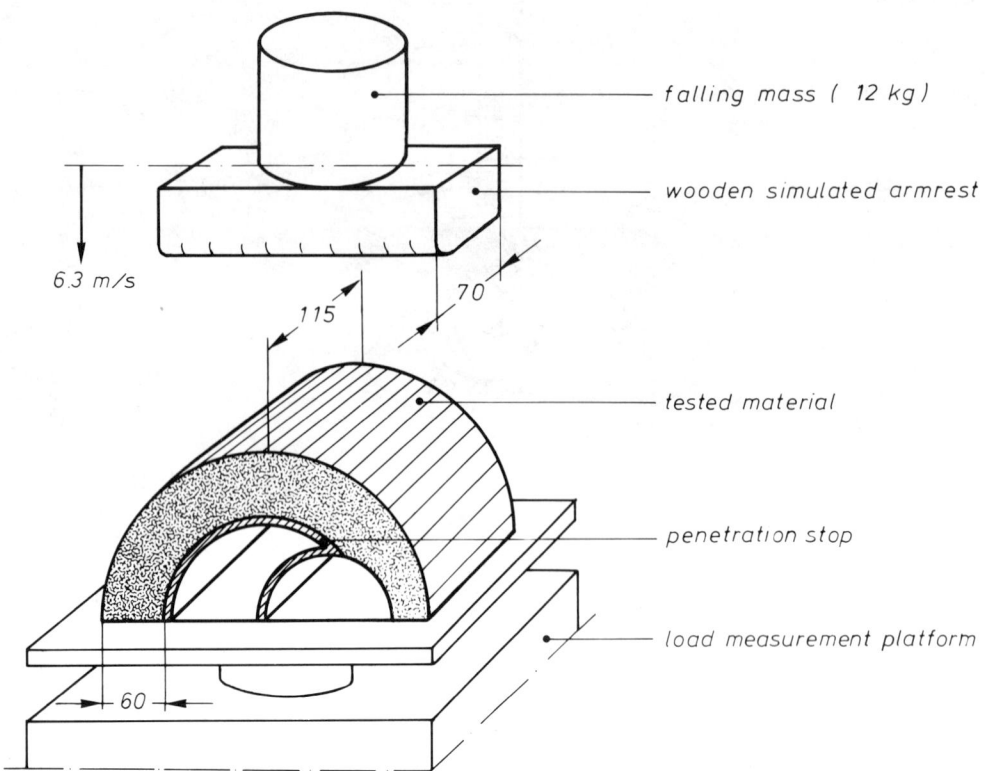

Fig. 4 - Dynamic impacts on foam specimen

From these preliminary tests it was found that even relative hard urethane and rubber foams gave too low a force response at the beginning of penetration. The desired force-penetration corridor could only be reached at higher penetrations, which was due to the bottoming effect (fig.5). The relative low force at low penetrations of the foam may be caused by three separate effects:
1. The flat simulated armrest in contact with the curved shape of the foam layers initially compresses only a small amount of material (the geometrical effect).
2. The relative low mass of the foam will cause only small inertial forces, necessary to accelerate this mass; this results in an initially low force (the inertial effect).
3. Absence of visco-elastic properties (the visco-elastic effect).

The geometrical effect is there and cannot be changed but the inertial effect could offer possibilities for improvement. The abdomen in reality consists of relative heavy muscles, fat layers, a blood filled liver and other organs, which could explain the initial higher force found in the cadaver tests.

So the desired dynamical characteristics could be achieved by making an outside layer of the dummy abdomen of a relative heavy but flexible material such as a metal-filled rubber carried by a softer underlayer that allows the necessary penetration. A rigid impactor on a rather rigid mass, like the metal-filled rubber on the outside, will, however, cause an "inertial spike" of a high level and short duration superimposed on the static response (fig. 6).

A smoothed inertial spike effect with a lower peak and longer duration could be obtained by adding another light foam layer on the outside of the abdomen (outside padding). The problem then was to find a composition of outside foam, mass carrying rubber and inside foam, which together would give the desired dynamical response (fig. 7).

COMPUTER MODEL FORMULATION - To avoid the making and testing of a large number of material compositions it was decided to use the possibilities offered by Computer Aided Design. The availability of and the experience with the general purpose MADYMO CVS program package was utilized to formulate a non-lineair dynamical finite segment model of the abdomen half (10). The heavy outside layer was simulated by an arched chain of 19 rigid joint connected elements each carrying a certain amount of mass (fig.8). The light underlayer of foam was modelled by 19 mass-less springs with some viscous damping, which transferred the load from outside elements to the rigid penetration stop. The impacting rigid armrest was a single mass system with a flat contacting plane and a initial velocity of 6.3 m/s, that could penetrate

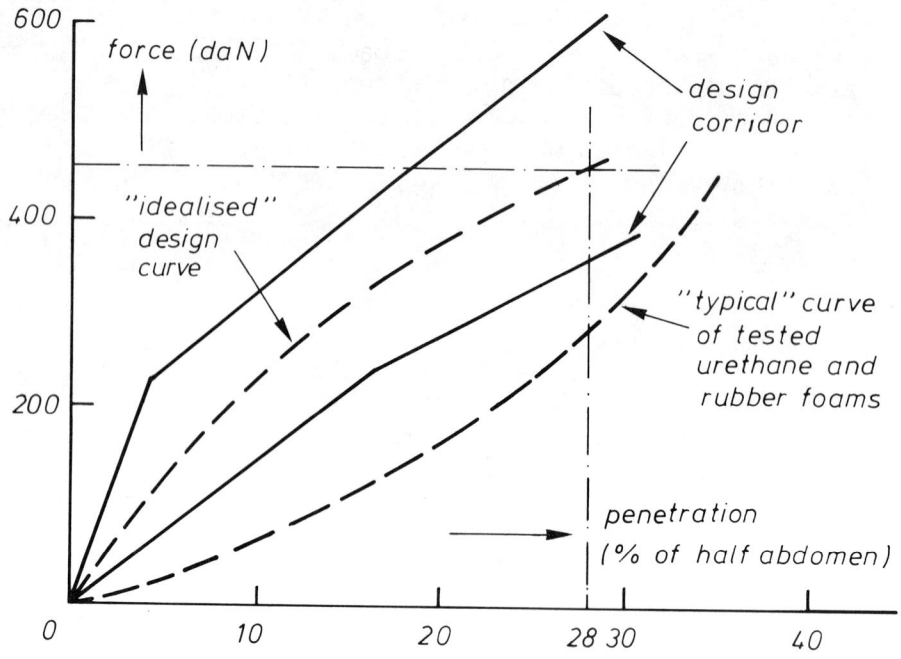

Fig. 5 - Preliminary test results

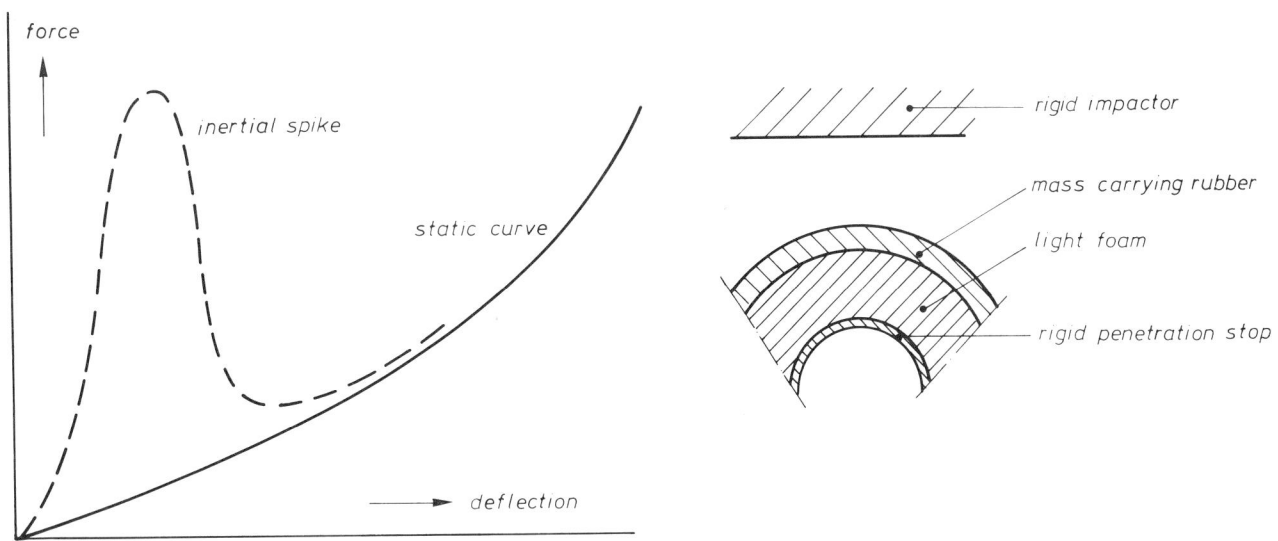

Fig. 6 - Theoretical inertial effect of a mass-carrying rubber outside layer

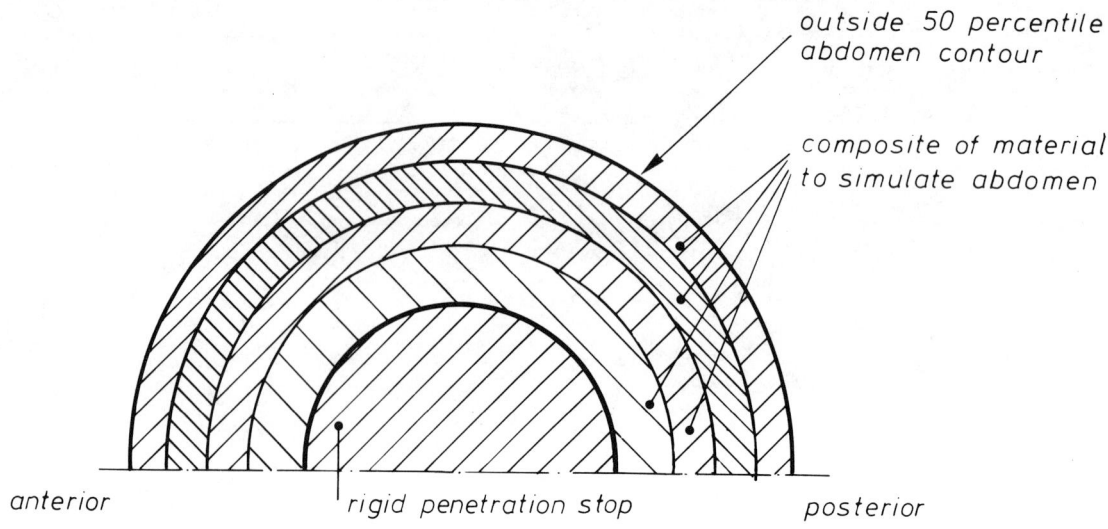

Fig. 7 - Material composite

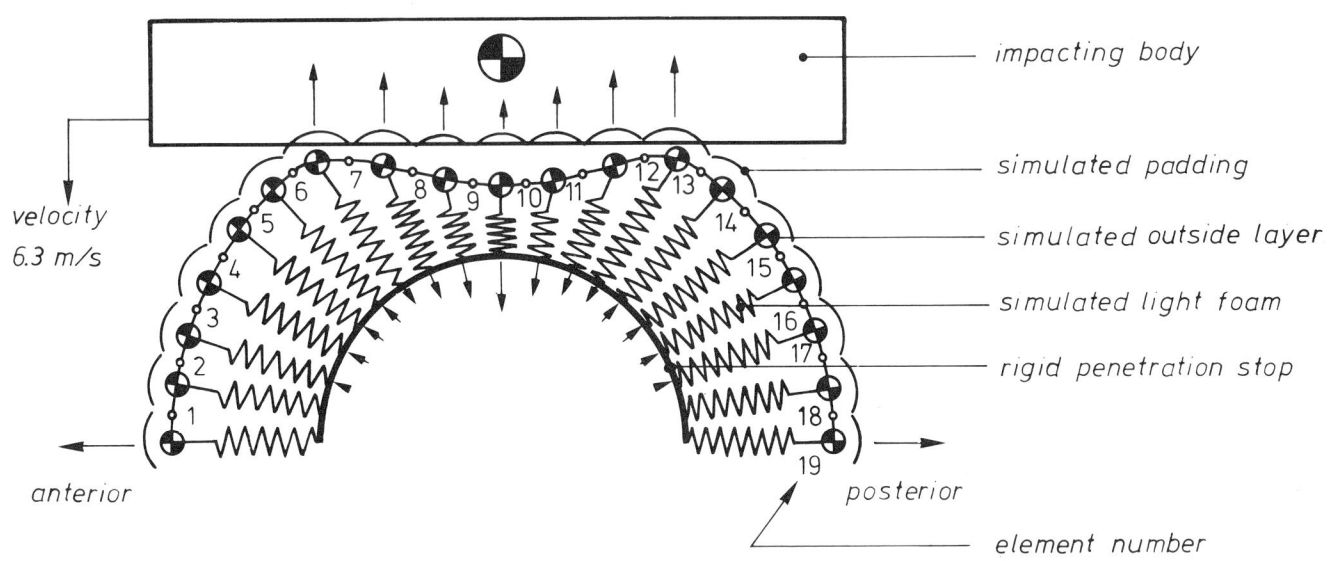

Fig. 8 - Concept of simulation model of abdomen half

any of the 19 contact sensing circles attached to the mass carrying elements. These contact sensing circles simulate the outside foam padding on the mass carrying layer by generating elastic and damping forces between impacting body and elements as a function of relative penetration and velocity.

COMPUTER MODEL PREDICTIONS - The input parameters for this MADYMO simulation model were initially obtained from static measurements on an abdomen half with a 6 cm thick layer of closed-cell rubber foam with a density of about 300 kg/m^3 (ASTM-D 1056-62 T SCE 42-42 CLMF). This rubber type for the soft underlayer was selected because of its appropriate mechanical properties. From these measurements the force-deflection curves were estimated for the coil springs and the padding in the model. Each rigid element carried a mass of 0.010 kg. The mass of the impacting body was 28 kg and its impact velocity 5.4 m/s. A few model runs were necessary with slight re-adjustments of spring and padding characteristics to obtain a model response in agreement with the static test (fig. 9, curve c). This model was used then to study the effect of adding mass in the outside foam layer. The first choice was a mass of 1 kg divided over the nine segments closest to the impacting body, so a mass of 0.111 kg each. The thickness of this rather rigid mass carrying layer is estimated to be 10 mm, which leaves 50 mm total for the outside padding and underlaying foam. The foam characteristics were corrected for this reduced thickness. A correct model behaviour without vibration or overshoot in the resulting force deflection curves, was obtained by using well adjusted damping coefficients for outside padding and underlaying foam. The values were estimated based on some rough calculations for critical damping. Again a few computer runs were necessary to find a realistic smooth response, the co-efficients found were 10 kg/s for outside contacts and 22 kg/s for the underlaying springs. These runs showed that the added mass of 1 kg was able to bring the abdomen response inside the design corridor during the first 25 mm of penetration (fig. 9, curve b). After these 25 mm all nine mass elements were accelerated and obtained a velocity equal to the impactor which causes the force deflection curve to drop until the curve raises again at 45 mm by "bottoming out" of the compressed foam. Based on this result it was decided to do another series of model simulations with an additional mass of 1 kg distributed over those elements that were hit by the impactor only after 25 mm of penetration. It was expected that the extra mass could eliminate the drop in the force response between 25 and 40 mm. The masses in the nine elements (nos 6-14) of 0.111 kg were maintained and masses of 0.100 kg were added on either side onto two sets of 5 elements centred at element 6 and 14, respectively (nos 4-8 and 12-16). After some re-adjustments in damping

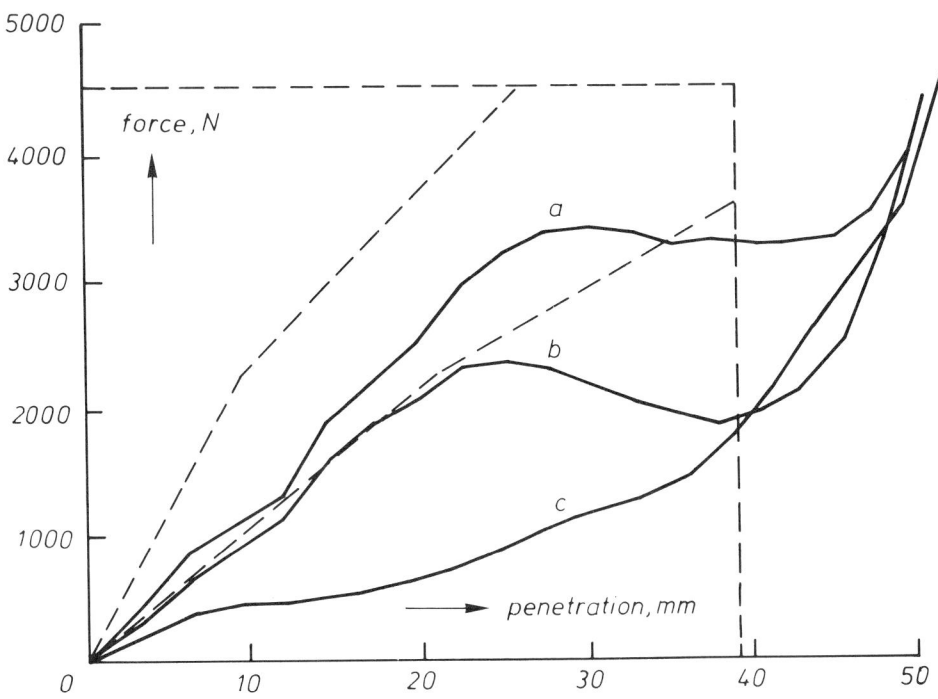

Fig. 9 - Model predictions of force penetration responses
a - foam with inserted mass of 2 kg
b - foam with inserted mass of 1 kg
c - foam layer only

coefficients these runs showed the positive effect of the added mass that resulted in a curve that was inside the design corridor, except for the last 5 mm of penetration (35-40 mm) (fig. 9, curve a). The last part of the curve could be easily raised, however, by selecting a thinner underlaying foam layer that gives the "bottoming" effect shortly before 40 mm of penetration is reached.

The kinematical response of this model is shown for one of the simulations in figure 10.

COMPUTER MODEL VALIDATION TESTS - In order to check the validity of these model predictions a series of pendulum impact tests with 5.4 m/s impact velocity was carried out on three specimens representing the model simulations described above. One specimen had a 60 mm thick layer of closed-cell-rubber only (A). One had 11 inserted steel rods of a diameter of 10 mm and a mass of 0.091 kg each, placed in a row that simulates the position of the 9 elements in the model and leaving an outside foam padding of 10 mm (B). One had the same 11 steel rods and 5 additional rods on either side of .100 kg each (C) (fig. 11). The measured force penetration curves of these experiments show good conformity with the model predictions which justifies the use of this model for design parameter variations, like number and values of masses, impact velocities and effect of padding bottoming (fig. 12).

MATERIAL SELECTION WITH AID OF THE MODEL - In reality the design procedure described above was done simultaneously, which means that the model was run during the tests to select new test conditions and the tests results were used to refine and improve the model. During this process the designer obtains much insight into the relative importance of the great number of design parameters. Owing to some practical limitations in the test set-up the first pendulum tests and consequently the computer simulations for validation were done with an impact velocity of 5.4 m/s (equivalent to 1.5 m dropheight). A first series of computerruns was done to study the effect of this dropheight based on abdomens with inserted masses totalling 1 and 2 kg. A more or less lineair correlation of peak force and dropheight was found for 1, 1.5 and 2 m range (fig. 13a). A second series was run with a varying number of mass carrying elements 5 (total 0.6 kg), 9 (total 1 kg) and 15 (total 1.6 kg) successively. These runs showed a decreasing effect of adding more mass carrying elements in the not directly impacted zone. Nine or eleven elements seemed to be close to optimal because the totally added mass must be kept as low as possible. Putting the mass more directly under the impactor, 1.5 kg divided over 9 segments, gives initially (to 30 mm penetration) the same response as a 2 kg mass distributed over 13 segments. The lower mass only causes the curve to drop easier in the 30 to 40 mm pene-

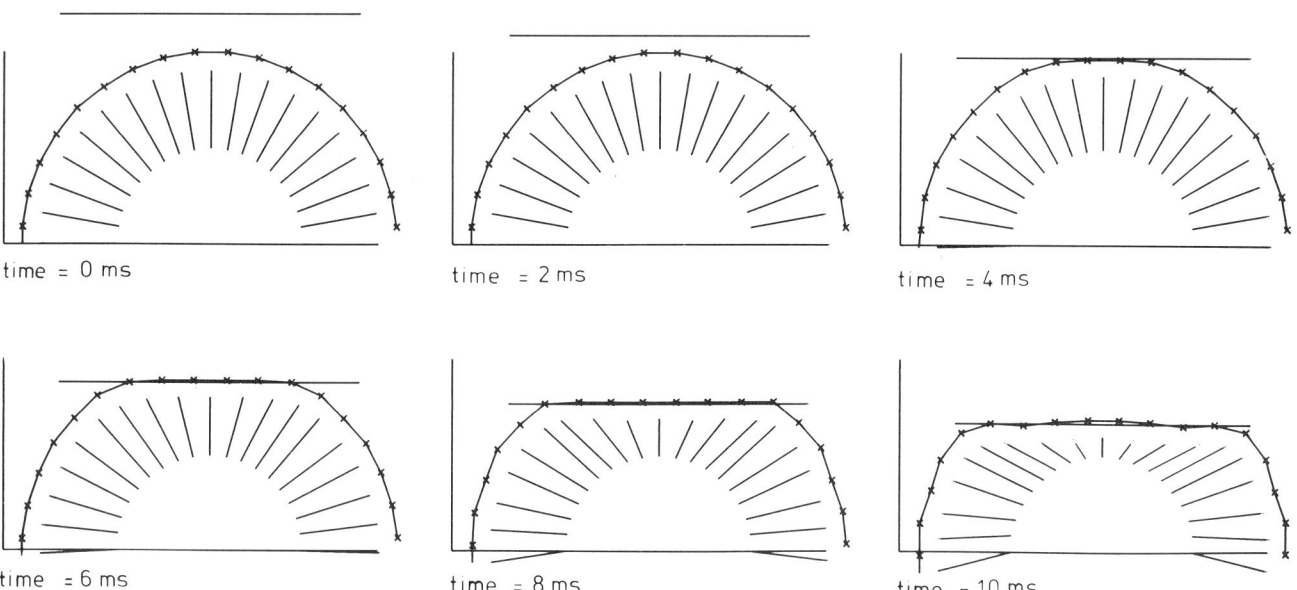

Fig. 10 - Kinematical response of abdomen simulation model

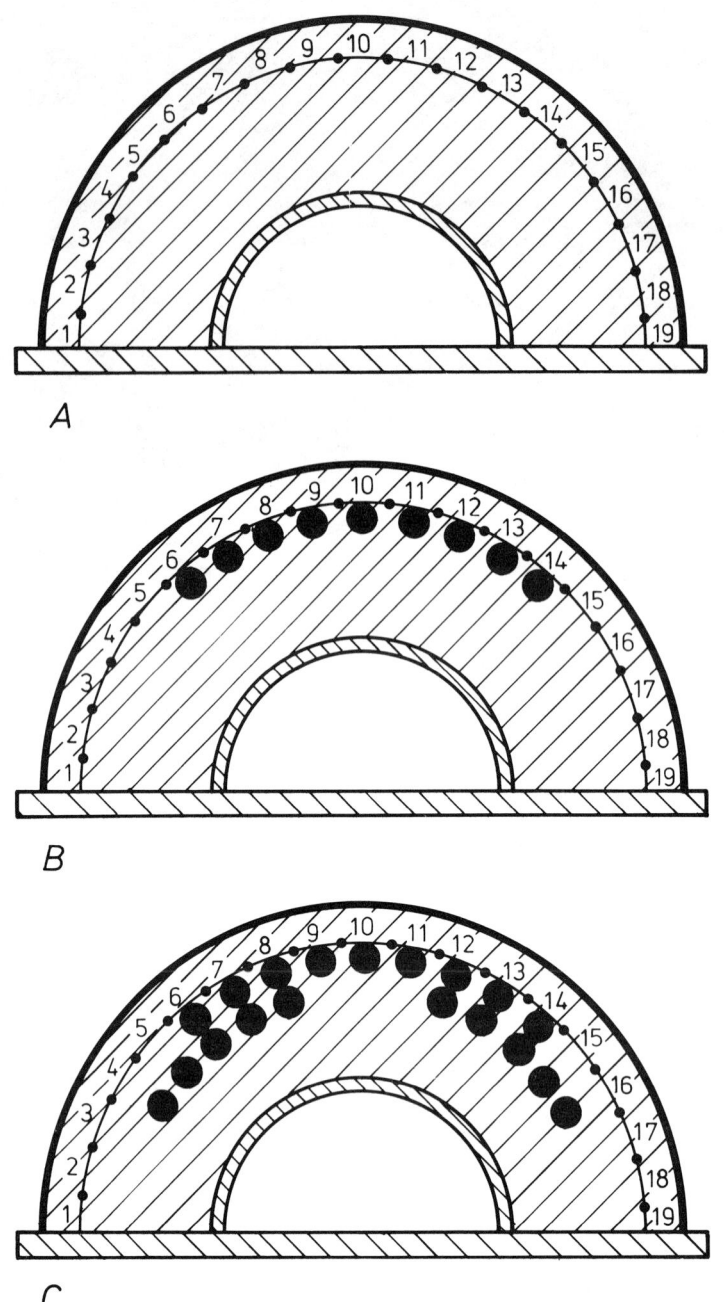

Fig. 11 - Test specimen A, B and C

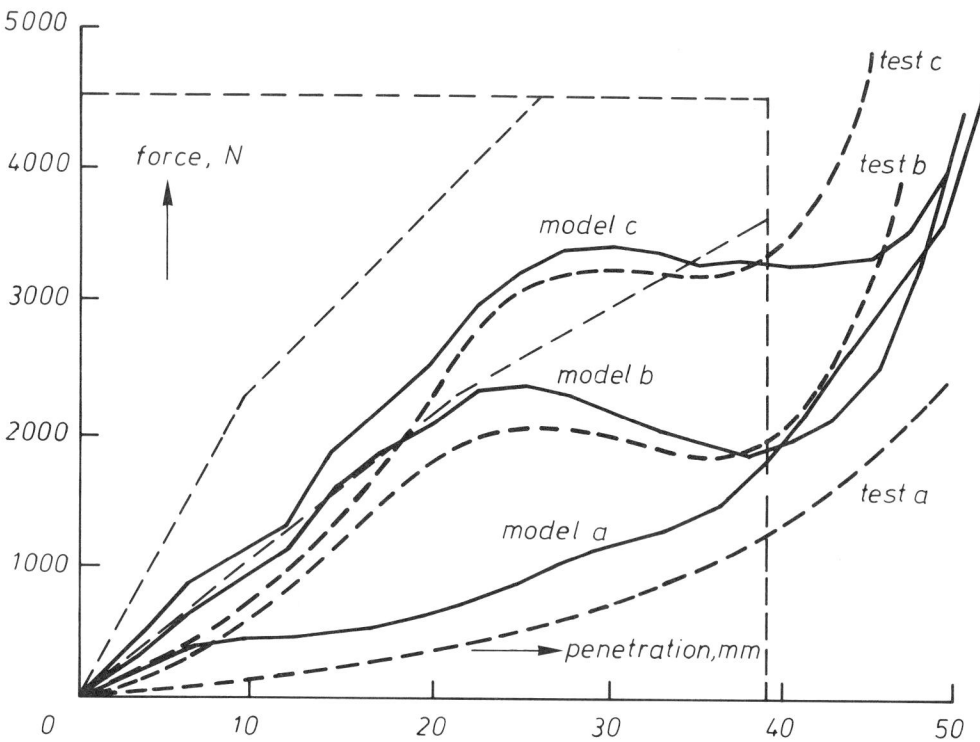

Fig. 12 - Model predictions compared with experimental results

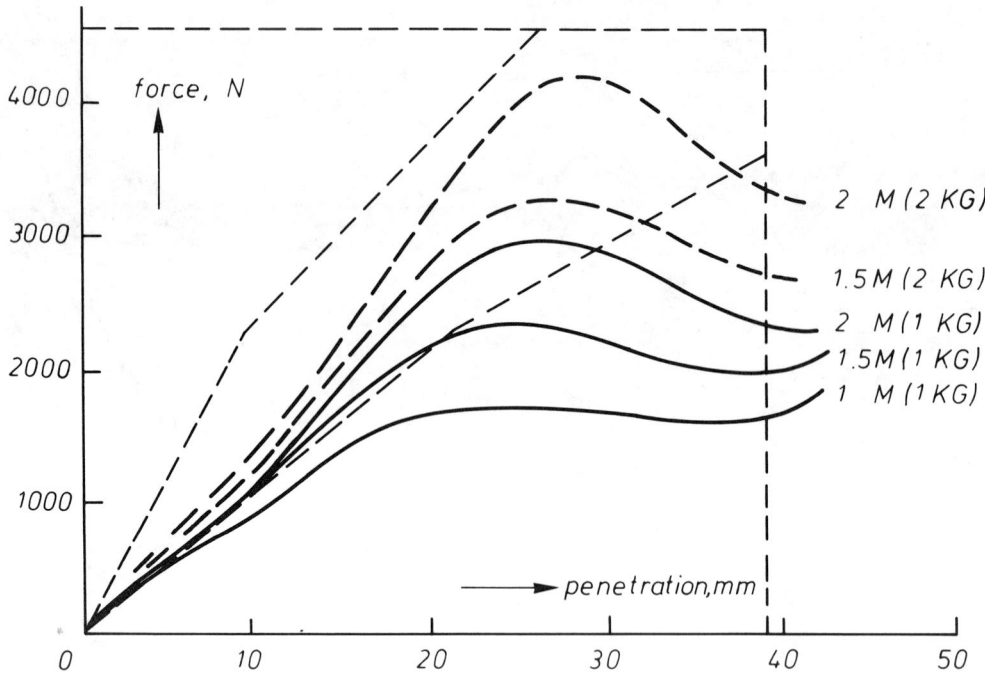

Fig. 13a - Effect of dropheight (impact velocity) for inserted masses of 1 and 2 kg

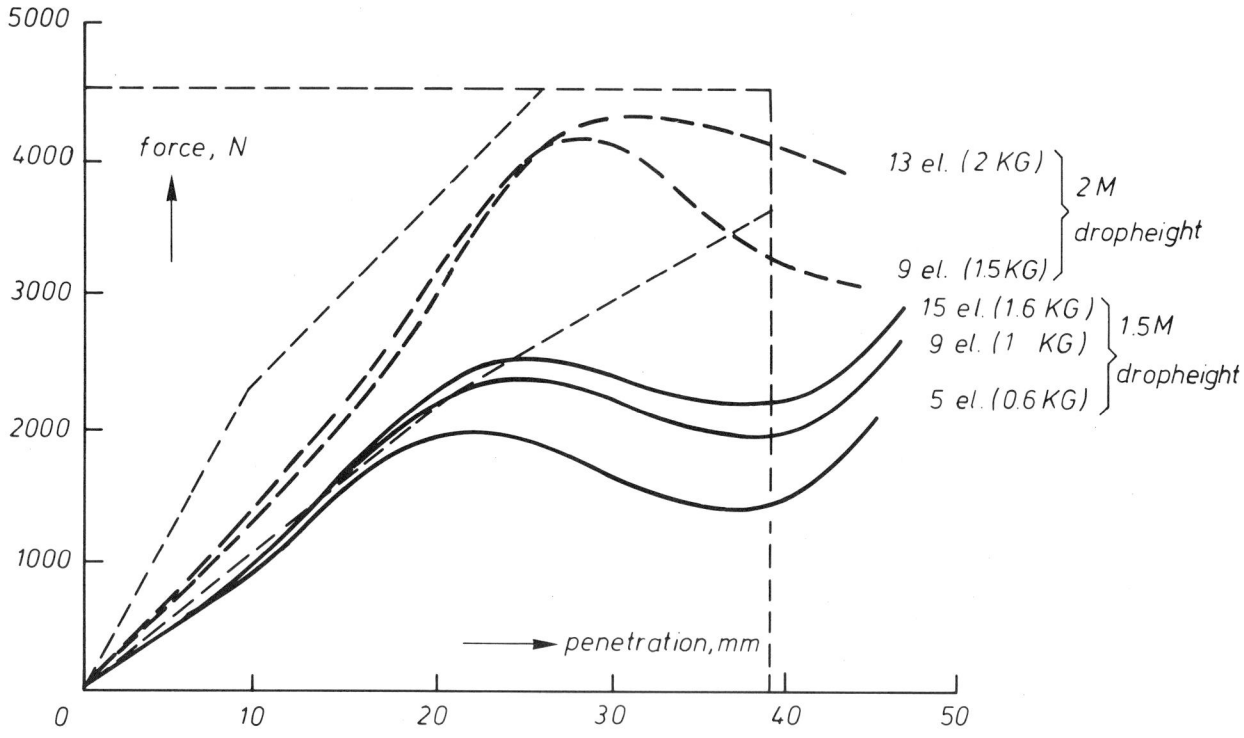

Fig. 13b - Effect of mass and mass distribution

tration region (fig. 13 b). From this study it was concluded that for the prototype a mass of about 1.5 kg in a section of the outside layer of about 200 mm long (corresponding to 11 elements in the model) would give the desired dynamical response. A global calculation of the space available for this mass resulted in 0.00024 m^3. This led for a total mass of 1.5 kg to a density of 6250 kg/m^3 which approximates those of steel. The problem was then to find a material with a density of steel and the flexibility and recovery capacity of rubber. The solution found was a vulcanised composite of rubber filled with small lead pellets of 1.2 mm diameter. The first specimen made showed that a density of 5730 kg/m^3 could easily be obtained. The heavy slab still had a good flexibility, this because the rubber formed the basic material matrix with only freely embedded lead pellets. This material was used for the mass carrying layer in the prototype. The rubber specification is NR-SBR, Shore A hardness 55/60. The thickness is 12 mm, the mass 1.6 kg, the outside layer is of 8 mm thick foam and the inside layer of 38 mm thick foam.

PENETRATION STOP CONSTRUCTION

The rigid penetration stop consists of a drum attached to the thorax-lumbar spine connection, which accomodates the penetration contact switches and the composite material covering. The main requirements for the drum were:
1. The construction must be rigid to avoid disturbing deformations.
2. The construction must be light because it should replace in most existing dummies an almost mass-less abdomen foam insert.
3. The construction should be easily interfaced with the thorax-lumbar spine connections of the Part 572 related constructions.
4. The construction must not interfere with the expected spine and pelvis motion during side-impacts.
5. Adaptions to other spine and pelvis constructions should be possible.

This resulted in a welded aluminium construction with a wall-thickness of 3 mm. The drum's outside contour was obtained from the external contour of the 50 percentile Part 572 dummy allowing a spacing for a 60 mm thick material layer. The Part 572 flange on top of the lumbar spine rubber cylinder is replaced by this construction, which provides a new integrated flange (fig. 14). The rim protruding at top and bottom of the construction serves two functions, firstly it carries the longitudinal compression load of the force measuring steel leaf springs and secondly it prevents the foam layer from shifting.

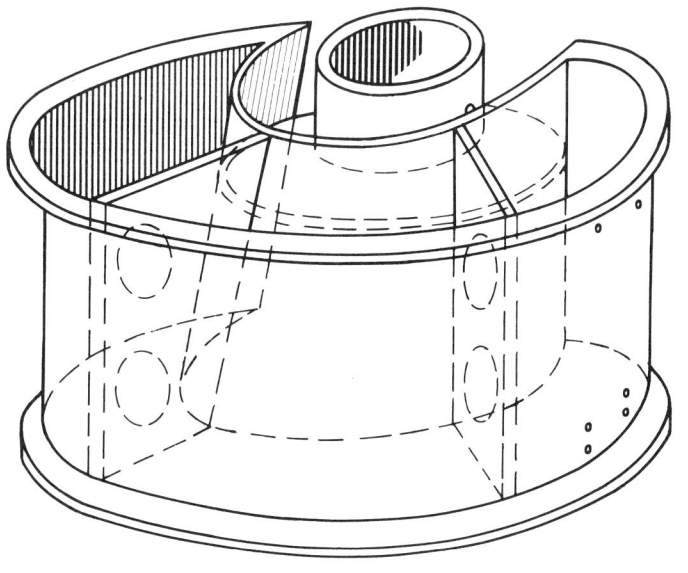

Fig. 14 - Rigid penetration stop assembly

SWITCHES CONSTRUCTION AND MEASUREMENT TECHNIQUE

Three tape contact switches are located on either side of the rigid drum to obtain a penetration measurement for $90° \pm 30°$ impacts. One is mounted centrally on the side of the drum and two others at radial angles of about $\pm 15°$ viewed from top. Each switch is protected by an arched steel leaf spring to assure a controlled and repeatable activating of the underlaying tape switches through the compressed foam when penetration and force limits are reached. When the load limit is reached, the spring pops in to a double wave form and presses on the tape switch. The arched form and clamped ends give a stiff spring that is able to withstand high loads and is somewhat insensitive to the direction and location of loading (fig. 15).

During the first impact tests with foam specimen on a half abdomen, a spring was mounted of 120 mm length, of 20 mm width and of 0.8 mm thickness and with a maximum spacing of 6 mm between arch and drum. The switch repeatedly closed at an external force of 2100 N applied through foam.

A separate test programme was set up to find correct design parameters for the leaf spring. Static tests were performed with a hydraulic tester on springs with thicknesses of 0.8, 1.0 and 1.4 mm, each with a width of 20 mm and a free arc length of 75 mm. The maximum spacing between spring-arch and drum was varied between 4.8 and 7.1 mm. The force was applied with the 7 cm wide wooden simulated armrest through a 45 mm thick closed cell rubber padding. The results of these tests are presented in Table 1. From these tests it was concluded that a high contact force could be obtained either by a thicker spring or by more arch spacing. A thicker spring with a low arch is preferred to a thinner spring with a high arch owing to a lower reproducibility of the latter as can be observed in tests 5 and 6 in 21, 22 and 23. Up and downward rotated armrests give lower forces, which is realistic because of the more concentrated force applied by the intruding edge of the armrest. An armrest only rotated forward or backward needs a higher force to activate the switch because it is only partially loading the spring. A uniform response is obtained by placing two identical springs on either side of the central one.

For the abdomen prototype springs of 1.4 mm with an arch spacing of 5.0 mm were selected, which activate the switch at a force of 4500 N.

The contacts made by each of the six switches are coded by a binary voltage, which ranges from 41 to 660 mV and are then added into a single channel output with a maximum of ± 1300 mV-DC to adapt for an analogue FM tape recorder. This system is built into a small converter module to be used in

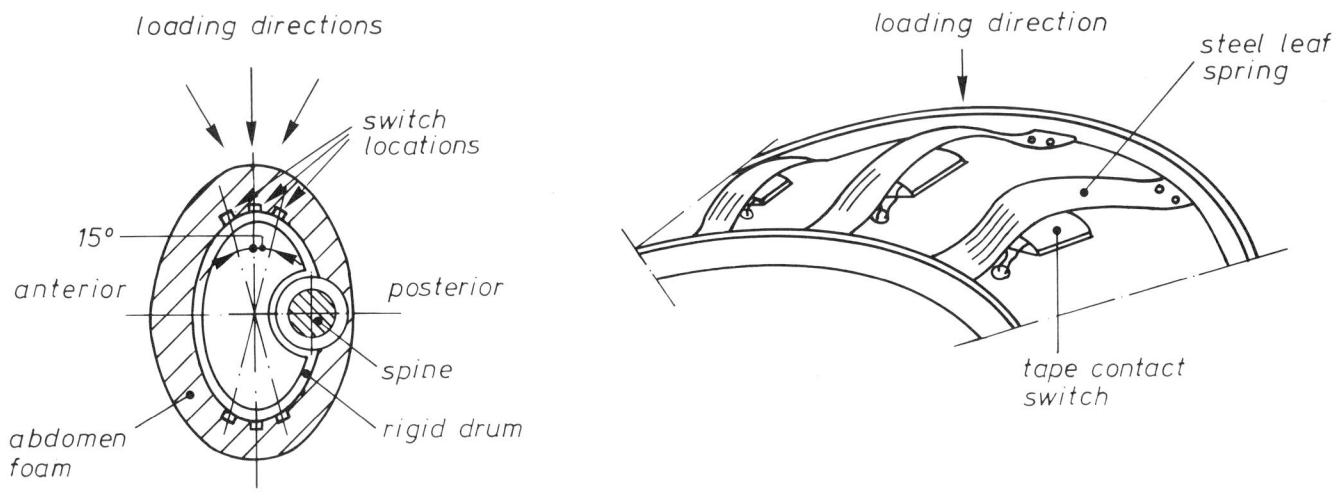

Fig. 15 - Switch construction

Table 1 - Contact Forces of Steel Leaf Springs

Test number	Spring thickness (mm)	Arch spacing (mm)	Loading direction	Applied force for switch contact (N)
1	0.8	4.8	centered	1660
2	0.8	4.8	"	1680
3	0.8	4.8	"	1660
5	0.8	7.7	"	2500
6	0.8	7.7	"	2360
18	1.0	5.7	"	3600
19	1.0	5.7	"	3500
20	1.0	5.7	"	3600
21	1.0	7.1	"	4350
22	1.0	7.1	"	4400
23	1.0	7.1	"	3900
24	1.4	5.8	"	4900
25	1.4	5.8	"	4500
26	1.4	5.8	"	4400
27	1.4	7.0	"	6400
28	1.4	7.0	"	6150
29	1.4	5.5	"	5000
30	1.4	5.5	"	4950
33	1.4	5.1	"	4800
34	1.4	5.1	"	4850
35	1.4	5.0	"	4500
36	1.4	5.0	"	4500
37	1.4	5.0	off-center 20 mm	4700
38	1.4	5.0	off-center 20 mm	4680
39	1.4	5.0	impactor rotated 15° downward	4200
40	1.4	5.0	impactor rotated 15° downward	4000
41	1.4	5.0	impactor rotated 15° forward	4680
42	1.4	5.0	impactor rotated 15° forward	4700

a high-g environment outside the dummy and requires ± 15 V input. The output voltage-time function gives the direct information about which specific tape switch is activated and at what time. More details are given by Stalnaker (8).

PERFORMANCE OF SYSTEM IN TESTS

To check the performance of the prototype system in realistic conditions a series of tests equivalent to the cadaver drop tests were carried out. Pendulum impacts closely resembling the Part 572 calibration procedure were selected to assure a well-defined and repeatable test programme. The front of the pendulum was equipped with a hardwood simulated armrest of 7 cm width, giving a total pendulum mass of about 25 kg. The pendulum hits the centre of the abdomen prototype mounted into a seated APROD 81 side-impact dummy and has a impact velocity of 5.7 m/s* (fig. 16). The APROD 81 is based on the Part 572 dummy and described by Stalnaker (1) and Fayon (2). The pendulum tests and the drop tests are equivalent because the strain-rates are almost constant and only dependent on the pendulum or drop velocity, which is due to the kinetic energy being some orders of magnitude higher than the energy initially absorbed by the abdomen construction.

Figure 17 presents some of these test results in comparison to a result from a static test obtained with a hydraulic tester. The three solid lines are from identical tests with the rectangular 7 cm wide wooden impactor centered on the abdomen side. The dashed line is from a test with a triangularly shaped impactor and the dashed-dotted line is from the static test. From these curves it was generally concluded that the bottoming of the material composite was in the desired 39 mm region, but that the dynamical load on the impactor was initially too low. The system showed a desired sensitivity to the shape of the impacting body.

The generally too low force response could only be partially explained by the lower impact velocity; most of it is probably be caused by too low a density of the lead filled rubber layer and too thick a layer of soft outside foam. The final abdomen version will have more mass in the rubber, less padding on the outside layer and consequently more on the inside layer.

During these tests the three tape switch readings were recorded while the one channel converter module was used.

---

* Owing to limitations in the test set-up, this impact velocity is somewhat lower than the equivalent value for two meters dropheight.

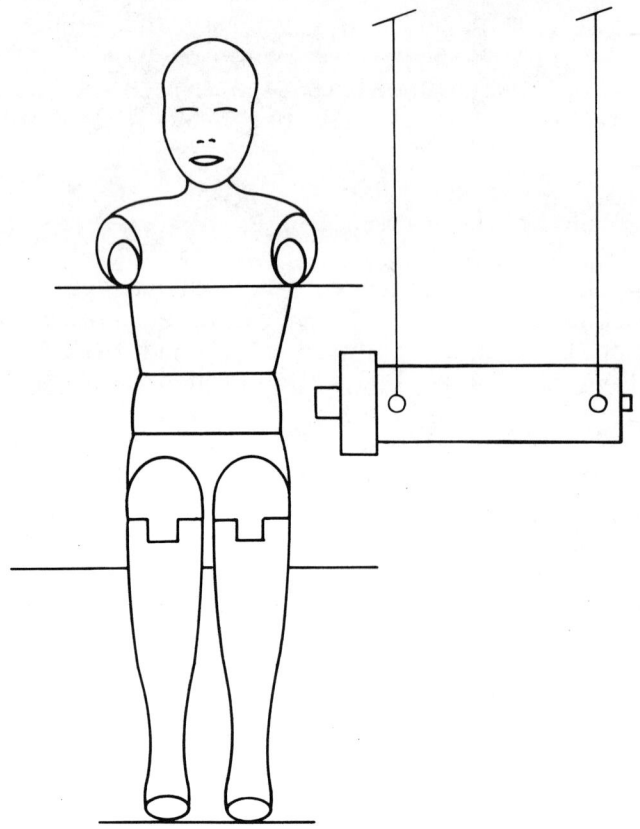

Fig. 16 - Pendulum test set-up

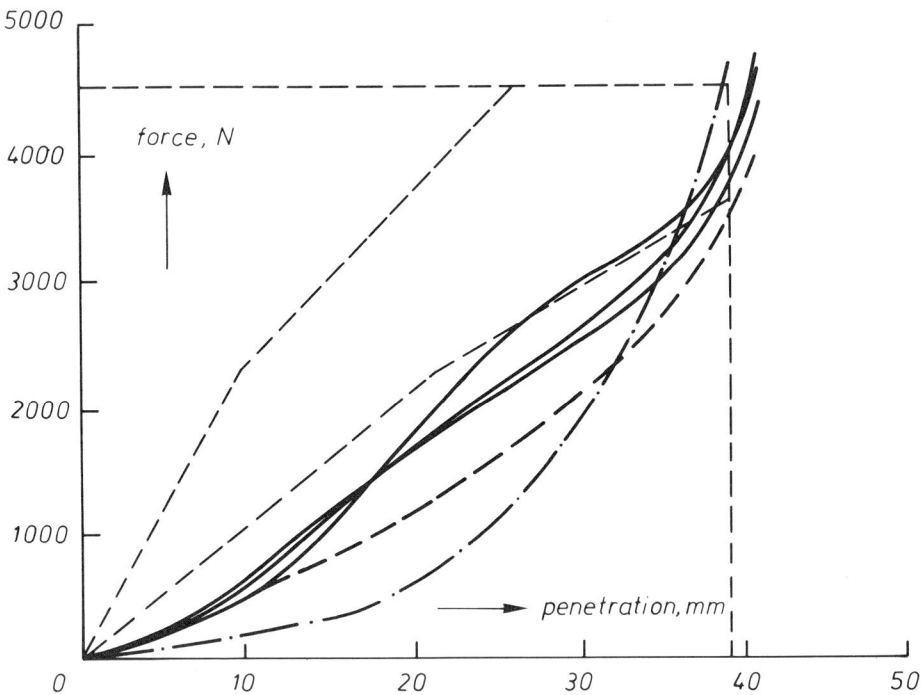

Fig. 17 - Results of pendulum tests
———— rectangular impactor (dynamical)
- - - - triangular impactor (dynamical)
-·-·- rectangular impactor (static)

The switches repeatedly closed when a certain load and penetration were exceeded. The load level, however, shifted to lower values after each test. The final value was about 1500 N, which was checked after the program by a static test. The reason found was that the highly longitudinal compression loads at the clamped ends of the leaf springs permanently deformed the aluminium drum, causing too small an arch spacing and stiffness of the spring. The final version will have a redesigned spring clamping with an adjustment possibility.

Some tests were done with the impact angles varied horizontally and vertically by 20^0. These tests showed that the system in general was rather insensitive to different loading directions.

DISCUSSION AND CONCLUSION

The design of a prototype and test results of a dummy abdomen for injury detection in side-impacts is presented. The design is based on built-in tolerance limits with a go/no-go detection for regulations testing of near-side collisions with intruding doors. The tolerance values and biomechanical performance were obtained from cadaver drop tests reported in previous studies. The design principally exists of a rigid penetration stop around the spine that is covered by a composite material, which in compression activates switches between material and stop whenever force and penetration limits are exceeded. The composite material is selected using Computer Aided Design together with a small series of specimen tests. The resulting structure can be build into any side impact dummy with a Part 572 derived thorax lumbar-spine connection. Because of the added abdomen mass the correction masses of chest and pelvis of the dummy should be reduced to maintain realistic 50 percentile mass distribution.

The prototype is tested with pendulum impacts, which shows the performance and repeatability capacities of the system and the need for some modifications. The same type of abdominal pendulum tests will be done in the second half of 1981 in the frame work of the EEC Biomechanics Programme phase 4, which is set up to compare the performance of four different side impact dummy prototypes (11). This programme also includes a considerable number of car-to-car accident reconstructions and rigid barrier-to-car tests to supplement the dummy parts comparisons. In a number of these full-scale tests the prototype abdomen will be incorporated and should prove its usefulness in realistic test conditions.

This abdomen, which is designed for injury detection

in side-impacts, principally allows extension to other than purely lateral impacts and even to frontal impacts. The primary injury mechanism for frontal injury may be penetration of the steering wheel, shoulder or lap belt parts. This is not too different from an armrest or a door reinforcement beam. There is also some evidence that a frontal abdominal protection criterion would not essentially differ from the lateral (12). This could enable the selection of different padding thickness on the abdomen frontal part and the design of other springs to be activated at an appropiate load.

The rigid penetration stop drum for side impacts is attached to the thorax-lumbar spine connection, which is felt to be adequate, because the relative motion between pelvis and thorax is low as a result of the translational nature of near-side lateral impacts. For frontal collisions larger rotations between thorax and pelvis must be expected, which makes the connection of the rigid penetration drum to the chest box unrealistic and probably causing problems. A possible solution could be a drum that is attached in the middle of the deformable rubber lumbar spine and so maintains a better abdominal position during the forward bending motion.

It is concluded that a prototype dummy abdomen could be constructed to measure the injury criteria derived from cadaver tests. The MADYMO CVS package proved to be a useful tool for formulation of the computer model used for selection of optimal design parameters and it considerably reduced the need of experimental tests. Results of the EEC phase 4 tests with the prototype will provide more information on the repeatability and durability of the system and its usefulness in real car collision tests.

ACKNOWLEDGEMENTS

This study is partially subsidized by the EEC-DG III in the framework of the Biomechanics Programme and partially by the Ministry of Science of the Dutch Government as a contribution to international dummy development. We gratefully acknowledge Dr. C. Tarrière and his staff of Association Peugeot/Renault for their work in establishing the protection criterion from cadaver tests and for their cooperation as regards the design principle. Mr. L.J.J. Wittebrood is thanked for doing the computersimulations and Mr. J.Th. Smit of the TNO Plastics and Rubber Institute for developing the rubber composite.

REFERENCES

1. R.L. Stalnaker, et.al., "Modification of Part 572

Dummy for Lateral Impact According to Biomechanical Data". Proceedings of the 23th Stapp Car Crash Conference, SAE Paper No 791011, 1979.

2. A. Fayon, et.al., "Presentation of a Frontal Impact and Side Impact Dummy, Defined from Human Data and Realized from a "Part 572" Basis". Proceedings of Seventh International Technical Conference on Experimental Safety Vehicles, Paris 1979. U.S. Government Printing Office, Washington, D.C. 20402.

3. J.W. Melvin, D.H. Robbins and J.B. Benson, "Experimental Application of Advanced Thoraric Instrumentation Techniques to Anthromorphic Test Devices". Proceedings of Seventh International Technical Conference on Experimental Safety Vehicles, Paris 1979.

4. J.W. Melvin, D.H. Robbins and R.L. Stalnaker, "Side Impact Response and Injury". Proceedings of Sixth International Technical Conference on Experimental Safety Vehicles, Washington, D.C., Oct. 1976.

5. A. Burgettano, J.R. Hackney, "Status of the National Highway Traffic Safety Administration's Research and Rules making Activities for Upgrading Side Impact Protection". Proceedings of Seventh International Conference on Experimental Safety Vehicles, Paris 1979.

6. F. Hartemann, et.al., "Occupant Protection in Lateral Impacts". Proceedings of the 20th Stapp Car Crash Conference, SAE paper No 760806, 1976.

7. G. Walfish, A. Fayon, C. Tarrière and J.P. Rosey, "Designing of a Dummy's Abdomen for Detecting Injuries in Side Impact Collisions". Proceedings of Fifth International IRCOBI Conference on the Biomechanics of Impacts. Sept. 1980, Secretariate 109 Ave. Salvador Allende, 69500 Bron, France.

8. R.L. Stalnaker and J.C. Bastiaanse, "Development of Anthropomorphic Test Dummies for Frontal and Lateral Collisions-Development of Abdominal Injury Detection". Final Report EEC-Biomechanics programme phase 2, June 1980, TNO-IW report 700120003-6, Delft, Netherlands.

9. R.H. Eppinger, "Prediction of Thoraric Injury using Measureable Experimental Parameters". NHTSA, Washington D.C.

10. J. Maltha and J. Wismans, "MADYMO - Crash Victim Simulations, A Computerized Research and Design Tool". Proceedings of Fifth International IRCOBI Conference on the Biomechanics of Impacts. Sept. 1980, Secretariate 109. Ave. Salvador Allende, 69500 Bron, France.

11. B. Aldman and T.E.A. Benjamin, "European Economic Community Support for Major Biomechanics Research Programme". Awaiting publication.

12. R.L. Stalnaker, V.L. Roberts and J.H. McElhaney, "Side Impact Tolerance to Blunt Trauma". Proceedings of 17th Stapp Car Crash Conference, SAE Paper No 730979, 1973.

821159

Pelvic Tolerance and Protection Criteria in Side Impact

Dominique Césari and Michelle Ramet
Laboratoire des Chocs et de Biomécanique

ABSTRACT

The protection of car occupants against side impact accidents needs a better knowledge of injury mechanisms and of tolerance which are necessary to propose protection criteria.

The results of the study reported in this paper give the values of pelvic fracture impact force and indicate the variation of this parameter in relation to the anthropometric parameters.

The injuries produced by these tests were compared to pelvic injuries sustained in side impact real accidents ; static tests made with half a pelvis have shown that the pubic rami were the deformed part of the pelvis.

According to these findings, we have tried to correlate the impact force values and the values of a parameter linked with the bending process. This relationship have been found very well correlated. These results allow to propose a pelvic human tolerance parameter from which a protection criterion for pelvis in side impact could be derived.

Protection of car occupants against side impact accidents can be considered as one of the main priorities in the field of passive safety (1).

Analysis of side impact accidents shows that they represent 15 % to 28 % of car traffic accidents (2, 3) and that their severity is clearly higher than the average severity of car traffic accidents.

Occupants seated near the impacted side are more often and more seriously injured and the injuries sustained by them are correlated with the intrusion of the side wall of the struck car (4). The areas which are the most frequently and the most severely injured are the head, the upper torso and the lower torso (5). The thorax and the pelvis are mainly injured by direct impact and thus the protection against these injuries depends from stiffness and damping characteristics of the impacted side.

The experimental study of injury mechanisms in side impact (6, 7) have shown the injuries sustained by nearside occupants are directly linked with the intrusion amount and with the impact between the occupant and the inside door panel. From these results it is obvious that a better protection in side impact can be ensured by minimizing the intrusion inside the struck car and by absorbing the energy of the impact between the inside door panel and the occupant.

Reduction of intrusion can be achieved by stiffening the side structures and possibly softening the front structures, whereas the inside energy absorption needs the knowledga of human tolerance in such impacts.

The aim of this study is the proposition of a pelvic protection criterion based on the tolerance of the human pelvis in side impact : even if the pelvic fractures are not very severe by themselves, they are often associated with abdominal injuries, especially at high speed impacts (8). Besides this the detailed analysis of side impact pelvic injuries has shown a high frequency of impacted side ilio and ischio pubic rami fractures and sometimes disjonction of sacro iliac and pubis symphysis junctions (9) whereas acetabulum fractures and dislocation are more frequent in frontal impact (dashboard injuries).

ANATOMICAL DESCRIPTION OF THE PELVIS

The pelvic girdle consists of a single bone by which the legs are connected to the trunck.

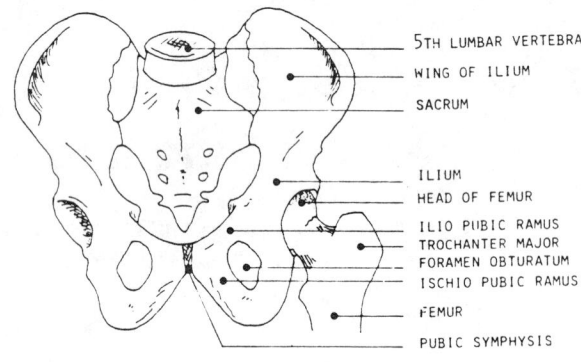

Fig. 1 - Anatomy of human pelvis

It is a large, irregularly shaped flat bone constitued by 3 parts : the ilium which includes a large articular surface, the acetabulum which is the pelvis articular part of the hip joint, by the connection which the femoral head, and the ischium which is the inferior part : it is open at the level of the foramen obturator. The banks of the foramen constitute the ilio and ischio pubic rami.

The pubis realizes the anterior part and is jointed in the middle line with the symetrical part of the pelvic bone. At the posterior part, the pelvis girdle is jointed to the sacrum which supports the vertebral spine.

The abdominal content is partially enclosed in the pelvic cavity.

Forces working transversally on the pelvis lateral part, bring closer the 2 parts of the pelvic girdle : there is then either a pubis symphysis disjunction, or a sacro-iliac or a posterior fracture of the iliac wing. But the compression works on the foramen obturatum sides and then there are the classical fractures of the ilio and ischio-pubic rami. The fractures of the acetabulum are not frequent although the compressive force works at the level of the trochanter major.

TEST METHODOLOGY

All the tests were performed using a device especially designed to reproduce impacts similar to those observed in real accidents. The procedure we used has been described in a previous paper (10) but it is briefly described hereafter. The device is made of a fixed frame and a mobile impactor, horizontally guided in order to hit a human subject seated on a rigid seat locked with the frame end. The mobile part is propelled by rubber extensible springs and the system is tightened through a small trolley guided on the same axis as the impactor and attache to a steel cable. It is possible to pull on the cable through a winch and then to move the trolley and the impactor back by tightening the rubber extensible springs. A bolt located between the trolley and the impactor releases the impactor which is then accelerated by the rubber extensible springs and hits the human subjects.

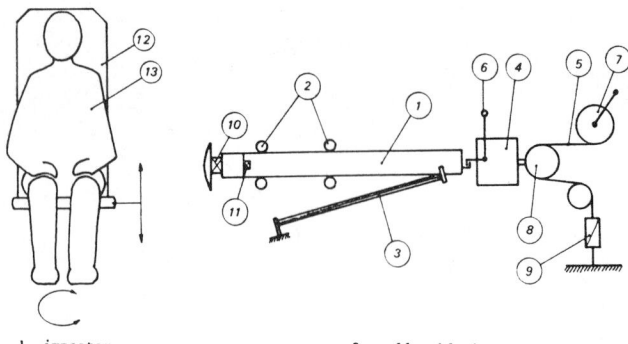

1. impactor
2. guiding rollers (2x3)
3. rubber extensible springs (3x3)
4. sled
5. pulling cable
6. locker
7. winch
8. pulley block
9. pulling force transducer
10. compressive force transducer
11. accelerometer
12. seat
13. human subject

Fig. 2 - Impactor Diagram

The impactor mass is 17.3 kg and the impacting system is the portion of a sphere (r = 600 mm, R = 175 mm). The impact force and impact acceleration are measured on the mobile system through transducers.

All the tests were performed with fresh human cadavers. They were incised along the iliac crest to expose the internal face of the wing of ilium. Three strain gauges were applied on this internal face : 2 below the iliac crest and 1 behind the acetabulum. These gauges were plastic sheathed, which made their fitting simpler. Then, the incision was sutured. A fourth gauge was placed on the same side on the upper face of the ilio-pubic ramus. Then, the cadaver was dressed up, weighted, measured and placed on the seat. The seat was centered on the trochanter major tuberosity.

The seat used gave the cadaver a posture identical to that of a car driver. The subject was unbelted and without lateral support.

In order to reach the pelvic fracture at a level as close as possible to the tolerance, several tests at increasing impact speed were conducted on the same cadaver. However, we performed only one impact test on 5 cadavers because the fracture happened at this first test. The results of these 5 tests would also allow to verify the influence of following tests on the same cadaver.

A X ray picture is taken after each test to verify wether it produced a fracture or not. Moreover, a X ray picture is taken before the tests to verify that there was no previous fracture or important osseous decalcification.

We decided to perform tests with unbelted subjects, because the analysis of car-to-car collisions shows that the safety belt is generally not sollicited in lateral impact, at least during the main phase of the impact.

60 impact tests on pelvis were performed for this study, using 22 cadavers. All the tests, excepted 5 which were performed with a padded impactor, were conducted using a rigid impactor described previously. Additional static tests have been conducted on five half pelvis in order to determine the force distribution inside the pelvic bone. Cortical area and inertia momentum of the two rami have been calculated for the pelvis of ten cadavers.

RESULTS

The results of impactor tests reported here are analysed in different directions :
- Injuries found by the autopsy,
- Dynamic tests results,
- Static tests results and bone mechanical properties.

RESULTS CONCERNING THE INJURIES : the injuries sustained by the cadavers during the impactor tests were carefully recorded by an autopsy made after the tests. During this autopsy the pelvis was removed and the pelvic fractures carefully analysed. This procedure allows us to set up a complete list of pelvic injuries sustained by the cadavers during the tests. The injuries recorded during autopsies are listed on table 1.

TABLE 1

Test N°	AIS	Injuries
A4	3	Fracture of the right ilio + ischio pubic rami sacro iliac disjunction. non complete fracture of sacrum
B3	3	Fracture of the right ischiopubic ramus. Fracture of the right femoral neck and collapse of the femoral head
C4	3	Fracture of the right iliac wing. Fracture of the right femoral shaft
D2	3	Fracture of the right ilio and ischio pubic rami, fracture of the right femoral neck, sacro iliac disjunction
E2	3	Fracture of ilio and ischio pubic rami. Sacro iliac joint disjunction
H4	2	Right femoral shaft fracture
I5	2	Fracture of the right iliac wing
J3	3	Fracture of the right ilio and ischio-pubic rami. Pubic symphisis disjunction.
M3	2	Fracture of the right iliac wing
N7	3	Fracture of the right iliac wing. Fracture of the right ilio and ischio-pubic rami. Right sacro iliac disjunction.
O6	3	Fracture of the right ilio and ischio-pubic rami and right sacro iliac disjunction.
R5	2	Fracture of the sacrum
S4	3	Collapse of the head of the right femur through the acetabulum. Fracture of the right and left ilio and ischio-pubic rami
T2	3	Fracture of the right acetabulum. Fracture of the right ilio and ischio-pubic rami
V2	3	Multiple fracture of the right ilio and ischio pubic rami. Fracture of the right femoral neck.
W2	2	Fracture of the right femoral shaft
X2	3	Fracture of the right and left ilio and ischio pubic rami. Bilateral sacro iliac disjunction.
Y2	2	Fracture of right ilio and ischio pubic rami
Z2	3	Fracture of the right ilio and ischio pubic rami. Right sacro iliac disjunction.

Pelvic injuries sustained in side impact real accidents are not generally described in details however an in-depth study of pelvic fractures in side impact accidents gives a description of injuries sustained by impacted side accident victims. The distribution of these injuries and those recorded on cadavers are listed in table 2.

TABLE 2

Number of fractures

Location	Tests (19)	Accidents (14)
Femoral shaft	3	4
Femoral neck	3	1
Acetabulum	2	1
Iliac wing	5	3
Pubic symphisis	1	1
Sacro-iliac symph.	6	3
Sacrum	1	1
One ramus	1	1
Two rami	10	5
Three rami	0	3
Four rami	2	3
Pelvic crush	1	1

Comparison of accident and test injuries shows a good correlation with nevertheless some minor differences. In both samples the fracture of pelvic rami is the most frequent injury (13 among 19 in tests and 12 among 14 in accidents). However the pelvic rami fractures are mainly on one side in tests whereas they involve as well one side as well both sides in accidents : these differences seem to depend from the severity of impact ; the tests were made at increasing speed until a pelvic injury is found, which limits the extension of injuries, whereas in accidents the energy dissipated by the impact between the occupant and the side parcel can be higher than the energy necessary to produce injuries, and then this impact can make extensive fractures.

The pubic rami fractures seem to be a typical injury of direct lateral impact in the sitting position (which corresponds to the position of car occupants). In tests conducted in similar conditions, but with cadavers having legs in line with the torso, i.e. like in standing posture, (11) the injuries found were completely different : they were mainly acetabulum (hip) fractures : but the energy to produce these injuries were in the same order of magnitude as the energy amount necessary to produce side impact pelvic injuries.

The other differences concern mainly the number of femoral neck fractures and of sacro-iliac disjunctions.

The femoral neck fractures are very rare even if we have found more in tests than in accidents. The femoral neck mechanical resistance decreases with age (the spontaneous femoral fracture of elderly is well known) and the cadavers used in these tests were older than the victims of car accidents.

The sacro-iliac disjunctions seem also more frequent in tests than in real accidents. These injuries have never been found isolated, but always associated with pubic rami fractures.

In two tests these disjunctions were very minor and were not found by X ray pictures analysis but only at the autopsy ; such injuries could be forgotten on human living.

In a general way cadavers sustained in a average, less pelvic injuries than human people involved in side accidents (51 pelvic injuries for 19 cadavers against 47 injuries for 14 accident victims). This increasing of the number of injuries can be associated with the higher severity of impacts in accidents compared to the tests.

DYNAMIC TEST RESULTS. For the purpose of this study 60 tests have been conducted. 55 of them were performed with a rigid impactor and 5 with a padded impactor. For all the tests the impactor was centered on the right great trochanler. They are analysed separately in this paper.

RIGID IMPACTOR TESTS. The results of the 55 tests performed with a rigid impactor are listed in table 3. These tests were made with 19 cadavers. 6 of them are female cadavers whose age varies from 59 years old to 84 years old with an average value of 71 years old. The age of the 13 male cadavers varies from 54 years old to 85 years old with an average value of 72 years old.

TABLE 3

TEST N°	SPEED KM/H	FORCE PEAK/3MS N	ACCEL. 3MS g	IMPULSE N.s	AIS
A1	21	4170/3355	-	63	0
A2	25.3	5800/4355	-	122	0
A3	30.0	6960/5220	-	163	0
A4	41.0	11140/8200	-	209	3
B1	21.0	5100/3240	-	71	0
B2	30.0	6260/5575	-	131	2
B3	34.9	8120/6200	-	161	3
C1	25.6	5620/5375	-	113	0
C2	32.0	10120/8070	-	136	0
C3	39.4	10140/8080	-	162	2
C4	47.5	13780/12920	-	232	3
D1	25.0	4410/3330	34	88	0
D2	30.8	5240/4720	45	115	3
E1	25.2	5520/4330	45	88	0
E2	31.1	5520/4440	34	112	3
F1	28.3	5610/4430	33	89	0
F2	31.1	3890/3330	24	90	0
F3	35.0	5610/4430	24	110	0
H1	25.5	6620/6390	27	82	0
H2	30.2	10760/10000	42	99	0
H3	34.6	11110/10440	40	128	0
H4	38.2	12690/10555		140	2
I1	25.5	10210/7330	39	77	0
I2	30.2	11040/7890	49	97	0
I3	35.5	11590/8440	49	115	0
I4	39.8	12690/8780	35	139	0
I5	40.1	13240/8935	80	157	2
J1	25.5	7730/6835	34	79	0
J2	30.6	6440/6110	30	124	0
J3	35.5	8270/6945	62	131	3
K1	25.0	5520/4665	34	73	0
K2	30.8	7170/4720	35	85	0
K3	35.0	8280/6720	40	102	0
L1	29.7	8330/8220	60	118	0
L2	35.0	11660/10275	60	130	0
L3	39.6	13330/11330	80	142	0
L4	44.6	15550/12770	120	174	0

M3	22.1	4330/3780	32	79	2
N5	33.0	8610/8390	59	110	0
N6	37.7	10000/9500	62	148	0
N7	41.1	10278/9580	72	163	3
O4	32.9	5695/5580	48	126	0
O5	37.8	6140/5890	51	142	0
O6	42.2	6830/6670	53	151	3
R1	36.5	9440/9280	68	163	0
R2	39.6	10694/10440	74	166	0
R3	43.4	10972/10750	81	168	0
R4	47.1	11806/11580	90	173	0
R5	50.6	12306/12080	95	177	2
S2	36.1	7083/6640	54	126	0
S3	40.7	6670/6500	60	137	0
S4	44.4	7140/6890	65	143	3
T2	34.6	4611/4445	33	107	3
V2	27.7	5740/4880	40	75	3
W2	30.0	7490/7165	56	98	2
X1	45.7				0
X2	53.2	7620/7220	52	172	3
Y2	53.9	11130/10750	65	225	2
Z1	45.5	7360/7150	25	158	0
Z2	52.0	9120/8760	79	180	3

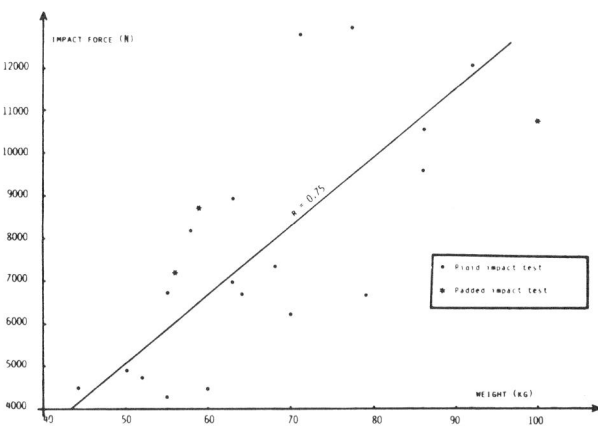

Fig.3 - Cadaver weight versus 3 ms injury producing impact force

The cadavers used in this study were carefully selected according to their antecedents and the medical treatment that they followed ; however, one cadaver (M) had very poor bone conditions, and the results of this cadaver should be cancelled.

Analysis of results shows that there is a large scatter of the results. The 3 ms impact force corresponding to pelvic fracture varies from 4880 N to 12920 N for male cadavers and from 4440 N to 8200 N for female cadavers.

If we consider the tests in which injuries occured, i.e. tests with an AIS 2 and an AIS 3, the average value of the 3 ms impact force is 5600 N for female cadaver and 8600 N for male cadavers. This value of 8.6 KN is higher than the acceptable limit proposed by TRRL to be measured on a side impact dummy (the proposal was 6 KN) (12). The tentatives to correlate the impact force with other parameters did not give interesting results except the correlation between the impact force and anthropometric parameters such as cadaver height or weight. The anthropometric parameters are correlated with bone sizes : taller and stronger persons have bigger bones, and the correlation found between impact force and height and weight seems to indicate a possible correlation between impact force and pelvic bone dimensions.

Fig.3 gives the value of 3 ms fracture producing impact force.

The versus the cadavers weight corpulence of the subjects can be evaluated by the use od the Livi index which is defined by :

$$Li = 10 \frac{\sqrt[3]{Weight}}{Height}$$

with weight in kg and height in m.

Based on statistical data the corpulence is defined as follows :
$Li \leq 22$: the subject is very thin,
$22 < Li \leq 23$: the subject is thin
$23 < Li \leq 24$: the subject is normal
$24 < Li \leq 25$: the subject is stout
$Li > 25$: the subject is obese.

The values of Li are listed in table 4.

These values can be used to correct the values of weight of cadavers. The proposed correction is :

$$W_c = W_a \frac{23.5}{Li}$$

in which W_c is the corrected weight, W_a is the actual weight, Li is the actual value of the Livi index. The coefficient 23.5 is the value of Livi index for a normal person.

The values of weight corrected according to Livi index values are also listed in table 4.

TABLE 4

CADAVER	SEX	AGE	HEIGHT cm	WEIGHT cm	LIVI INDEX	CORRECTED WEIGHT kg
A	F	70	167	58	22.9	39.5
B	F	84	154	70	26.4	62.3
C	M	69	173	78	24.3	75.4
D	F	63	160	52	23.0	53.0
F	F	59	152	55	24.7	52.3
H	M	69	175	86	24.9	81.0
I	M	65	181	63	21.7	68.2
J	M	75	177	63	22.2	66.7
K	M	75	171	55	21.9	59.0

L	M	71	175	85	25.1	79.6
M	M	68	165	62	24.0	60.7
N	M	54	184	86	24.0	84.2
O	M	70	160	79	26.8	69.5
R	M	80	180	82	25.1	86.1
S	M	79	164	64	24.4	61.6
T	F	79	144	44	23.7	43.6
V	M	61	162	50	22.7	51.8
W	M	85	170	68	24.0	66.6
X	F	54	162	56	23.6	55.8
Y	M	74	175	100	26.5	88.6
Z	M	67	167	58	23.2	58.8

If we draw the relationship between the 3 ms impact force of fracture producing tests, and the corrected weight we find a better linear correlation than with actual weight values, as indicated on fig. 4

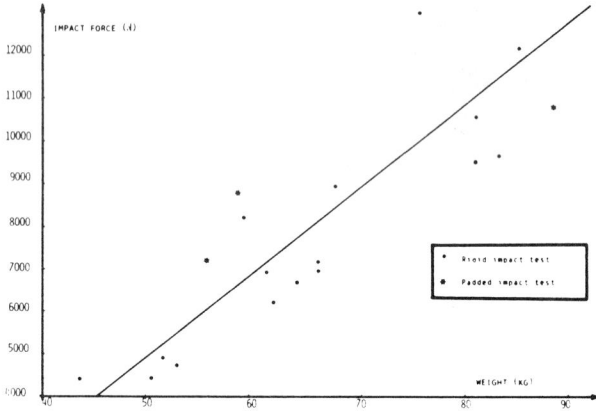

Fig. 4 - Corrected cadaver weight versus 3 ms injury producing impact force

. The correlation coefficient is .89 instead of .75 on fig. 3.

This better correlation confirms that the pelvic tolerance depends on the bone geometry which is linked to the anthropometry.

The value of impact force as a function of weight is given by the formula : impact force = 193.85 weight - 4710.6

The value of impact force calculated for a weight of 75 kg, which is the weight of the 50 th percentile male, is 9830 N, which is higher than the mean value for the cadavers used in this study.

During the test we recorded also pelvic acceleration ; the values of 3 ms pelvic acceleration are listed in table 2. All the values recorded are low and much under the proposed tolerance of 100 g's (13). This is probably due to the test methodology : in the impactor test only the pelvis is impacted and no other part of the body is restrained, whereas in drop tests and in sled or car tests, several areas of the body are involved by the impact.

The value of impact speed necessary to produce fractures is in the same order of magnitude as the door velocity change in car to car tests in which pelvic fractures occur (14). In these tests, the impact speed producing pelvic injuries varies from 22 km/h to 50 km/h.

19 cadavers sustained following impacts at increasing speed, until 5 of them got a pelvic fracture at the first impact. Comparison of results shows that several following tests at increasing speed do not change the capability of the cadaver to sustain impacts : the traces of recorded parameters are not changed after the first impact. The value of impact force always increases until the fracture occurs, and, in fact, the value of fracture impact force was lower for cadavers which sustained only one impact than for cadavers which got a pelvic fracture after several tests.

PADDED IMPACTOR TESTS. 5 tests with a padded impactor were performed on 3 cadavers. For these tests the impactor extremity was covered by a polyurethan foam parrallelepipedic block (14.5 cm thick, 24.7 cm long, 14.5 cm wide, density 130 kg/m^3). These blocks were developped by APR as paddings for side impact protection. Two of them sustained an AIS 3 pelvic fracture after the second test, whereas the third one sustained only one test which produces an AIS 2 injury. The impact force values recorded on the impactor were in the same order of magnitude as those recorded during rigid impactor test. But the impactor speed necessary to produce pelvic fracture is undoubtedly increased by the padding ; all the cadavers in padding tests sustained more than 52 km/h whereas the average value of impact speed in rigid impactor tests in which the injuries occured is 37.1 km/h. These results are summarized in table 5.

Table 5

	Rigid	Padded	Gain
Average impact speed (km/h)	37.1	52.6	40 %

STATIC TESTS. During the autopsy the pelvis of each cadaver was removed, cleaned and cut in the median plane. The half right pelvis (impacted side) was used to make the exact description of the injuries. In most of the tests, the left side was not brocken and we performed static compressive tests in 5 of these left half pelvis.

The half pelvis was fitted with 8 strain gauges as indicated on figure 5 and compressed through the great trochanter as shown on figure 6

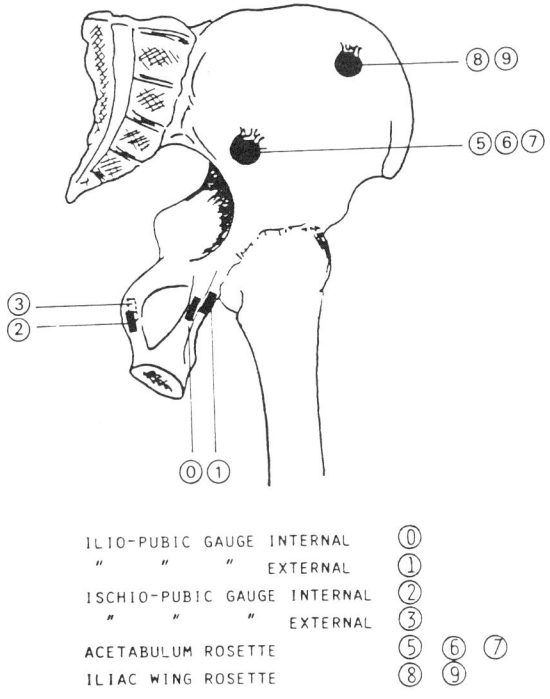

Fig 5. - Strain gauge location for static tests

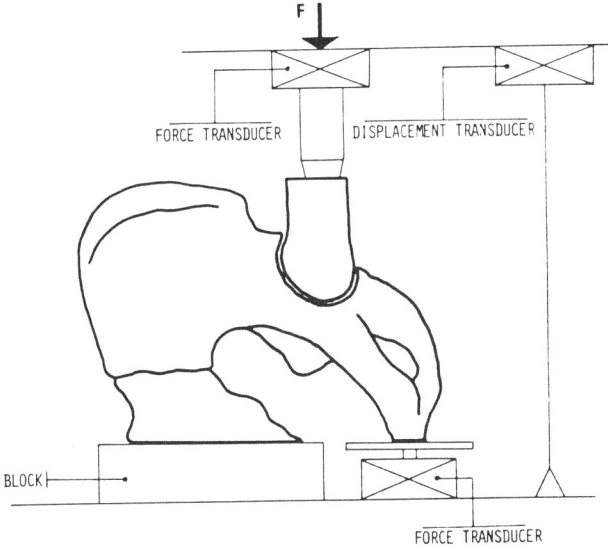

Fig. 6 - Force application on the pelvis in static tests

These tests were necessary to know the strain distribution in the pelvis. In each test we recorded the microdeformation versus impact force of each strain gauge. Figure 7 shows typical results of a static test : the two pelvic rami are the most strained parts of the pelvis and they sustain a bending process : one side is compressed whereas the other is in tension

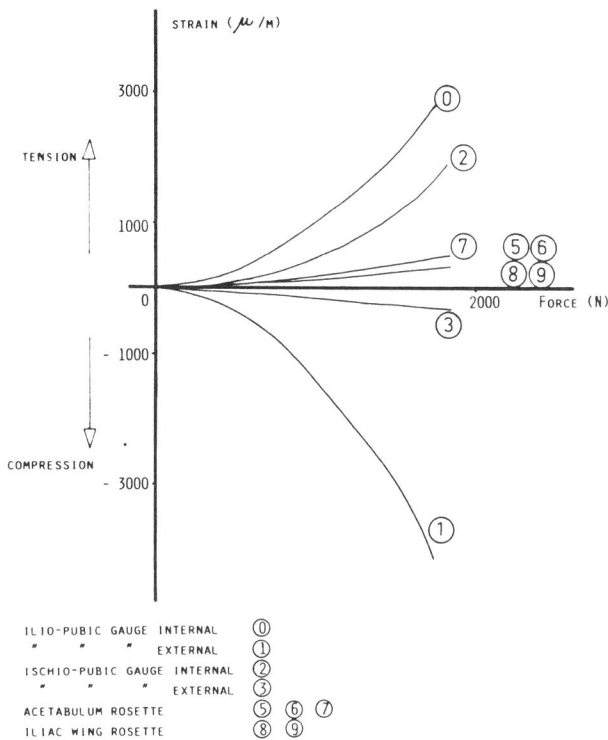

Fig. 7 - Typical strain gauges results of a static test

The comparison of the deformations of the two rami shows that the ilio-pubic ramus is much more strained than the ischio-pubic one at each compression level, even if the second one has a lower section than the first one. In fact, the ischio-pubic ramus is longer and more curved, which allows a lower stress in the sections for a specific compression.

This is in agreement with the impactor tests which produced mainly impacted side pubic rami fractures. In static tests, the other parts of pelvis on which strain gauges were fitted were not deformed by the test.

PELVIC BONE CHARACTERISTICS. For 10 of the 22 cadavers used in impactor tests, we have determined the value of parameters related to the bone structure. For this we have cut a slice of the 2 rami of half a pelvis. We took macro pictures of these bone slices and from the scaled pictures (figures 8 and 9) we determined the total and cortical bone sections and the inertia momentum of these sections

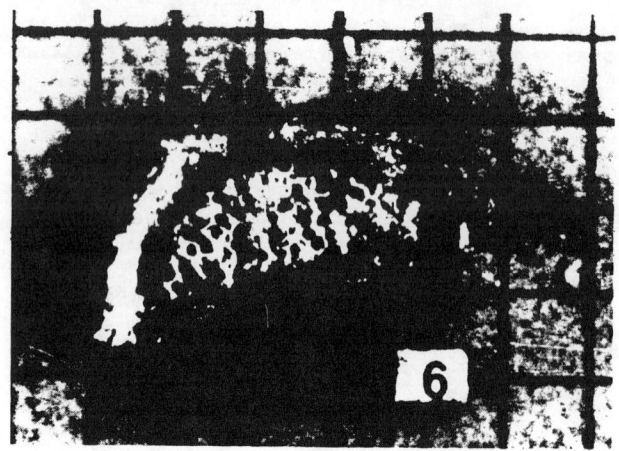

Fig. 8 - Picture of an ischio-pubic ramus cut

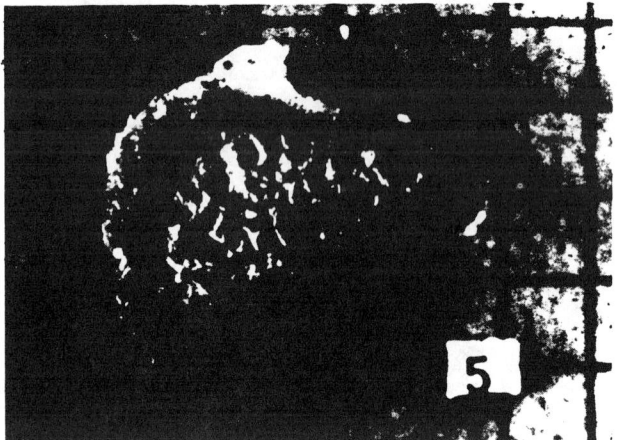

Fig. 9 - Picture of an ilio-pubic ramus cut

This was made with a computer which was used to digitize the outlines of the section and to make the calculations. The results of these parameters are included in table 6.

Table 6

TBF	Ramus	S_t mm2	S_c mm2	I_x mm4	I_y mm4	Ymini mm	$\frac{I_x}{Ymini}$ mm3
S	ilio	265.8	66	1748.2	3505.4	8.32	210
	ischio	165.6	43.3	687.5	1466.0	5.66	121
C	ilio	311.5	98.6	3349.8	4946.7	8.41	398
	ischio	281	85.3	1417.6	7175.7	5.64	251
H	ilio	250.2	86	2145.4	3193.3	7.32	293
	ischio	136.4	47.6	417.7	1713.4	4.30	87
K	ilio	217.5	66.7	1306.7	3048.9	5.65	231
	ischio	160.1	42.6	359.8	2615.5	3.58	100
N	ilio	256.5	96.7	2286.2	4496.2	7.82	292
	ischio	202.4	65.2	564.8	1170.6	5.59	101
O	ilio	159.3	53.3	1199.8	1530.4	6.32	190
	ischio	112.3	32.4	248.2	1013.3	3.44	72
T	ilio	139.9	45.5	672.1	1105.3	5.91	115
	ischio	100.2	32.7	193.2	1093.4	3.20	60
X	ilio	178.4	61.7	1166.9	1722.3	5.91	204
	ischio	148.7	43.4	381.8	1856.7	3.32	115
Y	ilio	248.4	94.5	2450.4	4284.8	7.93	309
	ischio	137.1	49.7	600	1288.1	5.66	106
Z	ilio	225.9	67.3	1790.5	3006.1	6.86	261
	ischio	167.3	44.9	761.6	2382.3	4.82	159

Table 6

DISCUSSION OF THE RESULTS. As the dynamic tests and the litterature indicate that the rami fractures are the most frequent injuries in side impact and as the static tests showed that the ilio-pubic ramus is the most stressed part of the pelvis, and that it is mainly bended, we tried to correlate the impact force with the value of the cross section inertia momentum divided by the distance between the center of mass and the external surface of the pubic ramus. We have choosen this parameter because it is the multiplying factor to determine the bending force from the strain value for a beam submitted to a bending process (15). This result is interesting because the rami fractures are the most frequent pelvic injuries and the static tests have shown that the pelvic rami were much more involved than any other pelvic area, in lateral compression. This means that the tolerance of the pelvis in side impact is directly connected with the geometry of the ischio-pubic ramus. These data are reported on figure 10 which indicates a good correlation of these two parameters.

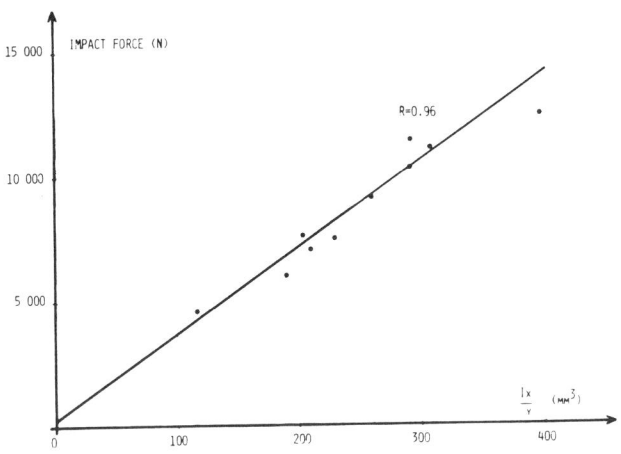

Fig. 10 - Injury producing impact force versus Ix/y of the ilio-pubic ramus

Analysis of dynamic test have shown a large scatter in test results ; this scatter can be reduced by a force correction related to the pelvis geometry. Nevertheless the female subjects seem to have a lower tolerance. Analysis of bone resistance have shown that female have a resistance equal to 4/5 of the male subjects (16). This has been established on the results of tests on several long bones but not on the pelvis itself.

The value of fracture producing impact 3 ms impact force varies greatly with anthropometry, and is for example for a normal person weighing 75 kg (which is the weight of the 50 th percentile male) 9830 N. For a person weighing 46 kg (which is the weight of the 5 th percentile female) this value is only 4260 N.

The relationship between impact force and either weight or ilio-pubic ramus geometry does not show any difference between male and female subjects : the female subjects have a lower pelvic tolerance in lateral impact because (generally) they are thinner and have a smaller ilio-pubic bone section.

In the same study, analysis of bone resistance variation versus shows a decreasing of resistance of the femur of 19 % for 60/69 years and 22 % for 70/89 years compared to the resistance of 20/39 years population. The values found on tests of other human bones are in the same order of magnitude.

PROPOSED PROTECTION CRITERION. On the basis of the test results described behind the tolerance for a cadaver weighing 75 Kg would be about 10 KN 3 ms impact force. This value would be the base for a protection criterion applied to a 50 th percentile dummy. The use of such a protection criterion implies that the side impact dummies are able to be fitted with a pelvic lateral force transducer. At the present time only one side impact dummy type, manufactured by the MIRA is fitted with pelvic force transducers. This pelvis is equipped with 3 force transducers needing 5 measurement channels and the use of this dummy in several test environments (car to car tests, sled tests, impactor tests) have shown the faisability of the measurement of pelvic lateral force in side impact ; but as most of the injuries are located on the pubic rami it seems possible to simplify the force measurement device, and to use only one force transducer located in the anterior part of the pelvis.

CONCLUSIONS

Analysis of these test results allows to conclude as follows :
- impactor tests reproduced realistic pelvic injuries at realistic impact speed
- these injuries are mainly impacted side ischio and ilio-pubic rami fractures
- the impact force seems more correlated to injury than pelvic acceleration
- the value of the tolerable impact force varies greatly with anthropometry
- the value of the tolerance is close to 10 KN of 3 ms impact force for the 50 th percentile male subjects and close to 4 KN for the 5 th percentile female
- static tests confirmed that pelvis rami are more stressed than any other pelvic part
- there is a correlation between the geometry of the ischio pubic ramus cross section and the tolerable impact force
- the use of a padding can protect efficiently by increasing the acceptable impact speed. A gain of 40 % has been found
- a protection criterion for pelvis based on the 10 KN tolerance could be used on a dummy fitted with a pelvic lateral force transducer.

REFERENCES

1. MALLIARIS A, HITCHOCK R. HEDLUND J.
Setting priorities in crash protection.
Presented at the 1982 SAE Congress.

2. MACKAY G.M.
Causes and effects of road accidents.
Dept. of Transportation & Environmental Planning. University of Birmingham, vol 3, 1969.

3. WOLF R.A
Causes of impact injury in automobile accidents. National Academy of Science, 1962

4. CESARI D., RAMET M.
Influence of intrusion in side impact
6th ESV, Washington, October 1976, 1-19

5. THOMAS P., LANSON S., GRIFFITHS S., BREEN J.
An investigation of a representative sample of real world side impacts to cars.
EEC Biomechanics programme final report of contract UK1, 1981

6. PADGAONKAR A.J., PRIYARANJAN PRASAD
Simulation of side impact using the CAL 3D occupant simulation model
23rd Stapp Car Crash conf. Oct. 17-19, 1979, 133-158

7. CESARI D., RAMET M., HERRY-MARTIN D.
Injury mechanism in side impact
22nd Stapp Car Crash conf. Oct. 24-26, 1978, 429-448

8. HARTEMANN F., FORET-BRUNO J.Y., THOMAS C., TARRIERE C., GOT C., PATEL A.
Influence of mass ratio and structural compatibility on the severity of injuries sustained by the near side occupants in car-to-car side collisions
23rd Stapp Car Crash conf. Oct. 17-19, 1979, 233-260

9. DEJEAMMES N.
Fractures du bassin au cours des chocs latéraux automobiles.
Thèse LYON 1978.

10. CESARI D., RAMET M., CLAIR P.Y.
Evaluation of pelvic fracture tolerance in side impact
24th Stapp Car Crash conf., 1980

11. CREYSSEL J., SCHNEPP J.
Fractures tanscotyloïdiennes du bassin,
MASSON Ed, 1961.

12. HARRIS J.
The design and use of the TRRL side impact dummy
20th Stapp Car Crash conf. Oct. 18-20, 1976, 77-106

13. LENZ K.H.
Joint biomechanical research project KOB
Unfall-und Sicherheitsforschung Strassenverkehr N° 34, 1982.

14. AVRIL J.
Encyclopédie Vishay d'analyse des contraintes
Vishay-Micromesures Ed., 1974

15. HIROSHI YAMADA
Strength of biological materials
F. GAYNOR EVANS Ed.
R.E. KRIEGER Publishing Company, 1973.

826036

Tolerance of Human Pelvis to Fracture and Proposed Pelvic Protection Criterion to be Measured on Side Impact Dummies

D. Césari, M. Ramet and R. Bouquet
O.N.S.E.R. France

INTRODUCTION

The problems of side impact protection have been extensively analysed in several countries in the world.

To make the evaluation of protection offered by cars against side impact, proposals of side impact tests using a mobile deformable barrier have been made as well in the United States (1) as in Europe (2).

The evaluation of car behaviour in side impact would be made through the values of injury parameters recorded on dummies. These injury parameters would be related to injury mechanisms of real side impact accidents.

This paper analyses the results of 60 cadaver tests conducted to determine the pelvis tolerance and to propose a protection criterion of pelvis in side impact.

TEST METHODOLOGY

All the tests were performed using a device especially designed to reproduce impacts similar to those observed in real accidents. The procedure we used has been described in a previous paper (3) but it is briefly described hereafter. The device is made of a fixed frame and a mobile impactor, horizontally guided in order to hit a human subject seated on a rigid seat locked with the frame end.

The mobile part is propelled by rubber extensible springs and the system is tightened through a small trolley guided on the same axis as the impactor and attached to a steel cable. It is possible to pull on the cable through a winch and then to move the trolley and the impactor back by tightening the rubber extensible springs. A bolt located between the trolley and the impactor releases the impactor which is then accelerated by the rubber extensible springs and hits the human subjects.

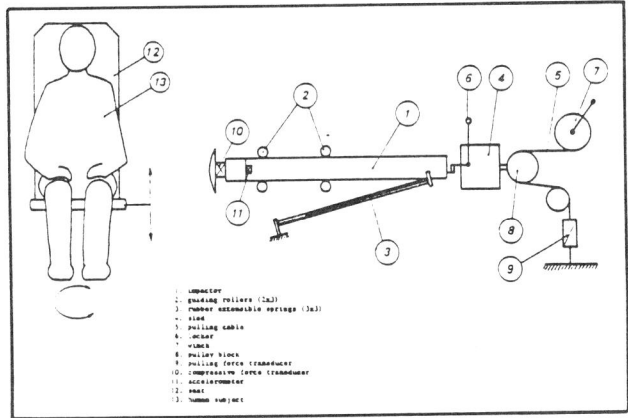

Figure 1. Impactor diagram.

The impactor mass is 17.3 kg and the impacting system is the portion of a sphere (r = 600 mm, R = 175 mm). The impact force and impact acceleration are measured on the mobile system through transducers.

All the tests were performed with fresh human cadavers. They were incised along the iliac crest to expose the internal face of the wing of ilium. Three strain gauges were applied on this internal face : 2 below the iliac crest and 1 behind the acetabulum. These gauges were plastic sheathed, which made their fitting simpler.

Then, the incision was sutured. A fourth gauge was placed on the same side on the upper face of the ilio-pubic ramus. Then, the cadaver was dressed up, weighted, measured and placed on the seat. The seat was centered on the trochanter major tuberosity.

The seat used gave the cadaver a posture identical to that of a car driver. The subject was unbelted and without lateral support.

In order to reach the pelvic fracture at a level as close as possible to the tolerance, several tests at increasing impact speed were conducted on the same cadaver. However, we performed only one impact test on 5 cadavers because the fracture happened at this first test. The results of these 5 tests would also allow to verify the influence of following tests on the same cadaver.

An X ray picture is taken after each test to verify whether it produced a fracture or not. Moreover, an X ray picture is taken before the tests to verify that there was no previous fracture or important osseous decalcification.

We decided to perform tests with unbelted subjects, because the analysis of car-to-car collisions shows that the safety belt is generally not solicited in lateral impact, at least during the main phase of the impact.

Sixty impact tests on pelvis were performed for this study, using 22 cadavers. All the tests, excepted five which were performed with a padded impactor, were conducted using a rigid impactor described previously. Additional static tests have been conducted on five half pelvis in order to determine the force distribution inside the pelvic bone. Cortical area and inertia momentum of the two rami have been calculated for the pelvis of 10 cadavers.

RESULTS

The results of impactor tests reported here are analysed in different directions:

—Injuries found by the autopsy,
—Dynamic test results,
—Static test results and bone mechanical properties.

Table 1.

Test N°	AIS	Injuries
A4	3	Fracture of the right ilio + ischio-pubic rami sacro iliac disjunction non complete fracture of sacrum
B3	3	Fracture of the right ischio-pubic ramus Fracture of the right femoral neck and collapse of the femoral head
C4	3	Fracture of the right iliac wing Fracture of the right femoral shaft
D2	3	Fracture of the right ilio and ischio-pubic rami, fracture of the right femoral neck, sacro iliac disjunction
E2	3	Fracture of ilio and ischio-pubic rami Sacro iliac joint disjunction
H4	2	Right femoral shaft fracture
I5	2	Fracture of the right iliac wing
J3	3	Fracture of the right ilio and ischio-pubic rami. Pubic symphisis disjunction
M3	2	Fracture of the right iliac wing
N7	3	Fracture of the right iliac wing. Fracture of the right ilio and ischio-pubic rami. Right sacro iliac disjunction
O6	3	Fracture of the right ilio and ischio-pubic rami and right sacro iliac disjunction
R5	2	Fracture of the sacrum
S4	3	Collapse of the head of the right femur through the acetabulum. Fracture of the right and left ilio and ischio-pubic rami
T2	3	Fracture of the right acetabulum. Fracture of the right ilio and ischio-pubic rami
V2	3	Multiple fracture of the right ilio and ischio-pubic rami. Fracture of the right femoral neck
W2	2	Fracture of the right femoral shaft
X2	3	Fracture of the right and left ilio and ischio-pubic rami. Bilateral sacro iliac disjunction
Y2	2	Fracture of right ilio and ischio-pubic rami
Z2	3	Fracture of the right ilio and ischio-pubic rami. Right sacro iliac disjunction

RESULTS CONCERNING THE INJURIES

The injuries sustained by the cadavers during the impactor tests were carefully recorded by an autopsy made after the tests. During this autopsy the pelvis was removed and the pelvic fractures carefully analysed. This procedure allows us to set up a complete list of pelvic injuries sustained by the cadavers during the tests. The injuries recorded during autopsies are listed on Table 1.

Pelvic injuries sustained in side impact real accidents are not generally described in details; however, an indepth study of pelvic fractures in side impact accidents gives a description of injuries sustained by impacted side accident victims (4). The distribution of these injuries and those recorded on cadavers are listed in Table 2.

Comparison of accident and test injuries shows a good correlation with nevertheless some minor differences. In both samples the fracture of pelvic rami is the most frequent injury (13 among 19 in tests and 12 among 14 in accidents). However the pelvic rami fractures are mainly on one side in tests whereas they involve both sides in accidents: these differences seem to depend from the severity of impact; the tests were made at increasing speed until a pelvic injury was found, which limits the extension of injuries, whereas in accidents the energy dissipated by the impact between the occupant and the side parcel can be higher than the energy necessary to produce injuries, and then this impact can make extensive fractures.

The pubic rami fractures seem to be a typical injury of direct lateral impact in the sitting position (which corresponds to the position of car occupants). In tests conducted in similar conditions, but with cadavers having legs in line with the torso, i.e., like in standing posture, (5) the injuries found were completely different: they were mainly acetabulum (hip) fractures: but the energy to produce these injuries was in the same order of magnitude as the energy amount necessary to produce side impact pelvic injuries.

The other differences concern mainly the number of femoral neck fractures and of sacroiliac disjunctions.

The femoral neck fractures are very rare even if we have found more in tests than in accidents. The femoral neck mechanical resistance decreases with age (the spontaneous femoral fracture of elderly is well known) and the cadavers used in these tests were older than the victims of car accidents.

The sacroiliac disjunctions seem also more frequent in tests than in real accidents. These injuries have never been found isolated, but always associated with pubic rami fractures.

In two tests these disjunctions were very minor and were not found by X ray pictures analysis but only at the autopsy; such injuries could be forgotten on human living.

In a general way cadavers sustained on an average, less pelvic injuries than human people involved in side accidents (51 pelvic injuries for 19 cadavers against 47 injuries for 14 accident victims). This increasing of the number of injuries can be associated with the higher severity of impacts in accidents compared to the tests.

DYNAMIC TEST RESULTS

For the purpose of this study 60 tests have been conducted: 55 of them were performed with a rigid impactor and 5 with a padded impactor. For all the tests the impactor was centered on the right great trochanler. They are analysed separately in this paper.

RIGID IMPACTOR TESTS

The results of the 55 tests performed with a rigid impactor are listed in Table 3. These tests were made with 19 cadavers. Six of them are female cadavers whose age varies from 59 years old to 84 years old with an average value of 71 years old. The age of the 13 male cadavers varies from 54 years old to 85 years old with an average value of 72 years old.

The cadavers used in this study were carefully selected according to their antecedents and the medical treatment that they followed; however, one cadaver (M) had very poor bone conditions, and the results of this cadaver should be cancelled.

Analysis of results shows that there is a large scatter of the results. The 3 ms impact force corresponding to pelvic fracture varies from 4880 N to 12920 N for male cadavers and from 4440 N to 8200 N for female cadavers.

If we consider the tests in which injuries occurred, i.e., tests with an AIS 2 and AIS 3, the average value of the 3 ms impact force is 5600 N for female cadavers and 8600 N for male cadavers. This value of 8.6 KN is higher than the acceptable limit proposed by TRRL to be measured on a side impact dummy (the proposal was 6 KN) (6). The tentatives to correlate the impact force with other parameters did not give interesting results except the correlation between the impact force and anthropometric parameters such as cadaver height or weight. The an-

Table 2.

Location	Number of fractures	
	Tests (19)	Accidents (14)
Femoral shaft	3	4
Femoral neck	3	1
Acetabulum	2	1
Iliac wing	5	3
Pubic symphisis	1	1
Sacro-iliac symph.	6	3
Sacrum	1	1
One ramus	1	1
Two rami	10	5
Three rami	0	3
Four rami	2	3
Pelvic crush	1	1

Table 3.

Test N°	Speed KM/H	Force Peak/3MS N	Accel. 3MS g	Impulse N.s	AIS
A1	21	4170/3355	—	63	0
A2	25.3	5800/4355	—	122	0
A3	30.0	6960/5220	—	163	0
A4	41.0	11140/8200	—	209	3
B1	21.0	5100/3240	—	71	0
B2	30.0	6260/5575	—	131	2
B3	34.9	8120/6200	—	161	3
C1	25.6	5620/5375	—	113	0
C2	32.0	10120/8070	—	136	0
C3	39.4	10140/8080	—	162	2
C4	47.5	13780/12920	—	232	3
D1	25.0	4410/3330	34	88	0
D2	30.8	5240/4720	45	115	3
E1	25.2	5520/4330	45	88	0
E2	31.1	5520/4440	34	112	3
F1	28.3	5610/4430	33	89	0
F2	31.1	3890/3330	24	90	0
F3	35.0	5610/4430	24	110	0
H1	25.5	6620/6390	27	82	0
H2	30.2	10760/10000	42	99	0
H3	34.6	11110/10440	40	128	0
H4	38.2	12690/10555		140	2
I1	25.5	10210/7330	39	77	0
I2	30.2	11040/7890	49	97	0
I3	35.5	11590/8440	49	115	0
I4	39.8	12690/8780	35	139	0
I5	40.1	13240/8935	80	157	2
J1	25.5	7730/6835	34	79	0
J2	30.6	6440/6110	30	124	0
J3	35.5	8270/6945	62	131	3
K1	25.0	5520/4665	34	73	0
K2	30.8	7170/4720	35	85	0
K3	35.0	8280/6720	40	102	0
L1	29.7	8330/8220	60	118	0
L2	35.0	11660/10275	60	130	0
L3	39.6	13330/11330	80	142	0
L4	44.6	15550/12770	120	174	0
M3	22.1	4330/3780	32	79	2
N5	33.0	8610/8390	59	110	0
N6	37.7	10000/9500	62	148	0
N7	41.1	10278/9580	72	163	3
O4	32.9	5695/5580	48	126	0
O5	37.8	6140/5890	51	142	0
O6	42.2	6830/6670	53	151	3
R1	36.5	9440/9280	68	163	0
R2	39.6	10694/10440	74	166	0
R3	43.4	10972/10750	81	168	0
R4	47.1	11806/11580	90	173	0
R5	50.6	12306/12080	95	177	2
S2	36.1	7083/6640	54	126	0
S3	40.7	6670/6500	60	137	0
S4	44.4	7140/6890	65	143	3
T2	34.6	4611/4445	33	107	3
V2	27.7	5740/4880	40	75	3
W2	30.0	7490/7165	56	98	2
X1	45.7				
X2	53.2	7620/7220	52	172	3
Y2	53.9	11130/10750	65	225	2
Z1	45.5	7360/7150	25	158	0
Z2	52.0	9120/8760	79	180	3

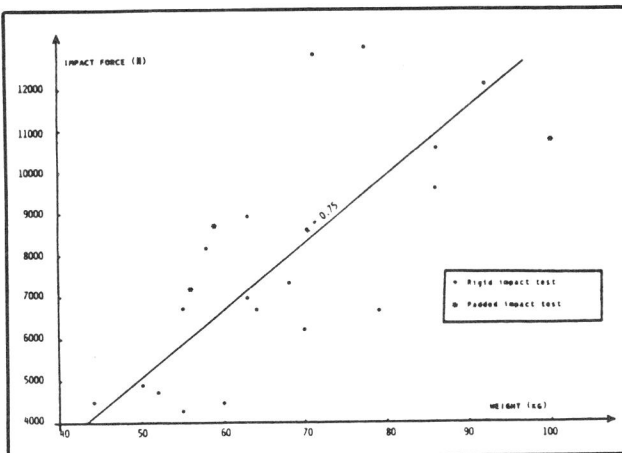

Figure 2. Cadaver weight versus 3 ms injury producing impact force.

thropometric parameters are correlated with bone sizes: taller and stronger persons have bigger bones, and the correlation found between impact force and height and weight seems to indicate a possible correlation between impact force and pelvic bone dimensions.

Figure 2 gives the value of 3 ms fracture producing impact force.

The corpulence of the subjects can be evaluated by the use of the Livi index which is defined by:

$$Li = 10 \frac{\sqrt[3]{Weight}}{Height}$$

with weight in kg and height in m.

Based on statistical data the corpulence is defined as follows:

$Li \leq 22$: the subject is very thin,
$22 < Li \leq 23$: the subject is thin
$23 < Li \leq 24$: the subject is normal
$24 < Li \leq 25$: the subject is stout
$Li > 25$: the subject is obese.

The values of Li are listed in Table 4.

These values can be used to correct the values of weight of cadavers. The proposed correction is:

$$W_c = W_a \frac{23.5}{Li}$$

in which W_c is the corrected weight, W_a is the actual weight, Li is the actual value of the Livi index. The coefficient 23.5 is the value of Livi index for a normal person.

The values of weight corrected according to Livi index values are also listed in Table 4.

If we draw the relationship between the 3 ms impact force of fracture producing tests, and the corrected weight we find a better linear correlation than with actual weight values, as indicated on Figure 4.

The correlation coefficient is .89 instead of .75 on Figure 3.

This better correlation confirms that the pelvic tolerance depends on the bone geometry which is linked to the anthropometry.

The value of impact force as a function of weight is given by the formula: impact force = 193.85 weight − 4710.6.

Table 4.

Cadaver	Sex	Age	Height cm	Weight kg	Livi Index	Corrected Weight kg
A	F	70	167	58	22.9	59.5
B	F	84	154	70	26.4	62.3
C	M	69	173	78	24.3	75.4
D	F	63	160	52	23.0	53.0
F	F	59	152	55	24.7	52.3
H	M	69	175	86	24.9	81.0
I	M	65	181	63	21.7	68.2
J	M	75	177	63	22.2	66.7
K	M	75	171	55	21.9	59.0
L	M	71	175	85	25.1	79.6
M	M	68	165	62	24.0	60.7
N	M	54	184	86	24.0	84.2
O	M	70	160	79	26.8	69.5
R	M	80	180	82	25.1	86.1
S	M	79	164	64	24.4	61.6
T	F	79	144	44	23.7	43.6
V	M	61	162	50	22.7	51.8
W	M	85	170	68	24.0	66.6
X	F	54	162	56	23.6	55.8
Y	M	74	175	100	26.5	88.6
Z	M	67	167	58	23.2	58.8

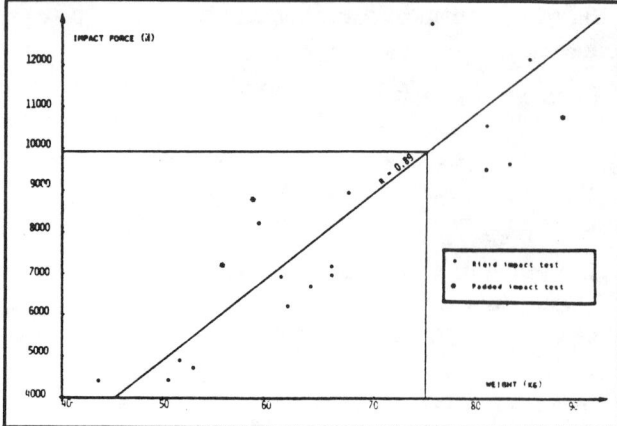

Figure 3. Corrected cadaver weight versus 3 ms injury producing impact force.

The value of impact force calculated for a weight of 75 kg, which is the weight of the 50th percentile male, is 9830 N, which is higher than the mean value for the cadavers used in this study.

During the test we recorded also pelvic acceleration; the values of 3 ms pelvic acceleration are listed in Table 2. All the values recorded are low and much under the proposed tolerance of 100 g's (7). This is probably due to the test methodology: in the impactor test only the pelvis is impacted and no other part of the body is restrained, whereas in drop tests and in sled or car tests, several areas of the body are involved by the impact.

The value of impact speed necessary to produce fractures is in the same order of magnitude as the door velocity change in car-to-car tests in which pelvic fractures occur (8). In these tests, the impact speed producing pelvic injuries varies from 22 km/h to 50 km/h.

Nineteen cadavers sustained following impacts at increasing speed, until five of them got a pelvic fracture at the first impact. Comparison of results shows that several following tests at increasing speed do not change the capability of the cadaver to sustain impacts: the traces of recorded parameters are not changed after the first impact. The value of impact force always increases until the fracture occurs, and, in fact, the value of fracture impact force was lower for cadavers which sustained only one impact than for cadavers which got a pelvic fracture after several tests.

PADDED IMPACTOR TESTS

Five tests with a padded impactor were performed on three cadavers. For these tests the impactor extremity was covered by a polyurethane foam parallelepipedic block (14.5 cm thick, 24.7 cm long, 14.5 cm wide, density 130 kg/m³). These blocks were developed by APR as paddings for side impact protection. Two of them sustained an AIS 3 pelvic fracture after the second test,

Table 5.

	Rigid	Padded	Gain
Average impact speed (km/h)	37.1	52.6	40%

whereas the third one sustained only one test which produces an AIS 2 injury. The impact force values recorded on the impactor were in the same order of magnitude as those recorded during rigid impactor test. But the impactor speed necessary to produce pelvic fracture is undoubtedly increased by the padding; all the cadavers in padding tests sustained more than 52 km/h whereas the average value of impact speed in rigid impactor tests in which the injuries occurred in 37.1 km/h. These results are summarized in Table 5.

PELVIC BONE CHARACTERISTICS

For 10 of the 22 cadavers used in impactor tests, we have determined the value of parameters related to the bone structure. For this we have cut a slice of the 2 rami of half a pelvis. We took macro pictures of these bone slices and from the scaled pictures we determined the total and cortical bone sections and the inertia momentum of these sections.

This was made with a computer which was used to digitize the outlines of the section and to make the calculations. The results of these parameters are included in Table 6.

The pubic rami are mainly involved in a bending process during a lateral impact; the stress at the fracture is defined by:

$$\sigma = \frac{P.L.Y}{Ix}$$

in which P is the force applied to the ramus, L the length of the ramus, Y the distance between the center of mass and the external surface of the ramus, and Ix the inertia momentum of the cortical area. As P is proportional to the impactor force and the variation of L is small the stress and the fracture could be written:

$$\sigma = KF \frac{Y}{Ix}$$

and then it would exist a linear relationship between F and $\frac{Y}{Ix}$. This relationship is drawn on Figure 4 which shows a good correlation.

However the values of geometrical parameters of the iliopubic ramus of the 50th percentile male have to be known to determine the human tolerance of this percentile. The geometry of human pelvis have been measured recently (9). The specific points for which coordinates

Table 6.

TBF	Ramus	S_t mm2	S_c mm2	I_x mm4	I_y mm4	Ymini mm	I_x/Ymini mm3
C	ilio	311.5	98.6	3349.8	4946.7	8.41	398
	ischio	281	85.3	1417.6	7175.7	5.64	251
H	ilio	250.2	86	2145.4	3193.3	7.32	293
	ischio	136.4	47.6	417.7	1713.4	4.30	87
K	ilio	217.5	66.7	1306.7	3048.9	5.65	231
	ischio	160.1	42.6	359.8	2615.5	3.58	100
N	ilio	256.5	96.7	2286.2	4496.2	7.82	292
	ischio	202.4	65.2	564.8	1170.6	5.59	101
O	ilio	159.3	53.3	1199.8	1530.4	6.32	190
	ischio	112.3	32.4	248.2	1013.3	3.44	72
S	ilio	265.8	66	1748.2	3505.4	8.32	210
	ischio	165.6	43.3	687.5	1466.03	5.66	121
T	ilio	139.9	45.5	672.1	1105.3	5.91	115
	ischio	100.2	32.7	193.2	1093.4	3.20	60
X	ilio	178.4	61.7	1166.9	1722.3	5.91	204
	ischio	148.7	43.4	381.8	1856.7	3.32	115
Y	ilio	248.4	94.5	2450.4	4284.8	7.93	309
	ischio	137.1	49.7	600	1288.1	5.66	106
Z	ilio	225.9	67.3	1790.5	3006.1	6.86	261
	ischio	167.3	44.9	761.6	2382.3	4.82	159

were measured were on the exterior surface and thus it is not possible to determine the inertia momentum of the ramus section but by comparing the external dimensions, the inertia momentum of the iliopubic ramus cross section can be evaluated. The found value is $I_x = 2300$ mm^4 and the distance between the center of mass and the external surface y = 7,8 mm, for the 50th percentile. The corresponding value of I_x/y would be 295 mm^3, which corresponds to approximately 10 kN for the 3 ms impact force.

PROPOSED PROTECTION CRITERION

On the basis of the test results described behind the tolerance for a cadaver weighing 75 kg would be about 10 KN 3 ms impact force. This value would be the base for a protection criterion applied to a 50th percentile dummy. The use of such a protection criterion implies that the side impact dummies are able to be fitted with a pelvic lateral force transducer. At the present time only one side impact dummy type, manufactured by the MIRA, is fitted with pelvic force transducers.

This pelvis is equipped with 3 force transducers needing 5 measurement channels and the use of this dummy in several test environments (car-to-car tests, sled tests, impactor tests) have shown the feasibility of the measurement of pelvic lateral force in side impact; but as most of the injuries are located on the pubic rami it seems possible to simplify the force measurement device, and to use only one force transducer located in the anterior part of the pelvis.

CONCLUSIONS

Analysis of these test results allows to conclude as follows:

— impactor tests reproduced realistic pelvic injuries at realistic impact speed
— these injuries are mainly impacted side ischio and ilio-pubic rami fractures
— the impact force seems more correlated to injury than other parameters
— the value of the tolerable impact force varies greatly with anthropometry
— there is a correlation between the geometry of the ischio pubic ramus cross section and the tolerable impact force
— the use of a padding can protect efficiently by increasing the acceptable impact speed. A gain of 40% has been found
— the value of the tolerance is close to 10 KN of 3 ms impact force for the 50th percentile male subjects
— a protection criterion for pelvis based on the 10 KN tolerance could be used on a dummy fitted with a pelvic lateral force transducer.

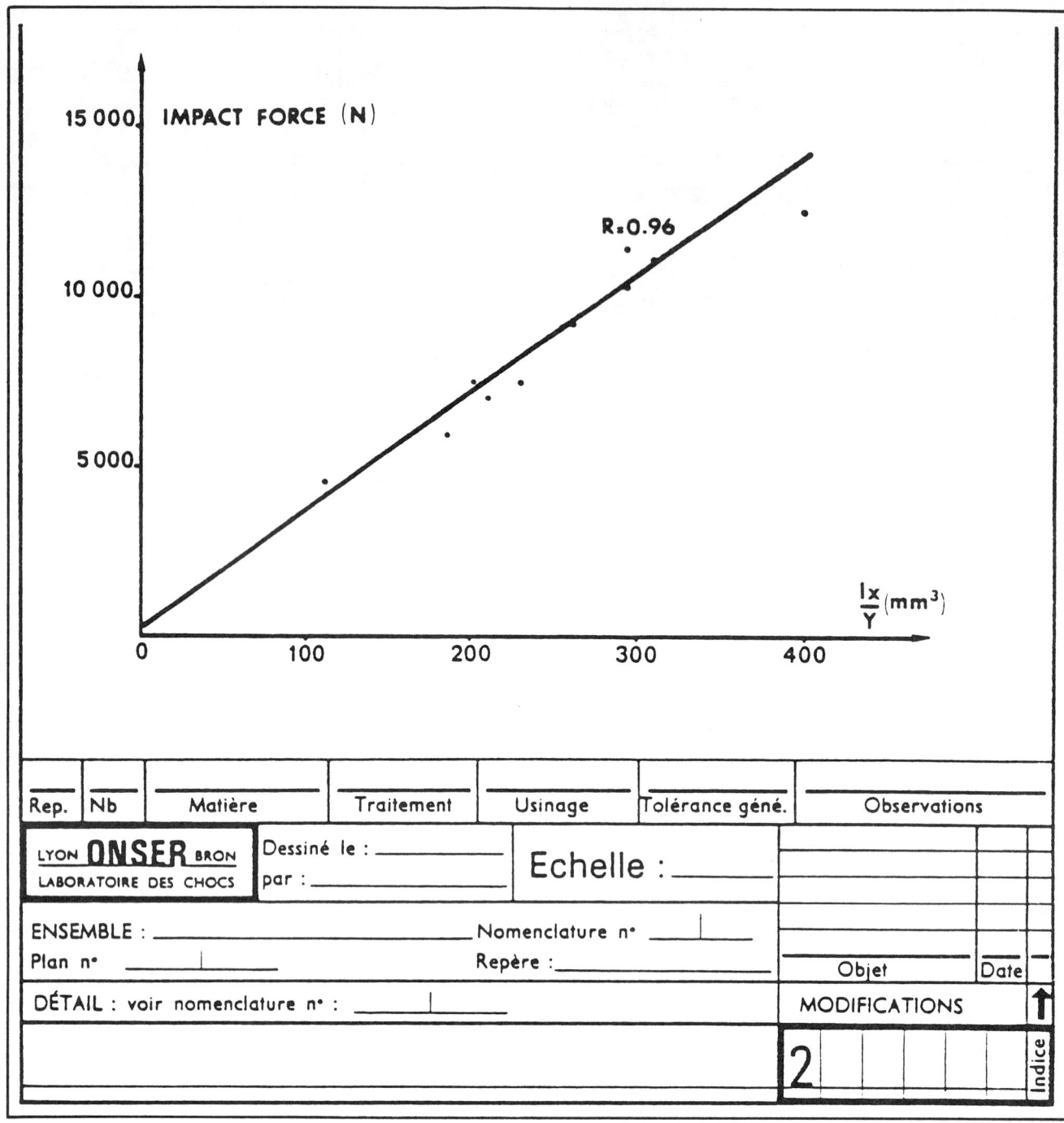

Figure 4. Injury producing impact force versus Ix/y of the ilio-pubic ramus.

REFERENCES

1. Davis, S., Ragland, C. Development of a deformable side impact moving barrier 8th International Conference on ESV, Wolfsburg 1980.
2. EEVC WG7 report-structures. Improved side impact Protection in Europe. 9th ESV Conference Kyoto—Nov. 1982.
3. Cesari, D., Ramet, M., Clair, P. Y. Evaluation of pelvic fracture tolerance in side impact 24th Stapp Car Crash conf., 1980.
4. Dejeammes, N. Fractures du bassin au cours des chocs latéraux automobiles. Thèse LYON 1978.
5. Creyssel, J., Schnepp, J. Fractures tanscotyloïdiennes du bassin, MASSON Ed, 1961.
6. Harris, J. The design and use of the TRRL side impact dummy 20th Stapp Car Crash conf. Oct. 18–20, 1976, 77–106.

7. Joint biomechanical research project KOB. Unfall-und Sicherheitsforschung Strassenverkehr. N° 34, BAST 1982.
8. Cesari, D., Ramet, M., Herry-Martin, D. Injury mechanism in side impact. 22nd Stapp Car Crash conf. Oct. 24–26, 1978, 429–448.
9. Reynolds, H. M., Snow, C. C., Young, J. W. Spatial Geometry of the Human Pelvis. Unpublished.

831634

Human Response to an Injury from Lateral Impact

Jeffrey H. Marcus, Richard M. Morgan, and Rolf H. Eppinger
National Highway Safety Administration

Dimitrios Kallieris, Rainer Mattern, and Georg Schmidt
University of Heidelberg

ABSTRACT

Lateral impacts have been shown to produce a large portion of both serious and fatal injuries within the total automotive crash problem. These injuries are produced as a result of the rapid changes in velocity that an automobile occupant's body experiences during a crash. In an effort to understand the mechanisms of these injuries, an experimental program using human surrogates (cadavers) was initiated. Initial impact velocity and compliance of the lateral impacting surface were the primary test features that were controlled, while age of the test specimen was varied to assess its influence on the injury outcome. Instrumentation consisted of 24 accelerometer channels on the subjects along with contact forces measured on the wall both at the thoracic and pelvic level.

The individual responses and resulting injuries sustained by 11 new subjects tested at the University of Heidelberg are presented in detail. An examination of the relationship between forces applied and responses observed in the thorax is discussed.

The average injuries for different sled test conditions are presented based on a total of 42 cadaver tests (11 of which are the ones discussed above). The comparison of rigid wall and padded wall sled tests is made based on these average injuries.

INTRODUCTION

Cadaver sled tests at 15-, 20-, and 25-mph (24-, 32-, and 40- km/hr) were reported by Melvin [1].* These were rigid wall sled tests. Based on that study, Eppinger [2] proposed a method for universal thoracic trauma prediction.

In 1979, a Side Impact Dummy (SID) was developed by the Highway Safety Research Institute (HSRI) based on biomechanical data [3]. Also, the Association Peugeot-Renault (APR) dummy was designed in France [4, 5]. Several injury criteria were proposed for side impact protection, including the "B parameter" computed from the rib acceleration data [6], power computed from the spine acceleration data [7], and deflection of the thorax [8].

The following year, work continued on the APR dummy and the thoracic deflection criteria [9],
and on the power and "B parameter" criteria [10]. There were comparisons of the SID and the APR dummy in experimental tests [10, 11].

Cadaver pendulum tests were conducted by a team led by Cesari [12]. Other research developed the "cumulative variance" technique [13] which allows objective judgment of a dummy's instrumentation signal magnitude and "signature" response to a test. Additional side impact sled tests with cadavers were conducted at the University of Heidelberg [14]. A dynamic characterization of the human thorax in the form of a digital impulsive response signature was obtained [15]. This signature linked the acceleration response of the struck side with the far side of the thorax under side impact conditions.

Burgett summarized the state-of-knowledge of side impact protection in a 1982 paper [16]. One of the French teams continued work on the development of a protection criteria and introduced a bone characterization factor as an indicator of thoracic injury resistance [17, 18].

Cesari conducted impactor tests (55 were with a rigid surface and 5 with a padded surface) against the pelvis of human cadavers [19].

---

*Numbers in brackets denote references cited at the end of paper.

The injuries were mostly impacted side pubic rami fractures. A protection criterion for the pelvis based on force was proposed.

Eppinger [20] proposed the use of fatality rate for use in the formulation of predictive equations for thoracic injury. Based on 30 cadaver tests, peak acceleration of the struck side rib along with age proved the best in predicting fatality rate, which is a function of the two highest AIS values in the body region.

DESCRIPTION OF CADAVER DATA SET

In the majority of the studies discussed in References 1 through 20, unembalmed human cadavers were impacted on the thorax, pelvis, or both. Those studies sponsored by the National Highway Traffic Safety Administration had the 12 accelerometer array [3] on the thorax but no deflection gauge or force measuring apparatus. The pelvis had a triaxis accelerometer array but no force measuring provisions. In this current paper, the data for eleven cadaver sled tests conducted at the University of Heidelberg--most of which measured force at the thorax and pelvis--are presented.

The sled is modeled after that designed by HSRI (now TRI) and is described in Reference 21. Load cells were placed in the wall fixture such that the only forces which could be measured by the load cells were those due to the test subject. (There is a small inertia force which is over by the time the cadaver contacts the plates.) There is a separate plate for both the thorax and the pelvis. Figure 1 shows the seat and plate dimensions for the University of Heidelberg sled.

The eleven new cadaver tests are summarized in Table 1. Force gauges were installed for all of the tests. Most of the headings in Table 1 are self explanatory. The symbol $AIS1_T$ means the most severe injury in terms of an AIS value for the thorax, i.e., that part of the body including the rib cage (but not the vertebral column, according to the AIS manual) and those organs and structures above the diaphragm. The symbol $AIS2_T$ denotes the second most severe injury for the thorax. The AIS hard thorax (AIS_{HT}) includes--in addition to the standard thoracic injuries--injuries to the thoracic spine and those abdominal structures that lie within the rib cage, specifically, the liver, spleen, and kidney [20].

For three of the cadaver impact tests in Table 1, APR padding was placed on the front of the thorax and pelvis force gauge plates. This padding and another of fiberglass material have been used to study the response of cadavers to force attenuating materials. The APR padding--supplied by the Association Peugeot-Renault--is an open cell foam approximately 5.5 inches in thickness. The fiberglass padding, made as a honeycomb structure, is approximately 3.5 inches thick. Force-versus-deflection curves of both these padding materials are found in Reference 22 (pp. 305, 322, and 323).

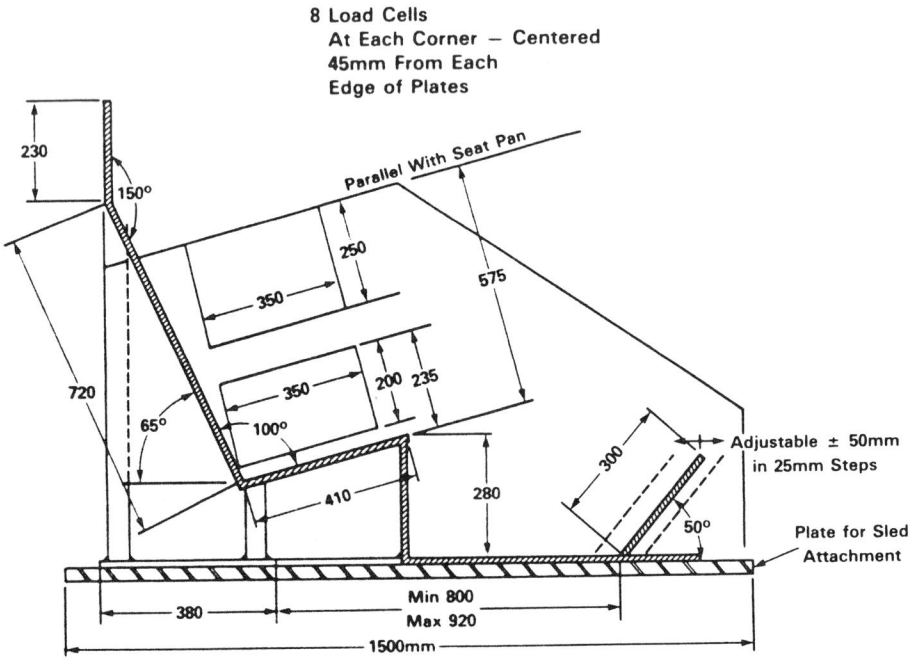

Figure 1 - University of Heidelberg force measuring sled

Table 1 - Eleven University of Heidelberg Side Impact Sled Tests

Test No.	Test Velocity (mph)&	Test Type*	Age (Years)	Sex	Weight (kg)	Height (cm)	AIS1T**	AIS2T	AIS1HT	AIS2HT	NFR***	AIS Pelvis
H-82008	19.6 (31.5)	PW	61	M	99	172	4	1	5	4	10	0
H-82009	25.3 (40.7)	RW	27	F	51	166	5	4	5	4	13	3
H-82012	25.3 (40.7)	RW	17	M	75	172	5	4	5	5	9	0
H-82014	20.3 (32.7)	RW	22	F	61	178	4	3	5	4	12	3
H-82015	14.6 (23.5)	RW	18	M	69	182	1	0	1	0	2	0
H-82016	19.6 (31.5)	RW	21	M	50	187	3	2	2	2	8	0
H-82018	14.6 (23.5)	RW	28	F	85	181	3	2	3	2	9	0
H-82019	14.6 (23.5)	RW	47	F	67	165	3	2	3	2	7	0
H-82020	19.6 (31.5)	RW	41	M	73	180	4	2	5	4	11	2
H-82021	20.3 (32.7)	PW	48	M	99	180	4	3	4	3	13	0
H-82022	20.3 (32.7)	PW	50	M	77	167	4	2	4	4	15	0

* - RW - Rigid Wall
    PW - APR Padded Wall
** AIS values in terms of 1980 manual.
*** NFR = Number of Fractured Ribs. Maximum possible value is 24.
AIS1T = most severe injury in thorax.
AIS2T = second most severe injury in thorax.
AIS1HT = most severe injury in hard thorax.
AIS2HT = second most severe injury in hard thorax.
& - Number in parenthesis is in units of km/hr.

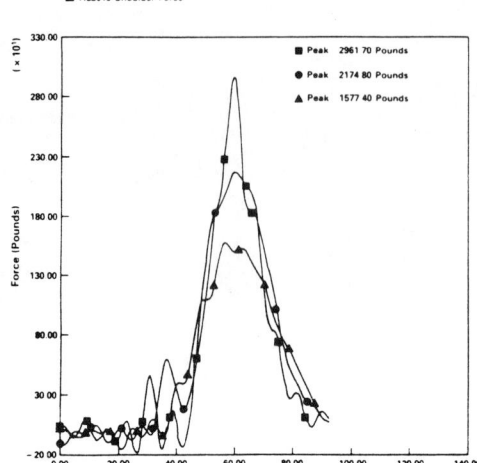

Figure 2 - Shoulder force for 15 mph rigid wall

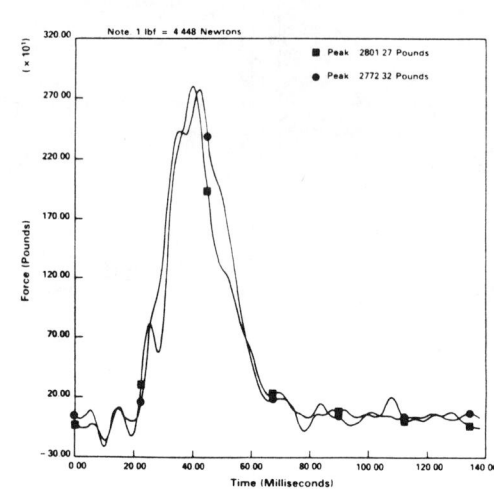

Figure 3 - Shoulder force for 20 mph rigid wall

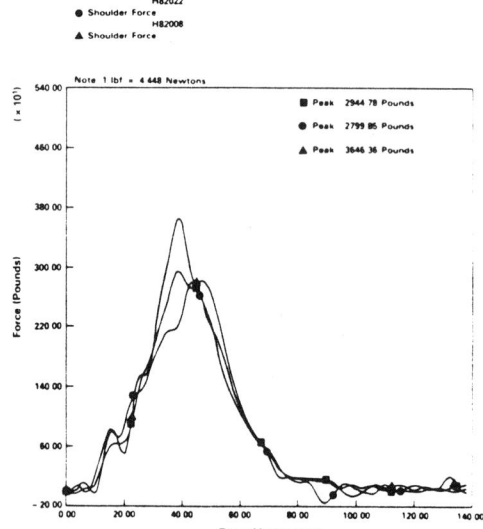

Figure 4 - Shoulder force for 20 mph APR padding

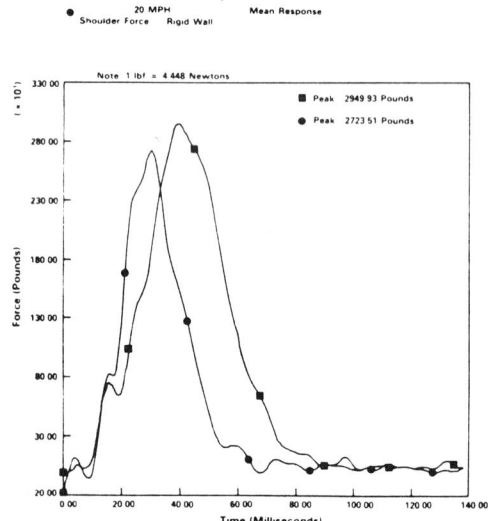

Figure 5 - Shoulder force for both APR padding and rigid wall at 20 mph

PRESENTATION OF CADAVER RESPONSES

The cadaver tests listed in Table 1 can be classified according to four sled test conditions: (1) 15 mph (24 km/hr) rigid wall, (2) 20 mph (32 km/hr) rigid wall, (3) 25 mph (40 km/hr) rigid wall, and (4) 20 mph (32 km/hr) APR padded wall. The force-versus-time readings for three 15 mph (24 km/hr) rigid wall tests are shown in Figure 2. The curves are actual observed data and are not scaled for either anthropometric or inertial differences among test subjects. The digitization and filtering used on these curves and throughout this paper are to the same specifications as described in References [10, 20] (100 Hz low pass filter, 1600 Hz sampling rate). The mean curve for these three signals has a peak value of 2,238 pounds.

The weight and anthropometry of test subject H82015 is almost identical to that of H82019. It shall be shown later in this paper that the percentage of total body mass which interacts with the shoulder force gauge and the pelvis force guage is the same between the two tests. The impulse $\int Fdt$ of these two curves is the same. However, the maximum value for these two shoulder forces is different.

The two shoulder force curves for the 20 mph (32 km/hr) rigid wall sled test are presented in Figure 3. (Force curves for test H82020 do not exist.) The mean force signal has a peak of 2,452 pounds. The three shoulder force curves in Figure 4 are for 20 mph (32 km/hr) sled tests with APR padding material. When the APR padding material was installed over the face of the rigid wall for the 20 mph (32 km/hr) sled test, the time for completion of the shoulder force curve was increased roughly 44 percent as can be seen in Figure 5.

Finally, the shoulder force versus time for one subject in a 25 mph (40 km/hr) rigid wall sled test is presented in Figure 6.

In general, the shoulder force curves in Figures 2 through 5 show large variability. In addition, the mean APR padding curve in Figure 5 shows a higher force level than the mean force curve for the rigid wall tests.

Examination of the weight and anthropometry shows that each of the APR padding test subjects is heavier and has greater anthropometric values (e.g., chest depth and chest circumference) than either of the rigid wall test subjects. Clearly, some form of scaling is in order to permit valid comparisons. A number of scaling procedures are available to normalize the cadaver data to represent a standard size occupant. One method of general geometric scaling using the subject mass and chest depth did successfully reduce much of the variability when scaled to the 50th percentile male. This scaling method, and its results will be discussed in a future paper.

Similarly, the force-versus-time records for the pelvis are presented in Figures 7 through 10. Figure 9 is interesting

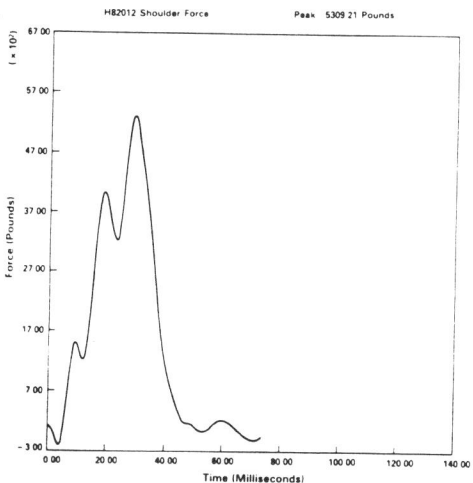

Figure 6 - Shoulder force for 25 mph rigid wall

because--based on the mass of the test subjects--it would seem that the peak pelvic force for test H82008 should be closer to 3000 pounds as test H82021 is. This is explained by calculations (to be shown later in this paper) that show 24 percent of the total body mass for H82008 interacted with the pelvic force gauge while 29 percent of the total body mass interacted for H82021.

Cesari [19], based on impacts to the pelvis of seated cadavers, developed a functional relationship between impact force at fracture and the cadaver weight, corrected by the Livi index. This relationship is:

$$F = 43.58 \left(\frac{23.5}{Li}\right) W_a - 1058.94, \quad (1)$$

where

F = impact force in pounds,
Li = Livi index = $10 \sqrt[3]{\frac{W_a}{Ht}}$,
W_a = actual weight in kg,
Ht = height in meters.

Cesari indicated that the region above the line defined by equation (1) should be the fracture region while the area below should contain the non-fracture region.

The Livi index and corrected weight for the University of Heidelberg sled tests are shown in Table 2. The Livi index is used to quantify how close a subject's weight is to normal for a given stature. Reference 19 uses the following

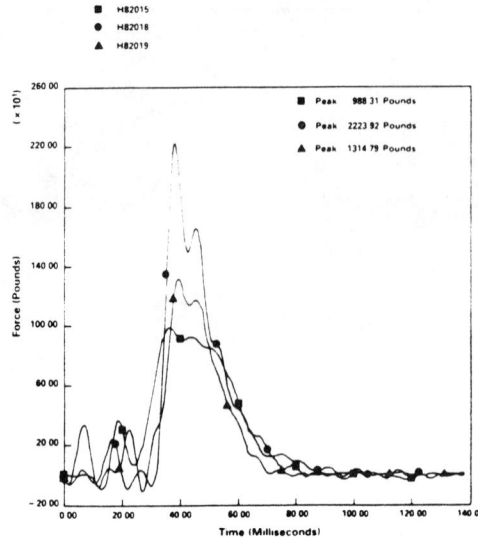

Figure 7 - Pelvic force for 15 mph rigid wall

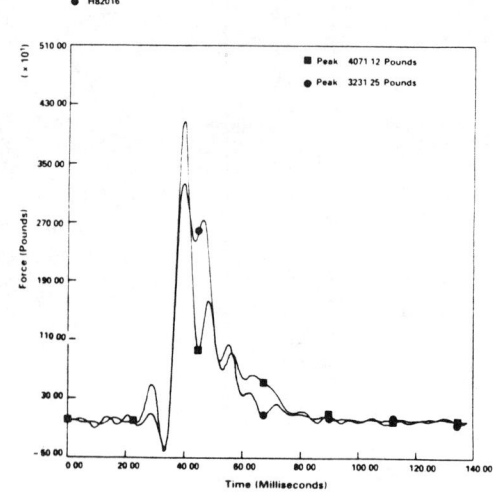

Figure 8 - Pelvic force for 20 mph rigid wall

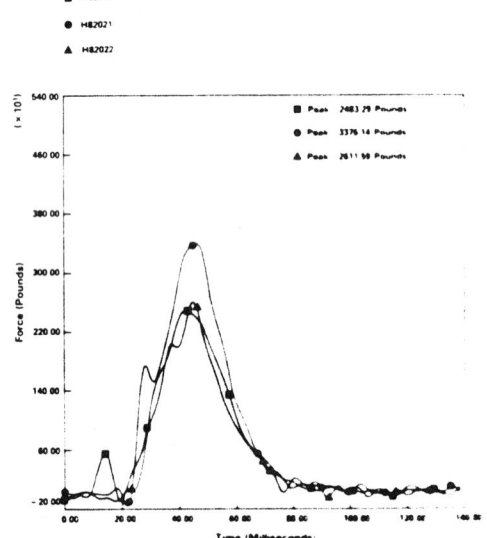

Figure 9 - Pelvic force for 20 mph APR padding

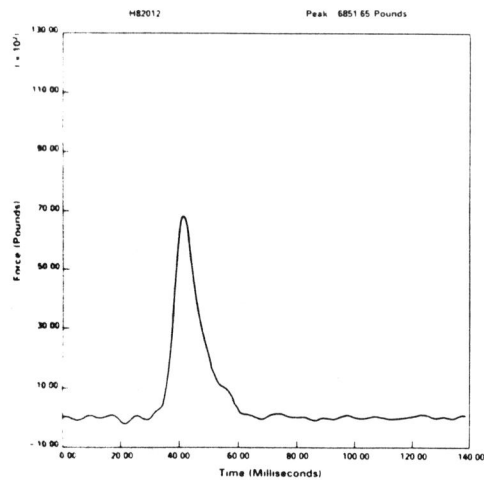

Figure 10 - Pelvic force for 25 mph rigid wall

ranges for the Livi index:

Li ≤ 22-subject is very thin;
22 < Li ≤ 23-subject is thin;
23 < Li ≤ 24-subject is normal;
24 < Li ≤ 25-subject is stout; and
Li > 25-subject is obese.

Figure 11 shows a plot of impact force on the pelvis versus corrected weight. (The force values shown in Figure 11 are derived from 3 millisecond clips of the "raw" data as specified in Reference 19.) The line from equation 1 is shown. Although it would be desirable to have more fracture data, Figure 11 suggests that the Cesari criterion may be conservative for the sled test condition. Cesari points out that in his methodology only the pelvis is impacted by the impactor and no other part of the body is restrained.

The cumulative effect of the wall force can be measured by integrating force over time, $\int F \, dt$, which produces the change in momentum. The integral of the shoulder force divided by the change in velocity ($\triangle V$) of the thorax should give an indication of what proportion of the total body mass is interacting with the shoulder force gauge. The same is true for the pelvic force guage. The results of these calculations are shown in Table 3. The $\triangle V$ of the body segment is based on the integral of the medial-lateral component of the acceleration. For the pelvis, this extraction is straight forward. For the thorax, at least three accelerometer locations were examined to estimate the one thoracic $\triangle V$ shown in Table 3. Approximately, 46 percent of the total body mass goes into the shoulder force gauge, and 28 percent of the total body mass goes into the pelvic force gauge. Thus, 74 percent of the total body mass impacts the shoulder force and pelvic force gauges. According to Reference 23, about 71.7 percent of the total body weight is found in the head, neck, torso, and total arm. As to the remaining body weight, the legs strike the sled wall and not a force gauge.

AVERAGE INJURY FOR SLED TEST CONDITION

Currently, the entire sled data base consists of 29 human cadaver subjects into rigid walls, 7 subjects into APR padding at 20 mph (32.2 km/hr), and 6 subjects into the fiberglass padding at 20 mph (32.2 km/hr).

Table 2 - Livi Index and Corrected Weight

Test No	Li	$W_c = W_a \frac{23.5}{Li}$ (Kg)
H82008	26.9	86.5
H82009	22.3	53.6
H82012	24.5	71.9
H82014	22.1	64.9
H82015	22.5	72.0
H82016	19.7	59.6
H82018	24.3	82.2
H82019	24.6	64.0
H82020	23.2	73.9
H82021	25.7	90.5
H82022	25.5	71.0

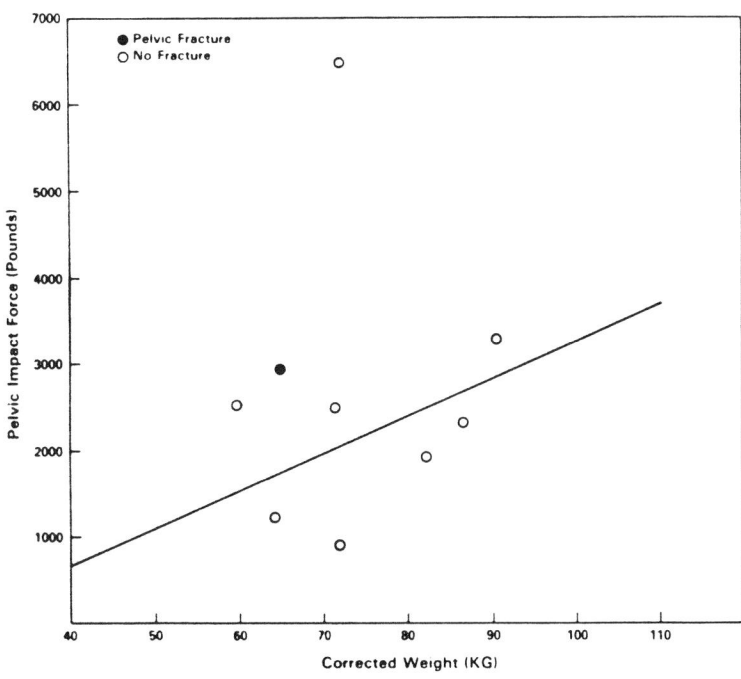

Figure 11 - Corrected cadaver weight versus pelvic impact force

Table 3 - Proportion of Total Body Mass Interacting with Force Gauges

Test No.	Test Velocity* (mph)	Thoracic ΔV^* (mph)	Pelvic ΔV^* (mph)	Calculated Shoulder Gauge Mass/ Total Mass	Calculated Pelvic Gauge Mass/Total Mass
H82008	19.6 (31.5)	24 (39)	32 (52)	.46	.24
H82012	25.3 (40.7)	29 (47)	37 (60)	.50	.27
H82014	20.3 (32.7)	24 (39)	28 (45)	.44	.27
H82015	14.6 (23.5)	18 (29)	19 (31)	.43	.24
H82016	19.6 (31.5)	20.6 (33)	25 (40)	.58	.39
H82018	14.6 (23.5)	19.5 (31)	18 (29)	.36	.26
H82019	14.6 (23.5)	16.6 (27)	18 (29)	.44	.25
H82021	20.3 (32.7)	22 (35)	34 (55)	.45	.29
H82022	20.3 (32.7)	26 (42)	28 (45)	.45	.31

*NOTE: Numbers in parenthesis are in units of km/hr.

A summary of pertinent data from these 42 tests is given in the Appendix in Table A1. (Most of these tests have been reported in detail in previous studies and shall not be discussed further herein.) Considering injury severity as the observed thoracic AIS (1980 manual) the average thoracic AIS for each test condition was calculated and is given in Table 4.

The injury severity values in Table 4 are not adjusted for age. However, accident statistics and experimental efforts suggest injury severity increases as age increases for the same impact level [24, 25]. Since, the average age in two of the five conditions (25 mph rigid wall and 20 mph fiberglass pad) is significantly less than the other, it appears that some form of age compensation of injury severity is required before definitive conclusions can be drawn about differences between the various test conditions.

Figure 12 is a scatter diagram presenting the thoracic injury severity of all 42 cadaver tests by age. Admittedly, there is a great deal of scatter in this figure. However, by considering the individual tests within a particular test type, an estimation of the sensitivity of injury severity with respect to age was made. It appears that there is an increase of approximately 0.025 $AIS1_T$ for each year of age. This is consistent with the results derived from accident data in Reference 24 for ΔV between 13 and 24 mph.

Table 4 - Average $AIS1_T$ for 5 Sled Test Conditions

Test Type	Average $AIS1_T$*	Standard Deviation	Ave Age
15 mph (24 km/hr) Rigid Wall	2.0	1.05	41.9
20 mph (32 km/hr) Rigid Wall	3.46	1.33	46.7
25 mph (40 km/hr) Rigid Wall	4.17	.98	32.3
20 mph (32 km/hr) APR Padding	2.43	1.62	43.4
20 mph (32 km/hr) Fiberglass Padding	.67	1.03	39.7

* $AIS1_T$ = most severe injury in thorax.

Using this trend and normalizing to 45 years following Neathery [26], adjusted cadaver injury level are presented in Table 5. The normalizing was accomplished by setting the normalized thoracic AIS equal to the actual AIS minus the expression .025(Age-45). Consequently, the actual thoracic AIS was adjusted upwards for younger subjects and downward for older subjects.

Table 5 - Average AIS1$_T$ for 5 Sled Test Conditions as Normalized to 45 Years

Test Type	Average AIS1$_T$*	Standard Deviation
15 mph (24 km/hr) Rigid Wall	2.08	1.05
20 mph (32 km/hr) Rigid Wall	3.42	1.12
25 mph (40 km/hr) Rigid Wall	4.48	.95
20 mph (32 km/hr) APR Padding	2.47	1.33
20 mph (32 km/hr) Fiberglass Padding	.81	1.09

*AIS1$_T$ = most severe injury in thorax.

Looking at Average AIS1$_T$ normalized to 45 years of age, it can be seen that the average injury level increases from 2.08 to 3.42 and 4.48 for the 15, 20, and 25 mph rigid wall test respectively. The addition of the APR pad to the 20 mph test condition, reduces the average injury level to almost the level observed in the 15 mph rigid wall. Remarkably, the average thoracic injury level for the 20 mph (32 km/hr) sled tests with fiberglass padding is slightly less than one, based on six subjects.

Using the standard Student's "t" distribution method [27] where one sample is considered superior to the other (one-tailed statistical test), the 20-mph sled tests were examined. The hypothesis that the population means for the APR and FBGIS are the same as the rigid wall could not be rejected at the 0.05 level. A similar hypothesis for the fiberglass pads and the rigid wall was rejected at greater than the 0.0005 level. Testing the sameness between the population means of the APR padding and the fiberglass padding tests resulted in the observed value of t falling in the rejection region at the 0.05 level. This suggests that, based on the available data and adjustments made to it, the fiberglass pad has greater injury attenuating capability than the APR pad. The impressive performance of the fiberglass pad indeed that additional testing be pursued to further substantiate these observed differences.

For completeness, a similar analysis is carried out in the Appendix for both number of fractured ribs and AIS1 for the hard thorax.

CONCLUSIONS

1. Force-versus-time curves were provided for the following side impact sled tests: (a) 15 mph (24 km/hr) rigid wall, (b) 20 mph (32 km/hr) rigid wall, (c) 25 mph (40 km/hr) rigid wall, and 20 mph (24 km/hr) APR padded wall. Because of the variability in the data and the fact that some test modes had significantly heavier subjects than others, some scaling procedure is needed to make direct comparisons between various test conditions. Work on an appropriate scaling procedure continues.

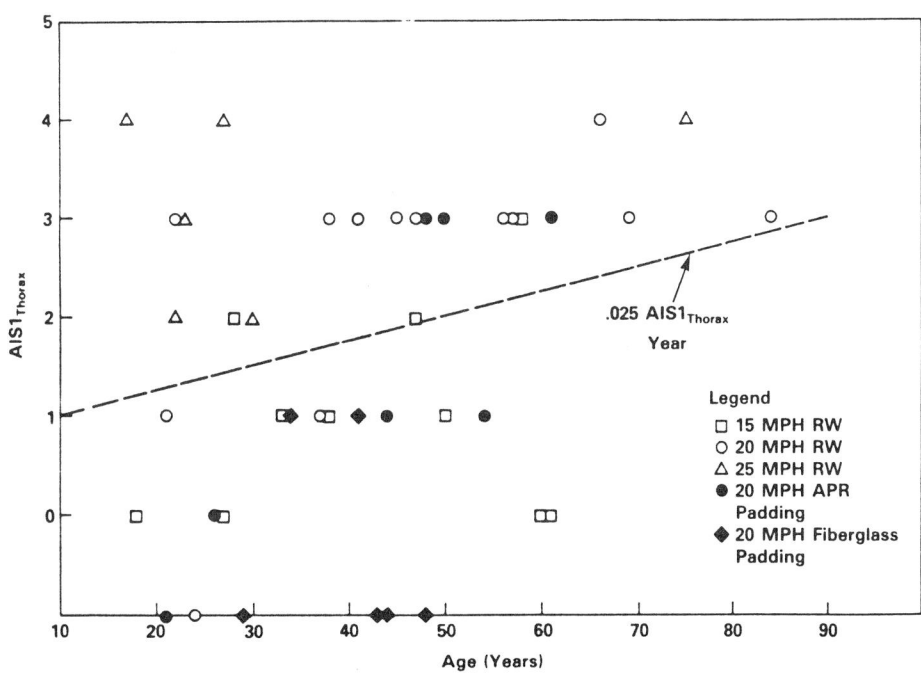

Figure 12 - Injury for 42 side impact cadaver tests

2. Impulse calculations suggest that 46 percent of the total body mass is picked up by the shoulder force gauge and 28 percent of the total body mass by the pelvic force gauge.

3. As would be expected when comparing a padded impact to an impact with a rigid wall at 20 mph the pulse length of the shoulder force from an APR pad test is longer than the pulse length from a rigid wall test.

4. Based on nine cadaver tests, it appears that the Cesari pelvic force criterion may be conservative for the side impact sled test condition.

5. When adjusted for age, the 15-, 20-, and 25-mph (24-, 32-, and 40- km/hr) rigid wall sled tests have an average cadaver thoracic AIS of 2.1, 3.4, and 4.5 respectively. When the wall is padded with APR padding or with fiberglass padding for 20-mph sled tests, the average cadaver thoracic AIS decreases to 2.5 and 0.8 respectively.

DISCLAIMER - The views presented are those of the authors and not necessarily those of the National Highway Traffic Safety Administration.

ACKNOWLEDGEMENTS - The efforts of Diane Carroll in organizing our test specification data, and Reginald McAllister in entering tests into the NHTSA data base are gratefully acknowledged. And finally, but not for the efforts of Beulah Evans, this document would never have been typed.

REFERENCES:

1. Melvin, J.W., Robbins, D.H., and Stalnaker, R.L., "Side Impact Response and Injury," Sixth International Technical Conference on Experimental Safety Vehicles, October 1976.

2. Eppinger, R.H., Augustyn, K., and Robbins, D.H., "Development of a Promising Universal Thoracic Trauma Prediction Methodology," Twenty-Second Stapp Car Crash Conference, October 1978.

3. Melvin, J.W., Robbins, D.H., and Benson, J.B., "Experimental Application of Advanced Thoracic Instrumentation Techniques to Anthropomorphic Test Devices," Seventh International Technical Conference on Experimental Safety Vehicles, June 1979.

4. Fayon, A., Leung, Y.C., Stalnaker, R.L., Walfisch, G., Balthazard, M., and Terriere, C., "Presentation of a Frontal Impact and Side Impact Dummy, Defined from Human Data and Realized from a 'Part 572' Basis," Seventh International Technical Conference on Experimental Safety Vehicles, June 1979.

5. Stalnaker, R.L., Tarriere, C., Fayon, A., Walfisch, G., Balthazard, M., Masset, J., Got, C., and Patel, A., "Modification of Part 572 Dummy for Lateral Impact According to Biomechanical Data," Twenty-Third Stapp Car Crash Conference, October 1979.

6. Robbins, D.H. and Lehman, R.J., "Prediction of Thoracic Injuries as a Function of Occupant Kinematics," Seventh International Technical Conference on Experimental Safety Vehicles, June 1979.

7. Burgett, A., and Hackney, J.R., "Status of the National Highway Traffic Safety Administration Research and Rulemaking Activities for Upgrading Side Impact Protection," Seventh International Technical Conference on Experimental Safety Vehicles, June 1979.

8. Tarriere, C., Walfisch, G., Fayon, A., Rosey, J.P., Got, C., Patel, A., and Delmas, A., "Synthesis of Human Tolerance Obtained from Lateral Impact Simulations," Seventh International Technical Conference on Experimental Safety Vehicles, June 1979.

9. Fayon, A., Tarriere, C., Walfisch, G., Duprey, M., and Balthazard, M., "Development and Performance of the APR Dummy (APROD)," Eighth International Technical Conference on Experimental Safety Vehicles, October 1980.

10. Morgan, R.M., and Waters, H.P., "Comparison of Two Promising Side Impact Dummies," Eighth International Technical Conference on Experimental Safety Vehicles, October 1980.

11. Mellander, H., and Bohlin, N., "A Comparison Between Different Dummies in Car-to-Car Side Impacts, "Eighth International Technical Conference on Experimental Safety Vehicles, October 1980.

12. Cesari, D., Ramet, M., and Bloch, J., "Influence of Arm Position on Thoracic Injuries in Side Impact." Twenty-Fifth Stapp Car Crash Conference, September 1981.

13. Morgan, R.M., Marcus, J.H., and Eppinger, R.H., "Correlation of Side Impact Dummy/Cadaver Tests," Twenty-Fifth Stapp Car Crash Conference, September 1981.

14. Kallieris, D., Mattern, R., Schmidt, G., and Eppinger, R.H., "Quantification of Side Impact Responses and Injuries," Twenty-Fifth Stapp Car Crash Conference, September 1981.

15. Eppinger, R.H., and Chan, H.S., "Thoracic Injury Prediction via Digital Convolution Theory," Twenty-Fifth Stapp Car Crash Conference, September 1981.

16. Burgett, A., and Brubaker, W., "The Role of the Side of the Motor Vehicle in Crash Prediction," SAE Publication No. 820245, International Congress and Exposition, Detroit, Michigan, February 1982.

17. Walfisch, G., Chamouard, F., Lestrelin, D., Fayon, A., Terriere, C., Got, C., Guillon, F., Patel, A., and Hureau, J., "Tolerance Limits and Mechanical Characteristics of the Human Thorax in Frontal and Side Impact and Transposition of these Characteristics into Protection Criteria," IRCOBI Conference, Cologne, Germany, September 1982.

18. Sacreste, J., Brun-Cassan, F., Fayon, A., Terriere, C., Got, C., and Patel, A., "Proposal for a Thorax Tolerance Level in Side Impacts Based on 62 Tests Performed with Cadavers Having Known Bone Condition," Twenty-Sixth Stapp Car Crash Conference, October 1982.

19. Cesari, D., and Ramet, M., "Pelvic Tolerance and Protection Criteria in Side Impact," Twenty-Sixth Stapp Car Crash Conference, October 1982.

20. Eppinger, R.H., Morgan, R.M, and Marcus, J.H., "Side Impact Data Analysis," Ninth International Technical Conference on Experimental Safety Vehicles, November 1982.

21. Melvin, J.W., and Benson, J.B., "Calibration Procedures of Test Dummies for Side Impact Testing," Report No. DOT-HS-803 253, PB No. 278 299, March 1977.

22. Monk, M.W., Morgan, R.M., and Sullivan, L.K., "Side Impact Sled and Padding Development," Twenty-Fourth Stapp Car Crash Conference, October 1980.

23. Chandler, R.F., Clauser, C.E., McConville, J.P., Reynolds, H.M., and Young, J.W., Investigation of Inertial Properties of the Human Body, Final Report, April 1, 1972, - December 1974, AMRL-TR-74-137, Aerospace Medical Research Laboratories, Wright-Patterson Air Force Base, Dayton, Ohio.

24. Eppinger, R. H., "Considerations in Side Impact Dummy Development," Seventh International Technical Conference on Experimental Safety Vehicles, June 1979.

25. Ricci, L., "National Crash Severity Study Statistics," Report No. DOT-HS-805-227, pg. 53, October 1979.

26. Neathery, R.F., Kroell, C.K., and Mertz, H.J., "Prediction of Thoracic Injury From Dummy Responses," Nineteenth Stapp Car Crash Conference, November 1975.

27. Mendenhall, W., Introduction to Statistics, Wadsworth Publishing Company, Inc., Belmont, California, pp. 187-191, 1965.

APPENDIX - This Appendix lists previously published data and the average injury level associated with the 42 cadaver tests is shown in Table A1.

The average AIS hard thorax is shown in Table A2.

Table A2 - Average $AIS1_{HT}$

Test Type	Average $AIS1_{HT}$*	Standard Deviation
15 mph (24 km/hr) Rigid Wall	2.1	.99
20 mph (32 km/hr) Rigid Wall	3.77	1.54
25 mph (40 km/hr) Rigid Wall	4.83	.41
20 mph (32 km/hr) APR Padding	2.86	1.46
20 mph (32 km/hr) Fiberglass Padding	.67	1.03

*$AIS1_{HT}$ = most severe injury in hard thorax.

The age normalization factor is again roughly .025 $AIS1_{HT}$ for each year (see Figure A1). The average AIS hard thorax normalized to 45 years is as shown in Table A3.

Table A3 - Average $AIS1_{HT}$ Normalized to 45 Years

Test Type	Average $AIS1_{HT}$*	Standard Deviation
15 mph (24 km/hr) Rigid Wall	2.18	1.03
20 mph (32 km/hr) Rigid Wall	3.73	1.41
25 mph (40 km/hr) Rigid Wall	5.15	.6
20 mph (32 km/hr) APR Padding	2.9	1.23
20 mph (32 km/hr) Fiberglass Padding	.81	1.09

*$AIS1_{HT}$ = most severe injury in hard thorax.

Table A1 - Injury Data for 42 Cadaver Tests

Test No.	Test Velocity* (mph)	Sled Test Type	Age (Years)	AIS1T	AIS1HT	NFR	Test No.	Test Velocity* (mph)	Sled Test Type	Age (Years)	AIS1T	AIS1HT	NFR
WSU487	20.7 (33.3)	APR	54	2	2	5	H81006	19.9 (32.0)	RW	37	2	2	8
WSU488	17.0 (27.4)	RW	58	4	4	7	H81011	19.9 (32.0)	FP	43	0	0	0
WSU489	20.0 (32.2)	APR	44	2	2	5	H81012	19.9 (32.0)	FP	33	2	2	4
WSU490	15.0 (24.1)	RW	50	2	2	10	H81015	14.6 (23.5)	FP	44	0	0	0
76T003	13.5 (21.7)	RW	60	1	1	1	H81016	25.3 (40.7)	RW	22	3	5	8
76T009	25.8 (41.5)	RW	75	5	5	20	H81021	15.2 (24.5)	FP	48	0	0	0
76T010	19.6 (31.5)	RW	84	4	4	13	H81022	25.3 (40.7)	RW	23	4	4	13
76T011	20.0 (32.2)	RW	69	4	4	12	H81025	20.3 (32.7)	RW	38	4	5	9
77T089	20.0 (32.2)	RW	66	5	5	9	H81027	25.3 (40.7)	RW	30	3	5	9
77T092	20.0 (32.2)	RW	45	4	4	21	H82002	20.3 (32.7)	RW	47	4	5	9
H80011	14.9 (24.0)	RW	27	1	2	1	H82008	19.6 (31.5)	APR	61	4	5	8
H80013	15.5 (24.9)	RW	33	2	2	7	H82009	25.3 (40.7)	RW	27	5	5	12
H80014	14.3 (23.0)	RW	60	1	1	3	H82012	25.3 (40.7)	RW	17	5	5	9
H80017	14.9 (24.0)	RW	38	2	2	6	H82014	20.3 (32.7)	RW	22	4	5	12
H80018	19.3 (31.1)	APR	21	0	2	0	H82015	14.6 (23.5)	RW	18	1	1	2
H80020	18.6 (29.9)	APR	26	1	1	3	H82016	19.6 (31.5)	RW	21	2	2	8
H80021	19.9 (32.0)	FP	29	0	0	0	H82018	14.6 (23.5)	RW	28	3	3	9
H80023	20.5 (33.0)	FP	41	2	2	8	H82019	14.6 (23.5)	RW	47	3	3	7
H80024	20.5 (33.0)	RW	24	0	0	0	H82020	19.6 (31.5)	RW	41	4	5	8
H81002	20.5 (33.0)	RW	57	4	4	14	H82021	20.3 (31.7)	APR	48	4	4	13
H81004	19.9 (32.0)	RW	56	4	4	16	H82022	20.3 (32.7)	APR	50	4	4	10

RW = Rigid Wall
APR = APR Padding on Wall
FP = Fiberglass Padding on Wall
NFR = Number of Fractured Ribs
* - Number in parenthesis in units of km/hr

The average number of fractured ribs is shown in Table A4.

Using the data plotted in Figure A2, the fractured rib data was normalized to 45 years by a factor of roughly .2 fractured ribs per year.

Table A4 - Average Number of Fractured Ribs

Test Type	Average NFR*	Standard Deviation
15 mph (24 km/hr) Rigid Wall	5.3	3.3
20 mph (32 km/hr) Rigid Wall	10.7	5.0
25 mph (40 km/hr) Rigid Wall	11.8	4.4
20 mph (32 km/hr) APR Padding	6.3	4.4
20 mph (32 km/hr) Fiberglass Padding	2.0	3.3

*NFR = Number of Fracture Ribs. Maximum possible value is 24.

The normalized fractured ribs are in Table A5.

Table A5 - Average Number of Fractured Ribs Normalized to 45 Years

Test Type	Average NFR*	Standard Deviation
15 mph (24 km/hr) Rigid Wall	6.1	4.0
20 mph (32 km/hr) Rigid Wall	10.7	4.8
25 mph (40 km/hr) Rigid Wall	14.4	2.0
20 mph APR Padding	6.6	3.1
20 mph (32 km/hr) Fiberglass Padding	3.2	3.7

*NRF = Number of Fractured Ribs. Maximum possible value is 24.

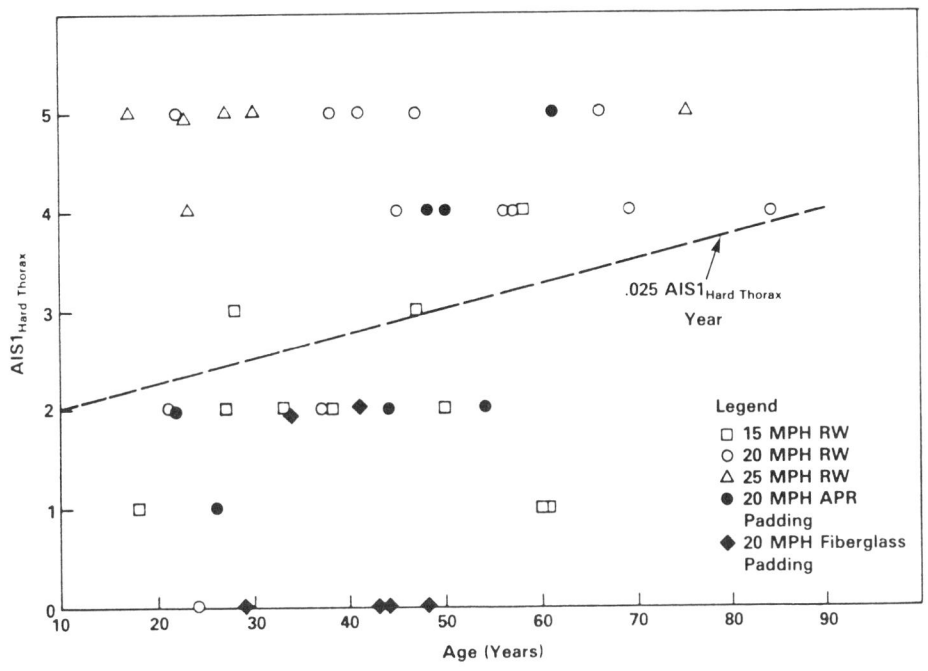

Figure A1 - AIS hard thorax for 42 cadaver tests

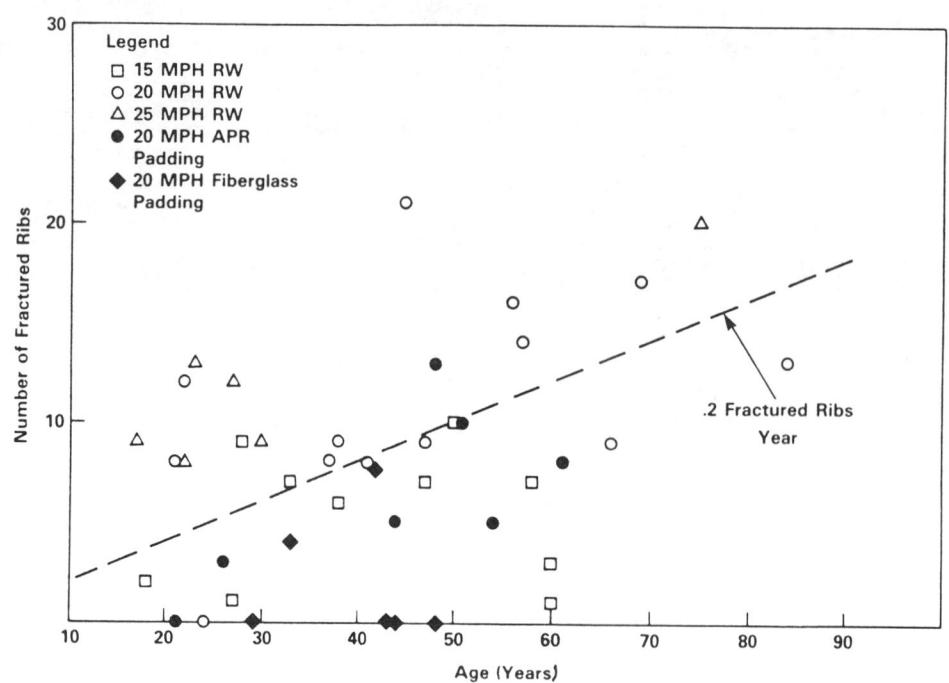

Figure A2 - Fractured ribs for 42 cadaver tests

851720

Abdominal Trauma—Review, Response, and Criteria

Richard L. Stalnaker
The Ohio State University

Marian S. Ulman
Transportation Research Center of Ohio

ABSTRACT

As an aid to designing an abdominal insert for anthropomorphic dummies, a study of abdominal trauma factors has been made. Questions regarding human impact response and tolerance were answered within the framework of primate scaling. Results of subhuman primate impacts and primate anthropometry were combined to produce injury criteria for frontal and lateral abdominal impacts. Impact response for the frontal and lateral directions was also defined for humans. The primate impact data used in the study was obtained in the early 1970's in laboratory tests utilizing a specially designed "air gun". This test set up emphasizes reproducibility and control. Human lateral abdominal impact data first published by Walfisch et al., in 1980 were reanalyzed and used to check the primate scaling. Significant differences in impact injury tolerances for various abdominal locations were noted and detailed. As a result of these analyses little difference was noted in the force-penetration response as a function of impact location. A design envelope is proposed which can be used in the development of a dummy abdomen, and an injury criterion first suggested by Viano and Lau in 1983 is validated against the set of data analyzed here.

INTRODUCTION

THE PURPOSE OF THE RESEARCH discussed in this paper was to develop design criteria for the abdomen of a dummy. This involved reviewing appropriate literature for data that could be used to establish performance requirements. At the same time the injury data was examined using a recently developed injury criteria to determine what dynamic properties must be measured within the abdominal area.

Through various studies, much has been learned about head and thorax impact response and tolerance. In contrast, little is known about the behavior of the abdomen when it is impacted. Although many animal abdominal impacts have been conducted, few have led to meaningful performance requirements.

LITERATURE SURVEY

The study of the mechanisms of injury in abdominal impacts has been pursued for many years. The research of the last 15 years includes a number of studies that contain data which may be analyzed for dummy design criteria.

In a 1971 study reported by Beckman et al., (1)* frontal impacts were conducted to determine abdominal injury mechanisms and a quantitative relationship between input mechanical parameters and the occurrence of trauma. It was also a goal to develop the criteria to recommend performance requirements for materials used in automotive fixtures which most frequently produce blunt abdominal injury. It was discovered that the lower abdomen can withstand impacts of greater velocity than can the middle or upper abdomen.

In the years 1970-1973, McElhaney and Stalnaker (2,3,4,5) conducted studies at the Highway Safety Research Institute (HSRI) of the University of Michigan on lateral abdominal trauma. Subjects used in this study included 5 types of primates. Animals were impacted in the upper side of the torso with a scaled, blunt, wedge-shaped impactor resembling

---

*Numbers in parentheses designate references at end of paper.

an armrest. In other experiments, a large flat impactor was used that contacted the animal over the entire torso. Sled tests were then performed to verify that the injuries sustained in controlled impacts resembled injuries received in a less controlled impact environment, which more closely resembled an actual automobile side collision. The surface contacted by the subject in each sled test was a door, scaled to the size of the animal being tested. This study revealed significant differences in the right and left side tolerances to impact, and it determined critical impact velocities at various body sites for several sizes and shapes of impactors.

In 1973, Trollope et al., (6) reported on two sets of tests. One of these series involved impacts directly to organs. The other series involved lateral abdominal impacts. In these impacts, velocity and depth of abdominal penetration were varied in an attempt to duplicate clinically observed injuries. Injuries were examined to evaluate the necessity for surgery. The findings of the study proved to be inadequate to analyze borderline injuries.

At the GM symposium on Human Impact Response in 1973, Stalnaker, et al., (7) reported a summation of all of the abdominal work done at HSRI to that date. The new research reported procedures and equipment similar to those used in the previous tests. Test subjects included squirrel monkeys, rhesus monkeys, and baboons, as well as 15 pigs. Various impactors, both rigid and padded, were used to simulate steering wheels, door handles, and arm rests, in order to reproduce common automotive injuries. A large surface area impactor was used to simulate passenger impacts with the dashboard and car-pedestrian accidents.

A significant finding of this study was that impacts with the narrow impactor into the body overlying the liver resulted in tearing and transection fractures. On the other hand, the liver burst when the impacts were made with a large impactor. This behavior was attributed to viscoelasticity of the liver. Other conclusions included the observation that relatively small forces were required to produce severe injuries of the abdominal viscera when the impact was made in the upper abdomen. Much greater forces were required to produce comparable injuries when the force was applied to the lower abdomen.

In an abdominal study presented in 1973 by Melvin et al., (8), impacts were applied directly to organs. The organ was surgically mobilized in an anesthetized rhesus monkey and then placed on a load cell while still being perfused by the living animal. Impact velocity and depth of penetration were varied to yield injuries of different types and severity levels. Seventeen tests were made on livers, and six on kidneys of three rhesus monkeys. Liver injuries produced by impacts included subcapsular hemorrhaging, tears, and fractures. In some static tests, the parenchyma was crushed while the capsule remained intact, a result of a different injury mechanism than that seen in dynamic tests. Kidney injury also showed a sensitivity to rate of loading, but the effect was less pronounced that it was for the liver.

Impacts in this study were made directly to the organs to minimize anatomical differences between their surrounding supporting tissue. The organ was tested while being perfused by the live animal to ensure a realistic physiological condition. Comparisons of the results of these tests with other animal abdominal impact studies show that approximately twice the average pressure is needed in whole body abdominal impacts to produce similar injuries. It was also found that the kidney withstood greater stresses than the liver. The injury levels caused by dynamic loading were similar to those observed clinically. An injury index resulting from this study was shown to correlate well with mechanical input parameters.

In a study published in 1977 by Gogler et al., (9) Gottingen minipigs were subjected to impacts with various rear body configurations of a Porsche 911. The study was directed at examining the possibility of a pedestrian receiving severe abdominal injuries from impact with the rear of the car. The impacts against rigid structural elements did yield high AIS injury levels. On the other hand, larger surface impacts caused injuries to multiple organs, but did not cause serious lesions to individual organs.

In 1980, Walfisch, et al. (10) published a study on the free fall of human cadaver subjects. They used 11 unembalmed human cadavers, allowing them to strike a rigid surface. The liver was most likely to be damaged in these impacts because of a protrusion on the rigid surface. The protrusion was designed to simulate a local intrusion such as that caused by an armrest in an automobile collision. The arm on the impacted side was arranged so that it would not interfere in the impact. A link was sought between severity of injury and various measured parameters. These parameters are the force applied by the simulated armrest, the average pressure, and the relative penetration of the armrest into the cadaver. The results of the study were used in designing an injury prediction system.

A 1980 study published by Nusholtz, et al., (11), used 10 canines, as well as 12 primates and three human cadavers to study abdominal injuries. Five of the monkeys and one of the canines were tested post-mortem, and the others were tested live under anesthesia. This research was directed towards studying shock mechanisms because hypovolemic shock frequently results from lesions incurred in abdominal impacts. Though few of the findings pertaining to shock apply to the current study, other results of this research are noteworthy. From the primate and canine studies, it was discovered that near body deflection is not directly related to the impactor stroke. Cadavers tested in this research were impacted in the right side, through the estimated c.g. of the liver, and the motions of internal organs were observed via X-ray cineradiography. Cineradiography was also utilized in some of the tests on post-mortem subhuman primates and on post-mortem canines.

In a 1981 study published by Lau and Viano (12), 26 New Zealand white rabbits were subjected to abdominal impacts. The purpose of this study was to define the threshold between crushing and impulsive injury mechanisms. From impacts using a 7.7-cm diameter flat rigid disk, it was discovered that minor hepatic contusions were produced at velocities of 8 to 10 m/s. Injuries of greater severity occurred at velocities greater than 12 m/s. Though spleen injuries were anticipated in these tests, none were encountered.

In another 1981 test by Lau and Viano (13), 12 beagles were impacted in the abdominal region by 2.5 cm wide nylon belts. Two belts were utilized in each test, one oriented transversely, and one diagonal. This testing was directed at studying hepatic injury mechanisms resulting from safety belt restraint systems. Four types of hepatic lesions resulted from these impacts, ranging in severity from minor lacerations to serious ruptures. Some of these injuries were more likely to be caused by one belt than the other, but the more severe wounds were caused by the loading of both belts.

In a 1984 study conducted at General Motors Research Laboratories by Rouhana et al., (14), 117 New Zealand white rabbits were subjected to abdominal impacts. Tests were conducted at 3 m/s to 15 m/s, with the impact centered on the 12th rib of either the left or the right side of the body. A modified Abbreviated InjuryScale was used to assess injuries. (The AIS was modified to include those injuries which might normally go unnoticed.) These experiments supported the results of previous studies in exhibiting a difference in injury tolerances between the right and the left sides of an animal. These tests showed though that only liver injuries were dependent upon side of impact; kidney injuries are independent of this consideration. The test results also showed good agreement with NCSS in percentages of serious injuries incurred by specific organs in lateral impacts. The risk of sustaining an abdominal injury was found to be a function of the impact velocity times the abdominal compression. This product, named the AIC (Abdominal Injury Criterion), was proposed as a measure of abdominal injury severity, although the relation between humans and animals must be determined.

Other previous research includes patient studies at hospitals. These give information on injury patterns, frequencies, and mortality rates. In a study reported by Frey, et al., (15), 139 patients were evaluated who were suffering from blunt abdominal trauma due to automobile accidents. The reported mortality rate for the 15 year study was 26%, but the deaths were not all directly attributable to the hepatic injury. Many of the patients who did die of their hepatic injury, died from hemorrhage.

Another hospital study conducted by Owens et al., (16), considered 150 cases of liver trauma. The study was not entirely limited to blunt trauma, nor was it limited to trauma resulting from automobile accidents. Automobile accidents, however, accounted for over half of the hepatic injuries and had the highest mortality rate. Blunt trauma was found to be more likely fatal than penetrating trauma.

A 1970 study conducted by Hardy (17) in Melbourne, Australia, examined the patterns of liver damage in 50 victims of fatal blunt trauma. Forty-four of these victims were involved in motor vehicle accidents. Hepatic injury either caused death or contributed to death. The most severe liver injuries were sustained by pedestrians in motor vehicle accidents.

Many other abdominal studies have been conducted since 1970 (18--30). Most of these examined clinical data, and their results contributed greatly to the knowledge of trauma management. Because the results are not directly applicable to the current study, this research will not be discussed any further here.

PROCEDURE

The data selected from the literature for this study were taken from three HSRI primate studies. For each test the original data files as well as the high-speed motion picture films were carefully reviewed to determine which tests were eligible for this study. The criteria used to pick these tests were as follows:

1. Quality of force data.

2. Quality of high-speed film.

3. Injury information.

4. Animal anthropometry.

5. Type and location of impact.

The first three points were essential considerations. The fourth point was waived in some cases if the anthropometry could be estimated in other ways, such as by film analysis or by scaling. Some tests were excluded because of the small data set for that impact condition.

The first study reviewed was a 1971 report by Beckman, et al., entitled, "Impact Tolerance -- Abdominal Injury," (1). Sixteen acceptable frontal impacts were found in this study. The 1971 and 1973, "Door Crashworthiness," reports by Stalnaker, et al., (3, 4) were reviewed next, and 17 right and left side impact tests were found to be useful. Two lateral and seven frontal impacts were extracted from a 1973 Journal of Trauma article by Trollope, et al., (6). The direct organ impacts in the Trollope study are inappropriate for the current study, so they are not used. The three data-sets yielded 42 usable tests using six impactor types and five impact locations on four primate species.

All impacts were carried out by a pneumatically operated testing machine especially constructed for impact studies. The machine consists of an air reservoir and a ground and honed cylinder with two carefully fitted pistons. The first of these, the transfer piston, is propelled by compressed air through the cylinder and transfers its momentum to the impact piston. An interchangeable striker plate, attached to the impact piston, travels a distance of about 10 cm. At this point, an inversion tube absorbs the energy of the impact piston and halts its movement. The stroke of the impactor is controlled by its initial positioning, and its velocity is controlled by the reservoir pressure. The impactor was instrumented with an accelerometer and an inertia compensated force transducer. High speed motion pictures from 1000 to 5000 frames per second were taken for photographic analysis.

Impacts were carried out using six types of impactors.

1. Rigid 8x.5: Magnesium bar 20.36 cm long and 1.27 cm wide.

2. Rigid 8x1: Magnesium bar 20.36 cm long and 2.54 cm wide.

3. Rigid 8x2: Magnesium bar 20.36 cm long and 5.08 cm wide.

4. Wedge 3x2.25: Wedge-shaped armrest with 90° rounded corner (hard rubber).

5. Wedge 3x3: Wedge-shaped armrest with 90° rounded corner (hard rubber).

6. Wedge 10x4: Wedge-shaped armrest with 90° rounded corner (hard rubber).

The contact force-time plot was obtained from oscilloscope traces. The force-time plots were electronically digitized and stored as files on the VAX-11/750. High speed movies of each test were digitized on an electronic film analyzer. This data was also stored on the VAX-11/750. The autopsy records for each test were reviewed, and the injury index used in the earlier studies was changed to AIS numbers using the following definitions (31):

1. AIS 1 - Minor

2. AIS 2 - Moderate

3. AIS 3 - Serious

4. AIS 4 - Severe

5. AIS 5 - Critical

6. AIS 6 - Maximum Injury, virtually unsurvivable by AIS-80

Four species of primate are represented in this data set and are listed below:

1. Saimiri sciurius, squirrel monkey (S).

2. Cercopithecus aethiops pygerythrus, vervet (V).

3. Macaca mulatta, rhesus (R).

4. Papio cynocephalus, baboon (B).

The primates in this data set were impacted in five abdominal locations. These locations are defined below:

1. UPPER-ABD - Frontal, highest point of the diaphragm.

2. MID-ABD - Frontal, midway between the highest and lowest points of the diaphragm.

3. LOWER-ABD - Frontal, just above the iliac crests.

4. RT-SIDE - Lateral, right side at the MID-ABD level.

5. LT-SIDE - Lateral, left side at the MID-ABD level.

RESULTS

A summary of the primate anthropometry and of the test conditions is given in Table 1. In Table 1, the "THE ORIGINAL RUN NUMBER" refers to the run numbers used in the original studies, and "OLD NUMBER" refers to the test numbers reported in the 1972 GM Symposium (5) paper.

NORMALIZATION -- In each of the four primate samples, variations in body weight and size were noted. It was decided to standardize on the average primate for each species group to minimize any dynamic or kinematic variations. The method chosen to normalize within the species group is based on standard scaling methods as described by Whittaker (32). This method has recently been suggested for animal scaling by Eppinger, et al., (33, 34). The average weight for each species was determined and used to standardize the linear dimensions of the test subject. Force and time were also standardized for each species group. Velocity remains unchanged by this normalization procedure. Normalization was achieved through the following equations:

TABLE 1 -- Impact Velocity and Primate Anthropometry for Data Set

	ORIGINAL RUN NO.*	OLD NUMBER	PRIMATE SPECIES	IMPACTOR TYPE	IMPACT LOCATION	ANIMAL WEIGHT kg	LAMBDA NORM. FACTOR	ANIMAL WIDTH AT IMPACT LOCATION cm	ANIMAL DEPTH AT IMPACT LOCATION cm	NORM. ANIMAL WIDTH AT IMP.LOC cm	NORM. ANIMAL DEPTH AT IMP.LOC cm	IMPACT VELOCITY m/s	DEPTH/ WIDTH
FRONT UPPER	71-02T	31	RHESUS	RIGID 8X1	UPPER-ABD	5.90	0.95	11.30	12.28	10.78	11.71	9.77	1.09
	71-03T	45	RHESUS	RIGID 8X2	UPPER-ABD	5.00	1.01	9.58	10.43	9.65	10.51	10.89	1.09
	71-04T	24	RHESUS	RIGID 8X.5	UPPER-ABD	5.60	0.97	10.96	11.66	10.63	11.31	14.47	1.06
	71-05T	23	RHESUS	RIGID 8X.5	UPPER-ABD	6.60	0.92	12.78	13.74	11.75	12.63	14.16	1.08
	71-06T	25	RHESUS	RIGID 8X.5	UPPER-ABD	6.40	0.93	12.66	13.32	11.75	12.37	12.77	1.05
	71-07T	21	RHESUS	RIGID 8X.5	UPPER-ABD	5.00	1.01	9.89	10.39	9.96	10.46	9.63	1.05
	71-08T	22	RHESUS	RIGID 8X.5	UPPER-ABD	4.60	1.04	9.00	9.58	9.32	9.92	11.11	1.06
	71-06AB	17	VERVET	RIGID 8X.5	UPPER-ABD	3.15	1.04	7.67	8.31	7.98	8.64	12.32	1.08
	71-10AB	43	VERVET	RIGID 8X2	UPPER-ABD	5.15	0.88	12.19	13.49	10.78	11.93	11.20	1.11
	71-13AB	34	VERVET	RIGID 8X1	UPPER-ABD	4.25	0.94	10.71	11.37	10.09	10.71	9.86	1.06
	71-15AB	33	VERVET	RIGID 8X1	UPPER-ABD	2.70	1.09	6.47	7.01	7.08	7.67	9.77	1.08
	71-17AB	42	VERVET	RIGID 8X2	UPPER-ABD	2.40	1.14	5.66	6.16	6.44	7.01	9.50	1.09
	71-18AB	32	VERVET	RIGID 8X1	UPPER-ABD	3.35	1.02	8.30	8.94	8.46	9.11	9.19	1.08
FRONT MIDDLE	71-07AB	18	VERVET	RIGID 8X.5	MID-ABD	3.75	0.98	8.27	8.62	8.12	8.47	11.35	1.04
	71-12AB	36	VERVET	RIGID 8X1	MID-ABD	3.60	1.00	8.26	8.57	8.22	8.53	12.61	1.04
	71-09AB	46	VERVET	RIGID 8X2	MID-ABD	4.60	0.92	10.49	10.87	9.63	9.98	12.65	1.04
	71-14AB	35	VERVET	RIGID 8X1	MID-ABD	2.80	1.08	6.34	6.63	6.86	7.17	8.40	1.05
	71-16AB	44	VERVET	RIGID 8X2	MID-ABD	3.55	1.00	8.28	8.42	8.28	8.42	8.76	1.02
FRONT LOWER	71-11AB	37	VERVET	RIGID 8X1	LOWER-ABD	3.80	0.98	8.66	8.81	8.47	8.61	12.07	1.02
	71-05AB	19	VERVET	RIGID 8X.5	LOWER-ABD	3.62	0.99	8.61	8.60	8.55	8.54	14.53	1.00
	71-36AB	20	VERVET	RIGID 8X.5	LOWER-ABD	3.30	1.02	8.05	8.02	8.25	8.22	15.56	1.00
	71-35AB	48	VERVET	RIGID 8X2	LOWER-ABD	3.60	1.00	8.47	8.63	8.43	8.59	15.69	1.02
	71-08AB	47	VERVET	RIGID 8X2	LOWER-ABD	3.25	1.03	7.72	7.77	7.95	8.00	12.25	1.01
RIGHT SIDE	70-38DCW	73	SQUIRREL	WEDGE 3X2.25	RT-SIDE	0.68	0.96	5.40	5.83	5.18	5.59	9.70	1.08
	70-40DCW	74	SQUIRREL	WEDGE 3X2.25	RT-SIDE	0.53	1.04	4.29	4.56	4.47	4.75	10.82	1.06
	70-33DCW	77	RHESUS	WEDGE 3X3	RT-SIDE	5.15	1.00	10.29	10.72	10.26	10.69	10.59	1.04
	70-31DCW	78	RHESUS	WEDGE 3X3	RT-SIDE	6.08	0.94	12.28	12.66	11.59	11.95	11.09	1.03
	71-10T	27	RHESUS	RIGID 8X.5	RT-SIDE	5.20	0.99	10.07	10.83	10.01	10.76	13.23	1.08
	71-13T	40	RHESUS	RIGID 8X1	RT-SIDE	4.75	1.02	9.89	10.39	10.12	10.64	13.41	1.05
	70-59DCW	83	BABOON	WEDGE 10X4	RT-SIDE	14.20	1.03	12.86	14.24	13.22	14.64	11.62	1.11
	70-68DCW	84	BABOON	WEDGE 10X4	RT-SIDE	15.80	0.99	16.40	17.77	16.28	17.64	12.52	1.08
	70-67DCW	85	BABOON	WEDGE 10X4	RT-SIDE	14.60	1.02	13.11	14.49	13.36	14.76	13.50	1.11
	70-73DCW	86	BABOON	WEDGE 10X4	RT-SIDE	21.60	0.90	20.89	22.89	18.70	20.49	14.26	1.10
	70-51DCW	90	BABOON	WEDGE 10X4	RT-SIDE	14.80	1.01	15.24	16.77	15.46	17.01	16.99	1.10
LEFT SIDE	70-39DCW	75	SQUIRREL	WEDGE 3X2.25	LT-SIDE	0.59	1.01	4.69	5.06	4.72	5.09	9.92	1.08
	70-35DCW	79	RHESUS	WEDGE 3X3	LT-SIDE	4.00	1.08	8.16	8.33	8.84	9.03	12.70	1.02
	70-32DCW	80	RHESUS	WEDGE 3X3	LT-SIDE	4.05	1.08	8.18	8.43	8.83	9.10	13.32	1.03
	70-37DCW	81	RHESUS	WEDGE 3X3	LT-SIDE	4.10	1.07	8.02	8.54	8.62	9.18	13.68	1.06
	70-36DCW	82	RHESUS	WEDGE 3X3	LT-SIDE	3.80	1.10	7.67	7.91	8.45	8.72	9.61	1.03
	70-60DCW	88	BABOON	WEDGE 10X4	LT-SIDE	11.70	1.10	10.89	11.93	11.94	13.08	14.31	1.10
	70-69DCW	89	BABOON	WEDGE 10X4	LT-SIDE	15.20	1.01	14.12	15.36	14.20	15.44	14.44	1.09
	70-72DCW	92	BABOON	WEDGE 10X4	LT-SIDE	19.40	0.93	18.21	20.12	16.89	18.66	15.74	1.10

* T-Trollope's Study,Ref.[6]; AB-Abdominal Impact Study,Ref.[1]; DCW-Door Crashworthiness Criteria,Refs.[3,4]

$$\text{Lambda } (\lambda) = (M_{ave}/M_i)^{1/3}$$

$$T_n = (\lambda) \times T_r$$

$$F_n = (\lambda)^2 \times F_r$$

$$L_n = (\lambda) \times L_r$$

Where:

Lambda - normalizing factor

M_{ave} - average weight of a given species

M_i - weight of specific subject in the species set

T - time

F - force

L - length

n - subscript indicating a normalized quantity

r - subscript indicating a non-normalized value

FORCE-PENETRATION -- The digitized force-time and the digitized piston displacement-time plots were synchronized by aligning the time at the very high acceleration spike of the impact piston caused by impact with the transfer piston, with the time that the piston starts to move. Since most of the tests were filmed at 5000 frames per second, this was found to be a very good method of synchronization. The time of initial animal contact, the maximum penetration and the time at maximum penetration were recorded from the film analysis and used to define the force-penetration curve for each test. These force-penetration curves were then normalized to the standard animal for that species. Area under the force-penetration curve was calculated and recorded as energy.

COMPRESSION -- The average weight, depth, and width at each impact location, and the abdominal aspect ratio for each of the five species are given in Table 2. The maximum abdominal compression was calculated by dividing the normalized depth of penetration by the average normalized width or normalized depth of that species at that impact location and then multiplying by a 100 to obtain a percentage.

The results of the impact analysis are shown in Tables 3 through 7. The AIS injury numbers are specified by individual organs.

ABDOMINAL TOLERANCE -- When the compression was plotted against the AIS numbers a strong correlation was seen for certain locations. A strong correlation was also found between impact velocity and AIS numbers for other locations. At still other locations no correlation was evident. Since the abdominal contents are approximately the same at most impact locations, some factor other than impact location is responsible for this variation in AIS correlations. Rouhana (14), with the team at the Biomedical Science Department of General Motors, has done a study with controlled impacts. In some of the GM tests, the velocity was fixed and the penetration varied; in others, the penetration was fixed and the velocity varied. Close examination of Rouhana's data shows results similar to those found in this study. That is, sometimes penetration correlates with injury and sometimes velocity correlates well with injury. Rouhana found that injury had a strong velocity dependence when the penetration was constant. On the other hand, he found a strong penetration dependence when velocity was constant. When the velocity was multiplied by the compression, and this product was plotted against the AIS numbers, good correlation was found for all impact locations. This product of velocity and compression for each test in this study is shown in Tables 3 through 7. The regression equations, correlation coefficient, and V*C for AIS=3 for each

TABLE 2 -- Anthropometric Measurements of Primate Species

SPECIES	AVG WEIGHT kg	UPPER AVG WIDTH cm	UPPER AVG DEPTH cm	UPPER AVG D/W	MIDDLE AVG WIDTH cm	MIDDLE AVG DEPTH cm	MIDDLE AVG D/W	LOWER AVG WIDTH cm	LOWER AVG DEPTH cm	LOWER AVG D/W
SQUIRREL	0.60±0.06	-	-	-	4.79±0.29	5.14±0.34	1.07±0.01	-	-	-
VERVET	3.55±0.67	8.47±1.54	9.18±1.69	1.08±0.02	8.22±0.88	8.51±0.89	1.04±0.01	8.33±0.21	8.39±0.24	1.01±0.01
RHESUS	5.10±0.86	10.55±0.90	11.27±0.95	1.07±0.02	9.59±1.02	10.01±1.08	1.04±0.02	-	-	-
BABOON	15.45±2.93	-	-	-	15.01±2.09	16.46±2.28	1.10±0.01	-	-	-
HUMAN*	76.00±4.54	30.60±2.30	22.00±1.60	0.72±0.02	28.60±3.50	20.90±3.80	0.73±0.02	28.30±4.35	21.25±4.15	0.75±0.02

* Dimensions were measured from Hybrid III and Part 572 Dummy.

TABLE 3 -- Results of the Impact Analysis for Upper Frontal Abdomen

RUN NO.*	MAXIMUM PENETRATION cm	NORM.MAX. PENETRATION cm	MAXIMUM COMPRESSION %	NORM. STIFFNESS N/cm	NORM. PLATEAU LOAD N	V*C m/s	AIS	AIS FOR INJURIES TO INDIVIDUAL ORGANS**
71-02T	4.19	3.98	35.30	358	588	3.45	3	L-3 K-0 SP-2 A-0 I-0 P-0 ST-0
71-03T	1.27	1.28	11.37	266	588	1.24	1	L-1 K-0 SP-0 A-0 I-0 P-0 ST-1
71-04T	6.11	5.93	52.58	358	588	7.61	6	L-6 K-1 SP-0 A-0 I-0 P-3 ST-0
71-05T	6.79	6.25	55.47	358	588	7.85	6	L-6 K-0 SP-4 A-0 I-0 P-0 ST-0
71-06T	4.38	4.07	36.13	173	725	4.61	4	L-4 K-0 SP-0 A-0 I-0 P-0 ST-0
71-07T	4.43	4.47	39.67	496	725	3.82	4	L-4 K-0 SP-0 A-0 I-0 P-0 ST-0
71-08T	5.32	5.53	49.04	496	725	5.45	5	L-5 K-1 SP-0 A-0 I-0 P-0 ST-0
71-06AB	3.90	4.06	44.18	153	350	5.44	5	L-2 K-0 SP-2 A-0 I-0 P-5 ST-2
71-10AB	5.99	5.27	57.38	311	650	6.43	6	L-6 K-1 SP-0 A-0 I-0 P-0 ST-0
71-13AB	5.27	4.95	53.88	153	350	5.31	6	L-6 K-2 SP-0 A-0 I-0 P-5 ST-0
71-15AB	3.77	4.15	45.16	153	350	4.41	5	L-5 K-0 SP-0 A-0 I-0 P-3 ST-0
71-17AB	4.59	5.23	56.93	217	450	5.41	6	L-6 K-0 SP-0 A-0 I-1 P-0 ST-0
71-18AB	4.06	4.14	45.08	217	450	4.14	5	L-5 K-0 SP-0 A-0 I-0 P-0 ST-0

* T-Trollope's Study,Ref.[6]; AB-Abdominal Impact Study,Ref.[1]; DCW-Door Crashworthiness Criteria,Refs.[3,4]
** L-Liver; SP-Spleen; P-Pancreas; K-Kidneys; A-Adrenals; ST-Stomach; I-Intestines

TABLE 4 -- Results of the Impact Analysis for Middle Frontal Abdomen

RUN NO.*	MAXIMUM PENETRATION cm	NORM.MAX. PENETRATION cm	MAXIMUM COMPRESSION %	NORM. STIFFNESS N/cm	NORM. PLATEAU LOAD N	V*C m/s	AIS	AIS FOR INJURIES TO INDIVIDUAL ORGANS**
71-07AB	3.54	3.47	40.74	199	662	4.62	3	L-0 K-0 SP-0 A-0 I-3 P-0 ST-0
71-12AB	5.07	5.07	59.51	250	400	7.50	5	L-2 K-0 SP-5 A-0 I-0 P-3 ST-0
71-09AB	5.10	4.69	55.09	144	625	6.97	5	L-0 K-0 SP-3 A-0 I-1 P-5 ST-0
71-14AB	3.77	4.07	47.87	83	--	4.02	3	L-0 K-0 SP-0 A-0 I-0 P-3 ST-0
71-16AB	1.18	1.18	13.92	144	200	1.22	0	L-0 K-0 SP-0 A-0 I-0 P-0 ST-0

* T-Trollope's Study,Ref.[6]; AB-Abdominal Impact Study,Ref.[1]; DCW-Door Crashworthiness Criteria,Refs.[3,4]
** L-Liver; SP-Spleen; P-Pancreas; K-Kidneys; A-Adrenals; ST-Stomach; I-Intestines

TABLE 5 -- Results of the Impact Analysis for Lower Frontal Abdomen

RUN NO.*	MAXIMUM PENETRATION cm	NORM.MAX. PENETRATION cm	MAXIMUM COMPRESSION %	NORM. STIFFNESS N/cm	NORM. PLATEAU LOAD N	V*C m/s	AIS	AIS FOR INJURIES TO INDIVIDUAL ORGANS**
71-11AB	4.13	4.05	48.29	239	462	5.83	1	L-0 K-0 SP-0 A-0 I-1 P-0 ST-0
71-05AB	4.75	3.91	46.64	239	375	6.78	1	L-0 K-0 SP-0 A-0 I-1 P-0 ST-0
71-36AB	4.24	4.32	51.45	181	288	8.01	3	L-0 K-0 SP-0 A-0 I-3 P-0 ST-0
71-35AB	4.70	4.70	55.96	239	462	8.78	4	L-0 K-0 SP-0 A-0 I-4 P-0 ST-0
71-08AB	3.69	3.80	45.25	250	875	5.54	0	L-0 K-0 SP-0 A-0 I-0 P-0 ST-0

* T-Trollope's Study,Ref.[6]; AB-Abdominal Impact Study,Ref.[1]; DCW-Door Crashworthiness Criteria,Refs.[3,4]
** L-Liver; SP-Spleen; P-Pancreas; K-Kidneys; A-Adrenals; ST-Stomach; I-Intestines

TABLE 6 -- Results of the Impact Analysis for Right Side Abdomen

RUN NO.*	MAXIMUM PENETRATION cm	NORM.MAX. PENETRATION cm	MAXIMUM COMPRESSION %	NORM. STIFFNESS N/cm	NORM. PLATEAU LOAD N	V*C m/s	AIS	AIS FOR INJURIES TO INDIVIDUAL ORGANS**
70-38DCW	1.39	1.33	25.63	286	238	2.49	1	L-0 K-1 SP-0 A-1 I-0 P-0 ST-0
70-40DCW	0.91	0.95	18.34	286	200	1.98	0	L-0 K-0 SP-0 A-0 I-0 P-0 ST-0
70-33DCW	4.25	4.25	40.50	194	238	4.29	5	L-5 K-2 SP-0 A-2 I-0 P-0 ST-0
70-31DCW	3.98	3.74	35.60	230	725	3.95	4	L-4 K-0 SP-0 A-1 I-0 P-1 ST-0
71-10T	3.03	3.00	28.60	311	350	3.78	3	L-3 K-0 SP-0 A-0 I-0 P-0 ST-0
71-13T	2.84	2.90	27.60	311	350	3.70	4	L-4 K-0 SP-0 A-0 I-0 P-0 ST-0
70-59DCW	3.59	3.70	25.90	326	862	3.01	2	L-0 K-0 SP-2 A-0 I-0 P-0 ST-0
70-68DCW	4.36	4.32	30.20	333	500	3.78	4	L-4 K-0 SP-0 A-2 I-0 P-0 ST-0
70-67DCW	3.86	3.94	27.60	333	500	3.73	3	L-3 K-2 SP-0 A-0 I-0 P-0 ST-0
70-73DCW	4.88	4.34	30.40	525	1710	4.34	5	L-5 K-3 SP-0 A-2 I-0 P-2 ST-0
70-51DCW	4.43	4.47	31.30	563	1750	5.32	6	L-6 K-3 SP-0 A-2 I-0 P-2 ST-0

* T-Trollope's Study,Ref.[6]; AB-Abdominal Impact Study,Ref.[1]; DCW-Door Crashworthiness Criteria,Refs.[3,4]
** L-Liver; SP-Spleen; P-Pancreas; K-Kidneys; A-Adrenals; ST-Stomach; I-Intestines

TABLE 7 - Results of the Impact Analysis for Left Side Abdomen

RUN NO.*	MAXIMUM PENETRATION cm	NORM.MAX. PENETRATION cm	MAXIMUM COMPRESSION %	NORM. STIFFNESS N/cm	NORM. PLATEAU LOAD N	V*C m/s	AIS	AIS FOR INJURIES TO INDIVIDUAL ORGANS**
70-39DCW	1.29	1.30	27.61	108	38	2.74	0	L-0 K-0 SP-0 A-0 I-0 P-0 ST-0
70-35DCW	1.93	2.08	23.89	414	575	3.03	1	L-1 K-0 SP-0 A-0 I-0 P-0 ST-0
70-32DCW	3.44	3.71	42.67	144	412	5.68	4	L-4 K-0 SP-3 A-0 I-0 P-0 ST-0
70-37DCW	1.56	1.68	19.37	145	738	2.65	0	L-0 K-0 SP-0 A-0 I-0 P-0 ST-0
70-36DCW	3.07	3.38	38.92	181	288	3.74	2	L-2 K-1 SP-0 A-0 I-0 P-0 ST-0
70-60DCW	3.74	4.11	28.64	765	1212	4.10	2	L-0 K-0 SP-2 A-0 I-0 P-0 ST-2
70-69DCW	3.88	3.92	27.31	774	1300	3.94	2	L-2 K-0 SP-2 A-0 I-2 P-0 ST-0
70-72DCW	5.04	4.69	32.67	759	1950	5.14	4	L-4 K-0 SP-0 A-0 I-0 P-0 ST-0

* T-Trollope's Study,Ref.[6]; AB-Abdominal Impact Study,Ref.[1]; DCW-Door Crashworthiness Criteria,Refs.[3,4]
** L-Liver; SP-Spleen; P-Pancreas; K-Kidneys; A-Adrenals; ST-Stomach; I-Intestines

TABLE 8 -- Injury Criteria For Various Abdominal Regions

LOCATION	a* m/s	b* m/s	CORRELATION COEFFICIENT	V*C FOR AIS=3 m/s	V*C FOR AIS=3** m/s
UPPER	0.01033	-0.12	0.923	3.02	---
MIDDLE	0.00803	-0.71	0.988	3.83	---
LOWER	0.01148	-6.22	0.970	8.03	---
RIGHT	0.01918	-3.77	0.977	3.53	3.10
LEFT	0.01388	-3.51	0.981	4.69	3.50

* Regression Equation: V*C = a + b·AIS   ** Rouhana(14)

body region are shown in Table 8. Figures 1 through 5 show the plots of velocity versus compression from the regression equation (AIS=3) for that body region. The points indicating test data are coded with AIS number and species type.

RESPONSE -- A typical normalized force-penetration curve is given in Figure 6. As can be seen in the plot, the force-penetration response can be characterized by three segments. First, there is a rapid rise in the force (Segment I). This is followed by a flat portion (Segment II), and the force once again rises in Segment III but not as rapidly as in Segment I. This type of response was seen, in one form or another, in all of the tests. The smaller animals and the lower speed impacts tended to have only Segment II or Segment III with a small bump near the front of the curve. The larger animals in high speed impacts tended to have very large forces early in the impact, but these fell rapidly to a plateau before increasing again.

Once this general characterization was realized, each force-penetration curve was analyzed by two parameters: first, by the Segment III stiffness, and secondly by the Segment II plateau load. The initial spike at the beginning of the pulse (Segment I) was governed by the abdominal mass and the impactor width. Because the force-penetration curves were normalized, they were found to be constant for each species group and directly proportional to the average mass of each species group. The average plateau load and stiffness for each species are shown in Table 9.

To define the characteristics of a human abdomen, regression equations were determined using the average mass, average plateau load and stiffness for

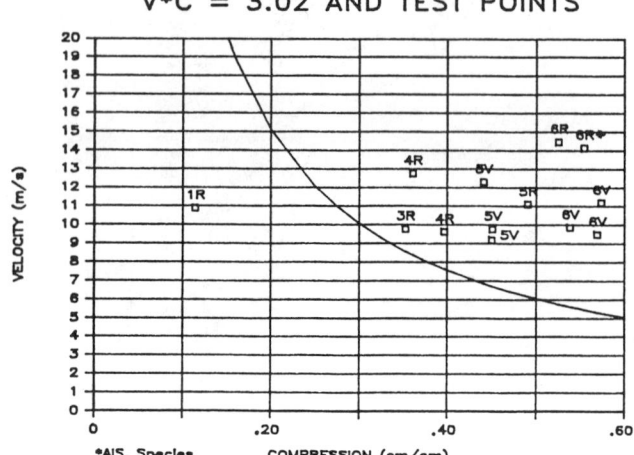

Fig. 1 - Front upper abdominal impacts

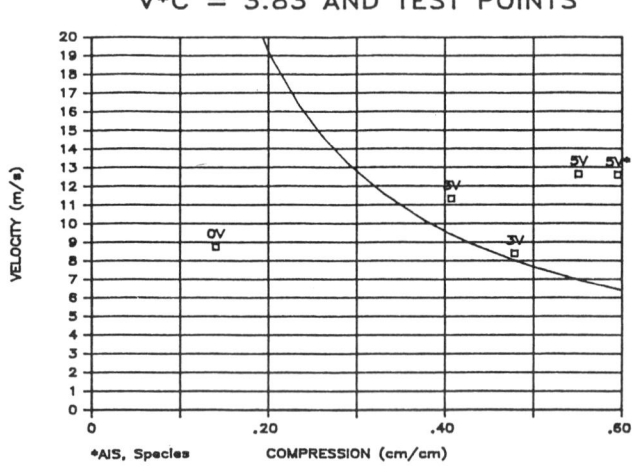

Fig. 2 - Front middle abdominal impacts

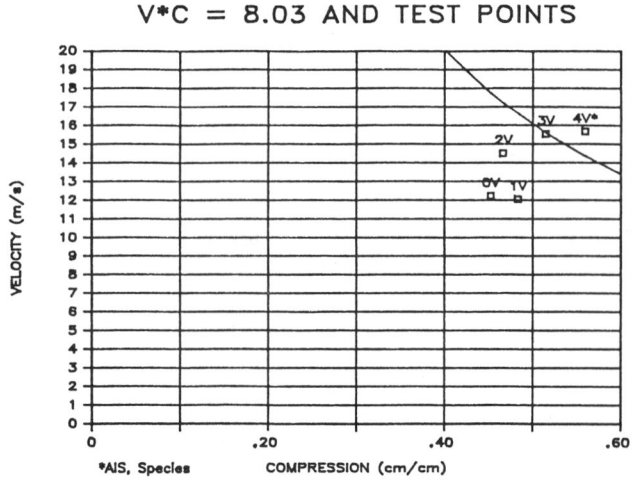

Fig. 3 - Front lower abdominal impacts

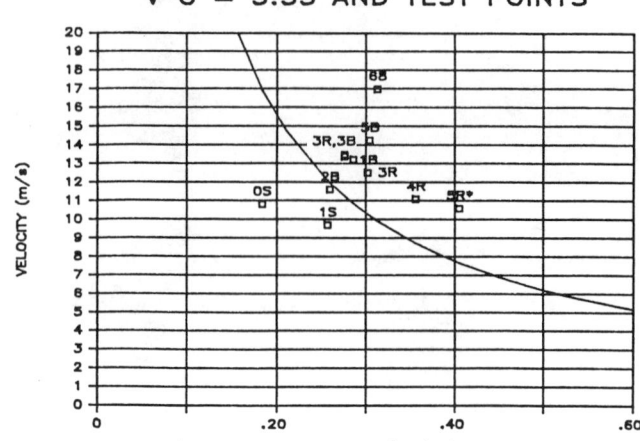

Fig. 4 - Lateral abdominal impacts - right

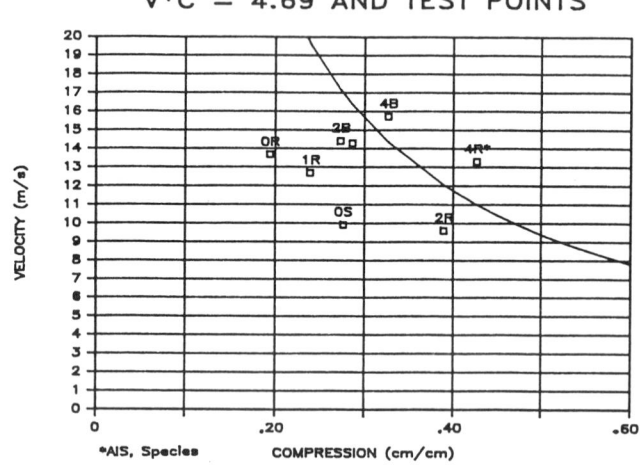

Fig. 5 - Lateral abdominal impacts - left

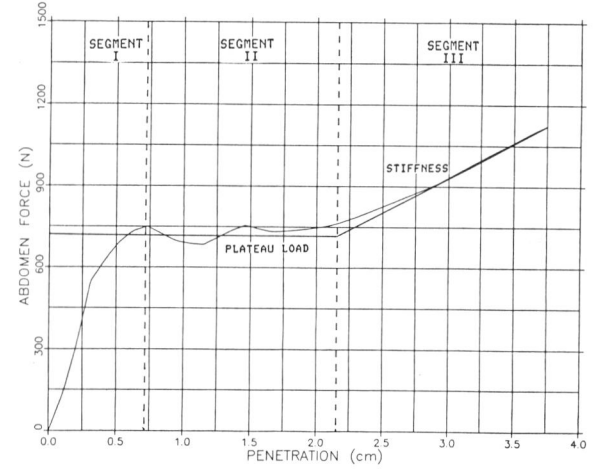

Fig. 6 - Typical force-penetration curve (70-31DCW)

TABLE 9 -- Abdominal Stiffness and Plateau Load

SPECIES	AVERAGE PLATEAU LOAD N	AVERAGE STIFFNESS N/cm	VELOCITY m/s
SQUIRREL	159 ± 87	197 ± 89	10.15 ± 0.5
VERVET	492 ± 172	210 ± 49	11.57 ± 2.3
RHESUS	547 ± 169	296 ± 114	12.03 ± 1.1
BABOON	1223 ± 527	547 ± 189	14.17 ± 1.7
MAN	5391 ± 2345	2047 ± 670	12.14 ± 2.1

each species. When an average human mass of 76 kg was used in the regression equations, human response properties were predicted. To determine appropriate standard deviations for the human, animal data regressions were again performed using the loads and stiffnesses with plus and minus one standard deviation from the averages. This then defines the standard deviations for human plateau load and stiffness. The plateau loads, stiffnesses, and velocities are presented in Table 9.

RESPONSE CORRIDORS -- In determining response corridors for human abdominal impacts, it was decided to consider the rhesus monkey data set first because it included the most impact directions and locations. When the set of data was subdivided into groups by impact location, the standard deviations of stiffness and plateau load were found to be greater than they were when the entire species data set was analyzed. This same analysis was performed for each of the other species groups with the same results. The abdominal contents for the frontal upper and middle regions and the right lateral regions are basically the same, i.e., the liver. The contents of the left lateral region and lower frontal region differ more, but overall, it is not totally unexpected that the impact responses for each of the impact areas are very similar.

Based on the above analysis, it was decided that only one corridor is necessary to encompass both frontal and lateral impacts. It was also decided to construct this corridor for only the middle abdominal region. Therefore, the animal and human mid-abdominal dimensions were used to set penetration limits for this corridor.

The first step in producing a human response corridor was to set penetration limits. This was achieved by noting the percentage of compression at which the spine is contacted. This occurred at 60% compression in the frontal direction and 45% compression in the lateral direction. These two limits represent human penetrations of 12.5 cm in the frontal direction and 12.9 cm in the lateral direction. Because these two numbers are very close, the average of 12.7 cm was selected as the penetration limit for humans in both frontal and lateral aspects.

Now that an absolute penetration limit has been defined for the human response corridor, other important points should be determined as well. The three segments of a typical response curve (Figure 6) have been described previously. The penetration values at which the slope of the curve changes most abruptly must be defined next. In animal tests, the break between curve segments II and III occurs at about 27% body compression in frontal and 23% compression in the lateral direction. The percentages represent a penetration of 5.6 cm in the frontal direction or 6.6 cm in the lateral direction for humans.

The change between Segments I and II occurs at about 9.6% or 2.0 cm for frontal impacts on humans and at 10.5% or 3.0 cm in lateral impacts and was determined the same way as above.

The load values and stiffness values needed to complete the corridor for the 12.14 m/s impact velocity are obtained from Table 9. That is, the average plateau value 5391 N sets the center of the corridor and the plus one standard deviation 7736 N sets the upper limit while the minus one standard deviation 3046 N sets the lower limit. The same is true for the stiffness levels. That is, the average stiffness 2047 N/cm sets the center stiffness while the upper stiffness is 2717 N/cm and the lower stiffness is 1377 N/cm.

All properties necessary to describe a corridor have now been calculated. The plateau load is utilized to define the Segment II corridor. To expand the corridor to accommodate both frontal and lateral impacts, the upper segment connects 2.0 cm to 5.6 cm (frontal penetration limits) while the lower line runs between 3.0 cm and 6.6 cm (lateral penetration limits). Stiffnesses are used to define the Segment III corridor. The upper stiffness of 2717 N/cm and the lower stiffness of 1377 N/cm each begins at the endpoint of the Segment II corridor and ends at 12.7 cm. The resultant corridor is shown in Figure 7.

After careful consideration of the corridor in Figure 7, it was noted that if the lower endpoints of the Segment III corridor were connected to zero - a point through which all the force-penetration responses must pass - the resultant envelope resembles a corridor for abdominal static-deflection response. This is shown by a dashed line on Figure 7.

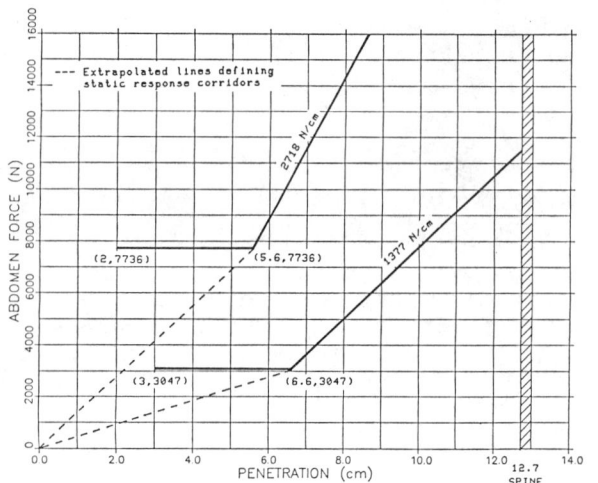

Fig. 7 - Human abdominal impact response corridor for 12.14 m/s

The corridor shown in Figure 7 did not accommodate Walfisch (10) lateral drop test results. It was then suggested by Dr. John Melvin that the plateau load of an impact response may be velocity dependent. To verify this theory, the Walfisch data was re-examined. First the Walfisch data was normalized to a 76 Kg man, so the results could be used for dummies. Next, the tests were checked to observe whether they exhibited a desirable Segment I-Segment II-Segment III form. Several of the tests were found to follow this pattern. Test 205, a one meter drop test (4.43 m/s velocity and 2037 N plateau load), and Test 217, a two meter drop test (6.26 m/s velocity and 3086N plateau load) were used to evaluate the velocity dependency of the plateau loads. Regressing the plateau loads with the impact velocities of the two Walfisch tests and the average human response calculated from animal impacts (12.14 m/s velocity and 5391 N plateau load) yielded a relationship between velocity and plateau load. A point of zero load and zero velocity was also inserted in the data to help force the equation through the origin.

$$PL = 445 V$$

Correlation coefficient 0.998

PL = Average Plateau Load (N)

V = Impact Velocity (m/s)

Using the regression equation given above and the static response portion of the curve in Figure 7, plateau loads, and the penetration range over which they are valid may be determined for a given velocity. A plateau load is calculated from the velocity first. Then, the corridor width of ± 43% of the average plateau load is determined. Forty-three percent was selected as a corridor width because it is the **coefficient of variation** calculated for human response (Table 9). Horizontal lines are drawn across the curve at the upper and lower load limits. The Segment II corridor ends and the Segment III corridor begins where the plateau load corridors intersect the static-deflection envelope. Segment II corridors begin at 2.0 cm and 3.0 cm as determined previously.

To check the procedure, Walfisch's tests were plotted as corridors defined for impacts of 4.43 m/s and 6.26 m/s. The results of this procedure are shown in Figures 8 and 9.

DISCUSSION

The V*C term was found to be a very good parameter for predicting abdominal

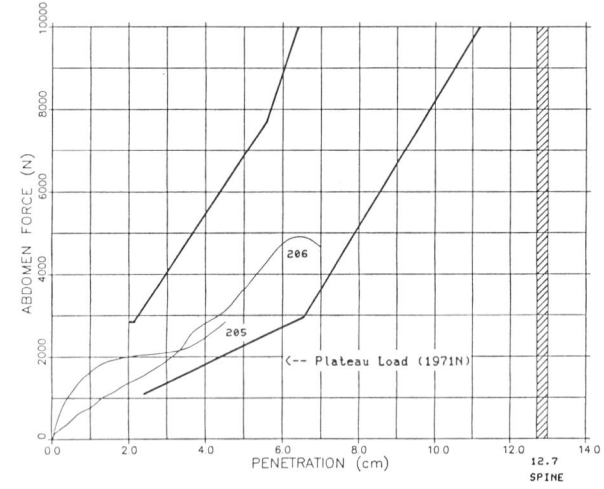

Fig. 8 - Human abdominal cadaver test and response corridor for 4.43 m/s

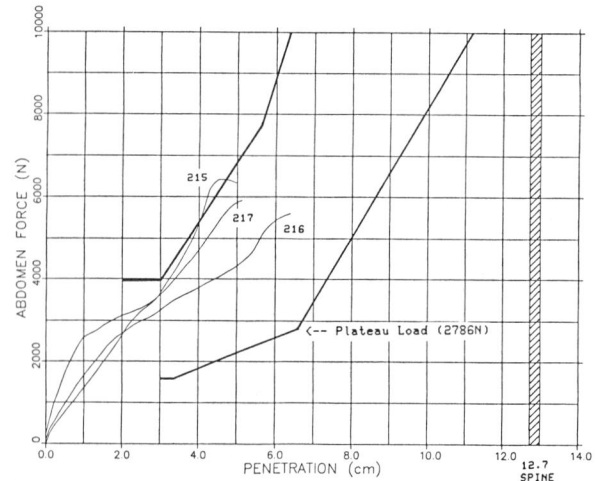

Fig. 9 - Human abdominal cadaver test and response corridor for 6.26 m/s

injury. In this study two types of injuries were observed. The first was tearing of organs from long impactor strokes. The second type of injury seen was the fracture type resulting from shorter, high velocity impactor strokes. A velocity of approximately 12.00 to 14.00 m/s is sufficient to cause the fracture type injury if the stroke is limited. It was not possible to find the lowest velocity causing fracture injuries due to the nature of this data set.

The frontal upper impact location was found to be the most susceptible to injury, whereas the lower abdomen was found to be the most tolerant impact location. The right side injury sensitivity was nearly the same as that of the front middle. Both of these locations showed less sensitivity than the upper impact region. This was due mostly to the severity of liver injuries. In the upper location the liver injuries were more severe because impacts to this location tended to damage the major vessels of the liver. Impacts to the middle location tended to tear off a piece of liver, but left the liver functional. The pancreas was also involved in many of the upper and middle location impacts. The lateral left location was more tolerant to impact than the front-upper, front-middle or right side. This was due to size, location and vulnerability of the spleen. The only injuries seen in the lower abdominal region were intestinal bruises and tears from penetration.

The squirrel, vervet, rhesus, and baboon all showed the same V*C versus AIS relationship. No species dependencies were seen. The mass ratio of the extremes of the test subjects was 25.75 to 1 and the mass ratio between the largest test subjects and the average man was 4.92 to 1. Because V*C versus AIS relationships was found to be invariant with species type and because the relative sizes of the abdominal contents of man are similar to that of lower primates, it is proposed that the abdominal injury criteria indicated here can be extrapolated to man. The proposed injury criteria for humans are shown in Figures 10 and 11.

The abdominal impact response in this study was found to be similar in shape to chest impact response. That is, an abdominal impact yields an inertial response in the beginning followed by a plateau and then an increase near the end of the impact. The way of looking at abdominal responses in this study was found to be significantly different from the way abdominal response has been looked at before.

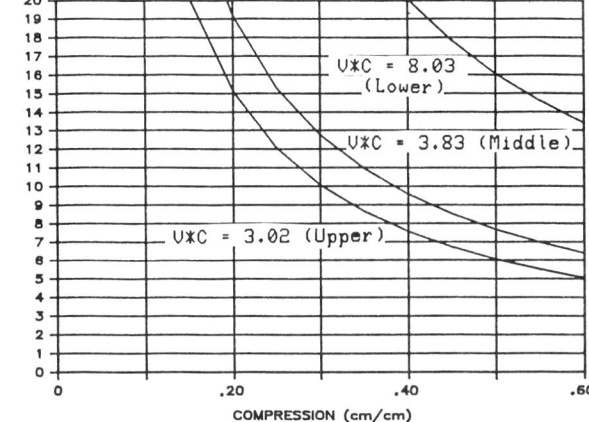

Fig 10 - Frontal abdominal impacts

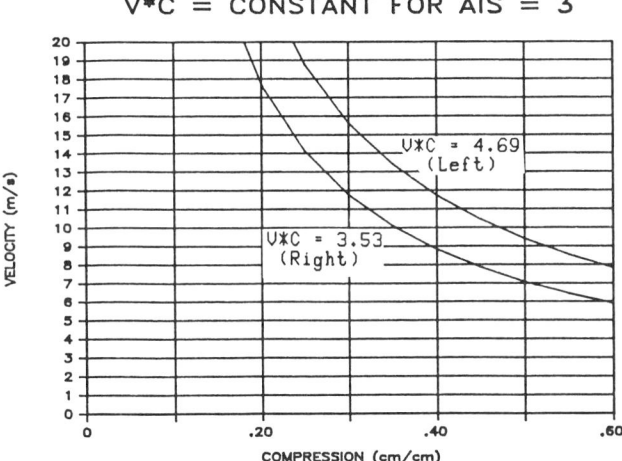

Fig 11 - Lateral abdominal impacts

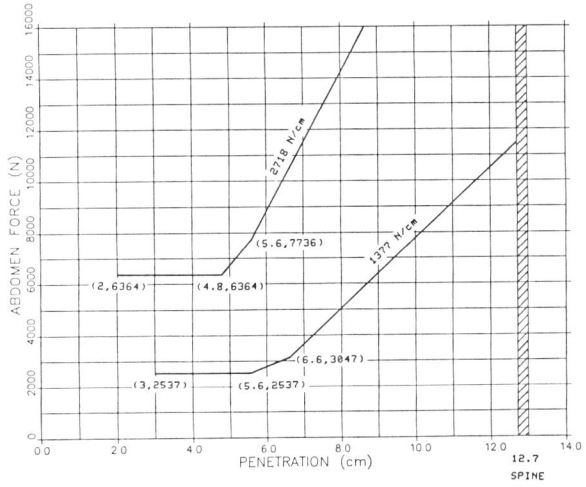

Fig 12 - Human abdominal impact response corridor for 10 m/s

747

Based on the 12.14 m/s (Figure 7) corridors defined in the Result section of this study and the plateau load as a function of velocity equation, a more meaningful abdominal impact response corridor can be defined. The corridor shown in Figure 12 was designed for an abdominal impact velocity of 10.00 m/s. This velocity was selected because it is approximately the impact velocity of the side door into an occupant for a 48.27 km/hr striking/24.14 km/hr struck standard accident configuration being studied for proposed FMVSS 214. This same velocity of 10 m/s was also found to be the approximate impact velocity of the steering wheel into a driver's abdomen for a 48.27 km/hr barrier test when the driver was unbelted.

Assumptions were made throughout this study such as:

1) Middle impact region only.

2) No differences between frontal and lateral response.

3) No differences in penetration between frontal and lateral impact.

4) Extrapolation from animals to man can be performed.

These assumptions were made so that just one response corridor could be defined. These assumptions, though not perfect, are thought to be minor when compared to variation in car size, variation in occupant size, and variation in crash conditions such as are seen in the real world.

Also, the response corridor is defined in terms of force (N) and penetration (cm) based on an average 76 kg man. The response corridor prescribed here is presented in terms of penetration and not in terms of percent penetration (compression) so the corridor can be used directly in dummy abdominal design.

CONCLUSIONS

1. V*C is a relevant parameter for predicting abdominal injury in subhuman primates.

2. V*C (AIS=3) values obtained from the lower primates appear to be useful in predicting abdominal injury in man.

3. The scaling of the abdominal impact response data from the subhuman primate tests led to a 10.00 m/s abdominal impact response corridor which can be used to design dummy abdomens.

4. One abdominal response corridor was defined for both lateral and frontal impacts to the upper and middle body regions.

5. In frontal abdominal impacts the region just below the sternum is the most susceptible to injury and the lower abdomen is the least susceptible.

6. In lateral abdominal impacts the right side was found to be more susceptible to injury than the left side.

7. The type of impactor used seemed to play a minor role in magnitude and type of injury and affected only the internal response in Segment I.

8. The abdominal impact force-penetration curves for this study have the same shape as the force-penetration curves for the classical frontal chest impacts.

9. Reanalysis of old data in view of new understandings of injury and response can be very useful.

ACKNOWLEDGMENTS

This work was supported by the Vehicle Research and Test Center, National Highway Traffic Safety Administration, U.S. Department of Transportation. The authors wish to especially thank Mr. Howard Pritz for his technical assistance in this project. The authors also acknowledge their appreciation to Mr. Jim Hofferberth for his guidance, assistance and support of this research. Thanks are also extended to Mr. Mike Monk and Mr. Roger Saul who contributed information and assistance and to Chichjung Alex Lin who processed much of the data presented in this paper.

REFERENCES

1. Beckman, D.L., McElhaney, J.H., Roberts, V.L., and Stalnaker, R.L., "Impact Tolerance -- Abdominal Injury," NTIS No. PB204171, 1971.

2. McElhaney, J.H., Stalnaker, R.L., Roberts, V.L., and Snyder, R.G., "Door Crashworthiness Criteria," _15th Stapp Car Crash Conference Proceedings_, 1971, pp 489-517.

3. Stalnaker, R.L., McElhaney, J.H., Snyder, R.G. and Roberts, V.L., "Door Crashworthiness Criteria," NTIS No. PB203721, 1971.

4. Stalnaker, R.L., Roberts, V.L., and McElhaney, J.H., "Door Crashworthiness Criteria," NTIS No. PB225000, 1973.

5. Stalnaker, R.L., Roberts, V.L., and McElhaney, J.H., "Side Impact Tolerance to Blunt Trauma," _17th Stapp Car Crash Conference Proceedings_, 1973b, pp. 843-872.

6. Trollope, M.L., Stalnaker, R.L., McElhaney, J.H., et al., "The Mechanism of Injury in Blunt Abdominal Trauma," _Journal of Trauma_, 13(11):962-970, 1973.

7. Stalnaker, R.L., McElhaney, J.H., Roberts, V.L., and Trollope, M.L.,

"Human Torso Response to Blunt Trauma," in King, W.F. and Mertz, H.J. (eds) _Human Impact Response: Measurement and Simulation_, New York: Plenum Press, 1973a, p. 181-198.

8. Melvin, J.W., Stalnaker, R.L., Roberts, V.L., and Trollope, M.L., "Side Impact Response and Injury," _17th Stapp Car Crash conference Proceedings_, 1973 pp. 115-126.

9. Gogler, E.A., Best, H.H., Braess, et al., "Biomechanical Experiments With Animals on Abdominal Tolerance Levels," _21st Stapp Car Crash conference Proceedings_, 1977, pp 713-751.

10. Walfisch, et al., "Designing of a Dummy's Abdomen for Detecting Injuries in Side Impact Collisions, _Fifth International IRCOBI Conference Proceedings_, 1980, pp. 149-169.

11. Nusholtz, G.S., Melvin, J.W., Mueller, G., et al., "Thoraco-Abdominal Response and Injury," _24th Stapp Car Crash conference Proceedings_, 1980, pp 187-228.

12. Lau, I. and Viano, D.C., "Influence of Impact Velocity on the Severity of Nonpenetrating Hepatic Injury," _Journal of Trauma_, 21(2):115-123, 1981a.

13. Lau, I. and Viano, D.C., "An Experimental Study on Hepatic Injury From Belt-Restraint Loading," _Aviation, Space, and Environmental Medicine_, October 1981, pp. 611-617.

14. Rouhana, S.W., Lau, I.V., and Ridella, S.A., _Influence of Velocity and Forced Compression on the Severity of Abdominal Injury in Blunt, Nonpenetrating Lateral Impact_. General Motors Research Publication, June 28, 1984.

15. Frey, C.F., Trollope, M.L., Harpster, W., and Snyder, R., "A Fifteen Year Experience With Automotive Hepatic Trauma," _Journal of Trauma_, 13:1039-1049, 1973.

16. Owens, M.P., Wolfman, E.F., and Chung, G.K., "The Management of Liver Trauma," _Archives of Surgery_, 103:211-215, 1971.

17. Hardy, K.J., "Patterns of Liver Injury After Fatal Blunt Trauma," _Surgery, Gynecology, and Obstetrics_, 134:39-43, 1972.

18. Bates, T., "Abdominal Trauma: A Repor of 129 Cases," _Postgraduate Medical Journal_, 49: 286-292, 1973.

19. Bondy, N., "Abdominal Injuries in National Crash Severity Study," _National Center for Statistics and Analysis Collected Technical Studies, Vol. II: Accident Data Analysis of Occupant Injuries and Crash Characteristics_, National Highway Traffic Safety Administration, Washington, D.C., 1980, pp. 59-80.

20. Crosby, W.M., King, A.I. and Stout, L.C., "Survival Following Impact: Improvement with Shoulder Harness Restraint," _American Journal of Obstetrics and Gynecology_, 112: 1101-1106, 1972.

21. Foley, R.W., harris, L.S., and Pilcher, D.B., "Abdominal Injuries in Automobile Accidents: Review of Care of Fatally injured Patients," _Journal of Trauma_, 17: 611-615, 1976.

22. Gallup, B.M., St-Laurent, A.M., and Newman, J.A., "Abdominal Injuries to Restrained Front seat Occupants in Frontal Collisions," _Proceedings of the 26th Conference of American Association of Automotive Medicine_, AAAM, Morton Grove, Illinois, 1982, pp. 131-148.

23. Gertner, H.R., Baker, S.P., Rutherford, R.B., and Spitz, W.V., "Evaluation of the Management of Vehicular Fatalities Secondary to Abdominal Injury," _Journal of Trauma_, 12: 425-431, 1972.

24. Grattan, E. and Clegg, N.G., "Clinical Causes of Death in Different Categories of Road User," _Proceedings of International Conference on the Biokinetics of Impacts_, IRCOBI, Bron, France, 1973, pp. 73-81.

25. Huelke, D.F. and Lawson, T.E., "Lower Torso Injuries and Automobile Seat Belts," SAE Paper No. 760370, Society of Automotive Engineers, Warrendale, PA, 1976.

26. Leung, Y.C., Tarriere, C., Fayon, A., Mairrese, P., and Banzet, P., "An Anti-submarining Scale Determined From Theoretical and Experimental Studies Using Three-dimensional Geometric Definition of the Lap Belt," _Proceedings of the 25th Stapp Car Crash Conference_, Society of Automotive Engineers, Warrendale, PA, 1981, pp. 685-729.

27. Leung, Y.C., et.al., "Submarining Injuries of Three-Point Belted Occupants in Frontal Collisions: Description, Mechanisms and Protection," _Proceedings of the 26th Stapp Car Crash Conference_, Society of Automotive Engineers, Warrendale, PA, 1982, pp. 173-205.

28. Mueller, W.F., "Nonpenetrating Injury of the Abdomen in landcraft Accidents," _Accident Pathology: Proceedings of an International Conference_, U.S. Government Printing Office, Washington, D.C., 1970, pp. 196-203.

29. Walt, A.J. and Grifka, T.J., "Blunt Abdominal Injury: A Review of 307 Cases," _Impact Injury and Crash Protection_, Ed. E.S. Gurdjian et al, Charles C. Thomas, Springfield, Ill., 1970, pp. 101-124.

30. Williams, J.S. and Kirkpatrick, J.R., "The Nature of Seat Belt Injuries," _Journal of Trauma_, 11: 207-218, 1971.

31. _The Abbreviated Injury Scale (1980 Revision)_, American Association for

Automotive Medicine, Morton Grove, Ill., 1976.

32. Whittaker, E.T., *A Treatise on the Analyticl Dynamics of Particles and Rigid Bodies*, Cambridge University Press, 1965.

33. Eppinger, R.H., Marcus, J.H., and Morgan, R.M., "Development of Dummy and Injury Index for NHTSA's Thoracic Side Impact Protection Research Program," SAE Publication No. 840885, Government/Industry Meeting and Exposition, Washington, D.C., May 21-24, 1984.

34. Eppinger, R.H., "Prediction of thoracic Injury Using Measurable Experimental Parameters," *Prceedings of the 6th Experimental Safety Vehicle Conference*, National Highway Traffic Safety Administration, Washington, D.C., 1976, pp. 770-780.

856028

Synthesis of Pelvic Fracture Criteria for Lateral Impact Loading

Mark Haffner
National Highway Traffic Safety Administration

Abstract

Two candidate functions for the prediction of pelvic fracture probability are created using lateral pelvic acceleration and age data from 84 cadaver impact experiments. These functions include measures of bone stress, bone strain, age, and load concentration factor. Data are analyzed using the maximum likelihood approach, and it is found that representation of the data by a Weibull distribution yields higher maximum likelihood than does the assumption of an underlying normal distribution.

Additional data are presented documenting pelvic force and acceleration responses for both cadavers and the Side Impact Dummy (SID). Systematic differences are noted and discussed.

Introduction

Lateral impact to the pelvis can result in injuries to the pelvic bone, to the hip joint, and to the soft tissue contents of the pelvic cavity. Bone fractures can occur at numerous sites on the pelvic ring: at the acetabulum, the sacro-iliac junction, the pubic symphysis, the pubic rami, and in the wing of the ilium. Within the pelvic cavity, fractures of the pelvis are associated with potentially severe injuries to the bladder and urinary tract.

Given this wide range of potential injury sites on the pelvic bone and within the pelvic cavity, it is most unlikely that a single parameter can be identified that is predictive of specific pelvic injury site and type. A more realistic goal, adopted here, is the identification of a parameter that is predictive of the occurrence of pelvic bone fracture, irrespective of fracture location.

In searching for a parameter predictive of pelvic fracture, we proceed on the assumption that a pelvic bone protection criterion will confer a large measure of protection on the contents of the pelvic cavity as well. Confirmation of this working hypothesis, however, remains for further study.

Data Resources

This analysis has drawn upon cadaveric lateral pelvic impact data from numerous sources. Table 1 presents a summary of these data resources and characterizes them by degree of applied load concentration, age range, average age of cadavers tested, and other variables of interest.

It is important for our purposes to note several significant ways in which the ONSER(A) data set differs from the balance of the data base:

1. The average age of ONSER(A) cadaveric specimens is higher than the average age for most other data sets included.
2. Loading in the ONSER(A) series was directed to the limited area of the greater trochanter via a hemispherical rigid impactor, as distinguished from the other test series in which both the iliac wing and trochanter could be loaded by larger impact surfaces.
3. The experimental design of the ONSER(A) test series differs from that of the other test series included. The ONSER(A) series sought to identify fracture threshold for each specimen, by repeatedly testing each specimen at increasing impact severity until fracture occurred. By contrast, the other test series in the data base tested each specimen once at known impact severity, with either fracture or nonfracture reported as outcome.

The fact that a markedly different experimental design was employed in the ONSER(A) series as compared to the other test series strongly suggests that these blocks of data be separated for analysis and that distinct methods of analysis be applied to the two resulting subsets.

With regard to transducer data available, it can be noted from Table 1 that input force data are available only for the ONSER(A) and the Heidelberg test series. Some observations will be made shortly with regard to the relationship of input force to measured pelvic accelerations for these two data sets; however, it is clear from Table 1 that the only common thread available in all data sets is pelvic acceleration and that only the y (lateral) component of pelvic acceleration is available in all data sets.

With regard to data processing procedures, digital data tapes were obtained for all test series so that uniform data processing procedures could be applied to them. Following a quality control process using the "raw" data, all remaining force and acceleration data were filtered, subsampled, and refiltered[1] before being entered into the project data base for further analysis.

Previously Proposed Injury Predictive Parameters

Previous investigators have proposed both maximum applied force and maximum pelvic acceleration fracture criteria for lateral pelvic impact. Cesari, et al.(2) have proposed a 10kN (3ms clip) limit on impact force for a 76kg male and 4kN (3ms) for a 5th percentile female. These values are based on the data obtained from their older subject population. Also, these limits are associated with the specific concentrated trochanter loading protocol of the ONSER(A) cadaver tests. Tarriere et al.(9) conducted a series of lateral drop tests using cadaver subjects and reported pelvic fractures associated with resultant peak pelvic accelerations of 62 to 120g. Peak resultant pelvic accelerations associated with nonfracture ranged up to 135g. Harris(10) discussed the potential interaction during impact of lateral loadings acting on

---

[1] Raw digital data were filtered with a 300Hz antialiasing Butterworth filter whose roll-off characteristics satisfied SAE J 211B. The data were then subsampled at 1,600SPS, and finally operated on with a finite impulse response filter with passband frequency = 100Hz, stopband frequency = 189Hz, passband ripple = 0225db, and stopband gain = 100db.

Table 1. Summary of data resources utilized in project data base

Organization	Description of Test Environment	Degree of Load Concentration on Pelvis	Number of Tests (Number of Fractures) male / female	Age Range male / female	Average Age male / female	Transducer Data Reported	References
Onser(A)	Rigid Impactor Strikes on Trochanter of Stationary Seated subjects	Concentrated	7 (4) / 5 (3)	61-85 / 63-79	71 / 70	Force & Pelvic ay	1,2,3
Heidelberg	Rigid and Padded Impacts with Sled Mounted Flat Wall	Distributed	23 (2) / 11 (2)	17-79 / 17-60	39 / 34	Force & Pelvic ax,ay,az	4
FAT	Moving Deformable Barrier into Opel Vehicles Nearside Impact	Distributed	29 (2) / 6 (0)	21-64 / 26-42	38 / 35	Pelvic ax,ay,az	5,6
Onser(B) (BMD Series)	Moving Deformable Barrier into Rabbit Vehicles Nearside Impact	Distributed	3 (0) / 2 (1)	43-55 / 39-40	50 / 40	Pelvic ay	7
HSRI	Rigid and Padded Sled Tests	Distributed	7 (0) / 3 (1)	62-84 / 45-75	71 / 59	Pelvic ax,ay,az	8

the iliac crest and on the hip joint. A tolerance value of 6kN for the sum of both the iliac crest and trochanter forces was proposed for specific use with the TRRL side impact dummy.

The EUROSID dummy now under development(3) employs three force transducers in the pelvic segment: one at the anatomical location of the pubic symphysis, and upper and lower transducers at the anatomical location of the junction between the iliac wing and the sacrum. Selection of one or a combination of outputs from these transducers for injury predictive purposes has not been finalized. The pelvis is also designed to accommodate a triaxial accelerometer for use with acceleration-based pelvic injury criteria.

Formulation of New Predictive Parameters

As has been pointed out by Nuscholtz, et al.(11), the interactions of the femur, pelvis, and associated soft tissue during lateral pelvic impact are complex. A fundamental source of variability appears to exist in the anatomy of the hip joint because rotation of the femoral head in the acetabulum during impact is a relatively unpredictable function of (a) initial femur and pelvic bone geometry, (b) degree of entrapment of the proximal femur by the impacting surface, and (c) variations in soft tissue thickness and distribution. Nuscholtz et al. properly caution that a generalized injury predictive parameter may be difficult to identify. Notwithstanding the variability inherent in pelvic response and injury patterns, however, we have attempted to isolate some of the confounding factors and quantify the extent of variability remaining in the data.

In formulating new fracture predictive parameters, we have elected to pursue two parallel analysis approaches. The first approach (denoted Approach 1) utilizes maximum bone stress as a primary explanatory variable, and also considers specimen age, specimen sex, and degree of applied load concentration for inclusion in analysis. The second approach (denoted Approach 2) substitutes maximum bone strain for maximum stress in the predictive function.

A brief discussion of the rationale for consideration of these variables follows.

1. Maximum Stress

Numerous solid material failure theories (e.g., maximum stress, maximum strain, maximum strain energy, maximum distortion energy, etc.) are available for application. For brittle materials, the maximum stress failure theory is generally favored. The maximum stress theory predicts failure when the largest principal stress reaches the uniaxial tensile or compressive failure stress. The efficacy of using a stress-related variable instead of raw applied force was suggested by Cesari(2). He hypothesized that many lateral pelvic fractures were linked to excessive bending stress in the frequently fractured pubic rami. In pursuing this hypothesis, he computed area moments of inertia of ilio-pubic ramus cross-sections (I_x) from undamaged portions of tested pelvic specimens, and successfully correlated fracture force (F) and (I_x) for fractured specimens (r = .96). The governing equation for simple bending is:

(1) $$\sigma = \frac{M}{(I_x/y)}$$

σ = ultimate tensile stress induced by bending of ramus

M = applied moment

I_x/y = area moment of inertia of ramus divided by offset from neutral axis

The moment applied to each specimen M = (F)(d), where d is a characteristic moment arm. Therefore, the above expression can be written:

(2) $$\frac{\sigma}{d} = \frac{F}{(I_x/y)}$$

The high linear correlation and near zero intercept reported by Cesari between F and (I_x/y) implies that:

(3) $$\frac{\sigma}{d} \cong \text{constant}$$

If d is a weak function of subject size and sex, the hypothesis advanced is upheld.

In the present effort, we have found it useful to invoke the equal stress-equal velocity scaling law to treat the experimental data (hereafter called subject data). The equal stress-equal velocity scaling law for geometrically similar models assumes that both density and modulus of elasticity are invariant and that the following relationships follow between subject data and data scaled for a specimen of standard size and mass. If we define:

(4) $$\frac{l_{sub}}{l_{std}} = \lambda$$

l_{sub} = characteristic length of subject

l_{std} = characteristic length of standard specimen

(5) then:

$$F_{std} = \frac{F_{sub}}{\lambda^2} \quad \text{for force}$$

(6) $\quad a_{std} = \lambda a_{sub} \quad$ for acceleration

(7) $\quad M_{std} = \dfrac{M_{sub}}{\lambda^3} \quad$ for mass

Using (4) and (5):

(8) $\quad \dfrac{F_{std}}{(l_{std})^2} = \dfrac{F_{sub}}{(l_{sub})^2} \equiv S$

Note in Equation (8) that the terms have units of force per unit area or stress, and thus that stress induced in the standard specimen and subject specimen are equal for the same test velocity (stress scales 1 to 1).

If, for convenience, we write equation (8) as:

(9) $\quad F_{std} = (S)(l_{std})^2$

we can observe that F_{std} is a measure of subject stress, adjusted only by a constant $(l_{std})^2$

Thus we would propose $F_{std} = F_{sub} \lambda^2$ as a measure of pelvic bone stress magnitude, which might have potential for fracture prediction.

For an isotropic specimen as assumed here:

λ is simply $\left(\dfrac{M_{sub}}{M_{std}}\right)^{1/3}$ from equation 7 and:

(10) $\quad F_{std} + F_{sub} \quad \left(\dfrac{M_{sub}}{76}\right)^{2/3} \quad \begin{cases} M_{sub} \text{ in Kg} \\ M_{std} = 76 \text{ Kg} \end{cases}$

In analogous fashion, using (6) and (7):

(11) $\quad a_{std} = \left(\dfrac{M_{sub}}{M_{std}}\right)^{1/3} (a_{sub})$

Multiplying the right hand side of (11) by the quantity we obtain:

$\dfrac{M_{sub}}{M_{sub}} = $ unity

(12) $\quad a_{std} = \left(\dfrac{1}{M_{std}}\right)^{1/3} \dfrac{(M_{sub} a_{sub})}{(M_{sub})^{2/3}}$

The quantity $M_{sub} a_{sub}$ has units of force, and $M_{sub}^{2/3}$ can be expressed as:

$[\rho_{sub} l_{c_{sub}}^3]^{2/3} = (\rho_{sub})^{2/3} l_{c_{sub}}^2$

where ρ_{sub} is subject density and $l_{c_{sub}}$ is a characteristic subject length.

Thus:

$a_{std} \approx \dfrac{1}{M_{std}^{1/3} \rho_{sub}^{2/3}} \left(\dfrac{F_{sub}}{l_{c_{sub}}^2}\right)$ (13)

Since M_{std} is a constant and ρ_{sub} is also invariant, equation (13) is of the form:

$a_{std} = (\text{constant})(\text{stress})$ (14)

We thus propose $a_{std} = \lambda a_{sub}$ as an alternative measure of pelvic bone stress. For an assumed isotropic specimen, Equation (11) may be used with $M_{std} = 76$ kg to yield:

$a_{std} = a_{sub} \left(\dfrac{M_{sub}}{76}\right)^{1/3} \quad \{M_{sub} \text{ in Kg}\}$ (15)

The above approach to the determination of λ does not, however, take into account variation in subject build; i.e., a short, stocky specimen and a tall, thin specimen each of equal mass would each yield the same λ. The following method is proposed to improve the estimation of λ when subject height and mass are known.

The body is considered as a cylinder of mass M, density ρ, height H, and diameter D. The diameter of a subject may be estimated as:

$D_{sub} = 2 \left(\dfrac{M_{sub}}{\pi \rho_{std} H_{sub}}\right)^{1/2}$ (16)

Similarly, the diameter of the standard specimen is:

$D_{std} = 2 \left(\dfrac{M_{std}}{\pi \rho_{std} H_{std}}\right)^{1/2}$ (17)

Then since $\rho_{sub} = \rho_{std}$

$\lambda = \dfrac{D_{sub}}{D_{std}} \left[\left(\dfrac{M_{sub}}{M_{std}}\right)\left(\dfrac{H_{std}}{H_{sub}}\right)\right]^{1/2}$ (18)

For $M_{std} = 76$ Kg and $H_{std} = 1.75$ m :

$\lambda = \left[\left(\dfrac{M_{sub}}{76}\right)\left(\dfrac{1.75}{H_{sub}}\right)\right]^{1/2} \quad \begin{cases} M_{sub} \text{ in Kg} \\ H_{sub} \text{ in m} \end{cases}$ (19)

and using (5):

$F_{std} = \dfrac{F_{sub}}{(M_{sub}/76)(1.75/H_{sub})}$ (20)

In analogous fashion, using (19) and (6):

$a_{std} = \left[\left(\dfrac{M_{sub}}{76}\right)\left(\dfrac{1.75}{H_{sub}}\right)\right]^{1/2} (a_{sub}) \quad \begin{matrix} M_{sub} \text{ in Kg} \\ H_{sub} \text{ in m} \end{matrix}$ (21)

Implementation of Equations (10) and (15) is denoted scaling method A. Implementation of Equations (20) and (21) is denoted scaling method B. Both methods have been used for processing subject data; results will be presented below in the Analysis section.

Since bone is a viscoelastic material, bone stress may be considered to be a function of both strain and strain rate. The strain rate dependence of bone has received considerable research attention. Evans(12) reports the experiments of McElhaney and Byars (1965) and McElhaney (1966). The experiments conducted were constant velocity compression tests on cattle and human femoral bone. At strain rates exceeding 1cm/cm/s, the investigators found that ultimate compressive stress and modulus of elasticity increased while strain at fracture decreased. (Ultimate compressive stress at 1cm/cm/s was 22 percent greater than at .01cm/cm/s; ultimate strain decreased 31 percent.

A lateral pelvic deflection of .5cm (.2in) in 20ms would correspond to a strain of approximately 2 percent and a strain rate of approximately 1.1cm/cm/s. Thus, it appears likely that the pelvic bone exhibits significant rate sensitivity in the automotive crash environment. The inclusion of strain rate sensitivity in a pelvic fracture model is, therefore, desirable.

2. Maximum Strain

A maximum strain failure criterion is also a likely candidate for consideration. In the present application, maximum strain will be calculated via a lumped parameter pelvic model as discussed under Approach 2 below.

3. Age Effects

Evans(12) reports the data of Messerer (1880), who investigated the static bending strength of fresh cortical bone specimens from the tibia, femur, and humerus of male and female subjects. Ultimate bending stress increased to a maximum in the range of 20 to 30 years of age and declined steadily thereafter. The ratio of male femur ultimate bending stress at 75 years of age to that at 24 years of age is approximately .81; the corresponding ratio for females tested was .85. Yamada(13) cites data for static bending of fresh cortical bone and reports maximum ultimate bending stress occurring for specimens in the range 20 to 40 years of age, with strength declining thereafter. The ratio of ultimate bending stress reported at 70 to 79 years of age to that at 20 to 29 years is .80.

Thus, it is concluded that age effects upon probability of pelvic bone fracture are significant and should be incorporated into our pelvic fracture model.

4. Sexual Differences

In the bending data of Messerer reported above, sexual differences in ultimate bending stress can be assessed. The ratio of female ultimate bending stress to male ultimate stress for a given age range is approximately .90 for the femur and 1.0 for the tibia. Yamada reports no significant sexual differences in compressive strength or bending strength in samples of cortical bone.

The absence of significant sexual difference in ultimate bending stress suggests strongly that the lower pelvic fracture forces reported by Cesari(2) for females as compared to males is largely due to smaller female pelvic bone cross-sectional areas. As was discussed earlier, when Cesari normalized the male and female fracture forces in terms of a measure of stress, the male and female data were observed to overplot.

Therefore, it is tentatively concluded that the use of a stress-related variable should permit male and female data to be merged for analysis.

The possibility exists, however, that the scaling laws we are proposing will not fully accommodate the differing pelvic geometries of male and female specimens. (The scaling law requires geometric similarity.) It is therefore proposed that the extent to which male and female data does overplot be observed before reaching a conclusion on the suitability of this scaling approach.

5. Degree of Load Concentration

The pelvic load concentration factor has been mentioned as an important potential influence upon fracture potential.

It may be recalled that two main load paths exist into the laterally impacted pelvis, through the acetabulum via the trochanter and through the iliac wing. The ONSER(A) data can be considered as defining the pelvic fracture tolerance for the trochanter load path. However, in the balance of the experimental data (and presumably in the vehicle environment), load is transmitted in some proportion through both paths. A pelvic accelerometer cannot distinguish which load path or paths are active but responds to net applied force. Thus, pelvic accelerations as measured from the ONSER(A) experiments should not be interpreted in the same way as pelvic accelerations measured in distributed load experiments.

A simplified schematic drawing illustrating this point is shown in Figure 1. The pelvis is shown assumed as a rigid body of mass M with crushable elements at the trochanter and iliac wing locations. Let us say that we know the "trochanter" will fail at force F_1, and that the "iliac wing" will fail at some force F_2. For argument, we will assume that these failures are independent. In case (a) similar to the ONSER(A) configuration, we would associate acceleration F_A/M with pelvic fracture. In case (b), where the iliac wing carries external load, we would associate pelvic acceleration $(F_A+F_B)/M$ with the same fracture. Clearly, the nature of load distribution is a significant input to the interpretation of an acceleration-based pelvic fracture criterion.

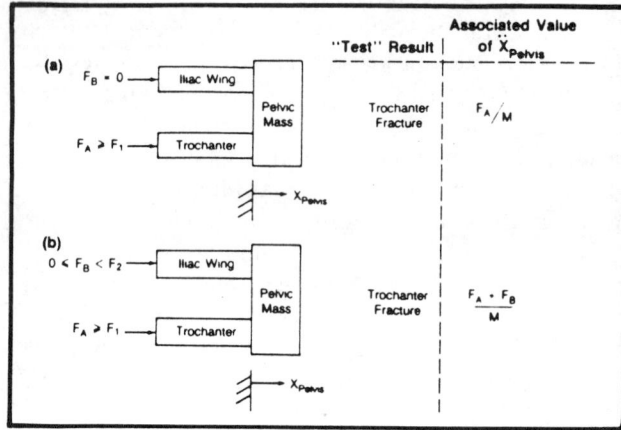

Figure 1. Schematic illustration of concentrated and distributed lateral pelvic loading

Summarizing our discussions relative to candidate parameters for inclusion in our fracture predictive function, it is postulated that probability of pelvic fracture is a function of the following variables:

1. A stress measure as quantified by a standardized (scaled) peak applied force or standardized (scaled) peak pelvic acceleration (Approach 1)
2. A strain measure as quantified by the output of a lumped parameter model (Approach 2)
3. Age of specimen
4. Degree of applied load distribution (concentrated or distributed)

Data Analysis and Results

Before proceeding with the analysis, it is of interest to look at the relationship between recorded force and acceleration for the limited number of ONSER(A) and Heidelberg tests in which both were recorded. (Only the lateral component of force F_y was measured. Also, only the y component of acceleration was utilized in analysis because (a) a_y is the only measurement available in all of the data, and (b) incorporation of resultant acceleration into the analysis was investigated and shown to yield no significant improvement in predictive capability.)

Typical overplots of force and acceleration traces from the ONSER(A) series are shown in Figures 2 and 3. (Note that the peaks of the force traces have been artificially scaled to match the peaks of the acceleration traces so that trace shapes can readily be compared.) As may be observed, there is lag in acceleration response initially, but force and acceleration peaks tend to coincide in time. Substantial differences exist, however, in the shapes of force and acceleration traces during the unloading phase.

Figure 4 shows the relationship between peak force and peak acceleration (scaled according to method A) for the 11 ONSER(A) tests in the data base for which both signals are available. The good correlation observed (r =

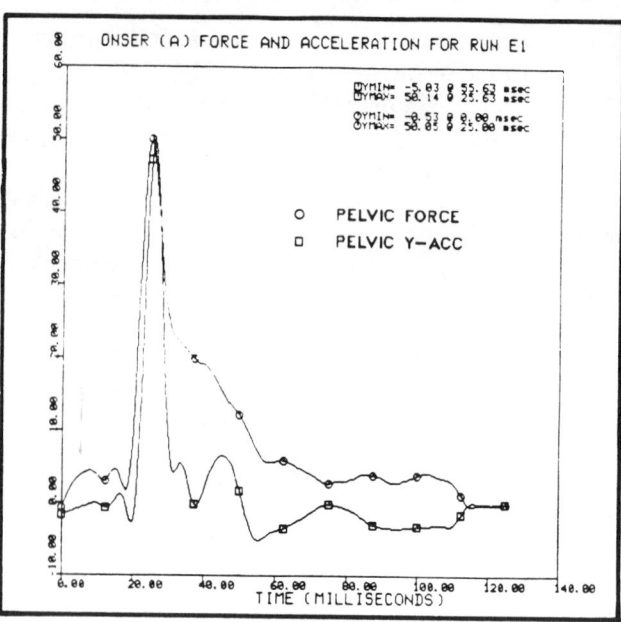

Figure 2. Pelvic force and pelvic Y-acceleration overlay for ONSER (A) test E1

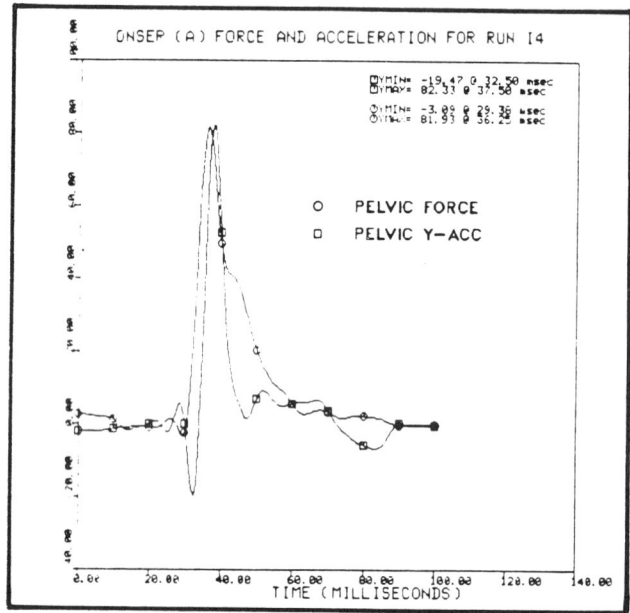

Figure 3. Pelvic force and pelvic Y-acceleration overlay for ONSER (A) test I4

.89) suggests that if (as has been proposed by Cesari) an injury criterion can be developed using peak applied force, then it should be possible to use pelvic acceleration to construct a similar predictive function.

Figures 5 and 6 present analogous overplots of force and acceleration for two Heidelberg tests—one rigid and one padded. The interesting and typical differences observed between these two tests will be discussed further in Appendix B, but for the moment we can observe that peak force and peak acceleration again tend to coincide in time. Figure 7 presents peak-scaled force vs. peak-

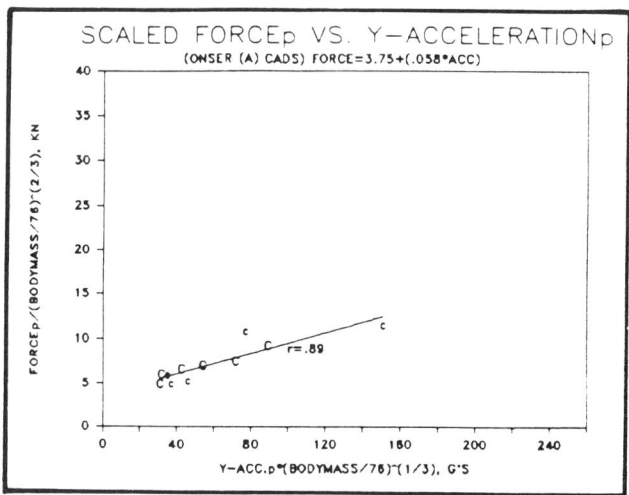

Figure 4. Scaled peak pelvic force versus scaled peak pelvic Y-acceleration for ONSER (A) tests

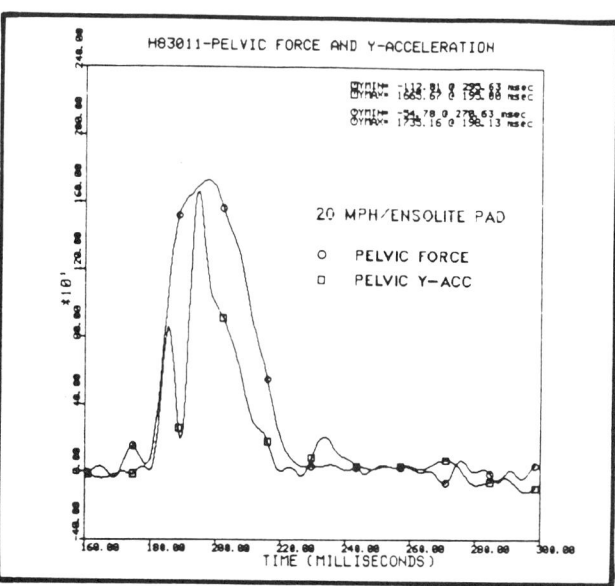

Figure 6. Pelvic force and pelvic Y-acceleration for Heidelberg test H83011

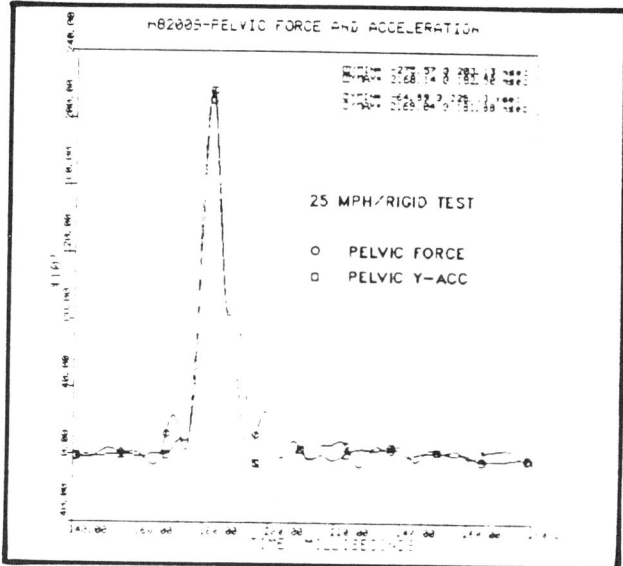

Figure 5. Pelvic force and pelvic Y-acceleration for Heidelberg test H82009

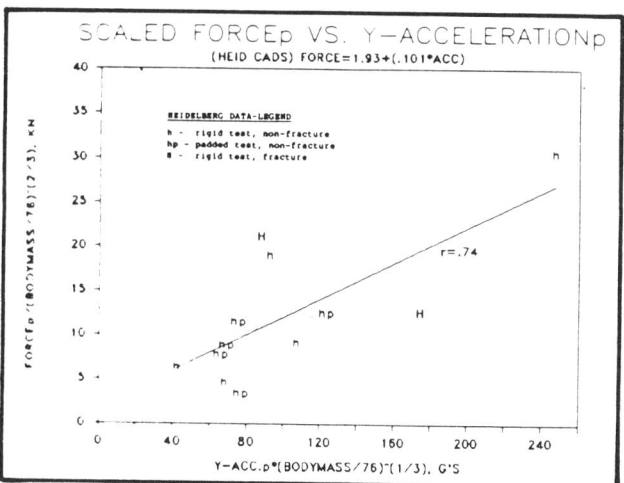

Figure 7. Scaled peak pelbic force vs. scaled peak pelvic y-acceleration for heidelberg tests.

scaled acceleration for available Heidelberg data. Correlation between them is not as high (r = .74) as the correlation found for the ONSER(A) data.

In general, it has not been possible to utilize force data to construct a predictive function from the non-ONSER(A) data. This is because excluding the ONSER(A) data, the number of cases of fracture for which force data is available is very small (0 male, 2 female). In any case, the force data as measured from the Heidelberg tests would not be comparable to the ONSER(A) force data, since the measured Heidelberg forces were applied via a large contact plate that spanned the pelvis and thigh.

As has been discussed, the ONSER(A) data have been separated from the other available data (see Table 1) for purposes of analysis. Analysis thus concentrated on the use of acceleration data as obtained from the Heidelberg, FAT, ONSER(B), and HSRI data sets.

Heidelberg, FAT, ONSER(B), and HSRI Data— Approach 1

The stress variable $a_{std} = (a_{subp})(\lambda)$ is plotted in Figure 8 against age, where we recall from Equation (19) that:

$$\lambda = \left[\left(\frac{M_{sub}}{76}\right)\left(\frac{1.75}{H_{sub}}\right)\right]^{1.2} \quad \begin{cases} M_{sub} \text{ in Kg} \\ H_{sub} \text{ in m} \end{cases}$$

757

and where a_{subp}, M_{sub} and H_{sub} are the peak y pelvis acceleration, body mass, and height for each test.

In Figure 8, each nonfracture test is plotted as a dot, while each fracture test carries the initial of its source according to the following code:

H—Heidelberg
B—ONSER(B)
F—FAT
S—HSRI

Based on the known decrease of ultimate bone strength with age presented earlier, a series of lines are drawn on Figure 8 with slope $m = -0.5g/yr$ corresponding to a 20 percent reduction in ultimate stress between the ages of 24 and 75 years. It is then postulated that the zone between each pair of lines represents a region of nearly constant fracture probability. Since the equation of each line is of the form:

(22) $(a_{subp})(\lambda) + (.5)(age) = $ constant

we further postulate that:

Probability of Pelvic Fracture
$= f[a_{subp} * \lambda + (.5)(age)]$

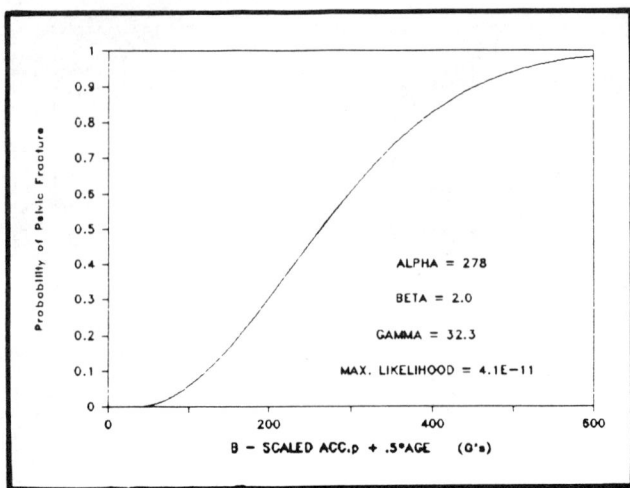

Figure 9. Probability of pelvic fracture from Weibull analysis of distributed load data—approach 1

recall, are for a specimen of mass = 76kg and height = 1.75m.

We may also note on Figure 9 the values of α, β, and γ as computed by the Weibull program for best fit to the data, and the maximum likelihood number of 4.1×10^{-11} associated with this computation. Figure 10 presents the computed probability density function. The fact that this function is not symmetrical confirms that the underlying distribution is not normal. However, we found it of interest to impose normality upon the data, observe the results, and compare them to the Weibull computations. (A probit analysis program was used for normal distribution computations.)

This comparison is presented in Figures 11 and 12, where it may be clearly seen that the Weibull distribution is right-shifted as compared to the normal distribution. Also of interest is the fact that the maximum likelihood number calculated for the imposed normal distribution

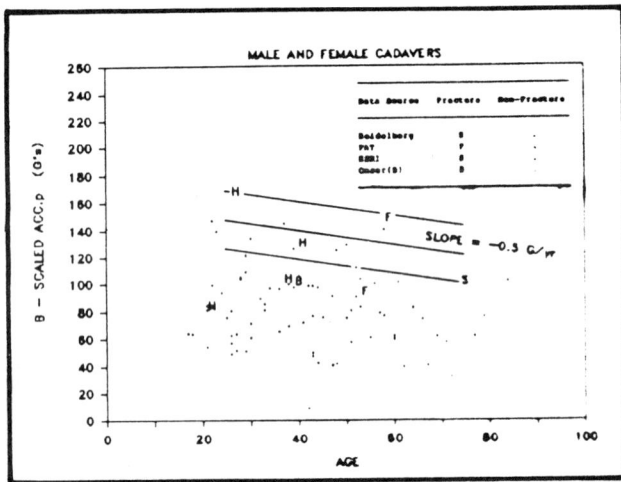

Figure 8. B-scaled acceleration versus specimen age—distributed load data

Since the data being considered are quantal or "censored," as defined by Ran et al.(14), we have applied the maximum likelihood approach discussed there, and have adopted a Weibull distribution as representative of the data. Figure 9 represents the result of analysis of the available distributed load data. For any selected fracture probability and age, a "tolerable" value of peak B-scaled acceleration = $a_{std} = \lambda a_{subp}$ can be read from the figure. For example, for a selected 20 percent probability of pelvic fracture at 40 years of age, we may find $a_{std} = 143g$. Similarly, for 10 percent fracture probability and 40 years of age, $a_{std} = 103g$. These "standard" values, we may

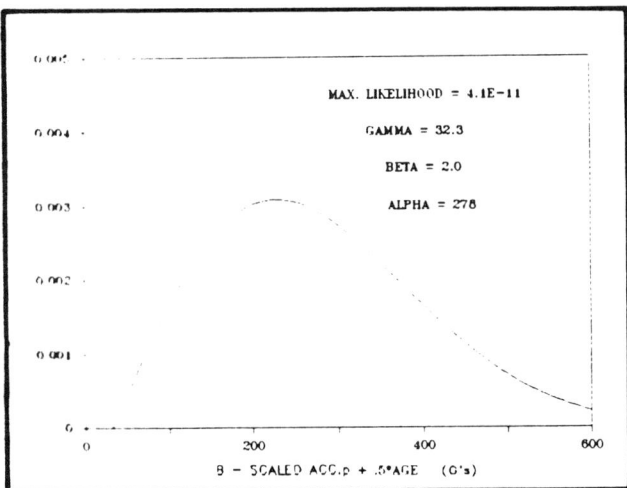

Figure 10. Weibull probability density function associated with Figure 9

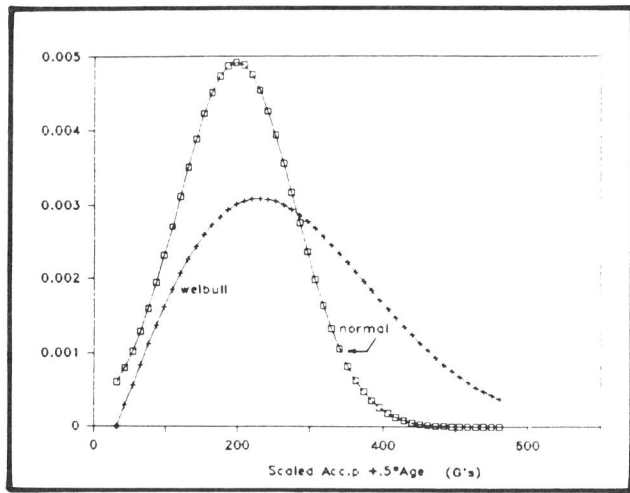

Figure 11. Comparison of Weibull and normal probability density functions calculated

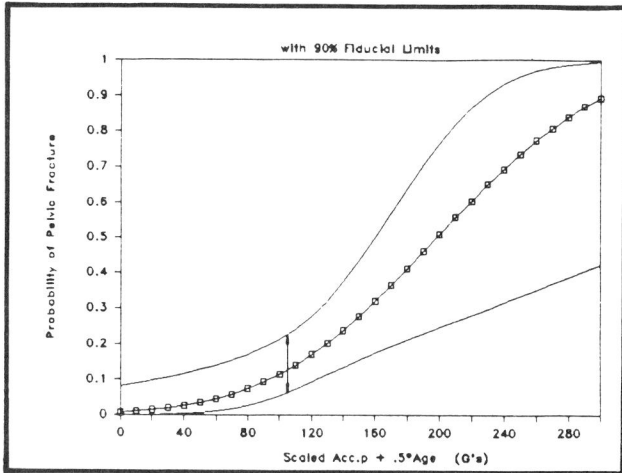

Figure 13. Fiducial limits on probability of pelvic fracture as computed from imposed normal distribution

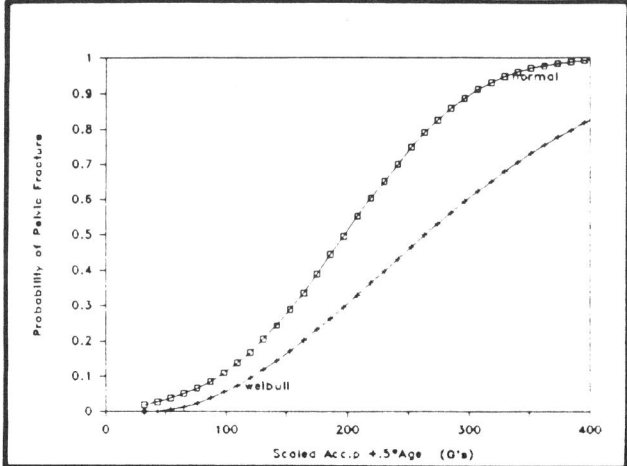

Figure 12. Comparison of pelvic fracture probabilities computed from Weibull and normal distributions—distributed load data—approach 1

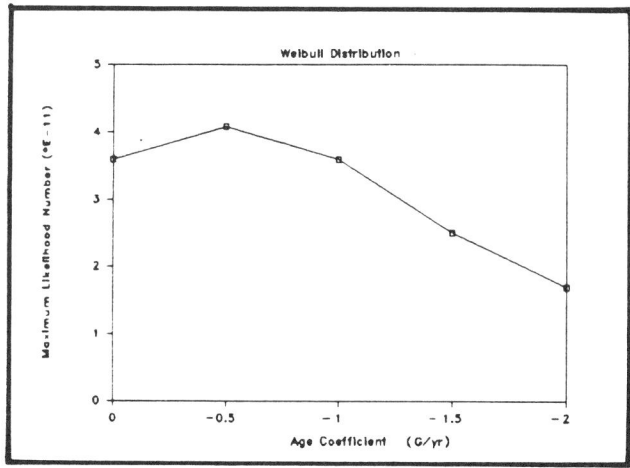

Figure 14. Maximum likelihood number versus age coefficient—Weibull analysis—approach 1

was 6.0×10^{-16}, lower than that for the Weibull computation, indicating that the Weibull function provides a better fit to our data.

With regard to confidence intervals, the algorithm for their computation is not presently available for the Weibull distribution. However, 90 percent fiducial limits have been computed for reference for the normal distribution assumption and are provided in Figure 13.

Further, as a check that the value of the coefficient on age m was correctly deduced as -0.5, a series of Weibull fits to the data were run for m = 0, -0.5, -1.0, -1.5, and -2.0. As indicated by Figure 14, maximum likelihood did indeed occur for m = -0.5, thus providing support for our selection process for m.

Heidelberg, FAT, ONSER(B), and HSRI Data— Approach 2

Approach 1 above operates on maximum pelvic acceleration as a measure of maximum stress. The utility of this approach tends to be limited, however, by the variability inherent in the measurement of a peak quantity. In Approach 2, a straightforward scheme was sought that would minimize dependence on this peak measurement. Toward this end, a lumped parameter one dimensional linear model was constructed as shown in Figure 15. Mass M_1 is associated with struck side upper leg mass, and M_2 is associated with the "pelvic mass" upon which the pelvic accelerometer is attached.

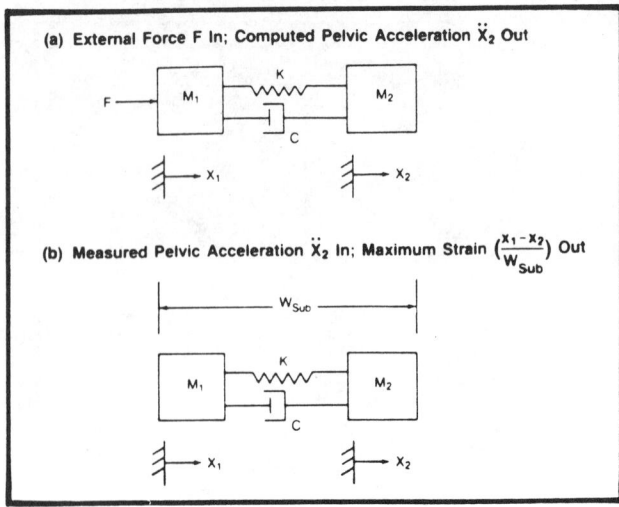

Figure 15. Model construct for pelvic injury assessment

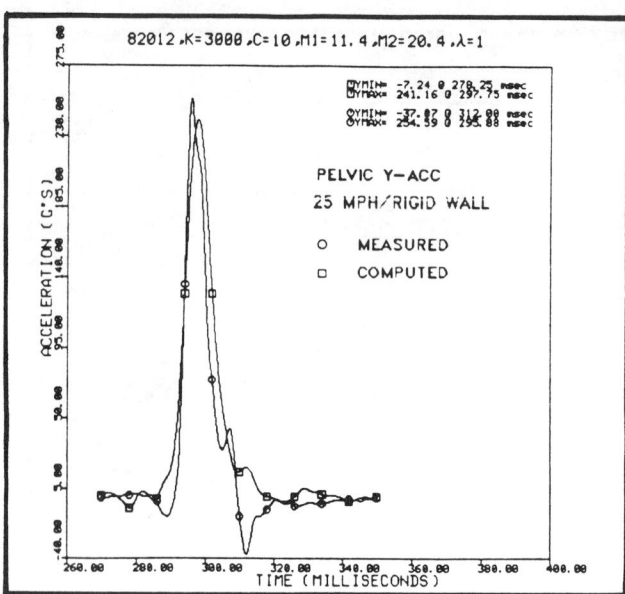

Figure 16. Comparison of measured pelvic Y-acceleration to that computed using two-mass model of Figure 15(a)—Heidelberg test H82012

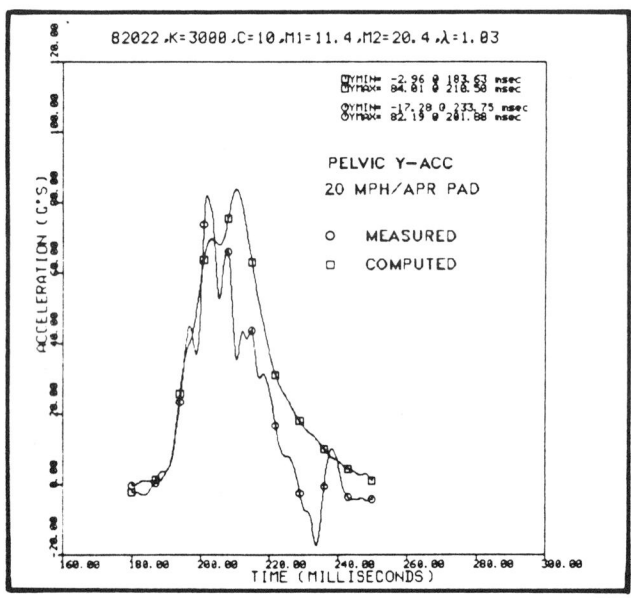

Figure 17. Comparison of measured pelvic Y-acceleration to that computed using two-mass model of Figure 15(a)

There is a basis for the formulation of a model in this configuration in the work of (11), wherein impedance plots for the laterally impacted pelves of three cadavers are reported. This simple construct should not be thought of as a literal model of the laterally impacted pelvis, but rather as a useful device for injury predictive purposes along the lines of the Brinn and Staffeld Effective Displacement Index(15) or the HSRI Maximum Strain Criterion(16).

Our operating premise is that if the model is "run backwards," i.e., if measured pelvic acceleration is provided as input to the model at M_2 (see Figure 15b), that a function of resulting maximum "pelvic" strain $(X_1-X_2)_{max}/W_{sub}$ can be utilized in a fracture predictive function (W_{sub} is subject pelvic width). Specifically, if we denote the quantity $(X_1-X_2)_{max}/W_{sub}$ as MPS or Maximum Pelvic Strain, we postulate that:

Probability of Pelvic Fracture = f[MPS÷(n)(age)]

where n is an age coefficient relative to reduction of ultimate strain with age.

To select reasonable values for parameters M_1, M_2, K, and C, the model was first exercised in the "forward" direction (see Figure 15a), using the 12 Heidelberg cadaver runs for which both force and acceleration data were available. (Parameters were scaled according to the mass and height of each specimen using scaling method B.) Initial parameter estimates were deduced from the impedance plots of (11); adjustment by trial and error then resulted in the determination of a parameter set for which observed and computed pelvic accelerations were reasonably matched for both a rigid case (H82012) and an APR padded case (H82022), as shown in Figures 16 and 17, respectively. The parameter set selected was as follows:

M_1 = 11.4 lb, M_2 = 20.4 lb, K = 3,000 lb/in, and C = 10 lb-s/in.

Because this model exercise showed output pelvic acceleration to be more sensitive to change in total mass than to change in K or C, and since the influence of strain on fracture predictive capability was being investigated, three sets of standard parameters were selected for further use, with three possible values for C, as shown in Table 2.

As a final preparatory step before exercising the model, the standard parameters of Table 2 were B-scaled

Table 2. Standard parameter sets chosen for exercise of MPS model

Set No.	M_1(lb)	M_2(lb)	K(lb/in)	C(lb-sec/in)
1	11.4	20.4	3000	5
2	11.4	20.4	3000	10
3	11.4	20.4	3000	20

for each subject in the data base to create a file of subject specific parameters using the following relationships:

$$(23) \quad M_{1\,sub} = \lambda^3 M_{1\,std}$$
$$(24) \quad M_{2\,sub} = \lambda^3 M_{2\,std}$$
$$(25) \quad K_{sub} = \lambda K_{std}$$
$$(26) \quad C_{sub} = \lambda^2 C_{std}$$

where the value of λ for each subject was obtained from Equation (19).

A listing of the calculated subject specific model parameters may be found in Appendix A.

As shown in Figure 15(b), and using actual subject pelvic acceleration data as input to mass M_2, the model was exercised three times for each qualifying subject in the data base, once for each of the three parameter sets of Table 2. For each model run, the quantities $V_{max} = (\dot{X}_1 - \dot{X}_2)_{max}$ and maximum strain were calculated (see listings in Appendix A). The maximum strain (MPS) for each subject was calculated as follows:

$$(27) \quad MPS_{sub} = \frac{(X_1 - X_2)_{max}}{\lambda W_{std}}$$

where W_{std} is the pelvic bispinous breadth for a standard specimen = 22.5cm (8.84in) and λW_{std} is therefore equal to W_{sub}, or subject pelvic width.

Using a method analogous to that employed in Approach 1, the MPS values calculated for each subject using the model were then plotted versus corresponding subject age data. Three plots were thus created corresponding to the three parameter sets of Table 2. Figure 18 presents the plot for parameter set 3. Again, using methods analogous to those employed earlier, three candidate fracture probability functions were created for the three parameter sets as follows:

For Set 1: Probability of Pelvic Fracture
= f (MPS + .035 * age)
For Set 2: Probability of Pelvic Fracture
= f (MPS + .030 * age)

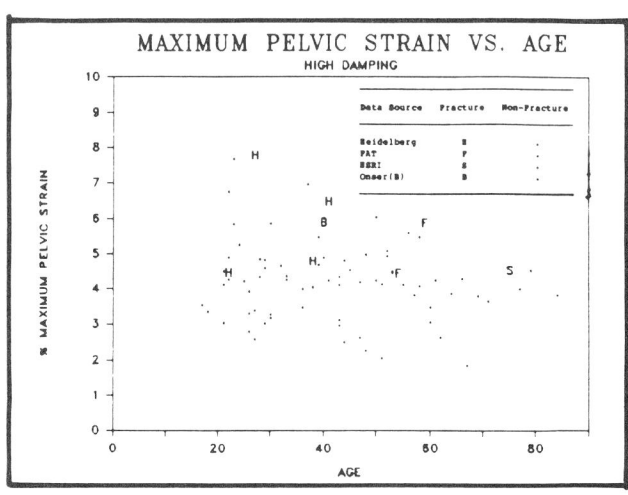

Figure 18. Computed maximum pelvic strain versus specimen age—parameter set #3—distributed load data

For Set 3: Probability of Pelvic Fracture
= f (MPS + .025 * age)

All three sets were submitted for Weibull analysis and computation of maximum likelihood numbers. The highest maximum likelihood, computed for parameter set 3, was 1.1×10^{-9}.

Figures 19 and 20 present the Weibull probability function and distribution, respectively, for parameter set 3 computations. We may note using Figure 19 that the value of MPS corresponding to 20 percent fracture probability at 40 years of age is approximately 6.1 percent, and that the corresponding value of MPS for 10 percent fracture probability and 40 years of age is approximately 4.8 percent.

It is also of interest to compare the best maximum likelihood number arising from Approach 2 to that computed from Approach 1. These are shown in Table 3.

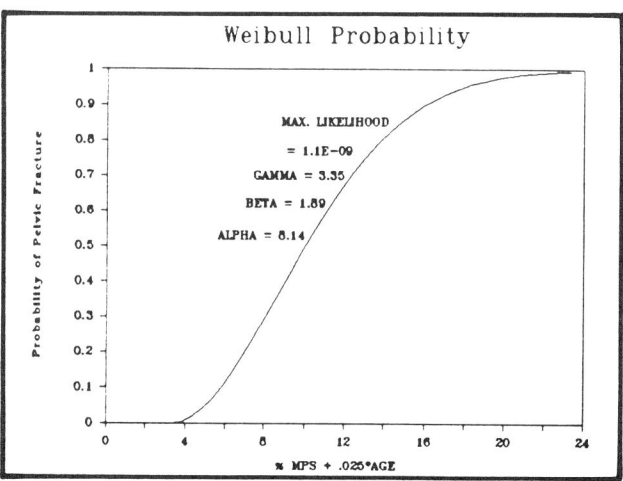

Figure 19. Probability of pelvic fracture from Weibull analysis of distributed load data, approach 2, parameter set #3 (M_1 = 11.4 lb, M_2 = 20.4 lb, k = 3,000 lb/in, C = 20 lb-sec/in).

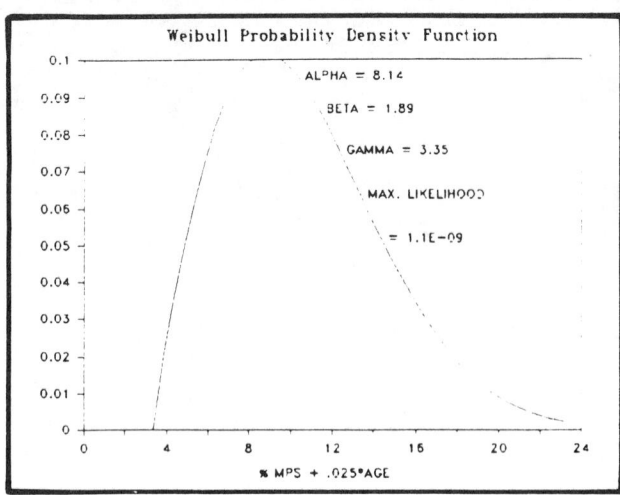

Figure 20. Weibull probability density function associated with Figure 19

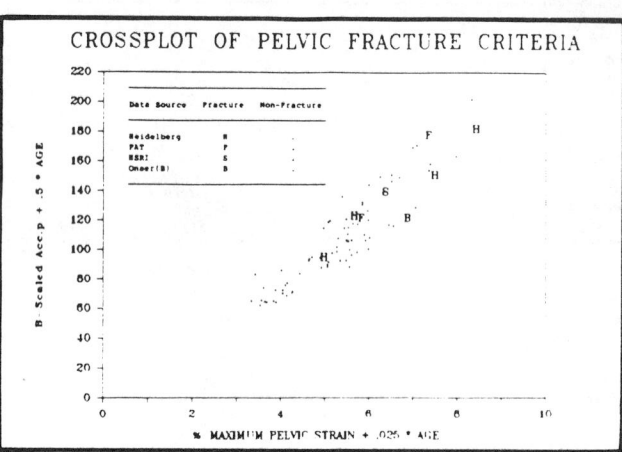

Figure 21. Crossplot of two candidate lateral pelvic fracture criteria

Table 3. Comparison of maximum likelihood numbers

Approach No.	Maximum Likelihood Number
1	4.1×10^{-11}
2	1.1×10^{-9}

It is concluded, based on the higher maximum likelihood number achieved for the MPS approach, that the incorporation of additional information from the acceleration pulse into the predictive function increases its predictive power.

Finally, we have cross-plotted the values of the predictive functions for the two approaches (Weibull computations) for all qualifying subjects and present the results in Figure 21. We may observe that differences do exist in the relative ordering of the data by the two approaches; however, these differences are not large.

Incorporation of ONSER(A) Data Into the Analysis

As has been previously discussed, the ONSER(A) data have been separated from the balance of the data for purposes of analysis because
- Unlike the other data sets, it is not quantal (or censored) in nature.
- Unlike the other data sets, concentrated loads were applied to the pelvis.

In subjecting each specimen to increasing impact severity until fracture occurred, Cesari sought to define the fracture tolerance of each specimen. For each specimen, we may presume that the severity of the last nonfracture test underestimates specimen tolerance, while the severity of the fracture-inducing test overestimates specimen tolerance to some degree. Therefore, we take as the best estimate of fracture tolerance for each specimen the average response of the last nonfracture test and the fracture test. Four test pairs are available for examination. Scaled acceleration data for specimens D, E, I, and J are presented on Figure 22 (results for E are anomalous in that last nonfracture response is higher than fracture response; the higher value is thus taken as the fracture response estimate). The range of estimates for scaled acceleration associated with fractures thus ranges from 41g (D) to 79g (I). Since all of these tests are narrowly grouped in age, we plot the above scaled acceleration range on Figure 8 at age = 69 years and present the result as Figure 23. It is immediately apparent that ONSER(A) fracture estimates plot very low in the distribution of other available data.

A similar presentation using MPS as the response variable is presented in Figure 24, and the corresponding fracture estimate range is plotted on Figure 18 as Figure 25. Again, the fracture range estimate plots very low in the distribution of the other data.

It is concluded that ONSER(A) fractures occurred at significantly lower measured pelvic accelerations than in the other data sets. In fact, the highest fracture estimate in the ONSER(A) set corresponds to about a 5 percent fracture probability level in the main data set.

Discussion

It is believed that a probable explanation for the result found in the previous section may be found in Figure 1. That is, for concentrated loading to the trochanter as schematically shown in 1(a), acceleration associated with fracture is minimized.

The fact, however, that the fracture distributions for the ONSER(A) data are so different compared to the balance of the data base points to the conclusion that the

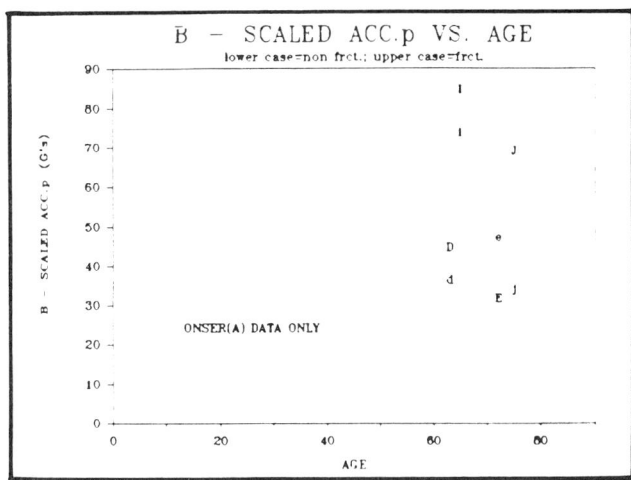

Figure 22. Nonfracture/fracture data pairs from ONSER (A) test series

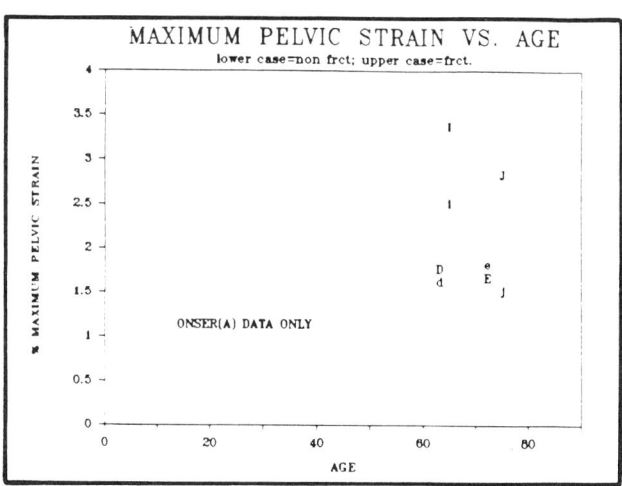

Figure 24. Nonfracture/fracture data pairs from ONSER (A) test series

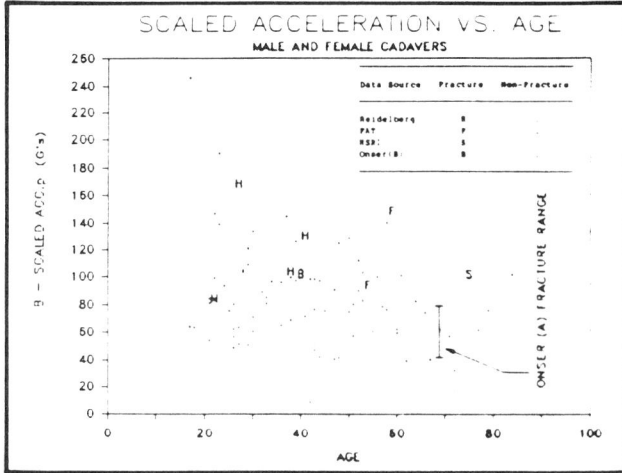

Figure 23. Superposition of ONSER (A) fracture range estimate on distributed load data—approach 1

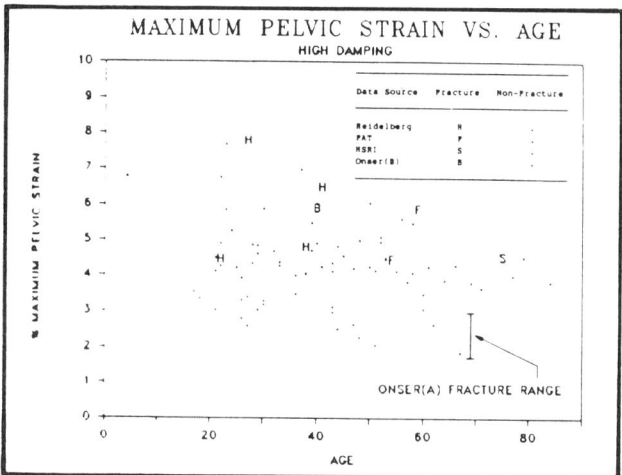

Figure 25. Superposition of ONSER (A) fracture range estimate on distributed load data—approach 2

ONSER(A) impact tests involved a degree of load concentration significantly higher than that realized in the vehicle environment. It will be recalled the tests used in our analysis involved rigid walls and three types of vehicle interiors (Opel, Rabbit, and Volvo). Yet in no case did a pelvic fracture occur at a response level as low as the estimated ONSER(A) fracture range.

The ONSER(A) data are, of course, most valuable in that the data define the load tolerance of one of the two major pelvic load paths. Investigation would also appear to be warranted into the load tolerance of the "other" load path through the iliac wing and into the effects of superposition of distributed loads as typically found in the vehicle environment.

It is recognized that any acceleration measure reflects the net force acting on the measured body. Thus, a pelvic acceleration measurement would be expected to be influenced to some degree by other forces acting on the pelvis during the impact event (e.g., horizontal seat interface force and horizontal shear force between the abdomen and pelvis). Some insight into the magnitude of this potential source of variability can be obtained by reference to Figure 4. Despite the presumed existence of seat and internal shear forces, a high correlation is obtained between peak applied force and peak pelvic acceleration. This result implies, for the ONSER(A) test condition at least, that the vector sum of the seat and shear forces is a predictable function of impact severity level. However, the extent of variability introduced into pelvic acceleration measurement in other environments more typical of the vehicle interior deserves further study before this observation can be generalized.

The data base is heavily biased toward nonfracture outcome. There is a need for additional fracture data to improve confidence in our fracture probability estimates, especially at higher fracture probabilities.

Male and female data have been merged for analysis, as have data from rigid and padded test conditions. The availability of further fracture data would permit a more detailed examination of the validity of this approach.

There is no doubt that a force-based approach to pelvic injury prediction exists as a strong alternative or adjunct to the acceleration-based proposals advanced here. The lack of a substantial body of comparable sets of force data have precluded our investigation of this alternative. When such data become available, a maximum likelihood analysis could provide a rational basis for ranking the effectiveness of the two approaches.

Summary and Conclusion

Two functions predictive of pelvic fracture due to distributed lateral impact have been synthesized from available data. The functions utilize the lateral component of pelvic acceleration as measured on 84 male and female cadaveric subjects from four major test series.

The second function, which incorporates the time history of measured acceleration, has been found to offer higher predictive power than does the first, which operates on peak acceleration magnitude alone. Age has been included as an explanatory variable in both approaches, and the value of its inclusion has been confirmed by the analysis.

All data have been analyzed using maximum likelihood methods. It has been confirmed that representation of the data by a Weibull distribution yields higher maximum likelihood than does the assumption that the data are normally distributed.

The degree of load distribution on the impacted pelvis has been identified as an important variable controlling pelvic tolerance to fracture. Acquisition of additional data defining the force tolerance of the pelvic bone under distributed loading conditions appears to be desirable.

Acknowledgments

Several individuals have made important contributions to the work reported here.

Deserving special mention, Margaret Hayden of Chi Associates painstakingly assembled the data base (see Appendix A) and artfully conducted innumerable queries of the data in the process of creating the presentations found throughout this paper.

Ranga Rangarajan of the Automated Science Group, Inc. implemented the MPS model under difficult time constraints and assisted in interpretation of early results.

Dominique Cesari of ONSER graciously provided a data tape of his [ONSER(A)] experiments for analysis, and Nabih Alem of UMTRI processed these data into the NHTSA format for our use.

Jeffrey Marcus and Richard Morgan of NHTSA developed many of the software routines that were extensively used on this project and that contributed materially to its progress.

Rolf Eppinger of NHTSA provided the benefit of many discussions during the course of the work.

Last, but certainly not least, Beulah Evans of NHTSA expertly prepared the manuscript for publication.

References

1. Cesari, D., M. Ramet, and P. Clair, "Evaluation of pelvic fracture tolerance in side impact," Proceedings 24th Stapp Car Crash Conference, SAE Paper 801306, 1980.
2. Cesari, D., and M. Ramet, "Pelvic tolerance and protection criteria in side impact," Proceedings 26th Stapp Car Crash Conference, SAE Paper 821159, 1982.
3. Cesari, D., R. Bouquet, and R. Zac, "A new pelvis design for the European side impact dummy," Proceedings 28th Stapp Car Crash Conference, SAE Paper 841650, 1984.
4. Kallieris, D., R. Mattern, G. Schmidt, and R. Eppinger, "Quantification of side impact responses and injuries," Proceedings 25th Stapp Car Crash Conference, SAE Paper 811009, 1981.
5. Klaus, G., and D. Kallieris, "Side impact—a comparison between HSRI, APROD, and HYBRID II dummies and cadavers," Proceedings 27th Stapp Car Crash Conference, SAE Paper 831630, 1983.
6. Klaus, G., R. Sinnhuber, G. Hoffmann, D. Kallieris, and R. Mattern, "Side impact—a comparison between dummies and cadavers, correlations between cadaver loads and injury severity," Proceedings 28th Stapp Car Crash Conference, SAE Paper 841655, 1984.
7. Cesari, D., and A. Johnson, "Evaluation of improved protection and dummy biofidelity in side impact," Proceedings Ninth International Technical Conference on Experimental Safety Vehicles, U.S. Department of Transportation, 1982.
8. Robbins, D., R. Lehman, and K. Augustyn, "Prediction of thoracic injuries as a function of occupant kinematics," Proceedings Seventh International Technical Conference on Experimental Safety Vehicles, U.S. Department of Transportation, 1979.
9. Tarriere, C., G. Walfisch, A. Fayon, J. Rosey, C. Got, A. Patel, and A. Delmas, "Synthesis of human tolerances obtained from lateral impact simulations," Proceedings Seventh International Technical Conference on Experimental Safety Vehicles, U.S. Department of Transportation, 1979.

10. Harris, J., "The design and use of the TRRL side impact dummy," Proceedings 20th Stapp Car Crash Conference, SAE Paper 760802, 1976.
11. Nuscholtz, G., N. Alem, and J. Melvin, "Impact response and injury of the pelvis," Proceedings 26th Stapp Car Crash Conference, SAE Paper 821160, 1982.
12. Evans, F. Gaynor, *Mechanical Properties of Bone*, Charles C. Thomas, Springfield, Illinois, 1973.
13. Yamada, H., *Strength of Biological Materials*, Williams and Wilkins, Baltimore, Maryland, 1970.
14. Ran, A., M. Koch, and H. Mellander, "Fitting injury versus exposure data into a risk function," 1984 International IRCOBI Conference on the Biomechanics of Impacts, IRCOBI Secretariat, Bron, France.
15. Brinn, J., and S. Staffeld, "The effective displacement index—an analysis technique for crash impacts of anthropometric dummies," Proceedings 15th Stapp Car Crash Conference, SAE, 1971.
16. Stalnaker, R., J. McElhaney, R. Snyder, and V. Roberts, "Door crashworthiness criteria," U.S. Department of Transportation, National Highway Traffic Safety Administration, DOT-HS-800 534, June 1971.

Key to Codes in Appendix A

General Table

NA	Data not available or rejected

Test No. Prefix Codes

H	HEIDELBERG
CES	ONSER(A)
F	FAT
BMD	ONSER(B)
7	HSRI

Test Type Codes

SLD	SLED
OPL	OPEL
BAS	ONSER (B) BASELINE RABBIT
MOD	ONSER (B) MODIFIED RABBIT
IMP	RIGID IMPACTOR

Impacted Surface Codes

RIG	RIGID
APR	APR PADDING
ENSO	ENSOLITE PADDING
VDR	VOLVO DOOR
MCI	MINICARS PADDING
SRL	FIBERGLASS HONEYCOMB PADDING
RAB	RABBIT DOOR
OPL	OPEL DOOR

Sex Codes

M	MALE
F	FEMALE
D	DUMMY

In AIS Column * = AIS 0

Appendix A. Lateral pelvic impact database, April 1985

Test No	Tst Typ	Speed MPH	Imp Surf	Sex	Age	Body Mass KG	Height Meters	ACC yP G's	Force yP (KN)	AIS	A-Scaled ACC(G's)	A-Scaled Force(KN)	Lamda	B-Scaled ACC(G's)	B-Scaled Force KN	M1 (lb)	M2 (lb)	K (lb/in)	C (lb-sec/in)	Max Strain (in/in #10 2)	VMAX (in/sec)
H82008	SLD	20 0	APR	M	61	99	1 73	90 0	NA	*	98 3	NA	1 149	103 4	NA	17 30	30 96	3448	26	4 33	72 42
H8106D	SLD	20 0	RIG	D	NA	76	1 75	114 9	NA	*	1 8	NA	1 000	1 8	NA	NA	NA	NA	NA	NA	NA
H8105D	SLD	20 0	RIG	D	NA	76	1 75	130 6	NA	*	1 8	NA	1 000	1 8	NA	NA	NA	NA	NA	NA	NA
H8103D	SLD	15 0	APR	D	NA	76	1 75	49 0	NA	*	1 8	NA	1 000	1 8	NA	NA	NA	NA	NA	NA	NA
H8102D	SLD	15 0	RIG	D	NA	76	1 75	50 8	NA	*	1 8	NA	1 000	1 8	NA	NA	NA	NA	NA	NA	NA
H81027	SLD	25 3	RIG	M	30	77	1 80	137 0	NA	*	137 6	NA	0 992	136 0	NA	11 14	19 94	2977	20	5 95	97 58
H81021	SLD	15 0	APR	F	48	57	1 65	48 7	NA	*	44 2	NA	0 892	43 4	NA	8 09	14 48	2676	16	2 36	25 98
H8101D	SLD	14 0	RIG	D	NA	76	1 75	45 2	NA	*	1 8	NA	1 000	1 8	NA	NA	NA	NA	NA	NA	NA
H81016	SLD	25 0	RIG	M	22	77	1 75	148 3	NA	*	148 9	NA	1 007	149 3	NA	11 63	20 80	3020	20	6 85	103 37
H81015	SLD	14 6	APR	M	44	73	1 73	44 8	NA	*	44 2	NA	0 987	44 2	NA	10 96	19 61	2961	19	2 58	16 21
H81012	SLD	20 0	APR	F	33	46	1 55	105 8	NA	*	89 5	NA	0 827	87 5	NA	6 44	11 52	2480	14	4 45	51 16
H81011	SLD	20 0	APR	M	43	59	1 65	111 3	NA	*	102 3	NA	0 907	101 0	NA	8 52	15 25	2722	16	4 42	7 15
H81006	SLD	20 0	RIG	M	37	82	1 70	139 4	NA	*	143 0	NA	1 054	146 9	NA	13 34	23 88	3162	22	7 05	81 01
H81004	SLD	20 0	RIG	M	56	80	1 65	97 1	NA	*	98 8	NA	1 057	102 6	NA	13 45	24 07	3170	22	5 67	62 87
H81002	SLD	21 0	RIG	M	57	65	1 65	85 2	NA	*	80 9	NA	0 953	81 2	NA	9 85	17 63	2858	18	3 89	51 55
H80024	SLD	21 0	RIG	M	24	65	1 75	104 0	NA	*	98 7	NA	0 925	96 2	NA	9 02	16 14	2774	17	5 33	4 15
H80023	SLD	21 0	SRL	F	41	82	1 60	68 0	NA	*	69 7	NA	1 087	73 9	NA	14 63	26 18	3260	24	4 33	55 6
H80021	SLD	20 0	SRL	M	29	63	1 80	58 7	NA	*	55 1	NA	0 898	52 7	NA	8 25	14 76	2693	16	3 12	27 88
H80020	SLD	19 0	APR	M	26	67	1 68	53 0	NA	*	50 8	NA	0 960	50 9	NA	10 08	18 03	2879	18	2 89	2 68
H80018	SLD	19 3	APR	M	21	61	1 65	61 0	NA	*	56 7	NA	0 923	56 3	NA	8 96	16 03	2768	17	3 12	32 46
H80017	SLD	15 0	RIG	M	38	70	1 75	74 3	NA	*	72 3	NA	0 960	71 3	NA	10 08	18 03	2879	18	4 11	37 53
H80014	SLD	14 0	RIG	F	60	84	1 68	60 2	NA	*	62 2	NA	1 075	64 7	NA	14 15	23 31	3224	23	3 14	49 61
H80011	SLD	14 0	RIG	M	27	89	1 88	51 5	NA	*	54 3	NA	1 045	53 8	NA	13 00	23 25	3134	22	2 67	26 72
FAT5D	OPL	31 1	OPL	D	NA	76	1 75	NA	NA	*	1 8	NA	1 000	1 8	NA	NA	NA	NA	NA	NA	NA
FAT4D	OPL	31 1	OPL	D	NA	76	1 75	NA	NA	*	1 8	NA	1 000	1 8	NA	NA	NA	NA	NA	NA	NA
FAT3D	OPL	31 1	OPL	D	NA	76	1 75	NA	NA	*	1 8	NA	1 000	1 8	NA	NA	NA	NA	NA	NA	NA
FAT2D	OPL	31 1	OPL	D	NA	76	1 75	NA	NA	*	1 8	NA	1 000	1 8	NA	NA	NA	NA	NA	NA	NA
FAT1D	OPL	31 1	OPL	D	NA	76	1 75	NA	NA	*	1 8	NA	1 000	1 8	NA	NA	NA	NA	NA	NA	NA
F8412	OPL	28 0	OPL	M	54	68	1 78	100 5	NA	3	96 8	NA	0 939	94 3	NA	9 43	16 87	2816	18	4 42	56 13
F8411	OPL	28 0	OPL	M	64	76	1 73	84 2	NA	*	84 2	NA	1 007	84 8	NA	11 65	20 85	3022	20	3 94	49 47
F8410	OPL	28 0	OPL	M	53	74	1 73	86 0	NA	*	85 2	NA	0 994	85 5	NA	11 19	20 03	2982	20	4 57	62 8
F8409	OPL	28 0	OPL	M	25	95	1 88	71 9	NA	*	77 5	NA	1 079	77 6	NA	14 33	25 65	32 38	23	4 31	53 06
F8407	OPL	28 0	OPL	F	27	61	1 60	70 1	NA	*	65 1	NA	0 937	65 7	NA	9 39	16 80	2812	18	3 48	43 41
F8406	OPL	28 0	OPL	M	30	60	1 75	70 7	NA	*	65 3	NA	0 889	62 8	NA	8 00	14 31	2666	16	3 36	44 8
F8405	OPL	24 8	OPL	M	60	64	1 70	66 2	NA	*	62 5	NA	0 931	61 6	NA	9 20	16 47	2793	17	3 57	43 33
F8404	OPL	24 8	OPL	M	51	60	1 68	90 8	NA	*	83 9	NA	0 908	82 5	NA	8 54	15 28	2725	16	4 21	54 51
F8402	OPL	31 1	OPL	M	33	73	1 88	88 0	NA	*	86 8	NA	0 946	83 3	NA	9 65	17 27	2838	18	4 35	49 52
F8041	OPL	31 1	OPL	M	36	91	1 75	90 2	NA	*	95 8	NA	1 094	98 7	NA	14 94	26 73	3283	24	4 07	91 66
F8329	OPL	24 8	OPL	M	38	77	1 78	102 4	NA	*	102 4	NA	0 999	101 9	NA	11 36	20 33	2997	20	4 14	9 18
F8328	OPL	31 1	OPL	M	44	88	1 85	95 5	NA	*	100 3	NA	1 047	99 9	NA	13 07	23 38	3140	22	4 89	87 27
F8327	OPL	31 1	OPL	M	53	62	1 70	115 4	NA	*	107 8	NA	0 916	105 8	NA	8 77	15 70	2749	17	4 53	76 93
F8326	OPL	37 3	OPL	M	32	82	1 70	86 8	NA	*	89 0	NA	1 054	91 5	NA	13 34	23 88	3162	22	4 74	51 69
F8319	OPL	24 8	OPL	M	40	82	1 83	147 0	NA	*	150 8	NA	1 039	152 7	NA	12 78	22 86	3116	22	6 1	11 52
F8318	OPL	31 1	OPL	M	26	63	1 83	92 7	NA	*	87 1	NA	0 891	82 6	NA	8 07	14 43	2673	16	4 01	45 12
F8317	OPL	37 3	OPL	M	50	85	1 72	122 7	NA	*	127 4	NA	1 067	130 9	NA	13 84	24 76	3200	23	6 12	91 17
F8315	OPL	24 8	OPL	F	36	60	1 64	73 6	NA	*	68 0	NA	0 918	67 6	NA	8 81	15 77	2754	17	3 55	56 13
F8314	OPL	37 3	OPL	M	23	80	1 92	196 5	NA	*	199 9	NA	0 980	192 5	NA	10 71	19 17	2939	19	7 74	157 62
F8313	OPL	24 8	OPL	F	26	51	1 59	68 7	NA	*	60 1	NA	0 859	59 0	NA	7 24	12 95	2578	15	3 4	30 12
F8306	OPL	31 1	OPL	M	59	60	1 83	164 3	NA	2	151 9	NA	0 904	148 6	NA	8 43	15 08	2712	16	5 87	137 97
F8305	OPL	31 1	OPL	F	42	60	1 62	109 0	NA	*	100 7	NA	0 923	100 7	NA	8 98	16 07	2770	17	NA	NA

Appendix A, continued

Test No	Tst Typ	Speed MPH	Imp Surf	Sex	Age	Body Mass KG	Height Meters	ACC yP G's	Force yP (KN)	AIS	A-Scaled ACC(G's)	A-Scaled Force(KN)	Lamda	B-Scaled ACC(G's)	B-Scaled Force KN	M1 (1lb)	M2 (1lb)	K (1lb/in)	C (1lb-sec/in)	Max Strain (in/in #10 2)	VMAX (in/sec)
F8304	OPL	31 1	OPL	M	28	61	1 72	117 0	NA	.	108 7	NA	0 904	105 7	NA	8 41	15 05	2711	16	4 94	73 25
F8303	OPL	31 1	OPL	M	52	68	1 72	120 3	NA	.	115 9	NA	0 954	114 8	NA	9 90	17 72	2862	18	5 03	68 45
F8302	OPL	31 1	OPL	M	22	65	1 75	109 3	NA	.	103 7	NA	0 925	101 1	NA	9 02	16 14	2774	17	4 97	60 17
F8301	OPL	31 1	OPL	M	39	57	1 73	147 4	NA	.	133 9	NA	0 871	128 4	NA	7 53	13 48	2613	15	5 55	98 73
F8213	OPL	31 1	OPL	F	47	90	1 70	84 4	NA	.	89 3	NA	1 104	93 2	NA	15 34	27 46	3312	24	4 27	66 97
F8211	OPL	31 1	OPL	M	29	59	1 77	127 1	NA	.	116 8	NA	0 876	111 4	NA	7 67	13 72	2628	15	4 91	77 06
F8210	OPL	31 1	OPL	M	29	70	1 84	131 9	NA	.	128 3	NA	0 936	123 5	NA	9 35	16 73	2808	18	4 68	118 61
F8207	OPL	31 1	OPL	M	58	68	1 65	146 3	NA	.	141 0	NA	0 974	142 5	NA	10 54	18 86	2922	19	5 55	100 93
F8206	OPL	31 1	OPL	M	23	63	1 75	155 3	NA	.	145 9	NA	0 910	141 4	NA	8 60	15 40	2731	17	5 94	112 23
F8205	OPL	31 1	OPL	M	43	77	1 78	79 2	NA	.	79 5	NA	0 998	79 0	NA	11 33	20 28	2994	20	4 2	51 73
H8405D	SLD	20 0	RIG	D	NA	76	1 75	225 7	NA	.	225 7	NA	1 000	225 7	NA	NA	NA	NA	NA	NA	NA
H8404D	SLD	20 0	RIG	D	NA	76	1 75	239 0	NA	.	239 0	NA	1 000	239 0	NA	NA	NA	NA	NA	NA	NA
H8403D	SLD	15 0	RIG	D	NA	76	1 75	47 3	NA	.	47 3	NA	1 000	47 3	NA	NA	NA	NA	NA	NA	NA
H8402D	SLD	20 0	RIG	D	NA	76	1 75	133 4	NA	.	133 4	NA	1 000	133 4	NA	NA	NA	NA	NA	NA	NA
H8401D	SLD	18 0	RIG	D	NA	76	1 75	100 7	NA	.	100 7	NA	0 998	100 7	NA	NA	NA	NA	NA	NA	NA
H84008	SLD	20 0	ENSO	M	79	64	1 68	83 4	NA	.	78 8	NA	0 938	78 2	NA	9 41	16 84	2814	18	4 59	47 52
H8306D	SLD	20 0	RIG	D	NA	76	1 75	204 2	37 16	.	204 2	37 2	1 000	204 2	37 16	NA	NA	NA	NA	NA	NA
H8305D	SLD	20 0	APR	D	NA	76	1 75	82 3	10 50	.	82 3	10 5	1 000	82 3	10 50	NA	NA	NA	NA	NA	NA
H8304D	SLD	15 0	RIG	D	NA	76	1 75	125 5	21 14	.	125 5	21 1	1 000	125 5	NA	NA	NA	NA	NA	NA	NA
H8303D	SLD	20 0	ENSO	D	NA	76	1 75	51 4	8 38	.	51 4	8 4	1 000	51 4	8 38	NA	NA	NA	NA	NA	NA
H83031	SLD	16 8	VDR	M	43	62	1 70	56 8	NA	.	53 1	NA	0 916	52 1	NA	8 77	15 70	2749	17	3 2	31 56
H83030	SLD	11 2	VDR	D	42	86	1 88	110	NA	.	115	NA	1 026	113	NA	12 32	22 05	3079	21	NA	NA
H8302D	SLD	22 4	ENSO	D	NA	76	1 75	701	11 48	.	701	115	1 000	701	11 48	NA	NA	NA	NA	4 78	81 06
H83021	SLD	15 0	VDR	M	38	58	1 65	115 6	NA	2	105 6	115	0 900	104 0	NA	8 31	14 87	2700	16	4 78	81 06
H83020	SLD	20 0	ENSO	F	17	52	1 52	74 7	6 06	.	65 8	78	0 887	66 2	7 71	7 95	14 22	2660	16	3 63	36 44
H8301D	SLD	16 8	ENSO	D	NA	76	1 75	65 7	8 98	.	65 7	9 0	1 000	65 7	8 98	NA	NA	NA	NA	NA	NA
H83016	SLD	22 0	VDR	M	52	68	1 70	96 7	NA	.	93 2	NA	0 960	92 8	NA	10 08	18 03	2879	18	5 16	56 5
H83012	SLD	20 0	ENSO	M	34	77	1 78	99 4	NA	.	99 8	NA	0 999	99 3	NA	11 36	20 33	2997	20	NA	NA
H83011	SLD	20 0	ENSO	M	26	61	1 88	74 3	7 69	.	69 0	NA	0 865	64 3	NA	7 37	13 20	2594	15	NA	179 19
H83010	SLD	16 8	ENSO	F	30	56	1 75	85 3	2 80	.	77 0	NA	0 858	73 2	NA	7 21	12 90	2575	15	3 27	53 35
H82022	SLD	20 0	APR	M	50	77	1 68	75 0	11 60	.	75 3	NA	1 029	77 2	NA	12 42	22 22	3087	21	4 32	49 11
H82021	SLD	20 0	APR	M	48	99	1 80	113 2	15 00	.	123 6	NA	1 125	127 4	NA	16 25	29 07	3376	25	5 06	115 79
H82020	SLD	19 4	RIG	M	41	73	1 80	135 0	NA	2	133 2	NA	0 966	130 5	NA	10 29	18 41	2899	19	6 48	179 19
H82019	SLD	14 4	RIG	F	47	67	1 65	43 9	NA	.	42 1	NA	0 967	42 5	NA	10 31	18 45	2901	19	2 72	22 14
H82018	SLD	14 4	RIG	M	28	85	1 80	103 1	NA	.	107 0	NA	1 043	107 5	NA	12 93	23 13	3128	22	4 42	81
H82016	SLD	19 4	RIG	M	21	50	1 88	106 4	14 37	.	92 5	NA	0 783	83 3	NA	5 47	9 79	2349	12	4 57	69 17
H82015	SLD	14 4	RIG	M	18	69	1 83	70 1	4 39	.	67 9	NA	0 933	65 4	NA	9 25	16 54	2798	17	3 43	34 43
H82014	SLD	22 0	RIG	F	22	61	1 77	94 4	18 18	3	87 7	NA	0 892	84 2	NA	8 09	14 47	2675	16	4 44	96 24
H82012	SLD	25 0	RIG	F	17	75	1 73	248 1	30 26	.	247 0	NA	1 001	248 2	NA	11 42	20 44	3002	20	9 9	202 2
H82009	SLD	25 0	RIG	F	27	51	1 65	199 6	9 68	3	174 7	NA	0 844	168 4	NA	6 85	12 25	2531	14	7 76	108 49
F8204	OPL	31 1	OPL	F	40	60	1 58	115 5	NA	.	106 7	NA	0 935	108 0	NA	9 32	16 68	2805	17	4 98	74 64
F8203	OPL	31 1	OPL	M	21	68	1 73	91 0	NA	.	87 7	NA	0 951	86 6	NA	9 82	17 57	2854	18	4 19	62 4
F8123	OPL	31 1	OPL	M	21	71	1 78	89 1	NA	.	87 1	NA	0 958	85 4	NA	10 03	17 96	2875	18	4 35	53 73
BMD05	BAS	40 0	RAB	F	39	64	1 70	107 0	NA	.	101 0	NA	0 931	99 6	NA	9 20	16 47	2793	17	4 77	61 16
BMD04	BAS	40 0	RAB	M	51	71	1 57	58 5	NA	.	57 2	NA	1 020	59 7	NA	12 11	21 68	3061	21	2 15	46 18
BMD03	MOD	40 0	RAB	M	55	73	1 74	64 2	NA	.	63 3	NA	0 983	63 1	NA	10 82	19 37	2949	19	4 19	34 01
BMD02	MOD	40 0	RAB	F	43	71	1 75	51 1	NA	.	50 0	NA	0 967	49 4	NA	10 29	18 42	2900	19	3 06	18 47
BMD01	BAS	40 0	RAB	F	40	59	1 67	112 8	NA	3	103 7	NA	0 902	101 7	NA	8 36	14 97	2706	16	5 89	71 78
77T098	SLD	20 0	MCI	M	71	59	1 68	65 8	NA	.	60 5	NA	0 901	59 3	NA	5 33	14 90	2702	16	3 72	26 02
77T095	SLD	20 0	MCI	M	77	93	1 83	59 2	NA	.	63 3	NA	1 083	64 1	NA	14 47	25 89	3248	23	4 07	41 01

767

Appendix A, continued

Test No	Tst Typ	Speed MPH	Imp Surf	Sex	Age	Body Mass KG	Height Meters	ACC yP G s	Force yP (KN)	AIS	A Scaled ACC(G s)	A Scaled Force(KN)	Lamda	B Scaled ACC(G's)	B Scaled Force KN	M1 (lb)	M2 (lb)	K (lb/in)	C (1lb-sec/in)	Max Strain (in/in #10 2)	VMAX (in/sec)
76T092	SLD	20.0	RIG	F	45	58	1.78	89.5	NA	.	81.8	NA	0.867	77.6	NA	7.43	13.29	2601	15	4.61	53.23
76T089	SLD	20.0	RIG	M	66	65	1.73	89.6	NA	.	80.4	NA	0.857	76.8	NA	7.17	12.82	2570	15	4.37	39.97
76T042	SLD	24.0	SLD	F	58	61	1.78	86.7	NA	.	81.9	NA	0.911	79.0	NA	8.61	15.41	2732	17	4.16	50.59
76T039	SLD	20.0	MCI	M	72	74	1.88	35.9	NA	.	35.6	NA	0.953	34.2	NA	9.85	17.63	2858	18	NA	NA
76T034	SLD	19.6	MCI	M	62	49	1.83	48.2	NA	.	43.3	NA	0.862	41.6	NA	7.31	13.08	2587	15	2.71	19.57
76T029	SLD	15.0	SLD	M	67	63	1.68	45.6	NA	.	42.8	NA	0.931	42.4	NA	9.19	16.44	2792	17	1.94	53.75
76T011	SLD	20.0	RIG	M	69	75	1.70	63.4	NA	.	63.1	NA	1.008	63.9	NA	11.67	20.89	3024	20	3.88	58.71
76T010	SLD	19.6	RIG	M	84	88	1.62	93.0	NA	.	97.7	NA	1.117	103.9	NA	15.89	28.43	3351	25	3.9	83.8
76T009	SLD	25.4	RIG	F	75	41	1.55	125.6	NA	.	104.7	NA	0.809	101.6	NA	6.04	10.80	2427	13	4.51	131.21
CFS22	SLD	12.3	RIG	M	67	48	1.67	NA	NA	3	NA	NA	0.894	NA	NA	8.15	14.59	2683	16	NA	NA
CFSZ1	IMP	28.8	RIG	M	67	58	1.67	NA	NA	3	NA	NA	0.894	NA	NA	8.15	14.59	2683	16	NA	NA
CFSY2	IMP	33.6	RIG	F	74	66	1.62	NA	NA	2	NA	NA	1.147	NA	NA	17.21	30.79	3441	28	NA	NA
CFSX2	IMP	33.0	RIG	F	53	63	1.53	NA	NA	3	NA	NA	0.892	NA	NA	8.10	14.49	2677	16	NA	NA
CFSX1	IMP	28.4	RIG	F	53	63	1.53	NA	NA	3	NA	NA	0.892	NA	NA	8.10	14.49	2677	16	NA	NA
CFSV2	IMP	24.6	RIG	M	85	65	1.77	NA	NA	2	NA	NA	0.960	NA	NA	10.08	18.03	2879	18	2.1	32.67
CFSS2	IMP	17.2	RIG	M	61	77	1.67	49.5	4.95	3	42.8	6.5	0.843	41.5	6.97	6.83	12.22	2529	14	1.52	54.14
CFST2	IMP	14.4	RIG	F	71	48	1.44	41.8	4.16	.	41.8	6.0	0.839	32.0	5.91	6.73	12.04	2516	14	1.7	13.74
CFSS3	IMP	25.5	RIG	M	72	70	1.77	NA	6.43	3	NA	7.2	0.892	NA	7.17	9.71	17.38	2844	18	NA	NA
CFSS3	IMP	25.5	RIG	M	72	70	1.77	NA	6.07	.	NA	6.8	0.948	NA	6.76	9.71	17.38	2844	18	NA	NA
CFSR6	IMP	23.4	RIG	M	80	81	1.81	NA	10.24	2	NA	9.7	1.024	NA	9.76	12.25	21.92	3073	21	NA	NA
CFSR4	IMP	29.1	RIG	M	80	71	1.81	NA	10.14	.	NA	9.6	1.024	NA	9.67	12.25	21.92	3073	21	NA	NA
CFSP2	IMP	20.2	RIG	M	70	72	1.81	NA	6.2	3	NA	6.0	1.066	NA	5.45	13.82	24.73	3199	23	NA	NA
CFSP1	IMP	23.6	RIG	F	70	72	1.81	NA	5.62	.	NA	5.5	1.066	NA	4.94	13.82	24.73	3199	23	NA	NA
CFSN7	IMP	25.5	RIG	M	53	68	1.81	NA	9.06	.	NA	7.7	1.037	NA	7.76	12.73	22.78	3112	22	NA	NA
CFSN6	IMP	23.4	RIG	M	54	68	1.81	NA	8.08	2	NA	7.0	1.037	NA	7.76	12.73	22.78	3112	22	NA	NA
CFSL1	IMP	27.7	RIG	M	71	85	1.81	154.4	12.44	3	150.9	10.7	1.058	NA	10.31	13.48	24.13	3173	22	NA	NA
CESK3	IMP	21.7	RIG	M	75	55	1.75	NA	NA	2	NA	NA	0.861	NA	NA	7.27	13.00	2582	15	NA	NA
CFSJ3	IMP	22.0	RIG	M	75	63	1.77	76.4	6.6	.	71.8	8.5	0.905	69.2	9.13	8.46	15.14	2716	16	2.83	44.33
CFSF3	IMP	21.5	RIG	F	59	63	1.77	37.7	5.28	.	35.4	6.8	0.905	34.1	7.30	8.46	15.14	2716	16	1.52	23.37
CESI5	IMP	24.9	RIG	M	72	60	1.81	94.7	8.16	2	89.0	10.5	0.895	84.8	11.54	8.18	14.64	2686	16	3.38	62.34
CESI4	IMP	24.7	RIG	M	65	63	1.81	82.3	9.58	3	77.3	12.3	0.895	73.7	11.95	8.18	14.64	2686	16	2.51	79.3
CESH4	IMP	23.7	RIG	M	69	86	1.75	NA	NA	.	NA	NA	1.064	NA	NA	13.72	24.56	3191	23	NA	NA
CESH3	IMP	21.5	RIG	M	69	86	1.75	NA	NA	3	NA	NA	1.064	NA	NA	13.72	24.56	3191	23	NA	NA
CESF3	IMP	21.7	RIG	F	59	55	1.52	NA	6.6	2	NA	8.5	0.913	NA	7.30	8.67	15.51	2738	17	NA	NA
CESE2	IMP	19.3	RIG	M	72	60	1.55	33.5	4.17	3	31.0	4.9	0.944	31.6	4.68	9.59	17.17	2832	18	NA	NA
CESE1	IMP	15.7	RIG	F	72	60	1.55	50.1	4.54	3	46.3	5.3	0.944	47.3	5.09	9.59	17.17	2832	18	1.81	38.14
CESD2	IMP	19.1	RIG	F	63	52	1.6	51.5	3.86	.	45.4	5.0	0.865	44.6	5.16	7.38	13.21	2595	15	1.76	36.78
CESD1	IMP	15.5	RIG	F	63	52	1.6	42.0	3.86	2	37.0	5.0	0.865	36.3	5.16	7.38	13.21	2595	15	1.62	24.72
CESC3	IMP	24.5	RIG	M	69	78	1.73	NA	7.28	2	NA	7.2	1.019	NA	7.01	12.06	21.58	3057	21	NA	NA
CESC2	IMP	19.9	RIG	F	69	78	1.73	NA	8.39	3	NA	8.2	1.019	NA	8.08	12.06	21.58	3057	21	1.66	24.29
CESB2	IMP	18.6	RIG	F	84	70	1.54	NA	NA	2	NA	NA	1.023	NA	NA	12.21	21.84	3069	21	NA	NA
CESB1	IMP	13.0	RIG	F	84	70	1.54	NA	NA	3	NA	NA	1.023	NA	NA	12.21	21.84	3069	21	NA	NA
CESA4	IMP	25.5	RIG	F	70	58	1.67	NA	NA	.	NA	NA	0.894	NA	NA	8.15	14.59	2683	16	NA	NA
CESA3	IMP	18.6	RIG	F	70	58	1.67	NA	NA	.	NA	NA	0.894	NA	NA	8.15	14.59	2683	16	NA	NA

Appendix B

Comparison of Cadaver and Dummy Lateral Impact Pelvic Data

1. Comparison of Peak Responses

A limited amount of data is available from the Heidelberg data set that permits comparison of cadaver and SID dummy force and acceleration responses. Figures B-1 and B-2 present peak force versus peak acceleration data for Heidelberg cadavers and Heidelberg SID dummies, respectively. It may be noted that the slope of the line fitting the dummy data (.196KN/g) is approximately twice the slope of the least squares fit to the cadaver data (.101KN/g). This result suggests that the dummy generates higher peak pelvic interface force for a given level of peak pelvic acceleration response.

To investigate this indication further, dummy and cadaver data were segregated by test speed and by impacting surface (rigid or padded), and the ratios of average dummy peak responses to average cadaver peak responses for each test condition were calculated and plotted. Figure B-3 presents these computed acceleration ratios. It may be noted that the ratio of peak dummy acceleration to peak cadaver acceleration ranges from 1.0 to 1.7 for rigid impacts and remains stable at a lower value of approximately .85 for padded impacts.

Figure B-4 presents corresponding computed force ratios. Although data are very limited and should be interpreted with caution, the dummy appears to generate

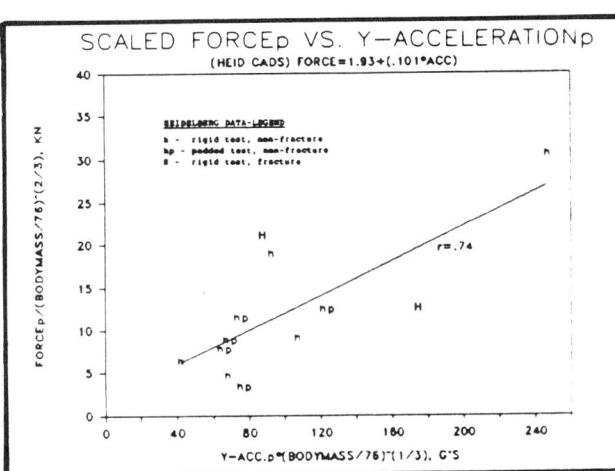

Figure B-1. Scaled peak pelvic forces versus scaled peak pelvic Y-acceleration for Heidelberg cadaver tests

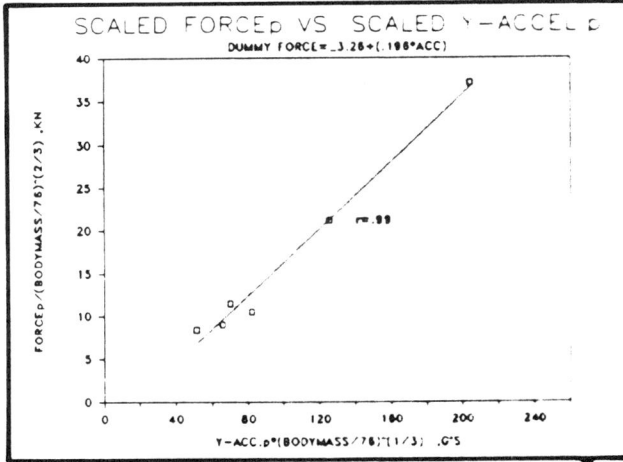

Figure B-2. Scaled peak pelvic force versus scaled peak pelvic Y-acceleration for Heidelberg SID dummy tests

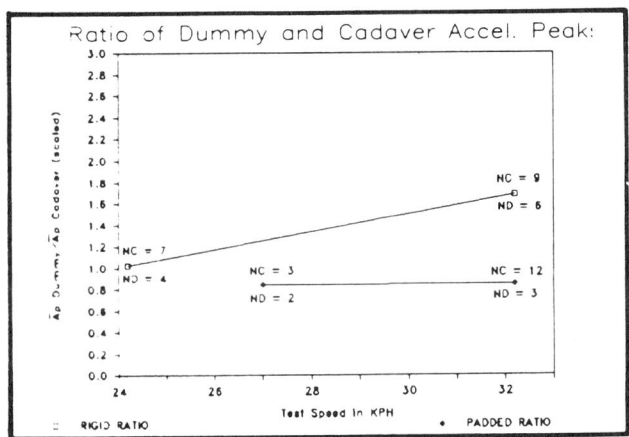

Figure B-3. Ratios of SID dummy and cadaver peak accelerations—Heidelberg data (NC and ND are number of cadaver tests and number dummy tests, respectively, included in ratio of determination at each data point)

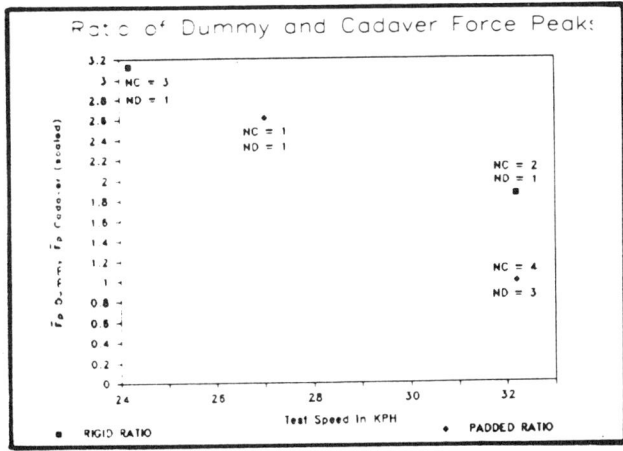

Figure B-4. Ratios of SID dummy and cadaver peak forces-Heidelberg data

higher interface force than does the cadaver at all test speeds. Also, the force ratio exhibits a trend toward reduction with increasing test speed. However, more data would be desirable to confirm these observations.

2. Comparison of Pulse Shape

Thus far, we have compared only the behavior of peak force and peak acceleration responses. It is also of interest to examine comparative pulse shapes for cadavers and dummies from the Heidelberg series, for both rigid and padded test conditions.

A. Rigid Interface

Figures B-5 and B-6 present overplots of pelvic force and acceleration data for a 15mph dummy test and a 20mph dummy test, respectively. (Traces have been artificially scaled to equalize plotted peak amplitudes so that curve shapes can be better compared.) Figures B-7 and B-8 present comparable data for 20mph and 25mph cadaver exposures.

For all dummy and cadaver rigid tests, excellent agreement of force and acceleration curve shape is seen, and rigid body behavior is approached.

B. Padded Interface

Figures B-9 and B-10 present typical dummy tests, at 17 and 20mph, into ensolite padding. Figures B-11 and B-12 are corresponding plots for two cadavers at 20mph into ensolite.

Distinctly different characteristic acceleration pulse shapes are evidenced by the SID and by the cadavers in the padded environment. Whereas the dummy exhibits good tracking of force and acceleration up to peak force, the cadaver accelerations are seen to track force well initially, but then to dip and rise again to meet the force curve. In all cases, as was observed in the main body of the paper, peak force and peak acceleration are closely coincident in time.

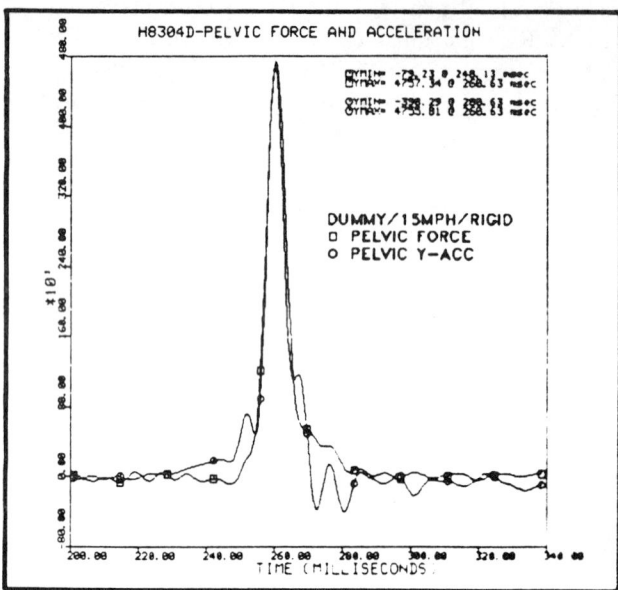

Figure B-5. Pelvic force and pelvic Y-acceleration overlay for Heidelberg SID dummy test H8304d

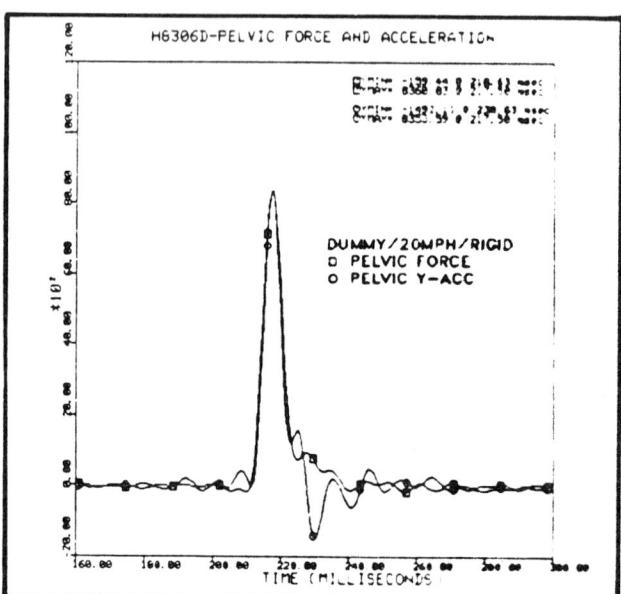

Figure B-6. Pelvic force and pelvic Y-acceleration overlay for Heidelberg SID dummy test H8306d.

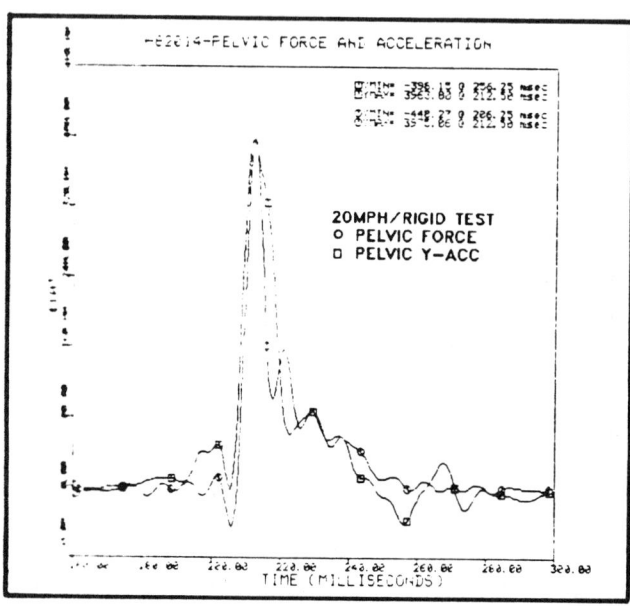

Figure B-7. Pelvic force and pelvic Y-acceleration overlay for Heidelberg cadaver test H82014

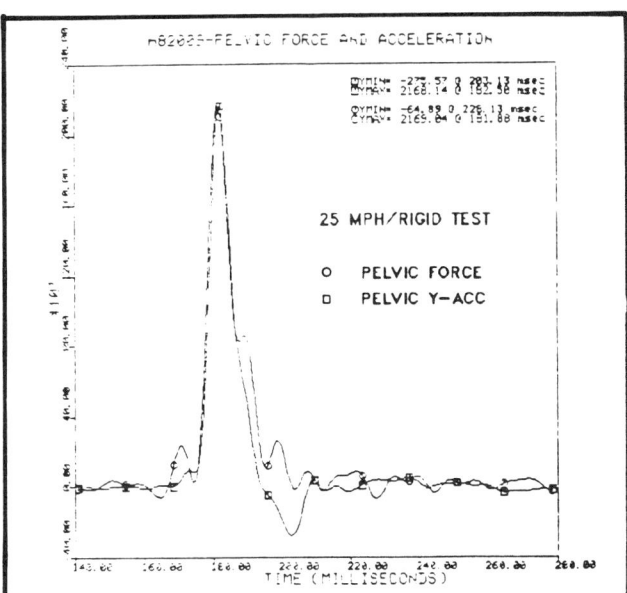

Figure B-8. Pelvic force and pelvic Y-acceleration overlay for Heidelberg cadaver test H82005

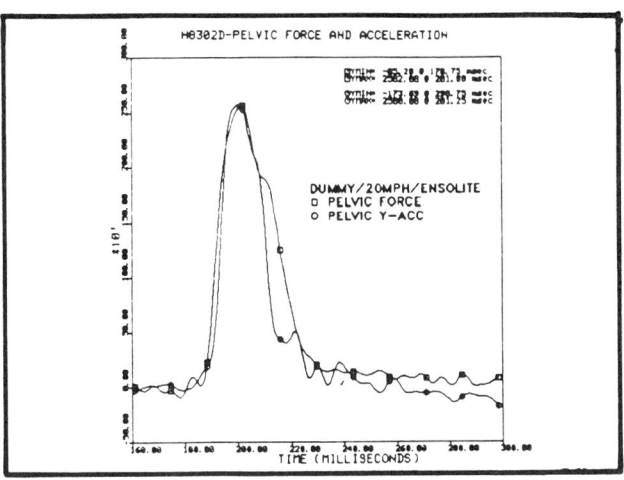

Figure B-10. Pelvic force and pelvic Y-acceleration overlay for Heidelberg SID dummy test H8302d

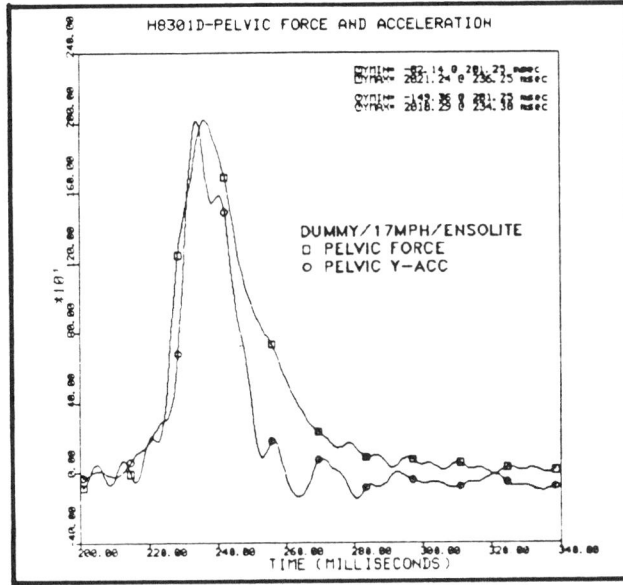

Figure B-9. Pelvic force and pelvic Y-acceleration overlay for Heidelberg SID dummy test H8301d

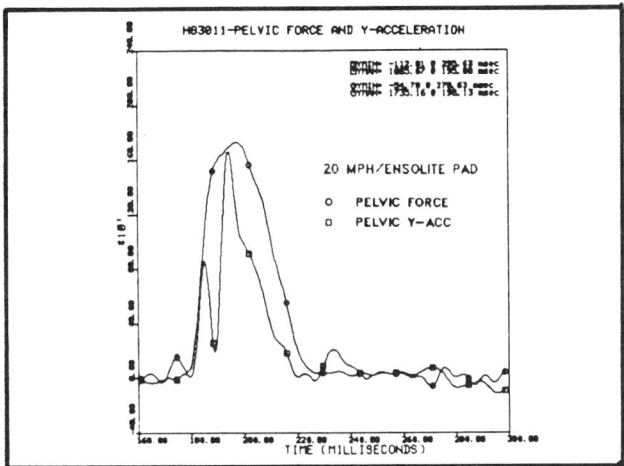

Figure B-11. Pelvic force and pelvic Y-acceleration overlay for Heidelberg cadaver test H83011

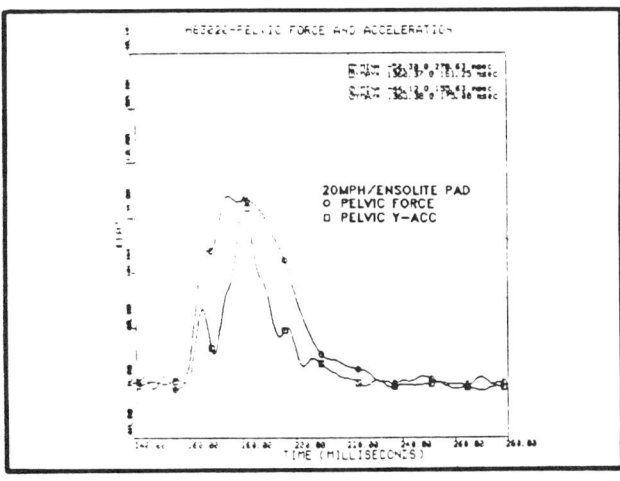

Figure B-12. Pelvic force and pelvic Y-acceleration overlay for Heidelberg cadaver test H83020.

It is interesting to speculate as to why the differences noted above occur in the padded environment and not in the rigid environment. This difference could be related to additional compliance in the structure of the human hip joint or could be due to differences in phasing of horizontal shear forces acting between the abdomen and pelvis.

Although not pursued here, these observed differences should be better understood for input to the development of advanced side impact dummy concepts.

861878

Lower Abdominal Tolerance and Response

John M. Cavanaugh, Gerald W. Nyquist,
Sarah J. Goldberg, and Albert I. King
Wayne State University

ABSTRACT

Twelve unembalmed human cadavers were tested for lower abdominal injury tolerance and mechanical response. The impacts were in an anterior-to-posterior direction and the level of impact was primarily in the lower abdomen at the L3 level of the lumbar spine. The impactor mass was either 32 kg or 64 kg. The impactor face was a 25 mm diameter aluminum bar, with the long axis of the bar parallel to the width of the cadaver body.

In this paper, mechanical response is presented in terms of force-time and penetration-time histories, and force vs. abdominal penetration cross-plots. Injury tolerance is described in terms of post-impact necropsy findings and AIS ratings.

Based on our studies, the lower abdomen of the unembalmed human cadaver is much less stiff than is suggested by previous research, and the stiffness is velocity and mass dependent, as is suggested by the correlation coefficients presented in this paper. Force-time history and force-penetration response corridors are presented.

INTRODUCTION

In the past twenty years, there have been a number of studies on abdominal impact, including accident surveys and laboratory tests. Accident surveys have shown that in lower torso injuries, the organs considered solid in a mechanical sense are more frequently injured than the hollow organs. Thus, the kidneys, liver and spleen are injured more frequently, overall, than the intestines or bladder. Bondy (1) has provided a breakdown of abdominal injuries occurring in vehicle occupants between 1977 and 1979 using the National Crash Severity Study (NCSS). In the study there were 1519 abdominal injuries in all ranges , representing only 2.6% of all injuries. However, for the AIS 3 to 5 range abdominal injuries represented 14.6% of all injuries.

According to Bondy, in frontal impacts there were 695 abdominal injuries in the AIS 1 to 5 range, and 314 for AIS 3 to 5. In frontal impacts, there were 120 injuries to the liver, 76 to the spleen, and 43 to the kidneys for AIS 3-5, but the digestive tract and urogenital organs sustained only 58 injuries in the AIS 3-5 range. For all impact directions the steering system was the most frequently contacted area, being involved in 30% of abdominal injuries. According to the Bondy study, few injuries occurred to restrained occupants. They sustained 7% of all abdominal injuries, and 2.6% of AIS 3-5 injuries.

A number of studies have attributed lower torso injury to the seat belt. Leung et al (2), using French accident data, reported on injuries to 1542 front seat passengers who wore three-point restraints. There were 35 abdominal injuries of AIS 3 through 5 , at least 68% of which were attributed to lap belt submarining.

There have been a number of laboratory studies on abdominal injury tolerance and response. Most of these studies have utilized animals as test subjects. A relatively recent cadaveric study was done by Walfisch et al (3), who conducted 1 and 2 meter lateral drop tests on eleven cadavers with a 70 mm wide impactor face simulating an arm rest. The impacts were to the right side of the abdomen. Three of the cadavers had cirrhosis of the liver. Six of the remaining eight sustained liver injury of AIS 3 to 5. The normalized force for AIS 3 injury to the liver was 4.5 kN. Load-deflection curves were presented in this study.

Recently, in an effort to shed more light on the actual biomechanical response of the abdomen, Stalnaker and Ulman (4) analyzed the response data of 42 sub-human primate test subjects extracted from four different studies, one by Beckman et al (5), two by Stalnaker et al (6,7) and one by Trollope et al (8). Altogether, the 42 tests included six types of impactor, five impact locations, and four primate species. Five of the 42 test subjects were impacted in the lower abdomen. Thirty-seven of the 42 test subjects were impacted in the lateral, middle and upper abdomen. One of the major conclusions of the study was that the force-deflection response of the abdomen is similar to that of many chest impacts, in that there is an initial spike (Segment I), followed by a plateau (Segment II) and then a final rise (Segment III) before bottoming out on the spine at about 60% of total abdominal depth. The actual numerical values of the different components of the curves were of course, found to be different than those for the chest. With the results from the primate tests an attempt was made to extrapolate to the human abdomen through a scaling method that used direct proportionality of masses between species. A response corridor for human abdominal response was proposed based on these findings.

The present on-going study at Wayne State University utilizes human cadavers* in evaluating abdominal response to impact. As will be discussed later, the use of cadavers presents shortcomings in the evaluation of injury tolerance, but has advantages in the evaluation of biomechanical response. A primary advantage is the minimization of the need for scaling techniques in analyzing the data. To date the study has concentrated primarily on impacts to the lower abdomen at the L3 level of the lumbar spine. There are several reasons for using this level of impact at this stage of the study. First, impacts concentrated at the L3 level involve little or no rib contact. In an erect anatomical position, L3 falls one vertebra below the lowest portions of the rib cage, as

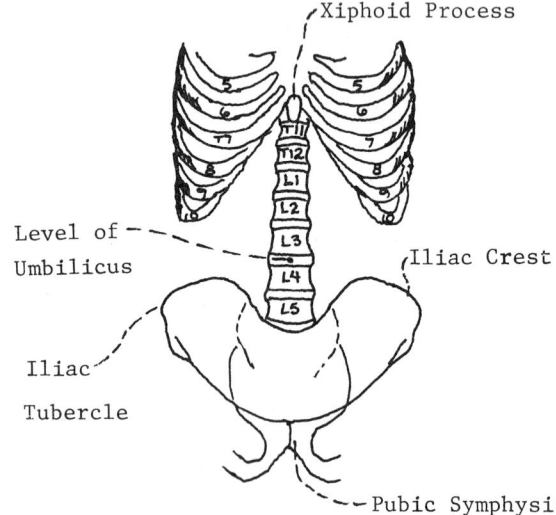

Figure 1. Drawing of the skeleton of the abdomen.

---

* This research complies with the provisions of the Uniform Anatomical Gift Act guidelines established by the National Academy of Sciences and others.

depicted in Figure 1. In a seated position, impacts at the L3 level may involve contact with the lowest portions of the rib cage, depending on the degree to which the torso is slumped forward. In this test series, the torso was kept in an erect position, to minimize this effect. The biomechanical response obtained at this level of impact involved primarily solid and hollow viscoelastic structures, with minimal influence from the overlying elastic and load distributing properties of the rib cage. Another reason for studying impacts at this level is that accidents involving an unbelted driver can result in forward translation of the body, with impact of the lower abdomen on the lower rim of the steering wheel. Abdominal impacts at the L3 level of the lumbar spine come in direct line with the lower portions of the head of the pancreas, the lower portions of the kidneys and duodenum, the inferior vena cava, and the abdominal aorta as illustrated in Figure 2. The use of a 25 mm diameter bar as an impacting device approximates the lower edge of a steering wheel rim.

In this paper, L3 is defined as being in the lower abdomen. This designation is based on the abdominal impact locations outlined in the Stalnaker and Ulman study (4), in which the lower abdomen is defined as being just above the iliac crests, and the mid-abdomen is defined as being midway between the highest and lowest points of the diaphragm. In a more classical division of abdominal regions, the abdomen is divided into nine regions using two horizontal planes, the subcostal and the transtubercular, and two vertical planes, one each at the right and left mid-clavicular line. Based on the more classical division, L3 lies in the middle zone (in the umbilical region).

The analyses of the results obtained thus far have focused on three different areas: i) analysis of the impact force-time history plots, ii) analysis of the abdominal force-deflection data, and iii) summary and evaluation of injury levels using the Abbreviated Injury Scale.

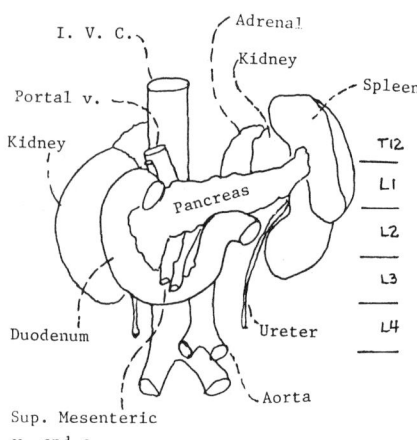

Figure 2. Drawing of abdominal organs and vessels and their vertebral levels.

METHODOLOGY

The cadavers used in this study consisted of eight males and four females ranging in age from 43 to 66 years and ranging in mass from 45 kg to 92 kg. For the males, the average age was 56.8 years, the average mass was 74.1 kg, and the average height was 1.77 m. For the females, the respective values were 50.5 years, 62.8 kg and 1.61 m. Pertinent test subject data are listed in Table 1.

Anthropometric data were compiled for each cadaver prior to the run. The standard used is the format recommended by the Department of Transportation for entering the subject data into the 3-dimensional Crash Victim Simulation Model. In addition, pre-test X-ray films of all skeletal structures were taken.

Prior to each test, the cadaver was instrumented with the following array of accelerometers:

Skull vertex: Nine accelerometer array in the 3-2-2-2 configuration
Occiput: Anteroposterior accelerometer
Ribs & Sternum: Standard eight accelerometer array
Spine: Triaxial accelerometers at T1, T12 and L3

Targets were affixed to the three spinal accelerometer mounts for the purpose of film analysis. A Foley catheter was inserted through the femoral artery such that its balloon was approximately 100 mm below the diaphragm. Another was inserted through the right carotid artery such that its balloon was at the level of the diaphragm. A pressure transducer was inserted such that its tip was between the two balloons at the approximate level of the hepatic artery. Methyl blue dye or heparinized sheep's blood was pumped through the upper catheter to pressurize the abdominal aorta to 100 mm of Hg in an attempt to perfuse the vasculature of liver and abdominal soft tissue organs to an approximately physiological state.

All cadavers were tested after rigor mortis had passed. In eight subjects the average time lapse between expiration and actual testing was ten days, with a range of seven to thirteen days. In the four other test subjects, there was a greater time lapse between expiration and testing. These subjects were frozen for a period of time. In the period prior to testing, the specimens were stored in a refrigeration unit at 35° F. No attempt was made to bring internal body temperature up to a physiologic temperature at time of testing. However, there was always a time lapse of several hours at room temperature prior to conducting the test.

All twelve abdominal impacts were carried out with the cadaver seated in an upright position, with legs parallel to and resting on a horizontal, hydraulically adjustable platform. The main axis of the torso was upright, at 90 degrees to the horizontal platform, and the anterior side of the torso was facing the impactor. The cadaver torso was held upright with suspension straps slung under the arms and connected above to an open-ended release hook which was hung from a pulley system. The back of the cadaver was unrestrained so that it was free to translate rearward on impact. In eleven of twelve runs the impact level was the L3 lumbar vertebra. In test No. 41 the impact level was at L1. Figures 3 and 4 show a Hybrid III dummy in the actual pre-impact test position.

The impactor itself is the Wayne State University Translational Impactor described by

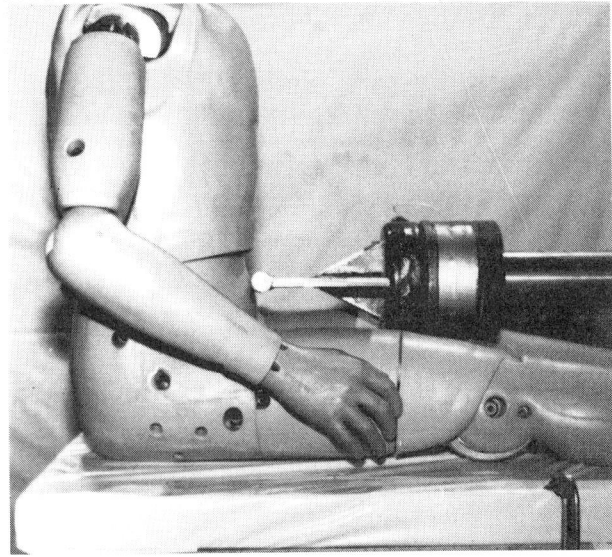

Figure 3. Lateral view

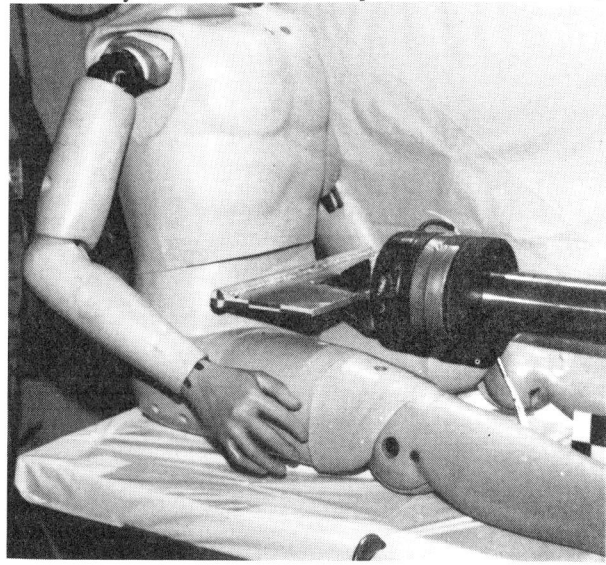

Figure 4. Oblique view

A Hybrid III dummy in the pre-impact test position. In the actual tests, unembalmed cadavers were used.

TABLE 1
Cadaver Characteristics

Test No.	Cadaver No.	Sex	Age (Years)	Stature (m)	Body Mass (kg)	Scaling Factor, Lamda*	Cause of Death
14	458	M	56	1.82	68	1.037	Small cell carcinoma of the lung.
19	473	F	43	1.59	53	1.130	Asphyxia due to carbon monoxide poisoning.
24	525	M	57	1.87	45	1.187	Ischemic anoxic brain injury, caustic material ingestion, diabetes mellitus, pneumonia.
28	578	F	57	1.63	75	1.002	Cardiopulmonary arrest
33	590	F	51	1.63	68	1.030	Congestive heart failure, arteriosclerotic heart disease, renal insufficiency.
37	684	M	50	1.69	88	0.954	Cardiac arrest, massive acute MI
41	712	F	51	1.59	55	1.115	Carbon monoxide poisoning
43	721	M	66	1.70	70	1.026	Cardiopulmonary arrest, arteriosclerotic heart disease, diabetes mellitus.
45	731	M	58	1.76	92	0.938	Cardiac arrest.
47	739	M	43	1.72	61	1.075	Cardiac arrest, end stage heart failure, cardiomyopathy.
57	751	M	64	1.84	90	0.945	Cardiac arrest.
61	786	M	60	1.80	79	0.987	Atherosclerotic cardiovascular disease.

* Lamda $= \left(\dfrac{76.0 \text{ kg}}{\text{Body Mass of Test Subject}} \right)^{1/3}$

Nyquist et al (9). The impactor mass used in the abdominal test series was essentially either 32 kg or 64 kg*. A magnetic pick-up passing over uniformly spaced metal teeth generated signals which were used to compute impact velocity. The assembly used on the impactor face was a 25 mm diameter, 381 mm long aluminum bar, oriented so that the long axis of the bar was parallel to the width of the body. The bar was reinforced with gusset and stiffening plates as depicted in Figure 4.

The impactor was instrumented with a uniaxial accelerometer and uniaxial load cell. Their sensitive axes were parallel to the direction of impact. The mass ahead of the impactor force transducer consisted primarily of the impactor bar assembly. The impactor load cell output was inertially compensated.

The electrical signals were prefiltered at 1000 Hz and the analog data were digitized at a 2000 Hz sampling rate using a 9-bit A/D converter and a PDP-8 computer. The digitized data were then processed on a main frame Harris computer.

The abdominal impact tests were filmed with a high speed camera operating at approximately 500 or 1000 frames per second. The film was analyzed with a Vanguard analyzer, primarily to obtain deflection data.

In analyzing the abdominal force-deflection and force-time response an equal stress - equal velocity scaling method was used to scale the data. The procedure has been described by Eppinger et al (10, 11). Normalizing the data in this fashion mitigates the difference in impact response among the various sized test subjects. The equal stress - equal velocity scaling method assumes equal mass density and equal moduli of elasticity between test subjects. The basic scaling factor, lamda, is obtained by taking the cube root of the mass ratio as the scaling factor for length scaling. The dimensional parameters are scaled as follows:

$$\text{Lamda} = \left(\frac{76.00 \text{ kg}}{\text{Body Mass. of Test Subject}}\right)^{1/3}$$

$T_n = \text{Lamda} \times T_r$

$F_n = (\text{Lamda})^2 \times F_r$

$L_n = \text{Lamda} \times L_r$

T = Time   F = Force
L = Length
n = subscript for normalized quantity
r = subscript for non-normalized quantity

Table 1 lists lamda for each test subject.

RESULTS AND DISCUSSION

FORCE-TIME HISTORY DATA: The 1000 Hz and 100 Hz non-normalized force-time history plots

---

* Precise values are listed in Table 4.

are shown superimposed on each other in Figures A1 through A12. Table 2 presents the force time-history characteristics of the impact data. Time from onset of impact to peak force and total impact duration are listed in both normalized and non-normalized fashion. Any plateau in the rising portion of the expanded force-time history plot is also noted. (Such a plateau would represent a viscous response consistent with the Segment II plateau described by Stalnaker and Ulman (4) for the abdominal force-deflection plots of various live primate species.) The average rise time was 25 ms with a range of 14 to 36 ms. The average duration of impact was 63 ms with a range of 51 to 90 ms. A review of Table 2 shows that normalization of the data did not reduce these ranges.

A plateau was noted in three of the twelve cadaver runs. An attempt was made to correlate the existence of the plateau with successful pressurization of the abdominal vasculature. Table 2 lists the peak abdominal pressures obtained. It was thought that there could be a relationship between viscous response and successful pressurization of the abdominal aorta; however, a review of Table 2 shows that the tests where a Segment II plateau occurs and the tests which show a dynamic abdominal pressure response do not correlate.

A review of Tables 2 & 4 also shows a trend toward higher peak force with higher impact velocity. There was a high correlation between impact velocity and peak force (r = 0.80). In addition, the duration of impact appears shorter with higher velocities. For the first five tests, the average velocity was 6.1 m/s and the average impact duration was 71 ms. For the last seven tests, the average velocity was 10.4 m/s and the average impact duration was 55 m/s.

Because of this apparent rate dependence, it was decided to construct two separate forc-time history response corridors as depicted in Figures 5 and 6. Figure 5 is based on the normalized force-time history data of the five lower velocity runs and Figure 6 on the seven higher velocity runs.

To obtain the average response the individual force-time histories were first aligned so that zero force occurred at the same time for all impacts. Each point on the average force-time history curve was obtained by using the equation:

$$F_{ave}(t) = \frac{\sum f_i(t)}{n} \text{ at each point in time, } t$$

Where $F_{ave}(t)$ = Average cadaver force response at time, t

$f_i(t)$ = Response at time t of the ith cadaver

n = Total number of cadavers in sample

Each response corridor was plotted by obtaining

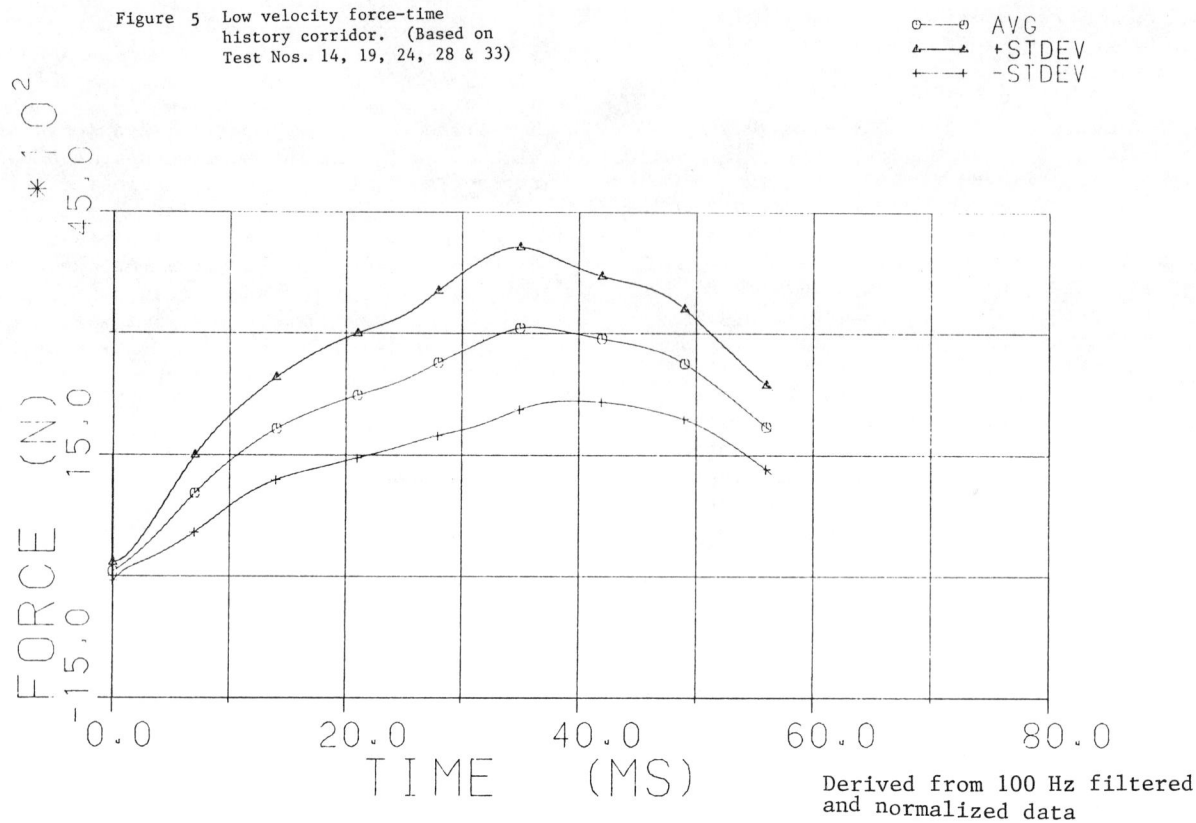

Figure 5 Low velocity force-time history corridor. (Based on Test Nos. 14, 19, 24, 28 & 33)

Derived from 100 Hz filtered and normalized data

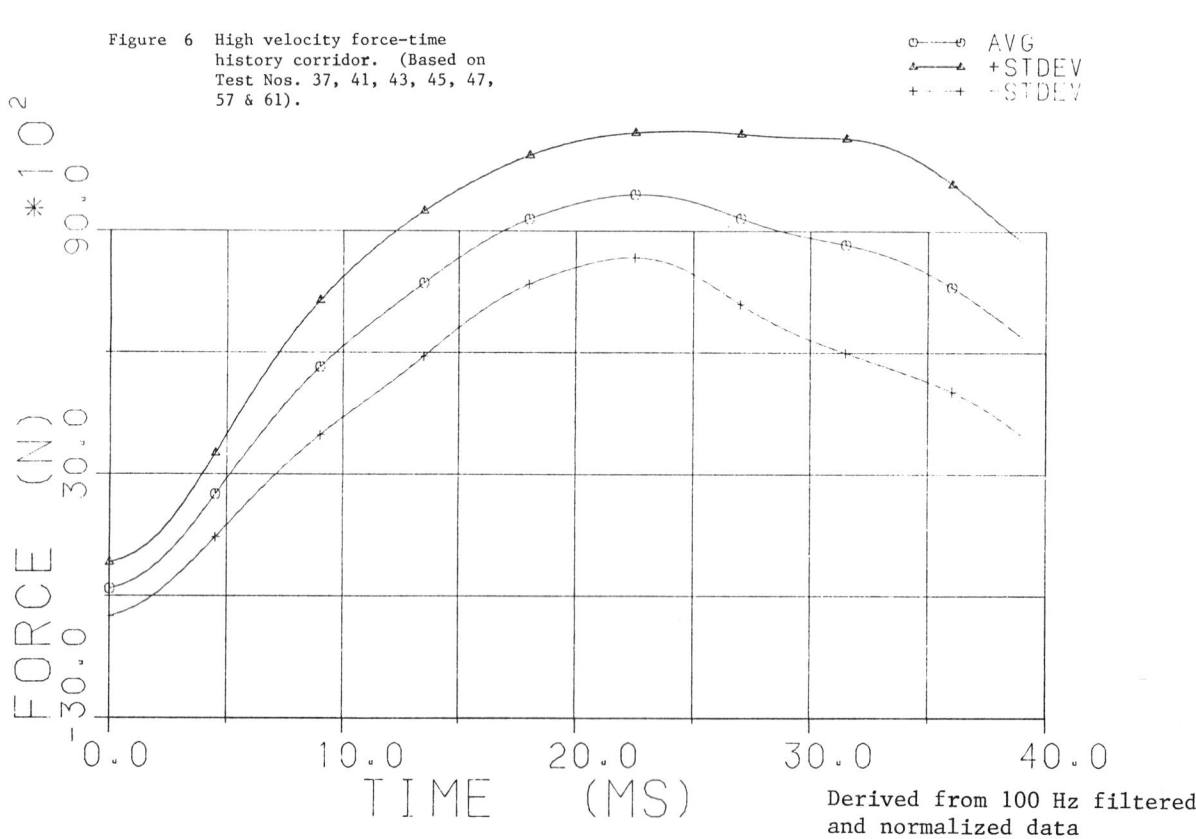

Figure 6 High velocity force-time history corridor. (Based on Test Nos. 37, 41, 43, 45, 47, 57 & 61).

Derived from 100 Hz filtered and normalized data

plus and minus one standard deviation of the average force (F ave) at each point in time, t.

For the low velocity corridor the average impact velocity is 6.1 m/s, the average the rise time is 36 ms, and the average peak force is 3.1 kN. The corresponding values for the higher velocity corridor are 10.4 m/s, 23 ms, and 10.2 kN. The standard deviations of these values are listed in Table 3.

FORCE-DEFLECTION DATA: Figures A13 through A24 are non-normalized abdominal penetration-time history plots. Figures 7 and 8 are normalized cross plots of impact force vs. abdominal penetration. Figure 7 shows the five lower velocity runs and Figure 8 the seven higher velocity runs.

In eleven of twelve cadaver tests the force data in the force-deflection cross plots were obtained by using impactor load cell data and inertially compensating for the impactor mass in front of the load cell. In Test No. 37, the impactor force was not available, so it was obtained by multiplying impactor mass by impactor acceleration. The deflection data were obtained by film analysis in ten of twelve tests. Abdominal penetration was taken as the difference in horizontal displacement between the impactor and the L3 target. Impacts at the L3 level caused rearward translation with minimal rotation in the lumbar area during impact. Consequently, vertical displacement of the L3 target was not used in obtaining abdominal penetrations. In Test Nos. 47 and 57 there was a lack of film data. Therefore, in these two tests, the horizontal displacement of the impactor and L3 target were obtained by double integration of impactor and L3-x acceleration data. The difference between these values was used to obtain abdominal penetration. (Good agreement was found between the two methods in other tests.) The final force-deflection plots were filtered at 100 Hz and normalized.

In reviewing Figures 7 and 8 it can be seen that the shape of the rising portion of the abdominal force-deflection curve varied somewhat from test to test. In Test Nos. 37 and 61 the rising portion of the curve was approximately a straight line. Test Nos. 33, 41, 43 and 45 had an irregular shape; but, overall, the rising portion of the curve appeared linear. The rising portion of the curve in Test No. 47 was concave upward. In Test Nos. 28 and 57 it was concave downward. In Test Nos. 14, 19, and 24 a Segment II plateau or at least the suggestion of such a plateau existed. Consequently, in analyzing the present data, it was decided to characterize abdominal stiffness by plotting a least-squares line through the rising portion of each force-deflection plot. The abdominal stiffnesses thus obtained are listed in Table 4. The stiffnesses ranged from 20.2 to 101.2 kN/m and, overall, increased as impact velocity increased. The hysteresis on unloading was approximately a vertical line.

Because there was an overall increase in abdominal stiffness with increasing impactor velocity, it was decided to correlate the two. For the eight impacts in which the impactor mass was 32 kg, the correlation coefficient relating impactor velocity to abdominal stiffness is r = 0.81. Using all twelve impacts and two impactor masses, there is still a good correlation between abdominal stiffness and impactor velocity (r = 0.71). A review of the stiffnesses in Table 4 suggest that abdominal stiffness may also increase with impactor mass. To account for the possible mass dependence, abdominal stiffness was correlated with impactor momentum and impactor kinetic energy. Using the data from all twelve runs, there is a high correlation between abdominal stiffness and impactor momentum (r = 0.85), and abdominal stiffness and kinetic energy at onset of impact (r = 0.87).

Based on this rate dependence, a lower velocity force-penetration response corridor, shown in Figure 9, and a higher velocity corridor shown in Figure 10, have been proposed. Figure 9 is based on Test Nos. 14, 19, 24, 28 and 33. Figure 10 is based on Test Nos. 37, 41, 43, 45, 47, 57, and 61. To construct the corridors, the average force-time history curves of Figures 5 and 6 were cross-plotted with average penetration-time history curves to obtain average force-penetration curves. A corridor was then established by taking plus and minus one standard deviation of the average curve. For the lower velocity corridor the average impact velocity is 6.1 m/s, the average kinetic energy at impact is 603 J, and the least squares stiffness is 20.8 N/mm. For the higher velocity corridor the corresponding values are 10.4 m/s, 2543 J, and 70.3 N/mm. Comparison of the average stiffnesses (20.8 N/mm vs. 70.3 N/mm) for the two corridors again illustrates the rate dependence of abdominal stiffness. For both response corridors plus and minus one standard deviation of average stiffness is given in Table 3. Because of the method used to align the curves, data only goes through the initial stages of the unloading portion of each response corridor. Based on the results of individual tests it can be predicted that each force-penetration corridor would continue to unload in an almost vertical hysteris to zero force.

One of the initial findings based on our series of tests is that the human lower abdomen did not necessarily follow the rise-plateau-rise force-deflection pattern described by Stalnaker and Ulman (4). Also, the force-deflection responses we have obtained are overall, much less stiff than their proposed corridor. There are several possible reasons for the difference in findings: 1) The Stalnaker and Ulman study included many impacts into upper and middle abdomen, thus involving more

TABLE 2: Time-History Data

Test No.	Rise Time (ms)**	Total Pulse Duration (ms)**	Non-Normalized Peak Force (kN) Filt 100 Hz	Plateau Duration (ms)	Peak Abdominal Pressure (kPa)
14	34 (35.3)	62 (64.3)	3.07	9 (9.3)	79.3
19	36 (40.7)	65 (73.5)	2.03	6 (6.8)	NA
24	25 (29.7)	51 (60.5)	2.37	4 (4.7)	22.1
28	24 (24.0)	87 (87.2)	2.38	-	29.6
33	34 (35.0)	90 (92.7)	4.23	-	NA
37	14 (13.4)	NA (NA)	8.18	-	0.0
41	22 (24.5)	57 (63.6)	7.63	-	103.4
43	23 (23.6)	53 (54.4)	8.61	-	NA
45	20 (18.8)	58 (54.4)	13.17	-	NA
47	30 (32.3)	53 (57.0)	12.65	-	65.5
57	21 (19.8)	53 (50.1)	12.30	-	441.3*
61	17 (16.8)	NA (NA)	9.12	-	275.8
Avg.	25 (26.2)	63 (65.8)			

* Saturated
** Normalized values are in parenthesis
NA Not available

TABLE 3: Response Corridor Parameters

	Avg Impact Velocity (m/s) (std dev)	Avg Impact K.E.(J) (std dev)	Avg Rise Time (ms)	Avg Peak Force(kN) (std dev)	Avg Stiff (kN/m) (std dev)
Low Velocity Corridor	6.1 (1.1)	603 (209)	36	3.1 (0.95)	20.8 (5.4)
High Velocity Corridor	10.4 (1.5)	2543 (525)	23	10.2 (1.3)	70.3 (5.9)

These values are based on 100 Hz filtered and normalized data.

TABLE 4: Impact Kinetics

Test No.	Impactor Mass (kg)	Impactor Velocity m/s (mph)	Impactor Momentum (kg-m/s)	Impactor Kinetic Energy (J)	Lower Abdominal Stiffness (kN/m)*	Peak Force (kN)*
14	31.24	6.84 (15.3)	214	731	34.2	3.30
19	31.24	5.00 (11.2)	156	391	25.5	2.59
24	31.24	4.87 (10.9)	152	370	25.2	3.34
28	31.52	6.66 (14.9)	210	699	20.2	2.39
33	31.52	7.24 (16.2)	228	826	26.9	4.49
37	31.30	10.59 (23.7)	331	1755	84.0	7.45
41	63.56	8.54 (19.1)	543	2318	61.3	9.49
43	63.56	9.07 (20.3)	576	2614	72.1	9.06
45	63.56	9.79 (21.9)	622	3046	101.2	11.59
47	63.56	10.15 (22.7)	645	3274	77.6	14.33
57	31.52	13.01 (29.1)	410	2667	54.3	10.99
61	31.52	11.62 (26.0)	366	2128	63.7	8.89

* 100 Hz filtered and normalized

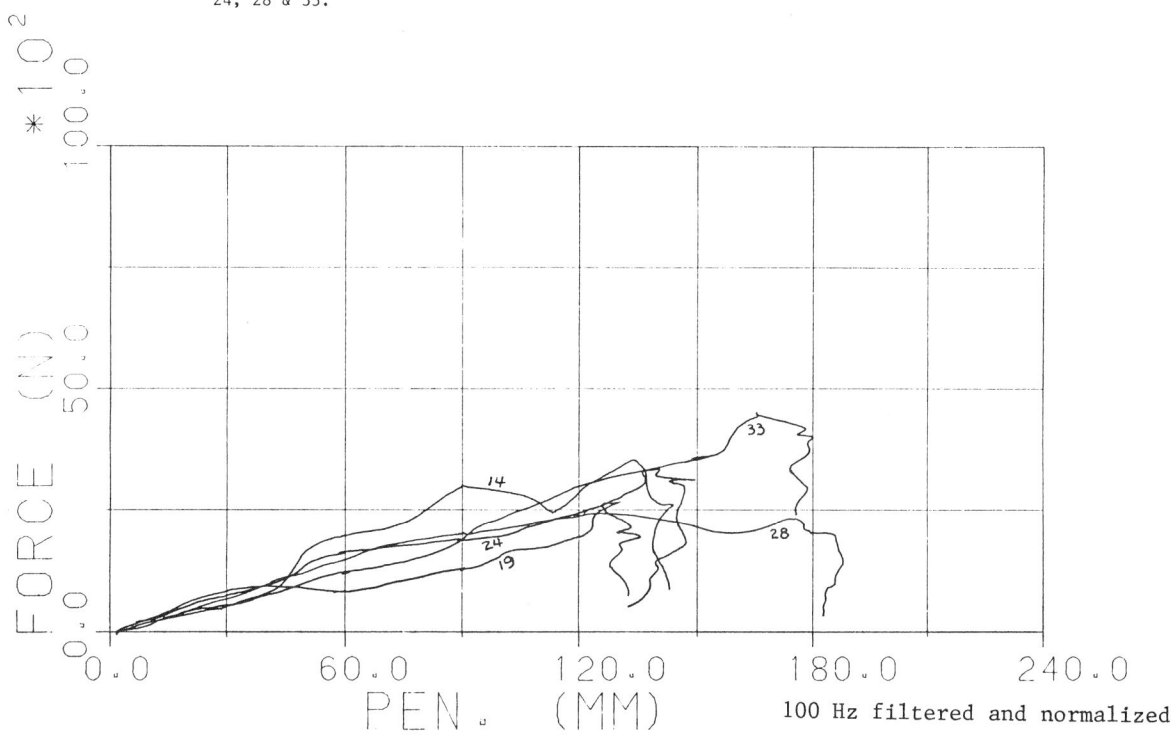

Figure 7 Normalized force-penetration curves for Test Nos. 14, 19, 24, 28 & 33.

100 Hz filtered and normalized

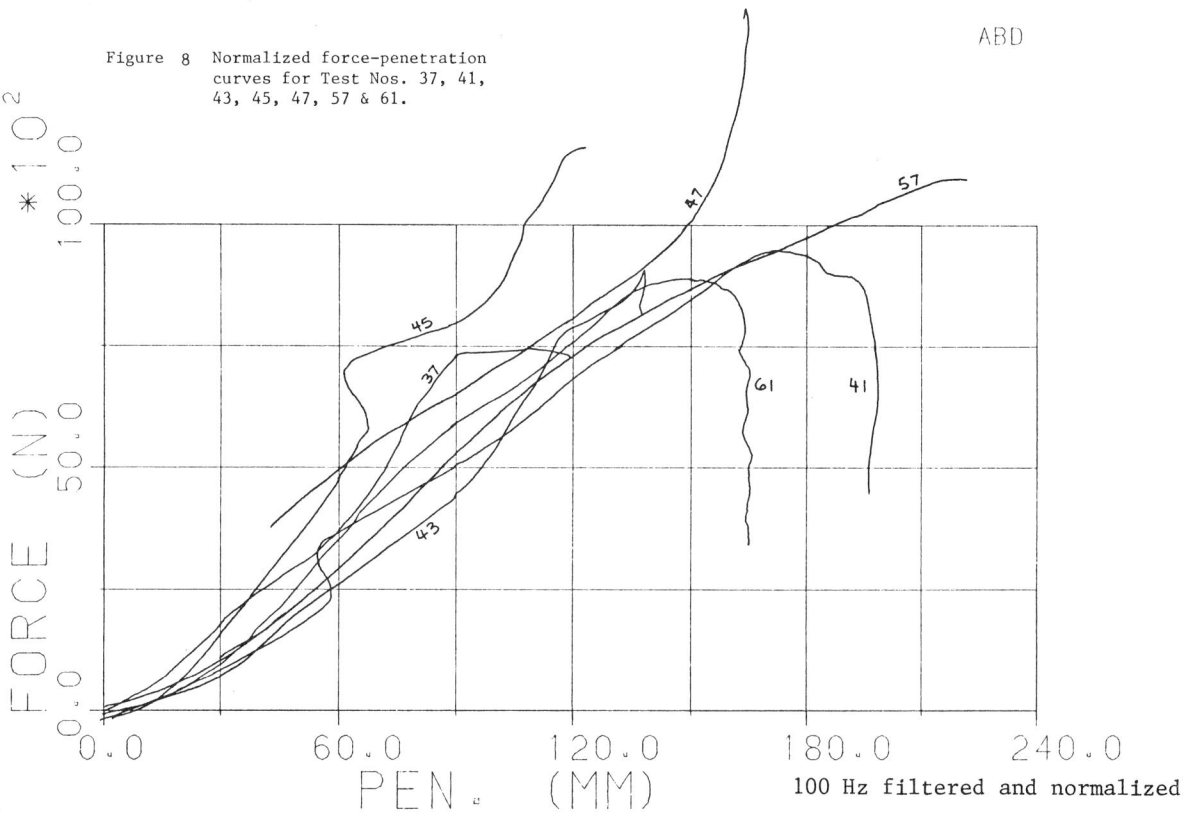

Figure 8 Normalized force-penetration curves for Test Nos. 37, 41, 43, 45, 47, 57 & 61.

100 Hz filtered and normalized

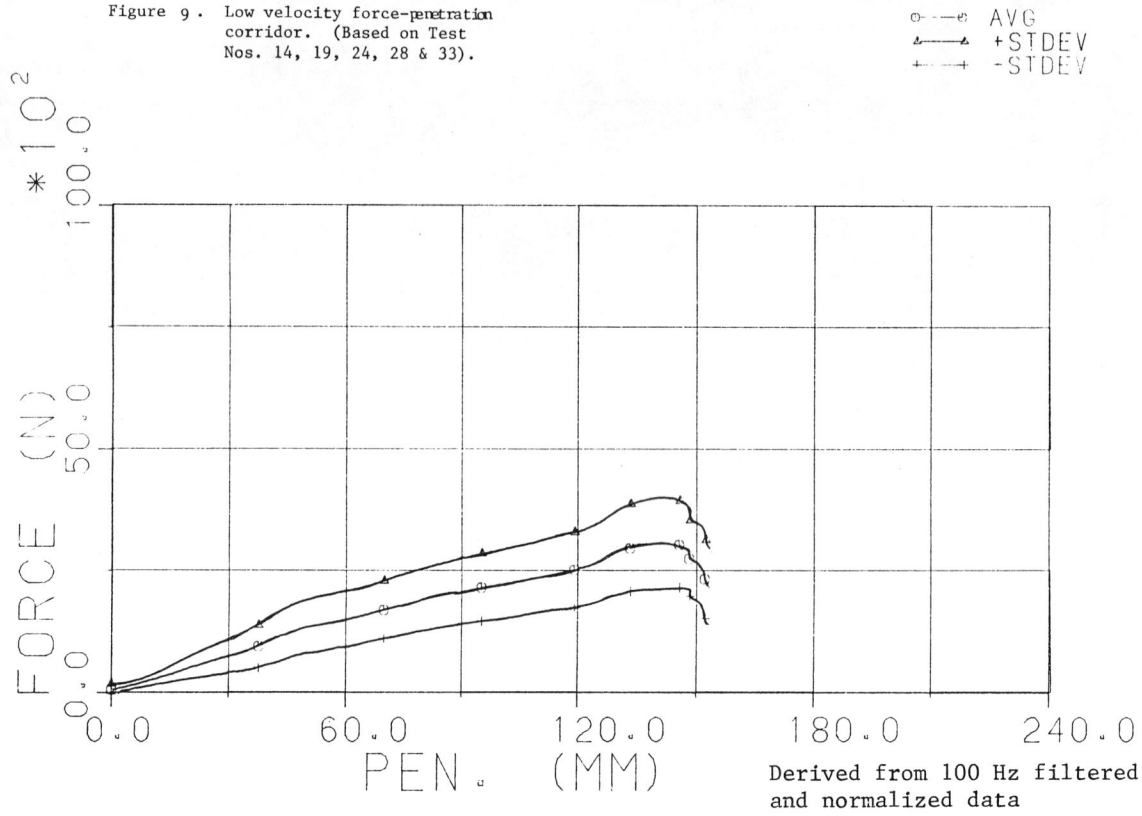

Figure 9. Low velocity force-penetration corridor. (Based on Test Nos. 14, 19, 24, 28 & 33).

Derived from 100 Hz filtered and normalized data

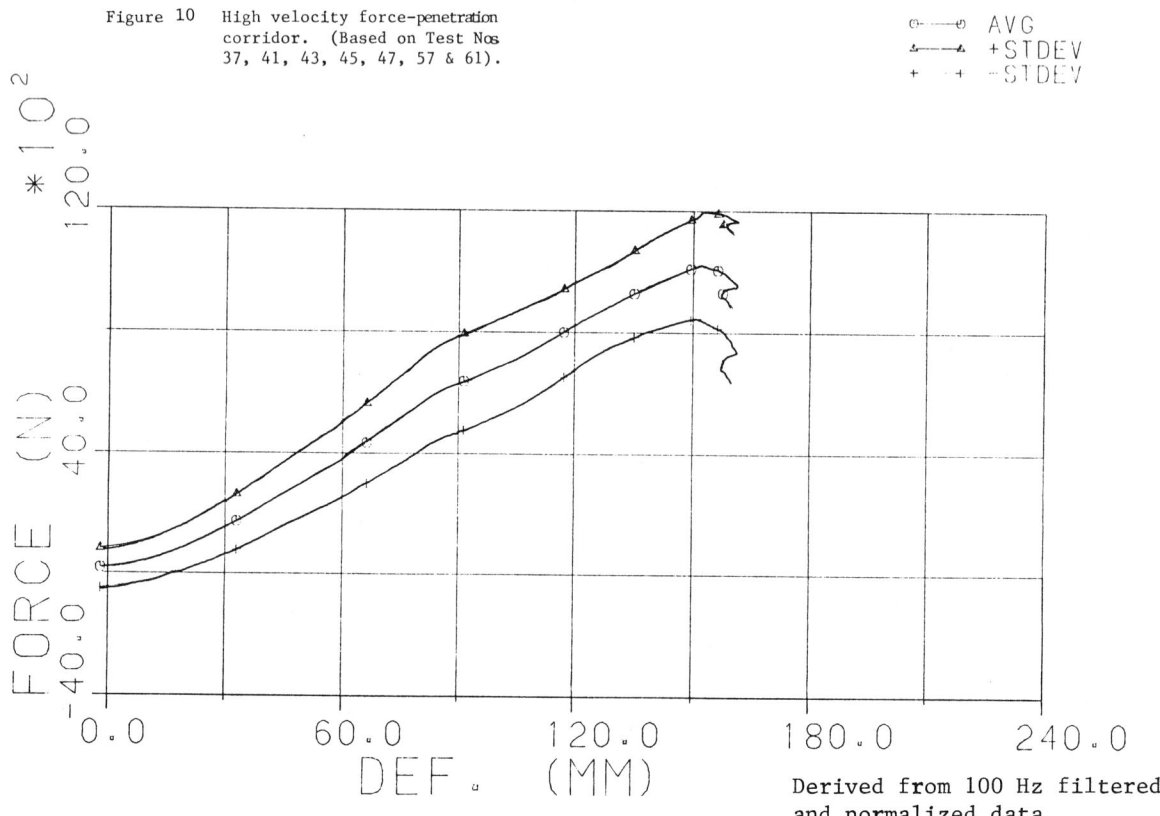

Figure 10 High velocity force-penetration corridor. (Based on Test Nos. 37, 41, 43, 45, 47, 57 & 61).

Derived from 100 Hz filtered and normalized data

rib contact than our impacts. 2) Our study used unembalmed cadavers with no muscle tone, and their study was based on live primate tests. 3) A narrow impactor face as in our test series may produce a less stiff response than wider impactor faces. 4) The proposed Stalnaker and Ulman corridor bottoms out on the spine at a depth of 125 mm. Our findings indicate that bottoming out occurs in the range of 170 to 190 mm in the lower abdomen. It appears that the paunch which develops in the sitting position increases total abdominal depth. 5) The scaling technique used in the Stalnaker and Ulman study utilized direct proportionality between animal species masses to extrapolate to the human. Equal stress - equal velocity scaling methods produce a less stiff human response. Comparison of our data to the Stalnaker - Ulman study is discussed in more detail in Appendix B.

ABDOMINAL TOLERANCE: There are inherent shortcomings in evaluating AIS injury level with cadavers as test subjects. A major problem is lack of soft tissue injury findings after cadaver impacts. Often, a similar impact would likely produce soft tissue injury in a live subject.

Contusion of an abdominal organ is an example of an injury achieved in live subjects, but unachievable in cadavers. Contusion, which is essentially bruising, requires perfusion of the local vasculature with blood, because the major observable sign of contusion, the local change in color, is caused by localized damage to blood vessels and consequent leaking of blood into extracellular spaces. In a cadaver, the smaller vessels are not being actively perfused with blood, even if the larger vessels are being artificially pressurized with fluid from an external source. Contusions of the duodenum, jejunum, ileum, pancreas, liver, spleen, kidneys, and adrenals are rated an AIS 2 or 3. Based on our experience, these are virtually unattainable in a cadaver test series.

In their review of abdominal impacts to 42 live primates, Stalnaker and Ulman (4), found good correlation between velocity times compression (V*C) and AIS injury level. In their study, regression equations were developed relating V*C to AIS numbers in each of five areas of the abdomen, including the lower abdomen. Table 5 in our study lists V*C and AIS injury for each of our cadaver runs. Injuries were assessed using the 1985 AIS (12). Because of the shortcomings in cadaver soft tissue injury evaluation, no attempt was made to correlate V*C with AIS injury level.

In reviewing Table 5 it is interesting to note that there were only two cases of laceration or rupture of abdominal organs in our tests run at the L3 level. In Test No. 14 rupture of the liver occurred, but autopsy findings showed the liver to be soft and friable due to metastatic carcinoma. In Test No. 61 a moderate laceration of the mesentery (AIS 3) occurred, but this may have been a pre-impact condition. In Test No. 41 an extensive laceration of the liver and spleen (AIS 4) occurred. The impact level here was at L1, which is in direct line with the lower portions of the liver and spleen.

Rib fractures were a common occurrence in this study, and the AIS results are summarized in Table 5. In only Test Nos. 41 and 43 were more than three adjacent ribs fractured, which resulted in AIS 3.

CONCLUSIONS

The following conclusions are based on the analysis of the twelve cadavers tested:
1. Overall, higher velocity impacts resulted in shorter impact durations. The low velocity force pulse of the Figure 5 corridor has an average rise time of 35 ms. The high velocity force pulse of the Figure 6 corridor has an average rise time of 23 ms.
2. Based on present data, the loading portion of the force-deflection curve of the lower abdomen of the human cadaver can be characterized by an almost linear rise from zero force to peak force.
3. The overall stiffness of the lower abdomen is both velocity and impactor mass dependent. Correlation coefficients suggest a strong relationship between abdominal stiffness and impactor velocity, momentum and kinetic energy.
4. The unloading portion of the force-deflection curve of the lower abdomen is approximately a vertical line.
5. Peak penetration of the lower abdomen was about 66% of total abdominal depth. This appears to be the depth at which the impactor bottoms out on the spine.
6. Based on the above findings two force-penetration response corridors have been formulated, one for low velocity, low energy impacts, and one for high velocity, high energy impacts. These corridors are depicted in Figures 9 & 10.
7. It is postulated that there may be a transition in response from chest to upper abdomen to lower abdomen. The chest often has a three segment response, often with a sharp initial spike of significant magnitude. Perhaps the upper abdomen responds as proposed by Stalnaker and Ulman (after rescaling as suggested by Melvin) with three segments as in the chest but, overall, with less stiffness. According to our studies, the lower abdomen responds in an even less stiff manner, showing viscoelastic rate dependence, but usually no clearly discernible transition between segments I, II and III.

ACKNOWLEDGEMENTS

The authors wish to acknowledge Warren Hardy for his assistance in compiling much of the data in this paper, Angela James for the preparation of the manuscript and Jo Ann Pepe

TABLE 5
Abdominal Compression and Injury Tolerance

Test No.	Max. Penet.(mm)[7] Normalized (Non-normalized)	Abdominal Depth(mm)[1] Normalized (Non-normalized)	Max.[2] Compress. (%)	V*C[3] (m/s)	MAIS[4]	AIS Indiv.
14	145.2 140.0	293 283	49.5	3.38	4	L 4 (5) SP 0 P 0 K 0 A 0 ST 0 R 0 S 0
19	135.6 120.0	261 231	51.9	2.60	0	L 0 SP 0 P 0 K 0 A 0 ST 0 R 0 S 0
24	150.0 125.5	305 257	48.8	2.38	0	L 0 SP 0 P 0 K 0 A 0 ST 0 R 0 S 0
28	185.0 184.6	276 275	67.0	4.46	0	L 0 SP 0 P 0 K 0 A 0 ST 0 R 0 S 0
33	177.9 172.7	269 261	66.2	4.79	0	L 0 SP 0 P 0 K 0 A 0 ST 0 R 0 S 0
37	113.9 119.4	317 332	36.0	3.81	0	L 0 SP 0 P 0 K 0 A 0 ST 0 R 0
41	198.5 178.0	301 270	65.9	5.58	4	L 4 SP 3 P 0 K 0 A 0 ST 0 R 3 S 3

(Continued on next page)

TABLE 5
Abdominal Compression and Injury Tolerance

Test No.	Max. Penet.(mm) [7] Normalized (Non-normalized)	Abdominal Depth(mm) [1] Normalized (Non-normalized)	Max. Compress. [2] (%)	V*C [3] (m/s)	MAIS [4]	AIS Indiv.	
43	138.3 134.8	251 245	55.0	4.99	3	L SP P K A ST R S	0 0 0 0 0 0 3 0
45	122.1 130.2	272 290	44.9	4.56	0	L SP P K A R S	0 0 0 0 0 0 0
47	203.4 189.2	345 321	59.0	5.99	0	L SP P K A ST R S	0 0 0 0 0 0 0 0
57	220 233	304 322	72.4	9.42	2	L SP P K A ST R S	0 0 0 0 0 0 2 0
61	165 167.2	273 277	60.4	7.02	3(6)	L SP P K A ST R S	0 0 0 0 0 0 2 0

L: liver; SP: spleen; P: pancreas; K: kidney; A: adrenal; ST: stomach; R: ribs; S: spine

(1) Abdominal depth is the total abdominal depth at the level of impact with the cadaver in a sitting position. In earlier tests, this value was scaled off of the high-speed film. In later tests, it is measured directly from the cadaver just prior to impact.
(2) Max. Compression = (Max. Penetration/Abd. Depth Sitting) x 100
(3) V*C is velocity (m/s) x maximum compression/100
(4) The AIS rating is based on the worst AIS injury found at necropsy.
(5) In test no. 14 the liver contained metastatic carcinoma and was described as soft and friable in autopsy report.
(6) AIS 3 in test no. 61 is due to laceration of mesentery near insertion on posterior abdominal wall.
(7) Maximum penetration was determined by film analysis except in Test Nos. 47 and 57, where double integration of impactor and L3-X accelerometer data was used to determine penetration.

for assisting in the statistical analysis of the data. The authors also wish to thank Frank DuPont, Gerry Locke, and John Ryan for their efforts in preparation and conduction of the impact tests. The authors wish a special acknowledgement to Dr. John Melvin for his recommendations on scaling the Stalnaker and Ulman data, and to Dr. Haresh Mirchandani for his expertise in conducting the autopsies. This research was supported by the National Highway Traffic Safety Administration, Contract No. DOT DTNH2283C27019.

REFERENCES

1. Bondy, N., "Abdominal Injuries in the National Crash Severity Study", National Center for Statistics and Analysis Collected Technical Studies, Vol. II: Accident Data analysis of Occupant Injuries and Crash Characteristics, NHTSA, Washington, D.C., 1980, pp. 59-80.

2. Leung, Y.C., Tarriere, C., Lestrelin, D., Got, C., Buillon, G., Pate, A, Hureau, J. Submarining Injuries pf Three-point Belted Occupants in Frontal Collisions: Description, Mechanisms and Protection", SAE Paper No. 821158, 26th Stapp Car Crash Conference Proc., SAE, 1982.

3. Walfisch, G., Fayon, A., Tarriere, C., Rosey, J.P., Guillon, F., Got, C., Patel, A. "Designing of a Dummy's Abdomen for Detecting Injuries in Side Impact Collisions," Fifth International IRCOBI Conference Proceedings, 1980, pp. 149-169.

4. Stalnaker, R.L., and Ulman, M.S. "Abdominal Trauma-Review, Response, and Criteria," SAE Paper No. 851720, 29th Stapp Car Crash Conference Proceedings, SAE, 1985.

5. Beckman, D.L., McElhaney, J.H., Roberts, V.L. and Stalnaker, R.L., "Impact Tolerance -- Abdominal Injury," NTIS No. PB204171, 1971.

6. Stalnaker, R.L., McElhaney, J.H., Snyder, R.G., and Roberts, V.L. "Door Crashworthiness Criteria," NTIS No. PB203721, 1971.

7. Stalnaker, R.L., Roberts, V.L., and McElhaney, J.H., "Door Crashworthiness Criteria," NTIS No. PB225000, 1973.

8. Trollope, M.L., Stalnaker, R.L., McElhaney, J.H., Frey, C. F., "The Mechanism of Injury in Blunt Abdominal Trauma," Journal of Trauma, 13(11):962-970, 1973.

9. Nyquist, G.W., Cavanaugh, J.M., Goldberg, S.J., King, A.I., "Facial Impact Tolerance and Response," SAE 30th Stapp Crash Conf. Proc., 1986.

10. Eppinger, R.H., Marcus, J.H., and Morgan, R.M., "Development of Dummy and Injury Index for NHTSA's Thoracic Side Impact Protection Research Program," SAE Publication No. 840885, Government/Industry Meeting and Exposition, Washington, DC, May 21-24, 1984.

11. Eppinger, R.H., "Prediction of Thoracic Injury Using Measurable Experimental Parameters," Proceedings of the 6th Experimental Safety Vehicle Conference, NHTSA, Washington, DC., 1976, pp. 770-780.

12. Abbreviated Injury Scale, 1985 Revision, American Association for Automotive Medicine, 1985.

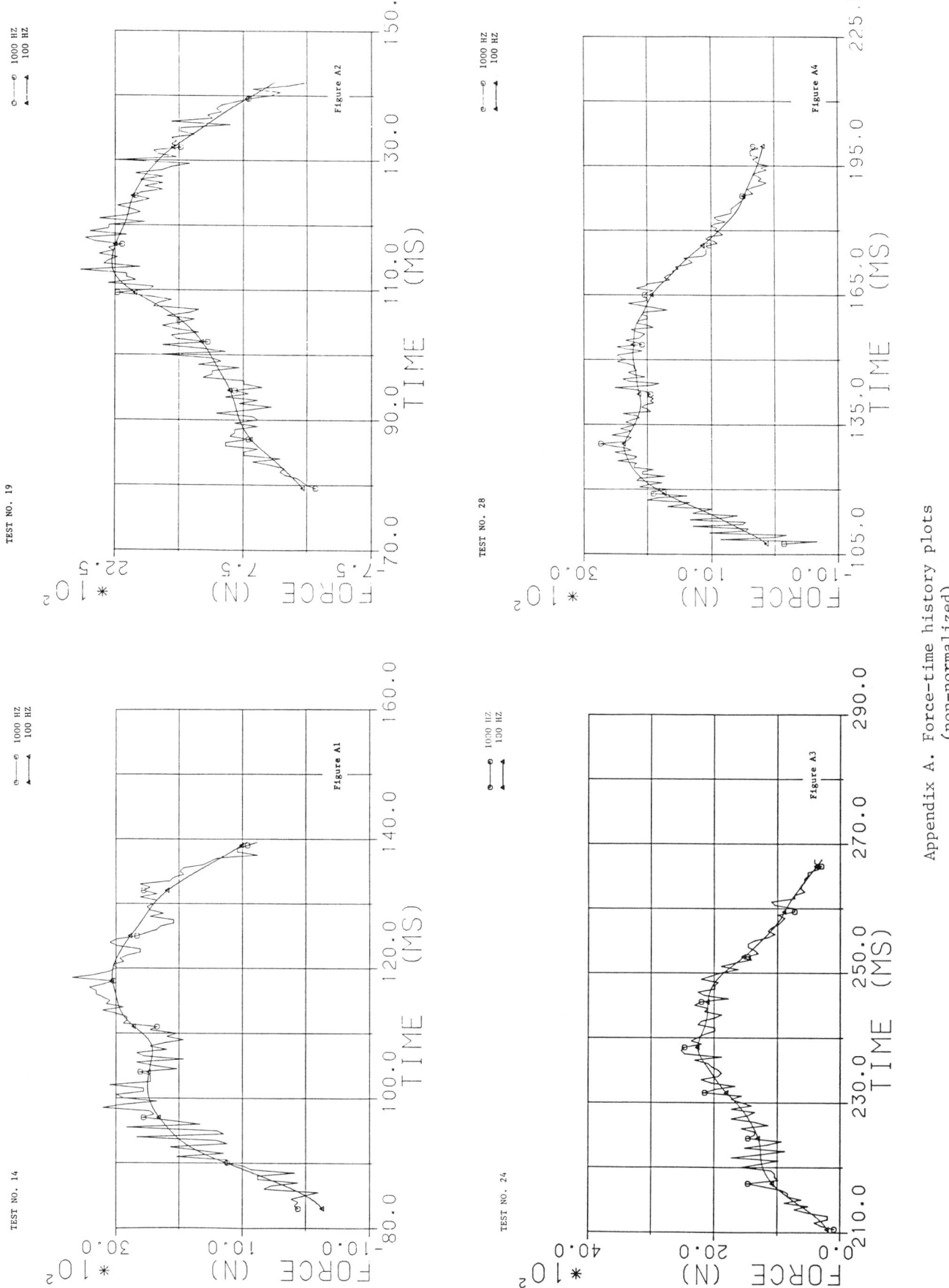

Appendix A. Force-time history plots (non-normalized)

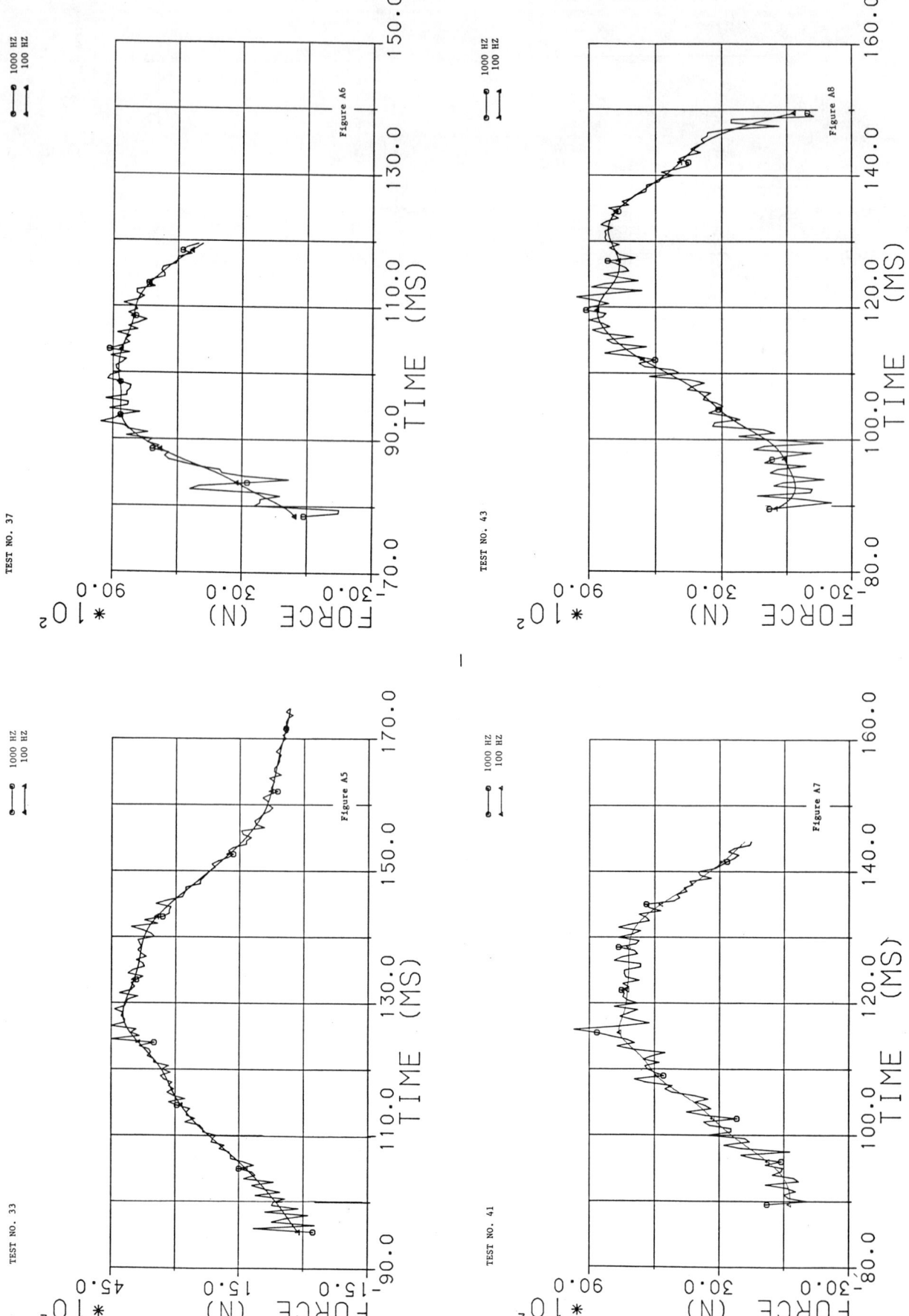

Appendix A. Force-time history plots (non-normalized)

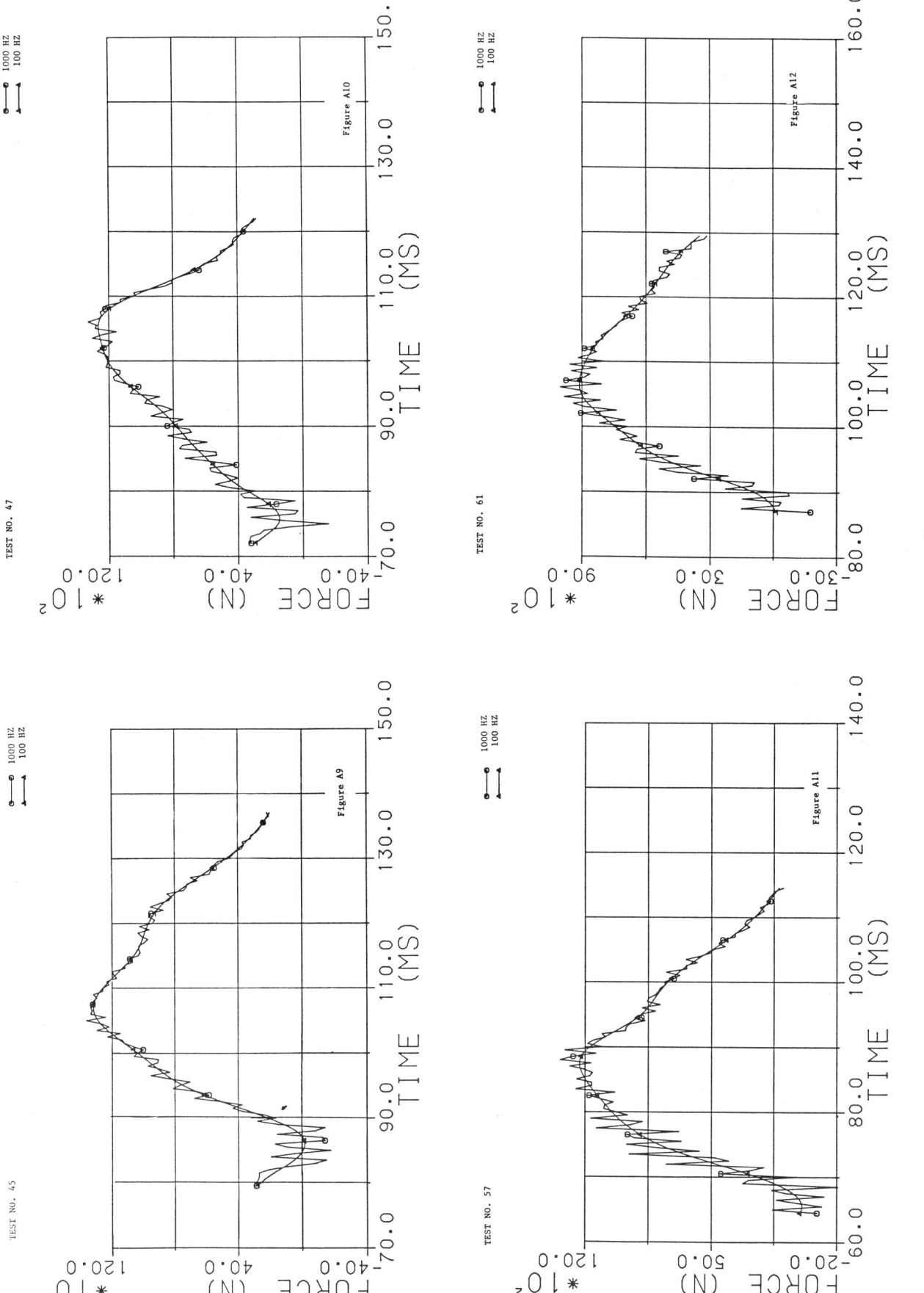

Appendix A. Force-time history plots (non-normalized)

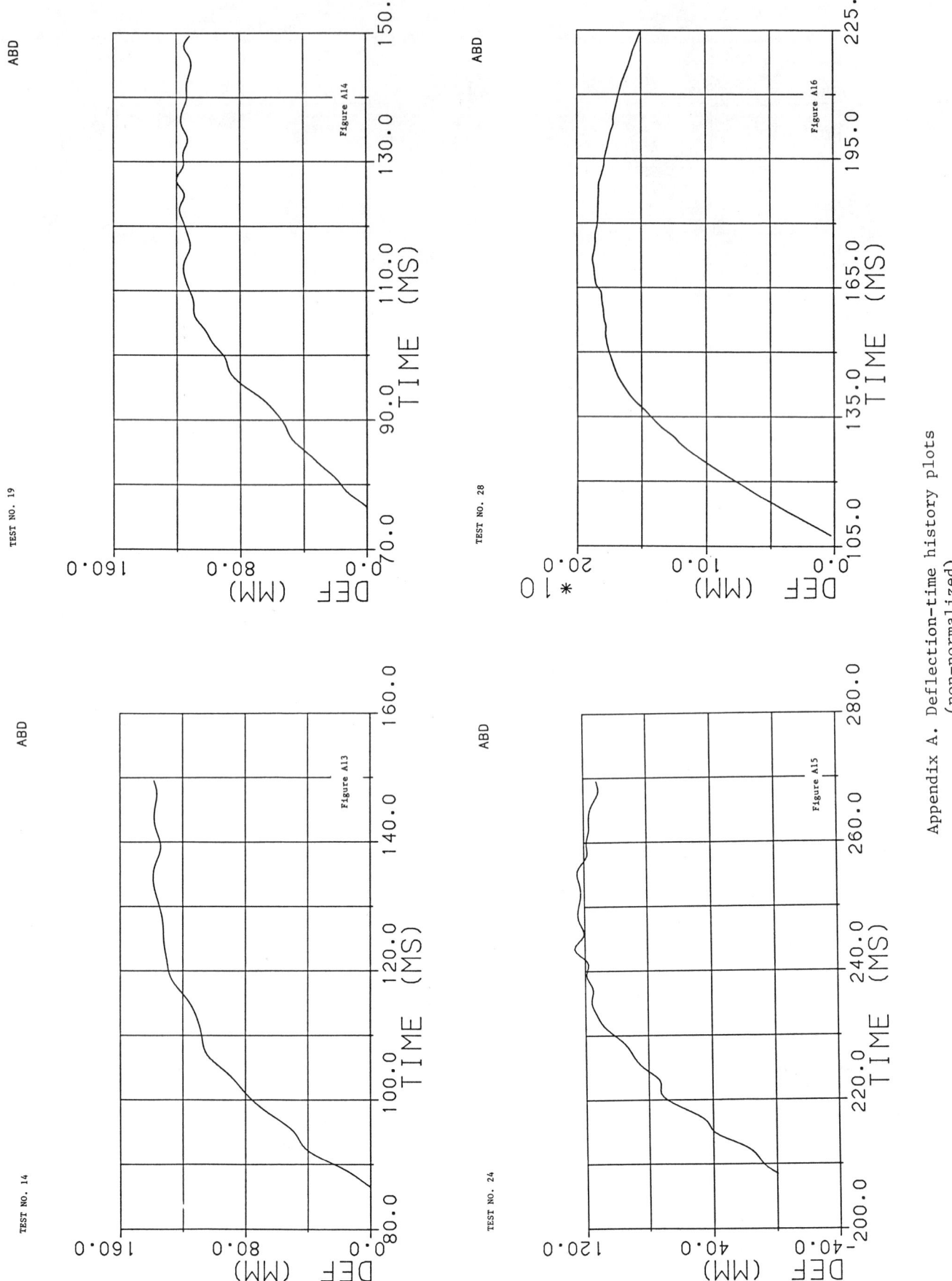

Appendix A. Deflection-time history plots (non-normalized)

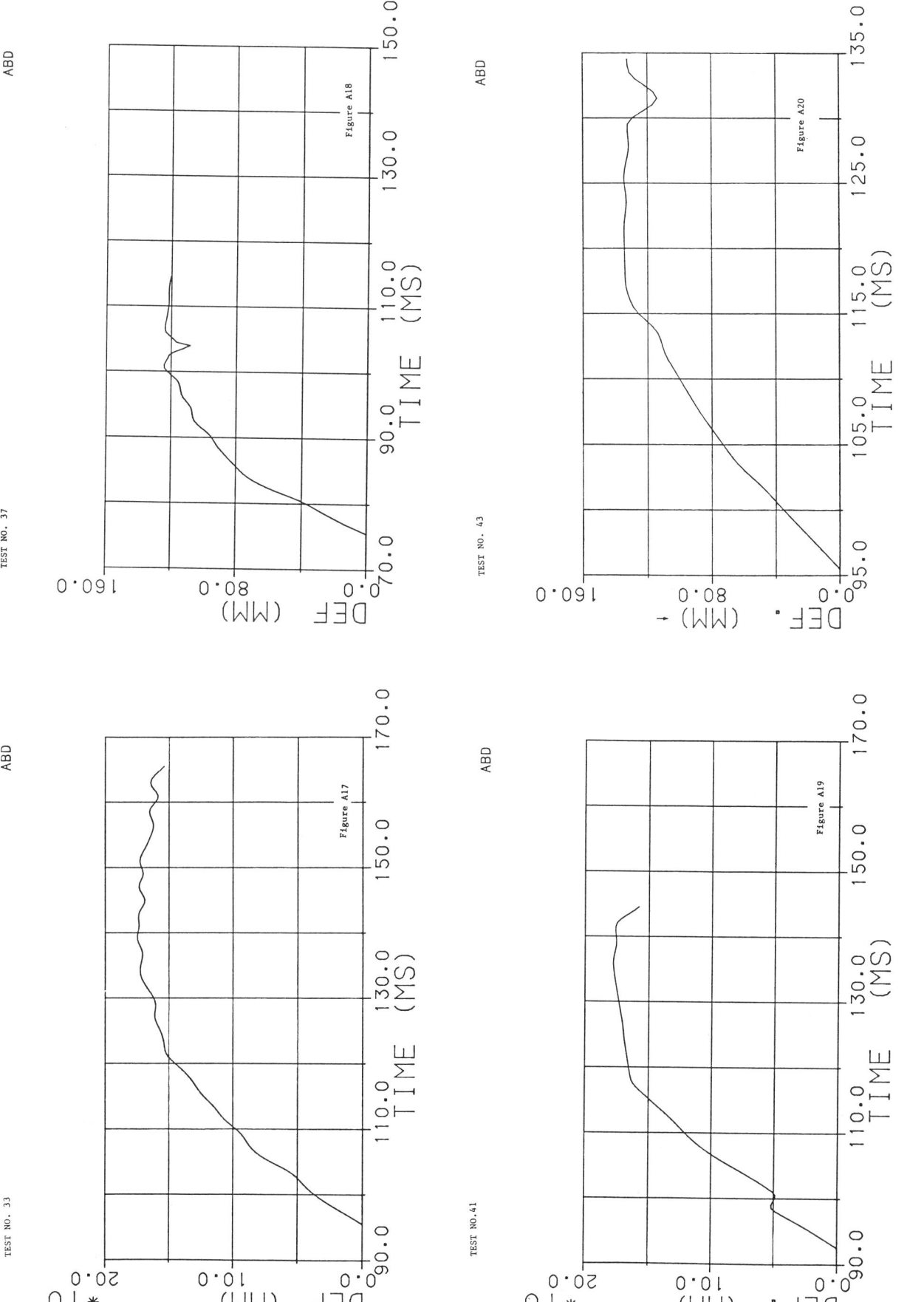

Appendix A. Deflection-time history plots (non-normalized)

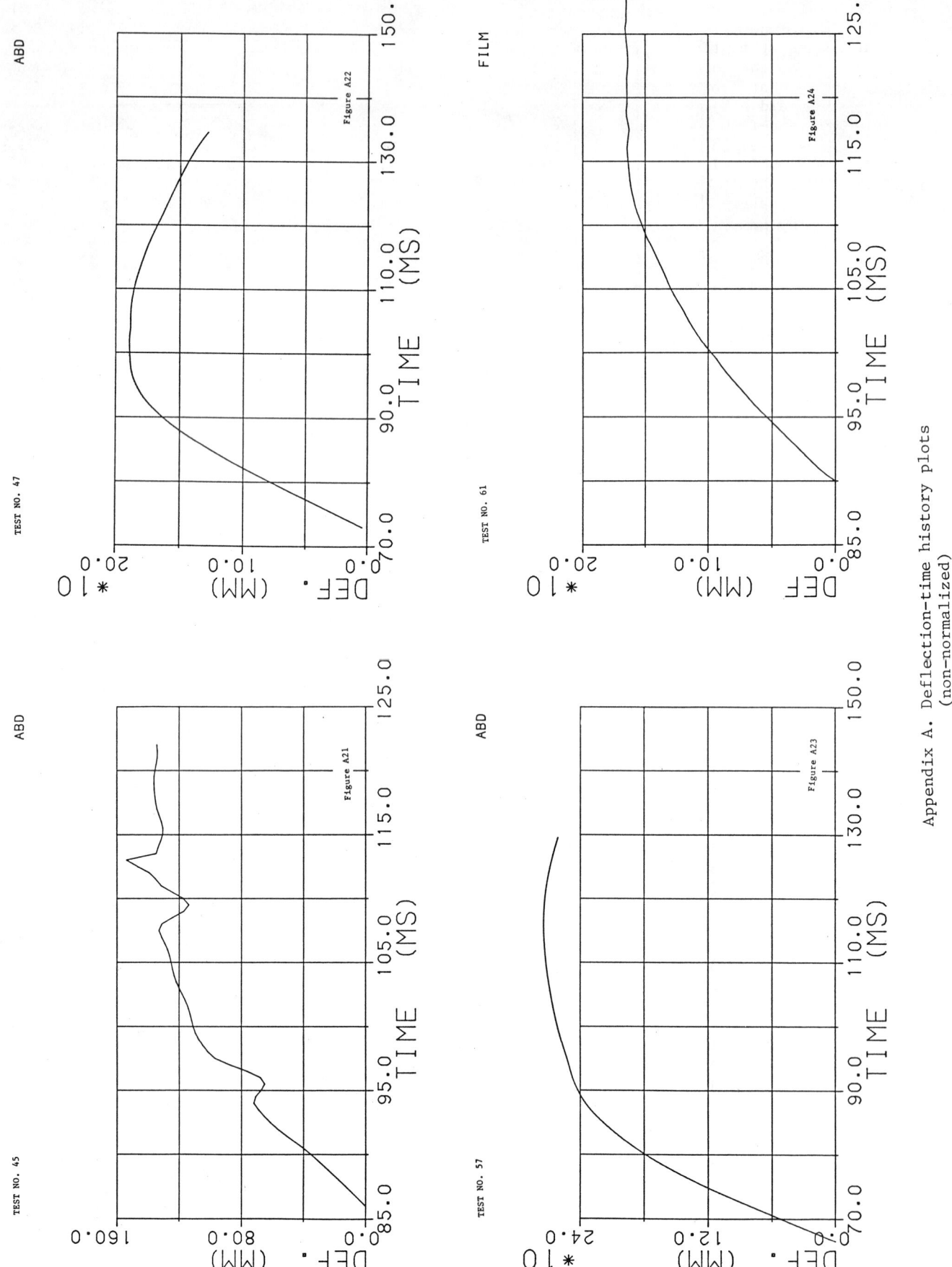

Appendix A. Deflection-time history plots (non-normalized)

APPENDIX B

Comparison of WSU Force Deflection Curves to Published Data: One of the initial findings based on our series of tests, is that the overall stiffness of the human lower abdomen was much less than that proposed by Stalnaker and Ulman (4), and did not neccessarily follow a rise-plateau-rise force-deflection pattern. There were several possible reasons for the difference in findings:

1) Thirty-seven of 42 of the subjects involved in the Stalnaker-Ulman (4) review were impacted in the upper, middle or lateral abdomen, and involved rib contact. The Walfisch (3) lateral drop tests cited in their review involved rib contact. In our tests, rib contact was minimal, which could explain why our force-deflection plots did not have the characteristic initial spike seen in chest impact studies and in the Stalnaker-Ulman review.

2) There could be no pre-tensioning of muscles in our cadaveric impacts. Previous findings in live subjects have shown that there is insufficient reaction time to pretense certain muscle groups in anticipation of high speed impacts. Muscle groups which are tensed for postural purposes may contribute to biomechanical stiffness during impact. This contribution was not available in our cadaver tests, while it could exist in live subjects.

3) Our impacts are made with a narrow impactor face which may produce a less stiff response than a broad impactor face. Biomechanical studies of frontal chest impacts indicate that the shape of the force - deflection curve appears to be dependent on the shape of the loading surface. Impacts to the chest with a circular flat - faced impactor tend to produce a sharp initial spike, then a plateau, then another rise, while a narrower impactor surface tends to produce a more gradual response.

4) The proposed Stalnaker and Ulman corridor bottoms out on the spine at 125 mm in frontal abdominal impacts (60% of a 209 mm abdominal depth). The average normalized depth at the level of impact in a seated cadaver in our test series was 289 mm. Using 60% of this value gives 173 mm as the depth at which the spine would be contacted. The increase in depth appears to be due to a change in abdominal girth as the body is moved from a supine to a seated position. In the seated position a discernible paunch develops, especially in the lower abdomen.

4) The linear regression techniques in the Stalnaker and Ulman (4) study used a direct proportionality between subject mass and the response parameters of plateau force and Segment III stiffness. As has been suggested by Dr. John Melvin, another method of approaching this is to use equal stress - equal velocity scaling methods. A review of Table B1 shows that the Segment II plateau load and the Segment III stiffness are considerably less in man if equal - stress equal-velocity scaling methods are used instead of scaling according to direct proportionality between subject masses. Figure B1 compares force-penetration responses using the two scaling methods. The construction of the plot based on equal stress-equal velocity rescaling is discussed below.

Stalnaker and Ulman considered the Segment II plateau to be rate dependent. After rescaling according to Table B1, their velocity versus force relationship becomes:

$$\frac{F}{V} = \frac{3.663 \text{ kN}}{11.98 \text{ m/s}} = 0.306 \frac{\text{kN-s}}{\text{m}} \quad (B1)$$

Thus, $F_p = 0.306\,V$, where F_p = plateau force (kN) and V = velocity at impact (m/s).

Based on the rescaled data in Table B1, Segment III has a velocity independent stiffness of 80.8 kN/m. The transition between Segments II and III in the Stalnaker and Ulman study occurred at about 27% compression in frontal impacts. The average normalized abdominal depth at the level of impact in the Wayne State University test series is 289 mm. The predicted transition between Segments II and III in a seated cadaver would then occur at a penetration of (27%)(289 mm)/100 = 78.0 mm.

A velocity-dependent Segment I stiffness can also be derived from the rescaled Stalnaker and Ulman data. To do this, the point of transition between Segments I and II must be known. Stalnaker and Ulman report that in the primate tests, the transition between Segments I and II occurred at about 9.6% compression in the frontal impacts. The predicted transition point is then (9.6%)(289 mm)/100 = 27.7 mm. The velocity dependent Segment I stiffness is then

$$S = \frac{306\,V\,(N)}{27.7\,(\text{mm})} = 11.05\,V \quad (B2)$$

where S = Segment I stiffness (kN/m) and V = velocity at impact (m/s).

The predicted force-deflection response based on the above relationships for Segments I, II and III can be compared to the actual response obtained in the Wayne State University cadaveric tests. In Figure B2 our lower velocity response corridor, with an average velocity of 6.1 m/s is superimposed on the rescaled Stalnaker-Ulman response for a 6.1 m/s impact. There is no good agreement between the two response curves, as the W.S.U. curve shows a softer response throughout. In Figure B3 our higher velocity response corridor, with an average impact velocity of 10.4 m/s, is superimposed on the rescaled Stalnaker-Ulman response for a 10.4 m/s impact. There is fairly good agreement between the two, except in the initial portions of the response, where the W.S.U. curve has no initial spike and no obvious plateau.

TABLE B1

SCALED ABDOMINAL IMPACT RESPONSE PARAMETERS

Subject	Average[1] Subject Mass (kg)	Lamda = $\left(\frac{76.0 \text{ kg}}{\text{Subj. mass}}\right)^{1/3}$	Average[1] Plateau Force (kN)	Scaled[2] Plateau Force (kN)	Average[1] Segment III Stiffness (kN/m)	Scaled[3] Segment III Stiffness (kN/m)	Average[1] Velocity (m/s)
Squirrel Monkey	0.60	5.02	0.159	4.007	19.7	98.9	10.15
Vervet Monkey	3.55	2.78	0.492	3.802	21.0	58.4	11.57
Rhesus Monkey	5.10	2.46	0.547	3.310	29.6	72.8	12.03
Baboon	15.45	1.70	1.223	3.534	54.7	93.0	14.17
Man	76.00	1.0	5.391	3.663 [4]	204.7	80.8 [4]	11.98 [4]

(1) Data from Stalnaker and Ulman, Ref. (4)
(2) Scaled Plateau Force = Lamda^2 x Average Plateau Force
(3) Scaled Segment III Stiffness = Lamda x Average Segment III Stiffness

(4) Scaled plateau force, scaled segment III stiffness and average velocity for man is obtained by taking the average of the values of the four other primate species

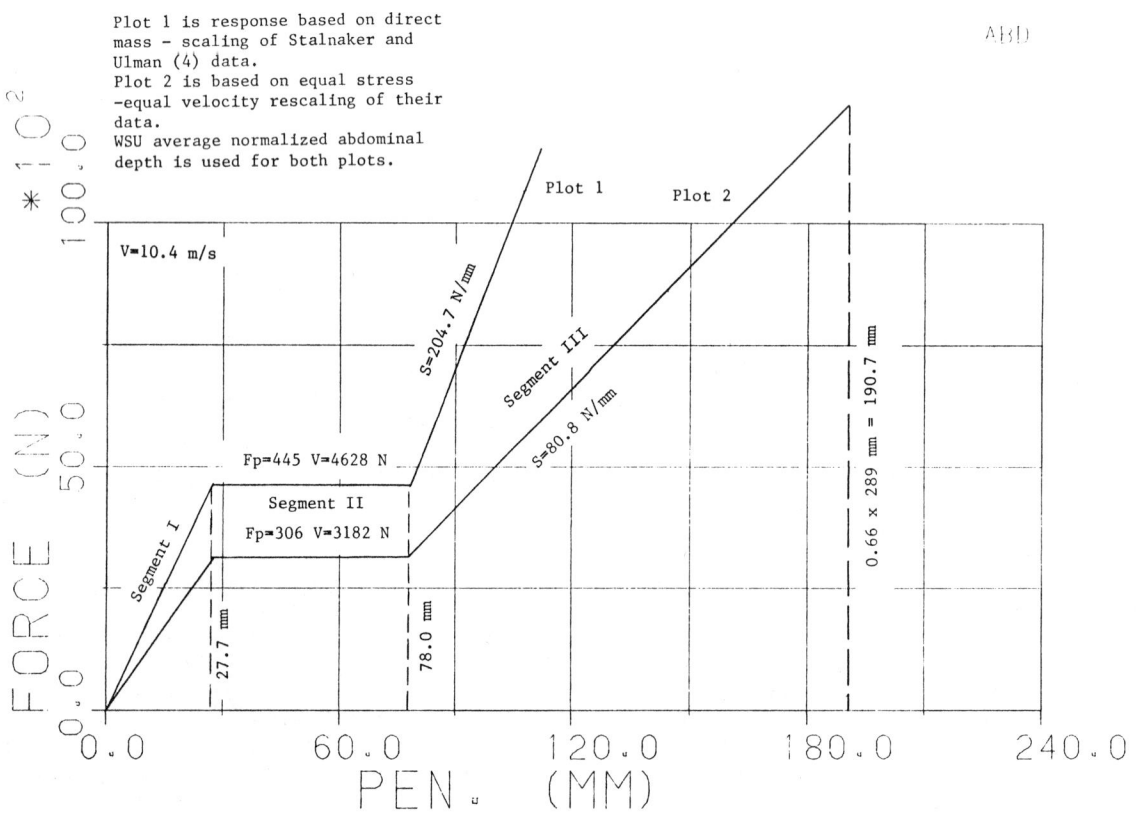

Figure B1

Plot 1 is response based on direct mass - scaling of Stalnaker and Ulman (4) data.
Plot 2 is based on equal stress -equal velocity rescaling of their data.
WSU average normalized abdominal depth is used for both plots.

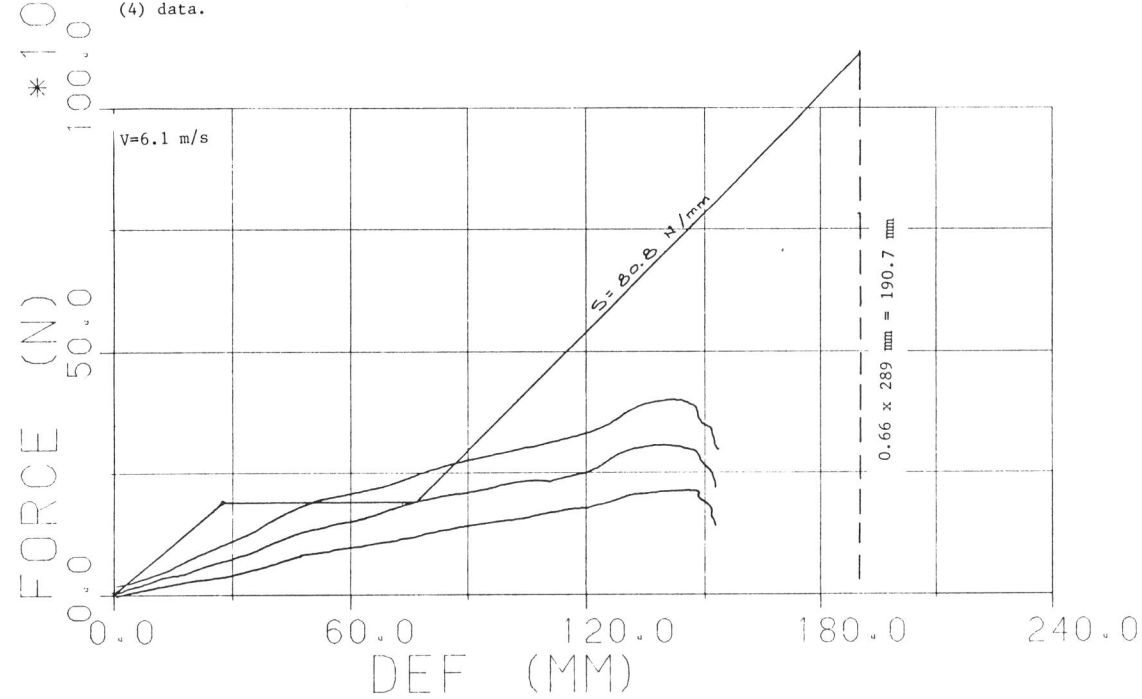

Figure B2
WSU low velocity corridor superimposed on response predicted by equal stress-equal velocity rescaling of Stalnaker and Ulman (4) data.

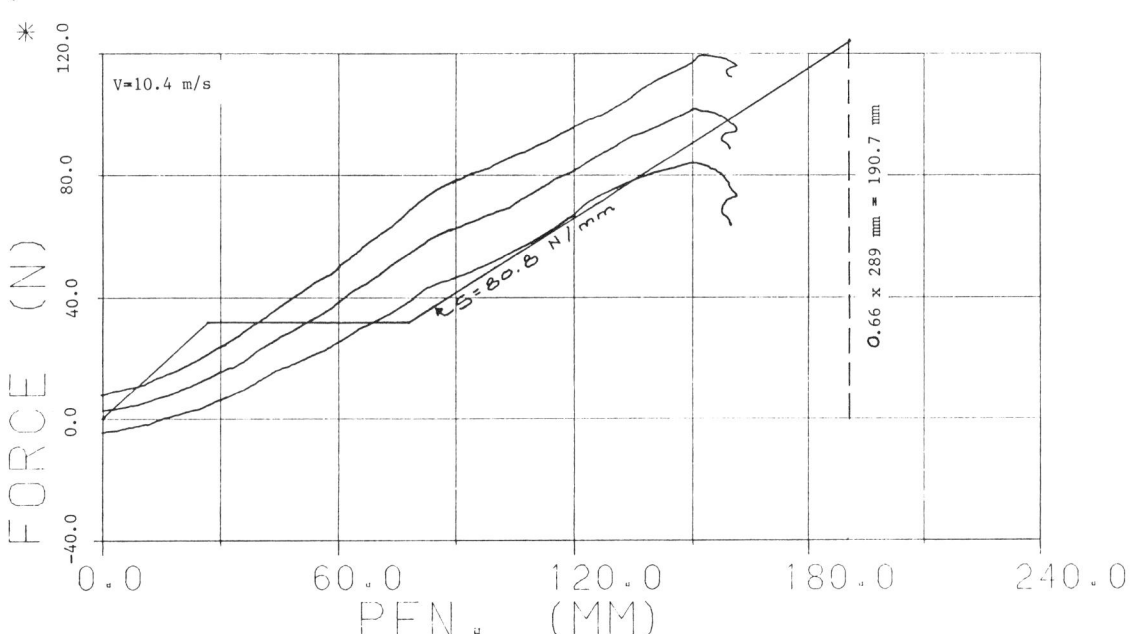

Figure B3
WSU High velocity corridor superimposed on response predicted by equal stress-equal velocity rescaling of Stalnaker and Ulman (4) data.

861879

The Effect of Limiting Impact Force on Abdominal Injury: A Preliminary Study

Stephen W. Rouhana, Stephen A. Ridella, and David C. Viano
General Motors Research Labs.

ABSTRACT

This report describes a series of experiments using Hexcel(TM) to limit the impact force in lateral abdominal impacts. Two hundred fourteen (214) anesthetized New Zealand White rabbits were impacted at 5 to 15 m/s using a pneumatic impactor. Injury responses from tests with a force-limiting impact interface (94 tests) were compared with the responses from tests with a rigid impact interface (120 tests) having the same level of lateral abdominal compression. The Hexcel had a length of 3 inches, the same diameter as the rigid impactor, and crushed at a constant force (pressure level of 232 kPa (33 psi)) once deformation was initiated.

The results of these tests showed that the probability of serious abdominal injury did not change significantly with the Hexcel, even though peak pressures were reduced to as little as one third of their previous values. The overall abdominal injury severity was dominated by hepatic injuries which remained as severe with Hexcel as the interface, although the probability of sustaining a renal laceration was three times lower with Hexcel. As seen in previous studies, the biomechanics of soft tissue injury appear to be dominated by the Viscous response.

IN ANTICIPATION OF INJURY MITIGATING EFFECTS from force-limiting or energy-absorbing materials, many studies have been done to determine whether such materials should be incorporated into automotive interiors in locations such as the side door, armrest, or instrument panel. Typical materials under consideration are open and closed cell foam padding materials, rubber, some polymers, expanded metals, and honeycombs. Some studies have evaluated the mechanical properties of these materials [1-3][1]; others have examined how these materials affect the severity of injury in tests with cadavers, animals, and anthropomorphic test devices [2-9].

The material used in this study was Hexcel™, an aluminum honeycomb material that crushes at a constant force or pressure as determined by the wall thickness and cell size of the Hexcel (Figure 1). The crush strength was independent of deformation rate in the range of impact velocity we used. Two crush strengths were used which will be referred to as low crush strength (232 kPa or 34 psi), and high crush strength (319 kPa or 46 psi). These limited the force to ≃1 kN (237 lbs) and ≃1.5 kN (327 lbs), respectively. In the first phase of this study which was previously published [10], at the threshold for serious abdominal injury in the rabbit, the pressure was approximately 280 kPa (40 psi). But, injury correlated better with the velocity and the extent of abdominal compression than with the force or pressure supporting the recent concept of a Viscous mechanism of soft tissue injury[2]. [10,20,21]

Values reported in the literature for the pressure tolerance of the abdomen associated with AIS >= 3 injury range from 214 kPa (31 psi) to 386 kPa (56 psi) [4,5,11,12], but the peak pressure has not proven to be a reliable correlate with injury [10,12]. More recent work has shown that the rate and the extent of compression are more reliable indicators of soft

---

[1] Numbers in brackets [] indicate references at the end of the paper.
[2] The Viscous mechanism of injury relates the injury sustained by soft tissues during impact with the mechanical environment they experience. The parameters which have been shown to describe the mechanical environment are the compression and the rate (velocity) of compression, and the functional relationship is the product of the instantaneous compression and rate of compression during the impact.

tissue injury, and particularly of abdominal injury [10,13,20].

FORCE (OR PRESSURE) AND ABDOMINAL INJURY - McElhaney et al. [4] and Stalnaker et al. [5] performed experiments on human cadavers and various species of monkey and observed that an "ESI=3" injury (moderate trauma to abdominal organs necessitating surgical repair) required 131 kPa (19 psi) with a blunt wedge shaped impactor, and 386 kPa (56 psi) with a "flat rigid striker of larger cross section than the animal struck".

Melvin et al. [11] performed tests on anesthetized rhesus monkeys and noted the onset of "moderate trauma" at 310 kPa (45 psi) when the test velocities were in the range of 2.5 to 5 m/s.

Stalnaker et al. [14] and Trollope et al. [15] observed that the pressure required to produce various levels of hepatic injury in baboons was dependent on the size and shape of the impactor. Trollope stated, that "... equal injuries were produced when a pressure of 87 psi was applied with a bar impactor and 22 psi was applied with a large-surface impactor." (The reader will note that this result conflicts with that reported by McElhaney and Stalnake

references 4 and 5.) From dimensional analysis, the authors concluded that the severity of abdominal injury is related to the peak impact force, impact duration, mass of the subject, and the contact area of the impactor. Trollope's study [15] showed that only a small percentage of the impact force is actually transmitted to any single organ in an abdominal impact. Their experiments with external blunt abdominal impacts required 1.6 kN (350 lbs) to produce the same level of injury as 0.7 kN (150 lbs) delivered directly to exposed organs. To minimize the number of variables in our study the impactor geometry and size were kept constant.

Melvin et al., in another study [6], examined the responses of 7 cadavers in sled impacts into rigid or padded walls. Abdominal injuries were observed only in the rigid wall impacts, but forces on the cadavers were not measured. Thoracic injury severity was reduced in high speed impacts into padded walls, but it increased in low velocity impacts.

Gogler et al. [12] found that for Gottingen minipigs impacted at 10 to 17 m/s, the threshold of force to produce "AIS = 3-4" injury was 1471 N (331 lbs). In these tests, the

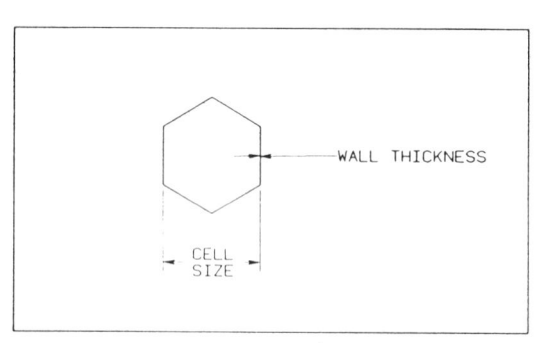
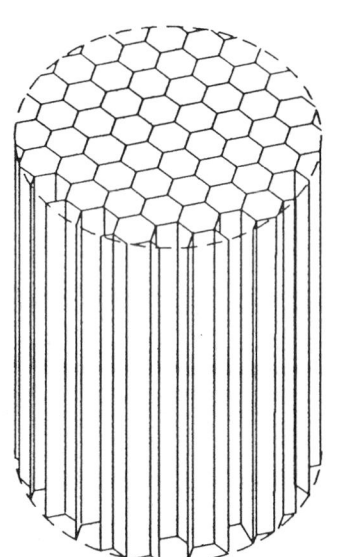

Hexcel Parameters				
Type of Hexcel	Material	Cell Size (inch)	Wall Thickness (inch)	Crush Strength (psi)
Lower Crush Strength	5056 Al	3/8	.0007	33.6
Higher Crush Strength	5052 Al	3/8	.0015	40.8

Figure 1 Diagram of typical Hexcel configuration, and parameters of the Hexcel used in this study.

subjects were propelled into the rear air spoiler of a Porsche 911, with impact occurring at the mid-abdominal region. The size of the spoiler was not stated, and had to be estimated from the scale drawings in the paper. We assumed that the width of the impact area was 25 cm and that the thickness of the spoiler was 2.5-5.1 cm. These dimensions would yield pressures in the range of 193-593 kPa (28-86 psi). The authors noted that "... the curves show that tolerance cannot be defined using the criterion of impact force and duration only...", further indication of the importance of the viscous mechanism of soft tissue injury.

Nusholtz et al.[7] used rigid and padded impact surfaces in a series of tests on 12 primates, 10 canines, and 3 human cadavers. Comparison of the padded versus rigid impacts was not done, but a review of the data shows that 4 out of the 5 padded impacts had AIS ≥ 3 kidney injury, while only 2 out of the five rigid impacts had a kidney injury. Serious abdominal injury (AIS ≥ 3) was observed in all of the primate tests, where the test velocities ranged from 8 to 13 m/s and the compressions from 60 to 80%. Examination of the tabulated forces shows that serious abdominal injury occurred with forces as low as 1.3 kN (292 lbs) when the primates were tested with padded surfaces.

Walfisch et al. [16], using cadavers in one and two meter drop tests, showed that the severity of liver injuries was correlated to "normalized" impact force (r=.98, p unknown). The cadavers were dropped onto hardwood, polystyrene, or phenospan simulated armrests. While a force-deflection corridor for lateral abdominal impacts was determined, the data was from only 8 cadavers. In addition, only two impact speeds were examined, although the authors acknowledged that the impact speed significantly affects the stiffness of the human abdomen. The force-deflection characteristics of the polystyrene and the phenospan were not given in the paper. The authors stated a value of 260 kPa (38 psi) as "...being associated with an AIS 3 for the abdomen". These force-deflection curves were then used in the design of a dummy abdomen by Maltha and Stalnaker [17].

Lau and Viano [18] studied hepatic injuries to beagles caused by belt-restraint loading (frontal). The study was restricted to a single velocity-compression combination of 1.7m/s and 60% compression. The average peak pressures were 340 ± 40 kPa (49 psi) and 330 ± 20kPa (48 psi) for transverse belt orientation and diagonal orientation, respectively. At that low velocity-high compression combination they noted that "...(the) injury was primarily caused by excessive tissue deformation via a crushing or tearing mechanism."

In our previous study [10] we observed that peak impact force was significantly correlated to injury, and the mean peak impact force producing AIS ≥ 3 injury was approximately 276 kPa (40 psi).

THE VISCOUS RESPONSE AND ABDOMINAL INJURY - McElhaney et al. [4] and Stalnaker et al. [5] also observed that "...small changes in velocity greatly change the injury level, ... (and) ... the depth of penetration ... is also an important variable..." indicating the importance of what we now know as the Viscous mechanism of soft tissue injury.

Melvin's study of rhesus monkeys [11] noted that "Both the liver ... and the kidney tests demonstrated the sensitivity of these organs to the rate of loading", but the "...rate of loading was most pronounced on the liver". The rate of loading may have been less significant for the kidney because the velocity range was below the threshold of serious kidney injury [10].

Lau and Viano [19] performed a series of frontal impacts to anesthetized rabbits in which the compression was held at a constant 16% of the abdominal thickness and the pre-impact velocity was varied from 8 to 16 m/s. They noted that "the liver showed a consistent increase in injury severity with impact velocity", with a transition from minor liver injury to lacerative liver injury at 12 m/s.

Viano and Lau [21] first proposed the concept of a Viscous Tolerance for soft tissues in the body from their analysis of frontal thoracic impacts on rabbits. The experiments included velocities of compression in the range of 5 m/s to 22 m/s, and maximum thoracic compressions of 4% to 55%. On the basis of occurrence of critical-fatal injury, the experiments confirmed a velocity and a compression sensitive tolerance to chest impact. The product of the maximum velocity and the maximum compression was shown to be a measure of the energy dissipated by the viscous elements in the thorax. Probit analysis allowed the determination of the 50% probability of critical-fatal thoracic injury at Vmax*Cmax = 4.0 m/s.

In our previous series of 117 lateral abdominal impacts [10], which comprised the first phase of these experiments, we noted that the probability of serious abdominal injury was well correlated to the product of the pre-impact velocity and the maximum abdominal compression (Vmax*Cmax), which we called the Abdominal Injury Criterion (AIC). The 50% probability of serious abdominal injury was determined to be at Vmax*Cmax = 3.3 m/s for left side impacts, and 2.7 m/s for right side impacts.

Stalnaker and Ulman [13] re-examined data previously published to determine an abdominal response corridor for dummy design. The three sets of data examined included that of Beckman et al, Stalnaker et al., and Trollope et al. A single force-deflection corridor was proposed for both lateral and frontal impacts to the upper and middle abdominal regions. The corridor was determined primarily from cadaver data of Walfisch et al., and has a stiffness quite similar to the thoracic stiffness which seems to be too stiff. The Viscous response of the abdomen (Vmax*Cmax) was validated and suggested to be independent of species.

Horsch et al. [21] and Lau et al. [22], in more recent experiments on upper abdominal injury in anesthetized swine with steering wheel contact, found the viscous response to be the superior predictor of the severity and the time of occurrence of liver injury. These studies showed that liver injury by steering wheel contact occurred prior to maximum compression of the abdomen or maximum acceleration of the spine, but at the same time as the peak of the abdominal viscous response. The average maximum viscous response for tests resulting in critical liver injury was [VC]max = 1.8 m/s.

Kroell et al. [24] also found the Viscous response to be the best indicator of cardiac rupture in high-speed blunt frontal impacts to anesthetized swine. In 41 tests, cardiac rupture showed no correlation with maximum chest compression, but was highly correlated with Vmax*Cmax and [VC]max. The 50% probability of cardiac rupture occurred at Vmax*Cmax $\simeq$ 3.7 m/s, and [VC]max = 2.0 m/s.

CURRENT THINKING ON SOFT TISSUE INJURY - It is clear from recent work that the extent of soft tissue injury is well correlated to the Viscous response of the tissue, i.e., the compression and the velocity (rate of compression) [10,20,21,22]. The Viscous response appears to apply in frontal and lateral impacts, to the thorax and to the abdomen. Lau et al. [20,21,22] have proposed that knowledge of the instantaneous Viscous response throughout the impact allows the determination of when injury occurs to specific organs, and allows new insights for occupant protection.

METHODS

Two hundred fourteen (214) New Zealand white rabbits (2.5-3.5 kg) were used in this study.* The study was separated into two phases, with phase one involving a rigid impact interface and 120 rabbits as previously published [10], and phase two involving the Hexcel interface with 94 rabbits. Each rabbit was fasted overnight prior to use, and then preanesthetized with ketamine hydrochloride (35 mg/kg IM) and xylazine (5 mg/kg IM). Deep surgical anesthesia was achieved and maintained with Sodium Pentobarbital (25 mg/kg IV, to effect). The animals were shaved from forelimbs to hindlimbs around their entire circumference to remove the fur from the impact area. Electrical leads were attached subcutaneously to monitor lead II of the ECG, and a pressure transducer (Size 5F,Millar PC-350) was inserted into the esophagus and advanced to the upper thoracic level (T4) to monitor the esophageal presssure. For phase one all rabbits also had a pressure transducer inserted into the femoral artery on the side opposite the impact location. Since no correlations were noted between injury and blood pressure, this invasive procedure was discontinued in phase two. Finally, the animals were placed in a sling in front of a high speed pneumatic impactor (Figure 2), zoometric measurements were taken, and a single controlled impact was delivered to the left or right side.

Hypothesis testing showed that the average mass of the animals tested with Hexcel as the impact interface (3.05 ± .29 kg), was the same as the average mass of those tested with a rigid impact interface (2.88 ± .34 kg).

To the face of the impactor, we attached a smooth aluminum disk in all phase one tests, or a single sample of Hexcel in each phase two test. The samples of Hexcel had been machined into cylindrical shape, with a diameter of 7.6 cm (3.0"), and a height of 7.0 cm (2.75") (Figure 1). (The diameter of the Hexcel was equal to that of the aluminum rigid impact disk.) Each Hexcel sample was mounted onto a base plate of aluminum (6.35 mm thick), and capped with an aluminum disk (1.58 mm thick). The mass of the base plate, cap, and Hexcel sample was 0.131 kg. Because of the Hexcel's momentum at the end of the impact stroke, a metal-filled epoxy was necessary to hold it onto the base plate. The base plate was screwed onto the impactor. The aluminum cap prevented injury by edge loading from the sharp cells. Before mounting, each Hexcel sample was precrushed 6.35 mm (1/4") quasi-statically on an MTS universal testing machine. During precrush, force-displacement curves were generated for each sample which demostrated that the crush strength values were very reproducible for both types of Hexcel used.

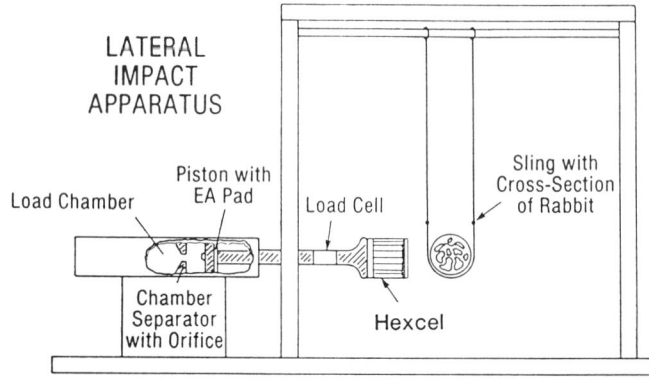

Figure 2 Schematic of the experimental apparatus, with a detailed view of the pneumatic impactor.

----

* The rationale and experimental protocol for the use of an animal model in this program have been reviewed by the Research Laboratories' Animal Research Committee. The research follows procedures outlined in the U.S. DHEW <u>Guide for the Care and Use of Laboratory Animals</u>, or the U.S. DHEW-NIH <u>Guidelines for the Use of Experimental Animals</u>, and complies fully with the USDA regulations in the Laboratory Animal Welfare Act of 1970 and 1976 (PL 89-544).

To examine the method of adding Hexcel to the pneumatic impactor, the mechanics of the impact event were analyzed. During impact the Hexcel did crush, but the mechanics of the impactor (captive piston) gave rise to sufficiently large decelerations to cause the Hexcel to uncrush as the piston was snubbed. That is, the force exerted on the Hexcel, due to the momentum change of the aluminum cap, was sufficient to uncrush the Hexcel that had just been crushed in the experiment.

Therefore, to determine how much the samples used in the experiments had crushed, we recrushed them on an MTS universal testing machine while recording force and displacement. Control samples were: (1) also crushed a known amount on the MTS, (2) uncrushed on the pneumatic impactor as if in an experiment (but without the animal), and (3) subsequently recrushed on the MTS. Hexcel used in an experiment required a lower force to produce the same amount of deflection as Hexcel that was not used in an experiment (never crushed). Comparison of the force-deflection curves from the samples used in experiments with those from the controls allowed determination of the amount the Hexcel crushed in the experiments.

In addition, the amount of sample crush showed linear correlation with the pre-impact piston velocity (Figure 3), with a correlation coefficient of R=.83, (p<.001). This is in good agreement with the results of the rigid impactor study which showed a linear correlation of the peak impact force with pre-impact velocity, with R=.95 (Figure 4). For high velocity impacts, it is reasonable to expect the impact force to remain high for a longer time than in low velocity impacts. Thus, there should be a progression to more crush of the Hexcel as the impact velocity (and hence the peak force) increases.

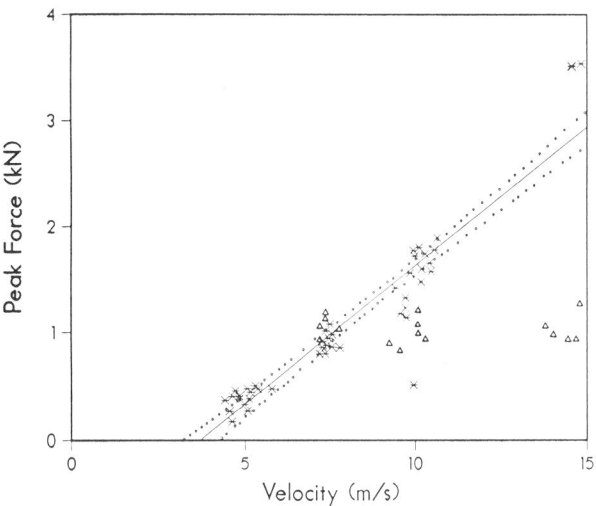

Figure 4 Peak force VS pre-impact velocity. (✱ = without Hexcel, △ = with Hexcel)

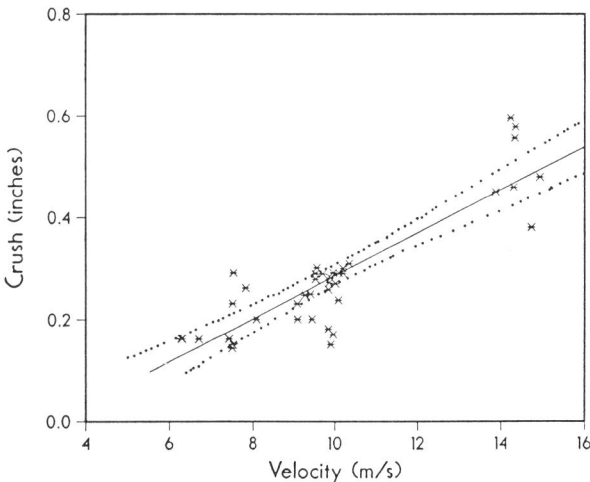

Figure 3 Amount of Hexcel crush during impact VS pre-impact velocity.

To examine the motion of the Hexcel/animal interface, high speed x-ray cineradiography was performed in several tests, because in visible light high speed movies of the tests the impact interface was obscured from view as the impactor compressed the animal. The uncrushing of the Hexcel appeared to take place in contact with the animal, before whole body motion started. Therefore, the Hexcel continued to compress the animal as it uncrushed to its original length. Then the preset compression was the actual compression we input to the animal since the pre-impact position of the animal was determined assuming that the Hexcel wouldn't crush. (The compressions in these experiments were from 10 to 50 percent of the abdominal diameter measured at the distal tip of the 12th rib.) Then, as measured in terms of compression, the exposure severities in the tests with Hexcel as the interface, were similar to those in the tests with the rigid impact interface. In contrast, although the pre-impact velocities were identical to those in the rigid interface tests, the velocity of the impact interface had to be lower during some phase of the Hexcel tests when the Hexcel crushed.

The velocities reported here are defined as the velocity of the front surface of the impactor immediately before impact (pre-impact velocity). It is measured for each experiment just prior to impact, by a photocell which records the transit time for two grooves with a known spacing on the piston shaft. The velocities used in phase I were from 3 to 15 m/s (6.6 to 33 mph), and in phase II were from 7.5 to 15 m/s (16.5 to 33 mph). The pre-impact velocities were upper bounds on the velocity because the crushing of the Hexcel could only have reduced the velocity of the Hexcel-rabbit interface.

Immediately following impact, euthanasia was administered to the animals by injection of T-61 Euthanasia Solution (1ml IV). A complete abdominal necropsy was then performed. The condition of the abdominal organs was determined from macroscopic examination, and classified according to the Abbreviated Injury Scale (AIS-80). The thoracic organs were also examined for laceration, severe contusion, and rib fracture, but were not included in the analysis.

The probability of injury with AIS ≥ 3 (contusive) and AIS ≥ 4 (lacerative) was determined from the necropsy results using Eq. (1).

$$\text{Prob of Injury}(AIS \geq n) = \frac{\text{number of subjects with AIS} \geq n}{\text{number tested at parameter}} \quad (1)$$

The input biomechanical variables were pre-impact velocity and maximum compression, and several tests were performed at each combination of these variables. Varying the pre-impact velocity and the maximum compression caused the peak impact force (which was measured by a load cell mounted between the piston and the Hexcel) to vary as well. The results of our experiments were sorted into groups, by velocity, compression, velocity times compression, and peak force to examine any correlations of these variables with injury severity. The probability of injury was determined at each value of the variable tested in each group. For example, the probability of injury at 5, 10, and 15 m/s with Hexcel as the interface, would each be calculated separately using the tests in each group.

The force on the animal was continuously recorded through a 44 kN (10,000 lbs) load cell which was attached to the impactor between the piston shaft and the Hexcel holder. During impact the load cell only senses the force due to the mass behind it, but the subject senses the entire mass of the impactor, including the load cell and the Hexcel assembly. Several attempts were made to compensate the load cell to account for the mass in front of it (the Hexcel assembly, which included the Hexcel, cap, and base). Compensation is usually possible using an accelerometer mounted on the mass in front of the load cell. Our attempts at compensation were not fruitful owing to the large decelerations experienced during snubbing of the piston. The stopping was so severe that a 100,000 g accelerometer and several lower range accelerometers were destroyed. (The mechanism of destruction was probably case deformation rather than overdriving the inertial mass.) While we could not compensate for added mass in front of the load cell, the load readings can be corrected using standard techniques. Assume that the total mass of the impactor, load cell, and Hexcel assembly is given by "M". Then the force the subject experiences (the interface force) while decelerating the piston with acceleration equal to "a" is M times a. If the mass in front of the load cell (the Hexcel assembly) is given by "m", then the force the load cell experiences during the impact, while it tries to decelerate the mass behind it, is equal to (M-m)a. Since the two accelerations are the same for a rigid body, then the two forces are related by Eq. (2).

$$\text{Load Cell Force} = \frac{(M - m)}{M} * \text{Interface Force} \quad (2)$$

The total mass in front of the load cell in these experiments was .332 kg, and the total mass of the impactor including the load cell and the Hexcel assembly was 2.10 kg. Then the load cell recorded forces were 84.2% of the actual forces experienced by the subjects.

The means of the peak force values recorded during pre-crush and during impact are given in Table 1 for the low crush strength Hexcel and for 32 samples of high crush strength Hexcel which were also used in these experiments. In addition, the forces recorded during impact have been corrected with Eq. (2) and are given in the Table. The results show no significant differences between the corrected forces recorded during impact and the pre-crush forces. The reader should note that the UNCORRECTED forces have been used in the rest of this analysis.

The force limiting action of the Hexcel is clear from Figures 4 and 5. Figure 4 compares the force recorded during impact with a rigid interface to the force recorded with Hexcel as the interface. They have been presented on the same graph to facilitate comparison. Note that linear regression yields r^2 = .90 for the rigid impacts and r^2 = .28 for the Hexcel impacts. Figure 5 compares the force-time history for a typical impact having low crush strength Hexcel as the interface with an impact having a rigid interface. Each test shown had pre-impact velocity equal to 15 m/s and maximum compression equal to 40%.

The aluminum plate which covers the Hexcel acts as a distributor of forces over the entire area of the sample and as such could prevent local crushing. If the initial contact area is small, the effective crush strength that the subject would experience could be much higher than the values obtained during pre-crush. To examine this possibility a study was done of rabbit zoometry with a typical subject in the impact sling. The elliptical shape of the rabbit abdomen was preserved in the sling and lead to a nearly flat impact interface. When the impact face was placed against the rabbit in the sling 95% of area of the impact face was in direct contact with the rabbit's abdomen. When pressure was applied to the impact face the interface was 100% coupled. The pressure was

Table 1
Comparison of Peak Force Values

Reading	Force ± s.d kN (pounds)	Pressure ± s.d. kPa (psi)	n
Low Crush Strength Hexcel			
Pre-crush	1.06 ± .07 (237.3 ± 15.17)	231.7 ± 14.5 (33.6 ± 2.1)	97 97
Impact	0.98 ± .17 (215.2 ± 36.6)	220.7 ± 37.6 (32.0 ± 5.3)	38 38
Impact Corrected	1.15 ± .20 (255.6 ± 44.4)	262.2 ± 43.2 (38.0 ± 6.3)	38 38
High Crush Strength Hexcel			
Pre-crush	1.45 ± .09 (326.9 ± 20.7)	318.6 ± 20.0 (46.2 ± 2.9)	32 32
Impact	1.28 ± .21 (288.2 ± 47.1)	281.4 ± 46.2 (40.8 ± 6.7)	17 17
Impact Corrected	1.54 ± .25 (342.2 ± 55.9)	341.4 ± 55.9 (48.5 ± 7.9)	17 17

only enough to compress the rabbit ≈1/4 inch. This lead us to conclude that the crush strength experienced by the subjects should be the same as the crush strength measured in pre-crush tests.

The method used to analyze the data invlolved regression analysis of injury probability in relation to the force, velocity, compression, and the Abdominal Injury Criterion or AIC. The AIC is a less rigorous and more specific form of the Viscous Criterion, [VC]max, proposed by Viano and Lau [10,20,21,22,23]. The AIC is the product of the pre-impact (or maximum) velocity and the maximum compression. In contrast, the [VC]max is the maximum of the product of the instantaneous rate of compression and the compression. (Eqs. 3 and 4).

$$AIC = V_{max} * C_{max} \quad (3)$$

$$[VC]_{max} = (V(t)*C(t))_{max} \quad (4)$$

When the velocity profile of the interface during impact remains constant, $V_{max}*C_{max} \simeq [VC]_{max}$. The experiments with the rigid impact interface are very good approximations to this constant velocity situation because the impactor piston is driven

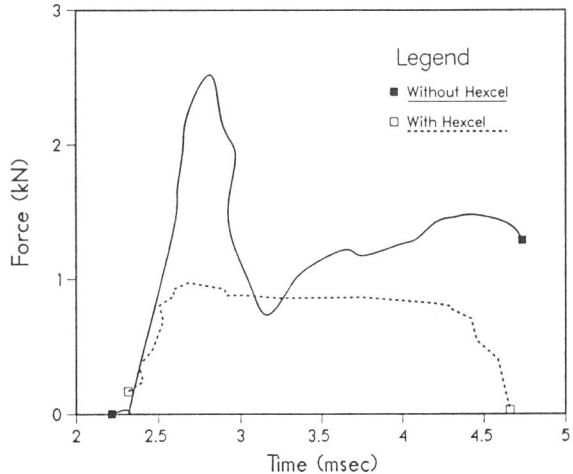

Figure 5 Typical force-time history with Hexcel and without Hexcel.

by the expanding gas from the load cylinder. In tests where the velocity profile changes, as in the experiments where the Hexcel crushed, [VC]max provides an instantaneous measure of the severity, whereas Vmax*Cmax only provides a measure of the maximum severity. Then if one uses [VC]max, it is possible to determine the approximate time that injury occurs from the position in time that the maximum occurs, but it is not possible to determine the time of injury if if one uses Vmax*Cmax. We did not monitor the interface velocity during impact and have used Vmax*Cmax as the biomechanical parameter to be tested.

To avoid confusion, the definitions associated with the Viscous mechanism of injury as given by Lau and Viano [23] are presented here:

<u>Viscous Criterion</u> = a biomechanical index of potential for injury in soft tissue based on its rate sensitivity.

<u>Viscous response</u> = VC, a function of time formed by the product of the instantaneous compression C(t), and the instantaneous rate (or velocity) of compression, V(t).

<u>Viscous tolerance</u> = the risk of soft tissue injury associated with a specific impact-induced Viscous response, VC. The maximum risk occurs at the peak Viscous response, [VC]max.

The Viscous criterion can also be misleading if it is used for impacts outside its range of applicability, such as very low velocity but high compression impacts. In low velocity impact, the dominant mechanism of injury is crushing and the Viscous response is not applicable. For example, if the impact velocity was 1 mm/s (.001 m/s) and the compression was 100%, the injury would definitely be serious but the Viscous response would indicate a low probability of serious injury.

RESULTS

The probability of injury with AIS $\geq$ 3 (contusive) and AIS $\geq$ 4 (lacerative) as determined by Eq. (1) is tabulated for the liver and the kidney in Tables 2 and 3. Comparisons were made of tests in identical ranges of Vmax*Cmax to ensure comparison of probability in exposures of nominally identical severity. The results were subjected to a chi-squared analysis, to determine if the probability of sustaining injury of a given severity was independent of the presence of Hexcel.

The probability of sustaining a serious renal or hepatic contusion, or a hepatic laceration was INDEPENDENT of the presence of Hexcel, at the 5% level of significance. However, the probability of sustaining a renal laceration was DEPENDENT on the presence of Hexcel, also at the 5% level of significance. That is, Hexcel reduced the probability of renal laceration by a factor of 3, but it did not reduce the probability of hepatic laceration, nor renal or hepatic contusion.

The probability of injury was graphed versus velocity, compression, Vmax*Cmax, and

Table 2
Probability of Renal Injury

Test Series	N	P(AIS $\geq$ 3)	P(AIS $\geq$ 4)
Rigid Interface	88	.44	.33
Low Crush Strength Hexcel	68	.31	.10
High Crush Strength Hexcel	21	.43	.10

Table 3
Probability of Hepatic Injury[1]

Test Series	N	P(AIS $\geq$ 3)	P(AIS $\geq$ 4)
Rigid Interface	43	.56	.56
Low Crush Strength Hexcel	45	.64	.60
High Crush Strength Hexcel	14	.71	.64

[1] Since previous experiments showed no liver injury from left side impacts (a result corroborated in these tests), hepatic injury was determined from right side impacts only.

peak force. Linear regression analysis was performed, and the correlations of probability of contusive and lacerative renal and hepatic injury with these biomechanical parameters were tabulated and graphed (Tables 4 and 5; Figure 6 a-d for AIS ≥ 3 liver injuries; Figure 6 e-h for AIS ≥ 3 kidney injuries; Figure 6i for AIS ≥ 4 kidney injuries). Each data point in these graphs represents the numerical average for all tests performed at that value of the biomechanical parameter being studied. The dotted curves above and below the regression line represent 95% confidence limits.

DISCUSSION

RENAL INJURY - Hexcel mitigated lacerative renal injury, but it did not affect contusive renal injury. When the impact interface was rigid, the probability of sustaining a renal injury correlated very well with Vmax*Cmax [10] and with the peak force, and was especially poorly correlated with the compression (Table 4). When the low crush strength Hexcel was the impact interface, the probability of injury was still well correlated to the peak force and Vmax*Cmax (Figure 6e & f), and poorly with compression alone and velocity alone. The correlation with peak force is due to the sharp transition from no injury at lower velocities when the Hexcel did not crush, to 50% probability of renal contusion at higher velocities when the Hexcel did crush. The probability of lacerative injury was 3 times lower with Hexcel (Table 2), and there was no correlation of AIS ≥ 4 renal injury probability with peak force because there were so few of these injuries (Table 4-b-2).

It appears that kidney injury occurred very early in lateral impacts, and at relatively high pre-impact velocities (and consequently at high forces). The peak force occurred at approximately 1-2 milliseconds into the impact. At that time, the impact interface was probably traversing the location of the kidney as seen in Figure 7. At a velocity of 10-15 m/s (10-15 millimeters/millisecond), the interface would require 1-2 milliseconds to move the ≃1.0 cm

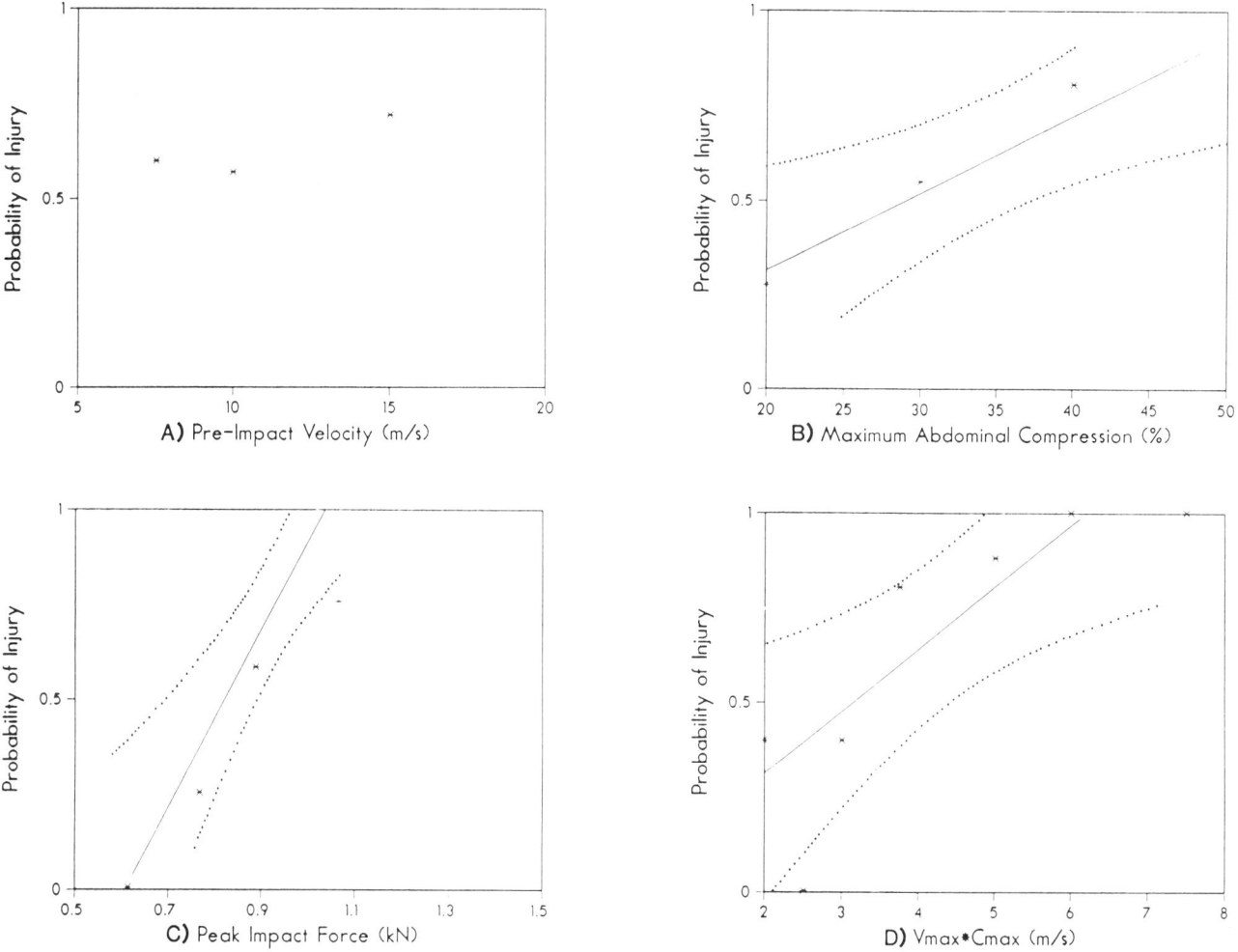

Figure 6 Probability of AIS ≥ 3 *LIVER* injury with a Hexcel interface VS: A) pre-impact velocity, B) maximum compression, C) peak impact force, D) Vmax*Cmax (AIC).

distance between the external abdominal skin and the lateral margin of the kidney.

The low crush strength Hexcel limited the peak abdominal impact pressure of the rabbits to less than ≃221 kPa (≃31 psi), and the high crush strength Hexcel limited the peak pressure to less than ≃281 kPa (≃41 psi). The probability of renal laceration was a factor of 3 lower with both types of Hexcel. Therefore, renal lacerations probably occur at pressures higher than 281 kPa.

Renal contusion did occur in these impacts, but it occurred at forces equal to the crush strength of the Hexcel (Figure 6e). It is clear from the figure that no contusion occurred at forces below ≃980 N (220 lbs), and in fact the probability of contusion increases to its maximum value of ≃50% at that value of the force. The 50% probability of renal contusion in the rigid impactor tests was at 1820 N (409 lbs). This is twice the maximum peak force possible with Hexcel as the interface. So, while the peak force is an indicator of the mechanical environment during impact, and limiting the peak force mitigated renal laceration, the peak force does not appear to be a reliable indicator of renal contusion, or other injuries.

HEPATIC INJURY - With the rigid impact interface, the probability of serious hepatic injury was very well correlated with Vmax*Cmax, and fairly well correlated with the velocity alone, regardless of the compression. With Hexcel as the impact interface, the probability of serious injury was well correlated to the peak force, and fairly well correlated with compression and the Vmax*Cmax. The correlation with peak force occurred because the probability of serious hepatic injury was already at its maximum before the force increased enough to cause the Hexcel to crush. In the rigid impactor tests, the probability of injury was 50% when the peak force was ≃900 N (200 lbs); in the Hexcel tests the probability of injury was 50% when the peak force was ≃870 N (195 lbs).

Note that the Vmax*Cmax for 50% probability of serious HEPATIC injury (≃2.7 m/s) was the same for both the rigid interface and the Hexcel interface. But, the Vmax*Cmax for 50%

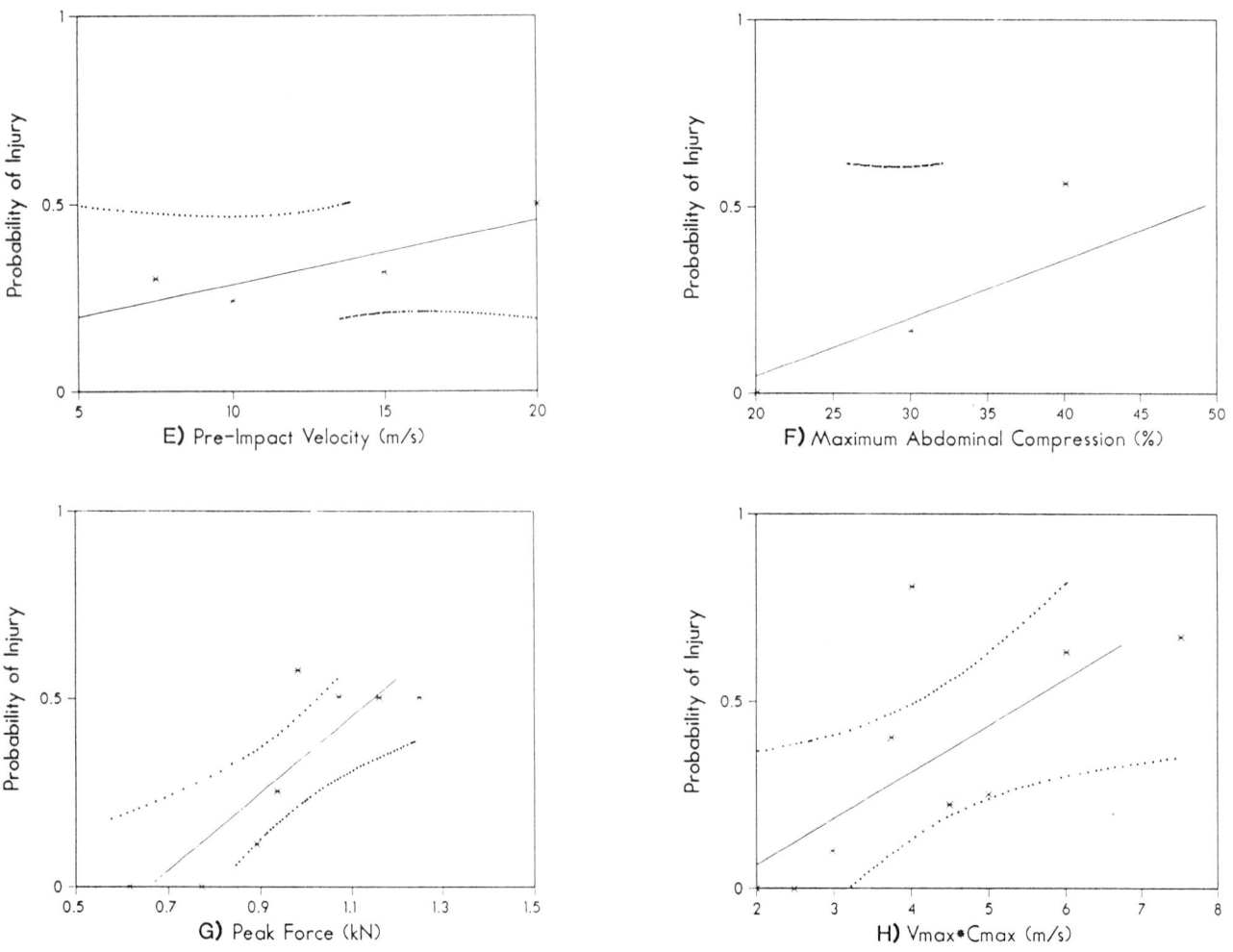

Figure 6 Probability of AIS ≥ 3 *KIDNEY* injury with a Hexcel interface VS: E) pre-impact velocity, F) maximum compression, G) peak impact force, H) Vmax*Cmax (AIC).

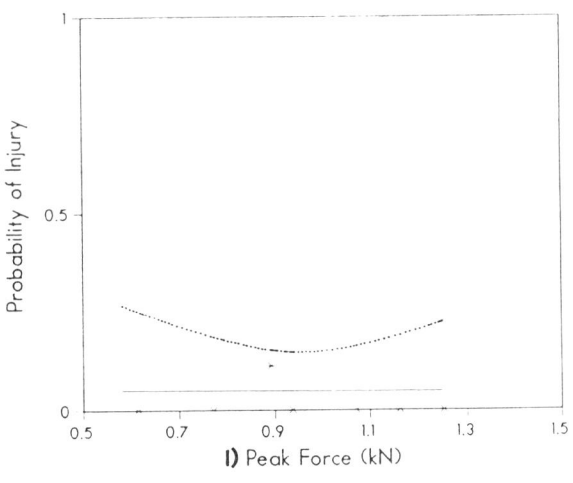

Figure 6I) Probability of AIS ≥ 4 *Kidney* injury with a Hexcel interface VS peak impact force.

TABLE 4
Probability of AIS ≥ 3 Renal Injury

a) Rigid Interface

Correlate	R =	p <	Significance
Vmax*Cmax	.84	.002	Highly Sig
Peak Force	.99	.006	Highly Sig
Velocity	.93	.02	Significant
Compression	.34	.55	Not Sig

b-1) Low Crush Strength Hexcel

Correlate	R =	p <	Significance
Peak Force	.86	.007	Highly Sig
Vmax*Cmax	.72	.03	Significant
Velocity	.86	.14	Slightly Sig
Compression	.82	.18	Slightly Sig

b-2) Low Crush Strength Hexcel & AIS ≥ 4

Correlate	R =	p <	Significance
Peak Force	-.009	.98	Not Sig

c) High Crush Strength Hexcel

Correlate	R =	p <	Significance
Vmax*Cmax	.87	.05	Significant
Compression	.68	.32	Not Sig
Peak Force	.68	.32	Not Sig
Velocity	.52	.65	Not Sig

probability of serious RENAL injury was increased to ≃5.8 m/s when Hexcel was used as the impact interface (compared to Vmax*Cmax = 2.7 m/s with a rigid interface).

THE IMPACT EVENT - While we could not monitor the velocity during impact, nor the motion of the impact interface, we can qualitatively describe the impact event through reasoning (Figure 8a-d). The basic principle in the following discussion is that if the Hexcel crushes during the impact, then the piston must have a greater velocity than the Hexcel cap. By definition if the Hexcel crushes, then the distance between the cap to which it is cemented and the base to which it is cemented must decrease. Since the piston cannot speed up during impact, the cap must slow down for the distance between the cap and base to decrease. Unfortunately, we could not determine quantitatively the change in the cap velocity. But regardless of the quantity, the following analysis should be qualitatively correct.

Figure 8a shows the force time history typical for Hexcel, and for our impacts. The time for the force to become large enough to initiate crushing of the Hexcel is less than one millisecond. The time at which the Hexcel crushes is called $t(c)$. Typically, after approximately 1-2 milliseconds, the force plateaus, followed by an increase much later if the compression of the subject is allowed to continue.

In Figure 8b, the interface velocity is shown as a function of time. While the interface is compressing the rabbit, a force is being applied to the rabbit which is proportional to the compression and the rate of compression due to the Viscous response of the tissues. The force increases as the compression increases in accordance with this response. When the force becomes greater than the amount of force the Hexcel can transmit (greater than the crush strength of the Hexcel), then the Hexcel crushes, $t(c)$, and the interface is decelerated rapidly. When the interface velocity drops, the rate of compression drops accordingly (Figure 8d). The piston however, continues with its initial velocity undiminished (Figure 8c). As the rate of compression drops, the force consequently drops until the Hexcel stops crushing, becomes a rigid body again, and the interface is rapidly brought back to the

TABLE 5
Probability of AIS ≥ 3 Hepatic Injury[1]

a) Rigid Interface

Correlate	R =	p <	Significance
Vmax*Cmax	.84	.0002	Highly Sig
Velocity	.89	.04	Significant
Peak Force	.78	.22	Not Sig
Compression	.65	.23	Not Sig

b) Low Crush Strength Hexcel

Correlate	R =	p <	Significance
Peak Force	.90	.003	Significant
Compression	.97	.03	Significant[2]
Vmax*Cmax	.81	.02	Significant[2]
Velocity	.87	.33	Not Sig

c) High Crush Strength Hexcel

Correlate	R =	p <	Significance
Compression	.95	.19	Slightly Sig
Vmax*Cmax	.81	.19	Slightly Sig
Peak Force	.33	.67	Not Sig
Velocity	.22	.86	Not Sig

[1] Since previous experiments showed no liver injury from left side impacts (a result corroborated in these tests), hepatic injury was determined from right side impacts only.

[2] When the difference between the p values is not significant, the order of the values is by correlation coefficient.

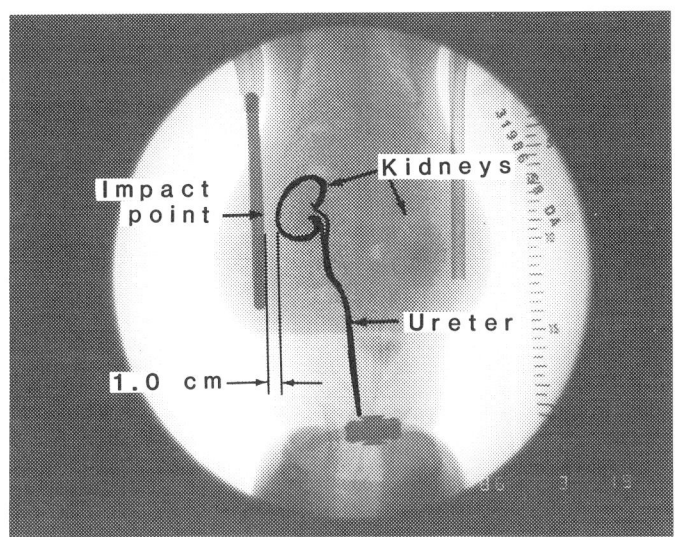

Figure 7 Radiograph of a rabbit abdomen. The anesthetized rabbit was given Renografin (IV, to effect), a radiopaque contrast agent, to permit visualization of the kidneys. One kidney has been highlighted for clarity. A compression band necessary to occlude the ureters caused the abdominal bulge. The true external surface at the level of the kidneys is marked by the metal bars seen lateral to the kidneys. As seen, the distance from the external surface to the medial surface of the kidney is approximately 1 cm. Thus, the time of peak force coincides well with the time of involvement of the kidney in the impact.

same velocity as the piston, t(r).

At some later time, t(s), the piston is snubbed so its velocity goes to zero (Figure 8c). Because the Hexcel cap has momentum, it attempts to continue on its trajectory and uncrushes the Hexcel that was just crushed (Figure 8b & c). The uncrushing takes place in contact with the animal which has not yet begun whole body motion (according to high speed movies). Finally at some point all of the previously crushed Hexcel has been uncrushed, and the cap tries to pull against uncrushed Hexcel, which snubs the cap.

At time t(c) the Viscous response would show a precipitous decrease, and this is the time we believe the interface is compressing the kidney as judged by the time the peak force occurs and the known position of the kidney. Kidney injuries are prevented as the Hexcel crushes due to the corresponding reduction of the interface velocity. At a later time, t(s), the compression of the animal continues at or near the pre-impact velocity. At t(u) the [VC]max and Vmax*Cmax would be in agreement, both being at maxima. We believe the injuries to the liver occurred in these experiments at some time between t(r) and t(u). The force is below that necessary to crush the Hexcel, but the compression has become so great that the organ begins to crush.

The Viscous response is a time varying function which we did not measure in these experiments, but we did approximate by knowledge of Vmax*Cmax which gives the maximum value of [VC]. So we conclude that while our measurement of Vmax*Cmax did provide useful information, knowledge of the time history of the Viscous response was shown to be another important factor in soft tissue injury. The time of peak Viscous response appears to correlate with the time of injury for the various organs at risk.

While these experiments were performed on rabbits, their tissue composition, structure, and function are similar enough to human tissue

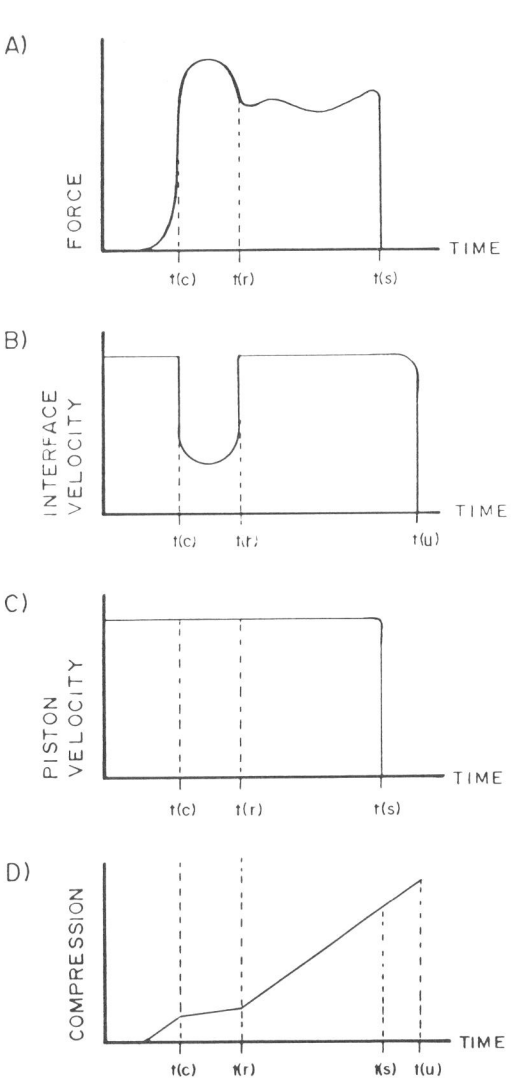

Figure 8 Ideal representation of the A) impact force, B) interface velocity, C) piston velocity, and D) compression during the impact event.

809

to make qualitative, and probably even quantitative extrapolation possible. The finding of Stalnaker and Ulman [13] that the threshold for serious injury as measured by Vmax*Cmax was species independent supports this position. However, the probability of injury to the spleen could not be accurately extrapolated from our results owing to the spleen's smaller size in the rabbit relative to the other abdominal organs.

In addition, while limiting the impact force in these experiments did mitigate renal lacerations, it was not enough to prevent all serious abdominal injury. Since the abdomen can be compressed at a very low force, the force-limitation necessary for mitigation of all serious abdominal injuries may not be achievable through padding.

SUMMARY AND CONCLUSIONS

In 94 lateral abdominal impacts, we successfully limited the impact force by using an impact interface of Hexcel™ which crushed when the force reached 1 kN or 1.5 kN depending on the type of Hexcel used. The resulting correlations between impact force, pre-impact velocity, maximum abdominal compression, and Vmax*Cmax were compared with correlations from tests with a rigid impact interface.

The results of these tests showed that the probability of serious abdominal injury was unchanged by the addition of Hexcel to the impact interface, even though the peak pressures were reduced to as little as one third of their previous values. The overall abdominal injury severity was dominated by hepatic injuries which remained as severe with the Hexcel interface, although the probability of sustaining a renal laceration was three times lower with Hexcel. This study suggests that:

(1) renal injury in the rabbit probably occurs at the time of peak force in the rigid impactor experiments, since the addition of Hexcel significantly reduced the number of renal lacerations.
(2) the crushing of the Hexcel caused a significant reduction in the velocity of compression as the interface loaded the kidney, and consequently the Viscous response was significantly reduced.
(3) for impacts with velocity above 5 m/s, compression alone is not an adequate indicator of abdominal injury severity; the velocity of compression is also important.
(4) a force-limiting material for abdominal protection may require a crush force well below that of the force-limiting materials used in this study.
(5) in abdominal injury studies one should measure the compression as a function of time if at all possible, but lacking that, one should measure Vmax*Cmax since it correlates well with the probability of abdominal injury.

ACKNOWLEDGEMENTS

Many people contributed in some way to this study, and we would like to express our gratitude for their assistance. In particular, the authors acknowledge the support of Ed Jedrzejczak, Joe McCleary, Yong Lee, Dick Madeira, Mary Foster, Bill Little, Kathy Smiler, Scott Webb, Nellie Tracy, John Hiben, Tom Terzo, and Dennis Andrzejak; and we appreciate the many helpful comments of Ian Lau, John Horsch, John Melvin, and Charlie Kroell.

REFERENCES

(1) Melvin, J. W., and Roberts, V. L.: Compression of Cellular Plastics at High Strain Rates. *J. of Cellular Plastics*, 7(2):1-4, 1971.

(2) Monk, M. W., Morgan, R. M., and Sullivan, L. K.: Side Impact Sled and Padding Development. *24th Stapp Car Crash Conference Proceedings*, pp. 255-326, 1980.

(3) Dynamic Science, Inc. Countermeasures for side impact - final report. DOT Contract No. DOT-HS-9-02177, 192 pp., August 1982.

(4) McElhaney, J. H., Stalnaker, R. L., Roberts, V. L., et al: Door crashworthiness criteria. *15th Stapp Car Crash Conference Proceedings*, pp. 489-517, 1971.

(5) Stalnaker, R. L., Roberts, V. L., and McElhaney, J. H.: Side impact tolerance to blunt trauma. *17th Stapp Car Crash Conference Proceedings*, pp. 377-408, 1973b.

(6) Melvin, J. W., Robbins, D. H., and Stalnaker, R. L.: Side impact response and injury. *Sixth International ESV Conference Proceedings*, pp. 681-689, 1976.

(7) Nusholtz, G. S., Melvin, J. W., Mueller, G., et al.: Thoraco-abdominal response and injury. *24th Stapp Car Crash Conference Proceedings*, pp. 187-228, 1980.

(8) Hollowell, W. T., Hackney, J. R., MacLaughlin, T.: The status of the National Highway Traffic Safety Administration Side Impact Research. *Ninth International ESV Conference Proceedings*, pp. 458-464, 1982.

(9) Hackney, J. R., Monk, M. W., Hollowell, W. T., et al.: Results of the National Highway Traffic Safety Administration's Thoracic Side Impact Protection Research Program. *SAE Technical Paper No. 840886*, 1984.

(10) Rouhana, S. W., Lau, I. V., and Ridella, S. A.: Influence of velocity and forced compression on the severity of abdominal injury in blunt, nonpenetrating lateral impact. *J. Trauma*, 25(6):490-500, 1985.

(11) Melvin, J. W., Stalnaker, R. L., Roberts, V. L., et al.: Impact injury mechanisms in abdominal organs. *17th Stapp Car Crash Conference Proceedings*, pp. 115-126, 1973.

(12) Gogler, E., Best, A., Braess, H. H., et al.: Biomechanical experiments with animals on abdominal tolerance levels. *21st Stapp Car Crash Conference Proceedings*, pp. 713-751, 1977.

(13) Stalnaker, R. L., and Ulman, M. S.: Abdominal trauma - review, response, and criteria. *29th Stapp Car Crash Conference Proceedings*, pp. 1-16, 1985.

(14) Stalnaker, R. L., McElhaney, J. H., Roberts, V. L., et al.: Human torso response to blunt trauma. *In* King, W. F., and Mertz, H. J. (eds.) *Human Impact Response, Measurement, and Simulation* New York, Plenum Press, 1973a, pp. 181-198.

(15) Trollope, M. L., Stalnaker, R. L., McElhaney, J. H., et al.: The mechanism of injury in blunt abdominal trauma. *J. Trauma*, 13(11):962-970, 1973.

(16) Walfisch, G., Fayon, A., Tarriere, C., et al.: Designing of a dummy's abdomen for detecting injuries in side impact collisions. *Fifth International IRCOBI Conference Proceedings*, pp. 149-164, 1980.

(17) Maltha, J., and Stalnaker, R. L.: Development of a dummy abdomen capable of injury detection in side impacts. *25th Stapp Car Crash Conference Proceedings*, pp. 651-682, 1981.

(18) Lau, I., and Viano, D. C.: An experimental study on hepatic injury from belt-restraint loading. *Aviat. Space and Environ. Med.*, pp. 611-617, Oct. 1981.

(19) Lau, I., and Viano, D. C.: Influence of impact velocity on the severity of nonpenetrating hepatic injury. *J. Trauma*, 21(2):115-123, 1981a.

(20) Viano, D. C., and Lau, I.: Thoracic impact: A Viscous Tolerance Criterion. *Tenth Conference on Experimental Safety Vehicles*, Oxford, England, June 1985.

(21) Viano, D. C., and Lau, I. V.: Role of impact velocity and chest compression in thoracic injury. *Aviat. Space Environ Med*, 54(1):16-21, 1983.

(22) Horsch, J. D., Lau I. V., Viano, D. C., and Andrzejak, D. V.: Mechanism of abdominal injury by steering wheel loading. *29th Stapp Car Crash Conference* pp. 69-78, 1985.

(23) Lau, I. V., Horsch, J. D., Viano, D. C., and Andrzejak, D. V.: Mechanism of liver injury by steering wheel injury. *GM Research Publication Number 5172*, 1986.

(24) Kroell, C. K., Allen, S. D., Warner, C. Y., and Perle, T.: Interrelationship of velocity and compression in blunt thoracic impact to swine II. Submitted for publication in the proceedings of the *30th Stapp Car Crash Conference*, 1986.

881714

How and When Blunt Injury Occurs—Implications to Frontal and Side Impact Protection

Ian V. Lau and David C. Viano
General Motors Research Labs.

ABSTRACT

The timing of liver laceration in swine during the course of a blunt impact was investigated. The swine were impacted on the upper abdomen by the lower segment of a steering wheel at 6, 9 and 12 m/s. The degree of compression in each impact was controlled independently from 10 to 50%. By varying when "the punch of an impact was pulled," we reproduced progressive segments of a longer duration blunt impact. Autopsy of the subjects demonstrated that lacerations were initiated after 8 ms of loading at 9 m/s and 6 ms of loading at 12 m/s. The time of injury was concurrent with the time when the Viscous response exceeded a threshold of 1.2 m/s in our specimens. The Viscous injury criterion, defined as the peak Viscous response, was found to be the best predictor of liver laceration. We conclude that the Viscous response relates to the actual etiology of injury, in addition to being an excellent correlative measure. Our deduction of the timing of injury occurrence was confirmed by an analysis of published cadaver data where skeletal injuries can be observed. Field data of occupant injury in a side impact were re-examined in light of these findings to determine the optimal side impact protection. We found evidence that injury from both a high speed impact and from slower crushing is possible in a side crash. Our computer simulations also suggest that an anthropomorphic test device (ATD) with human-like compliance is necessary if laboratory test results are to reflect field performance.

INTRODUCTION

Our previous studies have shown that reducing the viscous response of the abdomen by softening the tipping force of the steering wheel virtually eliminated the risk of serious liver injury in our tests. Those studies were sufficiently conclusive to promote the introduction of the *self aligning* steering wheel. We have conducted a variety of studies to challenge our hypotheses, but we have felt the need for an additional study to pinpoint the mechanism and timing of liver injury by steering wheel impact. Our additional experiments indicated that the Viscous response is predictive of the underlying cause of impact injury, although there is a very narrow distribution of injury tolerance within a tightly controlled population of test specimens, and a much wider distribution for real world occupants.

A sigmoidal relationship exists between the biomechanical cause, such as the Viscous response, and the probability of a particular severity of injury. In such a probabilistic relationship between biomechanical response and injury risk, there are two regions of response where the risk of injury is either very low or very high, with a steep transition between the two extreme outcomes (Fig 1). Within that transitional zone, the injury risk increases rapidly from 25% to 75%. Since a majority within a population of specimen will traverse from non-injury to injury within those levels of response, we define that transitional zone as the threshold region. Those injured at the lower response levels are the weaker samples of the population, and conversely the high tolerance specimens, the stronger samples. In real-world crashes, the weaker specimens may be represented by the older, more frail occupants, and the stronger samples, the young, robust adults.

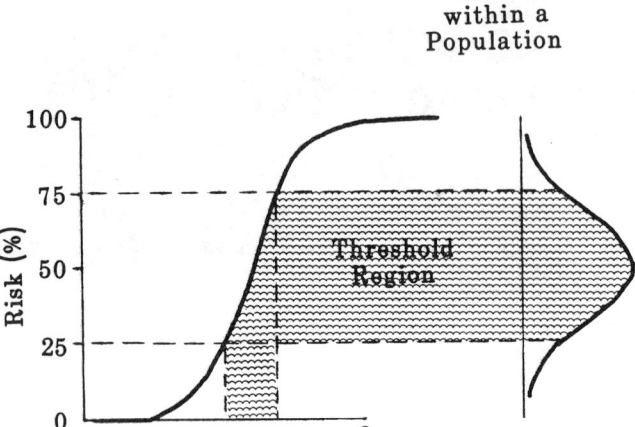

Fig 1: Threshold region defined by the sigmoidal relationship between injury risk and biomechanical response.

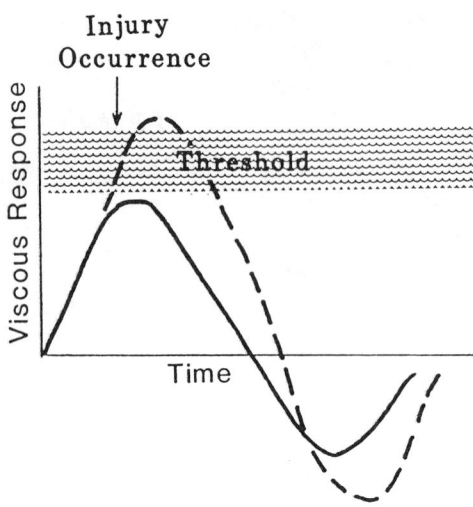

Fig 2: Hypothetical examples of the Viscous response in a non-injury producing versus an injury producing impact.

In our previous research we defined the biomechanical response at a 25% probability of critical injury outcome as the 'tolerance' for the population. This was selected recognizing the need to assure protection for the weaker occupants who were more than adequately represented in the cadaver data bases used to conduct the statistical analysis. In addition, we have standardized our analysis using the Logist function in the *Statistical Analysis System* package.

In a previous study of steering wheel induced liver injury (1 2), we demonstrated that the Viscous criterion, [VC]max, indicated the exposure severity for the upper abdomen in a sled test. The Viscous criterion (3 4 5) is defined as the peak Viscous response, which is a time function formed by multiplying the velocity of deformation and the compression of the torso. Using a programmable impactor, we then reproduced the time course of the injurious impact up to [VC]max and abruptly stopped the loading (2). Liver lacerations of similar severity as in the sled tests occurred in those impactor experiments. Additional experiments to be reported here demonstrated when injury was initiated between contact and [VC]max.

Since visceral injury cannot be readily observed as it happens, the event must be timed indirectly. In this report, we describe experiments in which we controlled and monitored the time course of impacts to the abdomen at different assigned combinations of velocity and compression, thereby reproducing selected segments of an impact event. By combining the results of the present tests with those from previous tests, we were able to isolate the biomechanical cause of the injury and deduce its time of induction with a high level of confidence.

In two very similar subjects, one Viscous response may have a peak value just below the threshold region, while another can rise above the the threshold region (Fig 2). This is typical of experiments in which injury did not occur in the first case, but did in the second. Our hypothesis would say that injury was initiated within the time when the response was in the transitional region. This study was set up to confirm or refute that hypothesis with regard to upper abdominal injury by steering wheel rim loading. In the process, we again challenged the predictiveness of the Viscous response by comparing it with other biomechanical responses against injury outcome, and by collating the timing of their peak amplitude.

Application of the injury functions identified from cadaver and animal experiments in an anthropomorphic test device requires biofidelity in the force-deflection response to impact. This is paramount since injury is caused by deflections associated with a viscous or crushing mechanism and assessment of injury risk in a dummy can only be done from a force-deflection response that closely follows the human reaction to impact. Proper reproduction of the force-deflection and deflection-time response is required to characterize ATD biofidelity. Adequate biofidelity is a prerequisite for realistic injury assessment, even with the correct injury criterion. The human chest can be characterized by an initial stiffness followed by a force plateau to maximum deflection (Fig 3). Such a response indicates that the impacted torso can be represented mechanically by an elastic spring and a viscous dashpot coupled between a front and a rear mass. A gradual

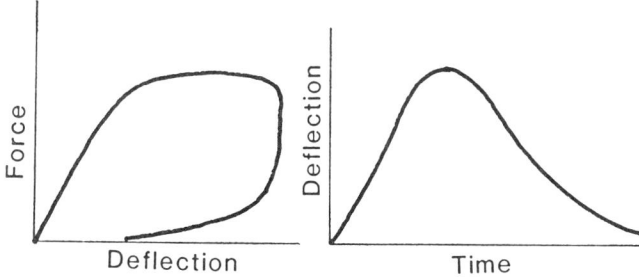

Fig 3: Biofidelity can be defined by Force-deflection and Deflection-time history.

force build up also reflects a low mass between the impactor and the viscoelastic elements.

Knowing the mechanism of injury and the instant of injury are an important prerequisite toward the design of an optimal countermeasure. Attention can then be focused on the occupant's interaction with the car interior during or before that time to reduce the injury hazard. This study seeks to pinpoint the mechanism and the timing of injury induction in an impact environment which resembles that of the typical unrestrained occupant in a frontal or lateral crash.

Given a valid injury criterion, a probabilistic risk function, and a test device with biofidelity, it is possible to conduct an assessment of safety design concepts. This effort is most realistic if laboratory performance of the concept is analyzed in relation to the real-world injury patterns it tries to prevent. The common link between the laboratory and real-world crashes is the severity of the exposure, most frequently reported as the change in velocity of the struck vehicle or the test velocity. This linkage is important because there are two competing effects in real-world crashes. First, the incidence of crashes decreases as the severity increases, *ie* there are more low severity crashes. Second, in contrasting fashion, the risk of occupant injury increases with the severity of a crash.

Another focus of the study was to apply the same principles to evaluate side impact protection. Previous studies (5 6) have shown that too stiff an ATD (7) could directly result in interior designs with negligible benefit in field accidents. Our data of lateral human impact response confirm that available ATDs are stiffer than and develop four times the plateau force of the human torso. A simulation study using the latest impact response data of the human and the ATDs demonstrates that a non-biofidelic ATD or a non-representative test severity can lead to designs that do not benefit the occupant in an impact, placing persons with low tolerance at particular risk.

EXPERIMENTAL MATERIALS AND METHODS

Nine swine,[1] weighing 46.7 ± 2.0 Kg, were restrained without excitement by a spring assisted injection of ketamine (20 mg/Kg,IM) and acepromazine (200 ug/Kg,IM) followed by atropine (0.08 mg/Kg,IM). The swine were then induced to a surgical plane of anesthesia with a mixture of fentanyl (40 ug/Kg,IM) and droperidol (2mg/Kg,IM) and maintained on an equal mixture of oxygen and nitrous oxide with 1-1.5% halothane. They breathed spontaneously in a dorsal recumbency on a V-shaped support for preparatory surgery, which was the same as in previous tests (2).

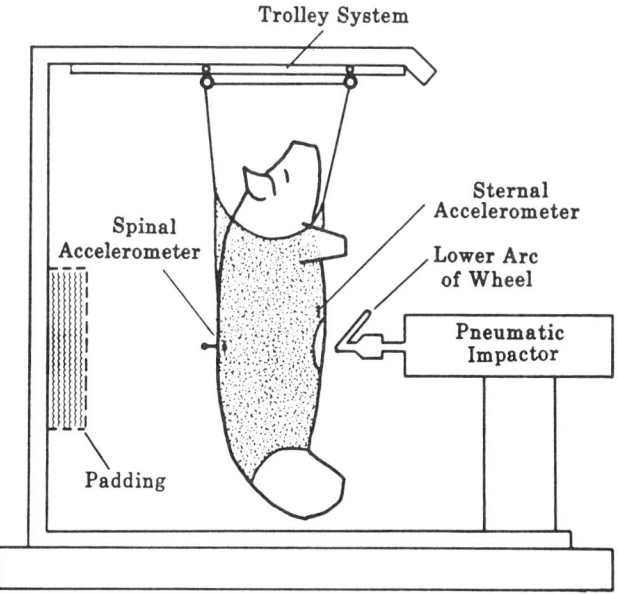

Fig 4: The experimental preparation with the required instrumentation.

[1] The rationale and experimental protocol for the use of an animal model in this program have been reviewed by the Research Laboratories' Animal Research Committee. The research follows procedures outlined in the *Guide for the Care and Use of Laboratory Animals*, U.S. Department of Health and Human Services, Public Health Service, National Institute of Health NIH Publication 85-23, Revised 1985, and Public Health Service *Policy on Humane Care and Use of Laboratory Animals by Awardee Institutions*, NIH Guide for Grants and Contracts, Vol.14, No 8, June 25, 1985, and complies with the provisions of the *Animal Welfare Act* of 1966 (PL 89-544), as amended in 1970 and 1976 (PL 91-579 and PL 94-270), and the Food Security Act of 1985 (PL 99-158).

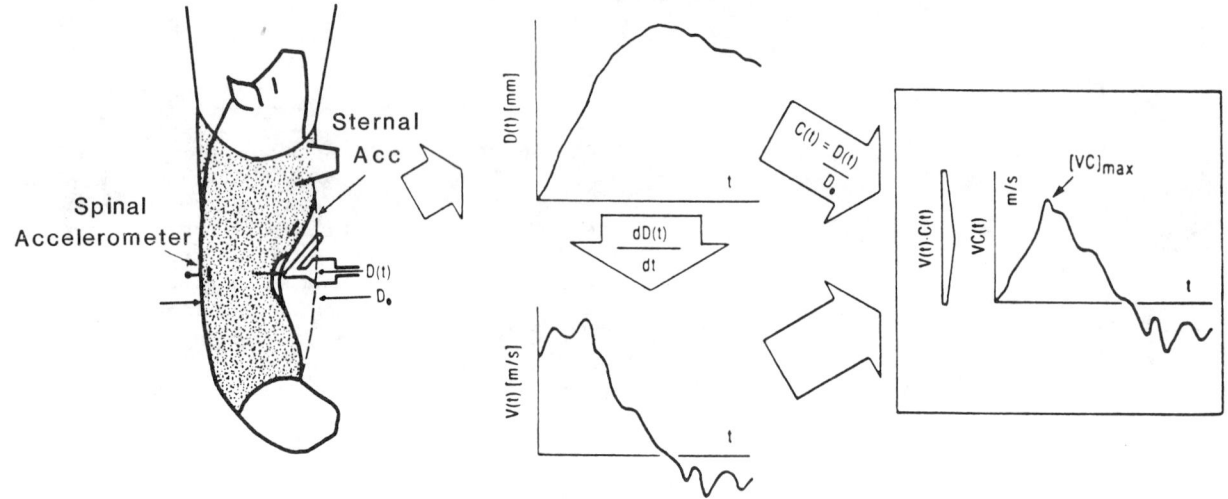

Fig 5: Derivation of [VC(t)] from instantaneous torso deformation [D(t)], which is derived from frame-by-frame analysis of high speed movies. Locations of the accelerometers relative to the principal direction of the impact is also shown.

The swine were maintained vertically in a sling during the tests. Particular adaptational aids required for a quadruped to maintain basal physiologic functions during vertical suspension were discussed and published previously (2). The test consisted of a direct impact of the swine at the xyphoid, or 50 mm below it, using the lower arc of the wheel as the impacting interface (Fig 4). A pneumatic impactor was programmed to strike at 6, 9 or 12 m/s for an assigned torso compression of 10 to 50%. The assigned compression may differ from the actual peak compression, since the back of the animal was free to move during the impact. To minimize the number of animals required, some of the swine were used in more than one test when we judged that injury had not occurred after a mild thump, consistent with the low injury risk observed in our previous experiments. A peritoneal lavage was always performed before the final, possibly injurious impact, which was applied only if the lavage was negative for blood in the peritoneum, confirming the absence of lacerative injury. We found no evidence for predisposition for lacerations in the milder impacts from petechiae or bruising. Those animals subjected to multiple impacts are identified in the results. In any given animal, only one injury producing impact was applied. High speed movies of the impact were taken at 1,000 frames per second. Frame-by-frame analysis of the impact event formed the basis for the instantaneous deflection data of the torso. The instantaneous deflection data were processed to derive the compression response and the Viscous response (Fig 5) based on an established algorithm (3). Midsternal acceleration and spinal acceleration at T12 along the direction of the impact were monitored by accelerometers. Contact was indicated by a flash on a movie frame and a simultaneous tick mark on an electronic data channel, generated by the same contact switch closure, which defined time zero. The acceleration channels were processed by a Channel Class 180 filter. The time of peak compression and Viscous response, and peak sternal and spinal accelerations were recorded for each test. In the film analysis, interpolation was made between adjacent frames to establish time zero where necessary. A summary follows of the injury criteria and injury functions which were examined. They were used as the basis to deduce the time of injury induction, which was collated against our empirical observations.

Injury Functions:

Viscous Response [VC(t)] - A time function produced by multiplying the instantaneous velocity of deformation and the compression response. (units in m/s, derived from film data)

Compression Response [C(t)] - The instantaneous deformation divided by the initial torso thickness along the axis of the impact. (dimensionless, derived from film data)

Sternal Acceleration Response [Gst(t)] - Instantaneous acceleration of the midsternum along the direction of the impact measured by the sternal accelerometer. (units in g's, derived from electronic data)

Spinal Acceleration Response [Gsp(t)] - Instantaneous acceleration of the spine along the axis of the impact measured by the spinal accelerometer on T12. (units in g's, derived from electronic data)

Injury Criteria:

Viscous Criterion [VC]max - The peak Viscous response.
Compression Criterion [C]max - The peak compression response.
Sternal Acceleration Criterion [Gst]max - The peak sternal acceleration response.
Spinal Acceleration Criterion [Gsp]max - The peak spinal acceleration response.

A thorough truncal necropsy for each of the animals followed established procedures (2). The focus of the necropsy was the presence and the severity of liver lacerations. Those observations were subdivided into three categories. When no tears were observed in the Glisson's membrane and the parenchymal tissues, ie absence of bleeding, the category of no lacerations was assigned. Simple tears of the Glisson's membrane no deeper than 5 mm anywhere in the parenchymal tissues were designated as superficial lacerations. Such lacerations usually would not require surgical intervention in a human. Tears deeper than 5 mm at its deepest point, stellate shaped lacerations, and junctional tears between liver lobes were all considered deep and extensive lacerations. Deep and extensive lacerations usually resulted in severe hemorrhage and might require surgical intervention in a human. Such an injury could be considered to be a severe or critical threat to life. Results from the present experiments were combined with those from previous experiments to determine when and if liver lacerations occurred. A Logist analysis was performed on each of the criteria to determine its correlation with, and the threshold for liver lacerations.

Previous experiments included in this data analysis are four impactor tests at 9 m/s using the same setup, and six Hyge sled tests. The previous tests are identified in the results section. The sled tests were performed at a velocity of 9 m/s, and were designed to evaluate the influence on abdominal injury of changing steering wheel stiffness. Abdominal impact of the swine in the sled test was also induced by the lower rim of the steering wheel. The sled would be traveling at test velocity by the time of the impact, and the unrestrained swine would interact freely with the steering system. Three liver injury producing sled tests using a stiffer wheel, and three non-injurious sled tests using a softer wheel (Table 1) were extracted from the complete sled data set (2). The four previous impactor tests (Table 3) were designed to simulate the initial rapid phase of abdominal compression in the stiffer-wheel sled tests. The lower rim of the wheel impacted the swine on the upper abdomen at 5 cm below the xyphoid in both the previous sled and impactor tests.

THE SLED TESTS

An understanding of the biomechanics of injury in the previous sled tests is pertinent to the new impactor study. Abdominal compression in a sled test can be subdivided into time segments based on torso interaction with the steering system (Fig 6). During the initial contact, the lower rim of the wheel compressed the abdomen at the highest rate encountered within the impact event. We are calling that period the rapid compression phase. [VC]max occurred at approximately the end of the rapid compression phase. Abdominal compression slowed down when column compression was initiated by hub contact of the thorax. We are calling that period the gradual compression phase. Decompression of the torso began as it rebounded and expanded toward its original shape. The subject then gained sufficient velocity from the impact to travel down the test track at sled velocity. We are calling that period the decompression phase. The pivotal difference based on wheel parameters between the lacerative and the non-lacerative sled tests was steering wheel stiffness (Fig 7). The stiffer wheel compressed the abdomen at the test velocity of the sled, whereas the softer wheel deformed during the rapid compression phase to shorten the rapid compression phase and reduce the velocity of abdominal deformation. The lacerative and the non-lacerative sled tests were best discriminated by [VC]max among the injury criteria (Table 1).

THE IMPACTOR TESTS

Among the injury criteria examined, [VC]max provided the most definitive laceration threshold (Fig 9). The level, or the effective dose of impact severity at which 50% of the subjects were injured, called [ED$_{50}$], was 1.2 m/s. As [VC]max increased beyond the threshold, deep and extensive lacerations were produced. Whereas liver lacerations could be induced with a [C]max of less than 20% at 12 m/s (Table 4), the tolerable [C]max exceeded 35% at 6 m/s (Table 2). Although [Gst]max and [Gsp]max were higher when the impact was applied to the xyphoid than to 5 cm below it, liver injury did not appear to depend on the 5 cm variation of impacting site. Neither correlated with liver lacerations, even if the contact location was kept constant for the analysis (Fig 9). In a Logist analysis, the sharpness of the transitional zone defines the sensitivity of a biomechanical response, and the injury discrimination by the criterion.

TIMING THE INITIATION OF INJURY

Since the sled tests were performed at 9 m/s, abdominal impact by the lower rim of the stiffer wheel in the sled test could be simulated by impactor tests at the same speed. Previous impactor tests (Table 3) were designed to simulate only the rapid compression phase and then retract abruptly (Fig 8). Those tests showed

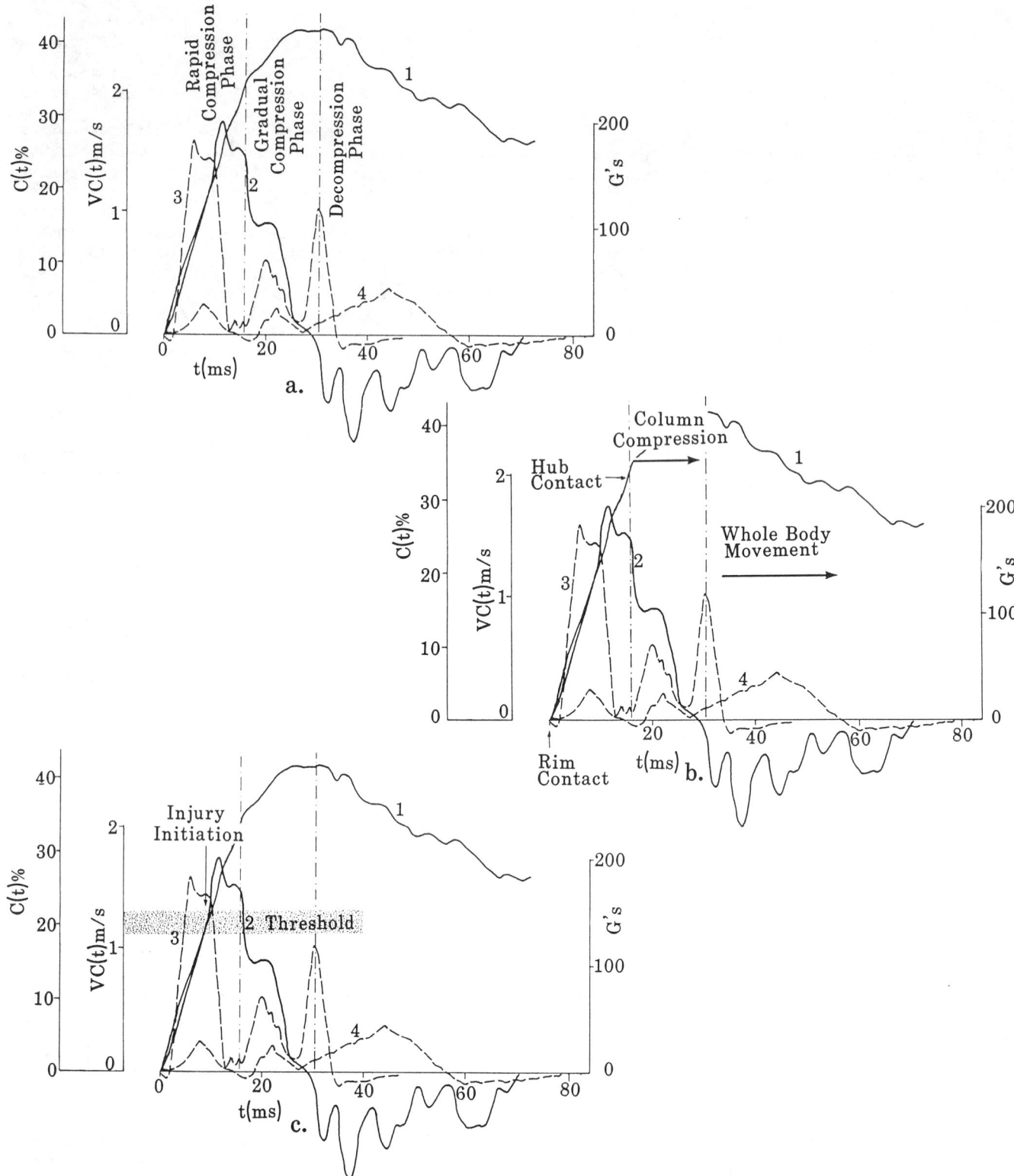

Fig 6: Time segments of a sled-induced impact to the upper abdomen (Test 1075) based on torso interaction with the stiffer steering wheel. Three identical figures are presented for clarity. a: The division of the impact event into the rapid compression phase, the gradual compression phase, and the decompression phase. 1 - Instantaneous compression of the upper abdomen [C(t)]. 2 - Viscous response [VC(t)]. 3 - Sternal acceleration [Gst(t)]. 4 - Spinal acceleration [Gsp(t)]. b: Rim contact of the upper abdomen defines time zero. c: Threshold region defined by impactor tests.

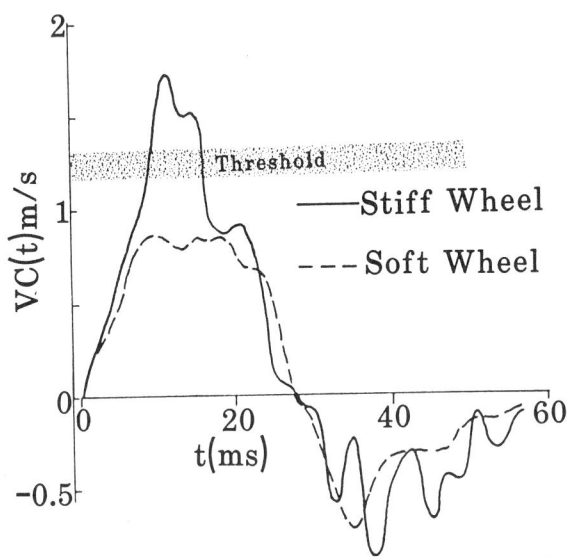

Fig 7: The Viscous response is reduced when a softer steering wheel (Test 1087) is used in an otherwise identical sled test. No liver injury was observed in the softer wheel test.

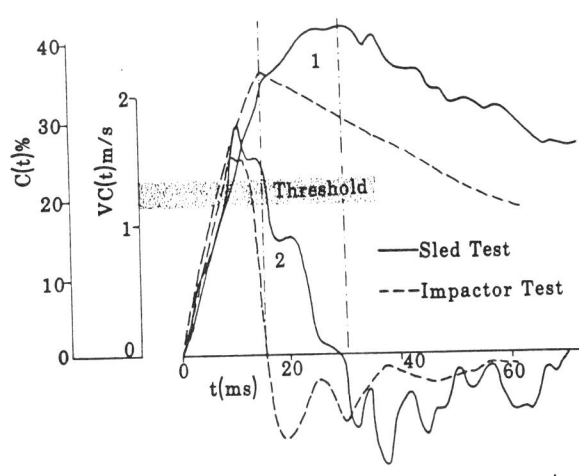

Fig 8: Impactor simulation at 9 m/s of the abdominal impact by the stiffer wheel on the sled. 1 - Instantaneous compression C(t). 2 - Viscous response VC(t). The compression of the upper abdomen by the impactor stopped abruptly at the end of the rapid compression phase of the sled test.

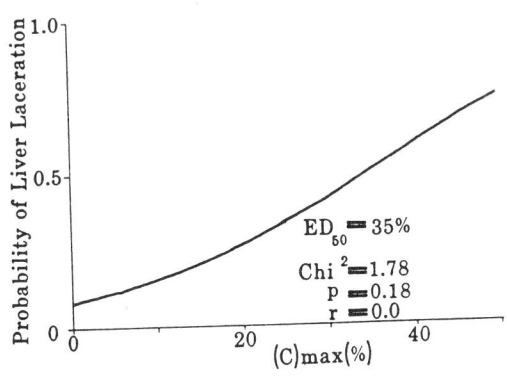

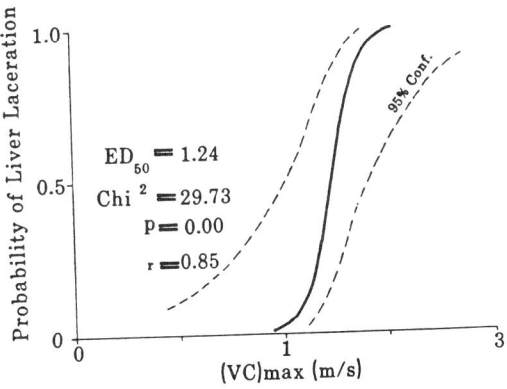

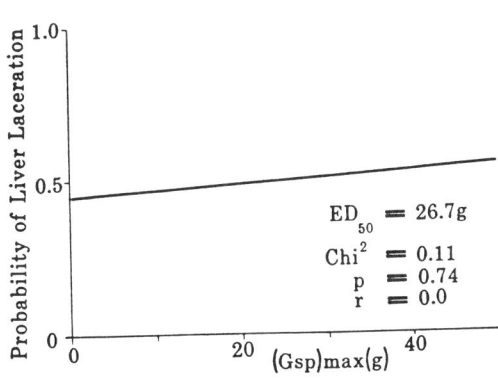

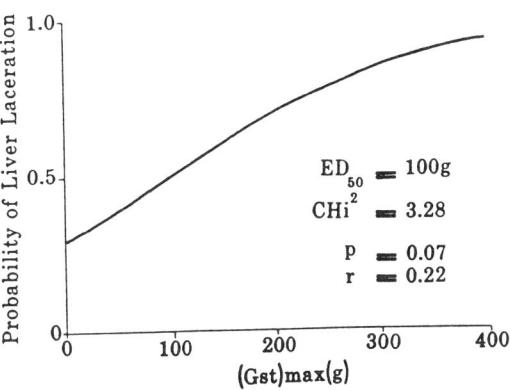

Fig 9: Logist analysis of liver lacerations based on [VC]max, [C]max, [Gst]max and [Gsp]max. All available data points were included for [VC]max and [C]max. Only impacts at 5 cm below the xyphoid were included for [Gst]max and [Gsp]max.

	STIFFER WHEEL			SOFTER WHEEL		
SWINE #	410	408	401	403	415	414
TEST #	1085	1082	1075	1079	1088	1087
[C]max (%)	36.0	41.0	42.0	34.4	32.6	36.0
0 time (ms)	23.8	28.1	31.0	32.8	31.7	26.3
[VC]max (m/s)	1.6	1.5	1.7	1.0	0.8	0.9
0 time (ms)	11.5	16.0	11.5	11.2	13.7	9.7
[Gst]max (g)	205	222	185	280	135	133
0 time (ms)	7.0	15.0	6.0	7.0	12.0	8.0
[Gsp]max (g)	46	66	43	54	53	50
0 time (ms)	19.0	24.0	44.0	29.0	20.0	21.0
No Liver Lacerations				*	*	*
Superficial						
Deep and Extensive	*	*	*			

Table 1: Selected sled test data at a sled velocity of 9 m/s (2). Time zero is defined by contact. The impact site was 5 cm below the xyphoid.

	SWINE #	4	10	11	12
	TEST #	12	17	16	18
ASSIGNED PARAMETERS:	COMPRESSION(%)	20	25	20	25
	IMPACTING SITE	-5	-5	-5	-5
MEASURED PARAMETERS:	[C]max (%)	18.7	25.5	18.8	28.1
	0 time (ms)	7.5	11.6	7.0	11.5
	[VC]max (m/s)	1.4	1.8	1.4	1.8
	0 time (ms)	5.0	8.4	4.6	8.3
	[Gst]max (g)	NA	170	350	430
	0 time (ms)	NA	4.0	3.0	4.0
	[Gsp]max	9	13	9	17
	0 time (ms)	4.0	6.0	4.0	5.0
LIVER INJURY SEVERITY	No Lacerations	*			
	Superficial Lacerations			*	
	Deep and Extensive Lacerations		*		*

Table 4: Impactor tests with a segmented wheel at 12 m/s.

	SWINE #	9	9	9	13	13	13
	TEST #	9	10	11	13	14	15
ASSIGNED PARAMETERS:	COMPRESSION(%)	30	35	35	40	40	50
	IMPACTING SITE	-5	-5	-5	-5	-5	-5
MEASURED PARAMETERS:	[C]max (%)	30.9	34.3	36.3	38.8	39.4	36.3
	0 time (ms)	24.4	39.8	41.8	49.5	52.3	45.5
	[VC]max (m/s)	0.7	0.8	1.1	1.1	1.0	1.0
	0 time (ms)	14.5	21.6	23.4	23.9	35.7	27.2
	[Gst]max (g)	23	22	64	74	NA	46
	0 time (ms)	9.8	16.0	15.6	15.3	NA	14.1
	[Gsp]max (g)	8	12	22	22	25	22
	0 time (ms)	14.1	23.0	26.2	27.0	25.5	25.6
LIVER INJURY SEVERITY	No Lacerations	*	*	*	*	*	*
	Superficial Lacerations						
	Deep and Extensive Lacerations						

Table 2: Impactor tests with a segmented wheel at 6 m/s. [C]max differs from assigned compression because of back movement. The impacting site was either -5, *ie* 5 cm below, or X, *ie* at the xyphoid. Multiple impacts of the same swine can be identified by the same swine number.

	SWINE #	1	1	1	2	2	3	3	4	416	428	429	430
	TEST #	1	2	3	4	5	6	7	8	1P	10P	11P	12P
ASSIGNED PARAMETERS:	COMPRESSION(%)	10	20	25	10	30	25	30	25	30	35	35	35
	IMPACTING SITE	X	X	X	-5	-5	X	X	X	-5	-5	-5	-5
MEASURED PARAMETERS:	[C]max (%)	13.9	17.7	26.5	11.2	28.7	24.4	33.6	25.8	31.0	36.0	35.4	35.1
	@ time (ms)	6.0	7.7	11.1	4.4	10.2	10.3	13.9	10.9	14.5	15.3	17.2	16.4
	[VC]max (m/s)	0.5	0.7	1.0	0.5	1.3	1.0	1.4	1.0	1.2	1.5	1.4	1.4
	@ time (ms)	3.7	5.1	6.9	2.6	6.6	6.8	8.1	6.9	7.0	9.7	11.7	12.6
	[Gst]max (g)	300	229	428	11	108	526	114	475	80	50	55	50
	@ time (ms)	2.5	3.0	2.4	12.5	9.1	2.6	7.9	2.7	10.2	11.6	10.7	9.8
	[Gsp]max (g)	38	43	49	3	41	47	37	49	16	20	22	17
	@ time (ms)	5.0	5.0	9.6	17.1	12.7	8.9	11.0	9.4	13.0	15.1	14.8	13.7
LIVER INJURY SEVERITY	No Lacerations	*	*	*	*		*		*				
	Superficial Lacerations					*		*		*			
	Deep and Extensive Lacerations										*	*	*

Table 3: Impactor tests with a segmented wheel at 9 m/s. Previous tests to simulate the initial rapid compression phase of the stiffer-wheel sled tests are designated by a P in the run number.

that liver injury was of similar severity as long as the full rapid compression phase of the sled-induced impact by the stiff wheel was reproduced. The gradual compression phase was less significant in injury causation despite the higher compression because the velocity of deformation was much slower. The time of injury initiation remains to be demonstrated by the new impactor experiments.

By supposition, exposure severity increases as an injury criterion increases. Since injury criteria are simply peak values of their respective time functions, injury potential is the highest at the peak of the injury functions. The demarcation between no-laceration and minor-laceration cases forms the most precise empirical indication of an injury threshold, which was computed mathematically by Logist analysis for the respective criteria. In those cases of minor laceration, each criterion was suggesting that the injury was initiated at the peak of the respective injury function as it narrowly exceeded the threshold. Therefore, one can pinpoint the time of injury induction by comparing the injury functions of the no-laceration versus the minor-laceration cases.

Based on impactor tests at 9 m/s (Fig 10a), one can establish that an impact to the abdominal viscera did not produce liver lacerations until [VC(t)] had attained at least 1.2 m/s after about 8 ms. Our empirical observation of a tolerance of 1.2 m/s certainly lies within that threshold region between 1.17 and 1.31 m/s respectively (Fig 9). Within the limitations of the test methodology, a subthreshold test at 9 m/s, by design, was the initial portion of an above-threshold test at the same speed, which in turn was the initial portion of the rapid compression phase in a sled test. In fact, the only difference among them was the amount of assigned stroke after contact, *ie*, when the punch was pulled. Therefore, the comparison between the subthreshold and above-threshold tests demonstrated that liver lacerations began after about 8 ms of loading for the 9 m/s impact as the Viscous response exceeded the lower boundary of the injury threshold. One can also deduce analogously that abdominal injury in the sled test was induced when and if the Viscous response exceeded threshold. [VC]max for the stiff and soft wheel tests were above and below the threshold region respectively (Fig 7).

At 6 m/s (Fig 11), the Viscous response required over 20 ms to attain its peak value, which remained below the threshold of 1.2 m/s. No liver laceration was produced among those impacts. By contrast, at 12 m/s the Viscous response exceeded threshold 6 ms after contact. Autopsy showed that minor liver lacerations were induced by the much quicker loading within a shorter stroke and duration in that test.

The logical deduction of the time of injury initiation can be extended to cases of extensive lacerations. One can conclude analogously that lacerations were initiated in those tests as the Viscous response exceeded threshold. Lacerations then became more extensive as the Viscous response continued to rise higher and stayed above the threshold. Those tests explained the extensive lacerations observed in the sled tests with the stiffer wheel.

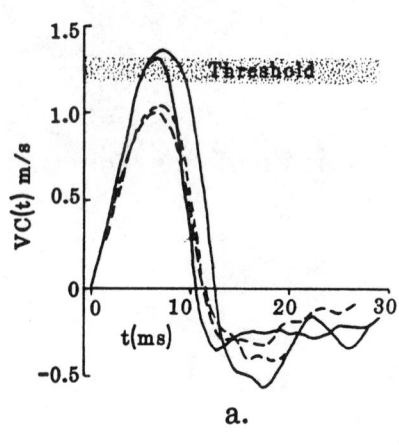
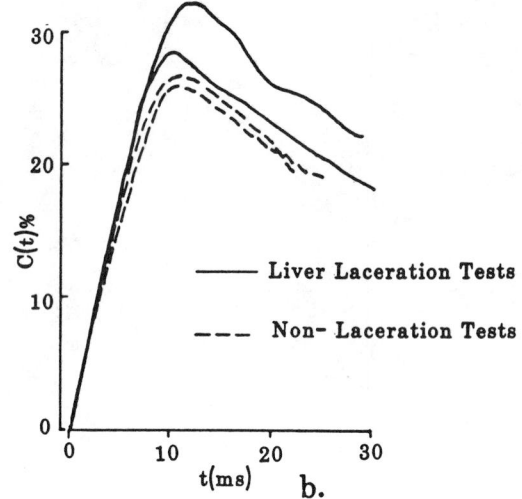

Fig 10: The Viscous response (a) and Compression response (b) of selected minor-laceration (Test #5, #7) versus non-injury cases (Test #3, #8) at 9 m/s.

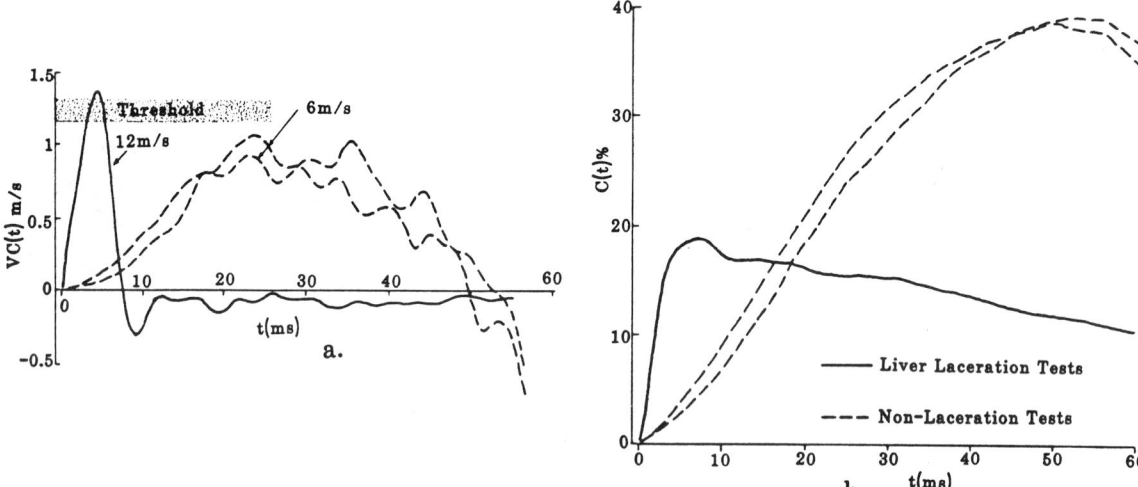

Fig 11: The Viscous response (a) and Compression response (b) of selected minor-laceration versus non-injury cases at 6 (Test #13, #14) and 12 m/s (Test #16).

Considerations for Compression, Acceleration and Power Criteria

Using [C]max as the basis to examine the same minor-laceration versus no-laceration cases at 9 m/s, one would have to conclude that laceration was initiated after about 12 ms of contact as a [C]max of 30% was attained (Fig 10b). Experiments at 6 m/s disproved that possibility because no injury was observed for a [C]max of 30% or higher (Fig 11b). As the compression response approached [C]max, the rate of torso compression was always approaching zero, and impacts at 6 m/s or 9 m/s were compressing the torsos of very similar subjects quasi-statically. Since injury was produced in one case but not the other, [C]max as an index of injury severity is only a correlative measurement within narrow ranges of impact velocity and cannot be used to determine the time of injury occurrence in a moderate to high speed impact. Injury by excessive compression alone in an impact remains possible. Those injuries, called crushing injuries, tend to be characterized by extensive rib fractures before soft tissues are involved in a chest impact (10). In our 6 m/s tests, the impactor could not induce sufficient torso compression to cause injury in the present experimental set up because whole body movement limited the actual abdominal compression to less than 40%.

The magnitude of [Gst]max and [Gsp]max depended on the load path between the impact site and the respective accelerometer. When impact was applied to the xyphoid, the sternum provided a

822

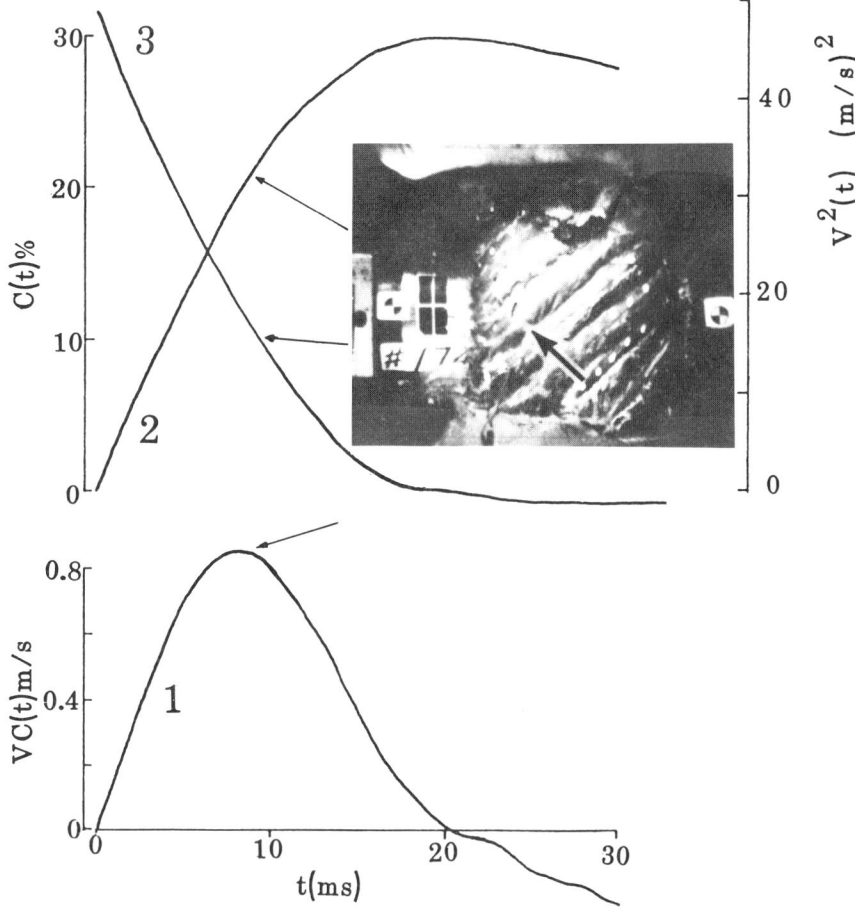

Fig 12: The Viscous response[1], compression response[2] and $V^2(t)$[3] of a test from a study by Kroell et al (9). Initiation of fractures was properly indicated by the Viscous response but not by the compression response, nor by $V^2(t)$.

direct load path from the contact point to the accelerometer resulting in a higher [Gst]max with a minimal time delay. Similarly, the force of an impact to the xyphoid was transmitted efficiently across the rib cage to the spine, which induced a higher [Gsp]max. By contrast, when the impact was applied only 5 cm lower to the abdominal viscera, soft tissues became an additional viscoelastic component of the load path, reducing the peak magnitude while inducing additional delay for both the sternal and the spinal accelerations. The 5 cm variation of impact site did not affect injury outcome because the sites stayed within the perimeter of the liver mass. Peak spinal acceleration always followed peak sternal acceleration in a given impact, reflecting transmission of the impact force across the mechanical impedance between the frontal structures and the spine.

The peak of the square of the instantaneous velocity of deformation, $[V^2(t)]$max, has been suggested as a proxy of the peak instantaneous power dissipated by the torso (11). Instantaneous power, like skeletal acceleration, impact force, and torso compression, may correlate with injury due to their common link to the overall severity of an impact. By isolating the biomechanical cause and the time of injury induction, one can determine that $[V^2(t)]$max is also an inadequate injury criterion. In these impactor tests, energy continues to be fed into the impactor pneumatically within the course of an impact. Therefore, the time of $[V^2(t)]$max is variably dependent on the assigned velocity of impact, the initiation of back movement, and the complex interaction between the torso and the impacting interface. However, $[V^2(t)]$max always precedes [VC]max and the time of highest injury risk. In a pendulum impact, the initial contact velocity always equals the highest velocity of deformation (Fig 12). However, injury risk is never the highest and internal trauma does not occur at contact.

Although our study has focused on liver laceration, the arguments apply equally well for injuries of other body regions. The basis of our contention follows that if an injury criterion is the peak value of an injury function, and if the function follows the causal impact response, injury is induced when the response, as well as the corresponding injury function, exceeds the tolerance of the subject synchronously. The Viscous response meets those requirements in frontal, side or oblique impacts (12 13).

An Observable Empirical Example

The study presented here is one of the first to investigate systematically the time of injury. We cannot find any other reference with its primary focus on the time of injury induction within a blunt impact. There is at least one paper in the literature that has followed the initiation of rib fractures anecdotally. Kroell et al (9) examined the dynamics of the human chest in a blunt impact. In a particular experiment, the fasciae were removed from a specimen, exposing the ribs. The subject was impacted at 7.2 m/s with a 23.1 Kg pendulum. In that test, rib fractures began at 9.2 ms after contact. Film data of the test were reanalyzed (Fig 12). [VC]max of 0.85 m/s in that test occurred at 8.3 ms. [C]max was at 20 ms, which confirmed the published data. Only two fractures were observed in that test. The exposure narrowly exceeded the subject's tolerance for rib fractures. In that test, the Viscous response properly indicated when fractures began; the compression response and $[V^2(t)]$ did not. In the larger cadaver data set (3), [VC]max of 0.85 m/s in a thoracic impact corresponds to only a 6% chance of acquiring an AIS4 injury and a 40% chance of acquiring an AIS3 injury. Injury of that particular specimen was an AIS2.

Impactor versus Sled Test Environments

In an impactor test, the subject is stationary before an impact. The impact induces only minimal whole body movement before it returns to rest. The subject in a Hyge sled test is also stationary before an impact. Within the course of the impact, and indifferent to injury causation, the subject always accelerates to sled velocity. The difference between those test environments has profound influence on acceleration measurements and criteria, but minimal effects on injury criteria based on torso deformation.

Since torso deformation is defined as displacement of the point of contact relative to the opposite side of the subject, whole body movement will not influence its interpretation. However, whole body acceleration in the sled environment, which does not affect injury outcome, can increase skeletal acceleration. Maximum sternal acceleration is usually not affected because it peaks within the initial few milliseconds before whole body acceleration begins (Fig 6). However, peak spinal acceleration is generally increased and delayed because the largest component of the spinal acceleration is often attributable to the whole body acceleration of the subject as it seeks to attain sled velocity. The initial pulse of spinal acceleration, which corresponds to torso deformation within the rapid compression phase, is sometimes neglected because it can be lower than the pulse induced by whole body acceleration. The disparity between those test environments explains

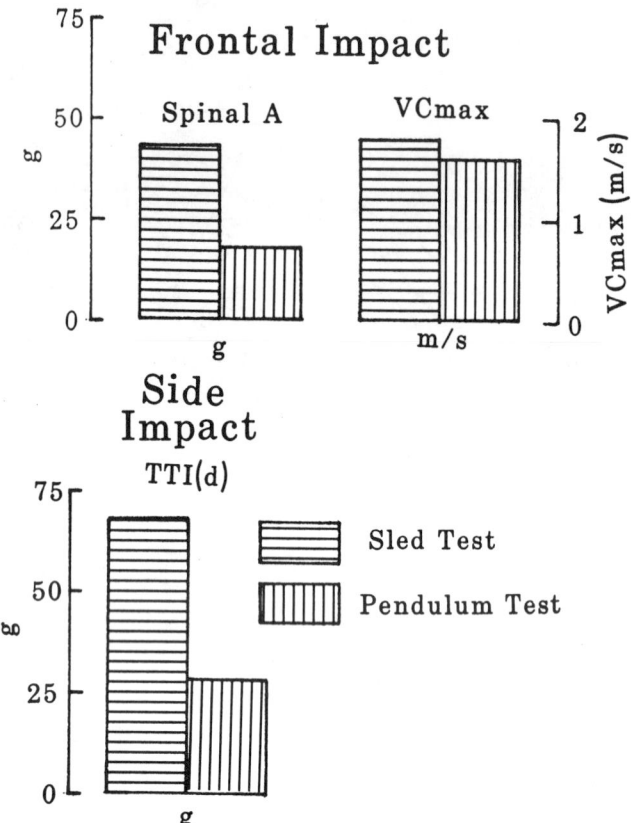

Fig 13: Spinal acceleration and [VC]max from impactor tests and sled tests in a frontal upper abdominal impact of swine by a steering wheel rim at 9 m/s (3). The tests produced severe liver lacerations. TTI(d) from pendulum tests and sled tests in a side impact of cadavers (14). The pendulum and sled tests produced AIS 3 injuries.

the doubling of the peak spinal acceleration from an impactor test to a sled test for similar injury severity in a frontal impact (Fig 13a). Since the Viscous criterion follows the causal injury response, it indicates injury potential independently of the impact environment.

Similar characteristics of the respective test environment are also evident in side impact based on data published by the NHTSA (14). TTI, a side impact injury criterion proposed by the NHTSA, is the sum of two components: a skeletal acceleration based portion, and a second component based on the subject's age. The two components accounts for 60 and 40% of TTI's magnitude respectively in the original cadaver data set. Since age cannot be measured in a dummy, TTI has evolved into TTI(d) by omitting the age component of TTI. However, for similar injury severity (AIS ≥ 3), the acceleration-based criterion TTI(d) is three times higher in a sled test than a pendulum test (Fig 13b) in the NHTSA data set, for the same reasons as in frontal tests. TTI(d), like other correlative

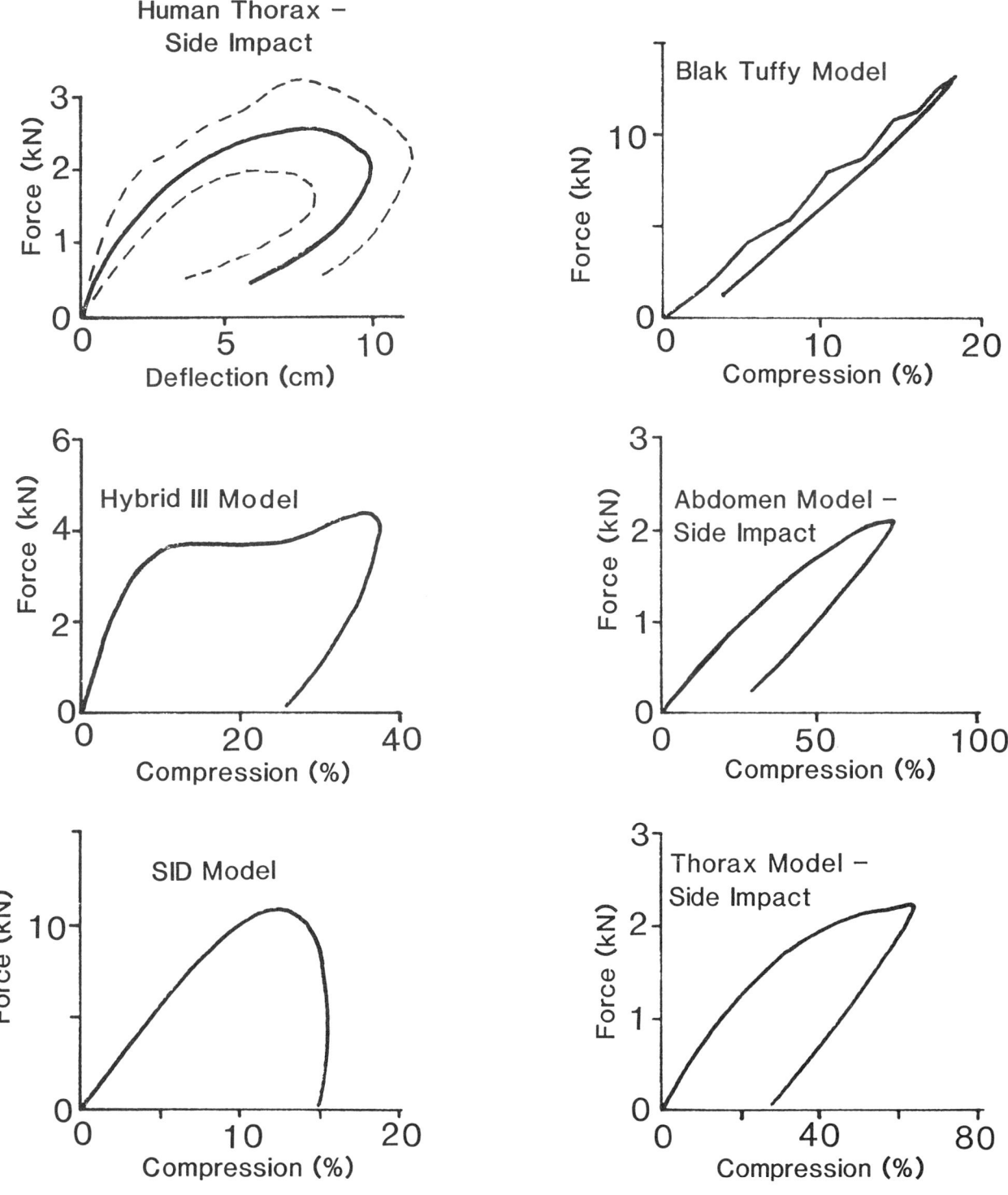

Fig 14: Force-Deflection characteristics of the human chest and the Lobdell model representing the Blak Tuffy, the SID, the Hybrid III, and the human chest and abdomen.

indicators of injury risk, is highly dependent on the impact environment. Delta V of the struck car will significantly influence TTI(d) in a test, regardless of injury causation.

INFLUENCE OF TEST VELOCITY AND ANTHROPOMORPHIC TEST DEVICE ON THE CHOICE OF COUNTERMEASURE

Animal tests provide the most definitive model of occupant injury because of their physiological vitality. The imposed homogeneity of the test subjects, such as similar size and age, provides a group of specimens with very similar thresholds of injury. Animal tests, therefore, are an important and powerful safety research tool. However, animal tests must only be used judiciously when alternatives are unavailable. To minimize the number of swine needed for this study, some of them were subjected to multiple impacts of increasing severity. In a parameter study, the best approach is computer simulation.

We simulated the force-deflection characteristics and the force-acceleration history of the J944 Blak Tuffy, the SID, the Hybrid III, and the human lateral thorax and abdomen by varying the parameter values of the original Lobdell model of the chest (Fig 14). A matched dynamic force-deflection characteristics, along with a matched deflection-time history, is the best indicator that the proper impedance of the ATD or the human torso is mathematically reproduced. The models were impacted by a 100Kg mass, which would not underestimate the inertia of the supporting structures of the steering system in a frontal impact, or the struck door with the front end of the striking car in a side impact. With those models, we examined how changing the impact velocity and the ATD could affect the optimal choice for crushable EA structures or materials. The optimal choice was based on the most appropriate injury criterion associated with that ATD or the human. These hypothetical crushable EA structures or materials, with a 5 cm available stroke, was characterized by a constant crush force.

Effect of Test Velocity

The simulation indicated clearly that the optimal crush force of the EA structure or material increased as the impact speed increased, regardless of the ATD or the choice of injury criterion (Figs 15, 16). Therefore, to optimize a countermeasure in a high speed test, an engineer would choose a high crush force structure or material. However, if the test speed were driven much higher than the injury threshold region or the the speed at which most field accidents occurred, those countermeasures that performed well in the severe laboratory tests would be ineffective in reducing human injury risks appreciably in the field. Thus, it is most effective to design countermeasures in the steep, threshold region of the sigmoidal probability function. Fig 17 shows such a sigmoidal function along with the test speed at which

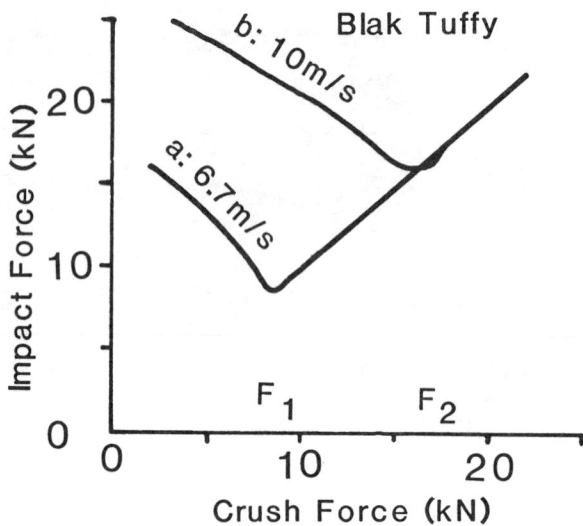

Fig 15: The peak impact force when the Blak Tuffy is struck by a 100Kg mass at 6.7 m/s (a) and 10 m/s (b) with a crushable interface. The constant crush force on the abscissa is indicative of the material properties of the interface. Peak force is the criterion used here because it is specified in J211 to measure steering system performance.

those criteria may be derived. Note that a 25% reduction at the high exposure region represents less than 10% in injury risk. In contrast, a 25% reduction in the steep region of the sigmoidal response results in a 50% reduction in injury risk. In the plateau region of over exposure, reduction in the injury criterion can represent zero reduction in injury risk.

Based on the Blak Tuffy test for a steering wheel, an engineer would design the steering system structure to yield at 8.5 kN or 16.0 kN if the test were at 6.7 m/s or 10 m/s respectively. However, he must also consider that the stiffer structure would provide no energy absorption even for the Blak Tuffy - a stiff, non-human like ATD, when the impact velocity was below 7 m/s (Fig 18). Therefore, in an accident of moderate severity, the occupant would derive no benefit from that countermeasure. The more susceptible occupants with lower injury thresholds, such as children and the elderly, would be among the first to be injured.

The Effects of ATD

The dynamic stiffness of an ATD has an even more profound effect on the choice of countermeasure. Since the Hybrid III chest is much softer than the Blak Tuffy, the proper countermeasure indicated by the Hybrid III is also much softer than that indicated by the Blak Tuffy at the same speed (Fig 16). For example, the optimal steering system for chest protection indicated by the

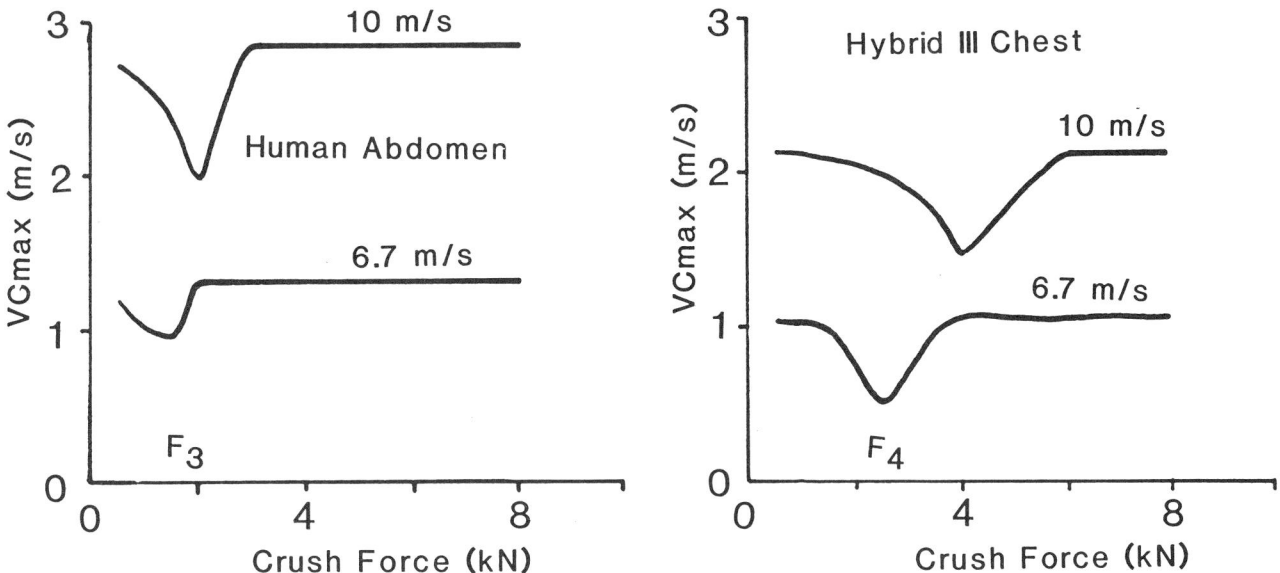

Fig 16: The Viscous criterion, [VC]max, when the Hybrid III chest is struck from the front or the human abdomen is struck from the side by a 100 Kg mass at 6.7 m/s or 10 m/s with a crushable interface. [VC]max is the criterion used here because it is the most predictive criterion for impact exposure at those velocities.

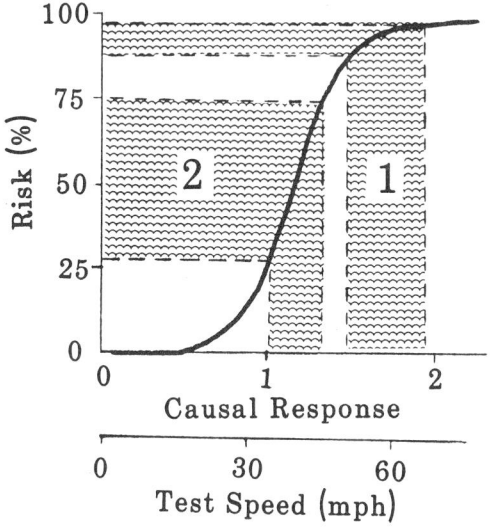

Fig 17: Interrelationship between injury risk, injury criteria, and test speed. Zones 1 and 2 represent 25% reduction of biomechanical response, but 10% and 50% reduction of injury risk respectively.

Hybrid III at 6.7 m/s yields at 2.5 kN, which is less than one third the crush force as that indicated by the Blak Tuffy. In fact, Hybrid III tests indicate that the optimal choices suggested by the Blak Tuffy tests at 6.7 m/s or 10 m/s have no effect on Hybrid III response and will not reduce human injury risk over the full range of impact velocity (Fig 19a). Those EA structures simply behave like rigid ones in a Hybrid III test. Since the human abdomen in a lateral impact is even softer than the Hybrid III chest, countermeasures suggested by the Blak Tuffy are also irrelevant for abdominal protection (Fig 19b).

APPLICATIONS IN STEERING SYSTEM DESIGN

Based on the Viscous criterion, the sled and impactor experiments demonstrated that abdominal organ injury was induced within the rapid compression phase before the energy absorbing column began to compress. Since the upper abdomen was interacting with the steering wheel at that time, countermeasure must also be focused on the wheel, and not the column. In contrast, had peak chest compression or spinal acceleration been chosen as the criteria to guide the development of a countermeasure, attention could have been focused on column compression characteristics. An opportunity to improve abdominal protection would have been missed.

Changing the steering wheel characteristics was thus the appropriate countermeasure for abdominal injury. Softening the spokes to yield on impact could reduce the velocity of deformation, the abdominal Viscous response, hence the injury risk for the abdomen. However, that same design could concentrate the load on the thorax to an area no bigger than the hub of the wheel, as the wheel plane retreats behind the hub. Such a design could reduce chest protection in the more severe impacts. These understanding, in concert with the knowledge that injury was induced within the rapid compression phase, had lead to the introduction of the GM *self aligning* steering

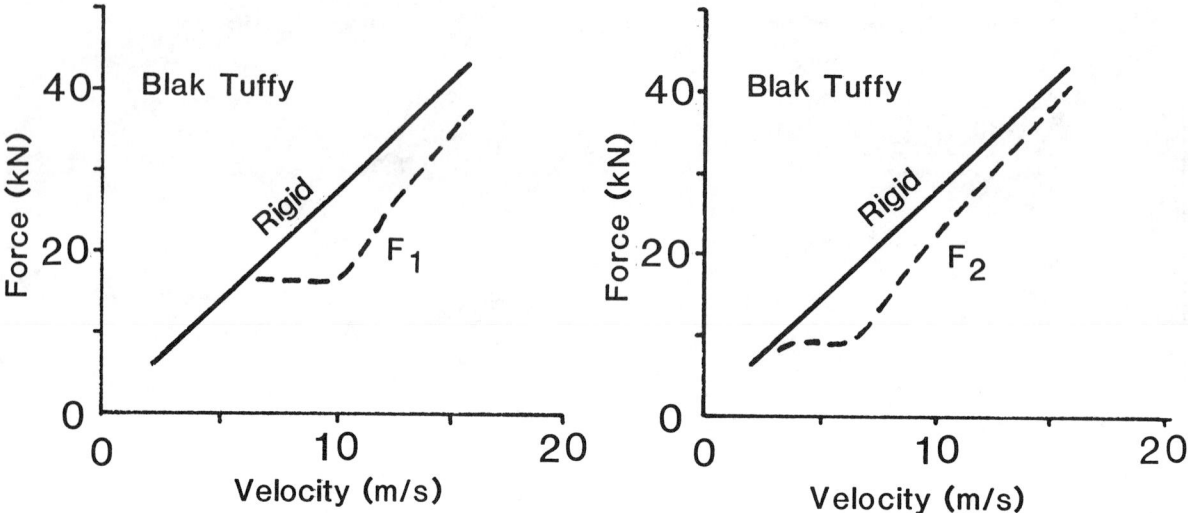

Fig 18: Comparison of Peak impact force in a Blak tuffy test over a range of impact velocity for a rigid impact, and impacts with paddings optimized for 6.7 m/s (Crush force F_1 = 8.5 kN) and 10 m/s (Crush force F_2 = 16.0 kN).

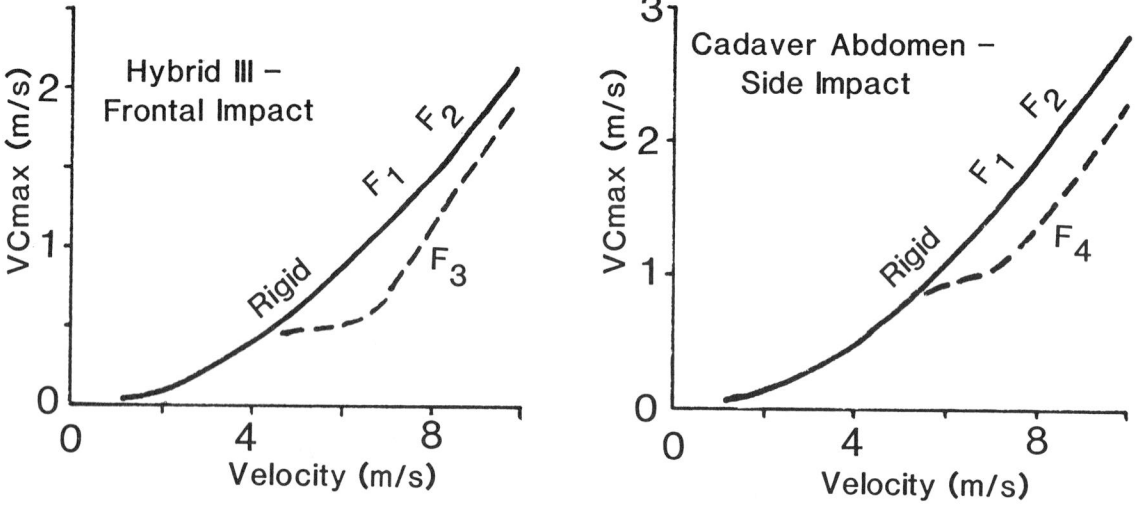

Fig 19: [VC]max for a rigid impact and the F_1 and F_2 (Fig 15) padded impacts are identical over the range of impact velocity for a frontal impact of the Hybrid III (a) or a side impact of the human abdomen (b). However, padding optimized at 6.7 m/s for the Hybrid III (Crush force F_3 = 2.5 kN) and the human abdomen (Crush force F_4 = 1.8 kN) show substantial reduction of [VC]max in the critical range between 1 to 2 m/s.

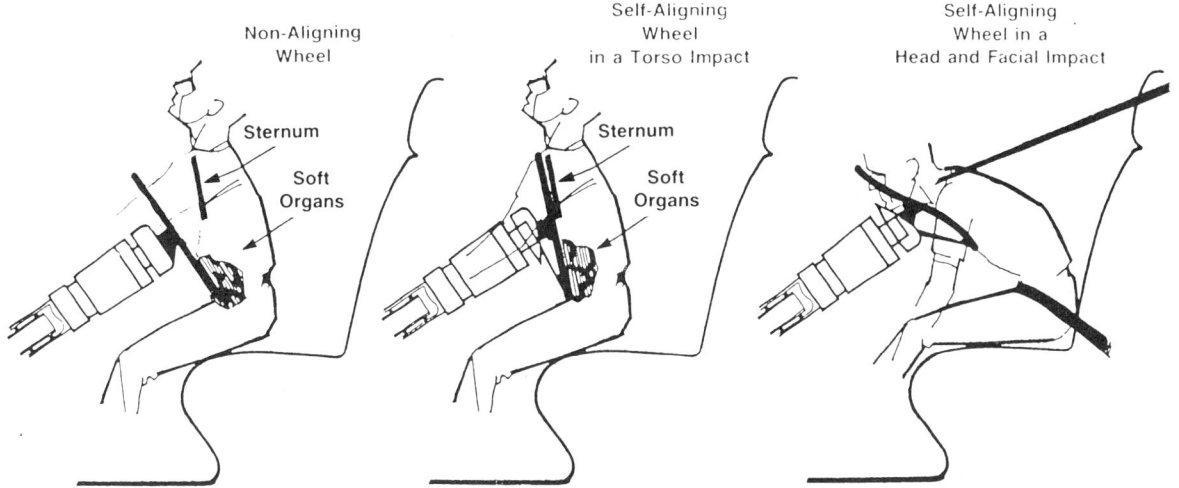

Fig 20: *Self Aligning* steering wheel which conforms its wheel plane to the torso. The new design was developed based on the torso Viscous response.

wheel, which aligns its wheel plane to the torso of an occupant, reducing abdominal injury risks in the initial phase of impact. And the wheel maintains its shape and load transfer to the chest and shoulder in a chest impact (Fig 20).

SIDE IMPACT

The human chest and abdomen in a side impact are compliant structures. Unlike the spine of the SID, the human spine deforms readily upon impact along with the rest of the torso (Fig 21). We examined the efficacy of a soft padding suitable for protection of the human thorax, and tested the padding on the SID (Fig 22a). We also examined the efficacy of a stiff padding effective in reducing TTI(d) in the SID, and tested the padding against the human thorax (Fig 22b). Due to the high inertial forces generated by the SID rib mass, the soft padding crushed very early. From then on, rib acceleration in the padded test reversed to that of a rigid impact. TTI(d) was reduced only marginally. However, that same padding was most effective in mitigating human injury within the impact environment where the potential pay off was high (1 m/s < [VC]max < 2 m/s). Based on TTI(d) in a SID test, an engineer would choose the stiff pad, which reduces TTI(d) to below 80g over a wide range of impact velocity. Such a stiff pad performed well because it could sustain the high, non-human like, inertial forces generated by the SID thorax. Peak rib acceleration was, therefore, reduced over a wide range of impact velocity. Unfortunately, the same pad would have zero benefit over a rigid impact at any velocity for an actual occupant.

The NHTSA explained that the SID was designed to be used with TTI(d) as the injury criterion, and within that context, the SID was an adequate ATD. The simulation here demonstrates that the

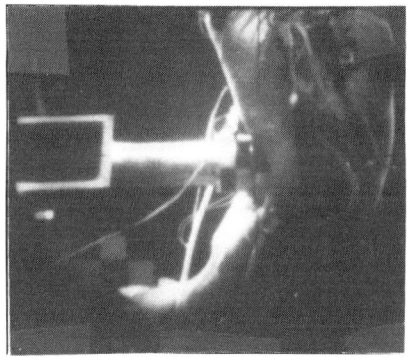

Fig 21: Deformation of the human spine in a side impact: Unlike the spine of the SID, the human spine is made of vertebrae linked by muscles and tendons, and it deforms freely upon impact.

SID/TTI(d) combination might lead to ineffective designs. The claim to biofidelity for the SID was made on the basis of skeletal acceleration or force alone. However, reproducing the peak acceleration at some skeletal locations simply implies that the aggregate response to peak input force at those locations has been reproduced. Those forces include variable components of whole body acceleration and torso deformation. Furthermore, a non-human like, inertial chest might be tuned to provide similar peak acceleration for a few test conditions by padding the dummy.

An injury criterion alludes to a mechanism of injury by its physical meaning. We are concerned with the lack of physical basis of TTI, the predecessor of TTI(d). To illustrate a possible result of injury prediction based on statistics

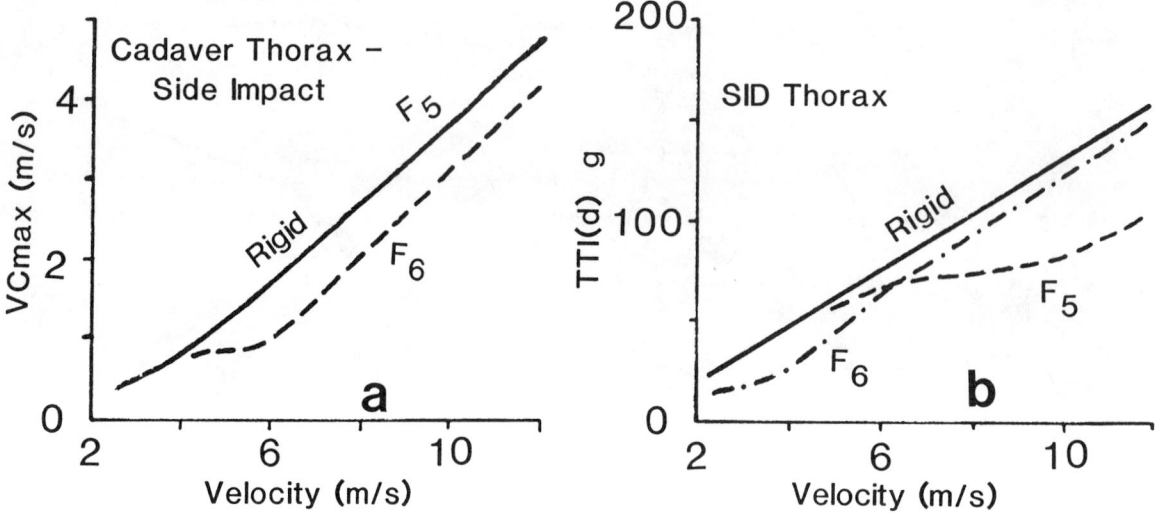

Fig 22: a: The human thorax in a rigid side impact, and side impacts with a stiff pad (Crush force $F_5 = 9$ kN) and a soft pad (Crush force $F_6 = 1.6$ kN). b: The SID in a rigid side impact, and side impacts with the same pads. Meeting the requirements for the SID does not ensure protection of the human thorax.

alone, a discriminate analysis was performed by GM's mathematics department to determine the best indicator of 'hard thorax' injury based on the published data from the University of Heidelberg (14). Pelvic acceleration was found to be the single, strongest correlate with chest injury. When the analysis examined all possible combinations of independent variables within the data set, it found the combination of age.mass, age.pelvic acceleration, and pelvic acceleration.rib acceleration to be the best discriminator of injury. That combination misclassified only twelve of the forty-one possible cases (29%) within the data set, whereas TTI misclassified twenty of the forty-seven possible cases (43%).

APPLICATIONS IN SIDE IMPACT

Before contemplation of countermeasure designs, it is essential to determine which injury mechanisms are pertinent in side crashes. We examined the injury pattern of the drivers in side crashes contained in the MIC files from 1981 to 1985. Both belted and unbelted drivers in left side crashes were included, but ejected drivers were excluded. We particularly examined the relationship between rib fractures and internal injuries of the thoracic and upper abdominal organs contained in the MIC files. As in any accident file, uninjured drivers accounted for the vast majority of the cases (Table 5). Among the drivers who were injured, the fifty-three cases of rib fractures only were the most common. They were mostly minor. There were two fatalities - possibly massively crushed chest, and three other cases of severe injuries (AIS=4). In eighteen other cases, internal injuries and rib fractures were observed in the

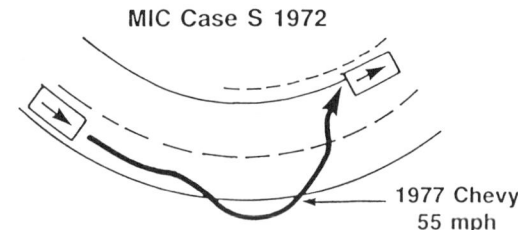

Driver: Male, 47 years, 170 lb, 71 in.

Injury: Laceration of the heart — AIS 6 Fatal
No rib fractures

Fig 23: Highlight of a case of fatal internal chest injury with no rib fractures.

Rib Fractures

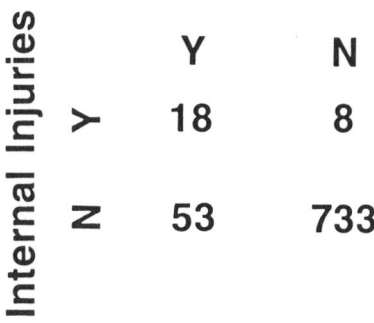

Table 5: Interdependence between rib fractures and internal torso injuries of drivers in side impacts. Based on MIC files from '81 - '85.

same occupant. Only three cases within that data subset might plausibly be classified as flail chest. In nine of the eighteen cases, the driver clearly incurred more severe internal injuries than skeletal injuries. There were eight cases of internal injuries with no rib fractures. In one of those eight cases, the driver had a fatal rupture of the heart, but no ribs were broken (Fig 23). We conclude that flail chest, or even rib fractures, is not a prerequisite for internal injury. Contrary to the hypothesis of Walfisch and Tarriere et al (15), we found in our studies that the severity of rib fractures were not an indicator of actual internal injuries. However, skeletal trauma remains to be an important indicator of the overall severity of trauma in cadaver tests. The lack of tissue function in cadaver subjects eliminates any patho-physiological trauma response and may also alter soft tissue injury response.

The cases of rib fractures alone, or rib fractures with minor internal injuries might have been induced by a viscous mechanism, a crushing mechanism, or their combination. The cases of internal injury alone, or internal injuries with minor rib fractures, were typical of injury induced by a viscous mechanism. Safety evaluation of a side crash should, therefore, be based on the Viscous criterion, which indicates the potential for internal and skeletal injury from a high velocity impact, and the occupant should be protected concurrently against crushing injury by a compression limit. Since the Viscous criterion and the compression criterion are based on the same chest deflection data, the countermeasures against the two mechanisms of injury are complimentary.

As in the case of frontal impact protection, side impact protection can be optimized only after the instant of maximum injury risk is identified. Based on barrier tests using the NHTSA procedure (Fig 24), the moving barrier impacts the struck car 20 - 30 ms before the door contacts the surrogate. Door velocity at contact is estimated to be 60 - 70 % of the coasting velocity of the barrier. Intrusion of the door into the passenger compartment continues after the peak torso Viscous response. With reference to the struck car, the surrogate will appear to be struck by the door. Those observations of a barrier test suggest that padding can potentially be an effective countermeasure for a given structure. Further stiffening of the side structure may effectively reduce the velocity of door contact on the occupant. However, a systems engineering of the side structure is needed to assure that the occupant does not impact the stiffened structure at a the same severity. Those observations also suggest why injury may not correlate with maximum door intrusion since injury by a viscous mechanism will occur well before maximum door intrusion. Any relationship between maximum door crush and injury is also

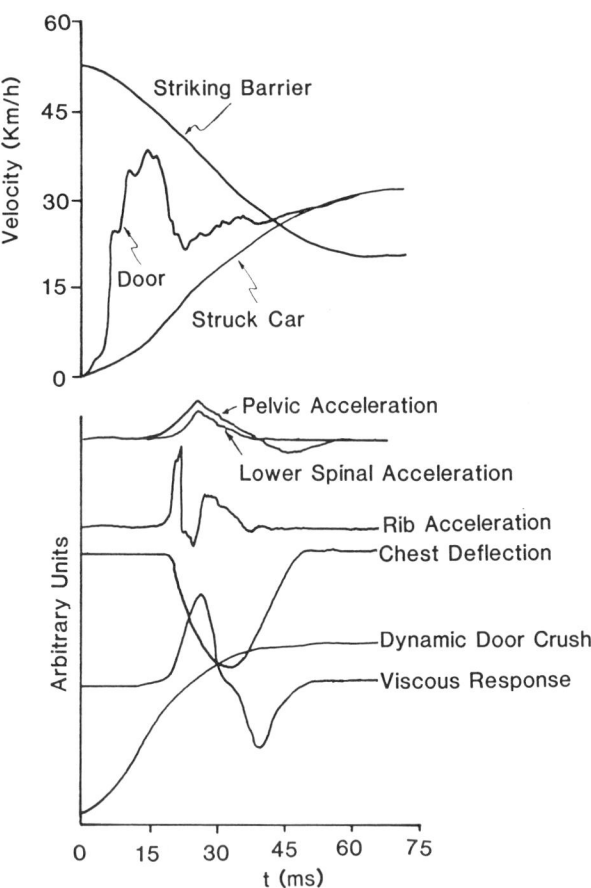

Fig 24: Composite representation of a parked car struck by a NHTSA barrier. a: Velocity of the barrier, the struck car, and the struck door. b: Impact of the pelvis and the rib cage.

due to their common link to the overall crash severity, and no cause-and-effect relationship exists. Similar misunderstanding of the relationship between steering system deformation and occupant injury was discussed elsewhere (16).

SUMMARY AND CONCLUSIONS:

1. Injury is induced in a blunt impact when the Viscous response of the subject exceeds its tolerance.

2. The Viscous response underlies the etiological injury event, and is highly correlative with injury outcome.

3. A valid injury criterion is most meaningful if it is applied to a biofidelic dummy.

4. Due to the SID's inertial properties, it will not lead to optimal side impact countermeasures. Additional development is needed.

5. In a side impact, the occupant needs to be protected against skeletal and internal injury by a high velocity impact and by a slow crushing impact.

6. A well-designed laboratory test should represent the typical field accident.

ACKNOWLEDGEMENTS

The authors thank Dennis Andrzejak for his participation in the surgical preparation, Franco Gamero of the Safety Research and Development Laboratories for the MIC data, Tom Lorenzen of GM's Mathematics Department for his discriminant analysis, and Corbin Asbury for his contribution in the data analysis. We also thank John Horsch, John Melvin and Mary Miller for their discussion and review of the manuscript.

REFERENCES

1. Horsch J.D., Lau I.V., Viano D.C., Andrzejak D.V.: Mechanism of Abdominal Injury by Steering Wheel Loading. *Twenty-ninth Stapp Car Crash Conference.* SAE Paper 851724, 1985.

2. Lau I.V., Horsch J.D., Viano D.C., Andrzejak D.V.: Biomechanics of Liver Injury by Steering Wheel Loading. *J. Trauma* 27: 225 - 235, 1987.

3. Lau I.V., Viano D.C.: The Viscous Criterion - Bases and Applications of an Injury Severity Index for Soft Tissues. *Thirtieth Stapp Car Crash Conference.* SAE Paper 861882, 1986.

4. Viano D.C., Lau I.V.: A Viscous Tolerance Criterion for Soft Tissue Injury Assessment. *J. Biomechanics* In press, 1988.

5. Viano D.C.: Evaluation of the Benefit of Energy-Absorbing Material in Side Impact Protection: Part I. *Thirty-first Stapp Car Crash Conference.* SAE Paper 872212, 1987.

6. Viano D.C.: Evaluation of the Benefit of Energy-Absorbing Material in Side Impact Protection: Part II. *Thirty-first Stapp Car Crash Conference.* SAE Paper 872213, 1987.

7. Viano D.C.: Evaluation of the SID Dummy and TTI Injury Criterion for Side Impact Testing. *Thirty-first Stapp Car Crash Conference.* SAE Paper 872208, 1987.

8. Lau I.V., Viano D.C.: Influence of Impact Velocity on the Severity of Nonpenetrating Hepatic Injury. *J. Trauma* 21: 115 - 123, 1981.

9. Kroell C.K., Schneider D.C., Nahum A.M.: Impact Tolerance and Response of the Human Thorax II. *Eighteenth Stapp Car Crash Conference.* Society of Automotive Engineers, 1974.

10. Viano D.C.: Thoracic Injury Potential. Proceedings of the *International Research Committee on the Biokinetics of Impact,* Lyon, France. 1978.

11. Di Lorenzo F.A.: Power and Bodily Injury. *Automotive Engineering Congress and Exposition* SAE Paper# 760014, Detroit, Michigan, 1976.

12. Kroell C.K., Allen S.D., Warner C.Y., Perl T.R.: Interrelationship of Velocity and Chest Compression in Blunt Thoracic Impact to Swine II. *Thirtieth Stapp Car Crash Conference.* SAE Paper 861881, 1986.

13. Rouhana S.W., Lau I.V., Ridella S.A.: Influence of Velocity and Forced Compression on the Severity of Abdominal Injury in Blunt, Nonpenetrating Lateral Impact. *J. Trauma* 25: 490 - 500, 1985.

14. Eppinger R.H., Marcus J.H., Morgan R.H.: Development of Dummy and Injury Index for NHTSA's Thoracic Side Impact Protection Research Program. *Government/Industry Meeting (Sponsor: SAE)* SAE Paper# 840885, 1984.

15. Walfisch G., Chamouard F. et al: Tolerance Limits and Mechanical Characteristics of the Human Thorax in Frontal and Side Impact and Transposition of these Characteristics into Protection Criteria. Proceedings of the *International Research Committee on the Biokinetics of Impact,* Cologne, Germany pp. 122 - 139, 1982.

16. Horsch J.D., Petersen K.R., Viano D.C.: Laboratory Study of Factors Influencing the Performance of Energy Absorbing Steering Systems. *SAE Paper#* 820475, 1982.

892433

The Effect of Door Topography on Abdominal Injury in Lateral Impact

Stephen W. Rouhana
General Motors Research Labs.

Charles K. Kroell
General Motors Research Labs.

ABSTRACT

Seventeen left lateral impact experiments were performed using anesthetized swine to determine the biomechanics of injury production in this impact mode. Two series of eight animals were used and one animal served as a control. In the first series of experiments, rigid thoracic and pelvic loading surfaces were separated by an "interplate gap" of 20.3 cm (8"). In the second series of experiments, the interplate gap was filled by a rigid plate mounted flush with the thoracic and pelvic loading surfaces. Impact velocities ranged from 7.2 to 15.0 m/s (about 15 to 30 mph).

Injury patterns for the liver, spleen, and rib cage were significantly different in the two series of experiments (level of significance > 90%). The causative factor responsible for the different injury outcomes was the interplate gap.

The conclusion of this report is that loading-surface discontinuities can cause significant injury. Therefore, in design of side doors and interiors, consideration should be given to the location of surface indentations (such as map pockets) as well as surface protuberances (such as armrests).

THE MECHANISMS AND MITIGATION OF INJURY in lateral impacts have been the focus of recent research by the automotive safety community. Much of that research is directed toward improved designs of anthropomorphic test devices. The original intent of this study was to further develop an experimental model for lateral impact induced injury using whole body sled tests with a porcine surrogate. The present paper describes an analysis of 17 experiments with 2 different loading surfaces. The test environment chosen was similar to that used in the side impact cadaver tests performed at the University of Heidelberg [see 9,10]*, and thus should allow comparison with an existing data base. The results of these experiments highlight the importance of loading conditions on side impact injury. They emphasize the need for additional research on side door and interior designs from the standpoint of biomechanical criteria, in addition to the traditional customer acceptance criteria of styling and function.

It has been well documented that injury to nearside occupants in lateral impact is primarily a consequence of contact with the side door surface [See for example, 11,15,19]. Similarly, it has been shown [11,17,18,20] that the shape, size, and compliance of the loading area influences the resulting injury.

The above mentioned studies report the effects of surface <u>protuberances</u> which cause injury when they are forcefully propelled into the thorax or abdomen. As will be shown, the analysis of the experiments performed in this study indicates that the inverse loading situation can also be injury producing. That is, surfaces with areas into which localized portions of the body can *extrude*, such as pockets in side doors, are also potentially injurious.

These results may become increasingly more significant as side door padding becomes a standard feature on vehicles since many of the proposed schemes suggest incorporation of zones of varying stiffness [5,7,8,12,21,22,23,24]

MATERIALS AND METHODS

Seventeen experiments were performed using a single porcine subject in each.* The 17 subjects were Landrace-Yorkshire crossbred males with an average mass of 50.9 ± 5.0 kg (112.0 ± 10.9 lbs). The subjects were pre-anesthetized by intramuscular injection of Acetylpromazine Maleate (0.37 mg/kg) and Ketamine HCl (33 mg/kg). They were then shaved and induced into deep surgical anesthesia by inhalation of Nitrous Oxide (50% for induction, 30% for maintenance) and Methoxyflurane (3% for induction, .75% for maintenance). Depth of anesthesia was assured by monitoring of heart rate, respiration rate and volume, blood pressure, and

---

* Numbers in brackets indicate references listed at the end of the paper.

---

* See footnote on next page.

neurological reflexes.

After surgical anesthesia was achieved via mask inhalation, a tracheostomy was performed and an endotracheal tube inserted to provide closed circuit anesthesia. A respiration rate sensor was attached to the endotracheal tube, and ECG leads were connected to the subject to monitor lead II. A Millar® pressure transducer was inserted into the right carotid artery and advanced to a position approximately one inch above the aortic valve in the arch of the aorta. Next, the subject was instrumented with accelerometers and photographic targets as follows: A uniaxial accelerometer was placed in the intercostal space between ribs 5 & 6 or 6 & 7 on the left side of the subject. The transducer mount was a bridge configuration similar to those used by Nusholtz [13] (Fig. 1a). Installation required blunt dissection of the muscles over the 5th intercostal space, where the interspace intersects a transverse plane through a point halfway between the palpated center of the xiphoid and mid-sternum. Following the dissection, the periosteum of each rib was elevated around its entire circumference. The accelerometer mount was then wire wrapped to the two exposed ribs using .025 " stainless steel safety aircraft wire. After the wire was tightened with an aircraft wire twister, four to eight pointed set screws were screwed through tapped holes in the mount. This caused the entire mount to rise and removed any slack in the safety wire while simultaneously anchoring the mount in the periosteum of the ribs via the cone points on the screws. With this procedure, fixation of the accelerometer mount was accomplished without penetration of the thoracic wall, thereby precluding pneumothorax.

Another uniaxial accelerometer (Fig. 1b) was screw mounted to the 6th rib on the right side of the subject, directly opposite the left side accelerometer. Since the impacts were to the left side of all subjects in this study, the left side will be called *nearside*, and the right side will be called *farside* throughout the remainder of this report. Two uniaxial accelerometers were also attached to the spinous process in the same transverse plane as the rib accelerometers using a clamp-on mount (Fig. 1c). These accelerometers were mounted orthogonally such that one axis of sensitivity was oriented ventro-dorsally and the other transversely (i.e., in the direction of sled travel). The spinal and farside rib mounts also served as bases for photographic targets.

---

* The rationale and experimental protocol for the use of an animal model in this program have been reviewed by the Research Laboratories' Animal Research Committee. The research follows procedures outlined in the <u>Guide for the Care and Use of Laboratory Animals</u>, U.S. Department of Health and Human Services, Public Health Service, National Institutes of Health NIH Publication 85-23, Revised 1985, and Public Health Service <u>Policy on Humane Care and Use of Laboratory Animals by Awardee Institutions</u>, NIH Guide for Grants and Contracts, Vol. 14, No. 8, June 25, 1985, and complies with the provisions of the <u>Animal Welfare Act</u> of 1966 (P.L. 89-544), as amended in 1970 (P.L. 91-579) and 1976 (P.L. 94-270), and the Food Security Act of 1985 (P.L. 99-158).

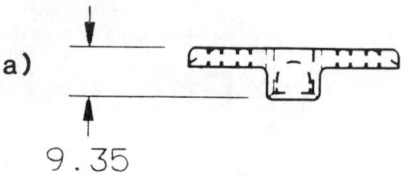
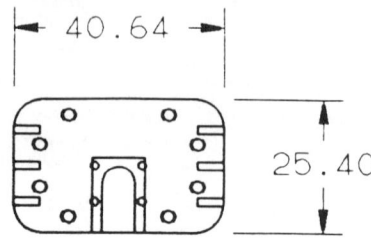

Figure 1a. Nearside rib accelerometer mount wire wraps onto ribs 5&6 or 6&7 after periosteal elevation. Cone pointed screws are then advanced into contact with the rib to provide traction and grips which keep the mount from moving.

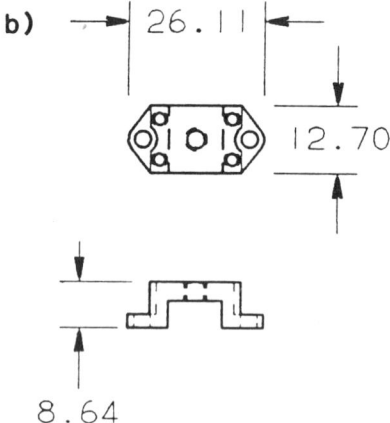

Figure 1b. Farside rib accelerometer mount screws onto rib 5 or 6. Cone pointed screws are advanced as in a).

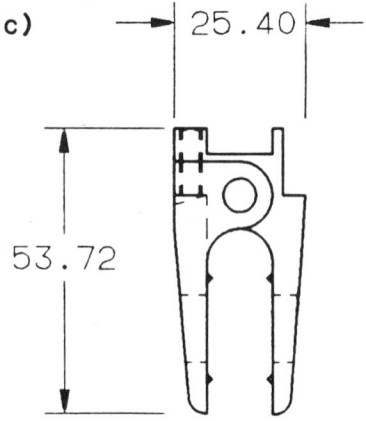

Figure 1c. Spinal accelerometer mount clamps onto spinous process dorsal to the location of the rib mounts and in the same transverse plane.

In eight of the experiments, the subject had a trans-thoracic rod surgically implanted and fixed to the accelerometer mount on the nearside ribs. The purpose of the rod was to serve as a photographic target which would allow accurate measurement of the absolute skeletal deflection as it moved relative to another target fixed to a rib on the opposite side of the subject. This measurement was necessary to determine the effects of skeletal compression on the organs within the ribcage. The rod was made of stainless steel tubing (.148" O.D.) with a round nylon tip. It was inserted through the intercostal muscles after the periosteal elevation mentioned previously, but before the rib mount was wired on.

The rod was pushed through the intercostal muscles and parietal pleura using just enough force to break through the pleura. When it was just inside the thoracic cavity, a purse-string suture was tightened and tied around it to effect a seal and prevent pneumothorax. The rod was then laid down along the original incision line pointed in a caudal-ventral direction, and advanced cautiously until it contacted the diaphragm. After contact with the diaphragm, the direction of motion of the tip was changed to medial-ventral. The tip was "walked" along the left diaphragm to the mediastinum, pushed through, and "walked" along the right diaphragm until it contacted the farside thoracic wall. It was then "walked" along the farside ribs until perpendicular to a sagittal plane at which point it was pushed through the farside wall. The rod was ball joint connected to the nearside accelerometer mount, which was then wire wrapped to the nearside ribs. (See the appendix in [16] for additional details concerning this trans-thoracic rod and its installation procedure.)

After implanting the instrumentation, the subject was transported under anesthesia and placed in a lateral impact fixture on a Hyge Sled. The fixture consisted of a smooth surface on which the subject was placed, an impact wall made up of two load plates (similar to those used in [9] and [10]; see below), and a rebound net to manage the subject's post-impact motion (Fig. 2). The subject was placed on the sled fixture oriented transversely and positioned 18" from the loading surface.

In these experiments, the sled was used as a velocity generator. That is, the fixture was designed so that the impact took place after the primary acceleration of the sled, while it was traveling at nearly constant velocity. As the sled accelerated, inertia and low surface friction kept the subject virtually stationary until struck by the loading plates. When impact occurred, the sled was moving at the preselected velocity which was nominally 15, 20, 25, or 30 mph. The compression and kinematic response of the subject was monitored by an overhead camera mounted on the sled and by two offboard cameras at the same height as the subject with a view perpendicular to the direction of sled travel.

The surviving subject was reconnected to the anesthesia machine and monitored immediately after impact, followed by administration of euthanasia using T-61 or an overdose of Methoxyflurane, or both. A gross thoraco-abdominal necropsy was then performed, and in the last 9 experiments tissue samples from the lungs, heart, liver, spleen, kidneys, and intestines were also collected and sent to a pathology laboratory for microscopic analysis. Necropsy consisted of exposure of the abdominal cavity by midsagittal incision, followed by exposure of the thoracic cavity by excision of the sternum. The character and severity of each thoracic and abdominal injury was then noted and documented according to the Abbreviated Injury Scale (AIS-85) which was developed for coding injuries to humans.

The experiments were performed in two series. The first series of experiments consisted of 8 subjects. The sled fixture had two load plates separated by a gap (Fig. 3). Each plate was mounted to an array of three load cells, which were in turn mounted rigidly on the impact wall. The larger load plate was intended to measure the force against the subject's thoracic region, and the smaller load plate to measure the force against the subject's pelvic region. The gap between the plates was 8" wide, 3.25" deep, and 13" high. This load plate arrangement was chosen because it resembled the arrangement used in the NHTSA sponsored experiments at the University of Heidelberg upon which the Thoracic Trauma Index is based [see 9,10]. The load plates were geometrically

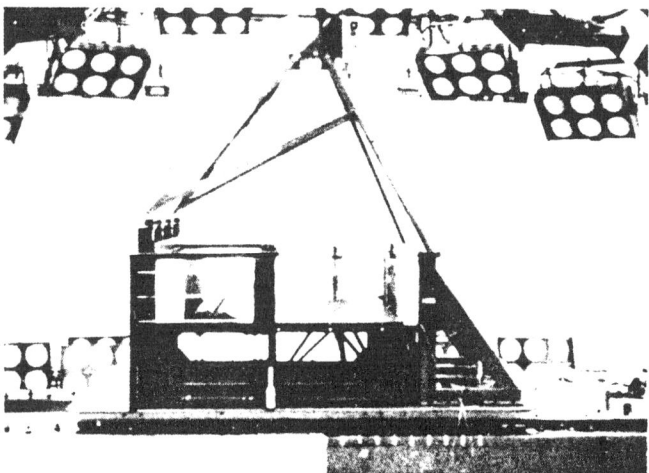

Figure 2. Schematic of lateral impact sled fixture used to generate the impact velocity desired. The impact wall is on the right, with the direction of sled travel towards the left

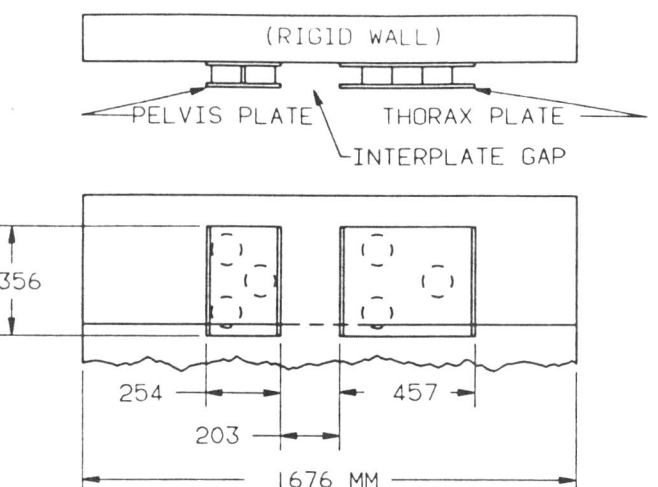

Figure 3. Load measuring arrangement with the interplate gap.

scaled so the ratio of the length of the porcine rib cage to the length of the thorax plate used in these experiments, was the same as the ratio of the 50th percentile human male rib cage to the length of the thorax plate used in the Heidelberg experiments. This would allow comparison of our results with an established human cadaver data base. In addition to the interplate gap, the subjects in the first series each had a transthoracic rod implanted.

The second series of experiments consisted of 8 subjects and a control subject which was instrumented exactly as the others but not subjected to impact. The interplate gap was filled in this series by a rigid steel plate which was mounted flush with the thoracic and pelvic plates (Fig. 4). Forces imposed on the plate filling the interplate gap were not recorded, and none of these subjects had a trans-thoracic rod.

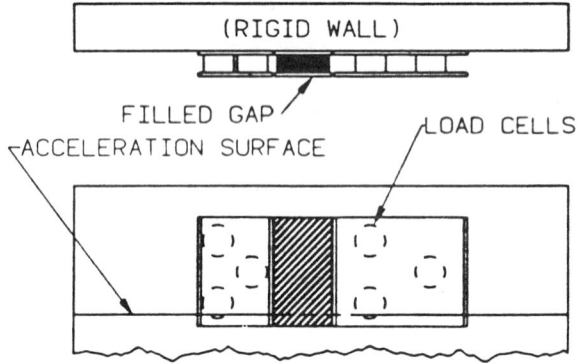

Figure 4. Load measuring arrangement with the filled interplate gap.

RESULTS

Chi-squared analysis was performed on the injury outcomes from the two series of experiments (Table 1). The Chi-squared test determines if two groups of data are independent of common factors. The results showed that the number of AIS $>= 3$ injuries to the liver, spleen, and ribs was significantly greater in the gap/rod series than in the no-gap/no-rod series of experiments. The level of significance was 90% for injury to the liver and ribs, and 97.5% for injury to the spleen (Table 2).

The closest organs to the rod were the lungs, heart, and dome of the diaphragm (Fig. 5). When implanted, the rod was situated across the thorax approximately 2.5-4 cm (1-1.5 inches) cranial from the dome of the diaphragm. The lacerations in all three of the livers that were seriously injured in the first series of experiments were remote from this location. One laceration occurred at the hilar junction of the caudal vena cava with the right lateral lobe; another laceration was noted in the left lateral lobe on the visceral surface of the liver (the side opposite the rod); the other two lacerations were in the left lateral lobe on the parietal surface of the liver, but these were at the lateral edges away from the dome of the diaphragm. Minor hepatic injuries occurred mainly on the visceral surface of the liver, but in two cases occurred on the parietal surface (one subject had a superficial laceration in the right lateral lobe, and another subject had two contusions with one in the right medial lobe and another in the left medial lobe). Therefore, there was only one case in which the rod was in the vicinity of an injury and was a possible causative factor of the injury. In addition, most of the liver lacerations occurred in the left lobes of the liver. That is consistent with being caused by the impact wall, and the edge of the thoracic load plate.

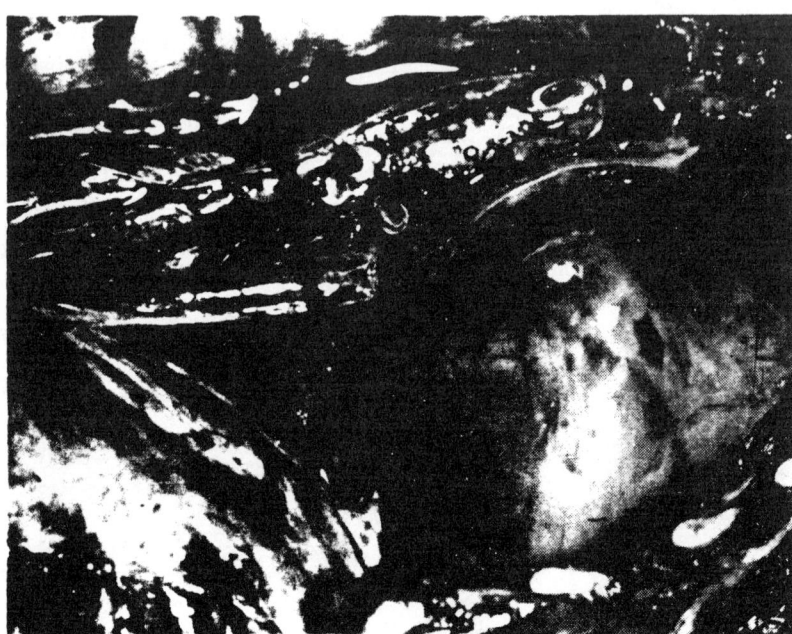

Figure 5. Typical positioning of the rod *in situ*. The rod lies just ventral to the caudal vena cava, posterior to the heart, and cranial to the diaphragm. The accessory lobe of the right lung (typically not seen in humans) can be seen wrapped around the rod

TABLE 1. Results of Experiments

Test No.	Velocity (mph)	Test Series	Kidney	Liver	Spleen	Intest	Rib	Lungs	Heart
1	21	Gap/Rod	0	4	2	0	1	0	0
2	21	"	2	0	2	0	4**	3	0
3	25	"	0	0	5	2	3	4	0
4	26	"	0	4	3	2	4	4	3
5	30	"	0	2	5	4	4	4	3
6	33	"	0	2	5	2	5	3	3
7	17	"	0	2	2	0	3	0	0
8	16	"	0	3	0	0	0	4	0
9	21	NoGap/NoRod	0	0	2	2	0	0	0
10	27	"	2	0	2	2	2	3	0
11	17	"	0	0	0	2	2	3	4
12	26	"	2	0	0	2	4	4	0
13	20	"	0	0	2	2	0	3	4
14	16	"	0	0	0	0	0	0	0
15	31	"	3	0	2	2	4	4	0
16***	0	"	0	0	0	0	0	0	0
17	25	"	0	0	2	2	0	4	2

* 1985 Version
** Rib fracture due to accelerometer mount
*** Control experiment - Subject instrumented but not subjected to impact

TABLE 2. Results of Chi^2 Analysis

Organ Injured	# AIS < 3 Tests 1-8	# AIS ≥ 3 Tests 1-8	# AIS < 3 Tests 9-17*	# AIS ≥ 3 Tests 9-17*	Significant Difference ?	Confid. Level
Abdomen	2	6	7	1	Yes	97.5%
Heart	5	3	6	2	No	90%
Liver	5	3	8	0	Yes	90%
Lungs	2	6	2	6	No	99.5%
Ribs	2	6	6	2	Yes	95%
Ribs(w/o Test 2)	2	5	6	2	Yes	90%
Spleen	4	4	8	0	Yes	95%

In the second series of experiments there were no injuries noted to any of the livers examined at necropsy. The liver from one of the subjects showed signs of hemorrhage microscopically, but did not show gross signs of injury. Therefore, it was considered to be uninjured for purposes of comparison.

The spleen is located on the left side, dorsal to the stomach. In this location it is farther removed from the rod than the liver, and as a result it is less likely to be injured by the rod. However, the anatomical position of the subject's spleen in these tests was exactly along the edge of the thoracic load plate (Fig. 6). The centerline of the spleen ran between ribs 13 and 14, right along the edge of the plate. The plate edge, therefore, seems to be the most likely candidate as the causative factor for injury to the spleen.

In the second series of experiments there were no serious splenic injuries. The spleen was contused in 5 of the 8 subjects examined. Splenic contusion in impacts at velocities between 15 and 30 mph is not surprising given the organ's anatomical location and proximity to the loading surface.

According to the Abbreviated Injury Scale, when 4 or more consecutive ribs are fractured, with or without hemothorax, the injury is considered to be serious (AIS ≥ 3). In 6 out of 8 experiments involving the gap, 4 or more consecutive nearside ribs fractured causing serious injury. The fractured ribs were in the range of ribs 10-15 (remote from the rod) with the closest fracture at least 4 ribs away from the location of the rod in all but one case. In experiment number 2, the two ribs on which the nearside accelerometer mount was attached and another adjacent rib fractured. It appears that this fracture was caused by a stress concentration at the edge of the accelerometer mount. Therefore, a second Chi-squared analysis was performed which excluded experiment number 2. The difference in injury potential between gap/rod tests and no-gap/no-rod tests, was still significant although only at the 90% level of significance instead of the 95% level.

In the second series of experiments, only 2 of the 8 subjects sustained serious injuries to the ribs (serious means ≥ 4 consecutive ribs fractured). In both cases the consecutive rib fractures occurred in the last 5 ribs and in close proximity to the junction of the rib with the vertebral body.

As seen in Fig. 6, the edge of the thoracic load plate was aligned between ribs 12 and 15 when the subject was positioned on the sled fixture. Therefore, it is reasonable to assume that the plate edge and interplate gap were responsible for the higher incidence of rib fractures.

DISCUSSION

Injuries to the spleen, liver, and ribs were of significantly greater severity in the series of experiments with the interplate gap and the trans-thoracic rod. Thus, either the presence of the rod, the presence of the interplate gap, or both were responsible for the difference. We believe the interplate gap was the causative factor and that the rod did not play a role in the aggravation of injury frequency or severity. The reasoning in support of this hypothesis lies in the similarity of pulmonary injury in the two series of experiments, and in the relatively large distance between the rod and the abdominal organs that were injured.

Although the rod traversed the thorax in contact with the lungs, the severity of pulmonary injury was unchanged when comparing injuries sustained with the gap and rod versus without. Since the rod did not injure the lungs with which it was in contact, it is unlikely that it injured abdominal organs located further away from it. Therefore, the increased injury severity to the organs not in contact with the lungs is more likely due to the impacting surface.

Examination of Tables 1 and 2 shows that with the interplate gap there was significantly greater risk of serious rib, liver, and spleen injury in these lateral impacts. As seen in Fig. 7, the subject's abdomen tended to *extrude* into the gap by virtue of its inertia and compliance. This filling of the gap was accomplished by bending around the edge of the load plates, which undoubtedly caused increased stress in the organs involved. Although the plate edges were rounded with a 1/2" radius and thus were not sharp, the stiffness discontinuity between the plate edge and the gap into which the organs extruded, probably caused stress concentrations which resulted in the injuries.

The limbs of the subjects in these experiments were positioned so that they were out of the way of the impact with the wall. The forelimbs were stretched out cranially and the hind limbs were stretched out caudally. Therefore, the influence of "arm" position on injuries caused by gaps is not known. Cesari, et al. [4] analyzed pendulum data which suggested that the human arm may protect the thorax at low speed, but noted that the type of injuries did not seem to be affected by an interposed arm.

As mentioned, these studies were designed to resemble the NHTSA sponsored studies at the University of Heidelberg upon which their side impact data are based. In some of those tests there was also a gap, but not enough injury information was available to determine any increased injury severity from that gap. In addition,

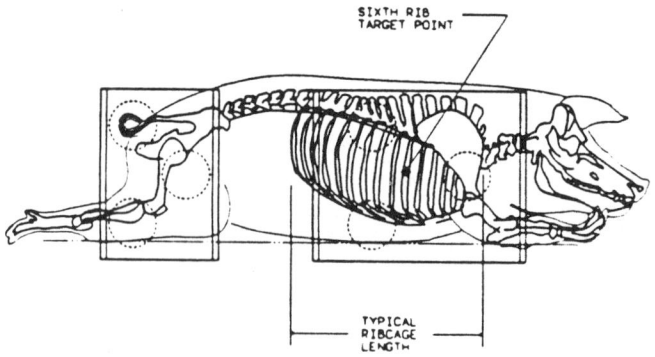

Figure 6. Relative position of the porcine thorax to the load plates and interplate gap. Thorax length has been geometrically scaled to the length of the thorax plate. In each experiment the subject was positioned so that the centerline of the thorax plate would contact the sixth rib.

the gap in our experiments was larger than that in the Heidelberg experiments since it was geometrically scaled to the larger porcine thoracic length. Thus there may be some critical gap size, above which increased injury production occurs, and below which no aggravation of injuries occurs.

All eight subjects in the first series of experiments died spontaneously. In the second series of experiments, the four subjects in the lower velocity impacts (< 24.6 mph) survived, and the four subjects in the higher velocity impacts (> 24.6 mph) died spontaneously. All cases of spontaneous death appear to be related to failure of the respiratory system. In the first series, the probable cause of death was pneumothorax induced around the transthoracic rod during impact. The rod entered the thorax through the intercostal muscles which were difficult to seal well enough to prevent the passage of air during the impact. In the second series, one possible cause of death was suffocation due to massive hemoptysis or coughing up blood (with the blood blocking the respiratory passages). Hemoptysis is a common symptom of pulmonary contusion but is usually not fatal in humans [1,6,14].

Alternatively, in studies of blast injuries to various species Benzinger [3] noted that "almost all animals exposed to blast near the lethal limit while (under anesthesia) died of respiratory paralysis. No other findings were made which would explain their death." Two of the four subjects which died spontaneously in these tests had respiratory arrest within 8 seconds of impact. One subject had respiratory arrest 52 seconds after impact, and one respirometer stopped functioning 4 seconds after impact but during a period of apnea that had lasted 1.5 seconds. In all four cases, blood pressure remained at pre-impact levels at least until after respiration ceased. (Blood pressure reached zero in 2-4 minutes for all 4 tests.) Therefore, respiratory arrest by some reflex mechanism or due to depressed respiratory centers while under anesthesia was the likely cause of death in the experiments in which the subjects died spontaneously.

Pulmonary, renal, intestinal, and myocardial injuries were indistinguishable between the two series of experiments. Typically the pulmonary, intestinal, and myocardial contusions were of minor severity, and there were no or very minor renal contusions. Then, in comparison to the experiments with the gap, those with the flat continuous wall produced relatively minor and fewer injuries.

It is striking that the injuries were not more severe in the experiments without the gap especially those performed at very high impact velocities (which are also subject delta-v's). This leads to the conclusion that in addition to reducing the impact velocity, it appears to be beneficial to preserve the shape of the impinging surface.

It has been shown that for the subjects of these experiments, lateral impact against a flat, rigid surface was less injurious than impact against a rigid surface which has the continuity of the surface broken by a gap. Therefore, indentations should be evaluated in the design of side door interiors. For example, from a biomechanical standpoint, the load distributing properties of doors in the area adjacent to a normally seated occupant's torso should be considered. When it is desired to incorporate pockets into door designs, a transition zone between regions of different stiffness may be enough to prevent the type of injury aggravation observed in these experiments. In contrast, since flat continuous surfaces have been shown to produce less severe injuries than those with

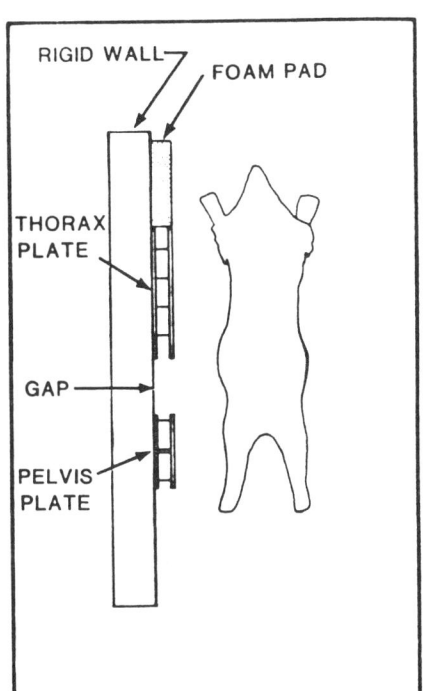
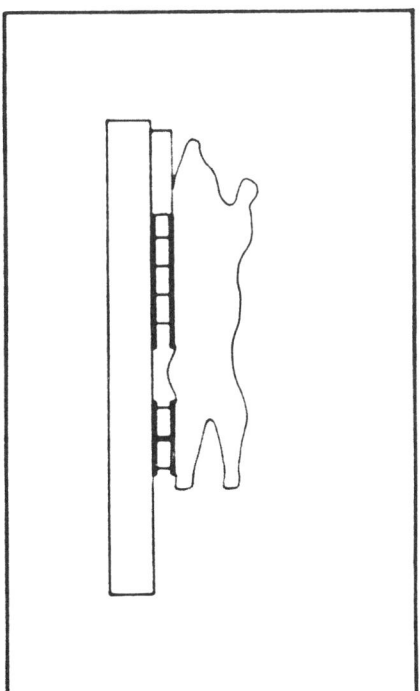
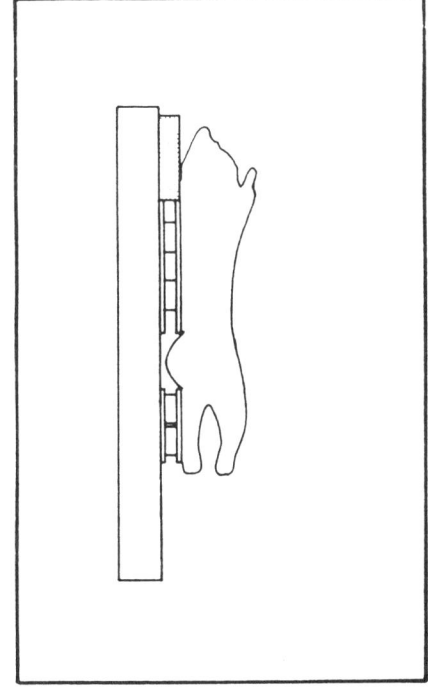

Figure 7. Line drawing of impact event showing an overhead view of the *extrusion* of the abdomen into the interplate gap. (Amount of extrusion has been exaggerated for demonstration purposes.)

sharp discontinuities in them, a possible side door design could be one that maintains a flat surface near the occupant despite external crush of the vehicle.

CONCLUSIONS

Injuries to the spleen, liver, and ribs were of significantly greater severity in the series of experiments with the interplate gap and the trans-thoracic rod than in the series with no gap and no rod. The injuries observed in the gap/rod test series were more likely due to edge of the impacting surface and the interplate gap and were not influenced by the rod. Therefore, surfaces with areas into which localized portions of the body can *extrude* are potentially injurious.

It is striking that injuries were not more severe in these tests, even at subject delta-v's of 30 mph. Therefore, in addition to reducing the velocity of an impinging surface, it appears to be beneficial to preserve a large, flat, continuous surface during impact.

ACKNOWLEDGEMENTS

A number of people contributed to the design and completion of these experiments. In particular the authors wish to acknowledge the contributions of: Stan Allen, Miriam Anvers, Don Barker, Howard Bender, Alexandra Brady, Dick Gasper, Jerry Horn, Ed Jedrzejczak, Richard Madeira, Joe McCleary, Kathy Smiler, and Tom Terzo for technical support; Ken Baron, Mary Foster, and Kerry Pellerino for computer support; Clyde Culver, and Ian Lau for helpful technical discussions.

The authors would also like to thank Dr. Guy Nusholtz for his kind assistance with accelerometer mounting techniques while at the UMTRI, and Drs. Rolf Eppinger, Jeff Marcus and Richard Morgan of the NHTSA for their FIR Filter, Weibull Programs, and detailed information on the tests sponsored by the NHTSA at the University of Heidelberg.

REFERENCES

1. Abbott, O.A.: "The Lung", In *Trauma to the Thorax and Abdomen,* (J.D. Martin, et al., Eds.), Charles C. Thomas, Springfield, 1969.

2. American Association for Automotive Medicine: "Abbreviated Injury Scale - 1985 Revision", Morton Grove, IL, 1985.

3. Benzinger, T.: "Physiological Effects of Blast in Air and Water" In *German Aviation Medicine - World War II,* Department of the Air Force, U.S. Government Printing Office, Vol. II, 1950.

4. Cesari, D., Ramet, M., and Bloch, J.: "Influence of Arm Position on Thoracic Injuries in Side Impact", Proceedings of the 25th Stapp Car Crash Conference, SAE Technical Paper 811007, 1981.

5. **Gabler, H.C., and Hackney, J.R.:** "The Safety Performance of Production Vehicles in Side Impacts", Proceedings of the 10th International Conference on Experimental Safety Vehicles, p. 607, 1985.

6. Guernsey, J.M., and Blaisdell, F.W.: "Pulmonary Injury", In *Cervicothoracic Trauma* (Vol. III of Trauma Management Series, Eds. F.W. Blaisdell and D.D. Trunkey), Thieme, Inc., New York, 1986.

7. Hackney, J.R., Monk, M.W., Hollowell, W.T., ullivan, L.K., and Willke, D.T.: "Results of the NHTSA's Thoracic Side Impact Protection Research Program", SAE Technical Paper 840886, 1984.

8. Huber, G.: "Aspects of Passive Safety in the Mercedes-Benz Research Car", Proceedings of the 9th International Conference on Experimental Safety Vehicles, p. 104, 1982.

9. Kallieris, D., Mattern, R., Schmidt, G., and Eppinger, R.H.: "Quantification of Side Impact Responses and Injuries", Proceedings of the 25th Stapp Car Crash Conference, SAE Technical Paper 811009, 1981.

10. Marcus, J.H., Morgan, R.M., Eppinger, R.H., Kallieris, D., Mattern, R., and Schmidt, G.: "Human Response to and Injury From Lateral Impact", Proceedings of the 27th Stapp Car Crash Conference, SAE Technical Paper 831634, 1983.

11. McElhaney, J.H., Stalnaker, R.L., Roberts, V.L., and Snyder, R.G.: "Door Crashworthiness Criteria", Proceedings of the 15th Stapp Car Crash Conference, SAE Technical Paper 710864, 1971.

12. Morgan, R.M., Marcus, J.H., and Eppinger, R.H.: "Side Impact - The Biofidelity of NHTSA's Proposed ATD and Efficacy of TTI", Proceedings of the 30th Stapp Car Crash Conference, SAE Technical Paper 861877, 1986.

13. Nusholtz, G.S., Melvin, J.W., and Lux, P.: "The Influence of Impact Energy and Direction on Thoracic Response", Proceedings of the 27th Stapp Car Crash Conference, SAE Technical Paper 831606, 1983.

14. Rossle, R.: "Pathology of Blast Effects", In *German Aviation Medicine - World War II,* Department of the Air Force, U.S. Government Printing Office, Vol. II, 1950.

15. Rouhana, S.W., and Foster, M.E.: "Lateral Impact - An Analysis of the Statistics in the NCSS", Proceedings of the 29th Stapp Car Crash Conference, SAE Technical Paper 851727, 1985.

16. Rouhana, S.W., and Kroell, C.K.: "The Biomechanics of Lateral Impact Injury in the Porcine Model", G.M. Research Report, In Press, 1989.

17. Stalnaker, R.L., McElhaney, J.H., Roberts, V.L., and Trollope, M.L.: "Human Torso Response to Blunt Trauma", In *Human Impact Response, Measurement, and Simulation*, (Eds. W.F. King and H.J. Mertz), Plenum Press, NY, 1973.

18. Stalnaker, R.L., Ulman, M.S.: "Abdominal Trauma - Review, Response, and Criteria", Proceedings of the 29th Stapp Car Crash Conference, SAE Technical Paper 851720, 1985.

19. States, J.D., and States, D.J.: "The Pathology and Pathogenesis of Injuries Caused by Lateral Impact Accidents", Proceedings of the 12th Stapp Car Crash Conference, SAE Technical Paper 680773, 1968.

20. Trollope, M.L., Stalnaker, R.L., McElhaney, J.H., and Frey, C.F.: "The Mechanism of Injury in Blunt Abdominal Trauma", J. Trauma, 13(11):962, 1973.

21. Tsujimura, H., Isobe, H., and, Maeda, K.: "Dummy Injury Values Obtained in Side Collision Sled Tests", Proceedings of the 9th International Conference on Experimental Safety Vehicles, p. 494, 1982.

22. Ventre, P., Provensal, J., and Stcherbatcheff, G.: "Development of Protection Systems for Lateral Impacts", SAE Technical Paper 790710, 1979.

23. Viano, D.C.: "Evaluation of the Benefit of Energy-Absorbing Material in Side Impact Protection : Part I", Proceedings of the 31st Stapp Car Crash Conference, SAE Technical Paper 872212, 1987.

24. Viano, D.C.: "Evaluation of the Benefit of Energy-Absorbing Material in Side Impact Protection : Part II", Proceedings of the 31st Stapp Car Crash Conference, SAE Technical Paper 872213, 1987.

896084
Comparison of EUROSID and Cadaver Responses in Side Impacts

E.G. Janssen, J. Wismans, P.J.A. de Coo,
TNO Road-Vehicles Research Institute

Abstract

The biofidelity of the production prototype European Side Impact Dummy—EUROSID—has been evaluated against requirements defined by ISO. Impactor tests, drop tests and sled tests have been conducted to assess the biofidelity of the head, neck, thorax, shoulder, abdomen and pelvis of the dummy.

Additionally, full-scale impact tests were performed to compare the responses of EUROSID with cadaver responses in identical tests. Special emphasis has been given to the comparison of protection criteria obtained from dummy tests and the injury severity of cadavers in impactor-, drop-, sled- or full-scale tests.

It appears that the response of the production prototype EUROSID in padded- and some rigid impact tests is in good agreement with the cadaver responses, while EUROSID appears to be too stiff in some other rigid impact tests. The injury assessment capabilities of EUROSID seem to be promising. It appears that the ISO requirements show inconsistencies and that the definition of some test set-ups should be improved.

Introduction

The European Side Impact Dummy—EUROSID—has been designed and constructed during 1983–1985 by a group of European research laboratories working together under the auspicies of the European Experimental Vehicle Committee—EEVC. The design and performance was based on biomechanical data. Four prototypes of EUROSID were built and evaluated in 1986 within the framework of an EEC Evaluation Programme (1).* The repeatability, reproducibility, sensitivity and durability of the four dummies have been evaluated by impactor tests, sled tests and full-scale car crashes. The dummy design was improved following this exercise and approximately 20 production prototypes have been evaluated during 1987–1988 by organizations in Europe, the United States of America, Canada and Japan.

In addition to requirements like sensitivity, repeatability and durability, a side impact dummy should also load the structural components of a car in a realistic way. Furthermore it should show a human-like response to this loading. Working Group 5 of ISO/TC 22/SC12 has defined a series of impact tests to assess the performance of these dummies. The impact test set-up and proposed dummy responses are based on cadaver and human volunteer impact tests and are described in documents ISO/DP 9790-1 to 9790-6. The TNO Road-Vehicles Research Institute has conducted a large number of the proposed tests to study the biofidelity of EUROSID. A description of the test set-up and test results is presented in this paper. In addition, cadaver injury severity and dummy protection criteria obtained from identical tests are compared.

In order to evaluate the performance of EUROSID in full-scale side impacts tests, the TNO Road-Vehicles Research Institute had conducted two series of three full-scale tests. The first series was based on the draft European test procedure, while the second series was based on the test procedure proposed by the United States Department of Transportation. The results will be presented in a FAT publication (2). The test set-up of the first series is similar to that used for a comprehensive FAT research programme to study the injuries of human cadavers in side impacts (see references (3) and (4)). EUROSID and cadaver responses are compared in this paper with respect to biofidelity and injury severity assessment.

The production prototype version of the European Side Impact Dummy has been used in the study presented in this paper. This dummy is described in an EEVC publication (5), as well as in the EUROSID User's Manual (6). EUROSID is designed to accept accelerometers, displacement and force transducers, as well as level detecting switches (see figure 1). Table 1 shows the location, type of transducer and channel filter class generally used.

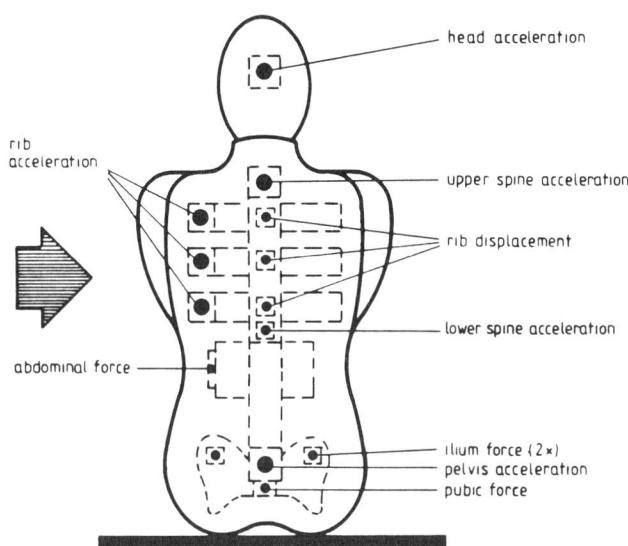

Figure 1. Overview of EUROSID's instrumentation.

This paper consists of three separate parts:

- Part 1: Biofidelity of EUROSID in ISO tests
- Part 2: Biofidelity of EUROSID in full-scale tests
- Part 3: EUROSID injury assessment.

Each part starts with an introduction and ends with a discussion. At the end of this paper a general discussion and conclusions are presented.

*Numbers in parentheses designate references at end of paper

Table 1. EUROSID instrumentation.

Location	transducer	SAE Channel Filter Class
Head	triax. accel.	1000
Upper spine T_1	triax. accel.	180
Upper rib	uniax. accel.	180
	displ. transd.	180
Middle rib	uniax. accel.	180
	displ. transd.	180
Lower rib	uniax. accel.	180
	displ. transd.	180
Lower spine T_{12}	uniax. accel.	180
Abdomen	3 switches	1000
Pelvis	triax. accel.	180
- pubic symphysis	force transd.	600
- iliac wings	strain gauges	600

Part 1—Biofidelity of EUROSID in ISO Tests

Introduction

A series of impact tests on all relevant body parts of EUROSID has been performed. The tests were based on the requirements described in documents ISO/DP 9790–1 to 9790–6. These documents propose a series of impact tests to assess the biofidelity of a side impact dummy, including impactor tests, drop tests and sled tests using the head, neck, shoulder, thorax, abdomen and/or pelvis of the dummy. The response of the dummy in these tests should be compared with cadaver responses in identical tests.

In a previous paper (7) the test set-up and test results were already presented. Partly based on recommendations presented in that paper the ISO documents have been changed, especially with respect to the required channel filter classes and normalization procedures. This paper presents the dummy responses, reanalyzed according to the latest version of documents ISO/DP 9790–1 to 9790–6 (8, 9, 10, 11, 12, 13).

For the test set-ups it is referred to the ISO documents, as well as to our previous paper (7). The lateral neck bending tests, which were not presented in that paper, are presented in more detail. Table 2 summarizes the ISO impact tests.

Table 2. Proposed ISO impact tests and number of tests performed by TNO and NBDL.

Impact test	Number of tests performed
Head	
1. 200 mm rigid drop test	4
2. 1200 mm padded drop test	4
Neck	
1. Ewing volunteer sled test	4*
2. Patrick/Chou volunteer sled test	-
3. Tarriere cadaver sled test	-
Thorax	
1. 1 m and 2 m drop tests	6
2. 24 km/h and 32 km/h sled tests	6
3. 4.3 m/s impactor test	3
Shoulder	
1. 4.5 m/s impactor test	3
Abdomen	
1. 1 m and 2 m drop tests	6
Pelvis	
1. 6 m/s - 10 m/s impactor tests	8
2. 0.5 m - 3 m drop tests	6**
3. 24 km/h and 32 km/h sled tests	6

* Performed by NBDL
** Only the 1 m and 2 m drop tests have been conducted

Test Set-up

General

The test set-ups described in the ISO documents have been used wherever feasible (7). The specific part of the body to be tested was instrumented according to the requirements laid down in the ISO documents. Additional transducers were used to "complete" the instrumentation as described in the previous section.

The channel filter classes prescribed in the ISO documents have been applied as well as the "standard" filter classes presented in table 1. High speed films have been made of the impact tests, except for the head drop tests.

Neck bending test No. 1

A series of four sled tests has been performed based on requirement No. 1 of document ISO/DP 9790–2 (9). The requirements in this document are based on human volunteer tests conducted by the Naval Biodynamics Laboratory (NBDL) in New Orleans. In order to reproduce the original volunteer test conditions as close as possible it was decided to perform the dummy evaluation tests at NBDL. Consequently the same sled pulse, sled test set-up, restraint systems, instrumentation, data processing facilities as in the human volunteer tests could be used. In this test set-up the dummy is seated in an upright position on a rigid chair with the right shoulder and hip against a vertical lightly padded wooden board. The dummy is restrained by shoulder straps, a lap belt and an inverted V-pelvic strap tied to the lap belt. In addition a 25 cm wide chest strap is used to minimize the load on the right shoulder. Figure 2 illustrates this test set-up.

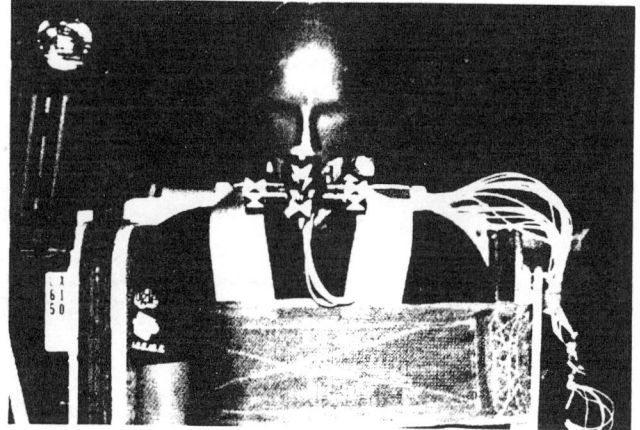

Figure 2. Test set-up for lateral neck bending test performed by NBDL.

Test Results

Introduction

To limit the amount of data to be discussed, only those responses which have to be compared with ISO-requirements are presented (see table 3).

Table 3. Summary of normalized EUROSID responses and requirements according to ISO/DP 9790.

ISO test		EUROSID responses mean	range	ISO requirements range	corridor
Head test no. 1					
- max. accel. (CFC 1000)	[g]	177	174.6 - 181.6	100 - 150	
Head test no. 2					
- max. c.g. accel. (CFC 1000)	[g]	414.4	396.7 - 424.1	217 - 265	
Thoracic test no. 1					
- max. impact force (CFC 180)					
• 1 m rigid	[kN]	16.2	15.5 - 16.8		Figure 4
• 2 m padded	[kN]	7.0	7.0 - 7.1		Figure 5
- average max. rib. defl. (CFC 180)					
• 1 m rigid	[mm]	43.4	41.8 - 45.6	25 - 35	
• 2 m padded	[mm]	50.0*	49.9 - 50.1*	38 - 48	
Thoracic test no. 2					
- max. impact force (FIR 100)					
• 24 km/h rigid	[kN]	9.7	9.3 - 10.2		Figure 6
• 32 km/h rigid	[kN]	15.5	15.3 - 15.8		Figure 7
• 32 km/h padded	[kN]	13.0	12.8 - 13.1		Figure 8
Thoracic test no. 3					
- max. impactor accel. (FIR100)	[g]	18.0	17.0 - 18.6		Figure 9
- max. upper spine accel. (FIR100)	[g]	18.1	17.7 - 18.6		Figure 10
Shoulder test					
- max. impact force (CFC180)	[kN]	2.9	2.8 - 3.0		Figure 11
- max. deflection	[mm]	95	93 - 97	34 - 41	
Abdomen test					
- max. impact force (CFC 180)					
• 1 m	[kN]	7.5	7.1 - 7.9		Figure 12
• 2 m	[kN]	13.1	12.6 - 13.7		Figure 13
- max. lower spine accel. (CFC 180)					
• 1 m	[g]	65.6	60.8 - 68.9	29 - 35	
• 2 m	[g]	128.1	118.5 - 140.9	75 - 92	
- max. lower rib accel. (CFC 180)					
• 1 m	[g]	282.2	239.4 - 331.7	100 - 125	
• 2 m	[g]	333.2	324.6 - 337.8	160 - 200	
Pelvic test no. 1					
- max. impact force (CFC 1000)	[kN]		Figure 14		Figure 14
Pelvic test no. 2					
- max. pelvic accel. (CFC 180)					
• 1 m rigid	[g]	74.7	72.8 - 77.6	63 - 77	
• 2 m padded	[g]	38.1	35.5 - 40.6	39 - 47	
Pelvic test no. 3					
- max. impact force (FIR 100)					
• 24 km/h rigid	[kN]	32.4	30.7 - 34.1	6.4 - 7.8	
• 32 km/h rigid	[kN]	54.5	54.2 - 54.8	22.4 - 26.4	
• 32 km/h padded	[kN]	20.7	20.6 - 20.8	11.6 - 13.6	
- max. pelvic accel. (FIR 100)					
• 24 km/h rigid	[g]	117.9	117.4 - 118.4	63 - 77	
• 32 km/h rigid	[g]	189.4	185.9 - 192.9	96 - 116	
• 32 km/h padded	[g]	64.7	64.0 - 65.3	61 - 75	

* Max. rib deflection = 50 mm

The dummy response requirements described in documents ISO/DP 9790–3 to 9790–6 (thorax, shoulder, abdomen and pelvis) are based on normalized cadaver responses. These cadaver data were normalized to represent the response characteristics of a 50th percentile adult male using the technique described by Mertz (14). From this procedure a so-called "effective mass" for the standard subject is selected for each type of impact test (see Appendix 1). ISO references (10, 11, 12, 13) require that the dummy data are also normalized in order to adjust for changes in effective mass due to slight differences in the position of the dummy on impact.

Head impact test No. 1

Table 3 summarizes the results of the 200 mm rigid head drop test. The response requirement described in ISO-reference (8) is that the peak resultant head acceleration on the non-impacted side of the head should be between 100 G to 150 G. Table 3 and figure 3 show that the actual response is approximately 18% above the upper response boundary.

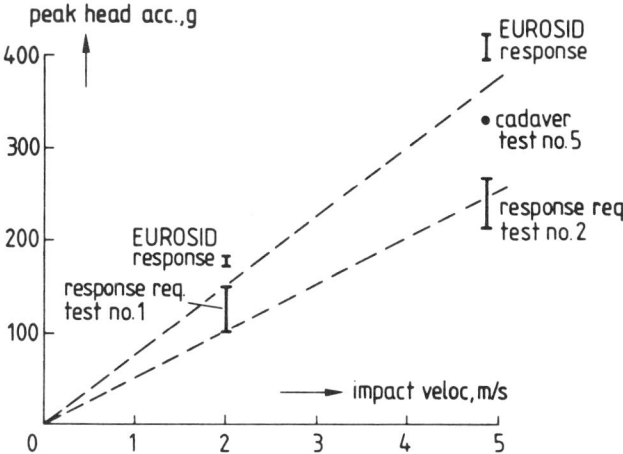

Figure 3. Peak head acceleration vs. impact velocity obtained from head impact test No. 1 (rigid drop) and head impact test No. 2 (padded drop); EUROSID responses compared with the ISO requirements.

Head impact test No. 2

Table 3 summarizes the results of the 1200 mm padded head drop test. The response requirement described in ISO-reference (8) is that the peak resultant head c.g. acceleration should be between 217 G to 265 G. Table 3 and figure 3 show that the actual response is approximately 56% above the upper response boundary.

Neck bending test No. 1

Table 4 summarizes the results of the NBDL sled tests. Only results are presented which were specified by ISO-reference (9). These results have been estimated from graphical time-histories provided by NBDL. Consequently for certain results the accuracy of the peak values might be smaller than if directly determined from electronic data. Head accelerations measured by NBDL are not included in table 4 since the results of NBDL were expressed in a laboratory fixed co-ordinate system rather than the head local co-ordinate system specified by ISO (9).

Table 4. Results of lateral neck bending test No. 1 (sled tests NBDL).

Test no. Responses		6163	6164	6165	6166	ISO requirements
Sled:						
- Velocity change	[m/s]	6.7	6.7	7.2	7.2	6.8 - 7.0
- Max. acceleration	[g]	6.8	6.8	7.7	7.8	7.1 - 7.3
- Rate of onset*	[m/s³]	1530	1467	1841	1767	- -
Dummy (max.):						
- Hor. T_1 acceleration	[g]	22	19	22	21	12 - 18
- Hor. T_1 displacement to sled	[mm]	90	90	100	100	46 - 63
- Head rotation angle	[°]	65	68	74	74	44 - 59
- Head twist angle	[°]	31	34	51	48	32 - 45
- Hor. c.g. displacement to T_1	[mm]	100	95	120	110	130 - 162
- Vert. c.g. displacement to T_1	[mm]	20	30	30	32	64 - 94
- Time of max. head excursion	[ms]	175	180	175	175	159 - 175

* Slope of the best square line fit of the rising position of the sled acceleration profile between 20% and 50% of the peak sled acceleration

C.g. displacements presented in table 4 are based on measurements of the trajectories of the dummies head anatomical origin. This origin is located about 10 mm posterior to the actual centre of gravity of the dummy. The effect of this difference is expected to be small. The time of maximum head excursion included in table 4 is based on the time of maximum head rotation. In general it can be seen that the repeatability of the responses is good. The slightly more severe tests 6165 and 6166 result in slightly larger values for most output parameters than the tests 6163 and 6164.

The first two requirements are related to the biofidelity of the shoulder rather than the neck. It follows that the average deflection of the shoulder is 50% above the upper boundary of the corridor, while the peak T_1 acceleration is just slightly above the upper boundary. The average head rotation angle is 20% above the upper boundary while the average head twist angle is within the corridor. The head twist definition used here (see reference (15)) varies slightly from the head twist definition used for the ISO requirements (see reference (16)); the effect of this is expected to be small. The average horizontal c.g. displacement is about 25% below the lower boundary of the corridor while the vertical displacement is about 50% lower. Finally it can be seen that the time of maximum head excursion is close to the requirement.

Thoracic impact test No. 1

Table 3 summarizes the results of the thoracic drop test. The dummy responses have to be normalized in order to compare them with the requirements described in ISO-reference (10); an impact force vs. time corridor for the 1 m rigid drop test (see figure 4) and a corridor for the 2 m padded drop test (see figure 5). Furthermore the normalized rib deflection should be 25 to 35 mm for the 1 m test and 38 to 48 mm for the 2 m test. It follows from table 3 that the rib deflections in the 1 m rigid drop tests appear to be 25% above the required upper response boundary. It can be concluded from the deflection responses presented in table 3 that the performance in the 2 m padded drop test is very close to the required upper boundary. Figure 4 shows the impact force vs. time response of EUROSID in the 1 m rigid drop test. The first peak is caused by the natural frequency of the rib/load platform system. The dummy response exceeds the cadaver corridor considerably (see also "*Discussion*"). Figure 5 shows the impact force vs. time response of EUROSID in the 2 m padded drop test. The amplitude of the response appears to be satisfactory, where the pulse duration is slightly longer than the cadaver response. However, it appears that the pulse duration of the corridor is wrong (see also "*Discussion*").

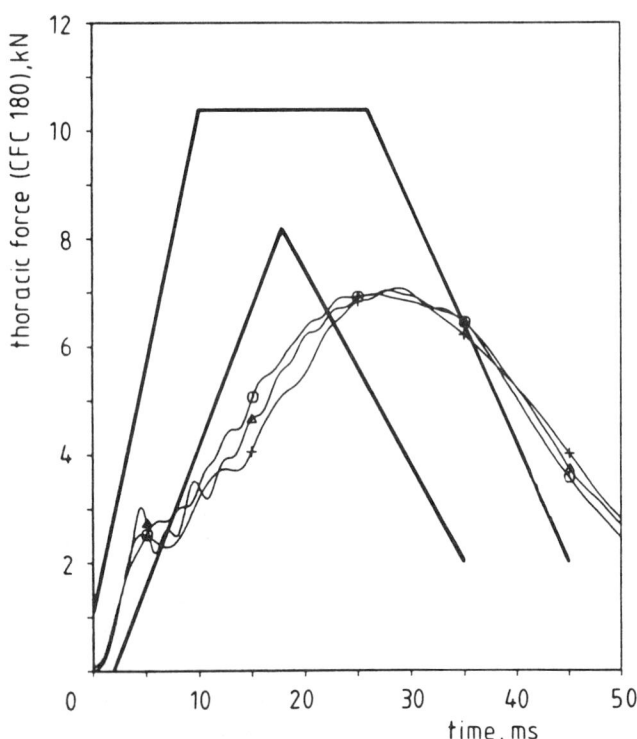

Figure 5. Normalized thoracic impact force versus time obtained from thoracic impact test No. 1 (2 m padded drop test); EUROSID responses compared with ISO requirement corridor.

Thoracic impact test No. 2

Table 3 summarizes the results of the thoracic sled tests. The dummy responses were normalized in order to compare them with the requirements described in ISO-reference (10); an impact force vs. time corridor for each test condition. Figures 6, 7 and 8 show the normalized impact force

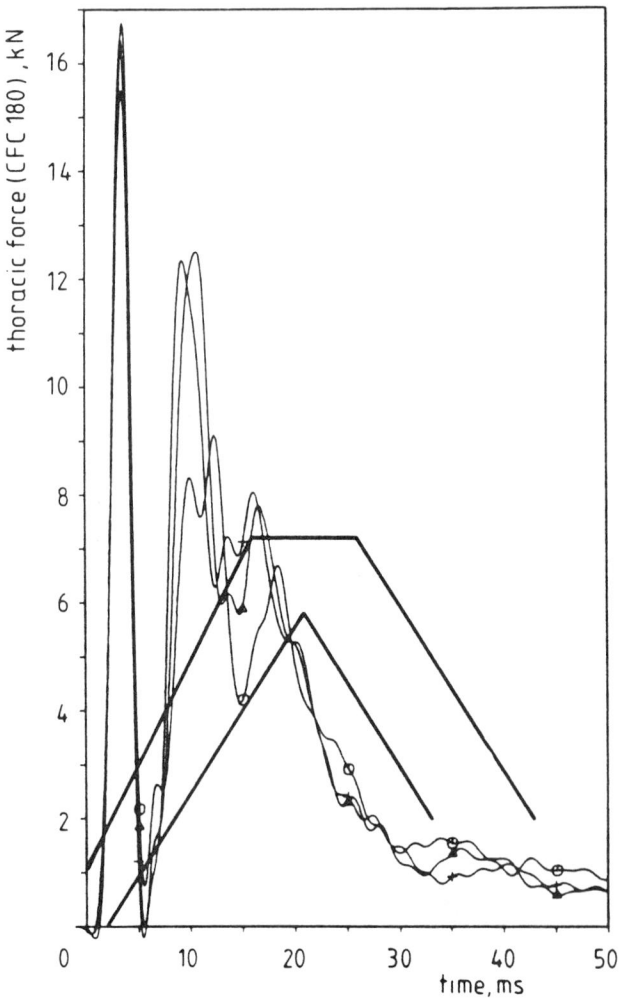

Figure 4. Normalized thoracic impact force versus time obtained from thoracic impact test No. 1 (1 m rigid drop test); EUROSID responses compared with ISO requirement corridor.

vs. time responses of EUROSID in the three different test conditions. It appears that the dummy responses are in good agreement with the cadaver corridors.

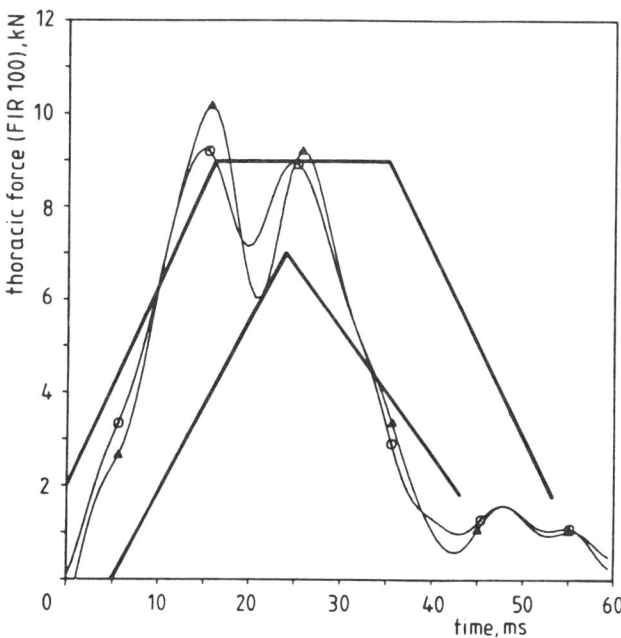

Figure 6. Normalized thoracic impact force versus time obtained from thoracic impact test No. 2 (24 km/h rigid sled test); EUROSID responses compared with ISO requirement corridor.

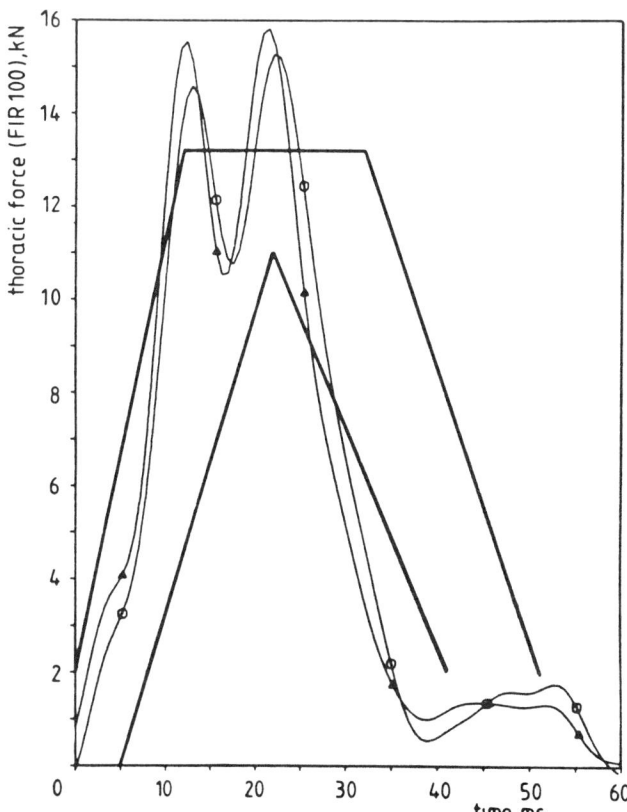

Figure 7. Normalized thoracic impact force versus time obtained from thoracic impact test No. 2 (32 km/h rigid sled test); EUROSID responses compared with ISO requirement corridor.

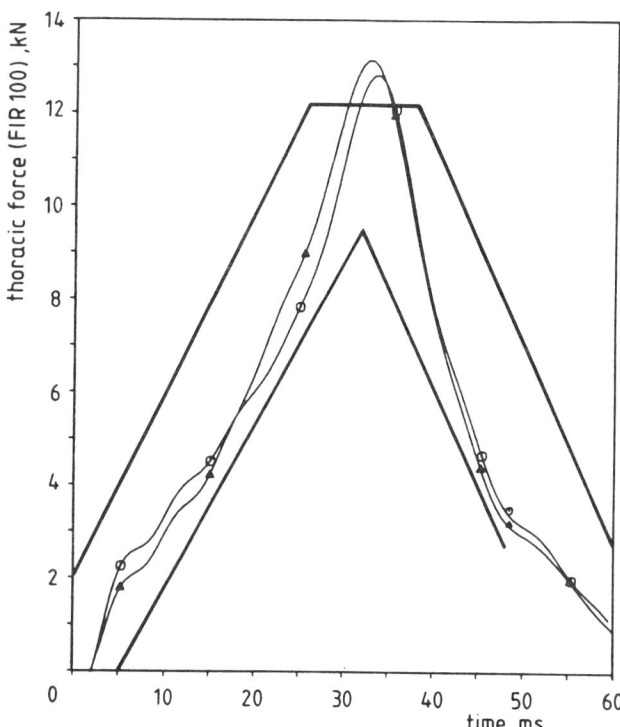

Figure 8. Normalized thoracic impact force versus time obtained from thoracic impact test No. 2 (32 km/h padded sled test); EUROSID responses compared with ISO requirement corridor.

Thoracic impact test No. 3

Table 3 summarizes the results of the thoracic impactor tests. The dummy responses were normalized using a standard effective mass of 32.7 kg as prescribed in ISO-reference (10). The normalized acceleration vs. time responses of the top spine (lateral T_1) and the impactor should lie within the corridors given in figures 9 and 10 respectively. It appears

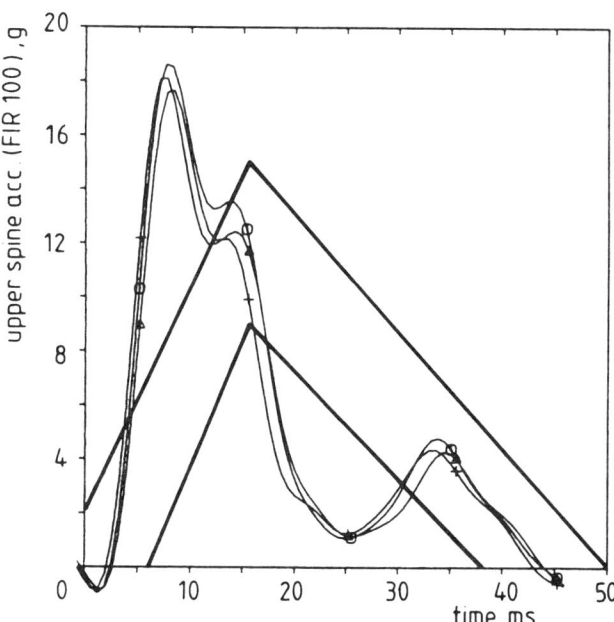

Figure 9. Normalized lateral upper spine acceleration versus time obtained from thoracic impact test No. 3; EUROSID responses compared with ISO requirement corridor.

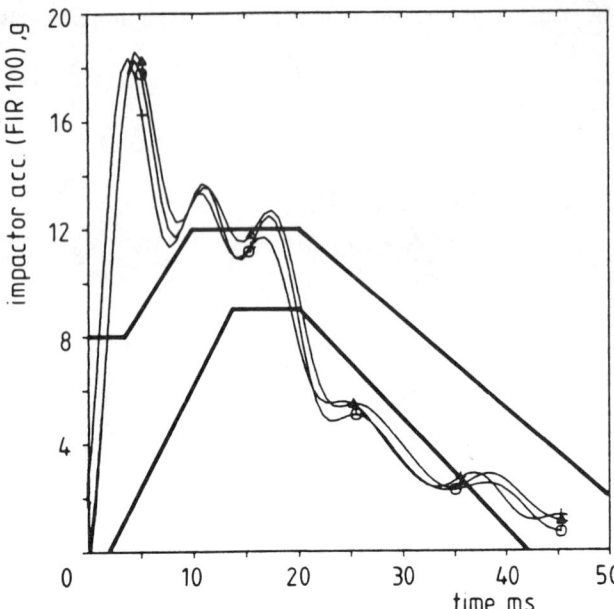

Figure 10. Normalized impactor acceleration versus time obtained from thoracic impact test No. 3; EUROSID responses compared with ISO requirement corridor.

that both responses exceed the corridor, especially in the rising part of the curves.

Shoulder impact test

Table 3 summarizes the results of the shoulder impactor tests. The CFC 1000 filtered responses (required by ISO-reference (11)) show high-frequency vibrations, which influence the repeatability of the results, especially the peak values. The repeatability of the CFC 180 responses appears to be satisfactory.

Since the shapes of the CFC 1000 and CFC 180 filtered impact force vs. time responses were identical, the latter has been used for comparison with the requirements of ISO-reference (11), because it has less high-frequency vibrations. Figure 11 shows the cadaver corridor together with the dummy responses. It appears that the EUROSID shoulder performance is in good agreement with the first require-

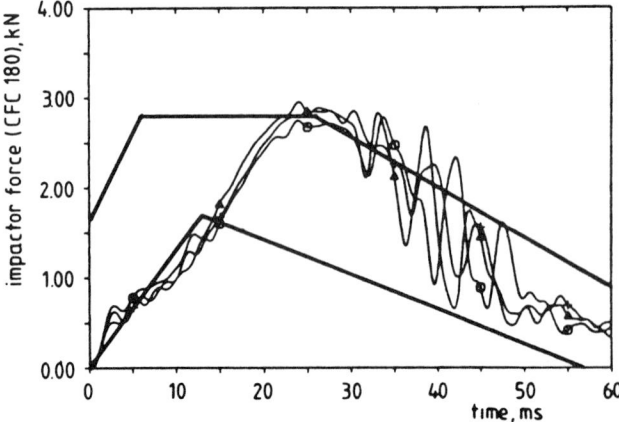

Figure 11. Normalized impactor force versus time obtained from shoulder impact test; EUROSID responses compared with ISO requirement corridor.

ment. However, the second ISO requirement is not fulfilled. The normalized deflections obtained from the current tests were 93 to 97 mm, rather than the required 34 to 41 mm.

Abdomen impact test

Table 3 shows the results of the abdomen drop tests. The test set-up for these tests appeared to be very difficult to repeat. This is especially true of the 2 m drop height, because the impact area is relatively small.

The dummy responses have to be normalized in order to compare them with the requirements described in ISO-reference (12); an impact force vs. time corridor for each drop height (see figures 12 and 13), as well as the required maximum lower spine and lower rib accelerations. Furthermore it is required that the abdominal penetration is at least 4.1 cm. The EUROSID abdomen has been designed to bottom out if a penetration of approximately 40 mm has been reached. Analysis of the high speed films showed that this value was exceeded in all tests and bottoming-out of the abdominal foam covering occurred. Figures 12 and 13 show the impact force vs. time responses of the dummy together with the cadaver corridors. It appears that the dummy response was too high. The acceleration requirements were also exceeded (see also table 3). However, it appears that these acceleration requirements are not appropriate (see "*Discussion*").

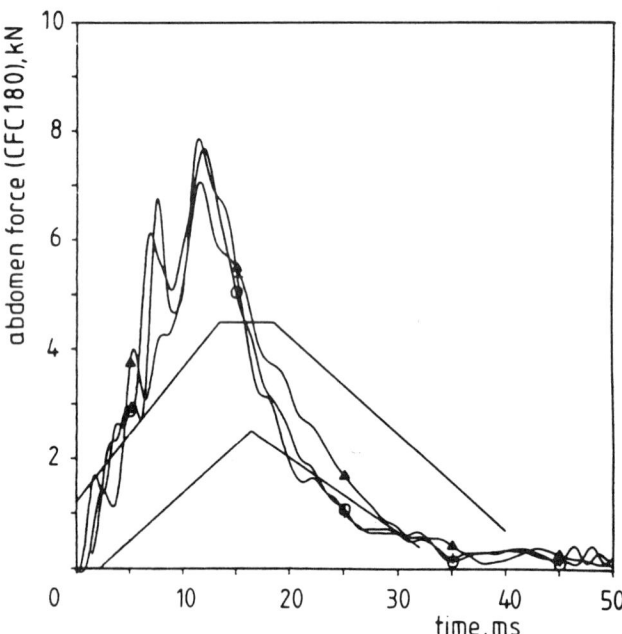

Figure 12. Normalized impact force versus time obtained from abdomen impact test (1 m rigid drop test); EUROSID responses compared with ISO requirement corridor.

Pelvic impact test No. 1

Table 3 summarizes the results of the pelvic impactor tests. The EUROSID responses have been normalized using the impact velocity. The normalized peak impact force vs. impact velocity response of the EUROSID pelvis shows a linear relationship, although it does have a considerable steeper slope than the cadaver corridor (see figure 14). This

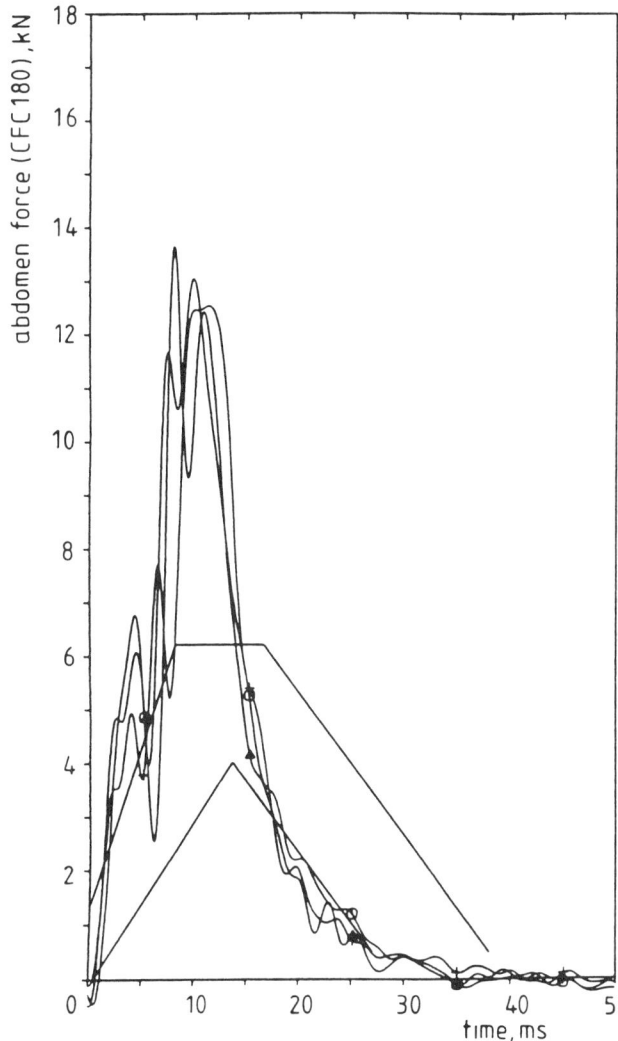

Figure 13. Normalized impact force versus time obtained from abdomen impact test (2 m rigid drop test); EUROSID responses compared with ISO requirement corridor.

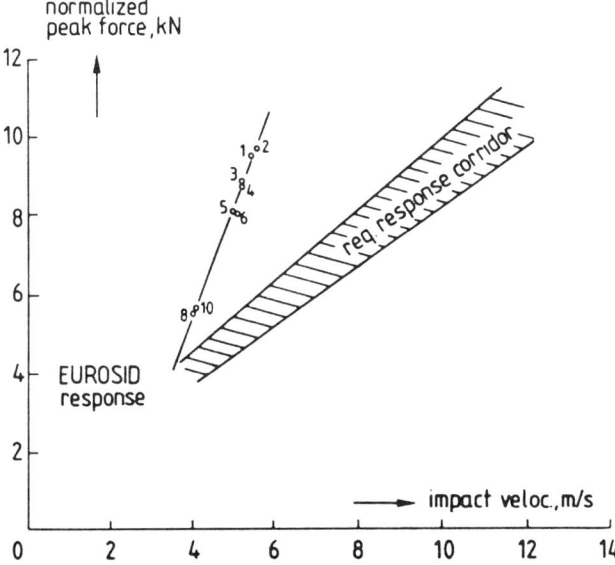

Figure 14. Normalized peak impact force versus impact velocity obtained from pelvic impact test No. 1; EUROSID responses compared with ISO requirement corridor.

results in too high a dummy stiffness at high impact velocities.

Pelvic impact test No. 2

Table 3 summarizes the results of the pelvic drop tests. The EUROSID responses have been normalized using a total dummy mass of 76 kg. The maximum normalized pelvic acceleration seems to be in good agreement with the requirements described in ISO-reference (13); 63 to 77 G for the 1 m rigid drop test and 39 to 47 G for the 2 m padded drop test.

Pelvic impact test No. 3

Table 3 summarizes the results of the pelvic sled tests. The normalized responses are based on a total dummy mass of 76 kg. ISO-reference (13) requires maximum normalized impact forces which appear to be considerably lower than the values obtained from the current rigid impact tests. Comparison with table 3 shows that the results obtained from the current tests are 2 to 4 times higher. The results obtained from the 32 km/h padded tests appear to be 50 percent higher than the upper boundary requirement (see table 3). The required maximum normalized pelvic accelerations are also shown in table 3. The dummy responses in the rigid tests are up to 60 percent higher than required, while the response in the padded test is within the requirements.

Discussion

A series of impact tests has been performed to assess the biofidelity of the European Side Impact Dummy. The test set-up was based on ISO proposals. The dummy responses have been normalized as required by documents ISO/DP 9790-1 to 9790-6.

The peak acceleration response of the EUROSID head in both drop tests appears to be too high compared with the cadaver responses. ISO-reference (8) prescribes an impact angle of 10 degrees, while the two cadavers in the tests performed by APR impacted the padded surface at angles of 5 degrees and 1 degree respectively (17). The response of the EUROSID head appears to be closer to that of APR cadaver test no. 5, impacted at 10 degrees, which resulted in a peak acceleration of 326 G (see also figure 3). This cadaver obtained a skull fracture and the test was therefore omitted from the ISO response requirements. In both cadaver test series complete cadavers were dropped, while the ISO test set-up requires that only the dummy's head be used. Since the responses were not normalized this could have influenced the results; 9% to 13% differences in peak head accelerations were found between head only tests and dummy tests (18).

The neck of the EUROSID is slightly too soft as far as head rotations are concerned and, on the other hand, too stiff with respect to the head c.g. excursions. Further it can be seen that time of maximum head excursion (i.e. maximum head rotation) is close to the requirement. The shoulder of the EUROSID appears to be too soft in comparison to the volunteers in the neck bending sled tests.

In these neck bending tests the original test conditions could be reproduced almost exactly since the same test equipment was used. The ISO requirements lack a detailed description of the test conditions particular as far as harness system and padding on the side board is concerned. Furthermore, in the ISO requirements a definition of the twist angle should be included.

The thorax of EUROSID appears to be too stiff in rigid impactor tests and in rigid drop tests, while the impact force vs. time responses in padded drop tests show a too long pulse duration. However the ISO response requirements for the drop tests are based on 9 cadaver tests with arm involvement and only 2 cadaver tests without arm involvement (19), while the ISO test set-up prescribes a direct impact on the dummy thorax. Furthermore, it was recently shown (e.g. references (20) and (21) that the pulse duration of some cadaver tests used to define the response corridor for the 2 m padded drop tests was twice as long than that presented in ISO reference (10). The normalization procedure is redone by APR, resulting in another standard effective mass (31.3 kg rather than 38 kg) and based on the velocity change ΔV rather than based on the impact velocity V_o. Moreover it is proposed to prescribe an impact with the arm positioned along the thorax (22). Figures 15 and 16 show the new corridors proposed by APR. TNO has performed a series of thoracic drop tests according to these proposals. Table 5 summarizes the test results. Figures 15 and 16 also show the EUROSID results. It appears that the EUROSID responses are in good agreement with these new corridors. The impact force vs. time responses in the rigid as well as padded thoracic sled tests appear to be in good agreement with the cadaver responses. If the standard effective mass for normalization of the cadaver and dummy responses would be also changed from 38 kg to 31.3 kg, the force (and time) responses presented in Figures 6, 7 and 8 would decrease by 9%.

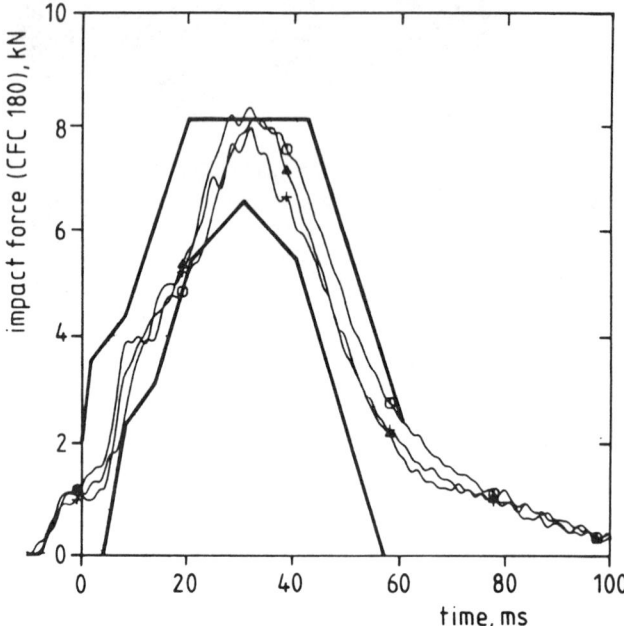

Figure 16. Normalized thoracic impact force versus time obtained from new proposed thoracic impact test No. 1 (2 m padded drop test with arm involvement); EUROSID responses compared with new proposed ISO requirement corridor (see reference (21)).

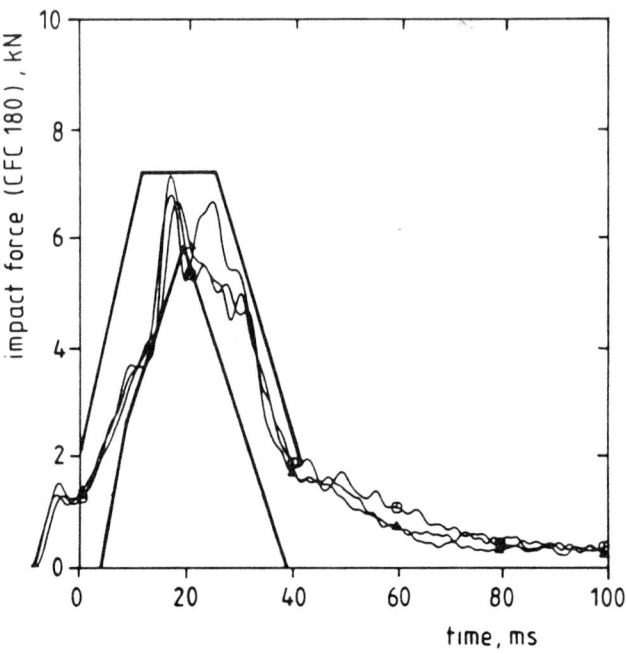

Figure 15. Normalized thoracic impact force versus time obtained from new proposed thoracic impact test No. 1 (1 m rigid drop test with arm/shoulder involvement); EUROSID responses compared with new proposed ISO requirement corridor (see reference (21)).

Table 5. Results of new proposed thoracic impact test No. 1 (drop test).

Test no.		1601	1603	1604	1605	1606	1608
Drop height	[m]	1	1	1	2	2	2
Impact surface		rigid	rigid	rigid	padded	padded	padded
Impact force (CFC 180)							
· max	[kN]	6.06	5.97	5.78	7.43	7.53	7.19
Rib deflections (CFC 180)							
· max upper rib	[mm]	27.7	32.7	32.2	40.7	37.7	43.2
· max middle rib	[mm]	24.0	29.5	25.3	44.7	41.7	43.7
· max lower rib	[mm]	25.0	27.5	24.9	46.5	41.5	42.5
Effective mass M_e	[kg]	21.90	23.51	22.88	25.88	25.16	25.27
Mass ratio R_m		1.43	1.33	1.37	1.21	1.24	1.24
Stiffness ratio R_k		1.0	1.0	1.0	1.0	1.0	1.0
Normalizing factors							
· force R_f		1.20	1.15	1.17	1.10	1.12	1.11
· deflection R_x		1.20	1.15	1.17	1.10	1.12	1.11
· time R_t		1.20	1.15	1.17	1.10	1.12	1.11
Normalized impact force							
· max	[kN]	7.25	6.89	6.77	8.17	8.39	8.00
Normalized rib deflections							
· max upper rib	[mm]	33.1	37.7	37.6	44.8	42.0	48.1
· max middle rib	[mm]	28.6	34.0	29.6	49.1	46.5	48.6
· max lower rib	[mm]	29.9	31.7	29.1	51.2	46.3	47.3

The impact force vs. time response of EUROSID in the shoulder impact tests appears to be in good agreement with the cadaver response corridor, while the shoulder deflection is twice as high as the required value. It is thought that the deflection in the cadaver tests was limited due to interference of the impactor face with the scapula (see e.g. test MS 201 in ISO-reference (11), which was omitted from the force-time response requirement due to the 'sudden' increase of force after 20 ms). In the dummy impacts only the clavicle was impacted. The deflection response of EUROSID appeared to be close to that of cadaver test no. 204, which was omitted from the ISO deflection response requirements because the impact angle was 15 degrees forward of the lateral position. The cadaver shoulder deflection in this test was approximately 100 mm (23).

The responses of EUROSID in the abdomen drop tests exceed the ISO requirements by a considerable margin. The abdomen has been designed to show a dynamic response within an impact force vs. deflection corridor based on cadaver drop tests. However if the proposed tolerance limits of 39 mm deflection and 4500 N force are exceeded, the flexible flesh-simulating material bottoms out and the impact force increases rapidly (24). In fact the abdomen was designed to show a human-like response up to the injury tolerance limits. Since the ISO response corridors are based on the same cadaver tests, this means a human-like response up to approximately 10 ms in figure 12 and up to approximately 7 ms in figure 13. The peak lower spine accelerations also occurred after these time 'limits', the rigid abdominal penetration stop being attached to the (lower) thoracic spine.

ISO/DP 9790-5 requires an impact on the abdominal region including 'the area of the 9th rib'. If the armrest is positioned on the abdomen section of EUROSID, the lower rib will impact the 'surrounding surface' which is not prescribed in DP 9790-5 with respect to dimensions and stiffness. The rib acceleration and spine acceleration responses are then a function of these surface characteristics. The biofidelity of the abdomen should not be assessed by these responses. If the armrest is positioned on the lower rib to cover 'the area of the 9th rib' as recently proposed (25), this would result in an impact response for the thorax rather than for the abdomen section of a dummy.

The peak impact force vs. impact velocity response of EUROSID in the pelvic (rigid) impactor tests appears to be quite reasonable in low velocity (4 m/s) impacts. This can also be concluded from the results of the 1 m rigid drop test (4.4 m/s) which had a satisfactory response. However in high velocity rigid impacts the pelvis appears to be too stiff, as can be seen from the rigid sled tests (6.7 to 8.9 m/s) in which the impact force and pelvic acceleration were much too high. In the high velocity padded tests (6.3 m/s drop test and 8.9 m/s sled test) the dummy responses appear to be in good agreement with the cadaver responses. It should be noted that a padded impact will be more typical of the occupant-to-door impacts experienced in side crashes than rigid impacts. Improvement of the ISO requirements appears to be necessary for the pelvic impact tests as well, for instance with respect to specification of the impactor face and seating surface in the pelvic impactor tests.

Part 2—Biofidelity of EUROSID in Full-Scale Tests

Introduction

Three tests were carried out according to the draft European procedure for side-impact collisions; a perpendicular impact (90°) with a Moving Deformable Barrier at 50 km/h (26). However, an alternative deformable element has been used in order to reproduce the test set-up used for cadaver experiments conducted by FAT (3, 4). A brief summary of the test set-up and test results is presented in the next sections. Finally, dummy and cadaver responses are compared.

Test Set-up

Vehicle

The tests were performed on Opel Kadetts D (2-door models 1982-1984). Triaxial accelerometers were mounted at the centre of gravity of the vehicle, on the non-impact side door sill and on the A- and B-pillars at impact-side. Displacement transducers were attached at the mid-door position and just behind the B-pillar. Seven high-speed cameras were used to cover the motions, including two cameras mounted to the vehicle. The total mass of the vehicles, including equipment and dummy was approximately 950 kg. The vehicles were positioned on a flat concrete surface with the handbrake disengaged and the gear lever in neutral position.

Barrier

The barrier front was provided with a CCMC deformable element consisting of eight blocks of PU foam, so as to represent the frontal stiffness of the average European car. The ground clearance of the front was 300 mm. The total mass of the barrier was 950 kg. The barrier impacted the left side of the vehicle (longitudinal axis of barrier aligned with R-point of vehicle) with an impact speed of 50 km/h, while the barrier was braked 200 ms after initial contact. The barrier was equipped with triaxial accelerometers, one at the centre of gravity and the other located just behind the impactor face.

Dummy

A production prototype EUROSID has been used for these tests. Besides the instrumentation shown in figure 1 and table 1 the dummy was equipped with uniaxial accelerometers mounted on the non-impact side of the ribs and on the frontal side of the upper and lower rib (upper and lower sternum position to measure frontal accelerations). The driver's seat was positioned in the mid-position and the seat back was set at an angle of 25°. The dummy was seated with free hand on the lower part of the steering wheel and the upper arm approximately parallel with the thoracic spine. Three-point automatic seat belts were used to restrain the dummy.

Test Results

Introduction

To limit the amount of data to be discussed, only the dummy responses are presented. Detailed results will be presented in a FAT publication (2).

Dummy

Table 6 summarizes the EUROSID results obtained from these tests. In general it appears that the repeatability is quite good. The responses in the third test seem to be somewhat higher than those of the other tests. The accuracy of the seating procedure as well as the status of the used vehicle could have influenced the dummy responses.

Table 6. Results of EUROSID in 50 km/h side-impact tests.

Test no.			Average	F87471	F87472	F87473
Head						
- result. accel.	max.	[g]	57	59 (49)	56 (48)	55 (47)
	3ms	[g]	55	58	54	53
	HIC	[s]	367	403	307	390
Upper spine (T_1)						
- lateral accel.	max.	[g]	62	57 (31)	57 (31)	71 (33)
	3ms	[g]	59	55	53	69
Upper rib left						
- lateral accel.	max.	[g]	156	157 (21)	162 (22)	149 (21)
	3ms	[g]	104	97	113	102
Middle rib left						
- lateral accel.	max.	[g]	138	142 (23)	135 (23)	136 (22)
	3ms	[g]	113	120	112	108
Lower rib left						
- lateral accel.	max.	[g]	194	199 (24)	176 (24)	206 (24)
	3ms	[g]	132	128	131	138
Upper rib right						
- lateral accel.	max.	[g]	76	75 (31)	70 (31)	84 (31)
	3ms	[g]	69	65	64	77
Middle rib right						
- lateral accel.	max.	[g]	86	87 (30)	78 (30)	94 (31)
	3ms	[g]	80	78	74	89
Lower rib right						
- lateral accel.	max.	[g]	95	99 (30)	84 (29)	102 (29)
	3ms	[g]	89	88	80	98
Upper rib sternum						
- long. accel.	max.	[g]	38	32 (34)	45 (21)	36 (20)
	3ms	[g]	16	24	11	14
Lower rib sternum						
- long. accel.	max.	[g]	83	87 (30)	78 (29)	83 (29)
	3ms	[g]	14	17	9	16
Lower spine (T_{12})						
- lateral accel.	max.	[g]	107	109 (30)	92 (30)	121 (31)
	3ms	[g]	99	97	88	111
Pelvis						
- lateral accel.	max.	[g]	137	125 (30)	127 (29)	160 (30)
	3ms	[g]	117	107	115	130
Pelvis						
- ilium force l.	max.	[kN]	4.2	3.9 (29)	3.9 (29)	4.8 (29)
	3ms	[kN]	3.5	3.3	3.2	4.0
- ilium force r.	max.	[kN]	1.1	1.0 (98)	1.0 (105)	1.3 (97)
	3ms	[kN]	1.1	1.0	1.0	1.0
- pubic force	max.	[kN]	9.3	6.4 (30)	9.0 (35)	12.4 (33)
	3ms	[kN]	6.8	5.6	7.1	7.7
Abdomen switches						
- front			.	.	*	.
- middle			.	.	*	.
- rear			.	.	*	.
Rib deflection						
- max. upper rib		[mm]	48	51	47	45
- max. middle rib		[mm]	45	47	44	45
- max. lower rib		[mm]	46	45	46	47
V*C max.						
- upper rib		[m/s]	0.85	0.94	0.85	0.77
- middle rib		[m/s]	1.01	0.99	1.03	1.01
- lower rib		[m/s]	1.37	1.37	1.33	1.41
TTI max						
- upper rib		[g]	121	122	116	124
- middle rib		[g]	119	121	112	123
- lower rib		[g]	142	141	133	151

( ) time in ms

It appears that the currently proposed protection criteria for the thorax (i.e. rib deflection ≤ 42 mm; $V*C \leq 1.0$ m/s) and the abdomen (deflection ≤ 39 mm and force ≤ 4500 N; i.e. no switch contact) are exceeded, while the average pelvic responses are just acceptable (ilium and pubic force ≤ 10 kN).

Discussion

The test set-up of these full-scale side impact tests is similar to that of a series of cadaver tests performed by the University of Heidelberg for FAT (3, 4). In the cadaver tests the vehicle body was mounted onto a trolley and the MDB was guided. However, a comparison of both test set-ups using dummies showed that they appear to be similar with respect to resulting vehicle deformations and door velocity (27).

Figure 17 summarizes some cadaver responses obtained from a series of 50 km/h left hand side impacts (4) together with the EUROSID responses. Mean values and standard deviations are shown. Rib deflections or pelvic forces were not available for the cadaver tests, while the head accelerations were not measured on the same location as in the dummies. It appears that the dummy responses are in good agreement with the cadaver responses. Only the maximum upper spine acceleration differs too much from the cadaver results. The response of EUROSID T_1 in a FAT study using the Heidelberg test set-up appears to be close to the cadaver upper spine acceleration (27). In references (3) and (4) the cadaver responses are compared with those of the APROD, SID and Hybrid II dummy. It appears that the biofidelity of EUROSID exceeds the biofidelity of these dummies.

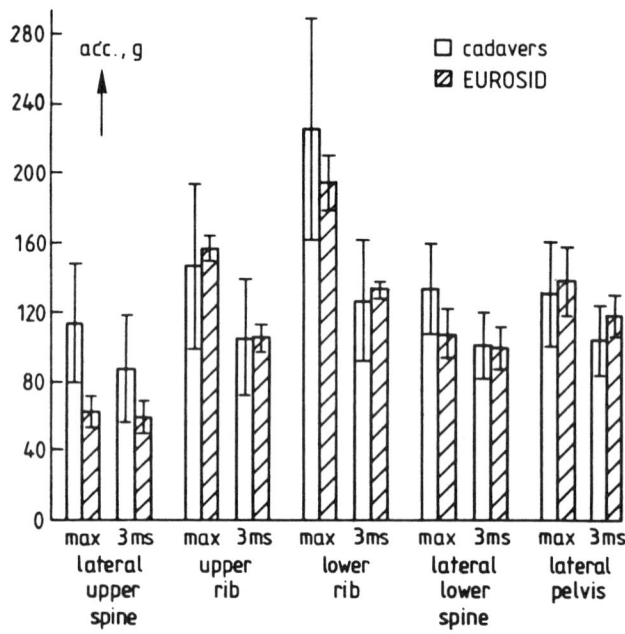

Figure 17. Comparison of human cadaver and EUROSID responses (mean values and standard deviations) obtained from full-scale vehicle impacts.

Part 3—EUROSID Injury Assessment

Introduction

In a previous paper (28) the protection criteria of the EUROSID thorax and pelvis have been compared with injury severities obtained from similar sled tests using human cadavers. Figure 18 shows as example a cross-plot of the cadaver thoracic injuries (i.e. Number of Fractured Ribs and AIS) versus the maximum V*C obtained from EUROSID. The cadaver injuries have been normalized for cadavers of 45 years, based on a study of Marcus et al. (29).

In this section the ISO- and FAT cadaver tests discussed in the previous sections are used to analyse the injury assessment capabilities of the thorax, abdomen and pelvis of EUROSID.

Thoracic Protection Criteria

ISO tests

Requirement no. 1 of ISO/DP 9790-3 (10) is based on a series of cadaver drop tests performed by APR. The thoracic injuries of the cadavers for the 1 m rigid drop tests (with and without arm involvement) and for the 2 m padded drop tests are summarized in table 7 (see also reference (30)). The results have been normalized for cadavers of 45 years; a correction of 0.025 AIS/year and 0.2 NFR/year was applied (see also reference (29)). The average EUROSID responses obtained from these tests are summarized in table 7 (note: dummy responses are not normalized). The influence of arm involvement appears to be obvious. The cadavers in the 1 m test without arm sustained a large number of fractured ribs.

Table 7. Average cadaver injury severity and average EUROSID protection criteria obtained from thoracic drop tests.

Drop height	[m]	1	1	2
Surface		rigid	rigid	padded
Arm involvement		no	yes	yes
Cadavers:				
- AIS		3.5	2.3	2.0
- NFR		11.5	4.0	4.3
- age		59	47	50
- normalized AIS$_{45}$*		3.2	2.2	1.9
- normalized NFR$_{45}$		8.7	3.6	3.3
EUROSID:				
- V·C max.	[m/s]	0.62	0.32	0.42
- TTI max.	[g]	114	77	51
- max. rib defl.	[mm]	42	31	44

* See text

Requirement no. 2 of ISO/DP 9790-3 is based on a series of cadaver sled tests conducted at the University of Heidelberg. In reference (28) the results of 42 similar sled tests have already been discussed. Cross-plots of cadaver injuries versus EUROSID responses were presented (see also figure 18). Table 8 summarizes the thoracic injury severity and dummy protection criteria respectively. The influence of impact speed and padding is clearly seen by all parameters, except for the maximum rib deflection. The average of the three maximum rib deflections appears to be a more discriminative parameter.

Table 8. Average cadaver injury severity and average EUROSID protection criteria obtained from thoracic sled tests.

Impact speed	[km/h]	24	32	32
Surface		rigid	rigid	padded
Cadavers:				
- AIS		2.0	3.5	2.4
- NFR		5.3	10.7	6.3
- age		42	47	43
- normalized AIS$_{45}$*		2.1	3.4	2.5
- normalized NFR$_{45}$		5.9	10.4	6.6
EUROSID:				
- V·C max.	[m/s]	1.01	1.42	1.17
- TTI max.	[g]	99	158	66
- max. rib defl.	[mm]	49	>50	>50

* See text

Requirement no. 3 of ISO/DP 9790-3 is based on a series of impactor tests conducted by HSRI. The injuries of the four cadavers are described in references (31) and (32). The mean severity and mean number of fractured ribs together with the EUROSID results are presented in table 9. The normalization of the injuries results in no fractured ribs for these tests.

Table 9. Average cadaver injury severity and average EUROSID protection criteria obtained from thoracic impactor tests.

Cadavers:		
- AIS		2.3
- NFR		1.5
- age		63
- normalized AIS$_{45}$*		1.9
- normalized NFR$_{45}$*		0
EUROSID:		
- V·C max.	[m/s]	0.34
- TTI max.	[g]	75
- max. rib defl.	[mm]	32

* See text

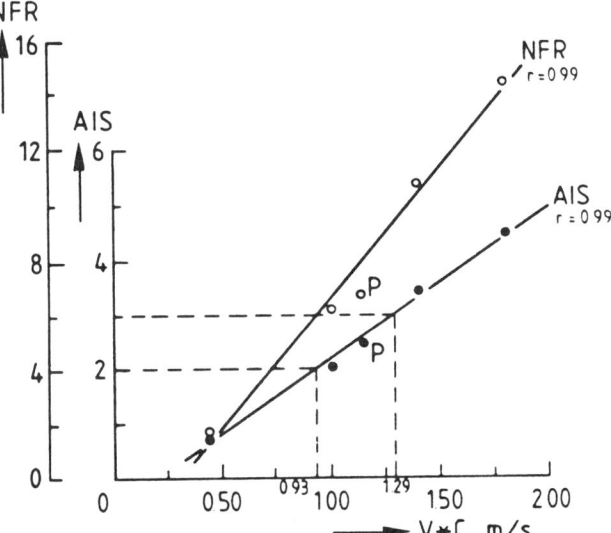

Figure 18. Cross-plot of thoracic cadaver injuries and maximum V*C of EUROSID obtained from rigid and padded ('P') wall sled tests (28).

FAT tests

In two FAT reports (3, 4) the test set-up and results of 58 full-scale side impact tests using human cadavers are presented. The cadavers were impacted from the left or right side, while the barrier impact speed was 40 km/h up to 60 km/h (the test set-up was already described in the previous section). The cadaver injuries for a 50 km/h left or right impact are summarized in table 10, together with the average EUROSID responses. The cadaver injury severity, as well as the EUROSID responses, indicate a severe impact.

Table 10. Average cadaver injury severity and average EUROSID protection criteria obtained from full-scale vehicle tests.

Cadavers:		
- AIS*		3.0
- age		39
- normalized AIS_{45}***		3.2
- NFR**		9.7
- age		37
- normalized NFR_{45}***		11.3
EUROSID:		
- V•C max.	[m/s]	1.37
- TTI max.	[g]	142
- max. rib defl.	[mm]	48

* See ref. [4]
** See ref. [3]
*** See text

Abdomen Protection Criteria

ISO tests

The requirements of ISO/DP 9790-5 (12) are based on a series of cadaver drop tests performed by APR. Recently APR reviewed these tests and the updated results are summarized in reference (33). Figure 19 shows the abdominal AIS as function of the maximum normalized force and maximum relative penetration. It appears that all injuries are found in the area where the penetration is larger than 36% (=50 mm for a 50th percentile dummy) and the force exceeds 4600 N. Figure 19 also shows the protection criteria of EUROSID; a built-in penetration criterion of 28% (=39 mm) and an adjustable force criterion (4500 N is currently proposed). Approximately 1 cm can be added to the penetration criterion to account for the thickness of the standard EUROSID jacket and the space between jacket and abdomen.

FAT tests

The relation between abdominal injury severity and barrier impact speed in the FAT full-scale side impact tests (see reference (4)) is shown in figure 20. It appears that a considerable influence of the impact side exists; right hand side impacts are more severe than left hand side impacts. This is caused by the position of the liver. The estimated severity for a 50 km/h side impact appears to be AIS = 1.3 for a left hand impact and AIS = 4.4 for a right hand impact.

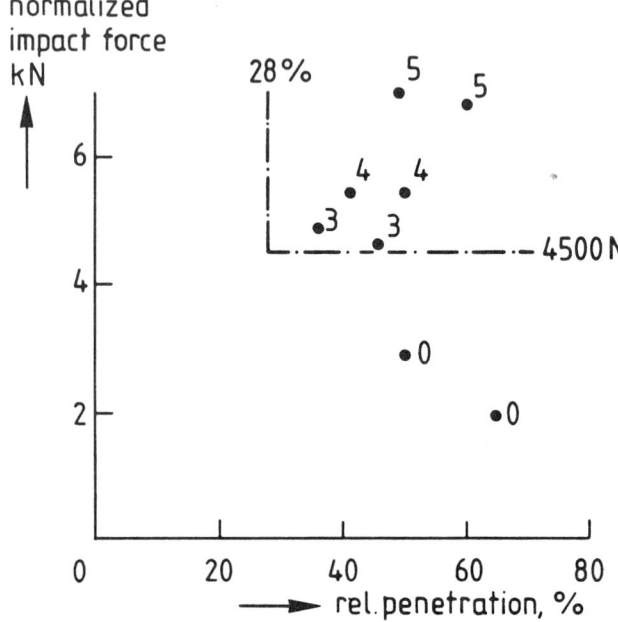

Figure 19. Abdominal AIS as function of normalized impact force and relative penetration in cadaver drop tests (see reference (33)). The protection criteria of the EUROSID abdomen are also shown.

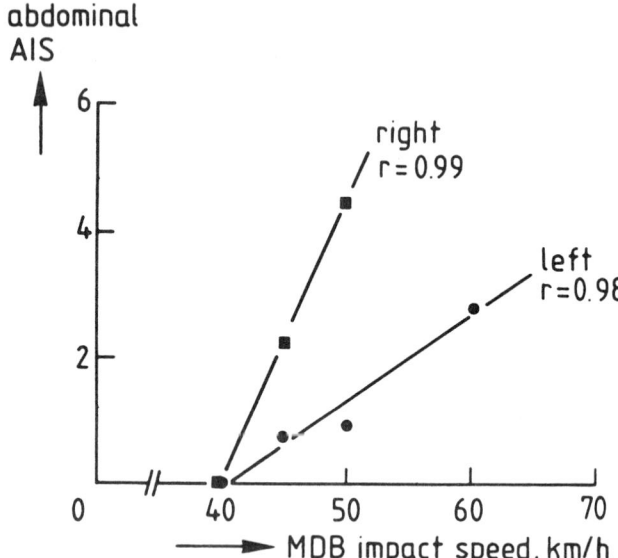

Figure 20. Abdominal AIS as function of impact speed in full-scale cadaver tests; comparison of left hand impacts and right hand impacts (see reference 4)).

Three 50 km/h side impact tests using EUROSID have been performed using similar vehicles as those in the above mentioned FAT cadaver tests (see previous section). In two tests the abdominal switches contacted (see also table 6), indicating an AIS ≥ 3 injury.

Pelvic Protection Criteria

ISO tests

Requirement no. 1 of ISO/DP 9790-6 (13) is based on a study of ONSER (=INRETS). The response of cadavers to lateral impacts delivered to the greater trochanter was analyzed. Each cadaver was impacted at increasing speeds until pelvic fracture was diagnosed. ISO analyzed only results where data for the first impact were given and the cadavers had acceptable bone conditions. So no pelvic fractures should be indicated in the dummy tests. The maximum impact speed in similar EUROSID tests was 5.6

m/s resulting in a maximum pelvic acceleration of 48 G and a 3 ms maximum of 41 G. The maximum pubic symphysis force obtained in this test series was 5.2 kN with a 3 ms maximum of 4.2 kN. So these values could be considered as non-injury producing dummy responses (see also table 11).

Table 11. Comparison of cadaver injury severity and EUROSID protection criteria in pelvic impact tests.

Tests	Cadaver AIS		EUROSID protection criteria*					
			accel. [g]		pubic force [kN]		ilium force [kN]	
	range	mean	max.	3ms	max.	3ms	max.	3ms
ISO impactor test (6 m/s)	0	0	48	41	5.2	4.2	-	-
ISO drop tests								
- 1 m rigid	0	0	75	69	6.9	6.2	3.3	2.7
- 2 m padded	0	0	40	38	4.2	3.4	1.2	1.2
ISO sled tests								
- 24 km/h rigid	0	0	127	100	13.9	10.8	4.4	3.2
- 32 km/h padded	0	0	67	64	8.5	6.8	2.6	2.5
- 32 km/h rigid	0-3	0.6	215	153	27.0	17.8	9.4	6.5
FAT full-scale tests	0-3	0.2	137	117	9.3	6.8	4.2	3.5

* Mean values

Requirement no. 2 of ISO/DP 9790-6 is based on a series of lateral drop tests performed by APR. The cadavers were dropped from heights ranging from 0.5 to 3.0 m on a padded or rigid surface. Only two cadavers out of twenty obtained a pelvic injury (AIS 2 or 3), both in the 3 m padded test configuration. So the 1 m rigid and 2 m padded dummy tests should not indicate pelvic injuries. The maximum pelvic acceleration using EUROSID in this test set-up appears to be 75 G with a 3 ms maximum of 69 G. The maximum and 3 ms maximum pubic symphysis forces are 6.9 kN and 6.2 kN respectively, while these values for the iliac wing force seem to be 3.3 kN and 2.7 kN respectively. So these values could be considered as non-injury producing dummy responses (see also table 11).

Requirement no. 3 of ISO/DP 9790-6 is based on a series of sled tests performed by the University of Heidelberg. The cadavers impacted a rigid or padded wall laterally at 24 km/h or 32 km/h. Only one pelvic injury (in a 32 km/h rigid test) was found in the 17 tests used by ISO to define the dummy responses. Therefore, the 24 km/h rigid and 32 km/h padded tests using EUROSID should not indicate pelvic injuries, while the 32 km/h rigid test should show a risk for injuries. The results for EUROSID are summarized in table 11. The difference in response between a 24 km/h and 32 km/h rigid sled tests appears to be remarkable. The influence of padding is clearly indicated by the dummy responses.

FAT tests

In 58 full-scale side impact tests using human cadavers, only 4 pelvic fractures (AIS 2 and 3) were observed (4). These 4 cadavers were 50 years or older, so the dummy tests should indicate a limited risk for pelvic injuries. The average responses obtained from the EUROSID full-scale tests (see also table 6) are presented in table 11.

Discussion

If the number of fractured ribs and the thoracic AIS of the cadavers presented in table 7 up to 10 are compared, an increasing test severity can be seen:

- impactor tests
- 2 m padded drop tests
- 1 m rigid drop tests (with arm)
- 24 km/h rigid sled tests
- 32 km/h padded sled tests
- 1 m rigid drop tests (without arm)
- full-scale vehicle tests (depending on vehicle)
- 32 km/h rigid sled tests.

It appears that V*C obtained from the EUROSID tests quite well estimates this severity order. However, both 1 m rigid drop tests are somewhat underestimated. It can be concluded from table 7 up to table 10 that TTI underestimates the severity of the padded drop- and sled tests. The remaining tests appear to be assessed in the above mentioned severity order. The maximum rib deflection underestimates the severity of both 1 m rigid drop tests, while the severity of the padded sled tests appears to be overestimated. It should be noted that the injury severity obtained from cadaver drop tests could be (too) high due to the specific (i.e. horizontal) position of the cadavers (e.g. internal organs are displaced towards the impact surface).

Figure 21 up to figure 26 show cross-plots of the thoracic injury severity from the cadaver tests and the thoracic protection criteria obtained from similar EUROSID tests. Linear regression has been applied to these results. It appears that the correlation between the protection criteria and the number of fractured ribs is quite good. Six fractured ribs would correspond to a maximum rib deflection of 42.5 mm, a maximum V*C of 0.80 m/s or a maximum TTI of 95 G. The correlation between TTI and AIS appears to be very

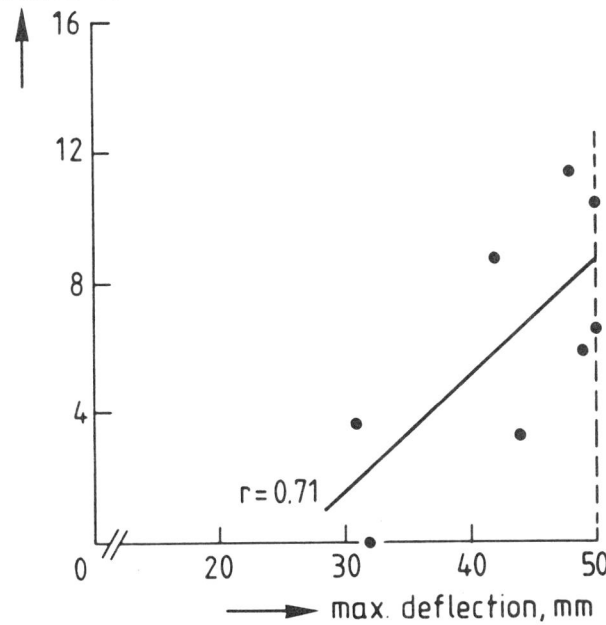

Figure 21. Cross-plot of thoracic cadaver injuries (number of fractured ribs) and maximum rib deflection of EUROSID obtained from full-scale and ISO impact tests.

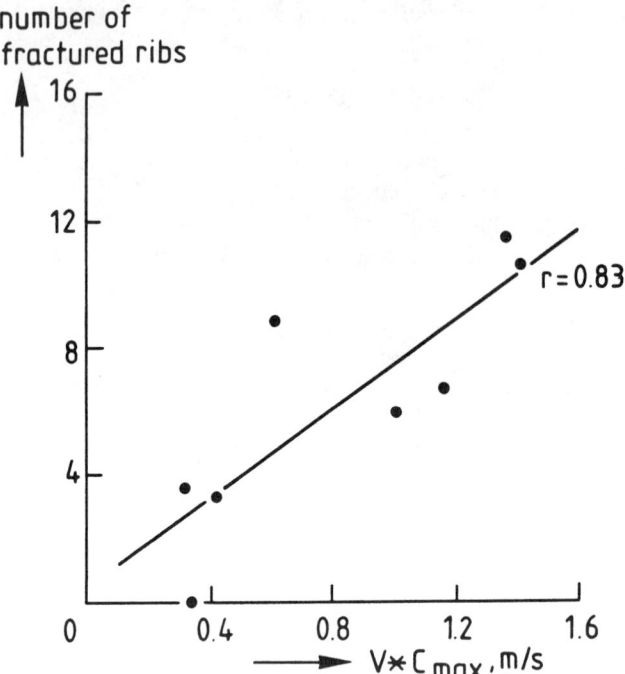

Figure 22. Cross-plot of thoracic cadaver injuries (number of fractured ribs) and maximum V*C of EUROSID obtained from full-scale and ISO impact tests.

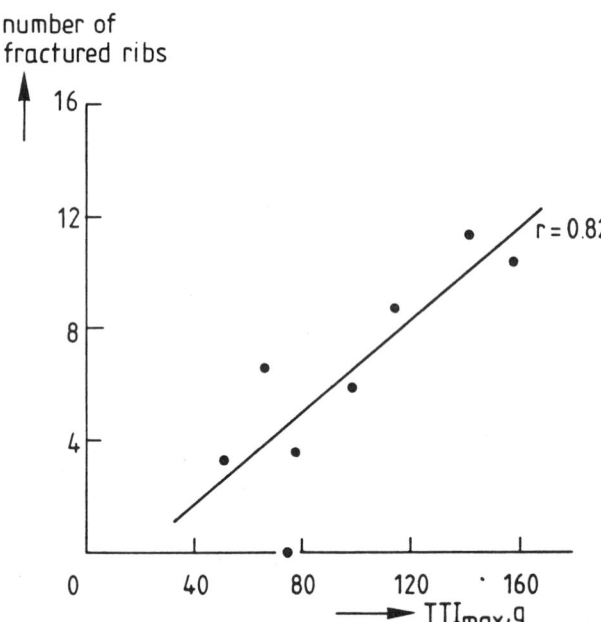

Figure 23. Cross-plot of thoracic cadaver injuries (number of fractured ribs) and maximum TTI of EUROSID obtained from full-scale and ISO impact tests.

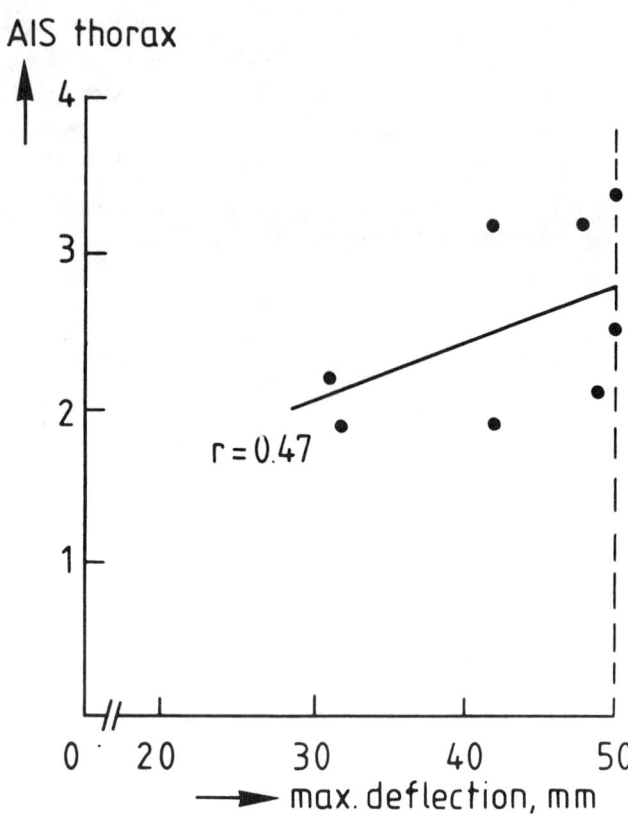

Figure 24. Cross-plot of thoracic cadaver injuries (AIS) and maximum rib deflection of EUROSID obtained from full-scale and ISO impact tests.

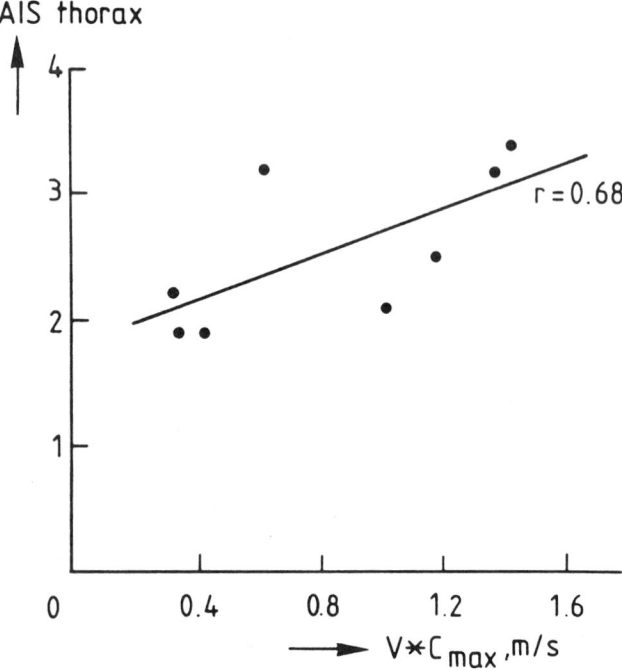

Figure 25. Cross-plot of thoracic cadaver injuries (AIS) and maximum V*C of EUROSID obtained from full-scale and ISO impact tests.

good, while that of V*C or the maximum rib deflection and AIS appears to be less obvious. AIS 2 and AIS 3 injuries would correspond with TTI levels of 60 G and 129 G respectively, with V*C levels of 0.24 m/s and 1.32 m/s respectively and with rib deflection levels of 29 mm and 55 mm respectively.

From figure 19 it can be concluded that the injury assessment capabilities of the EUROSID abdomen are quite good. It should be noticed that the moment of occurrence of the injuries is not known, so the force and deflection could continue after the injuries occurred. Therefore the presented maximum force and maximum penetration appear to be upper tolerance limits. The EUROSID abdomen is designed

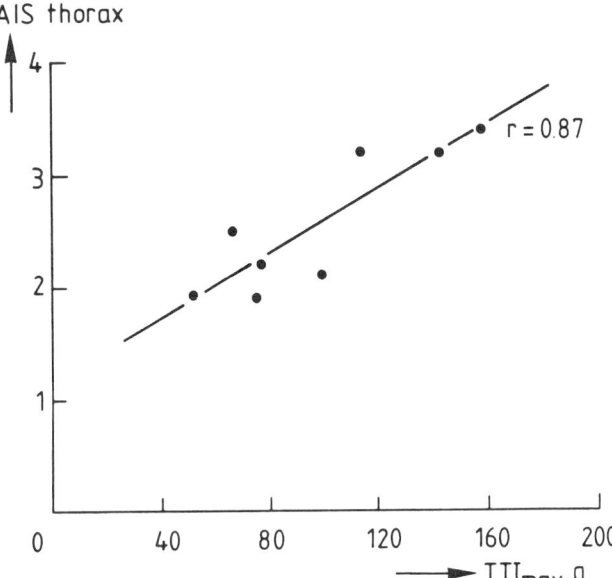

Figure 26. Cross-plot of thoracic cadaver injuries (AIS) and maximum TTI of EUROSID obtained from full-scale and ISO impact tests.

for the worst case; a right hand impact on the liver area. It appears from the full-scale test results that the abdomen quite well indicated the high risk for injuries in these tests.

Table 11 shows that most cadaver tests did not result in a pelvic injury. The highest non-injury producing EUROSID responses have been observed in the 24 km/h rigid sled tests. However, the pubic symphysis and ilium forces obtained from these tests are somewhat higher than the EUROSID responses obtained from the full-scale tests where some injuries did occur in similar cadaver tests. So a 3 ms maximum pelvic acceleration of 100 G and a maximum pubic symphysis force of 10 kN could be considered as non-injury producing limits for the production prototype EUROSID.

General Discussion

The objective of this study was to assess the biofidelity of the production prototype European Side Impact Dummy in impactor-, drop-, sled- and full-scale tests. A comprehensive series of impact tests has been performed by the TNO Road-Vehicles Research Institute. The test set-up of the full-scale tests was based on that of cadaver tests performed by the University of Heidelberg for FAT. The test set-up of the remaining tests was based on documents ISO/DP 9790-1 to 9790-6. The dummy responses have been normalized as required by ISO.

The responses of the EUROSID head in both drop tests exceed the cadaver responses. Now ISO considers the 1200 mm drop test too severe (34). Some improvement could be obtained by using silicone grease between dummy skin and skull.

In a vehicle test a range of possible head contact areas exist. Out of these many areas only one point is evaluated. It appears necessary to examine other possible areas with additional tests (35). EEVC considers 'the transfer of the correct inertial mass from the head to the thorax' the most important feature of the neck (35). In this respect the biofidelity of the EUROSID head-neck system appears to be acceptable.

The biofidelity of the thorax (and arms) in the new proposed drop tests, the sled tests and vehicle tests appears to be satisfactory. Only in the rigid impactor tests the ribs seem to be too stiff. However, these tests are not representative for vehicle tests. Some improvements with respect to the biofidelity of the thorax are proposed by EEVC (see reference (35)). It appears that a good correlation exists between the thoracic protection criteria (i.e. V*C, TTI, maximum rib deflection) and the number of fractured ribs. TTI also shows a good correlation with the thoracic AIS.

The shoulder should not be a major load path into the spine and therefore should not be too stiff (35). In this respect the biofidelity of the EUROSID shoulder appears to be satisfactory.

The biofidelity of the EUROSID abdomen seems to be acceptable up to the tolerance limits; if these are exceeded the design is too stiff. ISO now considers the 2 m drop test too severe (34). The injury assessment capabilities of the abdomen are satisfactory.

The pelvic responses in low velocity and/or padded impacts appear to be in good agreement with cadaver responses. The EUROSID pelvis is too stiff in high velocity rigid impacts and therefore improvements are proposed by EEVC (see reference (35)). Since not many cadavers sustained pelvic injuries, the injury assessment capabilities of the pelvis could not be analyzed in detail.

The tests discussed in this paper were performed using the production prototype EUROSID. Based on this and other studies some improvements with respect to biofidelity, but also with respect to durability, repeatability and instrumentation, are considered by EEVC (see reference (35)). These improvements will be included in the production dummy EUROSID-1.

In a previous paper (7) it was recommended to improve the ISO requirements with respect to definition of the test set-up, required filter classes and normalization procedures. Some improvements have been incorporated in the latest versions of these requirements (8, 9, 10, 11, 12, 13). However, it appears that some requirements still differ too much from the original cadaver tests (e.g. head drop tests and thoracic drop test). Moreover, still some test set-ups are not well defined (e.g. dimensions impactors or impact surfaces). Further improvement of the ISO requirements in this respect seems necessary.

The requirements for each ISO test condition are based on a relatively limited number of tests, sometimes two or three cadavers. It should be noted that many of these cadavers sustained considerable (skeletal) injuries, obviously indicating an overload condition. This raises the question whether a dummy should be able to reproduce the dynamic behaviour of a human being that is severely injured? ISO requirements should be applied critically if they represent overload conditions.

A large number of full-scale vehicle tests using human cadavers have been performed by FAT. The test set-up and test results appear to be well documented and therefore these full-scale cadaver tests could be considered for extension of (ISO) requirements to assess the biofidelity of side impact dummies.

Conclusions

1. A series of impactor tests, drop tests, sled tests and full-scale vehicle tests have been conducted to assess the biofidelity of the European Side Impact Dummy.

2. The test set-up of the full-scale tests is based on a FAT study, where the test set-up and response requirements of the other tests are based on documents ISO/DP 9790-1 to 9790-6.

3. In general the production prototype EUROSID appears to be an acceptable dummy with respect to the current biofidelity standards. Only in high velocity rigid impacts some body parts appear to be too stiff.

4. Minor improvements of the production prototype EUROSID with respect to biofidelity appear to be necessary.

5. A preliminary analysis showed a good correlation between several dummy protection criteria and cadaver injury severity. More detailed analysis is needed in future.

6. The proposed ISO requirements to assess the biofidelity of side impact dummies should be improved by a better definition of the test set-up and adoption should be critically reconsidered if the test set-up represents an overload condition.

References

(1) European Experimental Vehicles Committee (1985), The EUROSID Side Impact Dummy. Proceedings of 10th Conference on Experimental Safety Vehicles, Oxford.

(2) Forschungsvereinigung Automobiltechnik e.V. (1989), FAT Schriftenreihe—to be published.

(3) Forschungsvereinigung Automobiltechnik e.V. (1984), 'Belastbarkeitsgrenze und Verletzungsmechanik des angegurteten Fahrzeuginsassen beim Seitenaufprall. Phase I: Kinematik und Belastungen beim Seitenaufprall im Vergleich Dummy/Leiche.' FAT Schriftenreihe nr. 36, Frankfurt am Main.

(4) Forschungsvereinigung Automobiltechnik e.V. (1986), 'Belastbarkeitsgrenzen und Verletzungsmechanik des angegurteten Pkw-Insassen beim Seitenaufprall. Phase 2: Ansätze für Verletzungsprädiktionen.' FAT Schriftenreihe nr. 60, Frankfurt am Main.

(5) European Experimental Vehicles Committee (1987), 'The Development and Certification of EUROSID.' Presented to 11th Conference on Experimental Safety Vehicles, Washington.

(6) TNO Road-Vehicles Research Institute (1987), 'EUROSID User's Manual.'

(7) Janssen, E.G. and A.C.M. Versmissen (1988), 'Biofidelity of the European Side Impact Dummy—EUROSID.' Proceedings of 32nd Stapp Car Crash Conference, Atlanta.

(8) ISO/DP 9790-1 (1987), 'Road Vehicles—Anthropomorphic Side Impact Dummy—Lateral Head Impact Response Requirements to Assess the Biofidelity of the Dummy.' Technical Committee 22, Subcommittee 12, Geneva, Version November 1987.

(9) ISO/DP 9790-2 (1987), 'Road Vehicles—Anthropomorphic Side Impact Dummy—Lateral Neck Bending Response Requirements to Assess the Biofidelity of the Dummy.' Technical Committee 22, Subcommittee 12, Geneva, Version November 1987.

(10) ISO/DP 9790-3 (1988), 'Road Vehicles—Anthropomorphic Side Impact Dummy—Lateral Thoracic Impact Response Requirements to Assess the Biofidelity of the Dummy.' Technical Committee 22, Subcommittee 12, Geneva, Version July 1988.

(11) ISO/DP 9790-4 (1988), 'Road Vehicles—Anthropomorphic Side Impact Dummy—Lateral Shoulder Impact Response Requirements to Assess the Biofidelity of the Dummy.' Technical Committee 22, Subcommittee 12, Geneva, Version July 1988.

(12) ISO/DP 9790-5 (1988), 'Road Vehicles—Anthropomorphic Side Impact Dummy—Lateral Abdominal Impact Response Requirements to Assess the Biofidelity of the Dummy.' Technical Committee 22, Subcommittee 12, Geneva, Version July 1988.

(13) ISO/DP 9790-6 (1988), 'Road Vehicles—Anthropomorphic Side Impact Dummy—Lateral Pelvic Impact Response Requirements to Assess the Biofidelity of the Dummy.' Technical Committee 22, Subcommittee 12, Geneva, Version August 1988.

(14) Mertz, H.J. (1984), 'A Procedure for Normalizing Impact Response Data.' Presented to Government/Industry Meeting and Exposition, Washington, SAE Paper no. 840884.

(15) Wismans, J. and J. Spenny (1983), 'Performance requirements for mechanical necks in lateral flexion.' Proceedings 27th Stapp Car Crash Conference, SAE paper no. 831613.

(16) Wismans, J., H. van Oorschot and H.J. Woltring (1986), 'Omni-directional human head-neck response.' Proceedings 30th Stapp Car Crash Conference, SAE paper no. 861893.

(17) Laboratoire de Physiologie et de Biomécanique Peugeot S.A./Renault (1982), 'Lateral Dummy Comparison Testing.' Final Report EEC Biomechanics Programme Phase IV—Project F11.

(18) Bendjellal, F. et al. (1988), 'Comparative Evaluation of the Biofidelity of EUROSID and SID Side Impact Dummies.' Proceedings 32nd Stapp Car Crash Conference, SAE paper no. 881717, Atlanta.

(19) Tarrière, C. et al. (1979), 'Synthesis of Human Tolerances Obtained from Lateral Impact Simulations.'

Proceedings of 7th Conference on Experimental Safety Vehicles, Paris.

(20) Janssen, E.G. (1988), 'Evaluation of ISO Impact Response Requirements to Assess the Biofidelity of Side Impact Dummies—Thoracic Drop Test.' ISO/TC22/SC12/WG5—Anthropomorphic Test Devices, Document no. 228.

(21) Tarrière, C. (1989), 'Review of Data and Dummy Requirements Contained in ISO/TC22/SC12—Doc. DP 9790-3 Requirement 1 (July 1988).' ISO/TC22/SC12/WG5—Anthropomorphic Test Devices, Document no. 225.

(22) Mertz, H.J. (1989), 'Summary of APR proposed changes to requirement 1 of ISO/DP 9790-3.' ISO/TC22/SC12/WG5—Anthropomorphic Test Devices, Document no. 226.

(23) Tarrière, C. (1980), Letter and note on side impact dummy to Dr. Nyquist, 18 March 1980, and presented to ISO/TC22/SC12/WG5.

(24) Janssen, E.G. (1986), 'Abdomen Section of the European Side Impact Dummy.' In: The European Side Impact Dummy EUROSID, Proceedings of EEC Seminar held in Brussels December 1986, EEC Report EUR 10779.

(25) Tarrière, C. (1989), 'Observations related to the test set-up used by CCMC, TNO and GM in their respective evaluation of the biofidelity of the EUROSID abdomen.' ISO/TC22/SC12/WG5—Anthropomorphic Test Devices, Document no. 227.

(26) Commission of the European Communities, ad hoc working group "ERGA-Passive Safety" (1987), 'Side-Impact Collision Test.' Document ERGA S/65, Rev. 1A., based on TRANS/SC1/WP29/GRSC/R.58.

(27) Hoefs, R. (1988), 'Analysis of the EUROSID in 21 Full Scale Side Impact Tests.' Proceedings IRCOBI/EEVC Workshop on the Evaluation of Side Impact Dummies, Bergisch-Gladbach.

(28) Janssen, E.G. (1988), 'Evaluation of the European Side Impact Dummy in rigid wall and padded wall sled tests.' Proceedings IRCOBI/EEVC Workshop on the Evaluation of Side Impact Dummies, Bergisch-Gladbach.

(29) Marcus, J.H. et al. (1983), 'Human response to and Injury from Lateral Impact.' Proceedings of 27th Stapp Car Crash Conference, SAE paper no. 831634.

(30) Walfisch, G. et al. (1978), 'Determination des Tolerances Humaines et des Caracteristiques Necessaires a l'Optimalisation de la Protection en Choc Lateral.' Action Thematique Programmée 1978, Rapport Intérimaire No. 1.

(31) Robbins, D.H. et al. (1979), 'Prediction of Thoracic Injuries as a Function of Occupant Kinematics.' Proceedings of 7th Conference on Experimental Safety Vehicles, Paris.

(32) Morgan, R.M. and H.P. Waters (1980), 'Comparison of Two Promising Side Impact Dummies.' Proceedings of 8th Conference on Experimental Safety Vehicles, Wolfsburg.

(33) Brun-Cassan, F. et al. (1988), 'Clarification of APR Data on the Abdomen Tolerance of Human Beings Involved in Side Impact.' ISO/TC22/SC12/WG6, Document no. 277.

(34) ISO (1988), 'Summary of WG5 Evaluation of SID and EUROSID.' ISO/TC22/SC12/WG5, Document no. 218.

(35) Roberts, A.K. (1989), 'EEVC Working Group 9 Report on EUROSID 1989' Presented to 12th Conference on Experimental Safety Vehicles, Göteborg.

Appendix 1

Mertz (14) showed that for normalizing purposes a cadaver subject during impact with an impact surface can be replaced by a simple spring-mass system (see figure below). A mass, known as the "effective mass" M_e, can be determined that produces the same interaction impulse and velocity change as that experienced by the cadaver. Reference to impulse-momentum consideration gives,

$$\int_0^T F\,dt = W_e \Delta V / g + W_e T$$

$$\rightarrow W_e/g = [\int_0^T F\,dt] / (\Delta V + Tg) = M_e$$

where

F—load on subject due to interaction with impact surface
T—impact duration
g—acceleration of gravity
ΔV—velocity change
V_o—initial velocity
K—stiffness of subject
W_e—effective weight of subject
M_e—effective mass

For non-drop tests, e.g. impactor and sled tests, the equation reduces to:

$$M_e = [\int_0^T F\,dt] / (\Delta V)$$

Mertz selected an effective mass for a standard subject M_s by calculating the average percentage body mass involved in the cadaver tests. This percentage applied to the 50th percentile adult male's body mass (76 kg) is known as the standard effective mass M_s. The mass ratio used to normalize the cadaver data is,

$R_m = M_s/M_e$

The stiffness ratio is defined as:

$R_k = K_s/K_i$

where K_s is the stiffness of a standard subject and K_i of the i-th cadaver.

Mertz (14) calculated normalizing factors for force, acceleration, displacement and time using these mass and stiffness ratios:

$$R_f = (R_m)^{1/2} (R_k)^{1/2}$$
$$R_a = (R_k)^{1/2} (R_m)^{-1/2}$$
$$R_x = (R_m)^{1/2} (R_k)^{-1/2}$$
$$R_t = (R_m)^{1/2} (R_k)^{-1/2}$$

Documents ISO/DP 9790-3 to 9790-6 require that the dummy data be normalized in order to adjust for changes in effective mass due to slight differences in dummy position at impact. The velocity change ΔV for the calculation of M_e should be obtained from integration of the dummy acceleration-time curve:

$$\Delta V = \int_0^T a\, dt$$

For cases where the cadaver acceleration-time response was not available, the initial impact velocity V_o was used to approximate ΔV. For pelvic requirements 2 and 3 of DP 9790-6, neither the cadaver acceleration-time responses nor the force-time responses were available. For these requirements, the mass ratio R_m was calculated by:

$$R_m = 76\, kg/M_i$$

where M_i is the total cadaver mass. This relationship should be used to normalize the dummy data where M_i is the total dummy mass.

It is assumed that the stiffness ratio R_k for dummies is equal to 1, so the normalizing factors are based on R_m only.

Acknowledgements

The full-scale vehicle impacts have been sponsored by the Dutch Government and by the Forschungsvereinigung Automobiltechnik e.V. (FAT). The ISO thoracic drop tests based on the new proposed test set-up have been partly sponsored by the Laboratoire de Physiologie et de Biomécanique/APR. Ford Motor Company UK/USA partly sponsored the thoracic sled tests. The Naval Biodynamics Laboratory has performed the ISO neck sled tests.

896113

Biomechanics of the Human Chest, Abdomen, and Pelvis in Lateral Impact

David C. Viano, Ian V. Lau, and Corbin Asbury
General Motors Research Laboratories

Albert I. King and Paul Begeman
Wayne State University

Abstract

Fourteen unembalmed cadavers were subjected to forty-four blunt lateral impacts at velocities of approximately 4.5, 6.7, or 9.4 m/s with a 15 cm flat pendulum weighing 23.4 kg. Chest and abdominal injuries consisted primarily of rib fractures with a few cases of lung or liver laceration in the highest severity impacts. There were two cases of pubic ramus fracture in the pelvic impacts. Logist analysis of the biomechanical responses and serious injury, indicated that the maximum Viscous response had the best correlation with injury risk for chest and abdominal impacts. A tolerance level of VC = 1.5 m/s for the chest and VC = 2.0 m/s for the abdomen were determined for a 25% probability of serious injury. Maximum compression was similarly set at C = 38% for the chest and C = 44% for the abdomen. The experiments indicate that chest and abdominal injury can occur by a viscous mechanism during the rapid phase of body compression, and that the Viscous response is an effective measure of injury risk in side impacts. A compression tolerance is set to assess crushing injury risks. Pubic ramus fracture correlated with compression of the pelvis not impact force or acceleration. Pelvic tolerance was set at 27% compression.

The 1986 FARS indicates that 31.8% of passenger car fatalities occur in crashes with the principal direction of force lateral on the vehicle (figure 1). Two-thirds of the fatalities are in multi-vehicle accidents where the car is struck by a passenger car, truck, or other vehicle, while the other third involve single vehicle accidents into primarily fixed objects. Approximately an equal number of fatalities occur in driver side and passenger side lateral impact crashes, and the toll in human life is about 8,000 victims annually.

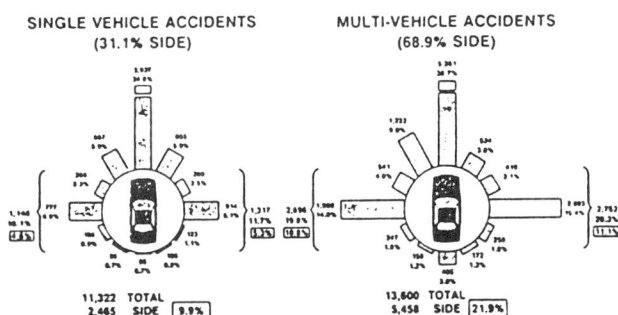

Figure 1. Distribution of impact by principle direction of force in 1986 FARS single and multi-vehicle fatal crashes.

A recent study (Viano 1989) of individual multi-vehicle side impact crashes indicates that a majority of the fatal crashes occur at an intersection and that the victim is primarily an older occupant. An evaluation of national statistics from NASS (table 1) indicates that when side and frontal impact crashes are compared, side impacts represent about half of the crashes involving serious to fatal passenger car injury. When crashes are separated into multi-vehicle (car-car) or fixed object impacts, the age of the occupant emerges as an important factor in side impacts. In particular, multi-vehicle side impact crashes are a major cause (40–54%) of injury to occupants over the age of 40, whereas occupants of this age range are infrequently involved in side impact crashes into fixed objects.

Table 1. Passenger car crashes from 1982–86 NASS with serious-fatal front seat occupant injuries.

Age	Side Impact Car-Car	Side Impact Fixed Object	Frontal Impact Car-Car	Frontal Impact Fixed Object	Total
20–	2,840 (21%)	4,829 (36%)	3,536 (27%)	2,072 (16%)	13,277
20–40	8,068 (25%)	6,718 (20%)	10,971 (33%)	7,110 (22%)	32,867
40–60	5,004 (40%)	761 (6%)	5,466 (43%)	1,417 (11%)	12,648
60–80	5,010 (44%)	165 (1%)	4,123 (36%)	2,110 (18%)	11,408
80+	819 (54%)	46 (3%)	369 (25%)	270 (18%)	1,504
	21,741 (30%)	12,519 (17%)	24,465 (34%)	12,979 (18%)	71,704

The current study simulates the forces of contact on the chest, abdomen and pelvis in a side impact crash. A pendulum impact mass is used to load an unembalmed cadaver over a range of impact speeds and follows a protocol that has been used previously to study frontal impact responses (Kroell 1976). This allows direct comparison of the lateral impact responses to the frontal data, and takes advantage of a proven methodology for research on impact biomechanics.

The study also addresses a range of candidate mechanical responses for injury assessment. These include the Viscous (Viano 1988b, Lau 1986) and compression (Nahum 1970) responses for the chest and abdomen since they are an effective measure of injury risk by impact and crushing mechanisms, respectively. The Viscous response is evaluated since it is proven to be the underlying mechanism of soft tissue trauma to internal organs and vessels in blunt impact. It has also successfully pinpointed the time of greatest injury risk in an impact. This has helped focus efforts on vehicle design changes to improve product safety. The Viscous response has also been shown to accurately measure the risk of serious and life-threatening trauma in cadaver and animal studies.

Based on Cesari (1982), hip acceleration is investigated for pelvic fracture. Although response and injury will be compared with peak acceleration measurements, peak acceleration is an insufficient correlate and not a causal factor in soft tissue chest and abdominal injury (Brun-Cassan 1987). In addition, the recent acceleration formulation TTI, has been criticized by many in the scientific community (Tarriere 1988, Viano 1987b, Lau 1988). Although acceleration criteria have a rich history in product safety testing, our current understandings of human injury indicate that body deformations are the causal factor of soft tissue chest and abdominal injury and such deformation is not adequately assessed by acceleration measures.

A scientific understanding of frontal impact injury biomechanics has been developed by using the pendulum impact methods of this study. This approach has successfully led to the development of human-like body deformation characteristics which include the force-deflection or compliance behavior of the chest and abdomen under impact loading. The data has enabled the development of the Hybrid III dummy which realistically simulates the human response in frontal impact, and enables a valid assessment of product safety improvements.

There has also been an advance in our understanding of the mechanisms of injury, and tolerance criteria of the human body to impact force. Much of this has been based on human cadaver tests, which help define body compliance and assess injury severity primarily based on skeletal trauma. Comparable research (Viano 1988b) has been conducted for frontal and lateral impacts with a physiological model to study life-threatening trauma, by laceration or rupture of internal organs and vessels or by interruption of normal cardiac or respiratory function. In frontal and lateral impact, the Viscous response has been shown to be the principal mechanical cause of soft tissue injury. This study aimed to assess its comparable tolerance level and risk function in lateral impacts of human cadavers.

Materials and Methods

Unembalmed cadavers were provided through the Department of Anatomy at Wayne State University Medical School as part of a willed-body program.[1] They had an average age of 53.8 ± 13.9 years and body weight of 67.2 ± 16.2 kg.

Specimen selection and handling

The specimen were selected on an age, condition, and cause of death criteria, which limited age to approximately 65 years unless the specimen was of good skeletal condition. All cadavers were tested after rigormortis had passed. In some of the specimen, the average time lapsed between expiration and actual testing was one to two weeks. In other specimen, the time lapse was greater between the expiration and testing, so the specimen was frozen (4°F) for a period of time. Prior to testing, the specimen were refrigerated at 35°F.

Instrumentation and preparation

The cadaver was instrumented with an array of accelerometers attached to the spine and pelvis. A triaxial accelerometer package was attached to the first, eighth and twelfth thoracic vertebrae and a similar package to the pelvic region at the second sacral vertebrae. Targets were attached to the triaxial clusters for photographic coverage and film analysis.

---

[1] The rationale and experimental protocol for use of human cadaver research subjects in this program have been reviewed by the Research Laboratories' Human Research Committee. The research complies with the provisions of the Uniform Anatomical Gift Act, follows guidelines established by the US Department of Transportation, National Highway Traffic Safety Administration and recommendations of the National Research Council of the National Academy of Sciences, and adheres to the provisions of The Declaration of Helsinki.

The cadaver's arterial system was pressurized by normal saline infused through a Foley catheter inserted in the aorta above the diaphragm. A vent tube was inserted in the brachial artery. Prior to an experiment, the catheter balloon was pressurized to block the flow below it and saline was pumped into the body until it flowed out of the vent tube. The vent was then clamped, ensuring pressure in the chest and upper abdominal organs. The lung was carefully drained of any fluid and then aerated repeatedly with room air prior to testing. The lung was pressurized.

Necropsy

Autopsy was performed by a board certified pathologist, and special attention was paid to injury of the chest, abdomen, and pelvis.

Data analysis

High speed movies of the impact were taken at 2,000 frames per second from the frontal and 500 frames per second from the posterior and overhead views. Frame-by-frame analysis of the impact event formed the basis for the instantaneous deflection data of the torso and hip. Deflection was processed to derive the compression and Viscous responses based on an established algorithm by Viano (1988a) and Lau (1986). The acceleration channels were processed by SAE or FIR filters.

Injury functions

Viscous Response [VC(t)]—A time function produced by multiplying the instantaneous velocity of deformation and compression responses (units in m/s, derived from film data).

Compression Response [C(t)]—The instantaneous deformation divided by the initial torso thickness along the axis of the impact (dimensionless, derived from film data).

Spinal Acceleration Response [Gsp(t)]—Instantaneous lateral acceleration of the spine measured by an accelerometer on T1, T8, T12 or pelvis at S3 (units in g's derived from electronic data).

Force [F(t)]—Impact force resulting from pendulum contact (units in kN's, derived from acceleration of the pendulum from electronic data multiplied by the pendulum mass).

Injury criteria

Viscous Criterion [VC]max—The peak Viscous response (Viano 1988a, Lau 1986).

Compression Criterion [C]max—The peak compression response.

Spinal Acceleration Criterion [Gsp]max—The peak lateral or resultant spinal acceleration response.

Force Criterion [F]max—The peak force acting on the body.

Statistical methods

Injury risk functions were computed using the Logist function in the Statistical Analysis Package. This function relates the probability of injury occurrence $P(x)$ to the magnitude of a response parameter x based on a statistical fit to a sigmoidal function $P(x) = [1 + \exp(\alpha - \beta\chi)]^{-1}$. The goodness-of-fit of the statistic is quantified by the chi-squared (χ^2), p-value (p) and correlation coefficient (R).

The impact

Experiments were conducted with a power-assisted pendulum impactor (figure 2). The 23.4 kg pendulum was freely suspended by guide wires and accelerated to impact speeds of approximately 4.5, 6.7 or 9.4 m/s in 5 cm by a pneumatically charged cylinder with thrust piston. The level of charge pressure determines the thrust velocity. The forward motion of the pendulum was abruptly stopped by a cable tether after 15 cm of contact.

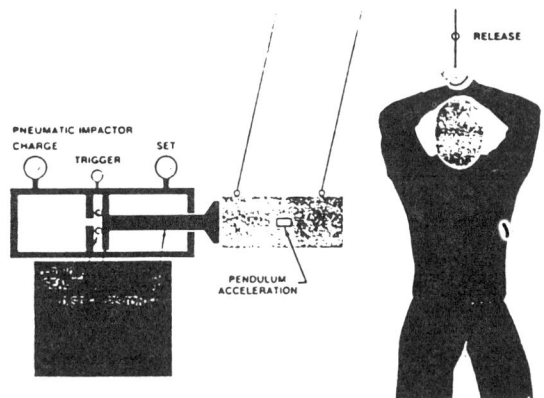

Figure 2. Experimental set-up with a pneumatic power-assisted pendulum and upright supported specimen.

The cadaver was suspended upright with hands and arms overhead. The specimen was rotated 30° so the point of pendulum contact was lateral on the thorax or abdomen. This protocol was used to assure that full lateral thoracic and abdominal impact occurred with the axis of force through the center of gravity of the torso. It resulted in controlled compression of the torso without coincident rotation of the body about the spine axis. The center of pendulum impact on the thorax was aligned with the xiphoid process (7.5 cm below midsternum). Abdominal impact was aligned 7.5 cm below the xiphoid (15 cm below midsternum). Pelvic impacts were conducted at 90° lateral with the impactor centered on the greater trochanter.

The pendulum interface was a smooth, flat, 15 cm diameter disc with the edges rounded. The axis of impact force was aligned through the center of gravity of the torso for chest and abdomen tests (approximately 2 cm anterior of the intrathoracic surface of the vertebrae). A uniaxial accelerometer was attached to the pendulum and its response was multiplied by the pendulum mass to give the force of impact. A suspension system released the arms at impact enabling a free torso response to impact. The off-side of impact was padded to gradually support the free body response.

Multiple tests were conducted on a specimen to increase biomechanical response data. This could include a low-severity left abdominal impact, an injurious high-severity thoracic test and a lateral pelvic impact.

Results

Three of six tests in the high velocity chest impact series resulted in lacerative injury of the lung, liver, diaphragm, kidney or spleen. In the high-velocity chest impact series, five of six specimen had flail chest with an average of 14 rib fractures. There were only two cases of severe upper abdominal injury in the high severity impacts and they consisted of laceration of the liver and diaphragm. In these impacts, only one of four specimen experienced more than eight rib fractures. There were six high velocity lateral impacts of the hip and, in spite of the high severity of loading, there were only two incidents of pubic ramus fracture. In terms of overall injury severity, each exposure was summarized by the number of rib fractures or skeletal injury, the maximum severity of skeletal trauma (SAIS), and the maximum overall severity of injury (MAIS).

The response and injury data were averaged in table 2 for the three pendulum impact speeds. Chest and abdominal impact responses increased as the severity of impact speed increased. The experimental protocol maximized the opportunity to define a correlation between injury and the measured response parameters but also set up the possibility that unrelated or weakly related parameters may also correlate with injury.

Table 2. Summary biomechanics and injury for lateral thoracic, abdominal and pelvic impact.

Thorax Response	Test Speed (m/s)		
	4.42 ± 0.86	6.52 ± 0.32	9.33 ± 0.71
Force (kN)	2.67 ± 0.99	3.10 ± 0.46	6.30 ± 0.90
Deflection (cm)	8.40 ± 1.30	11.20 ± 1.35	14.18 ± 1.79
Compression (%)	26.1 ± 4.1	34.9 ± 4.5	43.2 ± 3.9
VC (m/s)	0.62 ± 0.23	1.10 ± 0.18	2.05 ± 0.41
C_{T1-y}	14.0 ± 6.0		46.1 ± 8.3
C_{T8-y}	16.5 ± 6.5	33.6 ± 8.1	62.5 ± 20.4
C_{T12-y}	12.6 ± 8.5	25.4 ± 5.1	54.6 ± 25.3
MAIS	0.4 ± 0.9	2.8 ± 0.5	4.0 ± 0.6
SAIS	0.4 ± 0.9	2.8 ± 0.5	3.8 ± 0.4
Rib Fractures (#)	0.4 ± 0.9	5.2 ± 1.5	12.7 ± 4.5

Abdomen Response	Test Speed (m/s)		
	4.79 ± 0.77	6.83 ± 0.15	9.40 ± 0.87
Force (kN)	2.41 ± 0.49	3.71 ± 0.48	6.50 ± 1.10
Deflection (cm)	10.83 ± 2.30	11.43 ± 0.76	14.60 ± 2.36
Compression (%)	32.0 ± 6.6	36.2 ± 1.65	45.8 ± 3.1
VC (m/s)	0.77 ± 0.23	1.26 ± 0.12	2.22 ± 0.41
C_{T1-y}	6.9 ± 2.0	17.5 ± 1.9	37.5 ± 11.0
C_{T8-y}	10.8 ± 4.4	28.9 ± 7.1	29.1 ± 5.9
C_{T12-y}	11.6 ± 6.2	29.8 ± 12.4	44.3 ± 9.0
MAIS	0.7 ± 1.2	2.0 ± 1.4	2.0 ± 2.3
SAIS	0.7 ± 1.2	2.0 ± 1.4	1.8 ± 2.1
Rib Fractures (#)	0.8 ± 1.6	3.3 ± 3.0	3.8 ± 4.5

Pelvis Response	Test Speed (m/s)		
	4.83 ± 0.58	6.77 ± 0.10	9.65 ± 0.64
Force (kN)	5.45 ± 1.66	6.81 ± 1.60	11.20 ± 1.48
Deflection (cm)	4.90 ± 1.60	9.85 ± 1.34	7.83 ± 2.27
Compression (%)	13.5 ± 4.0	25.0 ± 0.3	22.9 ± 6.0
C_{T8-y}	7.7 ± 3.1		
C_{T12-y}	15.0 ± 12.6	18.5 ± 3.9	31.6 ± 8.5
C_{S3-y}	34.4 ± 15.0	23.6 ± 3.6	39.9 ± 26.8
MAIS	0	0	0.7 ± 1.0
SAIS	0	0	0.7 ± 1.0
Pelvic Fracture	0	0	0.3 ± 0.5

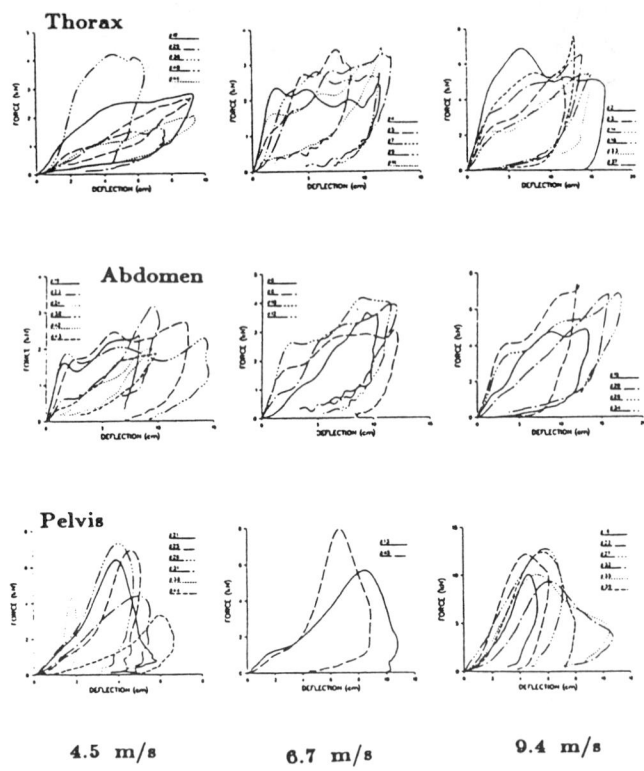

4.5 m/s   6.7 m/s   9.4 m/s

Figure 3. Grouped dynamic responses for applied force and body deformation in 4.5, 6.7 and 9.4 m/s pendulum impacts of the thorax, abdomen and pelvis.

A comparison of the chest and abdominal impacts indicates a similar level of peak force, deflection, and compression for each level of impact severity. The Viscous response was higher in the abdominal impacts probably because of less skeletal structure resisting the low-deflection response. A lack of vitality in the upper abdominal organs may have led to a lower average severity of abdominal injury than occurred in chest impacts of comparable impact severity. Internal chest injury was frequently associated with multiple rib fractures indicative of flail chest. For the pelvic impacts, the force increased with the increasing severity of impact speed.

Figure 3 summarizes the force-deflection responses for the experiments at the low, middle, and high severity impact of the chest, abdomen, and pelvis. The force-deflection response defines the compliance of the torso or pelvis under lateral impact and is a key biomechanical response of impact. The area under each curve represents the amount of energy absorbed by body deformation.

Logist analysis was applied to the biomechanical responses to identify risk functions for four or more rib fractures (MAIS 3+) or serious injury (MAIS 4+ or 9+ rib fractures). The Viscous response shows the strongest correlation with serious to critical injury for responses measured in the chest and abdominal impacts. Peak force had a higher correlation with serious injury but is an input parameter measured on the pendulum. Maximum chest compression was also a significant correlate with serious injury, whereas none of the responses correlated with the risk of moderate skeletal injury in the lateral abdominal impacts. Pelvic compression emerged as the only correlate with pubic ramus fracture.

The Viscous response emerged as the best and most descriptive measure of injury risk. Logist functions are plotted in figure 4 for the probability of serious injury as a function of the Viscous and compression response of the chest and abdomen. A 95% confidence interval is also given. The functions are sigmoidal in shape indicating three distinct regions. For low values of the response, there is a region of very low risk of injury. Similarly, for the very high values of the response, there is a flat high-risk of serious injury outcome. In-between is a region where injury risk is proportional to the associated response. The sigmoidal function is typical of a risk distribution with a biomechanical response from a population with weaker and stronger subjects.

Tolerance levels were determined for a 25% probability of serious injury in the chest, abdomen and pelvis. This probability level is consistent with previous studies of injury risk from human cadaver and animal impacts (Viano 1988a, 1988b, Lau 1986, 1987, 1988) and is at a risk level found in current crash protection standards. Tolerance to AIS 4+ injury is set at VC=1.5 m/s and C=38% for the chest and VC=2.0 m/s and C=44% for the abdomen. Pelvic tolerance is C=27%.

Discussion

This study has shown that the Viscous response is the best biomechanical parameter to assess impact injury in lateral impact of the chest and abdomen. The finding is consistent with previous research by Viano (1988a) and Lau (1986) on impact injury in frontal loading of the chest and similar research by Lau (1987) on the abdomen. In those studies the Viscous response was found to be the causal mechanism and strongest correlate with injury. More recent experiments by Lau (1988) have shown that serious injury to soft tissues and organs occurs at the time of peak Viscous response, well before maximum deflection. We expect that serious abdominal and thoracic injury from high-speed lateral impact will be similarly associated with the rapid compression phase of loading.

Experiments by Viano (1988b) with anesthetized swine show also that lateral impact injury is associated with a viscous mechanism. Serious internal thoracic and abdominal injury occurred with minimal skeletal damage. The research confirms in a physiologic model with organ sizes and weights similar to that of man that the Viscous response is an effective measure of injury risk in lateral impact.

The correlation of maximum deflection or compression with injury is consistent with relationships found in previous studies on the frontal impact response of human cadavers and anesthetized swine. However, a relationship was not found between compression and injury in recent lateral chest impacts of anesthetized swine (Viano 1988b). In those tests, a relationship existed between low and middle severity impacts but was not found between the middle and high severity tests. Spinal acceleration was higher between the middle and high severity tests as well as

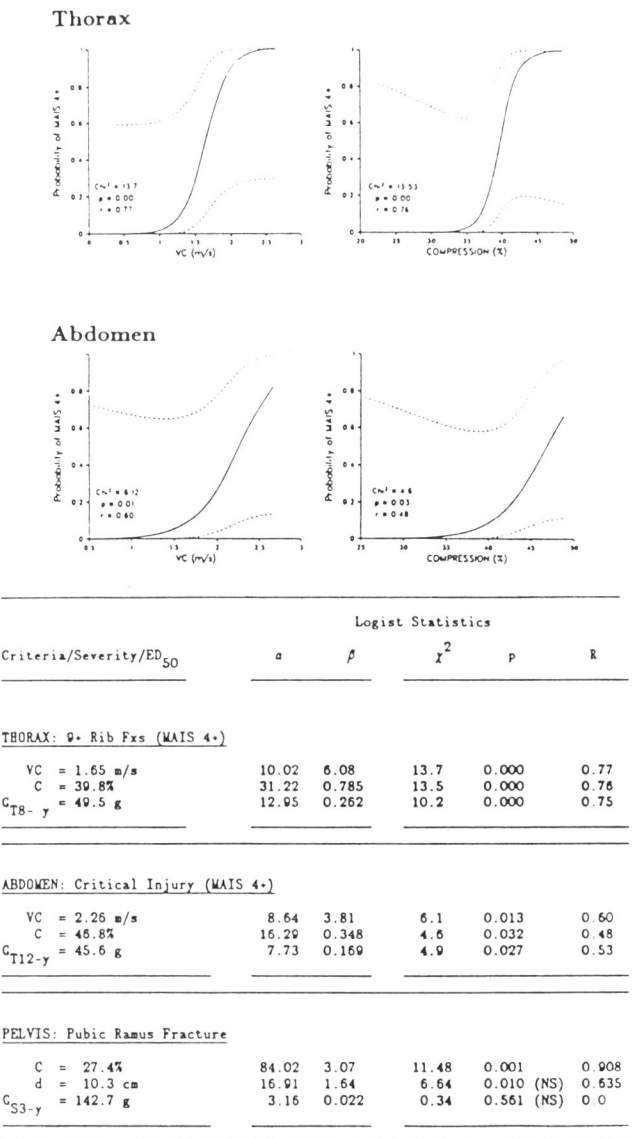

Figure 4. Logist functions and statistics for the probability of critical injury of the thorax and abdomen, and pubic ramus fracture of the pelvis.

impact force, resulting in more whole-body displacement of the animal. The failure of maximum compression to correlate with an increased severity of injury is further evidence that soft tissue trauma may be more associated with the rapid-phase of body deformation during impact. However, in some circumstances injury may occur by a slow crushing load on the body, and maximum compression would be an important factor.

Although acceleration measures correlate with some types of injury in this study, they have been shown in other research to be unrelated when a range of test-types are merged. In two studies by Lau (1986, 1988), pendulum and sled tests could be independently shown to correlate body accelerations with injury; but, when the data were merged no relationship existed between peak accelerations and injury. This situation has been shown for frontal impact and is a result of acceleration being the sum of two independent components: one associated with deflection of the body, and the other with whole-body displacement in response to force. Our studies have shown that body deformation is the key factor in impact injury and that whole-body acceleration primarily brings the body to a common velocity with the impactor or sled.

Our work is part of an effort to define the global biomechanics of the human chest and abdomen. It is possible to characterize the force-deflection response by an initial stiffness, and average plateau force in the mid-deflection region. This was done for the frontal and lateral chest impacts and is plotted in figure 5 by orientation from frontal (0°) through 60° lateral to 120° lateral. Solid lines connect the regions where test data are available and the dotted lines represent an estimate of what the full global biomechanical response may be when a complete set of responses is collected for the 6.7 m/s blunt impact condition.

The force-deflection characteristics of the human chest are an important response for the development of anthro-

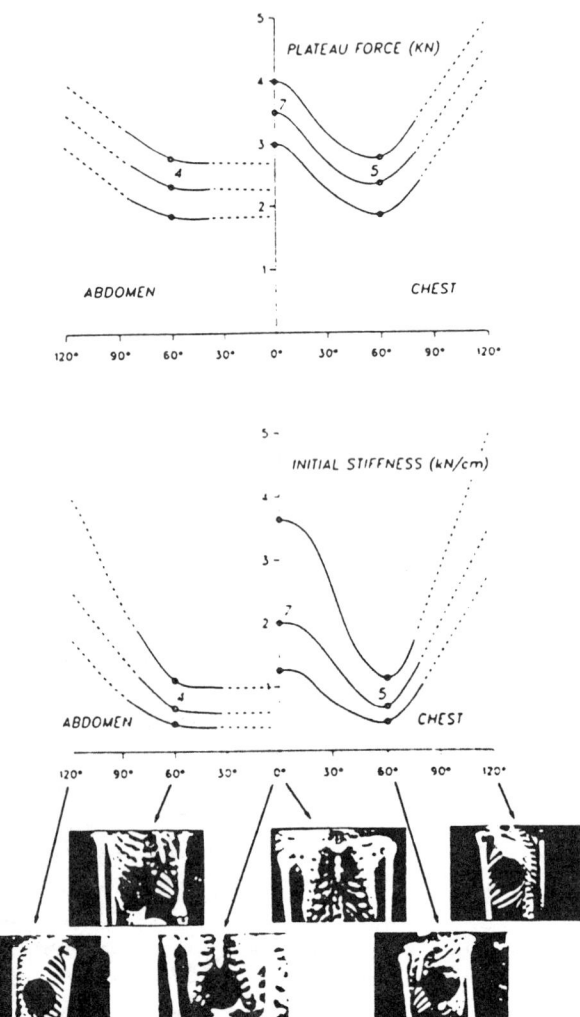

Figure 5. The global impact response of the human chest and abdomen is represented by the plateau force and initial stiffness (average ± 1 standard deviation). Solid lines connect known data and dotted lines represent estimates of the human response.

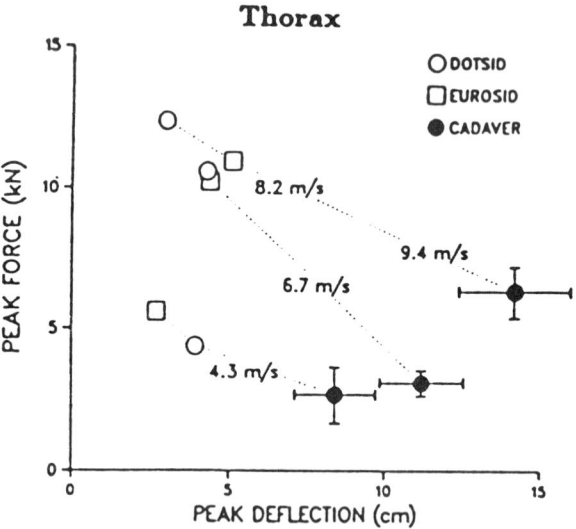

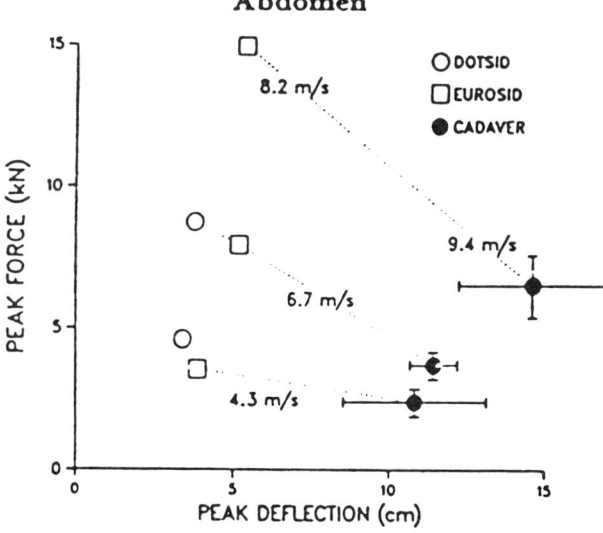

Figure 6. Peak force and deflection from blunt lateral impact of the human cadaver and current side impact test dummies at three levels of severity.

pometric test devices that simulate the human response to impact and assess injury risks. Figure 6 summarizes the peak force and deflection responses from lateral impacts of human cadavers at three test speeds as well as similar information from recent tests with the SID and EUROSID at similar speeds. These data indicate that current test devices develop significantly higher plateau forces and much lower deflections than the human cadaver and anesthetized swine. This lack of biofidelity in force-deflection response of the current side impact ATD's is a significant deficiency (Viano 1987a) in their ability to simulate the human response and injury in side impact tests.

Biofidelity is important because the design of side interior padding to optimize responses in the dummies will result in much stiffer materials to be compatible with the high force levels developed by the dummies. Stiff materials may essentially eliminate the safety potential for real occupants who develop much lower levels of force and thus need softer materials (Viano 1987b). The difference in compliance between current test dummies and the human will also result in significant differences in occupant kinematics during a side impact. In particular, the greater deflection experienced by the human chest and abdomen will allow the head to move more laterally with respect to the vehicle's side interior and will result in a significantly different trajectory of the head. This aspect is important to a system's engineering approach to improving side impact protection.

On the basis of this study and our previous research, we believe that the maximum Viscous response should be limited to protect against injury during the rapid phase of body deformation of the chest and abdomen during side impact loading. As shown in previous work by Viano (1988a) and Lau (1988), serious internal injury can occur without a significant number of rib fractures or rib cage injury at all. This evidence again supports the potential for the early occurrence of soft tissue injury at about the time of maximum Viscous response and where deflection or compression of the body has reached only about half of its maximum value. We also believe in the need to limit maximum chest compression during crash testing to protect against crushing injuries which may occur during slow or static deformation of the chest and abdomen. This is clearly a different mechanism of injury than the Viscous mechanism. Limiting the Viscous and compression response is a complementary approach to assessing safety systems (Viano 1988a, Lau 1986). Our data also indicate that compression of the pelvis may be a better predictor of hip fracture than pelvic acceleration.

References

(1) Brun-Cassan, F., Pincemaille, Y., Mack, P., Tarriere, C., "Contribution to the Evaluation of the Criteria Proposed for Thorax-Abdomen Protection in Lateral Impact." In *Proceedings of the 11th International ESV Conference*, Washington, DC, May, 1987.

(2) Cesari, D., Ramet, M., "Pelvic Tolerance and Protection Criteria in Side Impact." In *Proceedings of the 26th Stapp Car Crash Conference*, Society of Automotive Engineers Technical Paper #821159, pp. 145–154, Warrendale, PA, 1982.

(3) Kroell, C.K., "Thoracic Response to Blunt Frontal Loading." In *The Human Thorax-Anatomy, Injury and Biomechanics*. SAE Publication P-67, pp. 49–78, Warrendale, PA, Society of Automotive Engineers, 1976.

(4) Lau, I.V., and Viano, D.C., "The Viscous Criterion: Bases and Applications of an Injury Severity Index for Soft Tissues," In *Proceedings of the 30th Stapp Car Crash Conference*, SAE Technical Paper #861882 pp. 123–142, October, 1986.

(5) Lau, I.V., Horsch, J.D., Viano, D.C. and Andrzejak, D.V., "Biomechanics of Liver Injury by Steering Wheel Loading." *Journal of Trauma*, 27(3):225–235, April, 1987.

(6) Lau, I.V. and Viano, D.C., "How and When Blunt Injury Occurs: Implications to Frontal and Side Impact Protection." In *Proceedings of the 32nd Stapp Car Crash Conference*, Society of Automotive Engineers Technical Paper #881714, Society of Automotive Engineers, Warrendale, PA, October, 1988.

(7) Nahum, A.M., Gadd, C.W., Schneider, D.C., and Kroell, C.K., "Deflection of the Human Thorax Under Sternal Impact." SAE's International Automobile Safety Conference, Society of Automotive Engineers Technical Paper #700400, pp. 797–807, Detroit, MI, May 1970.

(8) Tarriere, C., Brun-Cassan, F. and Thomas, C., "Specific Highlights Relative to Injury Parameters in Side Impacts Including Unanimous Opinions of ISO SC12 Working Groups 5 and C." ISO/TC22/SC12/-GTG, No. 256, 1988.

(9) Viano, D.C., "Evaluation of the SID Dummy and TTI Injury Criterion for Side Impact Testing." In *Proceedings of the 31st Stapp Car Crash Conference*, SAE Technical Paper #872208, pp. 143–160, November, 1987a.

(10) Viano, D.C., "Evaluation of the Benefit of Energy-Absorbing Material for Side Impact Protection: Part II." In *Proceedings of the 31st Stapp Car Crash Conference*, Society of Automotive Engineers Technical Paper #872213, pp. 205–224, Society of Automotive Engineers, Warrendale, PA, November, 1987b.

(11) Viano, D.C. and Lau, I.V., "A Viscous Tolerance Criterion for Soft Tissue Injury Assessment." *J Biomech*, 21(5):387–399, 1988a.

(12) Viano, D.C., Lau, I.V., Andrzejak, D.V., and Asbury, C., "Biomechanics of Injury in Lateral Chest Impact in Anesthetized Swine." General Motors Research Report, Appendix to the GM Response to the Side Impact Notice of Proposed Rulemaking, Federal Docket, 1988b.

902305

Biomechanical Response and Injury Tolerance of the Pelvis in Twelve Sled Side Impacts

John M. Cavanaugh, Timothy J. Walilko, Anita Malhotra,
Youghua Zhu, and Albert I. King
Wayne State University

ABSTRACT

Twelve side impact sled tests were performed using a horizontally accelerated sled and a Heidelberg-type seat fixture. The purpose of these tests was to better understand biomechanical response and injury tolerance in whole-body side impacts. In these tests the subject's whole body impacted a sidewall with one of three surface conditions: 1) a flat, rigid side wall, 2) a side wall with a 6" pelvic offset, or 3) a flat, padded side wall. This paper presents the biomechanical response and injury tolerance data obtained for the pelvis. Peak values of sacral-y acceleration, pelvic force, compression and velocity x compression were evaluated as predictors of pelvic injury. Based on Logist analysis, Vmax x Cmax was the best predictor of probability of pelvic fracture in this test series, while peak pelvic force and peak compression also performed well.

INTRODUCTION

Pelvic ring fractures occur in 10-14% of nearside occupants in lateral impact (Cesari et al., 1980). Fracture can occur at several locations on the pelvic ring, including pubic rami, pubic symphysis, iliac wing, sacro-iliac junction and acetabulum. Internal organ injury (ie. to bladder) can also occur.

Maximum applied force, maximum pelvic acceleration, compression and velocity x compression have been proposed as fracture criteria in lateral pelvic impact. Cesari et al (1982) proposed a 10 kN limit on impact force for a 76 kg male and 4 kN for a 5th percentile female (3 ms clip). These data are for an older subject population, with pendelum impacts to the greater trochanter. Tarriere (1979), in a series of lateral drop tests to cadaveric subjects, reported pelvic fractures when pelvic accelerations were between 62 and 120 g. Viano et al (1989), performed lateral impacts to the pelvis with a 23.4 kg pendelum impactor, and analyzed compression, deflection and S3-y acceleration as injury risk functions using Logist analysis. Pelvic compression was the only correlate with pubic ramus fracture. Impact force and acceleration did not correlate with injury.

METHODS

The surrogates used in the lateral impact tests were unembalmed human cadavers donated to the University under the Willed Body Program. The cadavers were used shortly after rigor mortis had passed. The subjects were positioned on a Heidelberg-type seat fixture (illustrated in Marcus et al, 1983) which in turn was mounted to a horizontally accelerated sled. The sled was accelerated up to velocities of 6.7 to 10.5 m/s and then rapidly decelerated so that the cadavers would continue to translate laterally on a teflon seat into the wall of the seat fixture. The cadaver was instrumented with accelerometers and pressure transducers to record the kinetics and kinematics of impact. The impact side wall was instrumented with nine load cells to record impact forces (Fig. 1).

CADAVER PREPARATION AND INSTRUMENTATION - The cadavers had pre-test x-rays taken of all skeletal structures as well as abdominal and chest x-rays in order to determine existing skeletal and soft tissue anomalies. In addition to accelerometers mounted to the head and thorax the sacrum was instrumented with a triaxial accelerometer at the S2 level. Phototargets for pelvic film analysis were mounted at the sacral accelerometer site and the right (unstruck side) iliac crest.

The vascular system of the cadaver was repressurized in the thorax and abdomen with four balloon catheters fed through the carotid arteries and jugular veins into the thorax. Arterial pressure was measured with a pressure transducer fed from a carotid artery into the thoracic aorta. Placement was verified by x-ray. The femoral arteries and veins were tied off. Just before testing, a solution of India ink and normal saline was pumped into the vascular system from a pressurized tank. The areterial system was pressurized to 100 mm Hg, and the venous system to 50 mm Hg. The pressure tranducer monitored pre-impact and impact arterial pressure.

A tracheotomy was performed to permit access to the lungs, which were aerated five to seven times just before impact and left unpressurized.

SLED PREPARATION AND INSTRUMENTATION - The sled used was the horizontally accelerated WHAM III. The sled measures 2.0 m wide by 3.66 m long and is accelerated on a 40 m track. The system has a pneumatic propulsion device with a 22 m long acceleration stroke. At the end of this stroke the sled is disengaged from the propulsion mechanism and allowed to strike a hydraulic snubber. Snubber stroke was set at 0.203 m (8"). The sled was instrumented to measure sled acceleration and velocity.

IMPACT TEST PROCEDURE - The test subject was placed on the seat structure described above. In order to achieve a lateral impact where the subject approaches the impacting wall at a predetermined velocity, the subject was positioned parallel to and approximately one-half meter from the wall, with the left side (the struck side), facing the instrumented side wall. The subject sat against a two-bar seat back. In all tests the forearms were positioned slightly anterior to the mid-axillary line by tieing the arms together at the

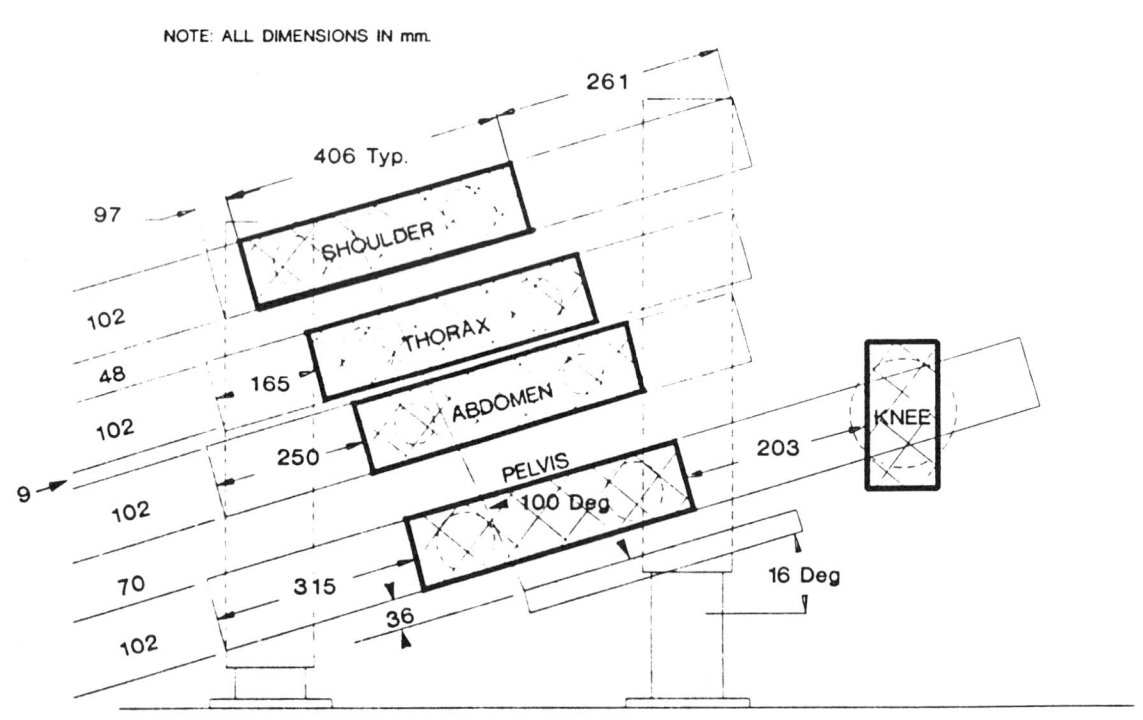

Figure 1. Diagram of impacted side wall showing beams at shoulder, thorax, abdomen, pelvis and knee instrumented with nine load cells.

wrists with duct-tape and letting the arms rest on the lap.

AUTOPSY - After the impact test post-impact x-rays were taken of all skeletal structures including the pelvis and femurs. A detailed autopsy was carried out by a board certified pathologist. The autopsy covered all regions of the body but special attention was focused on thoracic, abdominal and pelvic injuries.

Cadavers were handled with the infection control precautions we have developed as an extension of Centers for Disease Control guidelines (Cavanaugh and King, 1990).

DATA PROCESSING - Analog data was filtered at 1000 Hz (SAE class), digitized at 8000 Hz and uploaded to a Multiflow mainframe for further data processing.

FILM ANALYSIS - Two-dimensional film analysis was used in SIC 03, 04, 05, 06, 07, 10, 11 and 12 by tracking the sacral accelerometer target to measure half-pelvic width before and during impact to obtain pelvic compression of the half width. These data used a rear view camera at 1000 frames per second. These data were used to compute maximum compression (Cmax) and multiplied by maximum sled velocity (Vmax) to obtain Vmax x Cmax.

In SIC 08 and 09 rear view film was not available, so peak compression of the pelvic half width was estimated from the front view film (500 fps). Without a target to track, a compression-time history could not be obtained for these two runs. With only eight tests with compression-time histories, it was elected not to try to perform statistical analyses of VCmax, so VCmax is not presented in this paper. Ten data points were available for statisitcal analysis of Cmax and Vmax x Cmax. Also, data for 2-dimensional film analysis of the 9 m/s pelvic offset tests (SIC 01, 02) are not available, but oblique camera views are available for 3-dimensional analysis.

In the padded-wall tests (SIC 09-12), pelvic deflection was tracked by following a 25 mm target attached to a hollow metal rod which was attached to the struck face of the padding with a small metal plate (Fig. 2). In SIC 12 the rod broke free from the padding, so peak compression was estimated by measuring the deformation of the crushed pad after impact.

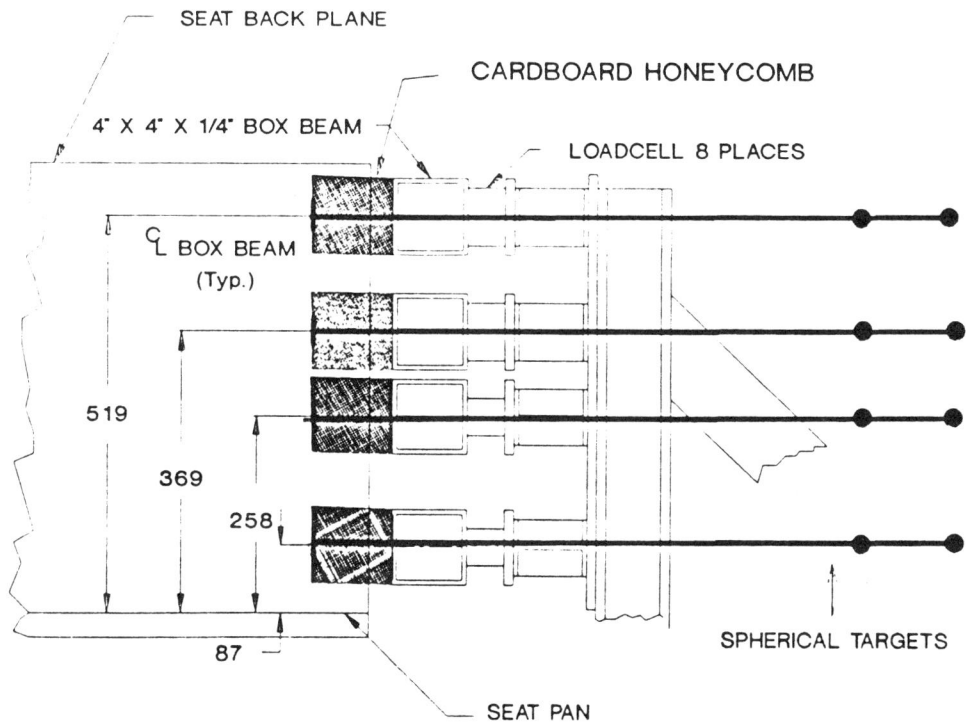

Figure 2. Diagram of side wall showing padding and rods with spherical targets used to measure padding deflection.

RESULTS AND DISCUSSION

A summary of the twelve tests is presented in Table 1. The acceleration data were digitally filtered at 180 Hz (SAE), digitally subsampled at 1600 samples per second and 100 Hz FIR filtered per the procedure outlined by Morgan et al (1986). The force data were processed the same way for the development of force-time corridors (see Appendix). The side wall force data were filtered with a 300 Hz Butterworth filter (BWF) for injury analysis. The data were normalized using the equal stress-equal velocity scaling procedure outlined by Eppinger et al (1984). Peak values of normalized pelvic beam force, normalized sacral-y acceleration, and compression along with Vmax x Cmax, are presented in Table 2.

BIOMECHANICAL RESPONSE

FORCES - The force-time histories at the pelvis were computed by summing the responses of the two load cells at the pelvic level (Fig. 1). The peak normalized pelvic forces (300 Hz BWF) averaged 11.68 kN in the 9 m/s pelvic offset tests, 11.81 kN in the 9 m/s flush wall tests and 7.43 kN in the 6.7 m/s flush wall tests. The average force responses (100 Hz FIR filtered, +/- one standard deviation) are presented as corridors in the Appendix.

SACRAL ACCELERATION - Peak normalized sacral-y accelerations (100 Hz FIR) ranged from 29 to 100 g. The average peak values were as follows: 66 g in the 9 m/s pelvic offset tests (SIC 01,02), 80 g in the 9 m/s unpadded flush wall tests (SIC 04,06), 50 g in the 6.7 m/s unpadded flush wall tests (SIC 05, 08), and 49 g in the padded wall tests (SIC 09-12). SIC 07 sacral-y acceleration failed quality checks and is not included.

COMPRESSION - The compression is defined here as the deflection of the struck side half-pelvis (measured at a target on the sacral accelerometer mount) divided by one-half of the pelvic width x 100. The average peak compressions were 32.1% in the three 6.7 m/s flush wall tests, 35.7% in the two 9 m/s flush wall tests, and 73.1% in the 10.5 m/s pelvic offset test. In the padded tests the values were as follows: 63.6% in SIC 09, 25% in SIC 10, 21.1% in SIC11, and 24.2% in SIC 12. Normalized time history plots of compression are shown in the Appendix.

INJURY TOLERANCE

The pelvic injuries are summarized in Table 3. The 1985 version of the Abbreviated Injury Scale was used in coding AIS injury level. The injuries occurred at inferior and superior left pubic rami and left sacro-iliac joint. The injury sites are illustrated in Fig. 3.

Of the twelve subjects, six sustained pelvic fractures. The most injury occurred in SIC 01 and 02, 9 m/s unpadded pelvic offset tests. Each sustained a left-sided sacro-iliac (SI) separation or fracture in addition to two pubic rami fractures. SIC 03, 06, and 09 each sustained two pelvic fractures. These tests were run at 10.3 m.s (SIC 03) and 9 m/s (SIC 06 and 09). None of the 6.7 m/s unpadded tests (SIC 05, 07, 08) sustained pelvic fracture. None of the 9 m/s tests using cardboard honeycomb sustained pelvic fracture (SIC 10-12), but SIC 09 using closed cell foam (ARSAN, trademark ARCO Chemical) sustained a pubic rami fracture.

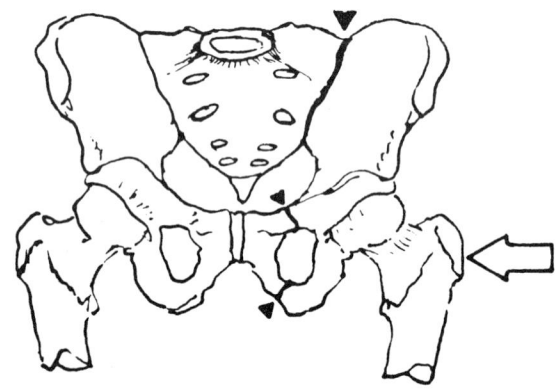

Figure 3. Illustration of human pelvis. Load vector (arrow) through greater troachanter of femur where pelvis impacted side wall. In six tests one or both left sided pubic rami were fractured (small arrowheads). Separation and fracture of the sacro-iliac joint occurred in two tests (large arrowhead). (modified from Clinically Oriented Anatomy, KL Moore).

TABLE 1

SUMMARY OF SIDE IMPACT TEST PARAMETERS

SIC = SIDE IMPACT CADAVER

RUN NO.	RUN DATE	PELVIC OFFSET (IN.)	WALL PAD?	PAD THICK. (IN.)	VEL. (MPH)	VEL. (M/S)	CADAVER NO.	MASS (KG)	HEIGHT (M)	AGE	SEX	LAMDA
SIC01	1-20-89	6	NO	0	19.94	8.91	UM6	70.5	1.76	67	M	1.021
SIC02	1-30-89	6	NO	0	20.29	9.07	187	49.5	1.63	64	F	1.148
SIC03	2-03-89	6	NO	0	23.43	10.47	188	70.0	1.75	37	M	1.023
SIC04	4-03-89	0	NO	0	20.25	9.05	215	57.6	1.63	69	M	1.092
SIC05	4-10-89	0	NO	0	15.00	6.71	216	44.0	1.72	67	M	1.194
SIC06	4-27-89	0	NO	0	20.23	9.04	217	61.2	1.84	60	M	1.070
SIC07	5-16-89	0	NO	0	14.92	6.67	206	74.8	1.70	66	M	1.001
SIC08	8-10-89	0	NO	0	14.74	6.59	UM12	73.9	1.62	64	F	1.005
SIC09	10-26-89	0	ARSAN	3	20.5	9.16	280	54.9	1.65	61	F	1.110
SIC10	01-17-90	0	15 CDB*	6	19.56	8.74	317	62.1	1.71	60	M	1.065
SIC11	02-22-90	0	15,23CDB*	4	19.98	8.93	330	55.3	1.65	54	F	1.107
SIC12	03-01-90	0	23,31CDB*	4	19.85	8.87	335	54.4	1.43	68	F	1.113

* SIDEWALL PADDING DESCRIPTION: CDB SIGNIFIES HONEYCOMB CARDBOARD.
15, 23, 31 ARE MANUFACTURER'S RATED COMPRESSIVE STRENGTHS IN PSI.
ACTUAL COMPRESSIVE STRENGTHS ARE LESS BECAUSE OF EDGE LOADING OF PAD.

SIC 09: PADDING 3" THICK 0.9 PCF CLOSED CELL FOAM ENTIRE HEIGHT OF SIDEWALL.
SIC 10: 6" THICK 15 PSI PADDING USED ENTIRE HEIGHT OF SIDEWALL.
SIC 11: 4" THICK 15 PSI PADDING USED AT THORAX & ABDOMEN BEAMS,
23 PSI AT SHOULDER & PELVIC BEAMS.
SIC 12: 4" THICK 23 PSI PADDING USED AT THORAX & ABDOMEN BEAMS,
31 PSI AT SHOULDER & PELVIC BEAMS.

TABLE 2

BIOMECHANICAL RESPONSE AT PELVIS

RUN NO.	FIR FIL VEL (M/S)	NORM FIR FIL SACR-Y ACCEL,G's	300 HZ NORM FORCE (kN)	CESARI PELVIC FORCE (kN)	COMPR. (%)	Vmax x Cmax (M/S)	PELVIC FX?
SIC01	8.91	81	12.16	8.97	---	---	YES
SIC02	9.07	50	11.20	5.31	---	---	YES
SIC03	10.47	99	16.50	8.83	73.1	7.65	YES
SIC04	9.05	59	12.92	6.33	33.7	3.05	YES
SIC05	6.71	62	10.67	5.06	26.0	1.74	NO
SIC06	9.04	100	10.69	8.31	37.6	3.40	YES
SIC07	6.67	---	6.68	9.01	33.6	2.24	NO
SIC08	6.59	37	6.20	8.25	36.9	2.43	NO
SIC09	9.16	58	7.90	6.15	63.6	5.83	YES
SIC10	8.74	29	5.40	7.51	25.0	2.19	NO
SIC11	8.93	36	5.77	6.17	21.1	1.89	NO
SIC12	8.87	71	8.04	5.42	24.2	2.14	NO

TABLE 3: PELVIC INJURY SUMMARY

6 INCH PELVIC OFFSET   N = 3

	VEL (M/S)	MASS (KG)	HT (M)	AGE	SEX	AIS	INJURY SUMMARY
SIC 01	8.91	70.5	1.76	67	M	2	FX INF PUBIC RAMUS
						2	FX SUP PUBIC RAMUS
						2	SEP LEFT S-I JOINT
SIC 02	9.07	49.5	1.63	64	F	3	SEP & FX LEFT S-I JOINT
						2	FX INF PUBIC RAMUS
						2	FX SUP PUBIC RAMUS
SIC 03	10.47	70.0	1.75	37	M	2	FX SUP PUBIC RAMUS X 2

UNPADDED FLUSH WALL   N = 5

	VEL (M/S)	MASS (KG)	HT (M)	AGE	SEX	AIS	INJURY SUMMARY
SIC 04	9.05	57.6	1.63	69	M	2	FX SUP PUBIC RAMUS
SIC 05	6.71	44.0	1.72	67	M	0	NONE
SIC 06	9.04	61.2	1.84	60	M	2	FX SUP PUBIC RAMUS
						2	FX LEFT ILIAC CREST
SIC 07	6.67	74.8	1.70	66	M	0	NONE
SIC 08	6.59	73.9	1.62	64	F	0	NONE

PADDED FLUSH WALL   N = 4

	VEL (M/S)	MASS (KG)	HT (M)	AGE	SEX	AIS	INJURY SUMMARY
SIC 09 3" ARSAN	9.16	54.9	1.65	61	F	3	SEP & FX LEFT S-I JOINT
						2	FX SUP PUBIC RAMUS
SIC 10 6" 15 PSI CARDBD.	8.74	62.1	1.71	60	M	0	NONE
SIC 11 4" 23 PSI CARDBD.	8.93	55.3	1.65	54	F	0	NONE
SIC 12 4" 31 PSI CARDBD.	8.87	54.9	1.54	68	F	0	NONE

INJURY CRITERIA

Scatter plots of the number of pelvic fractures versus four types of biomechanical response (Peak pelvic beam force, peak sacral-y acceleration, and Cmax and VmaxCmax) are shown in Figures 4a-d. Logist curves of the probability of pelvic fracture versus these same responses are shown in Figures 5a-d.

FORCE - Because of the placement of the pelvic beam just above the seat pan, load was transmitted to the pelvis primarily through the greater trochanter of the femur (Fig. 3). Six subjects sustained a peak normalized force > 10.6 kN and five of these had fractured pubic rami. Six subjects sustained a peak force of < 8 kN and only one had pelvic fracture, indicating that the fracture tolerance for the pelvis is between 8 and 10.6 kN, when the load path is through the greater trochanter. Figure 4a is a plot of peak pelvic force vs. number of pelvic fractures.

Cesari and Ramet (1982) developed an equation for pelvic tolerance with the region above this line a fracture region and below the line, non-fracture. This equation is

$$F = 43.58 \left(\frac{23.5}{Li}\right) Wa - 1058.94$$

where F = impact force in pounds, (3 ms clip)

Li = Livi index $10 \sqrt[3]{\frac{Wa}{Ht}}$

Wa = actual weight in kg,
Ht = actual height in meters

In eight of twelve tests the pelvic forces sustained were greater than the tolerance force calculated using Caesari's equation and six of these sustained pelvic fracture. In four tests the pelvic forces were less than the calculated tolerance force, and these sustained no fracture. This strongly suggests that the equation is a good predictor of pelvic fracture when the load path is through the greater trochanter. In the Heidelberg tests of Marcus et al (1983), pelvic fracture occurred less often, but with the larger pelvic force plate, the load path also included the iliac wing. Haffner (1985) has discussed how these two load paths result in different fracture tolerance limits.

Logist analysis of the probability of pelvic fracture vs. peak pelvic force gave the following values: chi-square = 8.59, p = 0.0034, and r = 0.629. Peak force was 7.98 kN at 25% probability of pelvic fracture.

ACCELERATION - Sacral-y acceleration had fair correlation with pelvic fracture. There was not a clear range of accelerations which marked the transition from no fracture to pelvic fracture (Fig. 4b). Logist analysis in which probability of pelvic fracture was analyzed as a function of peak sacral acceleration did not correlate as well as pelvic force (chi-square = 4.65, p = 0.0310, r = 0.418, Fig. 5b). Peak acceleration was 42.7 g at 25% probability of pelvic fracture.

In this test series pelvic fracture occurred at a much lower level of sacral-y accleration than seen in the FAT data (Klaus et al, 1981 and 1983). This is consistent with the load path in the CDC tests series being primarily through the greater trochanter of the femur. The FAT automobile tests probably included load through the iliac wing, as did the Heidelberg tests. Thus, the concentrated load of the CDC series may not represent the greater pelvic loading surface that appears to occur in the automobile environment.

COMPRESSION AND VELOCITY - Compression and Vmax x Cmax clearly marked the transition from no fracture to fracture. A review of Figure 4c shows that the transition from no fracture to fracture occurred at about 35% maximum compression (Cmax) of the struck half pelvis. Logist analysis shows Cmax was a good predictor of probability of pelvic fracture in this test series (chi-square = 7.63, p = 0.0057, r = 0.647, Fig. 5c). Peak compression is 32.6 % at 25% probability of pelvic fracture. In Viano et al (1989), 27% compression was the pelvic tolerance for fracture, but used the width of the whole pelvis rather than the struck half.

Vmax x Cmax gave the clearest transition from no fracture to fracture, which occurs between VmaxCmax of 2 and 3 m/s per Figure 4d. Logist analysis resulted in chi-square = 13.46, p = 0.0002 and r = 0.923 (Fig. 5d). VmaxCmax is 2.7 m/s at 25% probability of pelvic fracture, where Vmax is sled impact velocity.

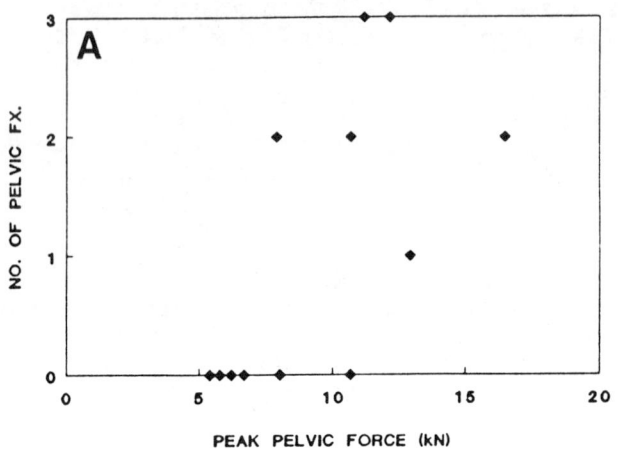
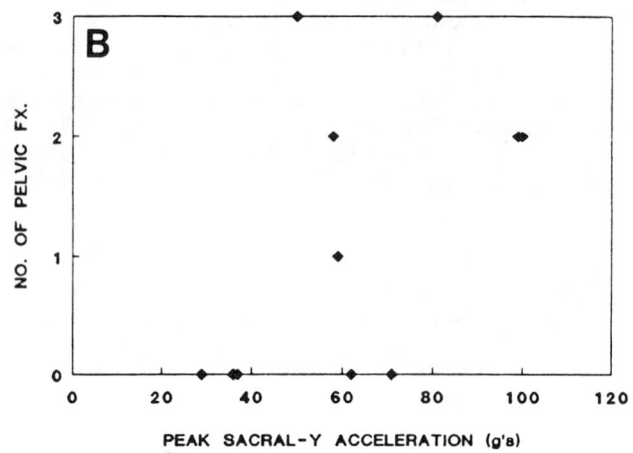
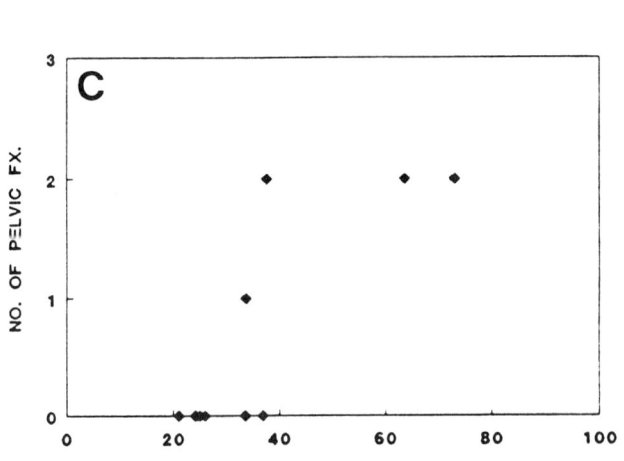
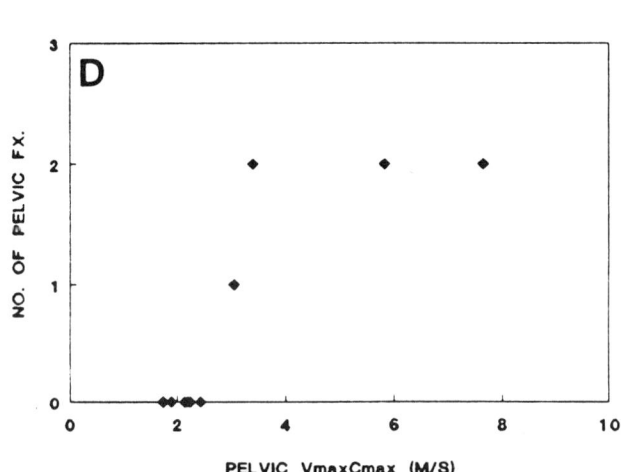

Figure 4a-d. Scatter plots of number of pelvic fractures vs. selected normalized biomechanical responses. The biomechanical responses are: a) peak pelvic force (300 Hz Butterworth filtered). b) peak sacral-y acceleration (100 Hz FIR filtered) c) peak compression of half pelvis, d) Vmax x Cmax of half pelvis. 95% confidence limits are shown with dotted lines.

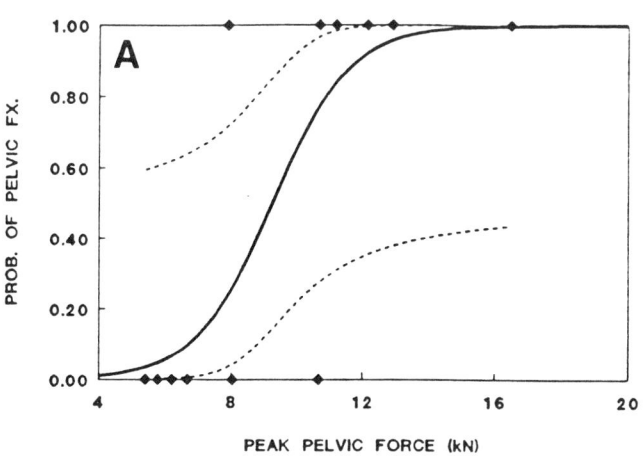
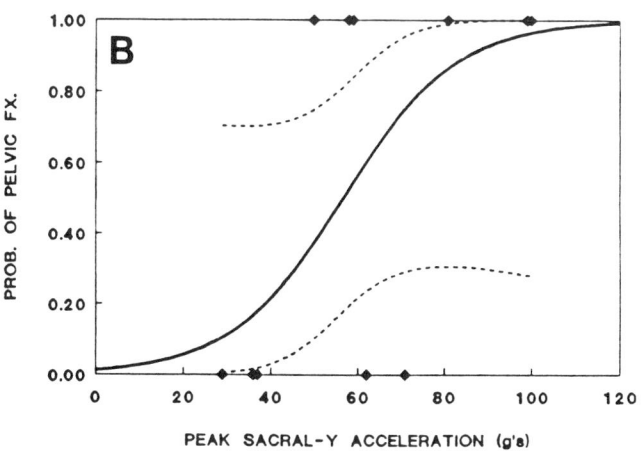
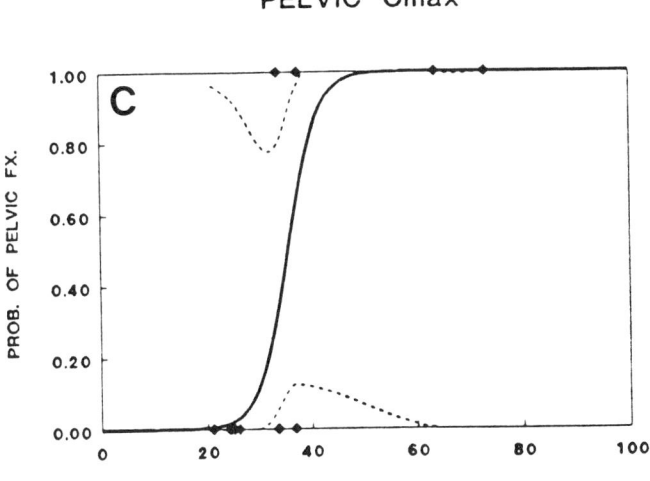
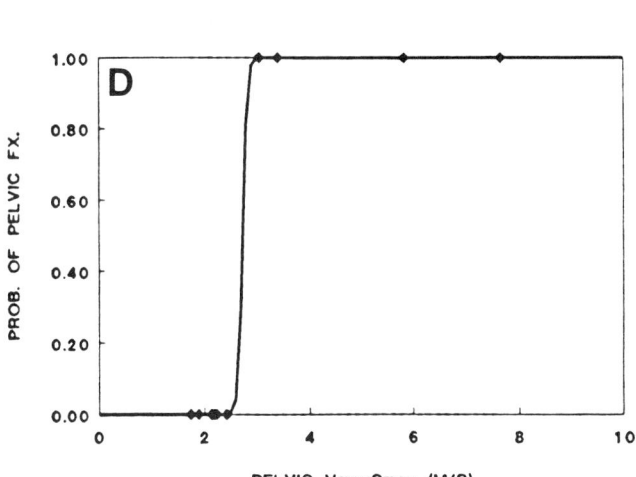

Figure 5a-d. Logist curves of probability of pelvic fracture vs. selected normalized biomechanical responses. The biomechanical responses are: a) peak pelvic force (300 Hz Butterworth filtered). b) peak sacral-y acceleration (100 Hz FIR filtered) c) peak compression of half pelvis, d) Vmax x Cmax of half pelvis. 95% confidence limits are shown with dotted lines.

CONCLUSIONS

1. Logist analysis indicates that peak force was a good injury predictor in this test series, while sacral-y acceleration did not perform as well.

2. Vmax x Cmax was the best injury predictor in this test series. VCmax was not evaluated.

3. With the load path primarily through the greater trochanter of the femur, pelvic fracture tolerance at 25% probability of fracture was as follows:

    8 kN peak force
    32.6 % compression of struck side half width
    2.7 m/s VmaxCmax of the struck side half-width

ACKNOWLEDGEMENTS

This work is supported by CDC Grant No. CCR 502347. We wish to thank Frank DuPont, Warren Hardy, Pradeep Balakrishnan, Annette Irwin, Chuck Jaggers, Mark Libich, Gerry Locke, John Ryan and the rest of the WSU Bioengineering Center staff who were an integral part of this study. We also wish to acknowledge Dr. Robert Kurtzman for performing the autopsies and for providing valuable insight into the injuries which occurred. We wish to thank Jeff Marcus and Rolf Eppinger of NHTSA for their cooperation and input into this project.

REFERENCES

Abbreviated Injury Scale (1985) American Association for Automotive Medicine.

Cavanaugh JM, King AI (1990) Control of HIV and other bloodborne pathogens in biomechanical cadaveric testing. J Orthop Res. Vol 8 (2): 159-166.

Cesari D, Ramet M and Clair P (1980) Evaluation of pelvic fracture tolerance in side impact. SAE Paper No. 801306. 24th Stapp Car Crash Conference.

Cesari D, Ramet M (1982) Pelvic tolerance and protection criteria in side impact. SAE Paper No. 821159. 26th Stapp Car Crash Conference.

Cesari D, Bouquet R, Zac R (1989) Improvements of EUROSID pelvis biofidelity. SAE Paper No. 890607, In: Side Impact: Injury Causation and Occupant Protection, 173-77.

Eppinger RH, Morgan RM, Morgan RM (1982) Side impact data analysis. Ninth International Conference on Experimental Safety Vehicles.

Haffner M (1988) Synthesis of pelvic fracture criteria for lateral impact loading. Proceedings of the Tenth International Technical Conference on Experimental Safetey Vehicles, U.S. Department of Transportation, 132-162.

Klaus G and Kallieris D (1983) Side impact - a comparison between HSRI, APROD, and HYBRID III dummies and cadavers. SAE Paper No. 831630, 27th Stapp Car Crash Conference.

Klaus G, Sinnhuber GR, Hoffmann G, Kallieris D, and Mattern R (1984) Side impact - a comparison between dummies and cadavers, correlations between cadaver loads and injury severity. SAE Paper No. 841655, 28th Stapp Car Crash Conference.

Marcus JH, Morgan RM, Eppinger RH, Kallieris D, Mattern R, Schmidt G (1983) Human response to injury from lateral impact. SAE Paper No. 831634, 27th Stapp Car Crash Conference.

Moore KL (1980) Clinically Oriented Anatomy.

Tarriere C, Walfisch G, Fayon A, Rosey J, Got C, Patel A, and Delmas A (1979) Synthesis of human tolerances obtained from lateral impact simulations. Proceedings of the Seventh International Technical Conference on Experimental Safety Vehicles, US Department of Transportation.

Viano DC, Lau IV, Corbin A, King AI, Begeman P (1989) Biomechanics of the human chest, abdomen and pelvis in lateral impact. 33rd Annual Proceedings of the Association for the Advancement of Automotive Medicine.

APPENDIX

Figures A1: Normalized force-time history corridors for the pelvic beam are shown for unpadded wall tests.

Figures A2: Compression-time histories for the struck-side half pelvis are shown for SIC 03-07.

APPENDIX

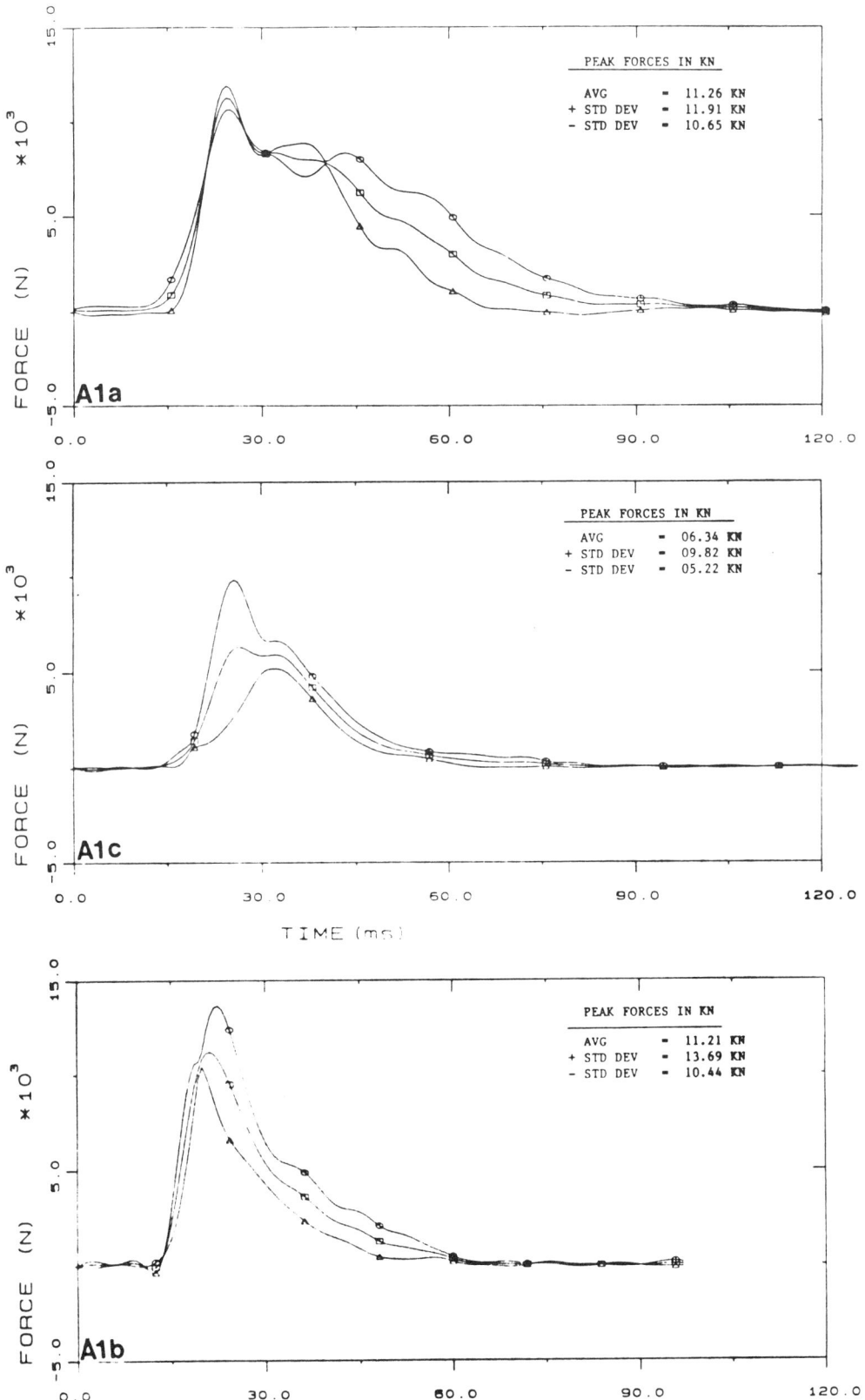

Figures A1. Force-time histories of normalized pelvic beam forces, 100 Hz FIR filtered. a. 9 m/s unpadded, 0.15 m pelvic offset tests. b. 9 m/s unpadded, flush wall tests. c. 6.7 m/s unpadded, flush wall tests. Average peak force and the peak force at plus and minus one standard deviation are shown to the right of each plot.

APPENDIX

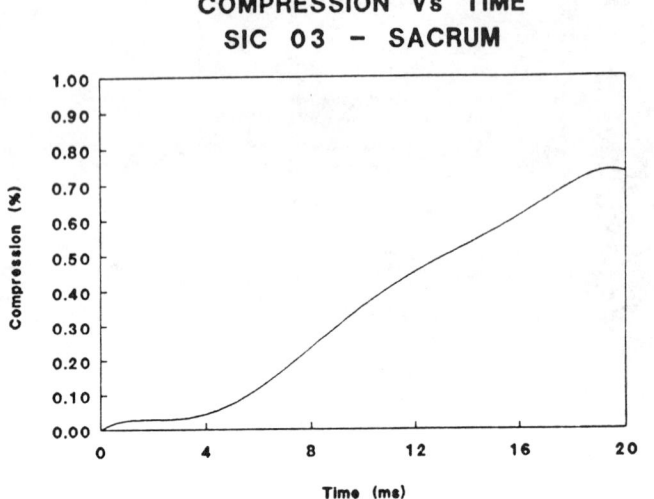
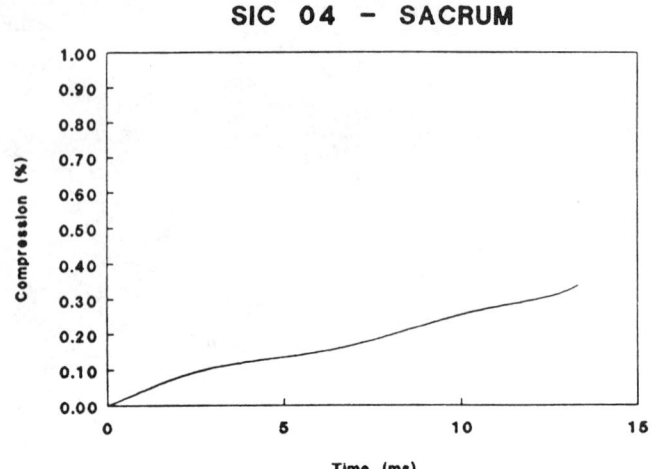
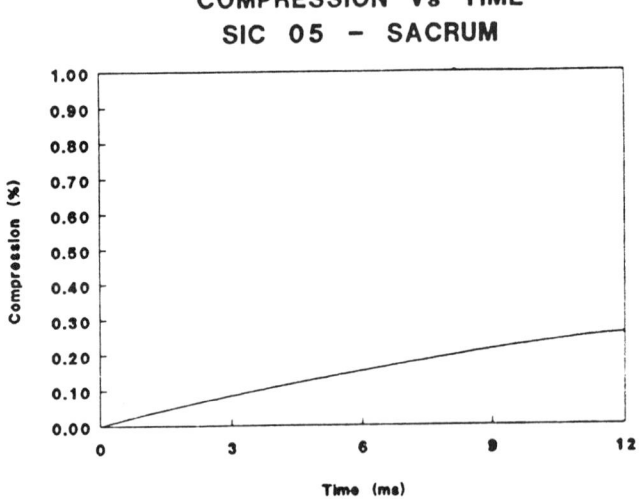
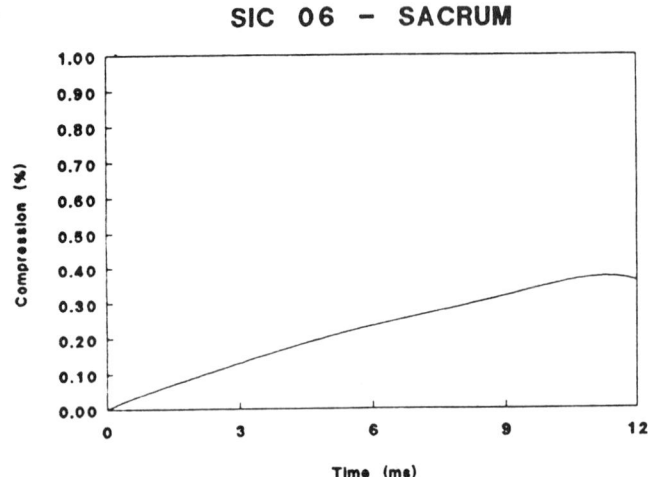
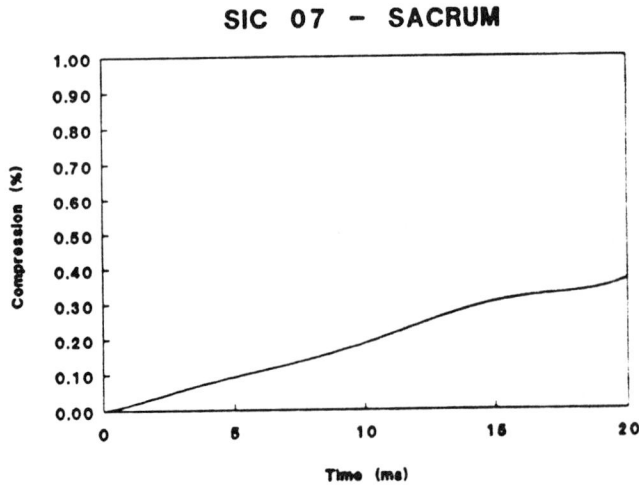

Figures A2. Compression-time histories of struck-side half-pelvis compressions for unpadded side impact tests SIC 03-07. Peak compressions occurred in the 12-20 ms range.

930435

Regional Tolerance of the Shoulder, Thorax, Abdomen and Pelvis to Padding in Side Impact

John M. Cavanaugh, Yue Huang, Yonghua Zhu, and Albert I. King
Wayne State University

ABSTRACT

Lateral impact testing has been performed on the shoulder, thorax, abdomen and pelvis of human cadavers by several investigators. The impacts have either been whole body impacts in sled tests or pendulum type impacts to the separate regions. Based on the forces produced in these tests and the accompanying injury, initial recommendations can be made on force-tolerance and padding tolerance to the various regions of the human body in side impact. The pelvis has the highest force tolerance, followed by the shoulder, abdomen and thorax. Padding crush strength tolerance based on these forces and estimated contact areas are presented. This information is of practical importance to engineers who design door interior trim for side impact safety.

INTRODUCTION

Side impact is a most serious automotive injury problem, second only to frontal impact in terms of injury and fatality in the United States. Docket 88-06, Notice 8 of the Federal Register (October 30, 1990) announced the new side impact standards, Federal Motor Vehicle Safety Standard No. 214 (FMVSS 214). According to this announcement about 8,000 automobile occupants are killed and 24,000 seriously injured each year in side impact collisions. This represents 30 % of all passenger car fatalities and 34% of serious injury. Side impact protection to chest and pelvis is addressed in the present federal rulemaking by requiring that accelerations in the chest and pelvis of SID, the side impact dummy, be kept below a specified limit in a test designed to simulate a 30 mile per hour broadside collision. The SID chest acceleration is called the Thoracic Trauma Index (TTI). TTI was developed by the National Highway Traffic Safety Administration (NHTSA) largely through data from 84 cadaver tests. Eppinger et al. (1984) and Morgan et al. (1986) analyzed the Heidelberg sled data and proposed the TTI which sums an age factor and the average of peak struck-side rib (RIBy) and lower spine (T12-y) accelerations scaled for mass. The equation is as follows:

$TTI = 1.4 \times AGE + (1/2) \times (RIBy + T12y) \times (MASS/MASS_{std})$
    for cadavers

For a dummy of standard mass (75 kg), there is no age factor and dummy TTI is defined as:

$TTI (d) = (1/2) \times (RIBy + T12y)$

Per FMVSS 214, the TTI(d) limit is 85 for four-door cars and 90 for two-door cars.

While side impact standards provide a performance specification for the thorax and pelvis, additional data is available to propose initial tolerance levels to the shoulder and abdomen. In addition, the available cadaveric data provide some insight into safe padding design limits at all four levels of the trunk: shoulder, thorax, abdomen and pelvis.

METHODOLOGY

The methods used to develop initial tolerance levels at various regions of the trunk utilize cadaveric force tolerance data of several investigators and projected contact areas of the various levels of the human trunk. The three sources for contact area used here are: the elliptical surface contact areas developed by Culver and Viano (1990), the full-scale anthropometric drawings developed by the University of Michigan Traffic Reserach Institute (1983) as part of the anthropometric studies of Schneider et al. (1985) and Robbins (1985a,b), and the review of deformation depth and contact area of paper honeycombs in the cadaveric side impact sled testing at Wayne State University (Cavanaugh et al., 1990a,b, 1992 a,b).

The force tolerance from the WSU/CDC data was derived by drawing two vertical lines through the scatter plots of injury vs. load plate force for each anatomical region. The lines indicate a transition from little or no injury to more severe injury. The upper force value of this transition zone was chosen as a tolerance level because the data are from unembalmed cadavers, which lack the muscle tone of live subjects and have more skeletal injury than real-world occupants under comparable impact conditions.

Forces were normalized using the equal stress-equal velocity scaling method described by Eppinger et al. (1984). The body masses used in scaling, and the basic scaling factors are shown in **Table 1**. Lamda is the scaling factor for length, and lamda^2 the scaling factor for area and force. Lamda^2 was used in scaling force tolerance from the mid-sized male to the small female and large male subjects in **Tables 2, 3, 4 and 5**. The masses were the mean values for these subjects in Schneider et al. (1985).

For pendulum impacts, the assumed body contact areas over which to distribute the force were the contact ellipsoids developed by Culver and Viano (1990). This may result in conservative values of tolerance since the forces in actual pendulum tests were concentrated over smaller areas. For WSU/CDC sled impact force data, body contact widths were measured from the lateral-view full-scale drawings of seated 5th, 50th and 95th percentile subjects developed at the University of Michigan Traffic Research Insititute (UMTRI, 1983). For the sled tests the contact heights were assumed to be the four inch (102 mm) load plate heights in the WSU/CDC sled fixture **(Figure 1)**. Body contact width was multiplied by load plate height to give the contact areas in **Tables 2, 3, 4 and 5**. The body contact widths measured from the deformed padding surfaces were actually somewhat higher than those measured in the UMTRI drawings. This could be due to increase in the posterior-to-anterior dimension of the body as it compresses in a lateral direction.

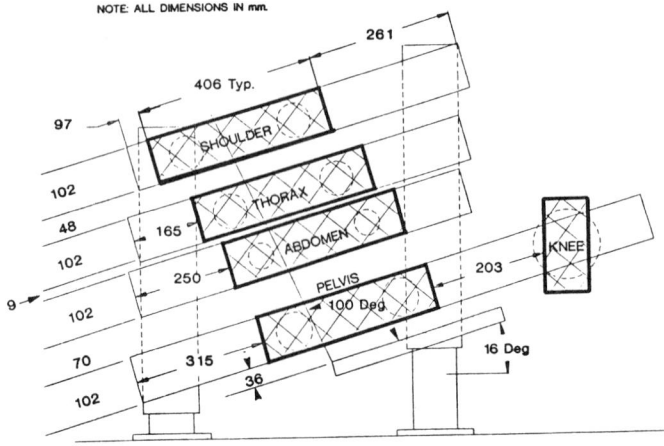

Figure 1. Diagram of impacted wall in the WSU/CDC test series showing load plates at shoulder, thorax, abdomen, and pelvis. Each load plate was instrumented with two load cells. (From Cavanaugh et al., 1990a). The peak loads generated at each level were used to develop regional load tolerance data presented in this paper.

RESULTS

SHOULDER:

The biomechanical response of the shoulder to lateral impact has not been extensively studied. Data can be obtained from the WSU cadaveric series in which whole body side impacts were performed and the body impacted a side wall divided into shoulder, thorax, abdomen and pelvic load plates **(Fig. 1)**. Peak shoulder forces were normalized and 300 Hz Butterworth filtered. The tolerable shoulder force of 3.5 kN was chosen from **Figure 2a**, a plot of maximum shoulder AIS (MAIS) vs. peak shoulder force in the tests. MAIS to the shoulder was 2, usually the result of acromio-clavicular separations or fractures of the struck-side clavicle. Only two subjects sustained shoulder injury below the 3.5 kN tolerance level chosen. Since peak force was not a good injury criteria, several tests which did not sustain shoulder injury had shoulder load plate forces greater than 3.5 kN.

The shoulder tolerance data is presented in **Table 2**. Using the estimated contact area and a 3.5 kN sustainable force, 27 psi (186 kPa) crush strength padding can be tolerated by the shoulder of a 50th percentile subject. Projected estimates for the 5th percentile female and 95th percentile male are also shown, using the equal stress-equal velocity scaling method to scale force from the 50th percentile to the larger and smaller subjects.

THORAX:

The most detailed data for lateral impact tolerance is available for the thorax and pelvis. In this study thoracic force tolerance data was obtained from 1) the WSU/CDC side impact sled tests and 2) the lateral impact tests to the thorax analyzed by Viano (1989). The Heidelberg side impact cadaveric sled tests analyzed by Marcus et al. (1983), Morgan et al., (1986) and Eppinger et al. (1984) were not used for the thorax tolerance estimate because in the Heidelberg tests the upper load plate included both shoulder and thorax loads, resulting in higher tolerable loads than to the thorax alone.

For the WSU/CDC sled data the estimated contact area is 36 square inches (232 cm^2). The peak tolerable force to this area is estimated to be 3 kN based on **Figure 2b**, where two vertical lines are drawn indicating the transition zone from moderate to severe thoracic injury. The resulting tolerable pad crush strength to the thorax is 19 psi (131 kPa) **(Table 3)**. If the lower value of the force transition zone of **Figure 2b** is used (2.5 kN), the tolerable pad crush strength is 16 psi (109 kPa).

Viano (1989) analyzed a series of impactor tests with unembalmed cadavers performed at Wayne State University. This pendulum data was generated with a six-inch diameter flat-faced impactor. The peak allowable force is 5.48 kN, the force for 25%

TABLE 1

SCALING FACTORS	WEIGHT (KG)	LAMDA	LAMDA SQUARED
5TH PERCENTILE FEMALE	46.9	1.18	1.39
50TH PERCENTILE MALE	76.7	1.00	1.00
95TH PERCENTILE MALE	102.6	0.91	0.82
CDC AVERAGE SUBJECT	62.9	1.07	1.14

TABLE 2

SHOULDER: LOAD TOLERANCE TO MINIMIZE AIS 2+	FORCE TOL. (KN)	AREA (SQ. CM)	AREA (SQ. IN)	PRESSURE TOLERANCE (PSI)
WSU/CDC SLED DATA				
5TH PERCENTILE FEMALE	2.52	155	24.0	24
50TH PERCENTILE MALE	3.50	187	29.0	27
95TH PERCENTILE MALE	4.25	212	32.8	29

TABLE 3

THORAX: LOAD TOLERANCE TO MINIMIZE AIS 4+	FORCE TOL. (KN)	AREA (SQ. CM)	AREA (SQ. IN)	PRESSURE TOLERANCE (PSI)
WSU/CDC SLED DATA				
5TH PERCENTILE FEMALE	2.16	175	27.2	18
50TH PERCENTILE MALE	3.00	232	36.0	19
95TH PERCENTILE MALE	3.64	258	40.0	20
PENDULUM DATA (MODIFIED FROM VIANO, 1989)	5.48	391	60.6	20

TABLE 4

ABDOMEN: LOAD TOLERANCE	FORCE TOL. (KN)	AREA (SQ. CM)	AREA (SQ. IN)	PRESSURE TOLERANCE (PSI)
WSU/CDC SLED DATA				
(TO MINIMIZE VISCERAL INJURY)				
5TH PERCENTILE FEMALE	2.16	187	29.0	17
50TH PERCENTILE MALE	3.00	258	40.0	17
95TH PERCENTILE MALE	3.64	310	48.0	17
PENDULUM DATA (MODIFIED FROM VIANO, 1989)				
(TO MINIMIZE ABDOMINAL INJURY, AIS 4+)				
	6.73	318	49.3	31
PENDULUM DATA (MODIFIED FROM VIANO, 1989)				
(TO MINIMIZE ABDOMINAL INJURY, AIS 3+)				
	3.00	318	49.3	14

TABLE 5

PELVIS: LOAD TOLERANCE FOR PELVIC FRACTURE	FORCE TOL. (KN)	AREA (SQ. CM)	AREA (SQ. IN)	PRESSURE TOLERANCE (PSI)
WSU/CDC SLED DATA				
TROCHANTER LOADING				
5TH PERCENTILE FEMALE	5.77	280	43.3	30
50TH PERCENTILE MALE	8.00	329	51.1	35
95TH PERCENTILE MALE	9.71	363	56.3	39
PENDULUM DATA (MODIFIED FROM CESARI AND RAMET, 1982)				
TROCHANTER LOADING				
5TH PERCENTILE FEMALE	4.38	176	27.3	36
50TH PERCENTILE MALE	10.16	266	41.3	55
95TH PERCENTILE MALE	15.18	339	52.6	65
PENDULUM DATA (MODIFIED FROM VIANO, 1989)				
TROCHANTER LOADING				
	12.00	266	41.3	65

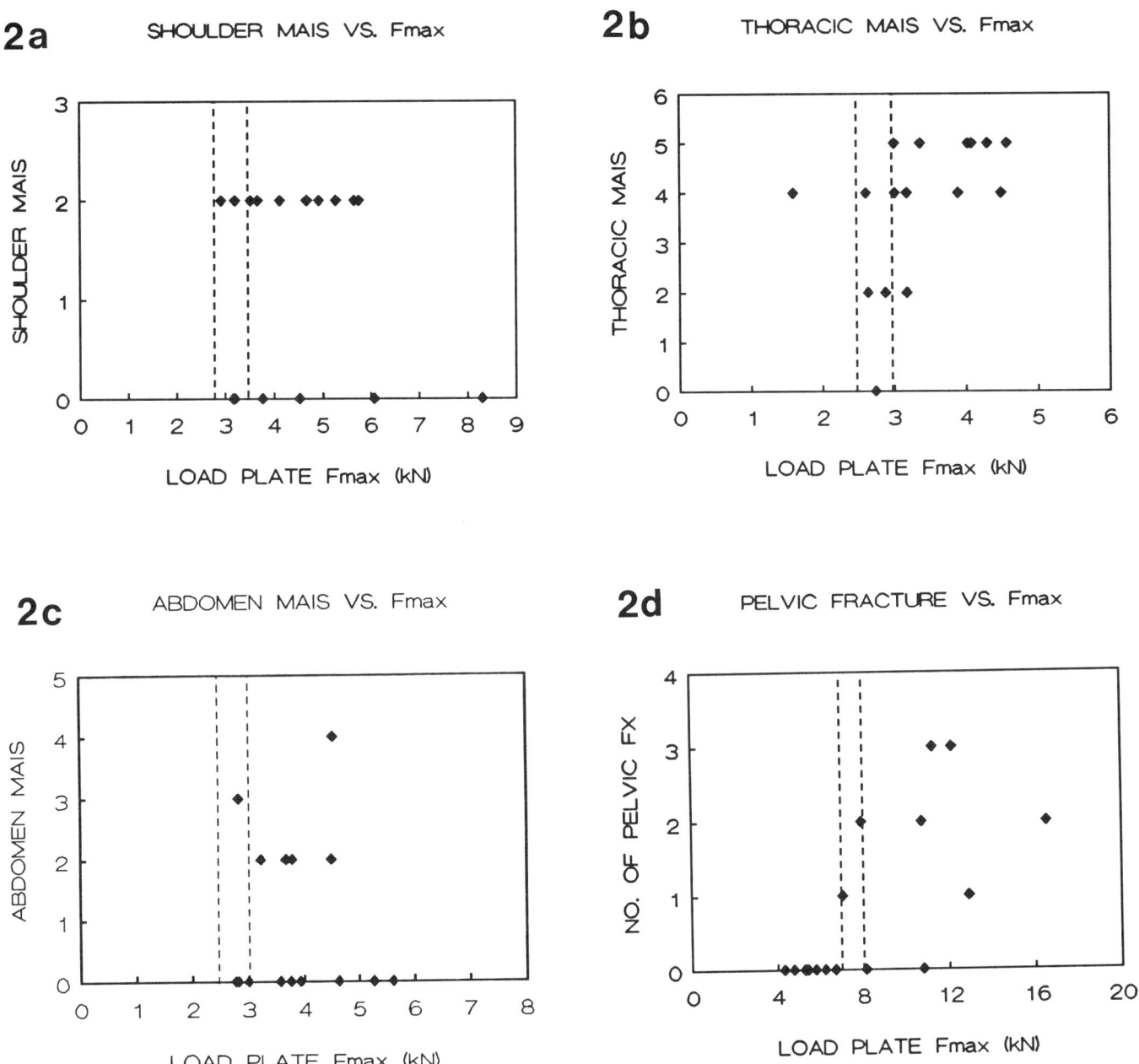

Figures 2a-d. Injury vs. peak force in the WSU/CDC cadaveric side impact sled tests for the four levels of measured load: shoulder, thorax, abdomen and pelvis. The vertical lines indicate force transition zones from little or no injury to injury which jeopardizes the structural integrity of each anatomical region. a. shoulder: 2.8 to 3.5 kN. b. thorax: 2.5 to 3 kN. c. abdomen: 2.5 to 3 kN. d. pelvis: 7-8 kN. Injury is graded per the Abbreviated Injury Scale (AIS) of the Association for the Advancement of Automotive Medicine (1990). Injury is plotted as maximum AIS (MAIS) on the y-axis of these plots.

probability of MAIS 4+ (Viano, 1989). The effective contact area for load resistance is assumed to be larger than that, and the contact ellipsoids generated by Culver and Viano (1990) are used here as the effective area to be matched with the pendulum-generated forces. This may be conservative. These data are summarized in **Table 3**. The tolerable pad crush strength based on these data is 20 psi.

Thus, 19-20 psi is the upper limit of pad crush strength tolerance at the thoracic level based on the above sled and pendulum data. If the 3 kN sled tolerance is reduced to 2 kN, the crush strength reduces to 13 psi. This is slightly higher than the crush strength of the soft paper honeycomb that resulted in minimum thoracic injury in the WSU/CDC series (Cavanaugh et al., 1992b).

ABDOMEN:

As with the shoulder, there is little data available on human abdominal lateral impact tolerance. The WSU side impact sled tests utilized an abdominal load plate, and normalized contact areas can be estimated from the UMTRI full-scale drawings and a load plate height of four inches. These force and contact area data are presented in **Table 4**. A force tolerance of 2.5 to 3 kN is estimated from **Figure 2c** and the higher value (3 kN) was chosen in determining padding tolerance. Since peak force was not a good injury criteria, many tests which did not sustain abdominal soft tissue injury had abdominal load plate forces greater than 3 kN. In only one test was there abdominal injury at a force less than 3 kN. The tolerable pad crush strength to the abdomen is 17 psi (117 kPa) based on these data. The abdomen is a more compliant region than the thorax, so a crush value less than the 19-20 psi tolerable to the thorax appears appropriate.

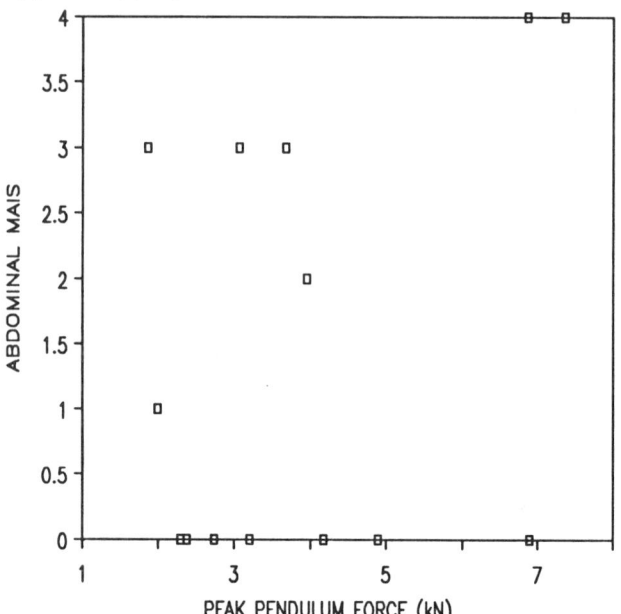

Figure 3. Maximum AIS (MAIS) to the abdomen vs. peak pendulum force from the data analyzed by Viano (1989). MAIS includes rib fractures.

Viano (1989) reported an abdominal impact tolerance of 6.73 kN based on 25% probability of MAIS 4+ to the abdomen in cadaveric pendulum impact tests. Using the contact ellipsoids of Culver and Viano (1990), a tolerable pad crush strength is 31 psi (214 kPa) **(Table 4)**. This is a crush value more twice as high as proposed based on the CDC sled data but is also the value for a higher level of injury. If the tolerance is chosen to minimize AIS 3 instead of AIS 4, 3 kN is an approximate tolerance level **(Figure 3)**. The allowable crush strength is then 14 psi, close to the 17 psi derived from the WSU/CDC data.

PELVIS:

The FMVSS 214 criterion for pelvic impact tolerance is a peak lateral pelvic acceleration of 130 g's. Pelvic force data was generated in the Heidelberg sled test series which was used to help set this criteria. The pelvic load plate appeared to load the whole pelvis, including the iliac wing and greater trochanter (Figure 4). Fracture tolerance levels could not be determined for this load path because only two subjects sustained pelvic injury (Haffner, 1985). The peak pelvic load plate forces in the two injury cases were 18.18 kN for a 61 kg female and 9.68 kN for a 51 kg female. In one case of a 75 kg male a peak force of 30.26 kN was sustained without pelvic fracture. Per Haffner (1985) the load plate spanned the pelvis and thigh.

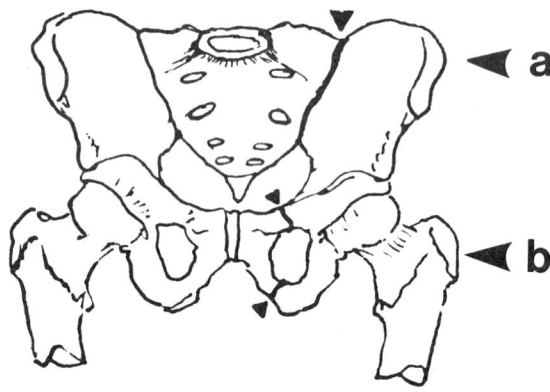

Figure 4. Diagram of the skeletal structure of the human pelvis. Arrow "a" indicates loading through the iliac wing, while arrow "b" indicates loading through the greater trochanter. Pubic rami (small arrowheads) are often fractured in pelvic impact. Separation and fracture of the sacro-iliac joint (large arrowhead) can also occur. (Modified from Cavanaugh et al. 1990a)

Pelvic load tolerance data is available from the WSU/CDC sled test series and is shown in **Table 5**. In this series, the pelvis was primarily loaded through the greater trochanter and not the iliac wing. With this load path, force tolerance is lower than in the Heidelberg series. The importance of the load path in determining force tolerance has been reviewed by Haffner (1985). With only the trochanteric load path the pelvic force tolerance is about 8 kN, as seen in **Figure 2d**. The contact area was not taken from the UMTRI drawings in this case, but instead was estimated from the deformed pad area in the WSU/CDC sled tests. The contact area includes the upper thigh. For an 8 kN allowable force the allowable pad crush strength is 35 psi (241 kPa) **(Table 5)**.

Loading through the greater trochanter without loading the iliac wing is probably not representative of most real-world side impacts. Haffner (1985) pointed out that cadaveric side impact tests involving vehicle interiors (Opel, Rabbit, Volvo) did not result in pelvic fracture at response levels as low as in the trochanteric impact study of Cesari and Ramet (1982).

Pelvic force tolerance based on pendulum data is greater than that based on sled testing. The force tolerance as generated by Cesari and Ramet (1982) and Viano (1989) were based on direct lateral impact to the greater trochanter in cadavers. Cesari and Ramet determined a force tolerance that varied with subject mass. In **Table 5**, their data is scaled using their scaling method rather than the equal stress-equal velocity method. Viano determined a force tolerance for 25% probability of pubic rami fracture. The force tolerances of both studies (10.16 and 12 kN) are shown in **Table 5**. Using the ellipsoid contact area generated by Culver and Viano, a pressure tolerance of 55-65 psi is obtained for pendulum impacts to the greater trochanter. It is probably conservative to use the ellipsoid contact areas for these impacts because the contact areas include the iliac wing, and the loading does not.

DISCUSSION

The contact pressure tolerances generated above are based on the peak tolerable forces for various anatomical regions and dividing by contact areas of those regions. These contact pressures can be considered an initial attempt at determining padding crush strengths tolerated by the human body in side impact to produce a force-limiting padding interface. By limiting forces to values at or below human tolerance, injury is reduced and the biomechanical responses that are correlated to injury are lowered. These include peak compression (Cmax), the peak viscous response (VCmax), and peak lateral accelerations.

By one argument it might be considered wise to lower padding crush strengths to values somewhat less than those generated above, to insure that pad compression is greater than human body compression during a side impact. On the other hand, the values generated above are from unembalmed cadavers, which do not have the muscle tone and skeletal strength of the general driving population.

At the thorax level, a reduction to 8-12 psi crush strength results in MAIS 2 or less if four or more inches of pad is used (Cavanaugh et al., 1992b). This thickness is probably only practically obtainable using a side-door air bag.

The incorporation of the shoulder load path should reduce injury at the thorax and abdominal levels. A MADYMO model incorporating the WSU/CDC data predicts that removing the shoulder load path (lowering the door sill) increases forces to the thorax and abdomen (King et al., 1992). If a lower door sill is used, a side door air bag that expands upward to engage the shoulder, as well as outward, could be beneficial.

The padding crush strength tolerances derived above and summarized below may be more representative of those tolerated by the middle-aged and younger occupant. Padding of about 20 psi crush strength was not tolerated by the thorax of the older subject in the WSU/CDC cadaver series (Cavanaugh et al., 1992b).

CONCLUSIONS

Proposed pad crush strengths were generated from human force tolerance data from various cadaveric impact studies. For the 50th percentile subject, the following values were derived:

shoulder: 27 psi
thorax: 19-20 psi
abdomen: 14-17 psi
pelvis: 35-65 psi (load to greater trochanter)

These pad crush strengths may serve as a guideline for designing door trim interior packages. Incorporating the shoulder load path appears to be important in reducing load and injury to the rest of the torso.

ACKNOWLEDGEMENTS

This work was supported by the Centers for Disease Control, Division of Injury Control, CDC Grant number CCR 502347.

REFERENCES

The Abbreviated Injury Scale (1990) Association for the Advancement of Automotive Medicine, Des Plaines, IL, 1990.

Cavanaugh JM, Walilko T, Malhotra A, Zhu Y, King AI (1990a) Biomechanical Response and Injury Tolerance of the Pelvis in Twelve Sled Side Impacts. SAE Paper No. 902305, 34th Stapp Car Crash Conference.

Cavanaugh JM, Walilko T, Malhotra A, Zhu Y, King AI (1990b) Biomechanical Response and Injury Tolerance of the Thorax in Twelve Sled Side Impacts. SAE Paper No. 902307, 34th Stapp Car Crash Conference.

Cavanaugh JM, Huang Y, King AI (1992a) SID Response data in a side impact sled test series. SAE Paper No. 920350, 1992 SAE International Congress and Exposition, Detroit, Michigan, Feb. 24-28, 1992.

Cavanaugh JM, Zhu YJ, King AI (1992b) Mechanical properties of various padding materials used in cadaveric side impact sled tests. SAE Paper No.

920357, 1992 SAE International Congress and Exposition, Detroit, Michigan, Feb. 24-28, 1992.

Cesari D and Ramet M (1982) Pelvic tolerance and protection criteria in side impact. SAE Paper No. 821159, 26th Stapp Car Crash Conference.

Culver CC and Viano D (1990) Occupant seating anthropometry: body ellipses and contact zones for side-impact protection research. ISPRS Journal of Photogrammetry and Remote Sensing, 45:267-284.

Eppinger RH, Marcus JH, Morgan RM (1984) Development of dummy and injury index for NHTSA's thoracic side impact protection research program. SAE Paper No. 840885, Government/Industry Meeting and Exposition, Washington, D.C.

FMVSS 214, 49 CFR Part 571 (1990) Federal Motor Vehicle Safety Standard No. 214, Side Impact Protection. Federal Register, Docket No. 88-06, Notice 8, RIN 2127-AB86, Vol. 55(210), Oct. 30, 1990.

Haffner M (1985) Synthesis of pelvic fracture criteria for lateral impact loading. Proceedings of the Tenth International Conference on Experimental Safety Vehicles, USDOT, 132-162.

King AI, Huang Y, Cavanaugh JM (1992) A mathematical model for the protection of car occupants in side impacts. ASME, PD-Vol. 47-2, Engineering Systems Design and Analysis, Vol. 2.

Marcus JH, Morgan RM, Eppinger RH, Kallieris D, Mattern R, Schmidt G (1983) Human response to injury from lateral impact. SAE Paper No. 831634, 27th Stapp Car Crash Conference.

Morgan RM, Marcus JH, and Eppinger RH (1986) Side impact - the biofidelity of NHTSA's proposed ATD and efficacy of TTI. SAE Paper No. 861877, 30th Stapp Car Crash Conference.

Robbins DH (1985a) Anthropometric specifications for mid-sized male dummy, Vol. 2, DOT HS 806 716.

Robbins DH (1985b) Anthropometric specifications for small female and large male dummies, Vol. 3, DOT HS 806 717.

Schneider LW, Robbins DH, Pflug MA, Snyder RG (1985) Development of anthropometrically based design specifications for an advanced adult anthropometric dummy family. Vol. 1, DOT HS 806 715.

University of Michigan Traffic Research Institute (1983) Anthropometry of Motor Vehicle Occupants - Specification Drawings. Sponsored by NHTSA. Contract No. DTNH22-80-C-07502.

Viano DC (1989) Biomechanical responses and injuries in blunt lateral impact. SAE Paper No. 892432, 33rd Stapp Car Crash Conference.

933128

Pelvic Biomechanical Response and Padding Benefits in Side Impact Based on a Cadaveric Test Series

J. Y. Zhu, J. M. Cavanaugh, and A. I. King
Wayne State University Bioengineering Center

ABSTRACT

The frequency of pelvic fractures is 10%-14% in side impact crashes. In this study, seventeen side impact sled tests were performed using a Heidelberg-type seat fixture. The pelvis along with the rest of the torso impacted a sidewall in these tests. This series of runs provided a good test of injury criteria performance for a variety of impact surfaces. Pelvic injury criteria based on force, acceleration, compression, and the viscous criterion were evaluated. Force was found to be a good criterion according to both the Weibull and Logist analysis. A promising new injury criterion tested was "Average Force" (Favg). It reflects the rate of momentum transfer to the pelvis during a side impact. The slope of the pelvic momentum trace, from 10 to 90% of its peak, is the time rate of change of momentum, and has the dimension of force. In a 32 km/h (20 mph) impact, Favg is 5 kN for a 25% probability of an AIS 2 pelvic injury (maximum likelihood 0.0135).

INTRODUCTION

Pelvic injury can occur at several locations on the pelvic ring during a side impact. Fractures of pubic rami, pubic symphysis, iliac wing, sacroiliac junction and acetabulum can occur (Haffner, 1985). Internal organ injury can also occur. Within the pelvic cavity, fractures are associated with potentially severe injuries to the blood vessels, bladder and urinary tract.

There have been several studies on the biomechanical response and injury tolerance of the pelvis to impact. Cesari et al. (1982) proposed a cadaver tolerance impact of 10 kN for 76 kg males and 4 kN for a 5th percentile female (3 ms clip). Haffner (1985) created two candidate functions for the prediction of pelvic fracture. These functions included measures of bone stress, bone strain, age, and load concentration factor. Tarriere et al. (1979) reported pelvic fractures occurring at pelvic accelerations of 62 to 120 g in a series of cadaveric lateral drop tests. Viano et al. (1989) performed lateral impacts to the pelvis with a pendulum impactor, and found that lateral compression was the only good correlate to pubic rami fracture, and that impact force and acceleration did not correlate well with injury. Cavanaugh et al. (1990) reported that VmaxCmax (maximum velocity times maximum compression) was the best predictor of pelvic fracture, while peak pelvic force and peak compression also performed well based on a Logist analysis of twelve tests. Based on review of various cadaveric studies, padding with a crush strength of 35-65 psi was recommended by Cavanaugh et al. (1993) for the protection of the pelvis. All of the candidate injury criteria for the pelvis were parameters associated with the biomechanical response of cadavers.

METHODS

This study is based on 17 cadaveric side impact tests conducted at Wayne State University. The test methodology and data processing have been described by Cavanaugh et al. (1990), including cadaver and sled preparation, autopsy and use of digital filters as well as film analysis. A 6-order polynomial was used to smooth the deflection curve obtained from film digitization.

Table 1 is a summary of the cadavic test conditions used, including the type of padding used for the pelvis. There were five types of impact:

1) 9 m/s (20 mph) with the pelvic load plate offset 150 mm toward the body from the rest of the load plates;
2) 9 m/s (20 mph) unpadded flat wall;
3) 6.7 m/s (15 mph) unpadded flat wall;
4) 9 m/s (20 mph) with 100 mm to 150 mm thick padding;
5) 9 m/s (20 mph) with 75 mm thick padding.

For injury evaluations, side-wall force data were digitally filtered at 300 Hz using a Butterworth filter (BWF).

Using FIR100 software provided by NHTSA, acceleration data were digitally filtered at 180 Hz (SAE), digitally subsampled at 1600 samples per second and 100 Hz FIR filtered according to the procedure described by Morgan et al. (1986). The data were normalized using the equal stress-equal velocity scaling procedure outlined by Eppinger et al. (1984). The procedure is based on the mass of each test subject. Lamda (λ), the basic scaling factor used in this method is shown in **Table 1**. The scaling algorithm works in the following manner:

$$\text{Lamda} (\lambda) = (M_s / M_i)^{1/3}$$

where: M_s = standard mass = 165 lbm = 75 kg
M_i = mass of test subject "i".

The magnitude of the digitized acceleration values is scaled by $1/\lambda$.

The magnitude of the digitized force values is scaled by λ^2.

The time interval between data samples is scaled by λ.

Table 2 presents the non-normalized raw data of the peak accelerations and forces, filtered at SAE CFC-1000 (SAE J211); the deflection data are the maximum values from film analysis without smoothing and without scaling.

RESULTS OF BIOMECHANICAL RESPONSE

Table 3 lists pelvic injury data as well as peak values of several potential injury criteria after normalization.

FORCES AND ACCELERATIONS - The peak impact forces listed in **Table 3** were obtained by summing the load cell responses of the two load cells at the pelvic level. Although the maximum forces varied from test to test, overall, they increased with increasing subject mass and sled velocity. Force-time histories of the pelvic beam are

TABLE 1: SIDE IMPACT CADAVER DATA AND TEST PARAMETERS FOR PELVIS

TEST TYPE SIC RUN NO & TYPE	SLED VEL. (m/s)	SLED VEL. (mph)	AGE	SEX	MASS (kg)	HEIGHT (m)	LAMDA	PAD TYPE	PAD THICK-NESS (mm)	PAD THICK-NESS (IN.)	PAD CELL SIZE (mm)	PAD CELL SIZE (IN.)	PAD CRUSH STRENGTH 35% THICKNESS (kPa)	(PSI)
UNPADDED PELVIC OFFSET														
SIC01	8.9	19.9	60	M	70.5	1.76	1.02	NONE	---	---	---	---	---	---
SIC02	9.1	20.3	64	F	49.5	1.63	1.15	NONE	---	---	---	---	---	---
SIC03	10.5	23.4	37	M	70.0	1.75	1.02	NONE	---	---	---	---	---	---
AVG	9.5	21.2	54		63.3	1.71	1.06							
UNPADDED, 9 m/s														
SIC04	9.1	20.3	69	M	57.6	1.63	1.09	NONE	---	---	---	---	---	---
SIC06	9.0	20.2	60	M	61.2	1.82	1.07	NONE	---	---	---	---	---	---
AVG	9.0	20.2	65		59.4	1.73	1.08							
UNPADDED, 6.7 m/s														
SIC05	6.7	15.0	67	M	44.0	1.72	1.19	NONE	---	---	---	---	---	---
SIC07	6.7	14.9	66	M	74.8	1.70	1.00	NONE	---	---	---	---	---	---
SIC08	6.6	14.7	64	F	73.9	1.62	1.00	NONE	---	---	---	---	---	---
AVG	6.7	14.9	66		64.2	1.68	1.07							
THICK PAD 9 m/s														
SIC10	8.7	19.6	60	M	62.1	1.71	1.06	PHC	152	6	25	1/1	55	8
SIC11	8.9	20.0	54	F	55.3	1.65	1.11	PHC	102	4	19	3/4	131	19
SIC12	8.9	19.9	68	F	54.4	1.43	1.11	PHC	102	4	16	5/8	193	28
SIC13	8.3	18.5	62	M	66.7	1.61	1.04	PHC	102	4	19	3/4	131	19
SIC14	9.4	21.1	60	M	55.3	1.74	1.11	PHC	102	4	19	3/4	131	19
SIC15	8.9	20.0	43	F	68.9	1.54	1.03	PHC	102	4	19	3/4	131	19
SIC17	8.9	19.9	65	M	93.0	1.70	0.93	PHC	152	6	19	3/4	131	19
AVG	8.9	19.8	59		65.1	1.63	1.06							
THIN PAD 9 m/s														
SIC09	9.2	20.5	61	F	54.9	1.65	1.11	ARSAN	76	3			152	22
SIC16	8.9	19.8	58	F	56.7	1.70	1.10	PHC	76	3	19	3/4	131	19
AVG	9.0	20.2	60		55.8	1.68	1.10							

LAMDA = SCALING FACTOR IN EQUAL STRESS–EQUAL VELOCITY SCALING   PHC = PAPER HONEYCOMB

provided in **Figure 1** for the unpadded 6.7 m/s (15 mph) and 9 m/s (20 mph) test conditions. The average peak force was 7.9 kN in the 6.7 m/s (15 mph) tests and 11.8 kN in the 9 m/s (20 mph) tests. The average peak acceleration of the pelvis was 74 g for the 6.7 m/s (15 mph) unpadded tests and 83 g for the 9 m/s (20 mph) unpadded tests. The average pelvic acceleration-time history is shown in **Figure 2**, bounded by ± 1 S.D. curves. The data were filtered at 180 Hz. The corridors of these curves are not as clearly defined as the force curves. The ratio of the peak force between the unpadded 6.7 m/s (15 mph) and 9 m/s (20 mph) tests was 67%, and that of the peak acceleration was 89%. Thus, the correlation between peak pelvic force and acceleration is low. The fact that peak accelerations in 9 m/s (20 mph) impacts were, on the average, only 13% higher than those in 6.7 m/s (15 mph) impacts, suggests that acceleration is not a good measure of pelvic impact severity. Peak forces appeared to be able to better reflect the difference in severity in the 17 tests conducted.

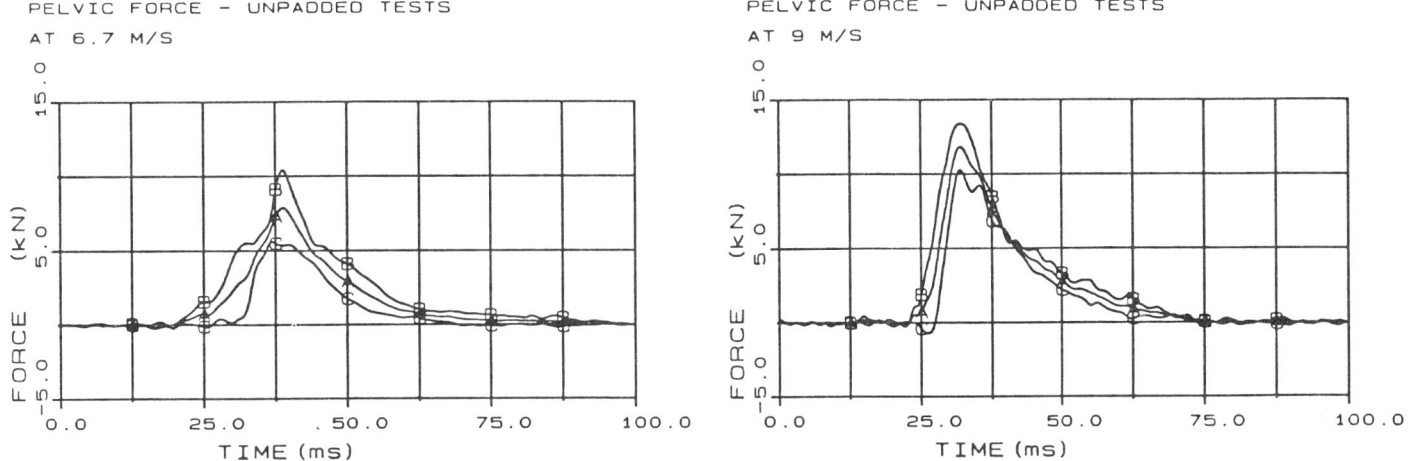

Figure 1. Pelvic force-time histories of unpadded 6.7 and 9 m/s tests (average and ±1 S.D. curves).

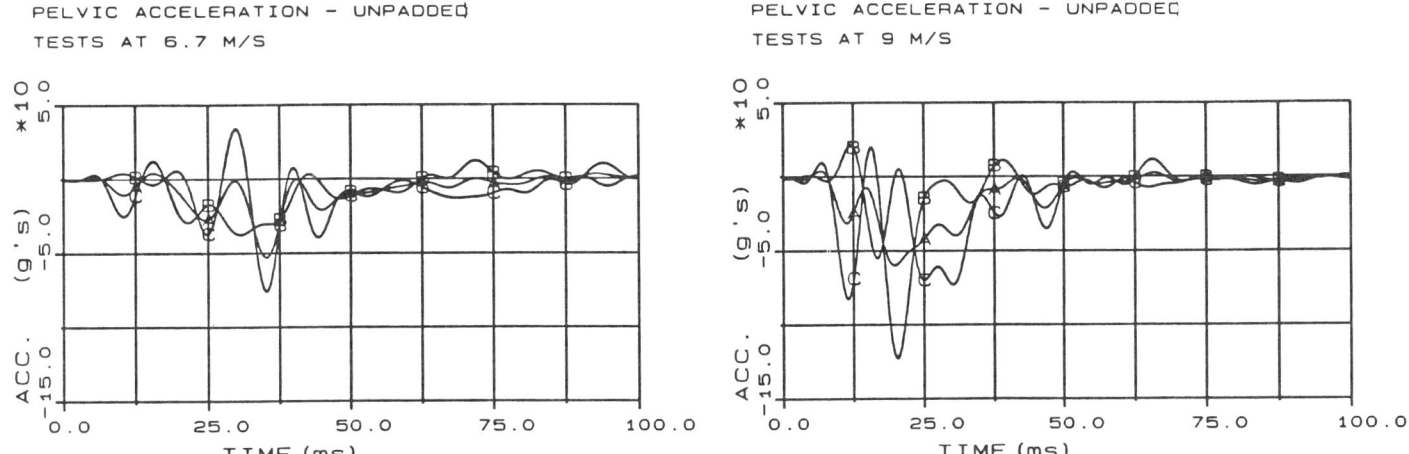

Figure 2. Pelvic acceleration-time histories of unpadded 6.7 and 9 m/s tests (average and ±1 S.D. curves).

TABLE 2: SUMMARY OF RAW DATA FOR PELVIS (NON-NORMALIZED, SAE CFC CLASS 1000)

TEST TYPE TEST RUN NO & TYPE	SLED VEL. (m/s)	SLED VEL. (mph)	CADAVER DATA AND INJURY MAIS	No. Fx.	MASS (kg)	HEIGHT (m)	SCALING CONSTANT LAMDA	LAMDA^2	1/LAMDA	RAW DATA ACCEL. (g's)	DEFL. (mm)	HALF BODY WIDTH (mm)	COMPRES SION (%)	MAX. FORCE (kN)
UNPADDED PELVIC OFFSET														
SIC01	8.9	19.9	2	3	70.5	1.76	1.02	1.04	0.98	134.6	---	---	---	12.31
SIC02	9.1	20.3	3	3	49.5	1.63	1.15	1.32	0.87	60.9	---	---	---	8.67
SIC03	10.5	23.4	2	2	70.0	1.75	1.02	1.05	0.98	317.2	134.0	200.3	66.9	16.56
AVG	9.5	21.2	2.3	2.7	63.3	1.71	1.06	1.13	0.94	170.9	134.0	200.3	66.9	12.51
UNPADDED, 9 m/s														
SIC04	9.1	20.3	2	1	57.6	1.63	1.09	1.19	0.92	107.2	45.3	137.9	32.8	11.22
SIC06	9.0	20.2	2	2	61.2	1.82	1.07	1.15	0.93	125.8	46.5	130.8	35.6	9.81
AVG	9.0	20.2	2.0	1.5	59.4	1.73	1.08	1.17	0.93	116.5	45.9	134.4	34.2	10.52
UNPADDED, 6.7 m/s														
SIC05	6.7	15.0	0	0	44.0	1.72	1.19	1.43	0.84	100.0	40.4	168.8	23.9	7.95
SIC07	6.7	14.9	0	0	74.8	1.70	1.00	1.00	1.00	132.7	63.9	190.5	33.5	6.82
SIC08	6.6	14.7	0	0	73.9	1.62	1.00	1.01	1.00	38.9	---	---	---	6.38
AVG	6.7	14.9	0	0	64.2	1.68	1.07	1.14	0.94	90.5	52.2	179.7	28.7	7.05
THICK PAD 9 m/s														
SIC10	8.7	19.6	0	0	62.1	1.71	1.06	1.13	0.94	46.0	48.0	181.7	26.4	6.39
SIC11	8.9	20.0	0	0	55.3	1.65	1.11	1.23	0.90	53.2	53.8	213.2	25.2	4.81
SIC12	8.9	19.9	0	0	54.4	1.43	1.11	1.24	0.90	141.3	56.9	195.9	29.0	7.26
SIC13	8.3	18.5	0	0	66.7	1.61	1.04	1.08	0.96	62.2	91.4	223.7	40.8	4.48
SIC14	9.4	21.1	0	0	55.3	1.74	1.11	1.23	0.90	116.9	73.9	175.2	42.2	4.49
SIC15	8.9	20.0	0	0	68.9	1.54	1.03	1.06	0.97	73.2	55.3	171.5	32.2	4.38
SIC17	8.9	19.9	0	0	93.0	1.70	0.93	0.87	1.07	71.6	78.4	186.5	42.0	6.28
AVG	8.9	19.8	0	0	65.1	1.63	1.06	1.11	0.95	80.6	65.4	192.5	34.0	5.44
THIN PAD 9 m/s														
SIC09	9.2	20.5	3	2	54.9	1.65	1.11	1.23	0.90	68.3	---	---	---	6.74
SIC16	8.9	19.8	2	1	56.7	1.70	1.10	1.20	0.91	81.6	86.8	194.1	44.7	6.16
AVG	9.0	20.2	2.5	1.5	55.8	1.68	1.10	1.22	0.91	75.0	86.8	194.1	44.7	6.45

LAMDA = SCALING FACTOR IN EQUAL STRESS-EQUAL VELOCITY SCALING

MAIS = MAXIMUM AIS

Fx = FRACTURES

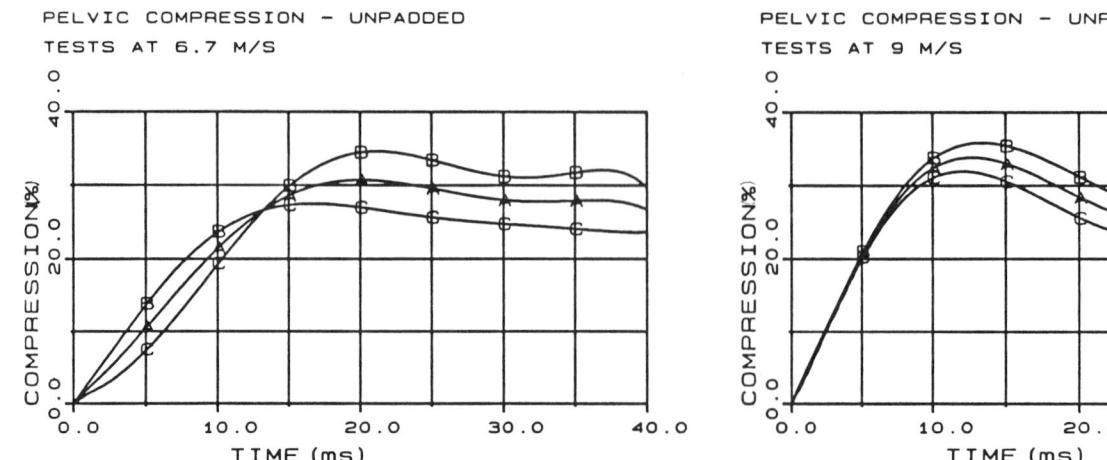

Figure 3. Pelvic compression-time histories of unpadded tests at 6.7 and 9 m/s (average and ±1 S.D. curves).

COMPRESSION - Pelvic compression, C, is defined as:

$$C = (D/W) \times 100$$

where D is the deflection of the struck side, and W is the half pelvic width.

These measurements were made at the level of the sacrum using film data. Peak compression data are summarized in **Table 3** along with VmaxCmax, FmaxCmax and VCmax. Compression-time histories for unpadded 6.7 m/s (15 mph) and 9 m/s (20 mph) tests are provided in **Figure 3** with average and standard deviation curves. The maximum values of C for the two velocities were almost similar, 31% for 6.7 m/s (15 mph) and 34% for 9 m/s (20 mph). There is thus an apparent limit to which the pelvis and its associated soft tissues can be compressed.

However, the time to maximum compression was very different, 20 ms in the 6.7 m/s (15 mph) tests and 12 ms in the 9 m/s (20 mph) tests, implying that the velocity of compression may play a role in pelvis ring fracture and injury.

PELVIC INJURY - The 1990 version of the Abbreviated Injury Scale (AIS) was used in coding the observed pelvic injuries. The principal injuries were fracture of the inferior and superior left pubic rami and separation of the left sacroiliac joint. The injury sites are shown in **Figure 4** (From Cavanaugh et al., 1993). A large arrow is used to indicate loading through the greater trochanter. Pubic rami, identified by two small arrowheads, were often fractured in pelvic impacts. Separation of the sacroiliac joint, identified by a medium-sized arrowhead, can also occur during more severe side impacts.

TABLE 3: SUMMARY OF IMPACT DATA FOR PELVIS

TEST RUN NO & TYPE	SLED VEL. (m/s)	SLED VEL. (mph)	MAIS	No. Fx.	MASS (kg)	HEIGHT (m)	LAMDA	ACCEL. (G'S)	COMPRESSION (%)	Vmax* Cmax (m/s)	VCmax (m/s)	MAX. FORCE (kN)	AVG. FORCE (kN)	Fmax* Cmax (kN)	Favg* Cmax (kN)
UNPADDED PELVIC OFFSET															
SIC01	8.9	19.9	2	3	70.5	1.76	1.02	81.7	---	---	---	12.17	7.45	---	---
SIC02	9.1	20.3	3	3	49.5	1.63	1.15	50.7	---	---	---	11.27	7.14	---	---
SIC03	10.5	23.4	2	2	70.0	1.75	1.02	99.6	63.9	6.7	4.2	16.52	9.95	10.56	6.36
AVG	9.5	21.2	2.3	2.7	63.3	1.71	1.06	77.3	63.9	6.1	4.2	13.32	8.18	8.51	5.23
UNPADDED, 9 m/s															
SIC04	9.1	20.3	2	1	57.6	1.63	1.09	62.9	29.8	2.7	0.9	12.92	6.68	3.85	1.99
SIC06	9.0	20.2	2	2	61.2	1.82	1.07	103.4	33.0	3.0	1.0	10.74	5.79	3.54	1.91
AVG	9.0	20.2	2.0	1.5	59.4	1.73	1.08	83.2	31.4	2.8	1.0	11.83	6.24	3.70	1.95
UNPADDED, 6.7 m/s															
SIC05	6.7	15.0	0	0	44.0	1.72	1.19	68.9	23.7	1.6	0.5	10.79	4.38	2.56	1.04
SIC07	6.7	14.9	0	0	74.8	1.70	1.00	116.1	33.4	2.2	0.9	6.68	4.85	2.23	1.62
SIC08	6.6	14.7	0	0	73.9	1.62	1.00	36.8	36.9	2.4	---	6.20	3.95	2.29	1.46
AVG	6.7	14.9	0	0	64.2	1.68	1.07	73.9	31.3	2.1	0.7	7.89	4.39	2.36	1.37
THICK PAD 9 m/s															
SIC10	8.7	19.6	0	0	62.1	1.71	1.06	30.0	25.6	2.2	0.5	5.40	4.38	1.38	1.12
SIC11	8.9	20.0	0	0	55.3	1.65	1.11	36.9	24.9	2.2	0.6	5.77	4.54	1.44	1.13
SIC12	8.9	19.9	0	0	54.4	1.43	1.11	74.5	29.4	2.6	1.0	8.12	6.14	2.39	1.81
SIC13	8.3	18.5	0	0	66.7	1.61	1.04	52.9	40.1	3.3	1.4	4.74	3.39	1.90	1.36
SIC14	9.4	21.1	0	0	55.3	1.74	1.11	59.3	42.7	4.0	1.1	5.26	4.17	2.25	1.78
SIC15	8.9	20.0	0	0	68.9	1.54	1.03	53.2	32.1	2.9	1.2	4.31	3.40	1.38	1.09
SIC17	8.9	19.9	0	0	93.0	1.70	0.93	63.1	41.5	3.7	1.2	5.30	4.14	2.20	1.72
AVG	8.9	19.8	0	0	65.1	1.63	1.06	52.8	33.8	3.0	1.0	5.56	4.31	1.85	1.43
THIN PAD 9 m/s															
SIC09	9.2	20.5	3	2	54.9	1.65	1.11	58.2	63.6	5.8	---	7.93	5.28	5.04	3.36
SIC16	8.9	19.8	2	1	56.7	1.70	1.10	59.9	43.4	3.8	1.8	7.04	5.46	3.06	2.37
AVG	9.0	20.2	2.5	1.5	55.8	1.68	1.10	59.1	53.5	4.8	1.8	7.49	5.37	4.05	2.86

LAMDA = SCALING FACTOR IN EQUAL STRESS–EQUAL VELOCITY SCALING

MAIS = MAXIMUM AIS

Fx = FRACTURES

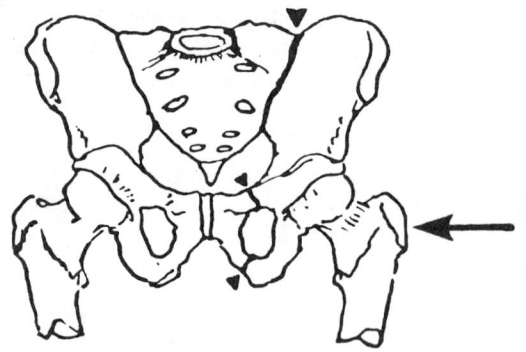

Figure 4. Lateral impact to the pelvis. The large arrow indicates loading direction and location. Two small and one medium-sized arrowhead indicate fracture locations.

There were no pelvic fractures in 6.7 m/s (15 mph) unpadded tests, but they always occurred in the 9 m/s (20 mph) unpadded tests (**Table 3**). Thus, the critical velocity of side impact is between 6.7 and 9 m/s (15 to 20 mph).

PADDING PERFORMANCE AND BENEFIT - There were nine padded tests. ARSAN 601 was used in SIC09. A variety of paper honeycomb pads was used in the other tests (SIC 10-17). Their material properties, shown in **Table 4**, were obtained from quasi-static tests on samples that were 150 mm square and 75 to 100 mm thick. The 25 mm (1 inch) cell size samples had initial peak compressive strengths of 97 kPa to 152 kPa (14 to 22 psi) with an average of 124 kPa (18 psi). At 35%

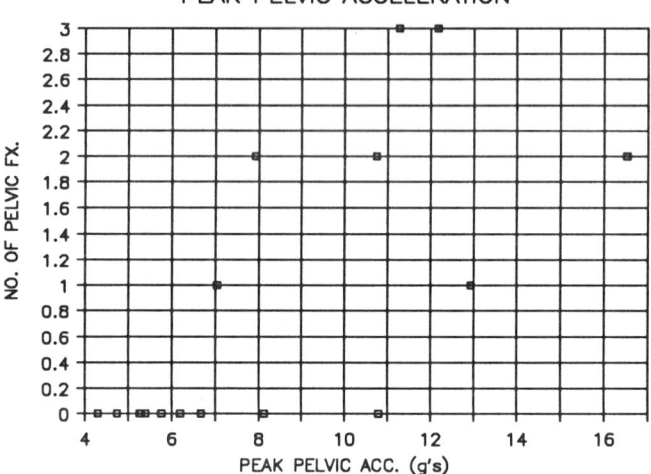

Figure 5. Scatter plot of pelvic fracture as a function of Acceleration

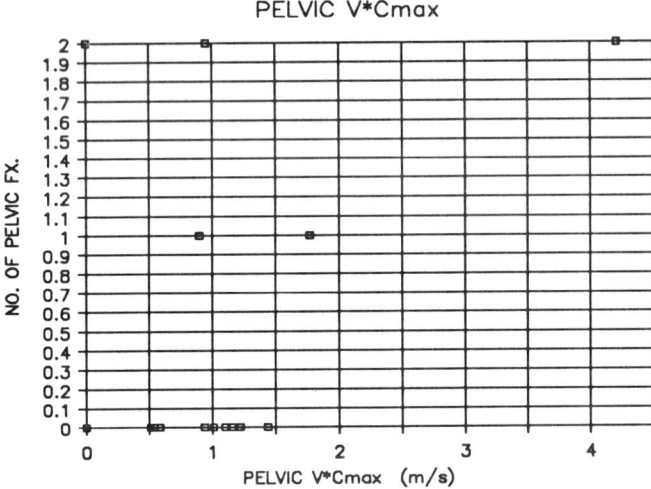

Figure 7. Scatter plot of pelvic fracture as a function of VCmax

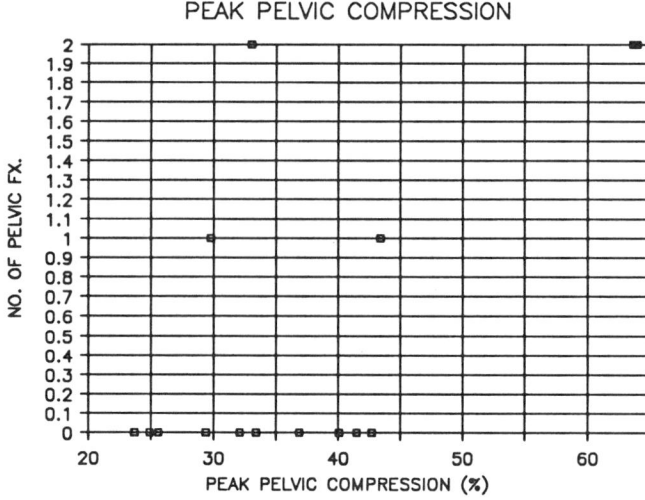

Figure 6. Scatter plot of pelvic fracture as a function of Cmax

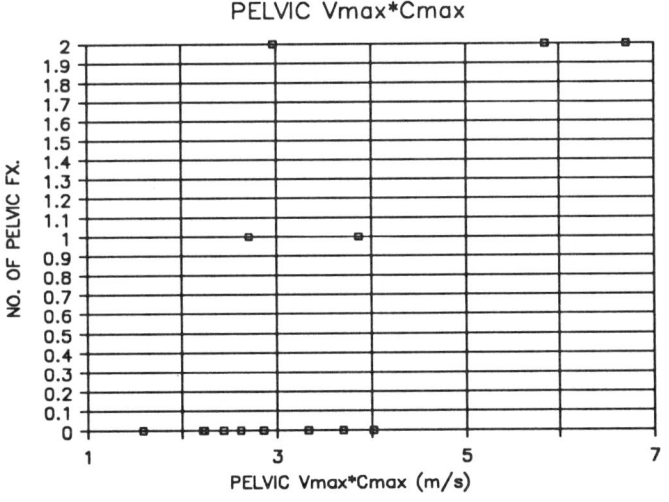

Figure 8. Scatter plot of pelvic fracture as a function of VmaxCmax

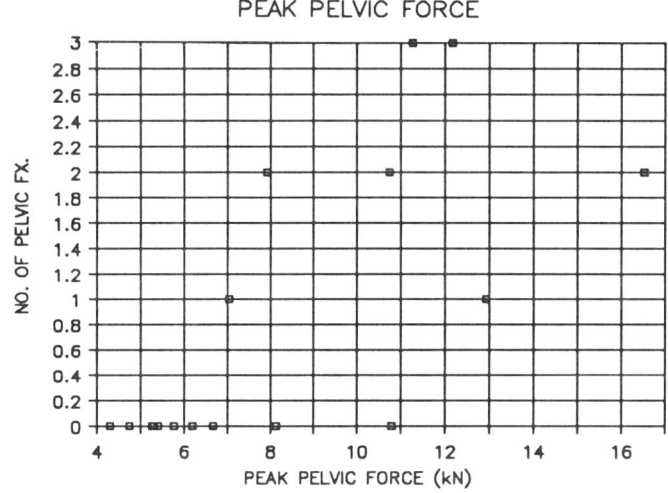

Figure 9. Scatter plot of pelvic fracture as a function of peak force (Fmax)

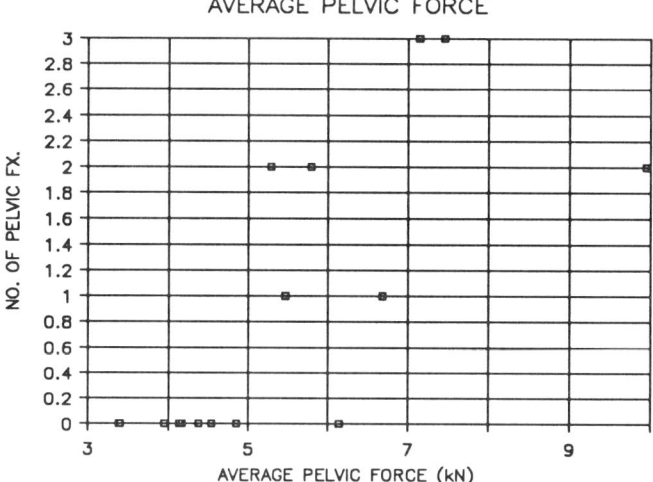

Figure 11. Scatter plot of pelvic fracture as a function of average force (Favg)

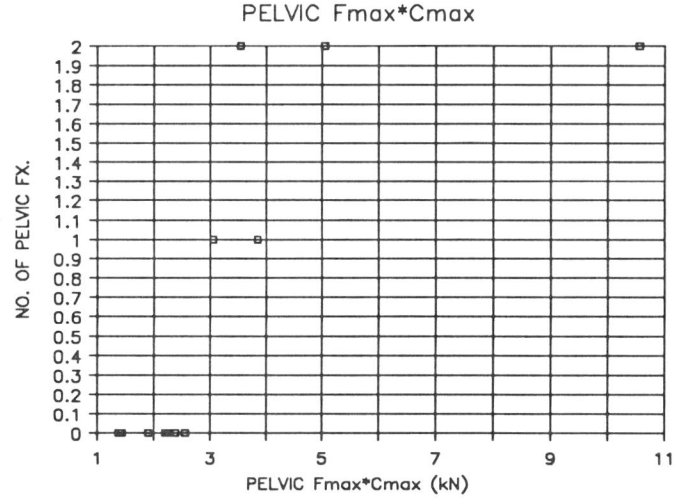

Figure 10. Scatter plot of pelvic fracture as a function of FmaxCmax

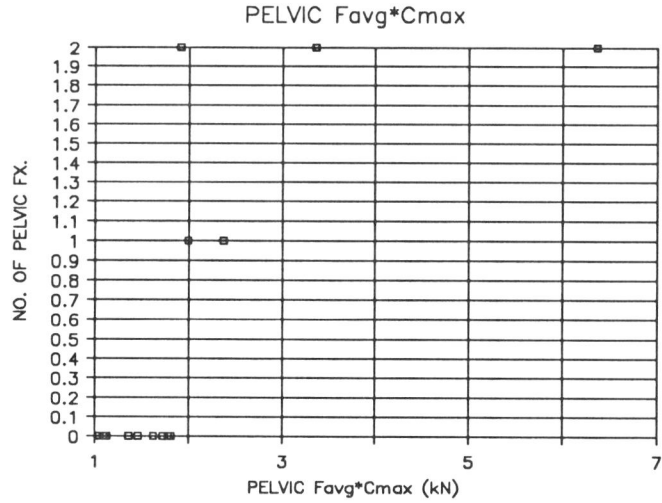

Figure 12. Scatter plot of pelvic fracture as a function of FavgCmax

TABLE 4. PADDING MATERIAL PROPERTIES   (QUASI-STATIC LOADING)

PELVIC IMPACT PADDING	CELL SIZE (IN.)	CELL SIZE (mm)	MANUFACTURER'S RATED STRENGTH (PSI)	(kPa)	WSU-TESTED INITIAL PEAK STRENGTH (PSI)	(kPa)	WSU-TESTED 35% CRUSH STRENGTH (PSI)	(kPa)
PAPER HONEYCOMB	1/1	25	15	103	18	124	8	55
PAPER HONEYCOMB	3/4	19	23	159	27	186	19	131
PAPER HONEYCOMB	5/8	16	31	214	45	310	28	193
VERTICEL HONEYCOMB	1/2	13	16	110	20	138	15	103
ARSAN 601	---	---	---	---	10	69	22	152

compression the strength was reduced to 48-76 kPa (7-11 psi) with an average of 55-62 kPa (8-9 psi). The padding had a manufacturer's rating of 104 kPa (15 psi) initial crush strength. The 19 mm (3/4 inch) cell size honeycomb had an initial peak strength of about 186 kPa (27 psi) and 131 kPa (19 psi) at 35% compression. The manufacturer's rating was 159 kPa (23 psi) initial crush strength. Verticel™ paper honeycomb with a 13 mm (1/2 inch) cell size was used in SIC 16 (75 mm or 3 in. thick). This padding had an initial peak compressive strength of 138 kPa (20 psi) and a crush strength of 97-110 kPa (14-16 psi) at 35% compression.

When 100 to 150 mm thick padding was used, pelvic AIS was reduced significantly. Injuries of the pelvis occurred in tests SIC09 and SIC16 in which a 75 mm thick padding was used. Pelvic fracture occurred in SIC09 with ARSAN 601 and in SIC16 with a 159 kPa (23 psi) paper honeycomb which bottomed out. There were no pelvic injuries in the other padded tests at 9 m/s (20 mph), in which thicker padding was used. The benefit of padding is to reduce the peak force and extend impact duration, thus reducing injury to the pelvis, if the padding is 100 mm (4 in.) thick or thicker.

DISCUSSION OF INJURY CRITERIA

The FMVSS 214 criterion (1990) for pelvic impact tolerance is a peak lateral acceleration of 130 g. This value appears to be too high based on these cadaveric tests. The average peak acceleration was 73 g for all of the pelvic injury cases. Other criteria need to be investigated.

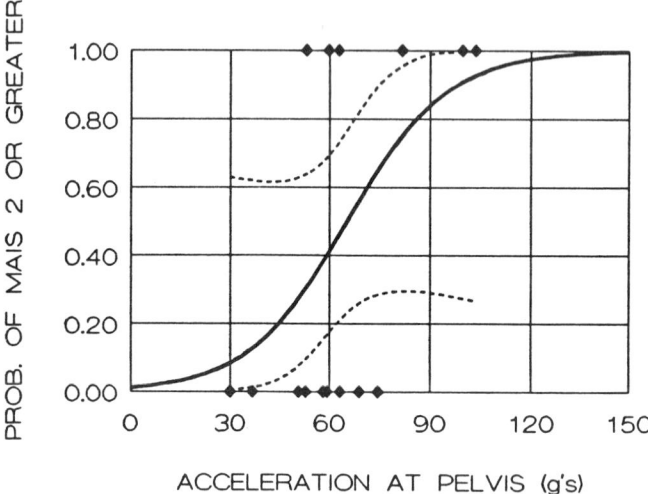

Figure 13. Logist curves for the probability of pelvic fracture as a function of peak acceleration

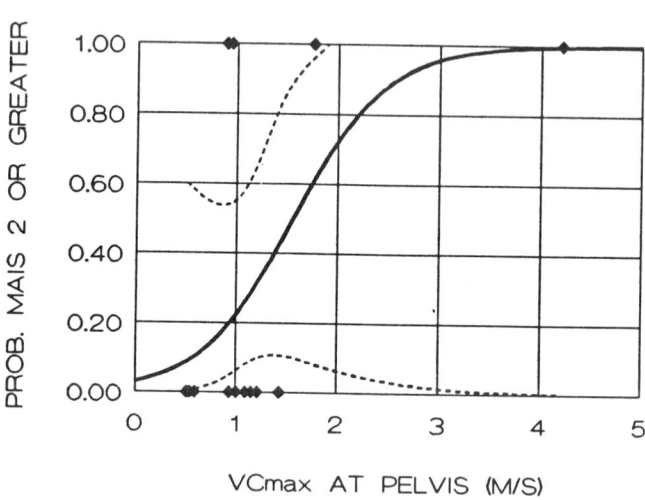

Figure 15. Logist curves for the probability of pelvic fracture as a function of VCmax

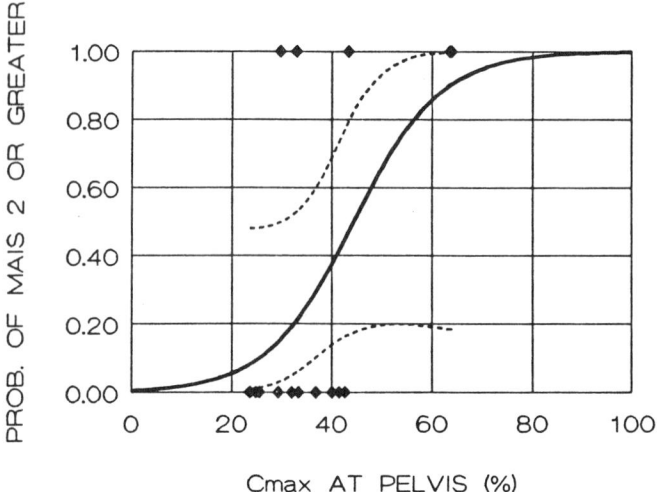

Figure 14. Logist curves for the probability of pelvic fracture as a function of Cmax

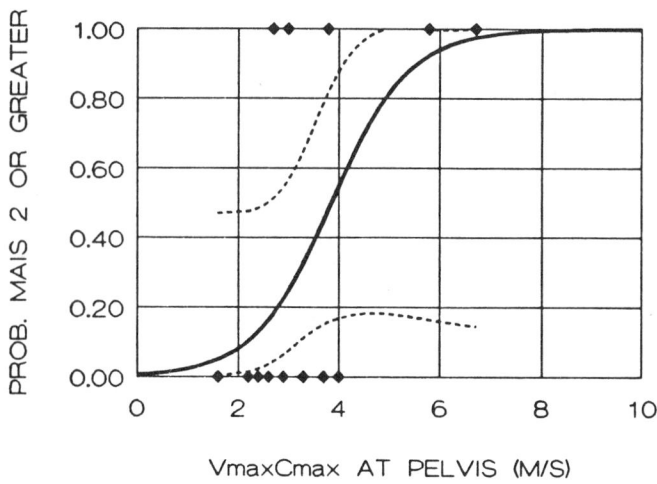

Figure 16. Logist curves for the probability of pelvic fracture as a function of VmaxCmax

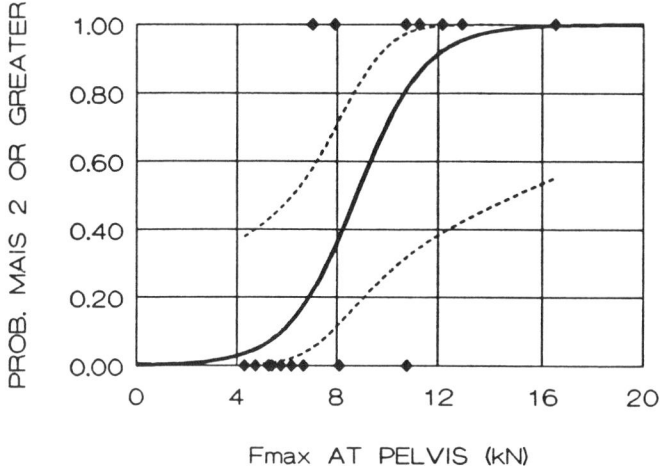

Figure 17. Logist curves for the probability of pelvic fracture as a function of peak force (Fmax)

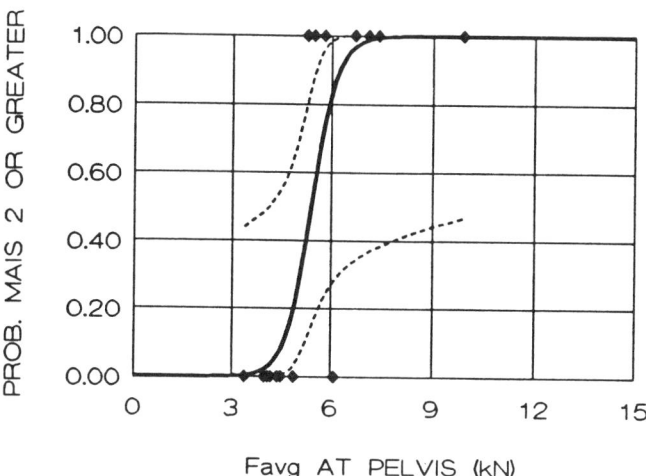

Figure 19. Logist curves for the probability of pelvic fracture as a function of average force (Favg)

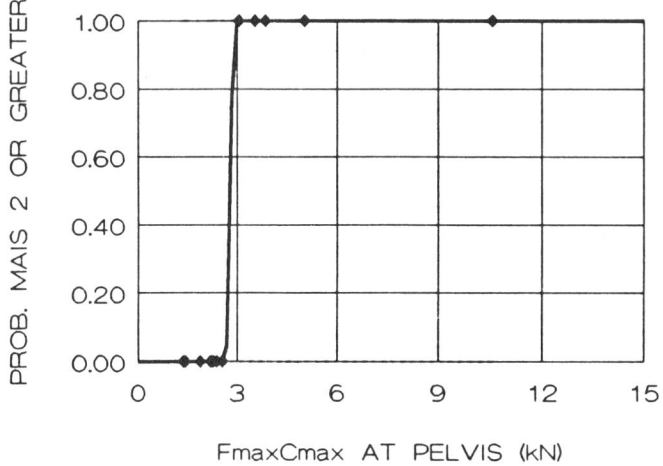

Figure 18. Logist curves for the probability of pelvic fracture as a function of FmaxCmax

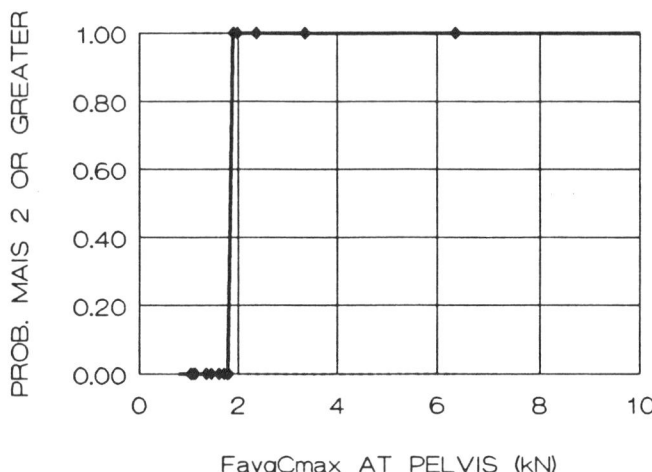

Figure 20. Logist curves for the probability of pelvic fracture as a function of FavgCmax

As shown in **Figure 15**, VCmax is a good, but not the best pelvic injury criterion in this sled test series. VmaxCmax (r = 0.444) is better than VCmax (r = 0.332), and Fmax is even better (r = 0.627). An attempt was made to search for an even better pelvic criterion.

A new parameter called "Average Force" (Favg) was derived from force-time histories of pelvic impact. It performed well as an injury parameter based on a Logist analysis (r = 0.734). Average force is a better parameter than peak force because the latter reflects a local contact phenomenon while the former is more representative of the entire impact. Average force was obtained by integrating the force-time curve to yield a new momentum curve, as shows in **Figure 21**. The momentum curve is almost linear between the 10-90% range. The slope of this momentum curve is the average force (Favg). It is a rate of change of pelvic momentum.

Average force is also effective in predicting injury reduction due to the use of padding. As shown in **Figure 21**, thicker (100 - 150 mm) padding reduces the rate of momentum change through padding deformation. Thus average force reflects the whole pelvic impact event, whereas a peak force is a response measure at only one point in time. The average forces derived from the momentum curves of **Figure 21**. The average force was 1.43 kN for the thick padding (100 - 150 mm) and 2.86 kN

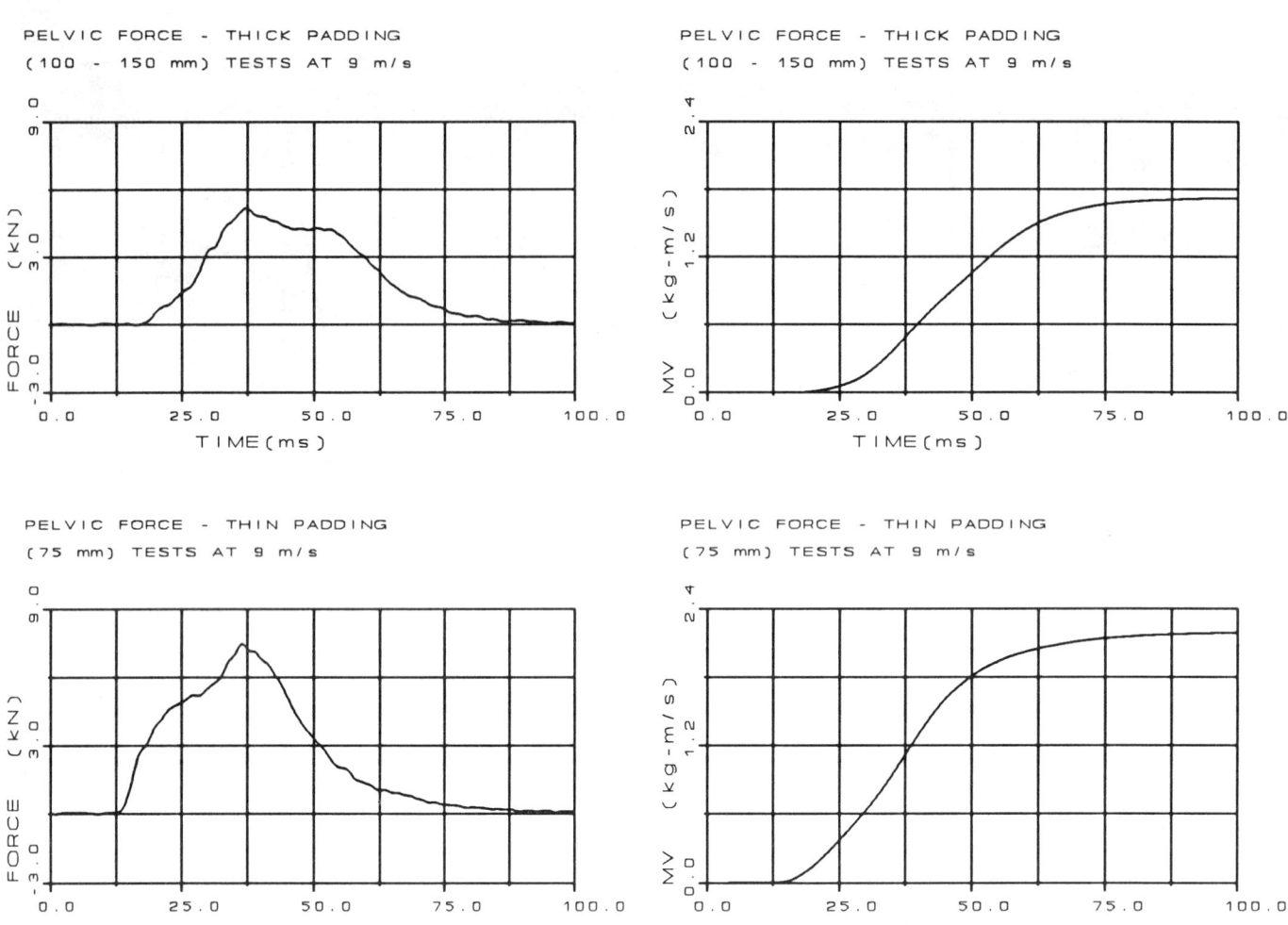

Figure 21. Force-time (left) and Momentum-time (right) histories for thick padding (100 - 150 mm) and thin padding (75 mm).

TABLE 5: CADAVER SLED TESTS: PROBABILITY ANALYSIS, CDC SIC01-17 FOR PELVIS

BIOMECHANICAL RESPONSE	UNITS	WEIBULL ANALYSIS MAXIMUM LIKELIHOOD	p 25% AIS 2	LOGIST ANALYSIS p 25% AIS 2	p 50% AIS 2	LOGIST ANALYSIS CHI-SQUARE	p	r	LOGIST ANALYSIS ALPHA	BETA
ACCELERATION	g's	0.0003	49.03	49.05	65.50	4.04	0.0444	0.314	-4.392	0.067
COMPRESSION	%	0.0007	34.83	35.00	44.70	4.59	0.0322	0.368	-5.158	0.116
VCmax	m/s	0.0027	0.98	1.07	1.57	3.77	0.0521	0.332	-3.450	2.195
VmaxCmax	m/s	0.0015	2.91	3.02	3.88	5.76	0.0164	0.444	-5.015	1.298
Fmax	kN	0.0037	7.02	7.30	8.78	11.07	0.0009	0.627	-6.463	0.735
Favg	kN	0.0135	4.94	5.01	5.43	14.41	0.0001	0.734	-14.340	2.642
FmaxCmax	kN	0.8418	2.70	2.77	2.81	19.09	0.0000	0.946	-82.015	29.221
FavgCmax	kN	0.2631	1.79	1.85	1.86	19.09	0.0000	0.946	-252.294	135.684

for the thin padding (75 mm), using the slope of the curve between 10 and 90% of maximum values.

The numerical results of the Weibull and Logist probability analyses are shown in **Table 4**. Acceleration and compression have a low level of likelihood, Chi-square and r values. The maximum likelihood value from the Weibull analysis was 0.0003 for acceleration and 0.0037 for force. This is more than a ten fold difference. Meanwhile, VCmax and VmaxCmax are slightly better than acceleration and compression while the force parameters have high maximum likelihood values, especially, average force (r = 0.734, Likelihood = 0.0135). Force or Average Force combined with compression of the pelvis (r = 0.946) is even better. However, compression is difficult to measure in a cadaver or dummy pelvis and force is thus a practical criterion. It is seen that average force is a better criterion than peak force. Tolerance in terms of average force is 4.94 kN from the Weibull analysis and 5.01 kN from the Logist analysis for a 25% probability of an MAIS 2 injury.

CONCLUSIONS

1. Average force (Favg), is a good predictor of pelvic injury based on data from this test series. Side impact tolerance for a 25% probability of fracture is 5 kN from both probability analyses.

2. Honeycomb material 100 mm (4 in.) thickness can markedly reduce pelvic injury in 9 m/s (20 mph) side impacts. No injury occurred in all 9 m/s (20 mph) tests with 100 mm of padding. For 75 mm thick padding, pelvic fracture occurred in both tests because Favg exceeded 5 kN. It was 4.3 kN for 100 mm thick padding. The honeycomb material 100 mm (4 in.) thick or thicker is effective in preventing pelvic injury in a 9 m/s (20 mph) side impact.

ACKNOWLEDGEMENTS

This work was supported by the CDC Grant No. 502347. We wish to thank Tim Walilko, Warren Hardy, Frank DuPont, Matt Mason, Yue Huang and the rest of the WSU Bioengineering staff who contributed to this work.

REFERENCES

Cavanaugh, JM; Walilko T; Malhotra, A; Zhu, Y; King, Al (1990) Biomechanical Response and Injury Tolerance of the Pelvis in Twelve Sled Side Impacts. SAE Paper No. 902305, 34th Stapp Car Crash Conference. (Reprinted in 1990 SAE Transactions, Passenger Cars, Sect. 6, pp. 1678-1693).

Cavanaugh, J; Zhu, YJ; King, Al (1992) Mechanical Properties of Various Padding Materials Used in Cadaveric Side Impact Sled Tests. SAE Paper No. 902354. In: Analytical Modeling and Occupant Protection Technologies, pp. 109-124. SAE International Congress and Exposition, Detroit, Michigan, Feb. 24-28, 1992.

Cavanaugh, J; Huang, Y; Zhu, Y; King, Al (1993) Regional Tolerance of the Shoulder, Thorax, Abdomen and Pelvis to Padding in Side Impact. 1993 SAE International Congress and Exposition, SAE Paper No. 930435.

Cesari, D; Ramet, M (1982) Pelvic Tolerance and Protection Criteria in Side Impact. 26th Stapp Car Crash Conference, SAE Paper No. 821159.

Eppinger RH, Marcus JH, Morgan RM (1984) Development of dummy and injury index for NHTSA's thoracic side impact protection research program. SAE Paper No. 840885, Government/Industry Meeting and Exposition, Washington, D.C.

FMVSS 214, 49 CFR Part 571 (1990) Federal Motor Vehicle Safety Standard No. 214, Side Impact Protection. Federal Register, Docket No. 88-06, Notice 8, RIN 2127-AB86, Vol. 55(210), Oct. 30, 1990.

Haffner, M (1985) Synthesis of Pelvic Fracture Criteria for Lateral Impact Loading. Proceedings of the Tenth International Technical Conference on Experimental Safety Vehicles, U.S. Department of Transportation, pp. 132-162.

Marcus JH, Morgan RM, Eppinger RH, Kallieris D, Mattern R, Schmidt G (1983) Human response to injury from lateral impact. Proc. 27th Stapp Crash Conference, pp. 419-432, SAE Paper No. 831634.

Morgan RM, Marcus JH, and Eppinger RH (1986) Side impact - the biofidelity of NHTSA's proposed ATD and efficacy of TTI. SAE Paper No. 861877, 30th Stapp Car Crash Conference.

Tarriere C, Walfisch G, Fayon A, Rosey JP, Got C, Patel A, Delmus A (1979) Synthesis of human tolerances obtained from lateral impact simulations. 7th International Conference on Experimental Safety Vehicles, Paris, France, pp. 359-373.

Viano DC, Lau IV (1983) Role of impact velocity and chest compression in thoracic injury. Avia. Space Environ. Med. 54: 16-21.

Viano DC and Lau IV (1985) Thoracic impact: a viscous tolerance criterion. Tenth International Conference on Experimental Safety Vehicles, Oxford, England, pp. 104-114.

Viano DC (1989) Biomechanical responses and injuries in blunt lateral impact. Proc. 33rd Stapp Car Crash Conference, pp. 113-142, SAE Paper No. 892432.

Section 4:
Biomechanical Response of Cadaveric Spine in Tension and Compression

760819

Static and Dynamic Articular Facet Loads

N. S. Hakim and A. I. King
Wayne State University

Abstract

Previous work on biodynamic response to whole-body +G_z (caudocephalad) acceleration gave ample evidence of facet loads in intact cadaveric spines. The computation of facet loads was based on an assumption that the total spine load was proportional to the measured seat pan load. In this study, the aim is to investigate the magnitude of the facet load during static and dynamic loading of an exised spinal segment. The applied loads resulted in a close simulation of those experienced by the intervertebral disc during whole-body impacts. An intervertebral load cell was used as the controlling mechanism in the duplication of the whole-body run in a testing machine. During these tests, both the total spine load and the intervertebral load were measured and thus the facet load was determined without relying on any assumptions.

Results from tests on 5 different cadaveric spinal segments, involving 32 static runs and 62 dynamic runs, show that facet loads exist under both static and dynamic loading and that these joints were capable of carrying up to 40% of the total spine load.

ANATOMISTS HAVE FREQUENTLY POSTULATED THAT THE VERTEBRAL body is the weight-bearing structure of the spine (Basmajian, 1, and Gray, 2)* Explicit statements were made by Fick (3) and Basmajian (1) to the effect that the posterior structures, specifically the articular facets, do not carry any load. Strasser (4) felt that the facets can have a load bearing role. Nachemson (5) measured intradiscal pressure in living humans and concluded that facets can be a load carrying member of the vertebral column. However, in 1963, he renounced his earlier conclusion (Nachemson, 6).

---

* Numbers in parentheses designate References at end of paper.

There is also collaborating evidence from animal studies to indicate that facets are indeed load-bearing structures. Kazarian et al. (7) have found that articular facet derangement can be made to occur in sub-human primates during $+G_z$ (caudocephalad) impact acceleration of short duration and high magnitudes. Recently, Kazarian (8) speculated that trauma to the neural arch was due to axial forces acting through the facets. He indicated that the mechanics of this injury mode was difficult to uncover in the clinical or operational literature. However, King et al. (9) have reported in the clinical literature the existence of a facet load during $+G_z$ acceleration, based on the work of Prasad et al. (10). Studies on the biodynamic response of seated cadaveric subjects which were subjected to $+G_z$ whole-body acceleration led to the conclusion that facets have a load bearing role.

In view of the intricate anatomy of the vertebrae and the small contact areas of the bony elements of the posterior spine, it is practically impossible to measure the value of the resultant (total) spine load at any level of the intact column. There was no known technique to measure directly the forces sustained by the anterior structure (the vertebral body-disc assembly), or the posterior structure (the neural arch interconnected by the articular facets). Preliminary evidence of the existence of a facet load was obtained from qualitative data, principally from strain data obtained from small strain gages located on the bony surface of the vertebra. In order to quantify these findings, an intervertebral load cell (IVLC) was designed and fabricated by Prasad et al. (11). This transducer is thin enough to completely replace the inferior portion of a lumbar vertebral body of a cadaveric subject, leaving the intervertebral disc virtually intact, and without damaging the pedicles. Recording the output of the IVLC during an impact run gives the vertebral body force as a function of time. An assumption still had to be made to compute the magnitude of the total spine load at the level of the IVLC in order to obtain the facet load. Prasad et al. (10) assumed that the total spine load was proportional to the seatpan load, with the proportionality factor equal to the ratio of the body weight above the IVLC to the total body weight. Conclusive evidence of facet load cannot be attained without removing the assumption for the calculation of the total spine load.

In this study, several preliminary dynamic runs were carried out on each of the human cadavers used. These tests were whole-body (<u>in situ</u>*) $+G_z$ acceleration

---

* The word "<u>in situ</u>" will be used to indicate whole-body experimentation on an intact spine.

runs performed on a vertical accelerator closely following the experimental procedure described by Prasad et al. (10). A realistic intervertebral load-time function was obtained for each run. The primary aim of this study was to simulate this intervertebral load in vitro* in a testing machine so that the total load and the intervertebral load could be measured directly. Hence, no assumption was necessary to calculate the facet loads. That is, at any level of the spine

$$TSL = IVL + FL$$

where

TSL = Total spine load at the IVLC level
IVL = Intervertebral axial load
FL = Facet load or load carried by the posterior structures of the vertebra

If the total spine load at the level of IVLC is measured, FL can be determined, without assumptions, from the above equation. This measurement is feasible only if the tests are made in vitro, by loading an excised segment in a testing machine. To be realistic, however, the applied loads should simulate the loads encountered by the intact spine during whole-body acceleration. Moreover, it was necessary to establish the existence of a facet load under static and dynamic loading conditions. The static part of the in vitro scheme was executed on a universal static testing machine. For the dynamic tests, an experimental technique was developed to simulate dynamic whole-body loading of a spinal segment in a testing machine. During whole-body caudocephalad acceleration of a cadaveric subject, the IVLC was used to measure the load sustained by a vertebral body. The excised segment containing the IVLC was then placed in an MTS testing machine which was commanded to load the segment so that the IVLC output matched the pre-recorded whole-body IVLC signal.

CADAVER PREPARATION

The procedure for cadaver selection and preparation has been described by Vulcan (12) and Prasad et al. (13). Age, cause of death, and body weight were the basis of selection. A careful roentgenographic examination of the vertebral column was then carried out to determine the suitability of the cadaver for $+G_z$ acceleration runs. Table 1 lists the relevant data for the six cadavers used in this work. To instrument the spine an anterior approach was used. Abdominal viscera below

---

* In the context of this paper, "in vitro" means experimentation on excised spinal segments.

the diaphragm were removed. The IVLC was thin enough to replace the inferior slice of a vertebral body just below the pedicles leaving the adjacent intervertebral disc virtually intact. A specially designed double-bladed rotary saw was used to cut the slot. X-ray measurements of vertebral body heights were made to ensure that the IVLC could be accommodated without damaging the pedicles. The slot was cut in L2 in 4 of the 6 specimens. It was in L3 for the other 2 cadavers. Figure 1 is a photograph of the IVLC. It has two channels; one measuring the axial force and the other the bending moment. The lip of the transducer was secured against the vertebral body and a strap held the load cell in place during the experimental runs. Neither the length nor the mobility of the vertebral column was affected when the IVLC was properly installed.

VERTICAL ACCELERATOR (IN SITU) RUNS

The in situ vertical accelerator runs were executed in order to determine realistic dynamic loads sustained by the spine. They were carried out at the vertical accelerator facility of Wayne State University which has been described by Patrick (14). A seat-pan load cell (SPLC) measured the axial force and bending moment at the seat pan level, while an accelerometer measured the sled acceleration. The instrumented cadaver was placed on the seat and was restrained by a lap belt and shoulder harness. Straps were used to tie the legs to the seat and the wrists to the seat pan. The control variable in the in situ runs was the impact acceleration profile. The most important dependent variable was the intervertebral axial load which had to be reproduced later on during the in vitro dynamic runs. Table 2 lists the runs executed on each of the specimens.

SEGMENT PREPARATION

After completion of the in situ runs on a cadaver, the vertebral column was carefully examined roentgenographically. If no fractures or dislocations were found, a segment containing at least two vertebrae above and below the IVLC was excised to be prepared for the in vitro runs. This segment also contained all of the soft tissue surrounding the vertebra. It was kept moist with embalming fluid at all times and was wrapped in a sheet of plastic so that the ambient relative humidity was approximately 100%. The only time it was exposed to room air was during strain gage installation. When not in use, the specimen was preserved in a cooler. Seg-

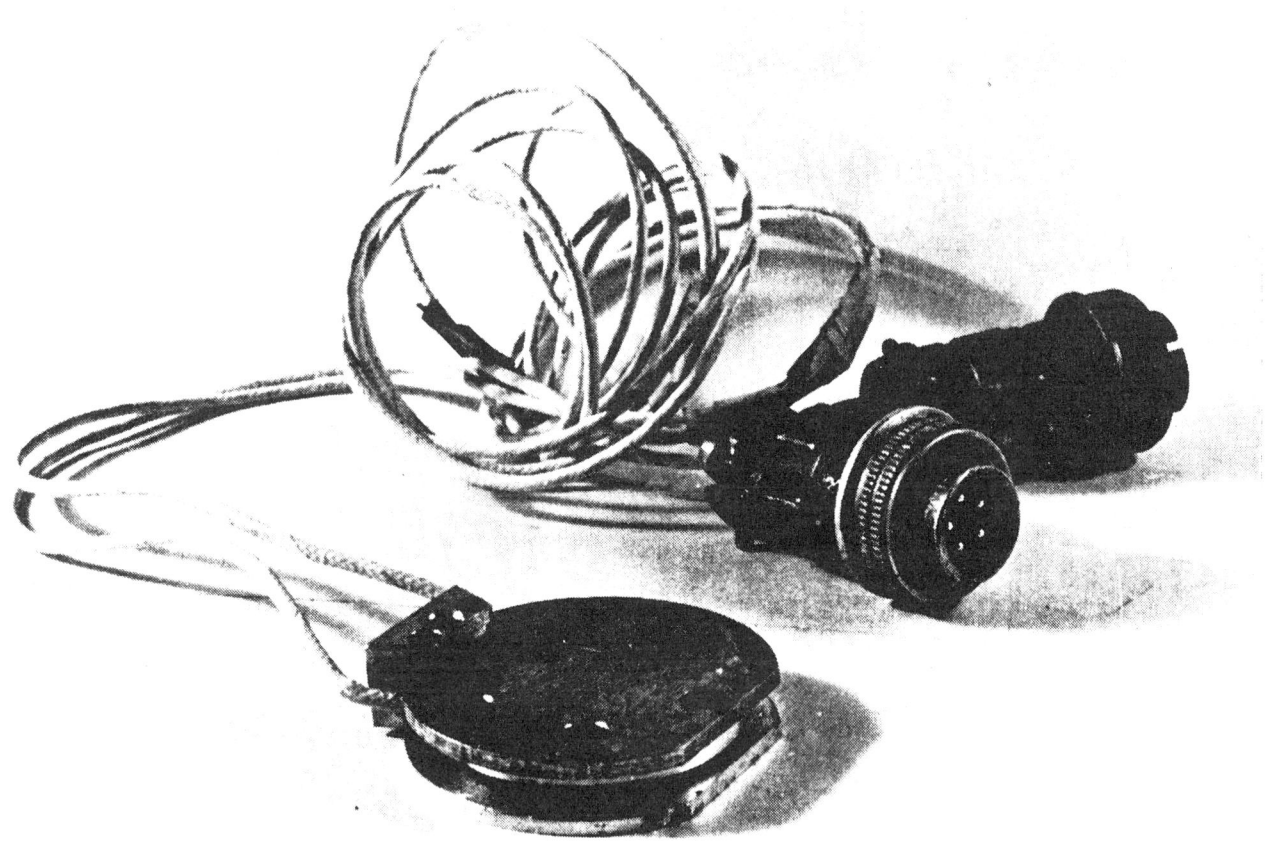

Fig. 1 - The intervertebral load cell

ment No. 1 (Table 1) was accidentally taken out of the cooler and partially dried out. It was resoaked in embalming fluid and left in the cooler for over 4 weeks before it was re-tested. Close observation during these tests did not reveal any characteristic differences peculiar to this segment, when compared with other specimens.

Procedures for segment preparation were the same for the static and the dynamic in vitro tests. First, a low melting point alloy (Ostalloy, m.p. = 47.3°C or 117°F) was used to cover both ends of the segment. The caudal end of the specimen was then embedded into a specially designed fixture using the same alloy. During the test this bottom fixture was fastened to a load transducer for measuring the total spinal load. The cranial end of the segment was also molded in a pipe flange of suitable diameter using the same alloy, providing an adequate loading surface for the specimen. Figures 2 and 3 show anterior and side views of the molded segment. During the molding process, two conditions had to be satisfied:
 a. The natural curvature of the segment should be the same as its in situ curvature.
 b. The top and bottom surfaces of the fixture must be parallel so that the testing machine can apply a normal load to the top surface.

STATIC IN VITRO RUNS

A universal screw-driven testing machine was used for the static tests. The load was applied at different eccentricities using an adjustable loading head designed for that purpose, as shown in Figures 2 and 3. This loading head permitted the application of load at any point on a transverse plane through the vertebra. The line of action of the total load applied by the testing machine was fixed for a given run and was changed only in the antero-posterior direction from one run to the next.

Several static runs were executed on each spinal segment at different eccentricities. The bending output of the intervertebral load cell was monitored to determine the run which had realistic bending when compared with the in situ dynamic runs.

A preload representing the weight of the body above the IVLC was first applied to the specimen. The load then was increased very slowly (quasistatically) to a specific value where it was maintained constant for about one minute before increasing it to the next higher value, usually in 111-N (25-lb) steps. After reaching the peak load, the same steps were followed during unloading.

Table 1 - Cadaver Data

Specimen No.	Sex	Age	Cause of Death
1	Male	57	Cardiorespiratory arrest
2	Male	37	Respiratory failure
3	Male	52	Hepatic coma; cardiac arrest
4	Male	52	Gastrointestinal bleeding
5	Male	45	Hepatic coma; ascites; jaundice
6	Female	53	Carcinoma of larynx

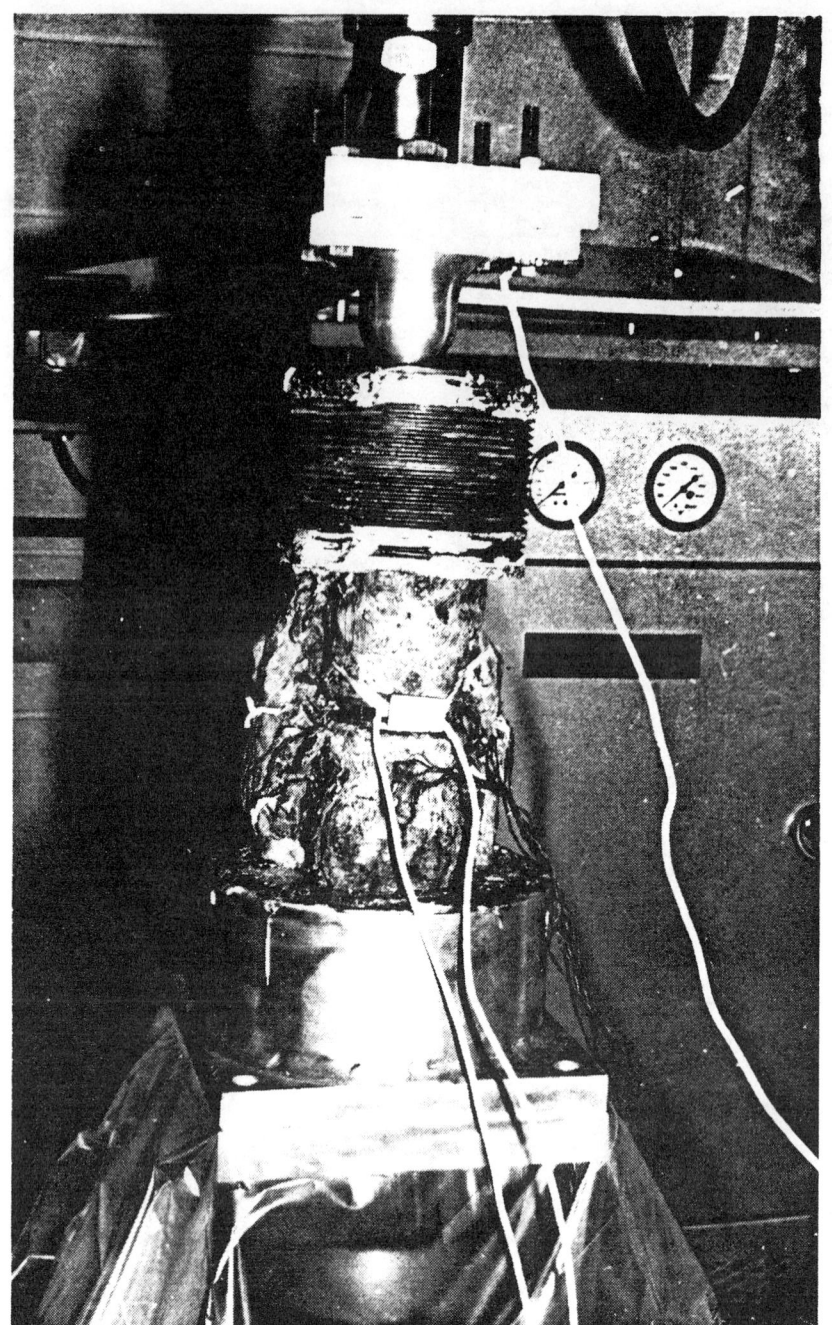

Fig. 2 - Anterior view of the molded segment

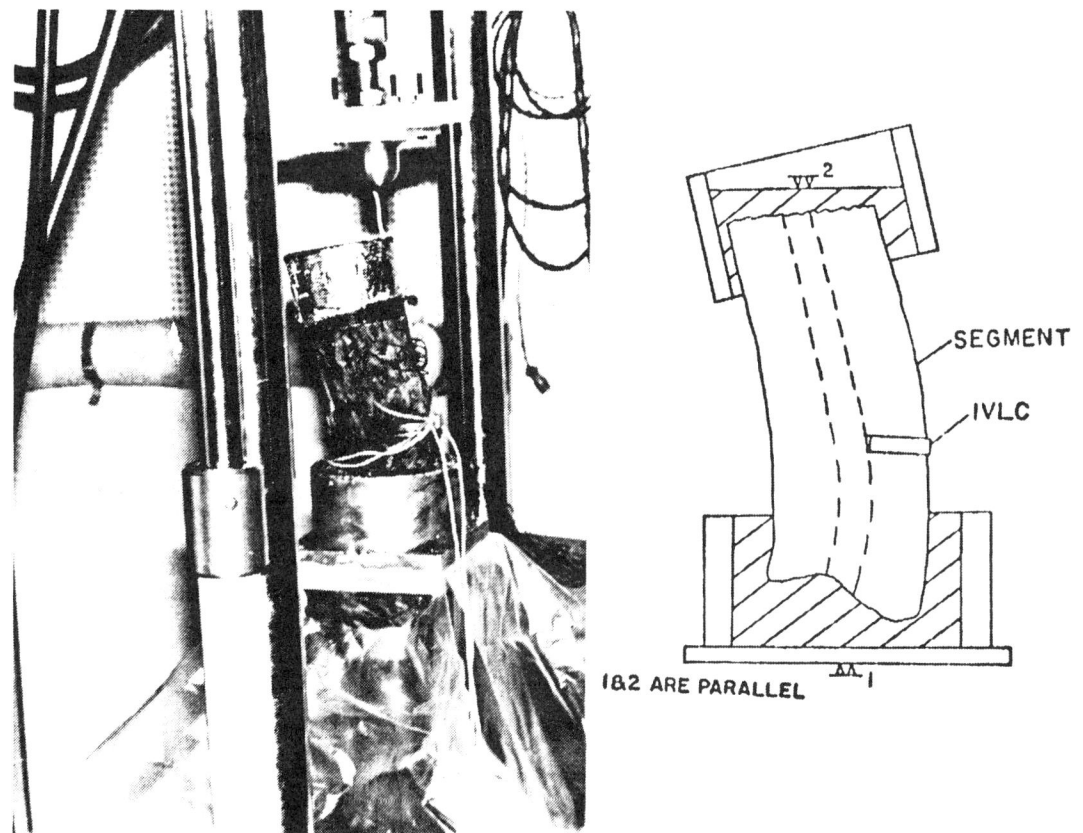

Fig. 3 - Side view and a schematic of the molded segment

DYNAMIC IN VITRO RUNS

The materials testing system (MTS) at Wayne State University has a single channel servo control mechanism with one linear hydraulic actuator and a function generator. The goal was to load the vertebral column segment in the testing machine to simulate the loading conditions experienced by the segment during whole-body accelerations. Figure 4 shows a schematic of the set-up used to achieve this purpose. As mentioned earlier, the intervertebral axial load signal was recorded during a whole-body run. During an MTS run, a static preload representing the weight of the body above the IVLC was first applied and the pre-recorded signal was then played back into the programmer of the system as the desired input command. The control transducer for the in vitro runs was, of course, the IVLC (axial). During the run, its output was conditioned and supplied to the servo controller as the feedback signal. A differential comparator in the servo-controller subtracted the input command and the feedback signal giving out a correction control signal (also called error signal or servo signal). Precise calculations and fine adjustments were necessary to ensure that both the input command and the feedback signals had the same scale in terms of physical units per volt. The correction signal was fed to a servo valve which controlled the hydraulic actuator through a high pressure hydraulic manifold. This instantaneous adjustment of the hydraulic actuator pressure effected continuous change in the total load applied to the segment so that the intervertebral feedback signal was the same as the pre-recorded programmer signal. A detailed description of the load duplication process was given by Hakim and King (15).

The system could only reproduce the magnitude of the intervertebral axial load. To replicate the whole-body in situ intervertebral loads it was necessary to simulate not only the magnitude but also the line of action of this load. Since a two-actuator servo control test system was not available, the same adjustable loading head used in the static test was utilized to effect changes in the line of action of the total load applied to the segment between runs. For a given vertical accelerator run, the magnitude of the intervertebral load at various eccentricities was duplicated. The selected in vitro run would then be the one with a bending output that most closely matched the bending output of the whole-body run. Since the moment arm was fixed for the entire duration of the MTS run, it was not expected to fully duplicate the bending moment encountered in the whole-body run. It was hoped, however, that some degree of resemblance would prevail.

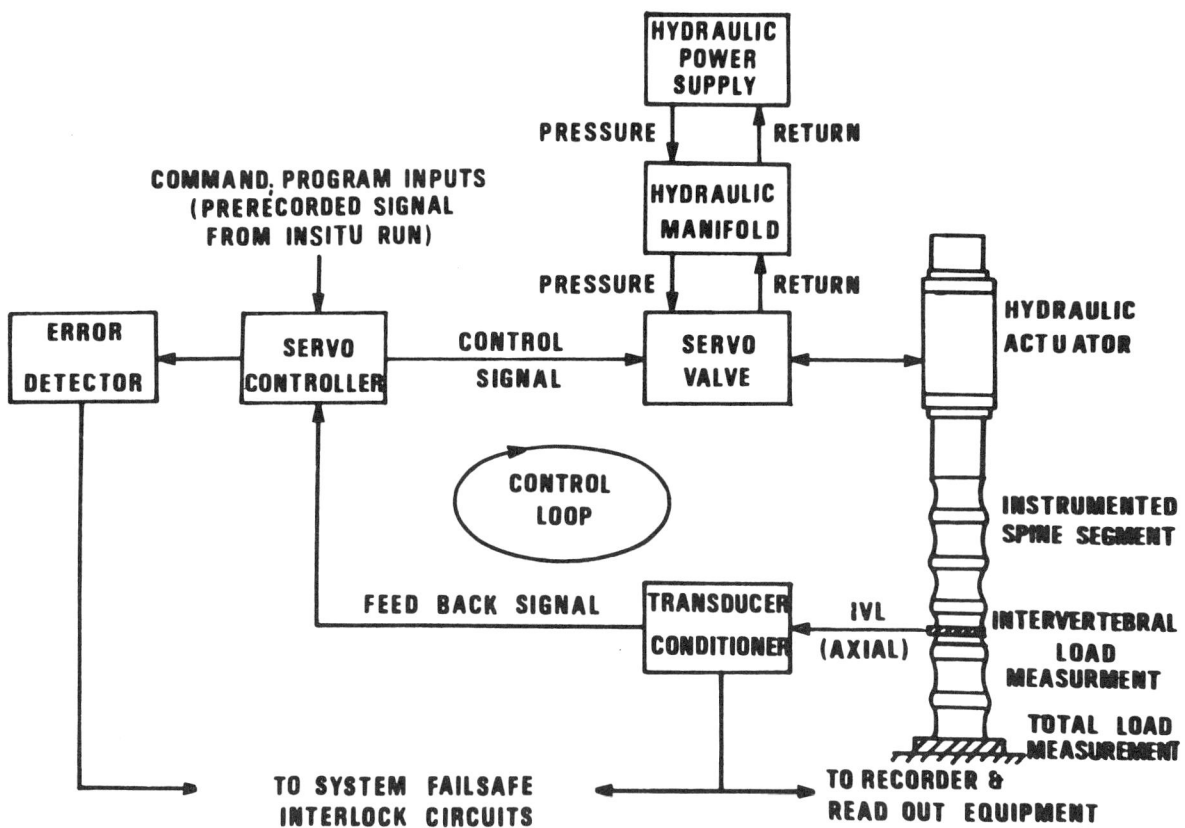

Fig. 4 - Schematic of the MTS servo-control loop

RESULTS

STATIC LOADING - A total of 32 static in vitro tests were made on three different segments as shown in Table 2. Figure 5 shows a typical plot of the total load versus the intervertebral body load (IVL) and the facet load (FL) for one of the segments (Specimen #3, Table 1). The bending moment (IVM) is also shown. Figures 6 and 7 are similar plots for the other two segments (Specimen #1 and #4), respectively.

In every case, the variation of the total load with the intervertebral body load was linear, as was that for the facet load and the intervertebral bending moment. The facets consistently bore 20 to 25% of the total load. The unloading phenomenon of the facets which was reported by Prasad, et al. (10) was not observed in these static tests.

DYNAMIC LOADING - A total of 62 dynamic in vitro tests were made on five different segments as shown in Table 2. In most of these tests the magnitude of the IVL was closely simulated. In some of the tests, however, the magnitude of the in vitro IVL was higher than that obtained during the corresponding in situ run to simulate a higher g-level whole-body run. The magnitude of the IVM was increased proportionately, but the moment arm or the line of action of the IVL was approximately the same as that in the in situ case. Figures 8 and 9 show the intervertebral load and moment respectively of an in situ run on Cadaver #5 which was to be duplicated. The in vitro replication is displayed in Figures 10 through 13. A comparison of the in vitro command signal or the IVL as recorded during the whole-body run, and the feedback signal or the corresponding IVL sustained by the excised segment is shown in Figure 10. Figure 11 shows the recorded total load and IVL as well as the facet load, which is the difference between the two. The facet load computed from in situ data was superimposed on this figure for comparative purposes. The intervertebral bending moment and moment arm are shown in Figures 12 and 13 respectively. It can be seen from Figure 11 that the facets were transmitting up to 28% of the total load carried by the spine during the simulated run. A comparison of Figures 9 and 12 reveals a surprising resemblence between the original and the reproduced intervertebral bending, despite the fact that this was achieved by manually adjusting the loading head without the assistance of a servo control. The moment arm shown in Figure 13 was evaluated as the ratio between the intervertebral moment to the IVL. It indicates that the IVL was acting at a point posterior to the anterior-most edge of the vertebra by about 57% of the total AP width of the

Table 2 - Summary of Experimental Runs

Specimen No.	Load Cell Location	No. of 'in situ' Runs	No. of Static Runs	No. of MTS Runs	Remarks
1	L2	21	12	18	
2	L2	20	--	--	Damaged segment
3	L2	10	11	8	Fracture at the top fixture
4	L3	11	9	8	Anterior wedge fracture
5	L2	6	--	17	
6	L3	6	--	11	

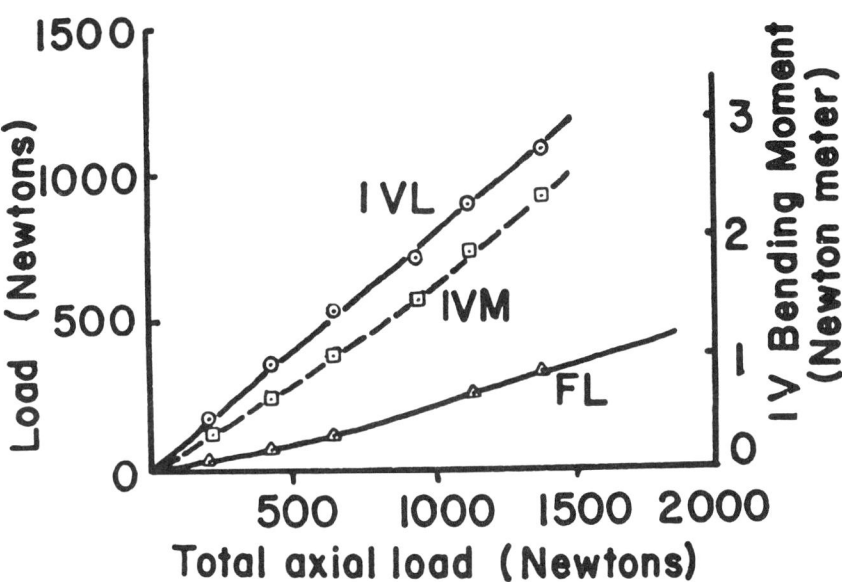

Fig. 5 - In vitro static spine loads of Specimen #3

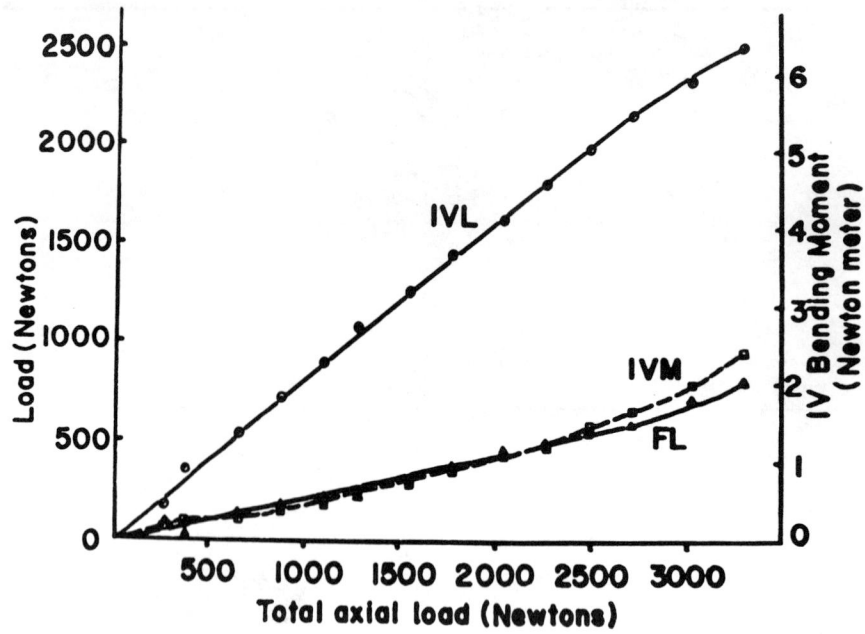

Fig. 6 - In vitro static spine loads of Specimen #1

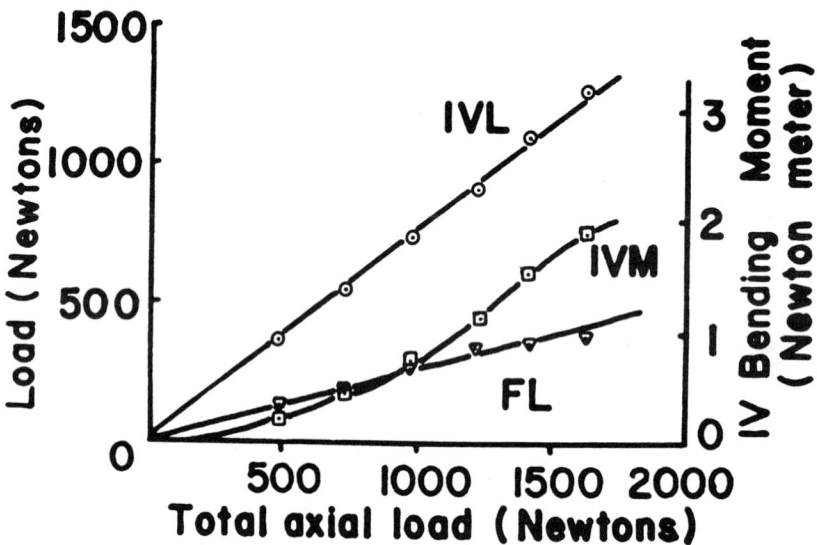

Fig. 7 - In vitro static spine loads of Specimen #4

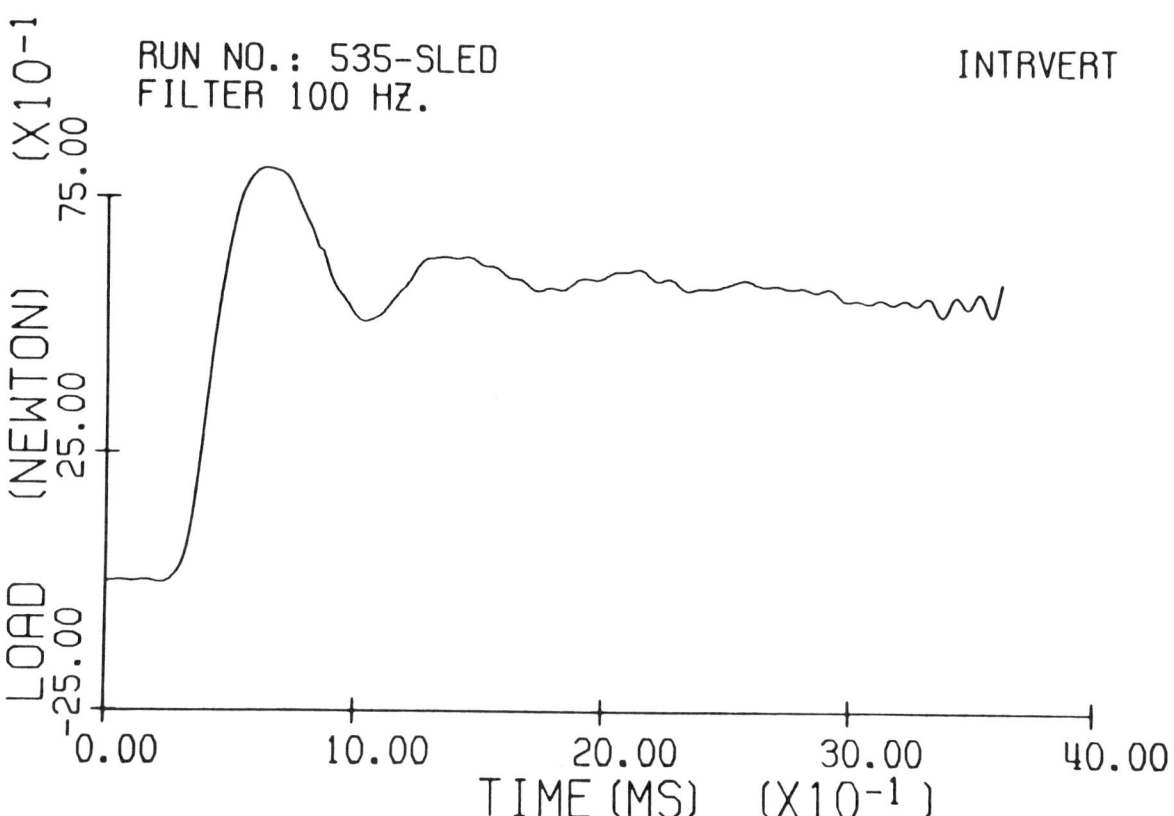

Fig. 8 - *In situ* intervertebral axial load of Run #535

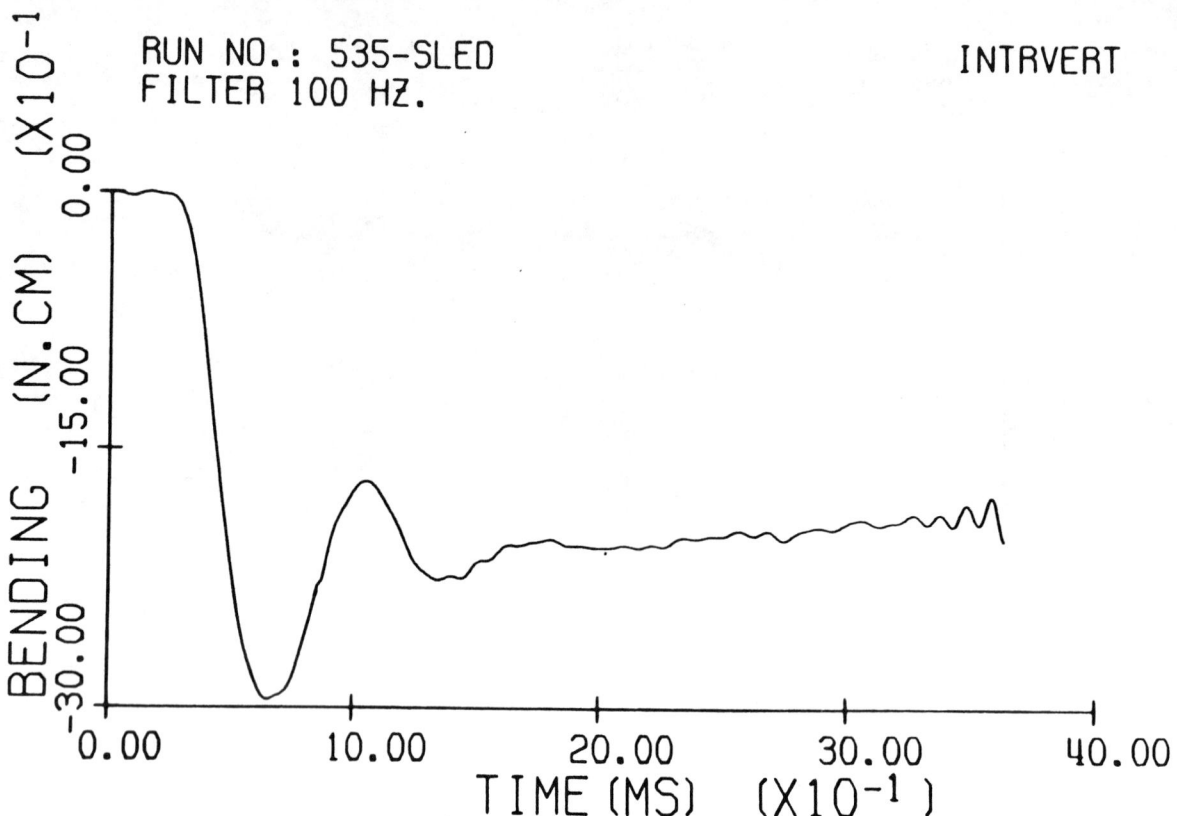

Fig. 9 - <u>In situ</u> intervertebral bending moment of Run #535

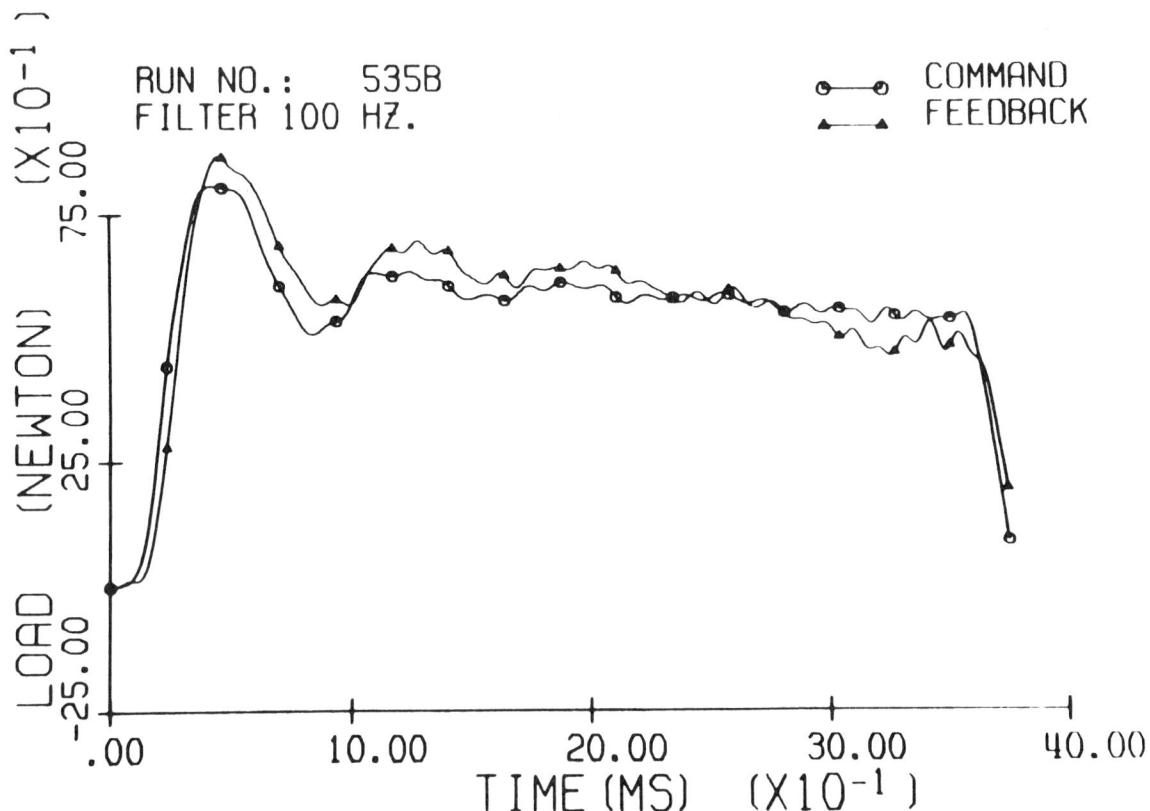

Fig. 10 - Comparison between in situ and in vitro intervertebral axial loads of Run #535B

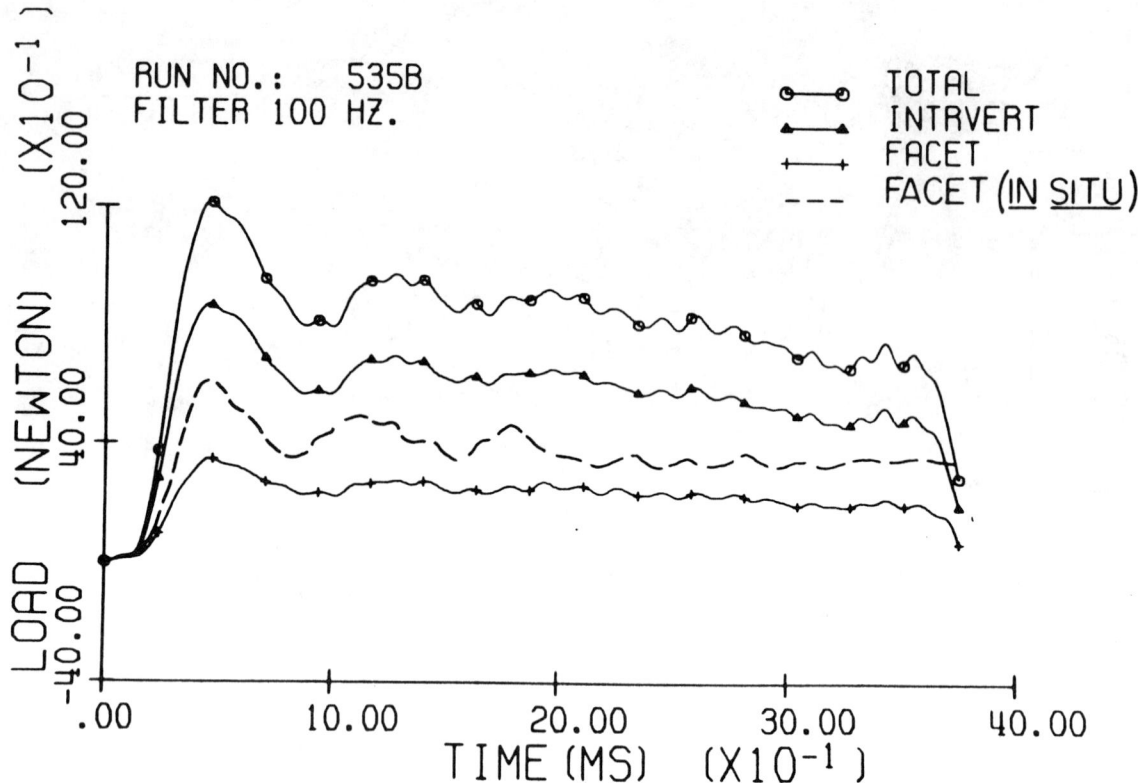

Fig. 11 - *In vitro* loads and *in situ* facet load of Run #535B

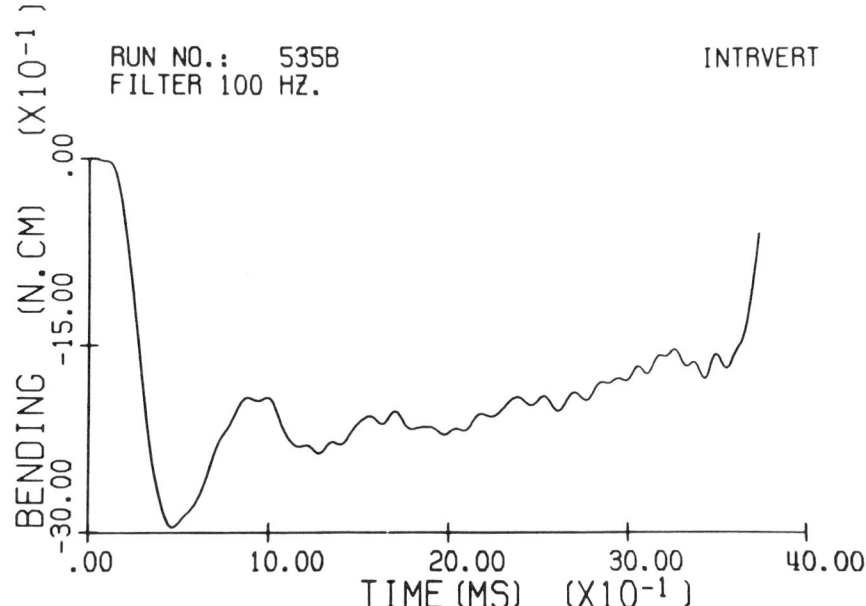

Fig. 12 - *In vitro* intervertebral bending moment of Run #535B

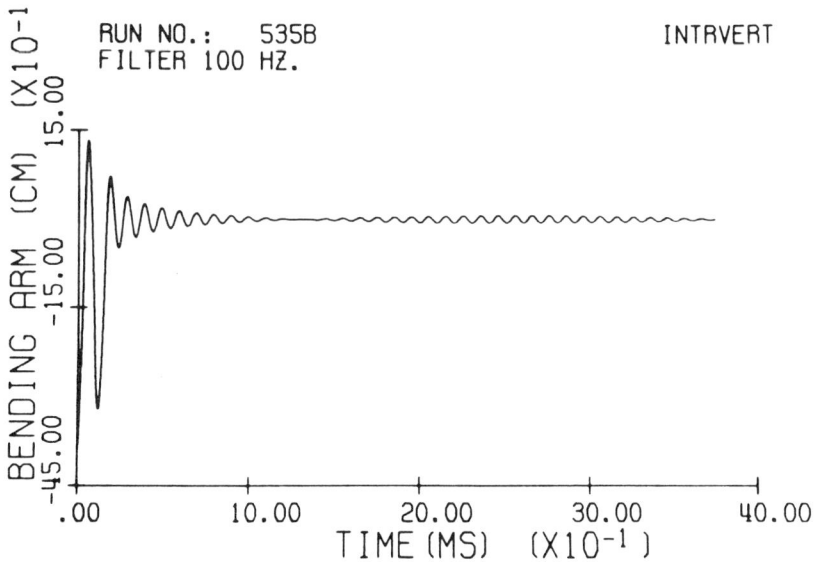

Fig. 13 - *In vitro* intervertebral moment arm of Run #535B

body. The large initial fluctuations were due to numerical errors when one small quantity was divided by another.

As shown in Figure 11 the calculated *in vitro* facet load was smaller than that estimated from *in situ* data. One reason which contributed to this difference is the assumption of equivalent dynamic response for the upper and lower torso. This was the assumption used for the *in situ* calculations. The *in vitro* duplication process can also be a possible cause. The intervertebral load and moment were duplicated but the total spinal moment at the level of the IVLC was not necessarily duplicated. The total spine load consists of an axial load and moment acting on both the centrum and the facets in a complex manner. The total and facet moments are not known or measurable. Duplicating the IVL and IVM could not guarantee that the facet loads and moments were automatically duplicated because there is no proof that these quantities are unique. A small spinal segment which is restrained in a loading fixture at both ends can very well be subjected to different bending characteristics when compared to those of an intact spine in a restrained cadaveric subject.

Another example of an *in vitro* duplication of a vertical accelerator run on the same segment is shown in Figure 14. The facet load was about 26% of the total load for this run and is shown in Figure 15. A comparison of *in situ* and *in vitro* intervertebral moment is shown in Figure 16. Although the moment was matched very well, with the difference in the peak value of only 52 N cm, the *in situ* facet load was again higher than that of the *in vitro* case, as displayed in Figure 15. Figure 17 demonstrates the duplication of the IVL for a third run on a different segment (Cadaver #6) and Figure 18 shows the facet load, which was 37% of the total spine load. The facet load for a fourth run on Cadaver #6 was duplicated on the MTS machine, as shown in Figure 19. It was about 38% of the total load. Simulation at higher g-levels was also carried out by changing the gain of the control signal (IVL). Figures 20 through 22 show three runs on three different segments at IVL loads about 65% higher than those measured *in situ*. The intervertebral moments were also higher and resulted in a low compressive facet load for one case (Figure 21, Cadaver #3), and a zero facet load for the third case (Figure 22, Cadaver #1).

CONCLUSIONS

It has been established that the articular facets support up to 40% of the total compressive spine load. No assumptions were made in the computation of the total spine load and the intervertebral load, both of

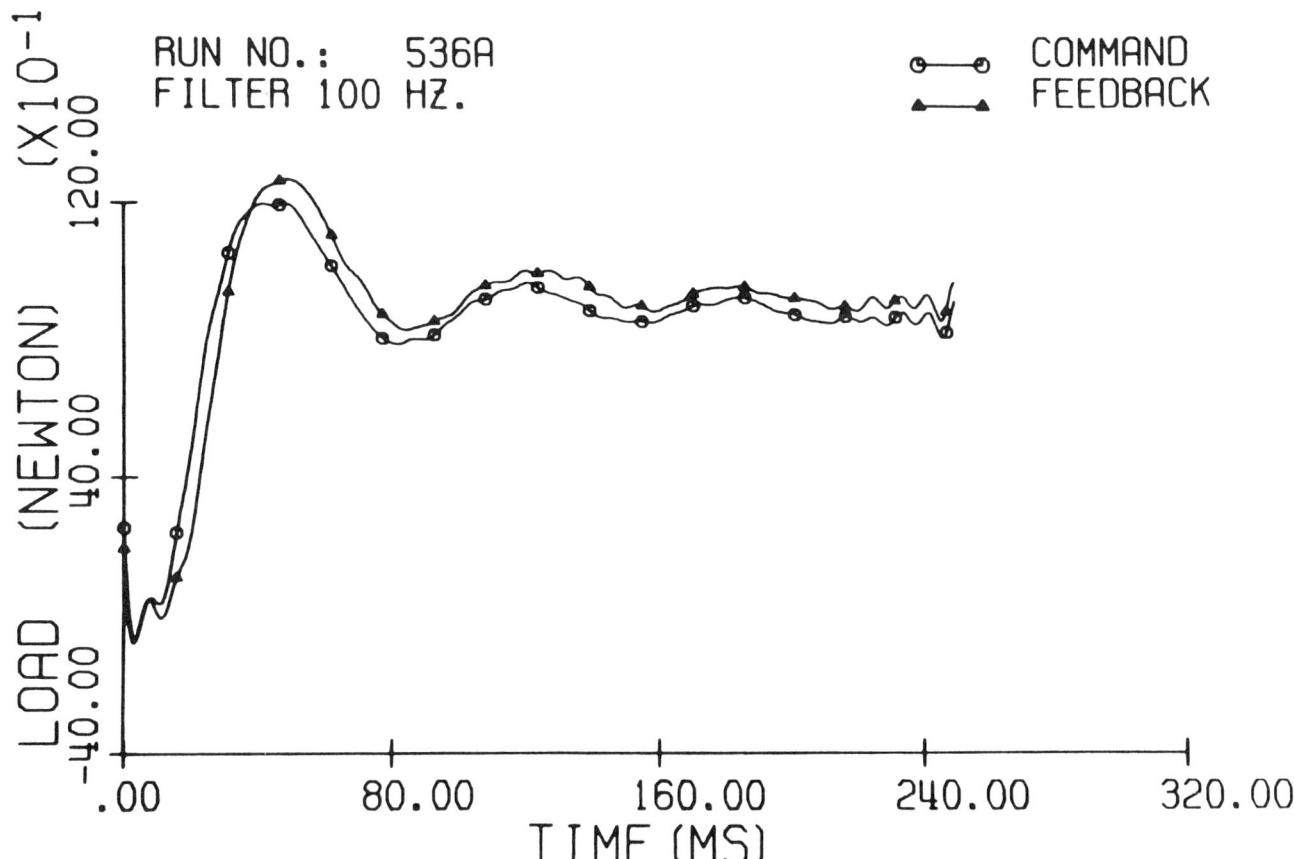

Fig. 14 - Comparison between in situ and in vitro intervertebral and axial loads of Run #536A

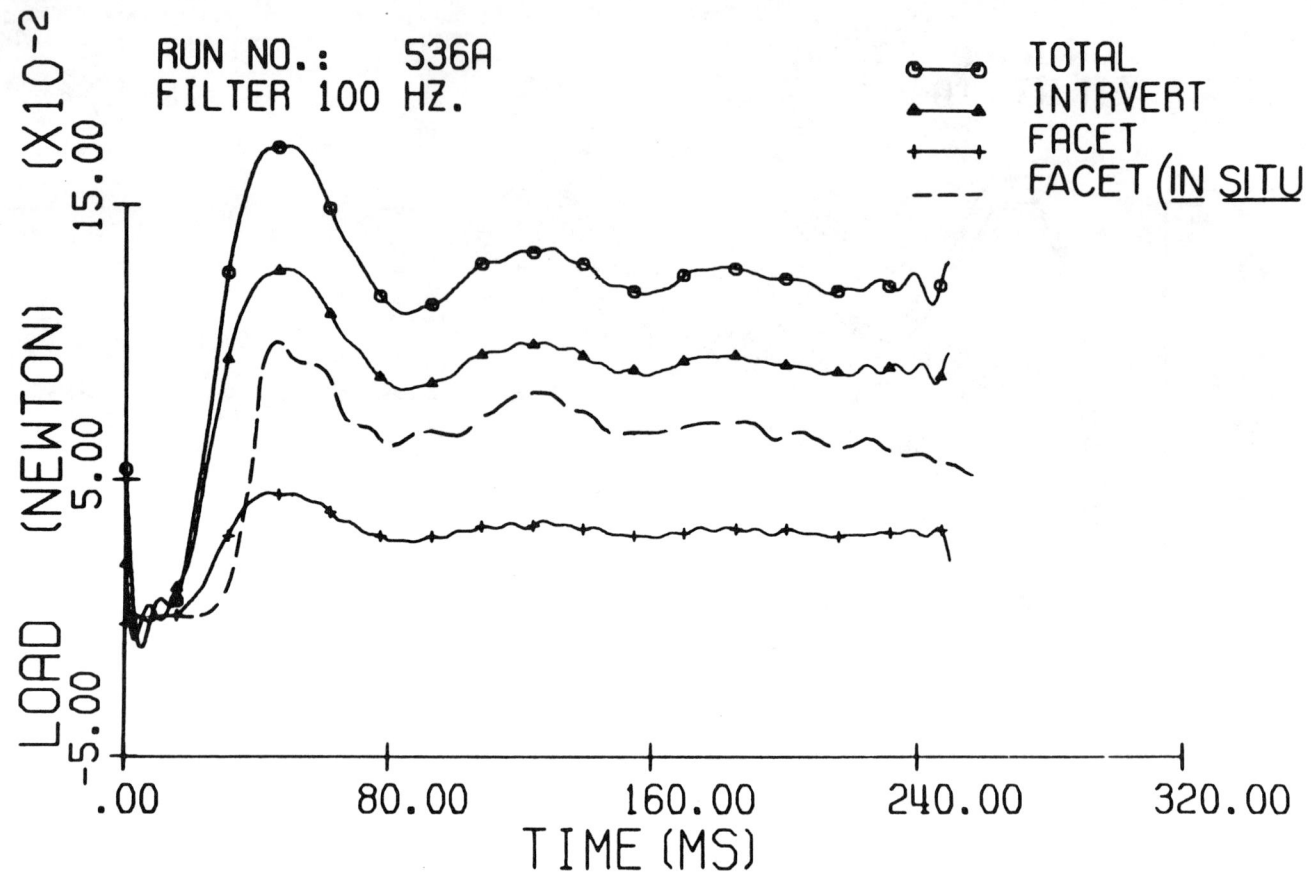

Fig. 15 - In vitro loads and in situ facet load of Run #536A

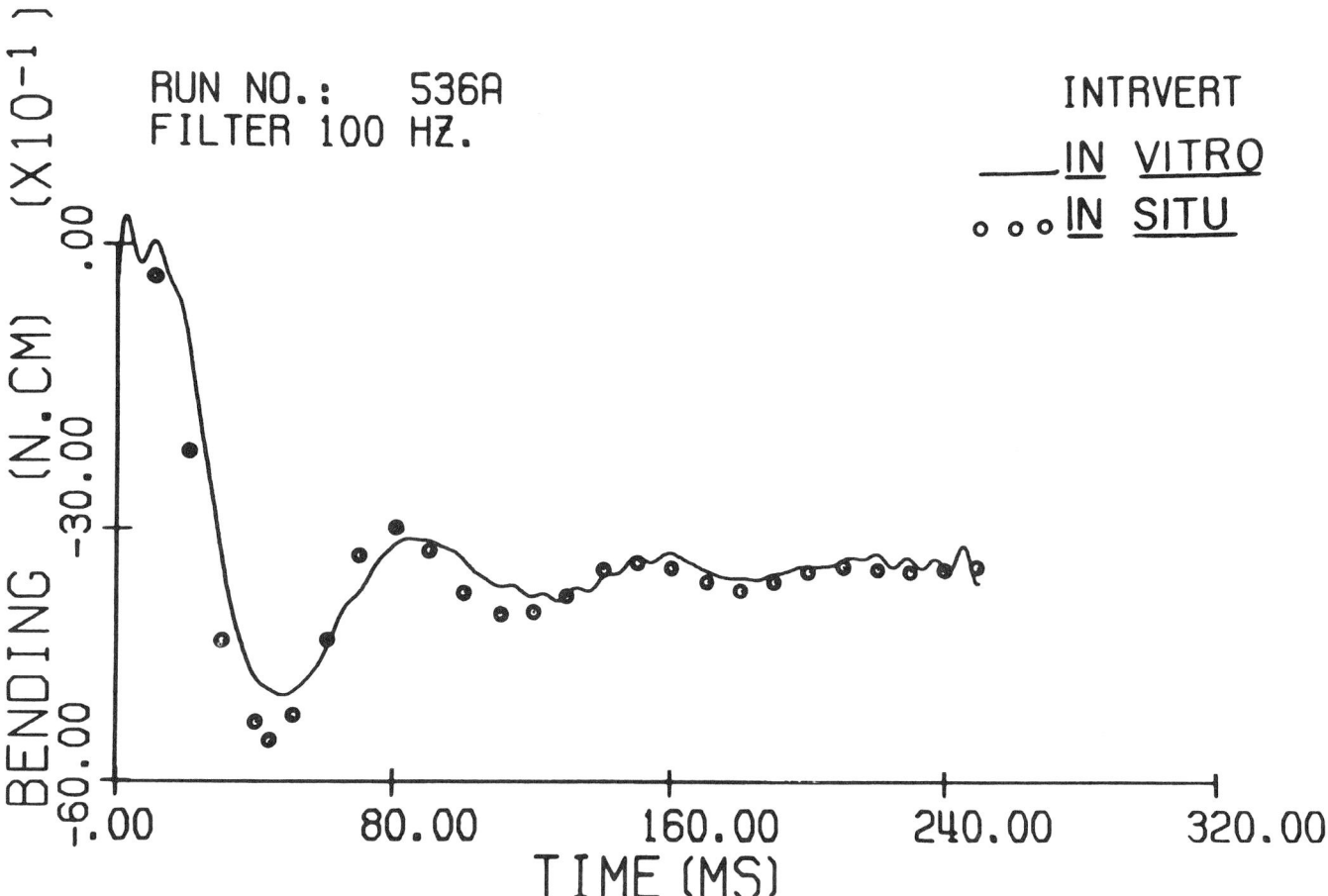

Fig. 16 - Comparison between in situ and in vitro intervertebral bending moment of Run #536A

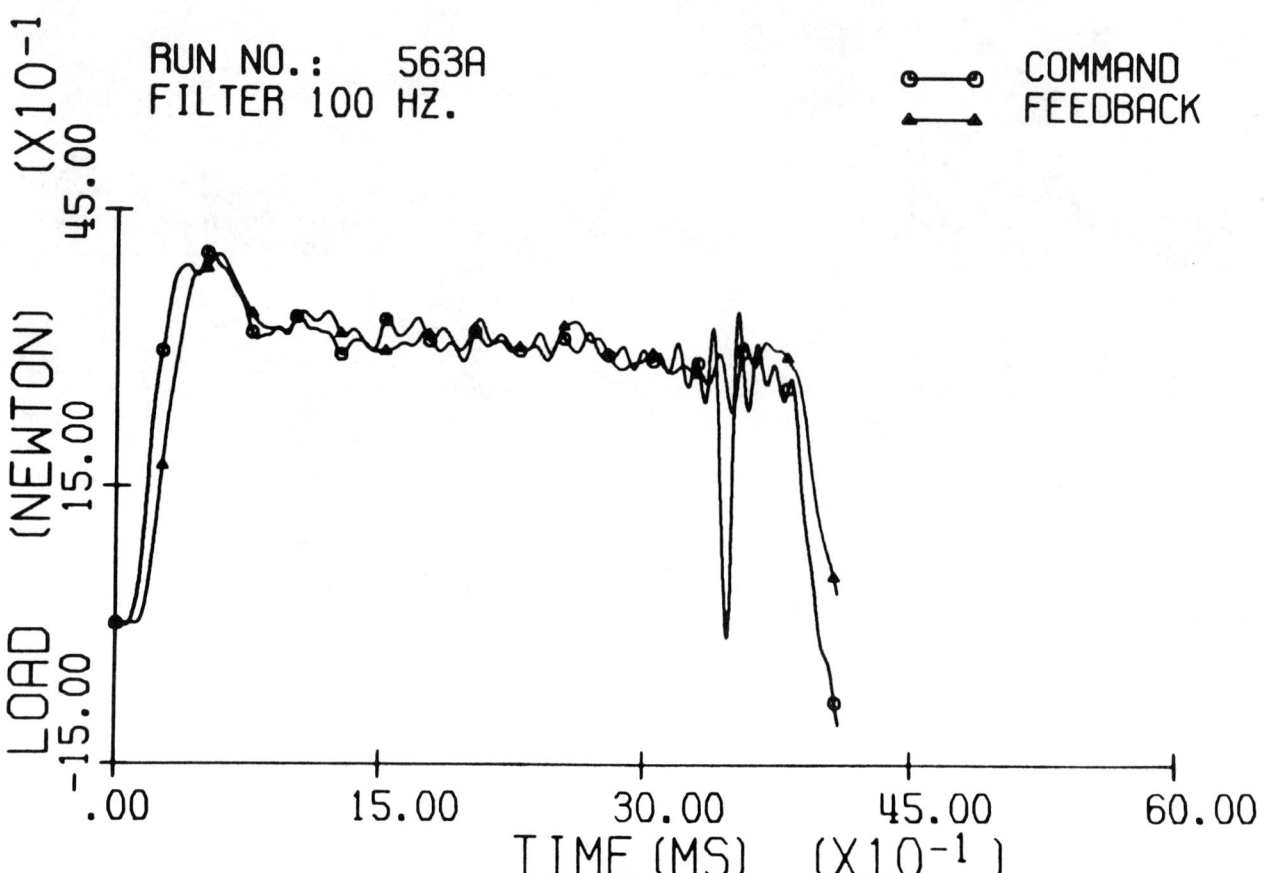

Fig. 17 - Comparison between in situ and in vitro intervertebral axial loads of Run #563A

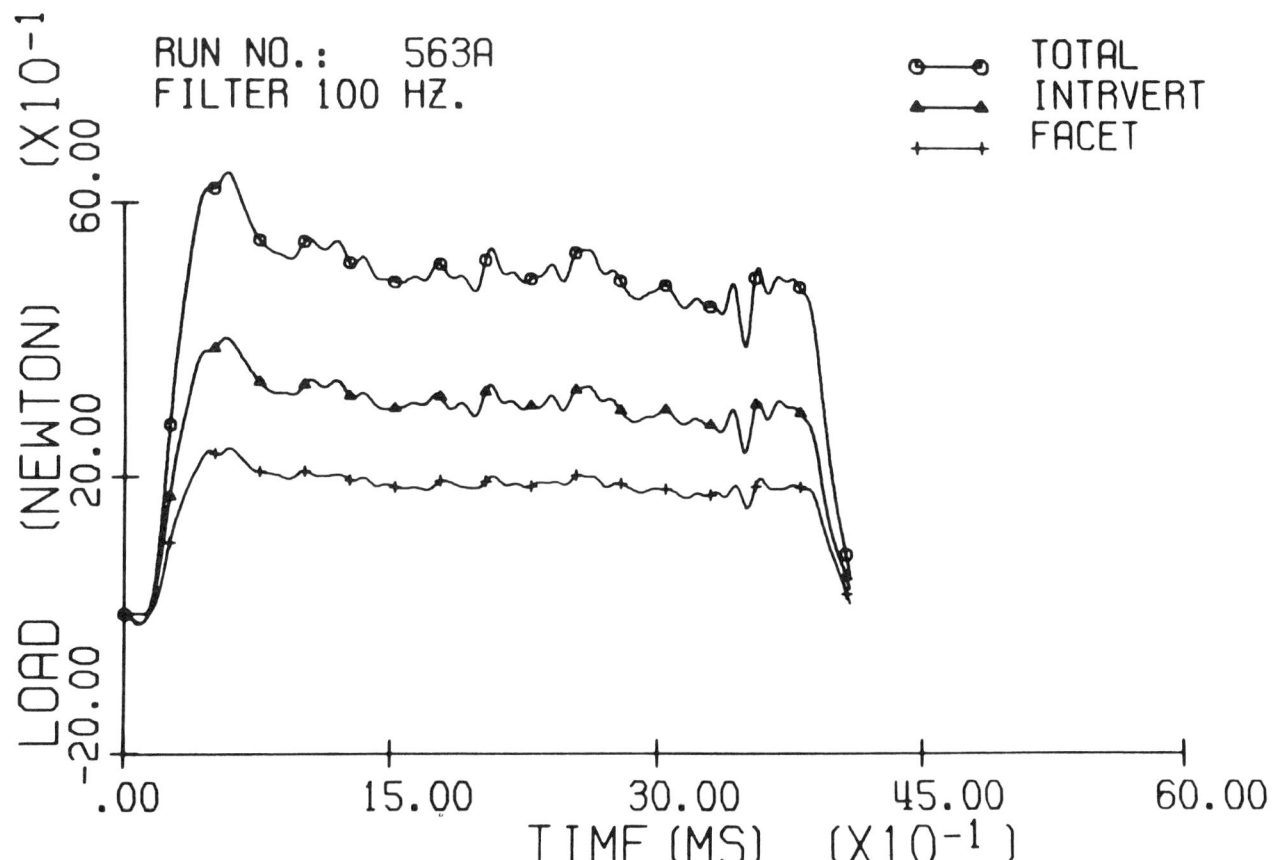

Fig. 18 - *In vitro* loads of Run #563A

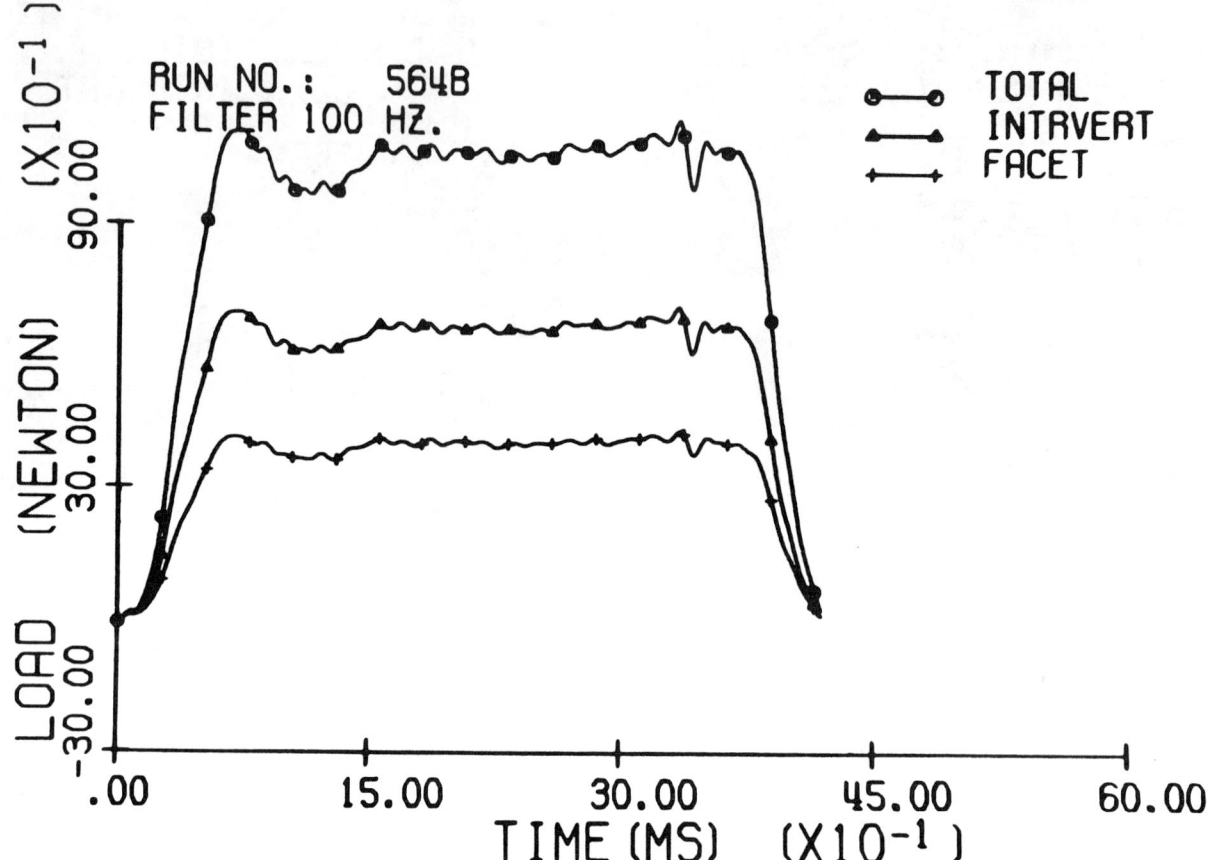

Fig. 19 - *In vitro* loads of Run #564A

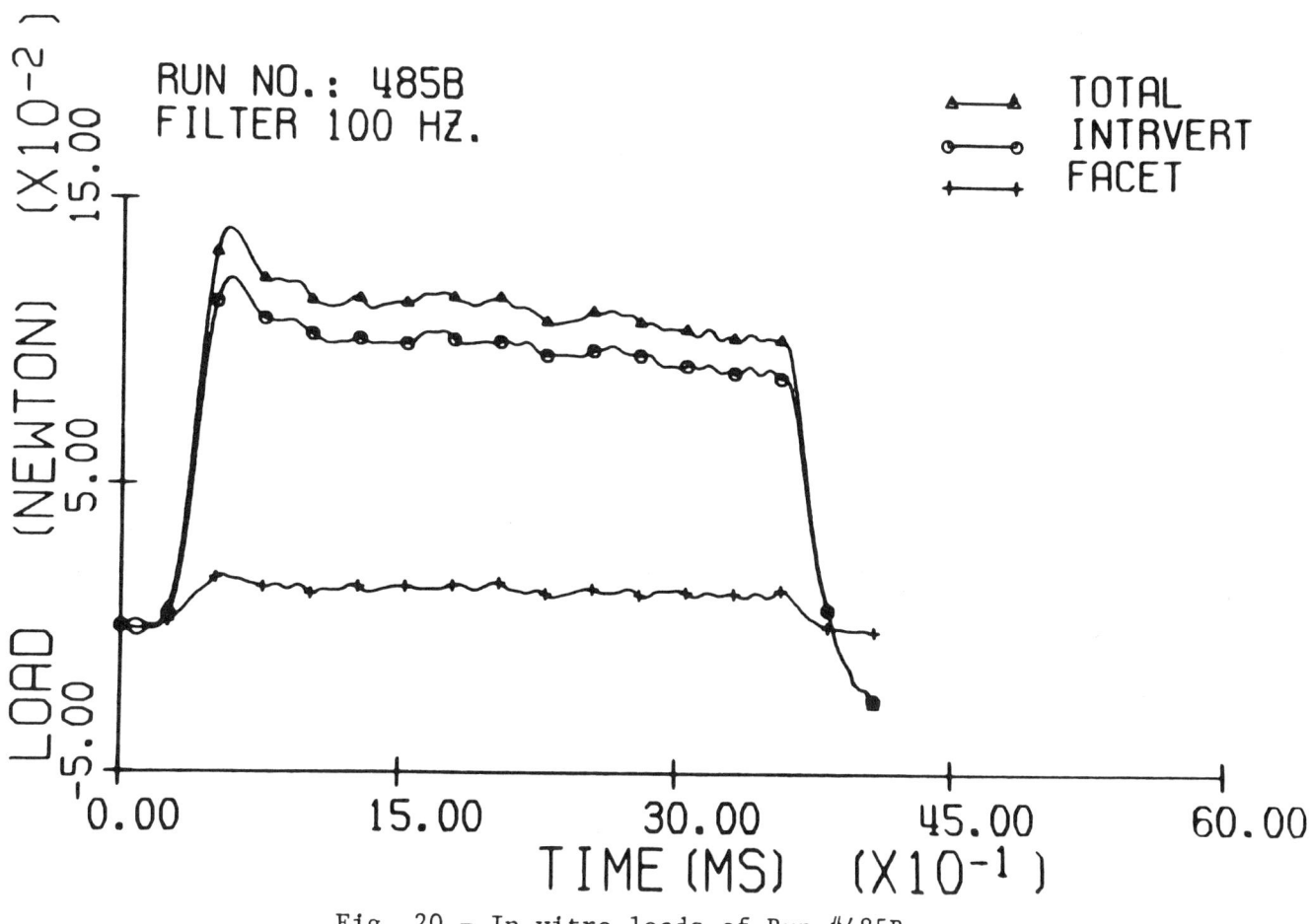

Fig. 20 - In vitro loads of Run #485B

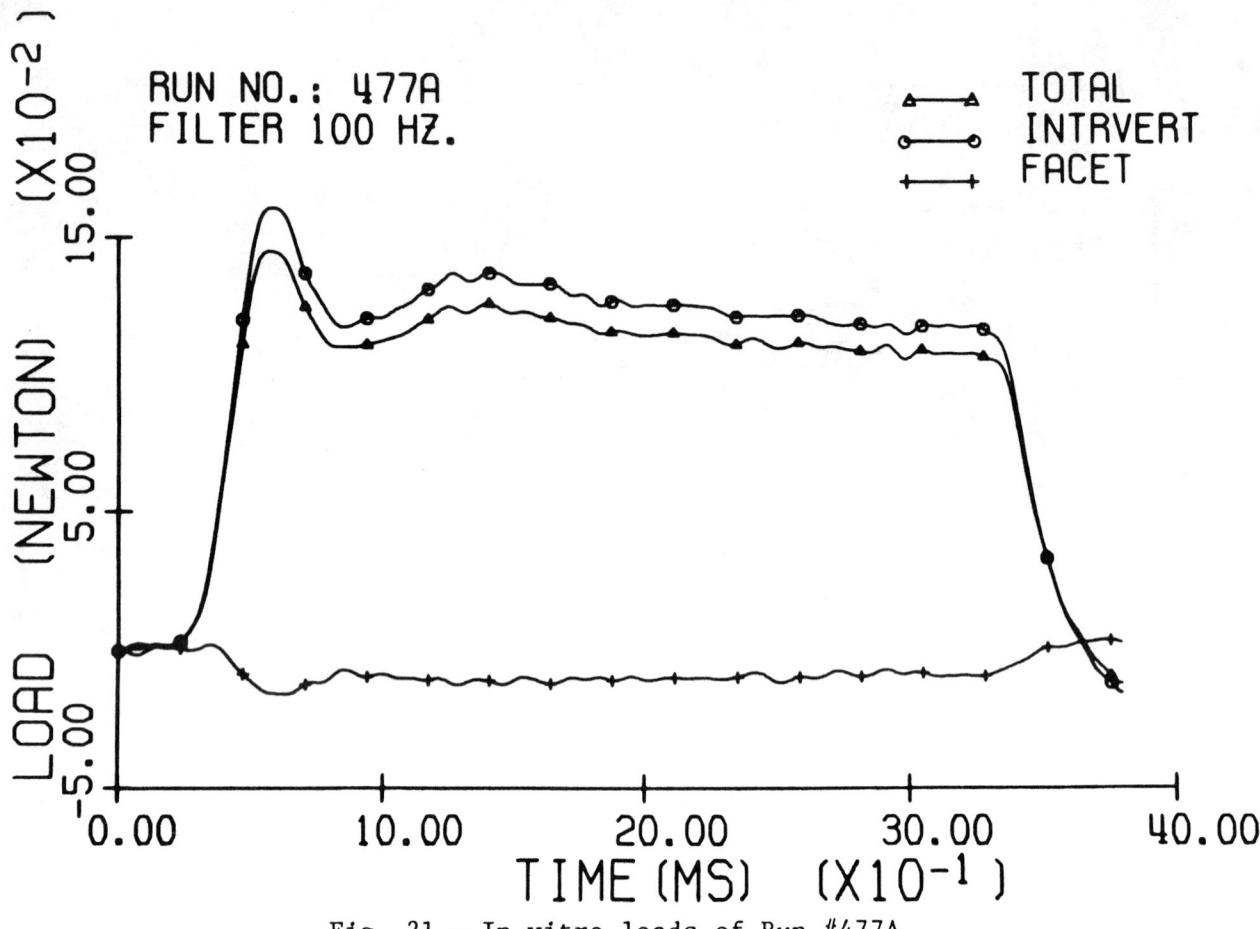

Fig. 21 - In vitro loads of Run #477A

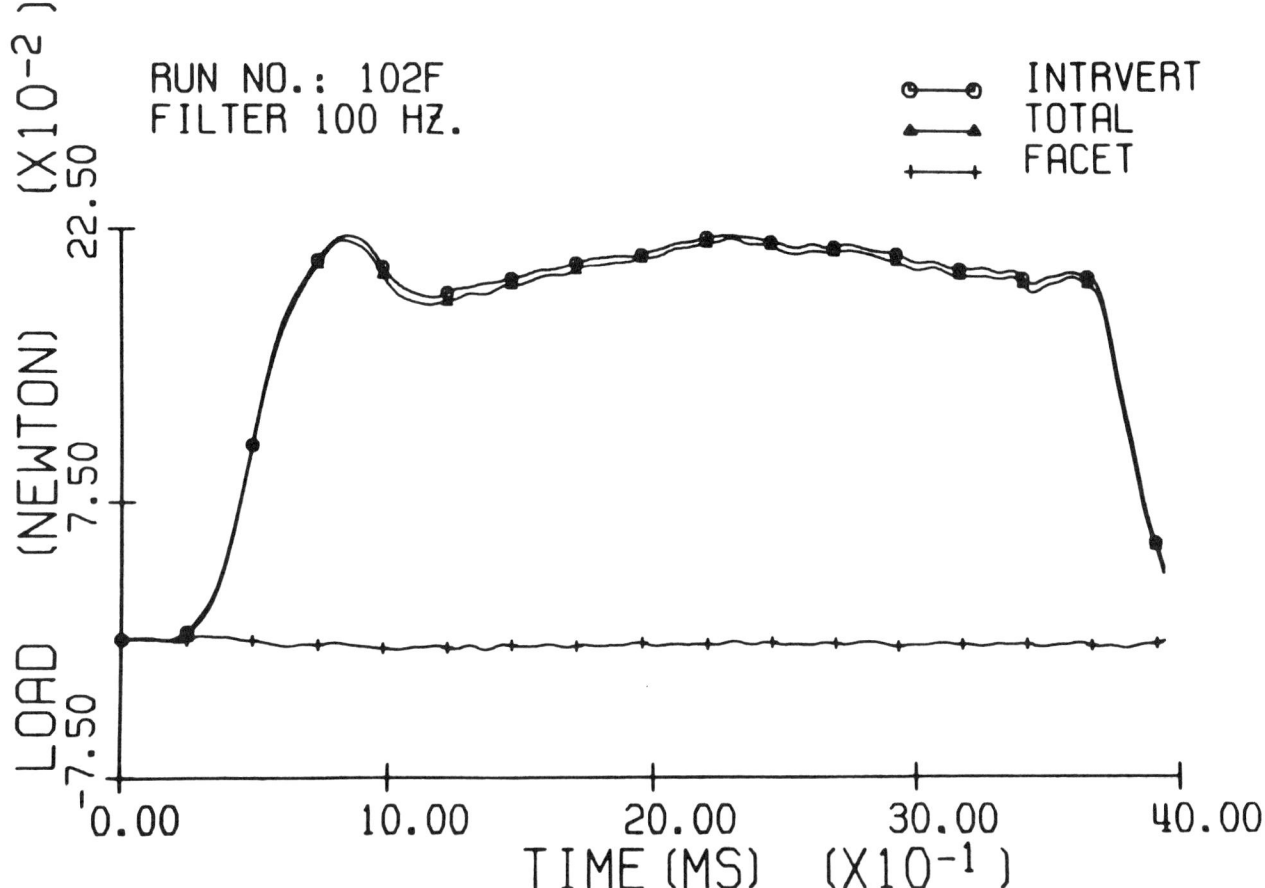

Fig. 22 - *In vitro* loads of Run #102F

which were measured experimentally. The unloading phenomenon which was reported by Prasad et al. (10) had been observed in two groups of tests, with one group only showing tensile facet loads of a magnitude in the range of 10% of the total load. More tests are needed to investigate the significance of this phenomenon.

ACKNOWLEDGMENTS

This research was supported in part by an NIH Grant No. GM20201-03 and by an NIH Career Development Award No. 5-K04-GM21145-05 (National Institute of General Medical Sciences).

The procedures used in this study conform to the code of ethics of the American Association of Physical Anthropologists and subscribed by the National Academy of Sciences National Research Board CHABA Committee.

REFERENCES

1. J. V. Basmajian, "Grant's Method of Anatomy," The Williams and Wilkins Company. Baltimore, p. 18, 1970.

2. H. Gray, "Gray's Anatomy." C. M. Goss, ed. Lea and Febiger, Philadelphia. 1973.

3. R. Fick, "Handbuch der Anatomie und Mechanik der Gelenke." Verlag Gustav Fischer, Jena. 1904.

4. H. Strasser, "Legrbuch d. Muskel und Gelenkmechanik." J. Springer. Berlin. 1913.

5. A. Nachemson, "Lumbar Interadiscal Pressure." Acta Orthop. Scand. Supp., Vol. 43. 1960.

6. A. Nachemson, "The Influence of Spinal Movements on the Lumbar Intradiscal Pressure and on the Tensile Stress in the Annulus Fibrosus." Acta Orthop. Scand. Vol. 33, p. 183. 1963.

7. L. E. Kazarian, D. D. Boyd and H. E. von Gierke, "The Dynamic Biomechanical Nature of Spinal Fractures and Articular Facet Derangement." AGARD Conference Proceedings No. 88 on 'Linear Acceleration of Impact Type.' AGARD-CP-88-71, Paper No. 19. (AD 737090). 1971.

8. L. E. Kazarian, "The Primate as a Model for Crash Injury." Proceedings of the 19th Stapp Car Crash Conference, pp. 931-963. 1975.

9. A. I. King, P. Prasad and C. L. Ewing, "Mechanism of Spinal Injury Due to Caudocephalad Acceleration." Orthopedic Clinics of North America. Vol. 6, pp. 19-31. 1975.

10. P. Prasad, A. I. King and C. L. Ewing, "The Role of Articular Facets During +G_z Acceleration." Journal of Applied Mechanics, Vol. 41, pp. 321-326. 1974.

11. P. Prasad, A. I. King, R. A. Denton and P. C. Begeman, "Intervertebral Force Transducer." Proceedings 10th International Conf. Med. Biol. Eng'r. Dresden, p. 137. 1973.

12. A. P. Vulcan, "Response of the Lower Vertebral Column and Caudocephalad Acceleration." Ph.D. Dissertation, Wayne State University. 1969.

13. P. Prasad, "Dynamic Response of the Spine During $+G_z$ Acceleration," Ph.D. Dissertation, Wayne State University, 1973.

14. L. M. Patrick, "Caudo-cephalad Static and Dynamic Injuries." Proceedings 5th Stapp Car Crash Conference. Univeristy of Minnesota, Minneapolis. 1962.

15. N. Hakim and A. I. King, "Programmed Replication of the 'In Situ' Loading Conditions During 'In Vitro' Testing of a Vertebral Column Segment." Journal of Biomechanics. (In press).

881331

Biomechanical Investigations fo the Human Thoracolumbar Spine

Narayan Yoganandan, Frank Pintar, Anthony Sances, Jr., Dennis Maiman and Joel Myklebust
Medical College of Wisconsin and V.A. Medical Center

Gerald Harris
Marquette University

Gautam Ray
Florida International University

ABSTRACT

In vitro biomechanical studies were conducted on fresh human cadaveric thoracolumbar spines to establish the limits of tolerance, explain the mechanism of failure, and investigate the effects of improvement in strength and stability of the injured column using Harrington distraction rods, Luque rods and modified Weiss springs. Quasistatic axial tensile loading on ligaments, compressive loads on vertebral bodies and intervertebral discs, and flexure and compression-flexion force vectors on ligamentous columns, intact torsos and injured spines were applied to delineate the biomechanical and functional patho-anatomic characteristics. Vertical drop tests were conducted with the Hybrid II manikin to predict the forces and accelerations on the vertebral column.

INTRODUCTION

The purpose of the human spinal column is to support and distribute the mechanical load. Although many factors contribute to dysfunction, finally, it is the ability of the structure to effectively withstand and transfer both static and dynamic loads (insult) that determines its integrity and mechanical stability. Insults to the spine occur routinely in vehicular accidents. A quantitative assessment of the functional changes secondary to the application of these adverse insults is an important step towards improved treatment of injury or improved design of vehicular environment. The study of isolated spinal components such as vertebral bodies, intervertebral discs and ligaments (micro-models) helps to delineate response of the structure without other variables such as spinal curvature. In addition, these studies can provide base line data to construct a detailed mathematical model of the spine [2]. On the other hand, experimental models employing the entire vertebral column (macro-models), isolated or intact, are essential to understand the mechanism of injury and the limits of tolerance under various injury producing force vectors [3]. The effects of stabilization can be best investigated using these models. In this study, we have determined the failure response and mechanism of injury to the human thoracolumbar spine using micro and macro-models.

* Numbers in parentheses designate references at end of paper.

ANATOMICAL OVERVIEW

The spinal column is composed of 24 individual vertebrae and 2 composite vertebrae, the sacrum and the coccyx. Of the 24 individual vertebrae, there are 7 cervical vertebrae in the neck, 12 thoracic vertebrae which support ribs, and 5 lumbar vertebrae (Figure 1). There are five fused vertebrae in the sacrum. The coccygeal vertebrae is formed by the fusion of four separate bodies.

The most prominent feature of the vertebra is the body located anteriorly, from which the vertebral arch extends posteriorly. This arch is composed of the pedicle which protrudes posteriorly from the body; the articular facets, having both superior and inferior portions; and the laminae, which come together posteriorly to close the arch. The vertebral foramen is thus formed, through which the spinal cord and its coverings pass. Extending laterally from the vertebral arch is the transverse process and extending posteriorly from the lamina is the spinous process. The vertebrae are interconnected anteriorly by the disc between each successive vertebral body, and posteriorly by a synovial joint between superior and inferior articular facets of adjacent vertebrae.

The thoracic vertebrae have the same prominent features as the lumbar vertebrae with a few exceptions. Since the thoracic vertebrae support the rib cage, there are facets for the ribs both on the vertebral body and on each transverse process. The vertebral bodies of the thoracic vertebrae are generally more heart-shaped and their spinous processes point in an inferior-posterior direction.

The spinal column is composed of 23 intervertebral discs. The discs, which together account for one-third to one-fifth of spinal column length, generally increase in geometry proceeding down the spinal column. Each intervertebral disc has two major components: the nucleus pulposus and annulus fibrosus. The nucleus pulposus is centrally located and is composed of a very fine network of fibers within a mucopolysaccharide gel. It has a very high water content, but is found to stiffen and degenerate with age. The nucleus is surrounded by the annulus fibrosus which is a composition of collagenous fibers arranged in helical bands. The fiber direction is such that it makes approximately a 30 degree angle to the disc plane, but in the adjacent bands the fibers run in the opposite direction to make a 120 degree angle with the fibers of the previous band.

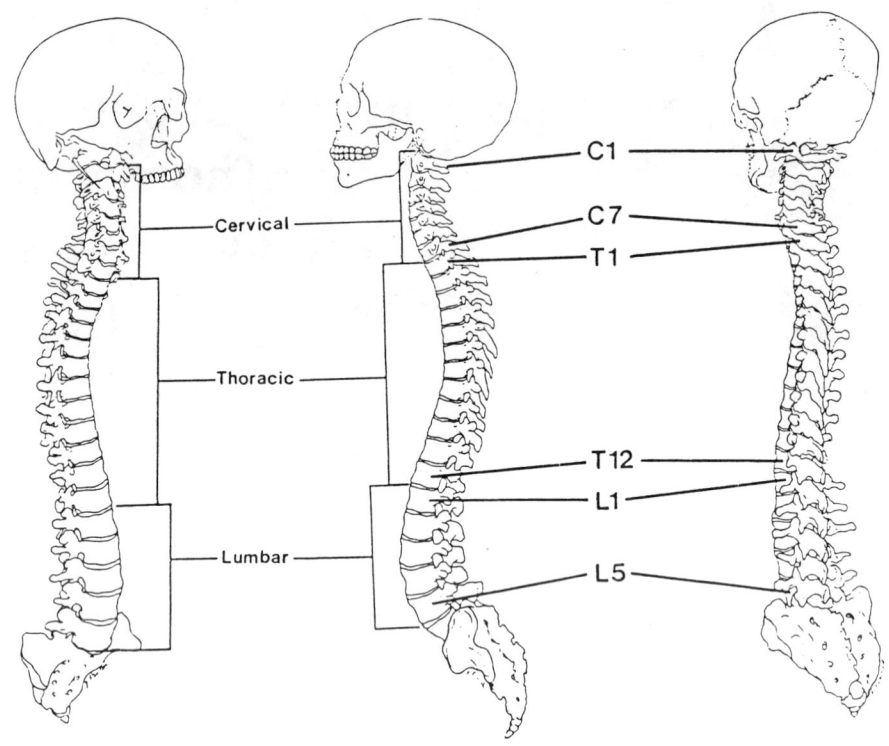

Figure 1 Antero-lateral (left), lateral (middle), and postero-lateral (right) views of the human spinal column. There are seven cervical, twelve thoracic, and five lumbar vertebrae, with 23 intervertebral disks.

Between the disc and the vertebral body lies a very thin (0.2 - 2 mm) cartilaginous endplate. The fibers of the annulus insert in the endplate to complete the intervertebral joint. Comparatively little is known about the cartilaginous endplate.

The anterior longitudinal ligament (ALL) and the posterior longitudinal ligament (PLL) are continuous ligaments that run the entire length of the spinal column. The ALL begins at the occiput and continues down to the sacrum covering one-quarter to one-third of the anterior circumference of the vertebral bodies and discs. The PLL begins at the second cervical vertebra and continues to the sacrum with fibers spreading out at the disc level and narrowing at the vertebral body. The PLL attaches to the posterior aspects of the vertebral body and disc just anterior to the spinal cord. Both PLL and ALL have a longitudinal (superior-inferior) fiber direction. The ligamentum flavum (LF) attaches to the superior and inferior surfaces of the laminae of adjacent vertebrae. It is generally V-shaped in cross section and is first seen at the C1 - C2 vertebral level and last seen at the L5 - S1 level. The interspinous ligament (ISL) joins the superior and inferior surfaces of the spinous processes of adjacent vertebrae. It begins at C2 - C3 and ends at L5 - S1 level. There has been some discussion as to the fiber direction of the ISL but Heylings [4] has shown by histological examination that the orientation is in the antero inferior to postero superior direction. The fibers of the ISL run into the fibers of the supraspinous ligament (SSL). The SSL begins at the most dorsal aspect of the C7 spinous process and is continuous into the lumbosacral region. The SSL is the continuation of the elastic ligamentum nuchae in the cervical spine. Researchers have reported the fibers to end any where between L3 and L5 spinal levels among the strong fibers of the lumbodorsal fascia [4,5]. The capsular ligaments (JC) attach to the vertebra adjacent to the facet joints. The fibers are perpendicular to the plane of the facets.

EXPERIMENTAL TECHNIQUE

SPECIMEN SELECTION - Micro-model studies were conducted on 58 fresh human male cadavers to determine the uniaxial failure, tensile strength of spinal ligaments, uniaxial compressive failure strength of vertebral bodies and intervertebral discs. Macro-model studies using 27 fresh human male cadavers were conducted to understand the mechanism of injury and effect of stabilization of intact and ligamentous thoracolumbar columns. Briefly, all specimens selected for the study were free of bone disease or metastatic cancer. Medical records were reviewed and plain radiographs were taken to select subjects without spinal disease or pre-existing fractures. The spinal column including the intact head and sacrum, was isolated carefully to avoid any soft tissue damage. All specimens were stored at -2 degrees Centigrade and thawed at room temperature 12 - 20 hours before testing. Handling and preserving in this manner is reported to have no effect on the mechanical properties of bone, disc and ligaments [6,7,8]. The isolated spinal columns, for micro-model studies (ligaments, vertebral bodies, and intervertebral discs), were further dissected to remove the ribs, the attached fat and muscles. The spinal column was then cut into manageable sections. Each ligament was isolated *in situ* or in its physiologic environment, i.e., it was not removed from its insertion zone [9]. At each disc level, the annulus and all other supporting structures except the ligament under study were transected using a disecting microscope. For isolated vertebral body compression studies, the vertebrae were isolated by transecting the ligamentous spine between bony segments. Soft tissues clinging to the vertebral body were carefully removed without damaging the endplates. The posterior elements were transected by sawing through the pedicles. Intervertebral disc experiments were carried out using the functional unit model, i.e., the vertebra-disc-vertebra structure was removed at different levels in the lumbar spine by transecting at the superior and inferior intervertebral disc level of the functional unit. Again, posterior elements were excluded. However, the anterior and posterior longitudinal ligaments remained intact. Isolated ligamentous columns from T3 - S1 levels were used for compression-flexion and flexure (three and four point bending) loading of the spine. Four intact cadaver torsos were also studied.

SPECIMEN MOUNTING

MICRO-MODEL STUDIES

Ligaments - The ligaments studied included ALL, PLL, LF, JC, ISL and SSL. The in situ preparation was mounted in a specially designed uni-axial tensile testing apparatus which allowed unobstructed movement for the ligament under test by firmly fixing the superior and inferior vertebral bodies (above and below the spinal level under test) with five Steinman pins. The top of the apparatus was attached to the piston of an electrohydraulic Material Testing System (MTS) device while the bottom was fixed to a rigid platform. The longitudinal axis of the ligament coincided with the central axis of the piston ensuring a pure tensile force.

Vertebral bodies - The isolated vertebral bodies were positioned between two cylinders with diameters significantly larger than the maximum exposed surface dimension of the structure. The vertebral bodies were compressed uniformly to 50% of original height using the piston of the MTS device.

Intervertebral discs - Both the superior and inferior vertebral bodies of the functional units were carefully embedded in polymethyl-methacrylate (PMMA) using a specially designed mold. Only one-third height of the vertebral body was fixed in PMMA. During mounting, care was taken to ensure that the plane at the mid height of the disc was parallel to the top and bottom surface of the prepared specimen. This was achieved by placing levels in two perpendicular directions on the top surface of the functional unit. ALL and PLL remained intact during the embedding operations.

MACRO-MODEL STUDIES

Ligamentous columns - The isolated spinal columns were fixed at the proximal and distal ends in 150 mm diameter aluminum rings using Steinman pins and blocked with PMMA reinforced with wire. The distal end of the preparation was then clamped firmly to the frame of the MTS device. The proximal end of the column was attached to the MTS piston to apply axial loading. The specimens were oriented at 15 degrees flexion.

In flexion experiments (three and four point bending tests), 20 mm diameter greased, stainless steel rods, were inserted through the neural foramina at the cephalad and caudad ends of the spinal column. These rods were then placed on a specially designed apparatus which permitted full movement of the spine to simulate simply supported ends for flexure loading.

To study the effect of improvement in the strength and stability of the spine, Harrington distraction rods (HR), Luque rods (LR) and modified Weiss springs (MWS) were used. After initial failure, the specimens were removed from the testing device and MWS were then inserted into the lamina two levels above and below the fractured segment. Then the specimens were repositioned beneath the piston of the MTS. Next, HR were placed three levels above and below the fractured level, and the test was repeated. Finally, the specimens were tested with 4.75 mm prebent LR segmentally wired using bilateral 18 gauge wire three levels above and below the fracture level. These three itechniques are standard surgical procedures. The devices were tested in the order described above (MWS, HR and LR) because preliminary studies indicated that failure of HR and LR induced comminuted lamina fractures which would not permit a proper placement of MWS for testing.

Intact Torsos - Intact cadavers were seated on a platform mounted to the MTS actuator device and fixed at the pelvis with belts. Lateral thoracic plates were used to restrain the rotation of the specimen. The specimens were preflexed with the upper thoracic vertebrae 50 - 100 mm anterior to the pelvis with an angle of 15 degrees to the horizontal plane. Axial forces were applied through the MTS piston to the T2 - T3 region using a 150 x 150 mm square plate.

Manikin Studies - Studies were conducted with a 50th percentile Hybrid II anthropometric manikin. The manikin was instrumented with a triaxial accelerometer in the region of the lumbar spine. The z-axis (principal direction) coincided with the superior-inferior direction, and x and y axes were along the lateral and antero-posterior directions, respectively. A Denton multi-axis force plate was used to record the axial and shear forces. The anthropomorphic manikin was dropped vertically from a height of 400 mm onto the force plate so that the buttocks of the Hybrid II contacted the surface. Three experiments were conducted. In the first two experiments, the manikin was positioned such that the buttocks of the manikin landed on the force plate vertically. In the third experiment, the dorsal aspect of the buttocks of the manikin contacted the force plate. These studies were conducted to simulate a direct vertical fall and a fall on the dorsal aspect.of the structure.

TESTING PROCEDURE - Before the start of loading geometrical data such as intervertebral disc height were measured using vernier calipers and x-rays were taken in both micro-model and macro-model studies. The testing was performed at a constant displacement rate of 2.5 mm/s. Failure in all the specimens was defined as the point on the mechanical response at which an increasing deformation resulted in a decreasing force. This coincided in ligamentous column compression-flexion load experiments with a wedge fracture of the most stressed vertebral body and disruption of posterior elements. In flexure load experiments on the thoracolumbar column the above definition of failure coincided with the disruption of posterior elements followed by minimal wedging of the bone. Immediately after failure, roentgenograms were taken with the specimen still experiencing the external load to determine the Cobb angles. Failure in the instrumented spines (MWS, HR, LR) was defined as hook extrusion or bending of the specimen to the appropriate initial fracture angle as estimated from a transparent grid incorporating angular markings. The actual angles were determined radiographically.

DATA COLLECTION - The loading head of the MTS device included a load washer (Kistler Model 9031) and a displacement transducer for load and deformation measurements, respectively. The applied load and deformations were recorded as a function of time on a digital oscilloscope (Norland Model 3001) capable of sampling at 1 µs, and a 18-channel visicorder (Honeywell Model 1858) with a frequency response of 2 kHz. The data were then transferred to a VAX 8600 computer for further analysis.

Fracture angles in the ligamentous column (macro-model) experiments were calculated radiographically using the Cobb method. Maximal bending moments in the compression-flexion loadings were calculated as the product of the applied load and the maximum eccentricity; the latter was measured as the distance from the fractured vertebral body to a vertical line dropped from the most cephalad vertebral body. In functional unit experiments intervertebral disc bulges were also recorded as a function of time using preloaded potentiometers placed at the outer periphery of the disc at its mid height.

In manikin experiments, data was collected using a modular data acquisition system (Trans Era MDAS model #7000) and a system of specially designed preamplifiers and filters. Class 1000 filtering (SAE J2116) at a sampling rate of 5 kHz was used. The sampled signals included the triaxial acceleration, and the vertical and shear force histories.

RESULTS AND DISCUSSION

MICRO-MODEL STUDIES

Ligaments - Typical force-elongation curves for the six ligaments tested (ALL, PLL, JC, LF, ISL, SSL) are illustrated in Figure 2. In general, the patterns of the load-deflection response were similar for a particular type of ligament (for example, ALL) at all levels of the thoracolumbar column. However, the magnitudes of the biomechanical parameters were different. Therefore, the entire spinal column data was grouped into three regions: upper thoracic (T1 - T6), lower thoracic (T6 - T12), and lumbar (T12 - S1). Table 1 includes the biomechanical data based on this classification. The force-elongation curves for all the ligaments with the exception of JC were non-linear and had a single peak. JC exhibited two peaks one followed by the other after 2 - 8 mm of additional extension. The magnitude of the axial tension was almost the same for these two peaks emphasizing purely uni-axial nature of the insult and the combined structural behavior of the individual capsules bilaterally.

From the force-deflection behavior, the maximum stiffness of the structure was also computed (Table 1). The mean maximum tensile forces for all the ligaments with the exception of PLL indicated an increase from cranial to caudal direction (T1 - S1). This agrees with published data [8,10]. ALL was the strongest ligament in resisting the tensile load and the ISL was the most flexible ligament (stiffness = 1.3 N/mm). The less dense structure of the ISL may be the cause for the least magnitude of its stiffness. Tensile deformations at failure indicated that the ligaments were more distensible in the lumbar region. In addition, the ligaments furthest away from the geometric center of the column (ALL and SSL) demonstrated greater

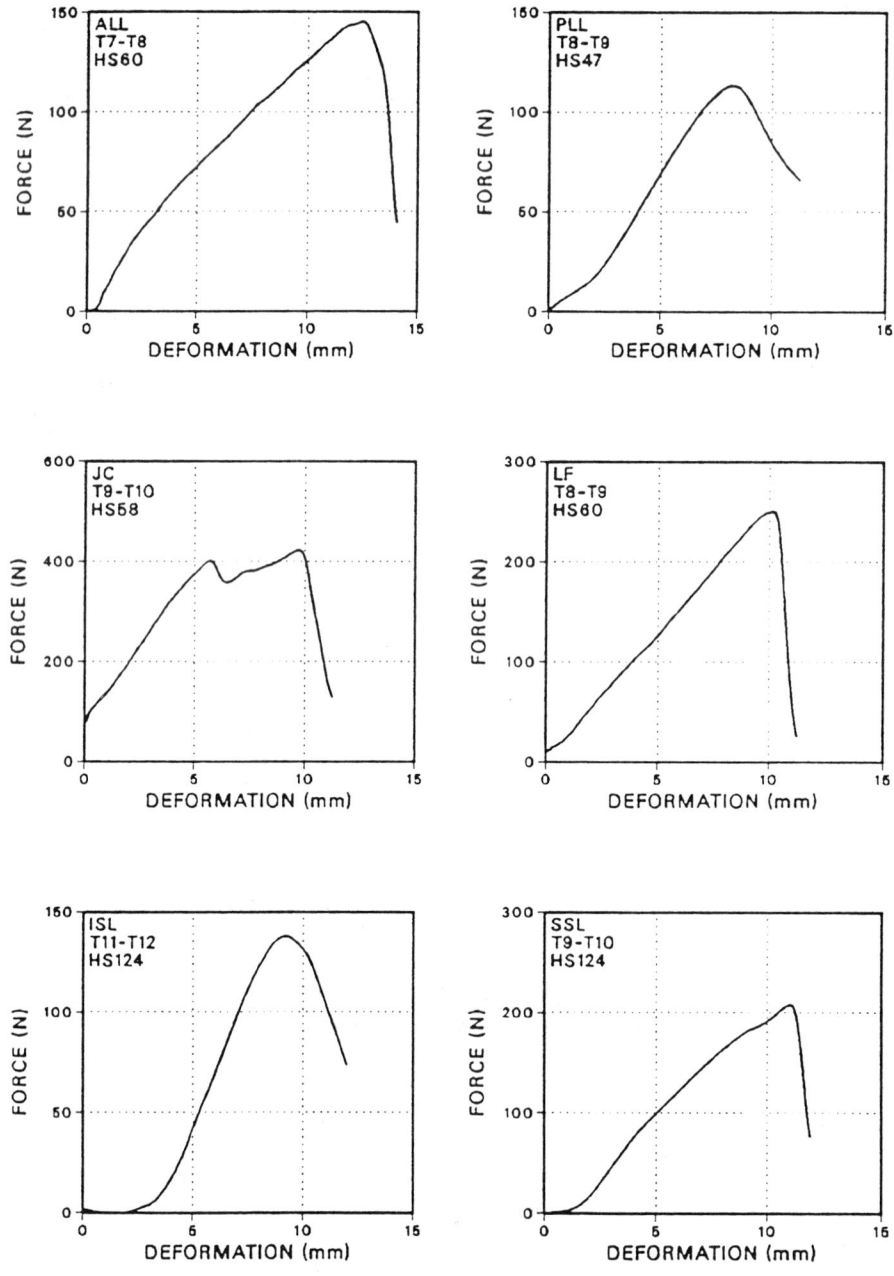

Figure 2   Representative force-deformation curves for thoracolumbar ligaments.

TABLE 1
Biomechanical parameters of human thoracolumbar spinal ligaments.
(Standard deviations are shown in parentheses).

Region	Ligament	n	Force (N)	Deformation (mm)	Energy (J)	Stiffness (N/mm)
UPPER THORACIC (T1-T6)	ALL	15	176 (74)	7.9 (3.9)	1.51 (1.33)	21.7 (9.4)
	PLL	16	91 (47)	4.1 (3.3)	0.26 (0.29)	26.5 (11.4)
	LF	14	150 (51)	7.2 (3.5)	0.79 (0.52)	24.6 (8.1)
	JC	19	196 (112)	6.8 (3.1)	0.82 (0.53)	28.4 (11.0)
	ISL	15	56 (39)	8.1 (5.5)	0.34 (0.35)	8.2 (6.9)
	SSL	7	189 (138)	12.3 (5.8)	1.69 (1.41)	20.0 (9.6)
LOWER THORACIC (T6-T12)	ALL	19	342 (157)	12.8 (4.7)	3.00 (2.05)	23.6 (10.7)
	PLL	17	95 (74)	4.9 (2.3)	0.42 (0.42)	24.9 (16.7)
	LF	21	235 (76)	9.2 (3.2)	1.33 (0.55)	32.6 (14.8)
	JC	21	218 (117)	6.9 (3.7)	1.24 (1.14)	34.4 (12.6)
	ISL	17	68 (58)	6.4 (4.6)	0.35 (0.38)	9.5 (6.1)
	SSL	18	227 (142)	14.6 (8.3)	2.23 (2.03)	22.6 (12.6)
LUMBAR (T12-S1)	AAL	19	444 (267)	14.9 (9.6)	4.53 (4.14)	33.1 (18.6)
	PLL	15	79 (62)	5.0 (3.5)	0.36 (0.40)	20.0 (13.8)
	LF	18	250 (118)	10.8 (3.9)	2.15 (1.49)	26.2 (8.7)
	JC	19	317 (96)	10.7 (3.7)	2.71 (1.59)	30.5 (11.0)
	ISL	15	128 (59)	13.7 (8.6)	1.27 (1.07)	1.3 (0.6)
	SSL	19	314 (223)	23.0 (9.5)	4.66 (3.96)	24.8 (14.2)

deformations to failure. PLL consistently had a lesser magnitude of failure elongation. Further, PLL, JC, and LF, the ligaments that are close to the geometric center indicated generally a higher trend in the stiffness than the ligaments which are further away (ALL, SSL, ISL).

Vertebral Bodies - Figure 3 includes typical axial force-compression characteristics of lower thoracic (T11 - T12), and lumbar (L2 - L5) vertebral bodies. The mechanical response exhibited non-linear and sigmoidal characteristics, representative of any biological material [11]. From the initial geometrical measurements (specimen height was obtained as an average of the four heights measured in the anterior, posterior and bilateral locations, and the cross sectional area was computed using the dimensions in the exposed superior and inferior transverse surfaces of the vertebral body with the assumption that the structure geometry is an ellipse), stress and strain at failure was also computed. Table 2 includes a summary of the biomechanical parameters of the thoracic and lumbar vertebral bodies grouped into upper thoracic (T1 - T6), lower thoracic (T7 - T12) and lumbar (L1 - L5) levels. These results are in general agreement with the values reported in literature [12-14]. Failure compressive loads cited by Yamada are slightly higher [14]. The discrepancy may be due to the population and method of testing [14].

Intervertebral Discs - Axial compressive force-deflection responses of the inter-vertebral discs, which were tested by including the adjacent vertebral bodies in the cranial and caudal directions (functional units), were also non-linear and sigmoidal. Nine functional units in the lumbar region were studied. Five of these samples had degenerated discs while the remaining four were normal. The degeneration levels were determined based on the macroscopic appearance of the disc according to the criteria reported in literature [15]. Normal discs had higher load carrying capacity (failure load = 11.03 ± 1.4 kN), higher energy absorption (energy to ultimate failure = 18 ± 3.4 J), and higher stiffness (maximum stiffness = 2850 ± 293 N/mm), compared to degenerated specimens (load = 5.3 ± 0.29 kN, energy = 5.8 ± 1.6 J, and stiffness = 1642 ± 447 N/mm). However, the compressive deformations at failure were not significantly different for these two types of specimens (normal disc = 4.0 mm, degenerated disc = 3.6 mm) although the failure loads were considerably lower for degenerated specimens. Therefore, from this preliminary analysis it appears logical to hypothesize that the intervertebral joint is a deformation sensitive structure, i.e., failure occurs when the structure experiences a deformation threshold. Therefore, to prevent the structure from experiencing trauma, it may be appropriate to limit the insult so that the deformations do not exceed its critical threshold.

MACRO-MODEL STUDIES

Flexure Loading - In three-point loading tests, failure was concentrated at the center of the spine, the region of maximum flexural moment. In four-point bending tests, failure generally occurred in the region of the spine between the two loading points where the specimen experienced a pure flexure moment without any accompanying shear force. However, in one experiment failure occurred near the support which may be due to an improper restraint on the fixation system. An interesting observation from these flexure loading experiments was that instability resulted from the tear of the posterior elements associated with very minimal anterior compression of the vertebral bodies. This type of trauma is not often seen clinically. Table 3 includes a brief summary of the maximum load, displacement, and bending moments from the three and four point bending experiments.

Compression-Flexion Loading - The principal advantage of flexure loading of the spinal column is that the initial failure can be controlled to occur in the thoracolumbar junction as most fractures of the thoracic and lumbar vertebrae are commonly seen between T10 and L2 [16]. However, these experiments preclude axial compressive forces on the thoracolumbar column which are primarily responsible for vertebral wedging. Therefore, it is necessary to use compression-flexion as the injury producing load vector to induce clinically relevant trauma to the spine. In these experiments, as expected, at the level of high moment the spinal column fractured resulting in wedging followed by the tear of the posterior ligaments depending on the level of axial load and degree of flexion moment. In two specimens, out-of-plane buckling was noticed. Table 4 summarizes the biomechanical data on these studies.

Table 5 compares the data between the intact (non-instrumented) spine and spines instrumented with MWS, HR and LR. When the isolated and intact cadavers were considered together, failure loads were higher in the MWS trials than in the HR trials at a significance level of $p<0.10$. The differences in failure load between the two was more significant in the intact spines ($p<0.01$) than in the isolated ligamentous columns ($p<0.15$). Failure loads for LR were not statistically different than those of initial injuries or MWS. However, the failure angles for the LR were lower than the initial injuries and MWS ($p<0.01$).

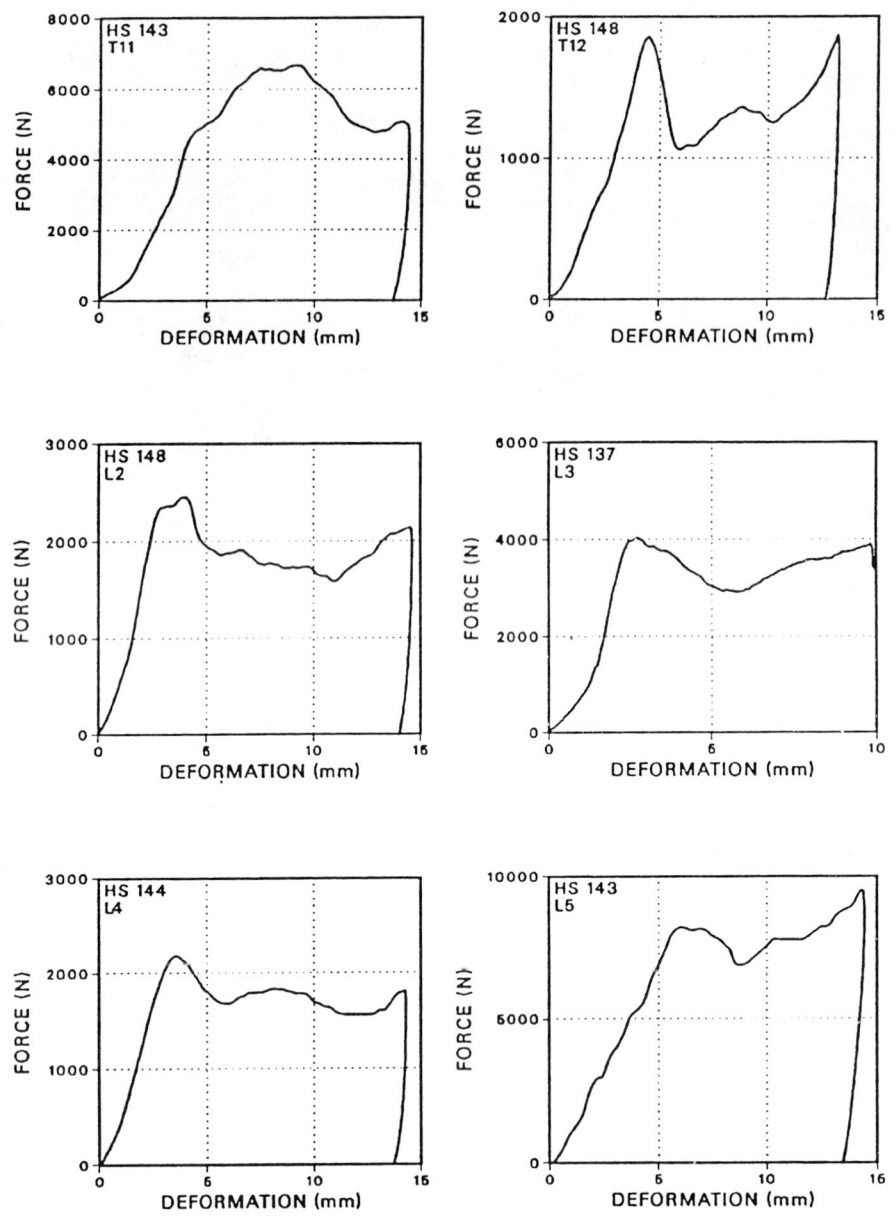

Figure 3   Representative compressive force-deflection characteristics of thoracolumbar vertebral bodies.

TABLE 2
Biomechanical vertebral body parameters at different regions of the spine.
(Standard deviations are shown in parentheses).

Spinal Region	n	Initial Height (mm)	Cross Sectional Area (Sq. mm)	Force at Failure (N)	Deformation at Failure (mm)	Stress at Failure (MPa)	Strain at Failure (%)
Thoracic (T1-T6)	12	19.0 (1.5)	667.8 (179.0)	2642 (555)	6.0 (1.8)	4.2 (2.7)	30.8 (9.0)
Thoracic (T7-T12)	15	20.9 (3.0)	1060.7 (240.3)	3264 (1211)	4.9 (1.7)	3.2 (1.4)	23.4 (9.5)
Lumbar (L1-L5)	11	27.7 (3.9)	1599.4 (365.9)	4590 (2061)	6.9 (3.2)	2.8 (1.4)	24.4 (9.5)

TABLE 3
Flexure loading on the human thoracolumbar spine.

Specimen #	Spinal Level	Length (cm)	Failure Level	Failure Load (N)	Failure Moment (cm)	Eccentricity (Nm)
Three-point bending
TB-64	T2-L3	26.0	T8	1681	12.0	109
TB-66	T3-L2	30.5	T10	2170	15.0	60
TB-70	T8-L3	22.0	T11	1432	9.0	76
Four-point bending
FB-37	T12-L5	30.0	L2	4893	5.0	245
FB-68	T4-L4	30.0	T8	1712	5.0	85
FB-69	T10-L2	33.0	T10	1544	5.0	77

TABLE 4
Compression-flexion loading on the human thoracolumbar spine.

Specimen #	Spinal Level	Length (cm)	Failure Level	Failure Load (N)	Eccentricity (cm)	Failure Moment (Nm)
IL-10	T3-L5	30.5	L1	1730	8.5	148
IL-11	T3-L5	31.0	T12	1113	8.5	95
IL-12	T2-L5	33.0	T9	967	8.0	78
IL-13	T3-L5	31.0	T7	2220	6.0	133
IL-16	T2-L5	30.5	T11	1668	8.0	133
IL-17	T2-L5	30.5	T9	801	6.5	52
IL-18	T4-L5	33.0	T12	4444	8.0	289
IL-27	C2-L5	38.0	T7	556	11.5	64
IL-28	C2-L5	40.0	T12	801	13.0	104
IL-29	T2-L5	33.0	T12	1330	10.5	134
IL-31	T3-L5	30.5	T10	2891	9.0	260
IL-32	T3-L5	34.0	T9	2000	9.0	180
IL-33	T3-L5	32.0	T11	1775	9.5	169
IL-38	T3-L5	34.3	T11	4220	7.0	295
IL-72	T3-L5	33.0	T9	2224	6.0	133
IL-74	T3-L5	34.0	T7	2927	6.0	176
IL-77	T6-L5	22.0	T12	5560	5.0	278
IL-78	T6-L5	24.0	T12	5275	5.5	290

TABLE 5
Comparison of fixation devices.
(Values in parentheses indicate the respective percentages from intact).

Description	Ligamentous Column Load (N)	Moment (Nm)	Cobb angle (deg)	Intact Torso Load (N)	Moment (Nm)	Cobb angle (deg)
Intact	1886	165	34.7	1737	188	32.8
MW	1290 (68%)	118 (71%)	31.0 (89%)	870 (50%)	74 (39%)	26.2 (80%)
HR	1112 (59%)	65 (39%)	17.6 (51%)	290 (17%)	18 (10%)	15.0 (46%)
LR	1490 (79%)	135 (82%)	26.1 (75%)	935 (54%)	79 (42%)	12.0 (37%)

The maximum bending moments for the LR and MWS were similar for the intact as well for the ligamentous column experiments. However, they were higher compared to the HR instrumented spines (p<0.01).

In our institutional experience, MWS has a failure rate of approximately 6% including hook slippage and failure to maintain the correction of deformity. Failure rate for HR has been about 15%, primarily related to hook extrusion. A high degree of spinal stability is produced by segmental spinal stabilization devices like LR. However, the potential for spinal cord or nerve root injury caused by placement of wires into the narrow canal of the thoracic spine must be given proper consideration [17,18]. Failures of stabilization and broken wires may injure the spinal cord resulting in neurologic deficit.

MWS was found to be biomechanically equal to or even superior to relatively more rigid devices such as HR for improving spinal stability. Other factors may also make the stiffened spring an optimal device for trauma induced by flexion-compression loading.

<u>Manikin Studies</u> - Figure 4 illustrates the resultant force history at the impact site and shows the corresponding resultant acceleration at the lumbar spine of the manikin. The results of the three drop experiments conducted are included in Table 6.

TABLE 6: Peak resultant force at the impact site and peak resultant acceleration at the lumbar region of the Hybrid II manikin for a 400 mm vertical drop.

RUN#	Resultant Force (N)	Resultant Acceleration (G)
1	9391.7	21.48
2	9236.5	23.43
3	11,444.7	29.20

In the first two experiments, the off-axis forces (shear force) and accelerations (anteroposterior and lateral directions) were an order of magnitude smaller than the data in the principal direction (vertical force and vertical acceleration). However, in the third test, the y accelerations were larger in magnitude than the x and z components. This was due to the orientation of the manikin during impact. The vertical force (z axis) on the force plate was again an order of magnitude greater than the shear force (y axis).

SUMMARY

The hallmark of mechanical insult to the human body is the application of force on the tissue causing rupture, weakening, tear or fracture. With particular emphasis to motor vehicle induced trauma, it is essential to quantify the thresholds of tolerance and understand the mechanism of load transfer and injury to the human spine. This will facilitate better treatment of the injured patient and it may assist the safety engineer in an improved design of the vehicular environment. In this investigation, we have studied the response of the human thoracolumbar spine subjected to mechanical insults.

Studies were conducted on isolated thoracolumbar components, ligamentous columns, and intact torsos. Among the six major ligaments, ALL was the strongest and PLL was the weakest structure. The most distensible ligaments were furthest away from the center of the spinal column. In general, all ligaments demonstrated an increase in strength from upper thoracic to lower lumbar levels. Similar behavior was observed in the physical and mechanical properties of vertebral bodies. Normal intervertebral discs tested using functional unit models indicated a higher load carrying capacity than degenerated specimens. However, the ultimate failure deformations did not exhibit this behavior. Although a study of these individual

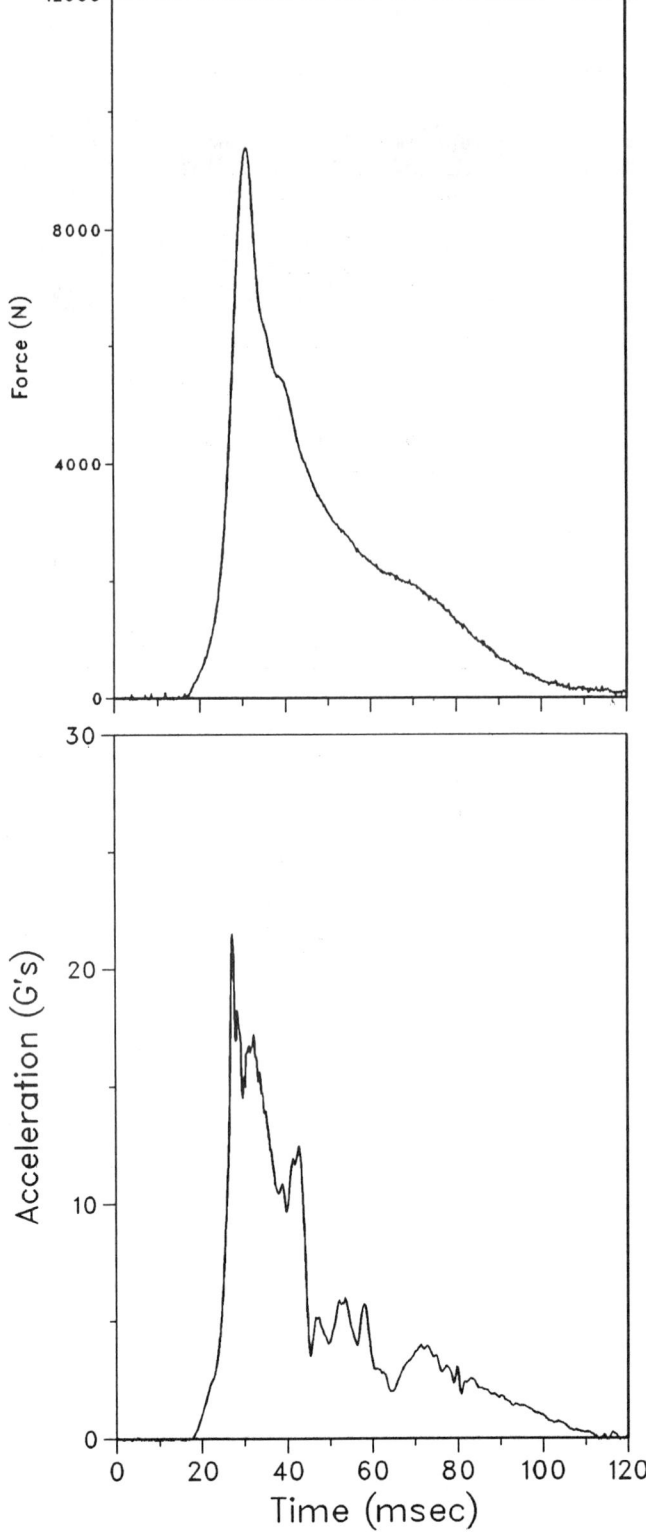

Figure 4   Resultant force history (top) at the impact site and resultant acceleration history (bottom) at the region of the lumbar spine in the Hybrid II manikin for a 400 mm vertical drop. A triaxial accelerometer measured the lumbar spine accelerations.

components establishes the limits of tolerance, it excludes other anatomic and structural features of the spine such as column buckling, and vertebral wedging accompanied by posterior element distractions. Studies using isolated ligamentous columns and intact torsos suggested that only compression-flexion loading produced anterior wedging and posterior element disruptions. Conventional flexure loadings demonstrated posterior disruptions with minimal anterior wedging. It was found that, under compression-flexion loads, all three devices stabilized the spine although recovery was below the strength of the intact spinal column. However, other factors such as size of spinal canal and level of degeneration which are crucial to the protection of the spinal cord, must also be considered before any particular device is recommended for the injured patient. At relatively low drop heights, manikin experiments produced higher forces and accelerations than the thresholds suggestive of injuries reported in the literature (19,20).

These studies on the uniaxial loading of thoracolumbar components, and compression-flexion and flexure loading of ligamentous columns and intact cadavers have provided base line biomechanical data and functional tissue changes under quasi-static force applications. Because traumatic injuries to the human spine in motor vehicle accidents are often associated with high rates of loading due to impact, it may also be necessary to investigate the effect of dynamic loads on the structural and pathological responses.

ACKNOWLEDGMENT

This research was supported in part by PHS CDC Grant R49CCR502508 and Veterans Administration Medical Research Funds.

REFERENCES

[1] Sances A Jr, Yoganandan N, Myklebust JB: Biomechanics and accident investigation. In Handbook of Biomedical Eng, J Kline, ed, Academic Press, 1988, pp 525-560.
[2] Yoganandan N, Myklebust JB, Ray G, Sances A Jr: Mathematical and finite element analysis of spinal injuries. CRC Crit Rev Bioeng 15(1):29-93, 1987.
[3] Yoganandan N, Sances A Jr, Maiman DJ, Myklebust JB, Pech P, Larson SJ: Experimental spinal injuries with vertical impact. Spine 11(9):855-860, 1986.
[4] Heylings DJA: Supraspinous and interspinous ligaments in dog, cat, and baboon. J Anat 130(2):223-228, 1980.
[5] Anderson JE: Grant's Atlas of Anatomy. 8th Ed., Williams and Wilkins, Baltimore, 1983.
[6] Sedlin ED, Hirsch C: Factors affecting the determination of the physical properties of femoral cortical bone. Acta Orthop Scand 37:29, 1966.
[7] Hirsch C, Galante J: Laboratory conditions for tensile tests in annulus fibrosus from human intervertebral discs. Acta Orthop Scand 38, 1967.
[8] Tkaczuk H: Tensile properties of human lumbar longitudinal ligament. Acta Orthop Scand, Suppl, 115, 69 pp, 1968.
[9] Pintar F: Biomechanics of spinal ligaments. Ph.D. Dissertation, Marquette University, Milwaukee, WI, 1986.
[10] Chazal J, Tanguy A, Bourges M, Gaurel G, Escande G, Guillot M, Vannenville G: Biomechanical properties of spinal ligaments and a histological study of the supraspinal ligament in traction. J Biomech 18(3):167-176, 1985.
[11] Yoganandan N: Biomechanical identification of injury to an intervertebral joint. Clin Biomech 1(3):149, 1986.
[12] Yoganandan N, Myklebust J, Wilson C, Cusick J, Sances A Jr: Functional biomechanics of thoracolumbar vertebral cortex. Clin Biomech 3(1):11-18, 1988.
[13] Kazarian L, Graves GA Jr: Compressive strength characteristics of human vertebral centrum. Spine 2(1):1-14, 1977.
[14] Yamada H: Strength of Biological Materials. Williams and Wilkins, Baltimore, MD, 1970, 297 pp.
[15] Rolander SD: Motion of the lumbar spine with special reference to the stabilizing effect of posterior fusion. Acta Orthop Scand, Suppl, 90, 1966.
[16] Larson SJ: The thoracolumbar junction. In The Unstable Spine, SB Dunsker, A Kahn, H Schmidt, and J Frymayer, eds, Grune & Stratton Inc, 1986, pp 122-152.
[17] Herring JA, Wenger DR: Segmental spinal instrumentation. A preliminary report of 40 consecutive cases. Spine 7(3):285-298, 1982.
[18] Sullivan JA, Conner SB: Comparison of Harrington instrumentation and segmental spinal instrumentation in the management of neuromuscular spinal deformity. Spine 7(3):299-304, 1982.
[19] Work practices guide for manual lifting. National Institute for Occupational Safety and Health, U.S. Dept of Health and Human Services, 1981.
[20] Aircraft crash survival design guide, Vol II. Aircraft crash enviornment and human tolerance. US Army Technology Laboratory, USARTL-TR-79-22B, Jan, 1980.

Section 5:
Biomechanical Data and Response of Children in Automotive Impact Environment

720442

Airbag Effects on the Out-of-Position Child

Lawrence M. Patrick and Gerald W. Nyquist
Wayne State University

EVALUATION OF THE SAFETY performance of the airbag safety system is unusual since there is no previous highway experience involving airbag systems. Consequently, it is necessary to evaluate these systems on an experimental basis. Dummies representing human adults and children, human volunteers, human cadavers, animals, and mathematical models have all been used to evaluate the airbag system experimentally and analytically.

Substantial knowledge of human tolerance for adults has been gained through experimental and clinical studies. However, there is a paucity of data on the tolerance of children to impact. The injury criteria that have been established for adults are of questionable value for evaluating potential injury to children. Known anatomical differences such as the larger size of the child's head in comparison to the rest of his body, the weaker neck, softer bones, and sutures (bone joints) only partly ossified (solidfied) are all complicating factors which make the methods used to evaluate safety systems from an adult standpoint unsuitable for use with children.

After carefully considering the various possibilities for evaluating the effect of the airbag on the out-of-position child,

---

*This research was sponsored in part by General Motors Corp.

it was decided that the use of primates of approximately the same weight as the child would provide the most realistic evaluation of potential injuries. The East African baboon was chosen as the animal for the experimental program from the standpoint of availability, internal organ similarity, and size. Twenty-two static deployment experiments have been conducted with four anesthetized, young, male baboons ranging in weight from 29-34 lb. The experiments were conducted with a prototype right front passenger airbag system. Similar experiments under dynamic conditions are being planned for the near future.

Five distinct positions were chosen to represent the out-of-position child. The normal seated position is included as one of the five with standing, kneeling, and sitting on the floor included as other positions which children assume voluntarily or are forced into during panic braking or other abnormal operating conditions.

TYPES OF INJURIES

After completion of a series of experiments, the animal was sacrificed for autopsy. Extensive observation, physiological records, and x-ray radiographs were made before and after the exposure. Palpation and reflex observations were taken on the anesthetized animal. A complete autopsy was per-

---

ABSTRACT

This paper describes experiments involving airbag systems. Because there is the least amount of data on the tolerance of children to impact, the out-of-position child was used in the experiments.

After careful consideration it was decided that a primate of approximately the same weight as a child be used, which would provide the most realistic evaluation of potential injuries. The animal chosen for the experimental program was the baboon.

Five distinct positions were chosen and this paper describes in detail the experimental physiological conditions and results.

formed if there was any suspicion of injury. Particular emphasis was placed on examining for the following injuries:

1. Potential brain injury with emphasis on concussion of a reversible nature as indicated by temporary loss of reflexes immediately after exposure, and more severe injuries as evidenced by the macroscopic and gross injury to the brain observed during necropsy (autopsy).

2. Neck injury from compression and/or hyperextension resulting from subjecting the animal to conditions which produce hyperextension (observation for possible injuries was made by palpation, observation, x-rays, and dissection).

3. Thoracic injuries from bag impact, including a search for contusions, bone fractures, and organ injuries.

4. Injuries to the abdominal viscera such as the stomach, gut, liver, spleen, heart, mesentery, and other internal structures.

5. Superficial soft tissue injury from direct bag slap and/or abrasive sliding action, including contusions, abrasions, and/or lacerations to the soft tissue in the bag contact area.

The injuries were recorded immediately after exposure, at specified time intervals thereafter, and during the autopsy.

EXPERIMENTAL SETUP

The experimental setup consisting of a production bench seat and a simulated instrument panel in correct relative position is shown in Fig. 1. The instrument panel in Fig. 1 is similar to some of the 1969 instrument panels, and was used in the first four runs. Thereafter, a prototype panel profile was used. The combined torso and knee airbag system is mounted under the instrument panel in the general knee impact area.

Fig. 1 shows the primary components of the airbag system including the gas bottle (approximately 4-1/2 in in diameter × 13 in long), the pipe leading to the manifold, the airbag cover, the plunger assembly, the operating solenoid, and a strobe light to synchronize timing between the electronic records and the high-speed cameras.

The components of the system include: high-pressure storage tank, diaphragm, spring-loaded, spear-type initiator with solenoid operation, orifice, manifold, airbag, and cover or door.

The highly stressed, dome-shaped diaphragm was punctured by the spring-loaded spear-type initiator operated by the solenoid. The diaphragm opened rapidly in four pie-shaped sectors when ruptured by the spear.

An orifice was placed in the pipe leading from the tank to the manifold. Two different circular orifices were used with areas of 0.285 and 0.675 in^2.

The anesthetized animal was maintained in position by two tethers. One of the tethers was taut to hold the animal in position, while the other was slack so it did not interfere with the animal during normal movement in the buck, but would stop the animal before it hit the floor outside the buck. After the first five runs, the slack tether was replaced by canvas nets placed around the body buck to catch the animal. The positioning tether (s) was released by a solenoid just prior to bag deployment in all runs.

Pressure measurements are made in both the main airbag and knee airbag. It should be pointed out that the long tubes from the airbag to the transducers could have resulted in a delay, phase shift, or modification of the pressure record. The pressure in the torso bag varied 32-52 psig peak during initial deployment and 0.8-1.8 psig sustained when measured by this method.

The major variables of the study are:

1. Two orifice sizes.

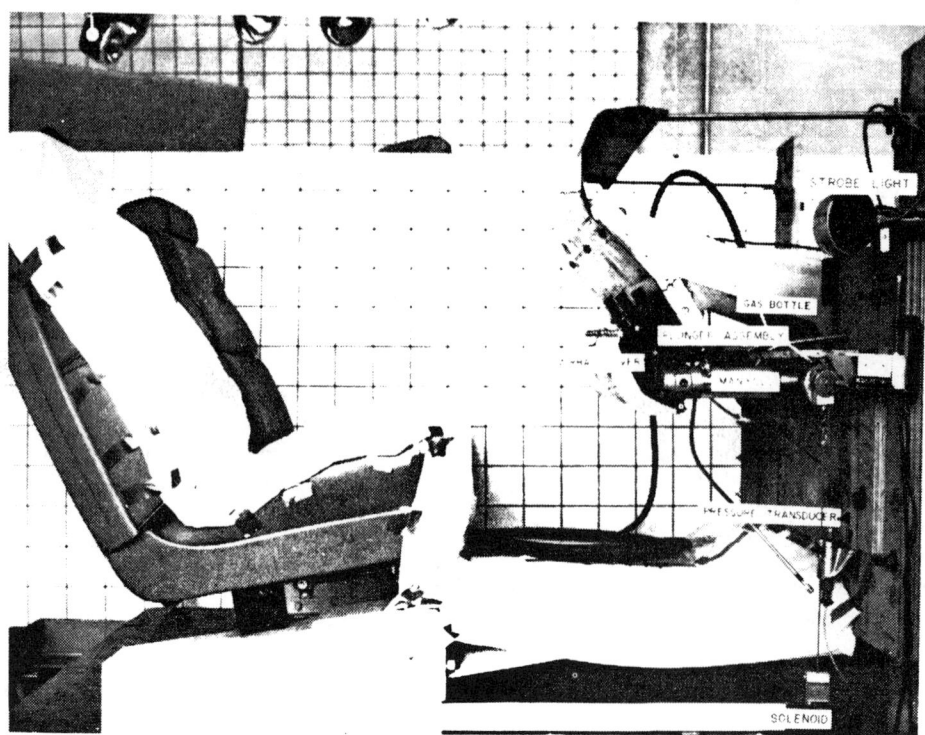

Fig. 1 - Experimental setup with first instrument panel

2. Two instrument panel designs.
3. Five exposure positions (with three variations to one of the positions).
4. Four different animals.

A summary of the conditions for the 22 runs including the aforementioned variables is presented in Table 1.

The airbag cover is a top-opening, bottom-hinged type with a tear-line molded into it across the top and down both sides. When the pressure in the bag is high enough, the cover is forced open by tearing along the tear-lines, after which it hinges downward along the bottom fabric hinge. A wire placed across the upper tear-line is broken as the cover opens to provide a signal on an oscillograph record at the instant of cover breakaway.

INSTRUMENTATION

No transducers were attached to the animal since it was considered inadvisable to introduce artifacts by any surgical tech-

Table 1 -
Summary of Experimental Physiological Conditions and Results

Experiment No.	Date (1971)	Baboon Position*	Baboon	Orifice Area, (in^2)	Eyelid Reflex**	Physiological Results†
1	3-26	1	A	0.675	Yes	Left clavicle dislocated at sternum
9	4-28	1	C	0.675	Yes	No apparent injury
13	5-4	1	C	0.285	††	No apparent injury
14	5-4	1	A	0.285	Yes	Abrasions on elbows
16	5-5	2	A	0.675	No	Abrasions—left upper arm and left nostril. Eyes closed for 40 s after impact
17	5-7	2	C	0.675	No	Eyes closed. Lid reflex returned 1 min after impact
2	3-29	2	A	0.262	††	No apparent injury
4	4-2	2	B	0.285	††	Lacerated eyebrow
15	5-5	2	C	0.285	No	Broken tooth, blood behind cornea—right eye; lacerated tongue; eyes closed for 25 min, no lid reflex for 8 min after impact
5	4-16	3	B	0.675	††	Fatal—ruptured liver (see autopsy report)
7	4-19	3	A	0.675	Yes	No apparent injury
8	4-23	3	C	0.675	Yes	No apparent injury
10	4-29	3	A	0.675	Yes	No apparent injury
3	3-31	3	B	0.285	Yes	No apparent injury
6	4-16	3	A	0.285	Yes	No apparent injury
11	5-3	3	C	0.285	Yes	No apparent injury
12	5-3	3	A	0.285	Yes	Abrasion—left elbow; broke tail
18	5-12	4	A	0.285	Yes	No apparent injury. Autopsy performed after this test
19	5-13	4	C	0.285	No	Eyes remained closed after test. No lid reflex for 6 min after impact
20	5-18	5a	D	0.675	Yes	Abrasion on anterior surface of upper arms and chin; lacerated tongue
21	5-19	5b	D	0.675	Yes	Abrasions on penis, right upper arm and right upper leg.
22	5-20	5c	D	0.675	Yes	Large abrasion on chest—approximately 4 in dia. Autopsy performed after this test. Lacerated or ruptured liver—not fatal

*See Table 2 for a description of positions.
**Immediately after impact.
†A log of Sernylan (drug) injections, blood pressure and pulse rate is available at Wayne State University.
††Not recorded.

nique or by strapping transducers to the animal. Fig. 2 is a typical record. Starting from the top of Fig. 2, the strobe flash synchronizes the timing of the high-speed movies with the electronic records. The second trace indicates the time at which the airbag cover opened. A wire which was part of a low-voltage galvonometer circuit was taped over the tear-line of the cover. When the cover opened, the wire was broken, causing a galvonometer trace deflection indicating the instant the cover opened on the record. The next two traces are the knee and torso bag pressure records. The last record at the bottom of Fig. 2 is a two-stage timing method used to further synchronize the records with the high-speed camera. At the instant the solenoid is actuated to rupture the diaphragm, the signal is changed from 1000 Hz to 100 Hz. The same record is put on the edge of the high-speed film to permit calculation of the exact time from the initiation of the solenoid to any part of the electronic record, or to any part of the high-speed film.

Photoinstrumentation included:

1. Close-up lateral coverage of the knee and airbag area with a Fastax camera at a nominal 3000 frames/s.

2. An overall lateral view with a Photosonics camera at approximately 500 frames/s.

3. Left-rear oblique, overall coverage with a Kodak camera at a nominal 3000 frames/s.

4. An overhead, overall coverage with a Fastair camera at approximately 300 frames/s.

5. A left-front oblique view with a Bell and Howell camera at 64 frames/s.

PROCEDURE

The bag was packed and installed prior to each experiment followed by calibration of the pressure transducers and a complete check of the entire system. After the system was ready, the baboon was anesthetized with Sernylan and transported from the animal quarters to the laboratory in the Engineering building. The blood pressure and heart rate were recorded at intervals before and after the run.

The animal was located in a predetermined position and held in place by tape and a tether. On the first five runs the slack, emergency tether remained in place during the run and the position tether was released by a solenoid. In run 6 and thereafter, the emergency tether was discarded, and the position tether was released at the instant the bag was inflated to eliminate any effect of the tether on the animal during the bag

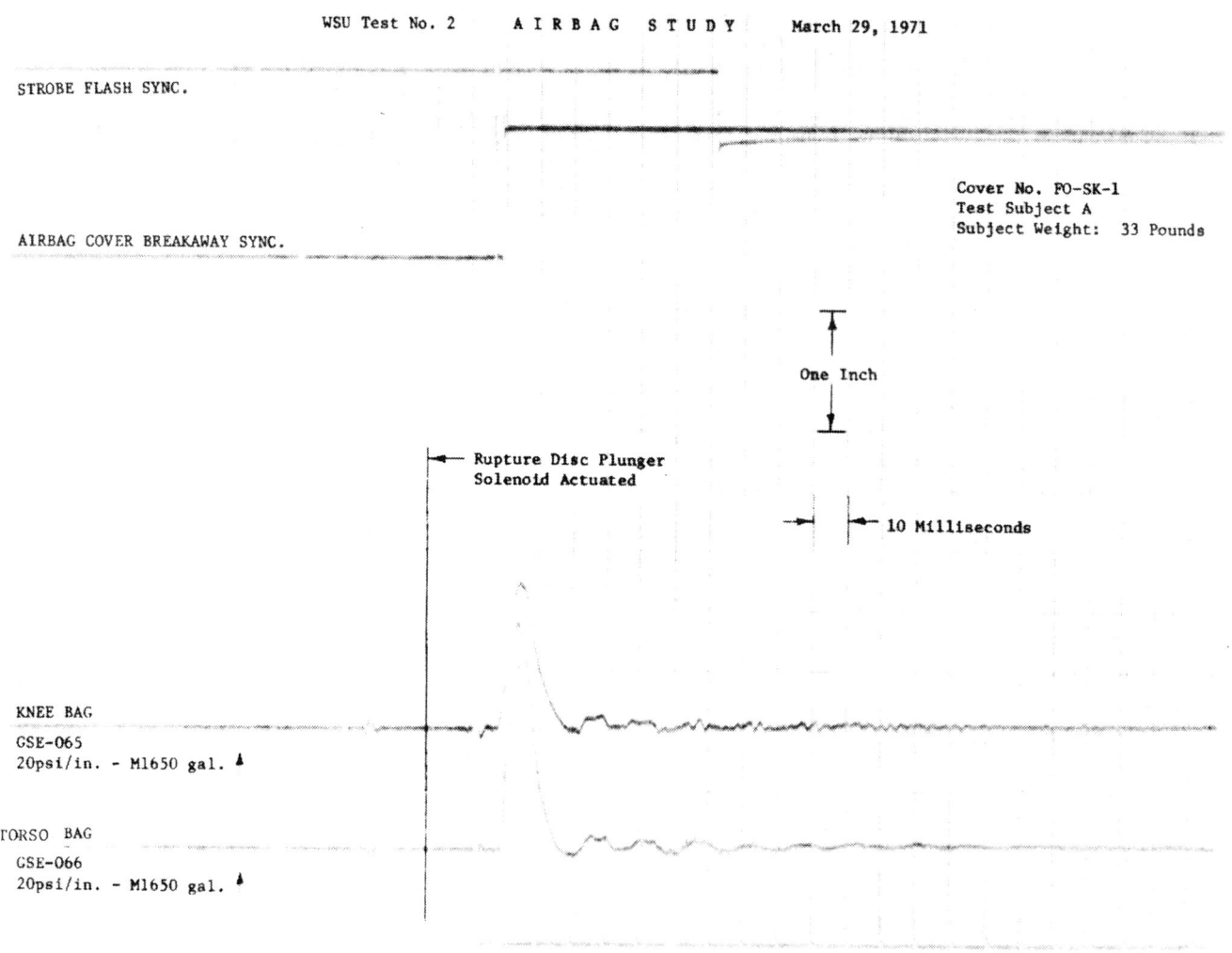

Fig. 2 - Record of run 2

deployment. Immediately after the run, the animal was checked for reflexes and then placed in the restraining chair for further recordings of blood pressure and heart rate to determine whether there was any observable effect from the exposure. If the vital signs were normal and there was no indication of any injury, the animal was observed for several days. It was then available for further experiments or autopsy depending on the number of exposures.

SIMULATED POSITIONS

The simulated positions are listed in Table 2 and shown in Figs. 3-9. Position 5 was essentially a normal seated position with three fore-and-aft seated positions included. The number of runs in each position is listed in Table 1. There were four runs in position 1, five in position 2, eight in position 3, two in position 4, and one each in positions 5a-c.

Table 2 -
Description of Occupant Positions Evaluated

Position Designation	Physical Position
1	Standing on floor
2	Crouching on seat, muzzle against cover
3	Kneeling on seat, arms and elbows on top of instrument panel
4	Sitting on floor
5a	Normal seating attitude, chest 6 in forward of aft end of inflated airbag
5b	Same as 5a, except 12 in
5c	Same as 5a, except 18 in*

*In this position, the anterior surface of the chest is approximately 1/2 in from the aft surface of the instrument panel.

Position 1 shown in Fig. 3 by a child dummy represents a child sitting on the forward part of the seat or standing on the floor. It is a rather common position, and one in which the lower part of the torso is exposed to the full impact of the airbag during inflation.

Position 2 shown in Fig. 4 represents a child bending over forward or lying on the seat with his head forward. In this position, the head is exposed to impact by the deploying airbag. With this particular installation, the airbag comes from slightly below the center of the head, exposing the face to the airbag inflation. Brain, neck, and soft tissue are all vulnerable in this position.

In position 3 (Fig. 5), the child is kneeling on the seat and leaning against the instrument panel. The lower part of the body is exposed to the airbag, and the upward component tends to propel the child upward and backward.

Position 4 in Fig. 6 is particularly hazardous to the face and neck. The child could be sitting on the floor playing, or could

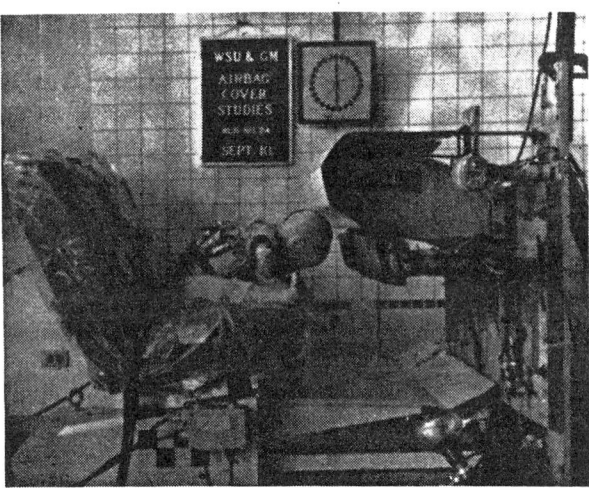

Fig. 4 - Child dummy test position 2

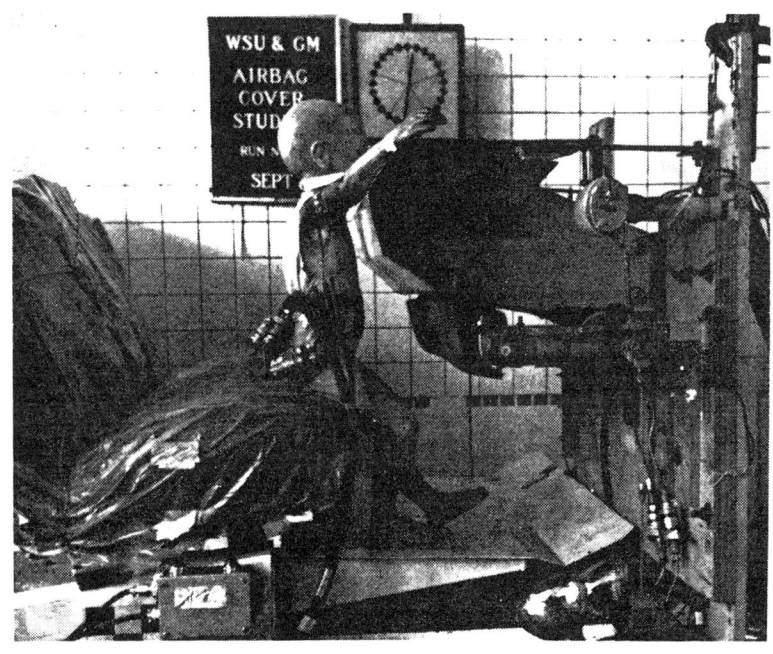

Fig. 3 - Child dummy test position 1

be forced into the position during a panic stop in which he might slide forward off the seat. The airbag cover, as well as the airbag, strikes the child in the face in this position. Hyperextension of the neck, injury to soft tissue of the face, injury to the fragile facial bones, and brain damage are all possible in this exposure.

Positions 5a-c are the normal seated configurations as shown in Figs. 7-9 for three different fore-and-aft locations. Position 5a is obtained when the child is sitting on the seat and forward far enough so his chest and face are approximately 6 in forward of the most aft position of the bag when inflated. Position 5b is the same except that he is moved forward 6 in, resulting in a position 12 in forward of the rearmost position of the bag. Position 5c is similar to positions 5a-b except that he is 18 in forward of the rearward position of the bag

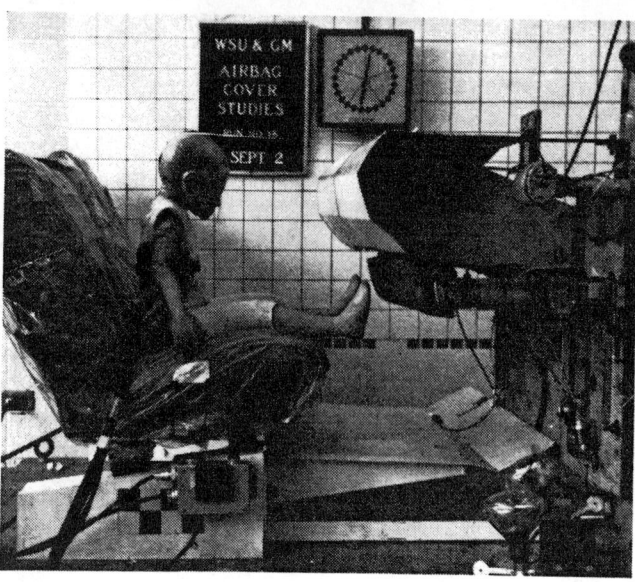

Fig. 7 - Child dummy test position 5a

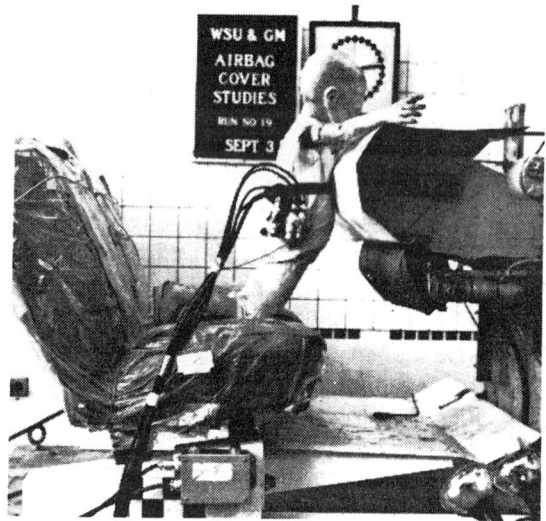

Fig. 5 - Child dummy test position 3

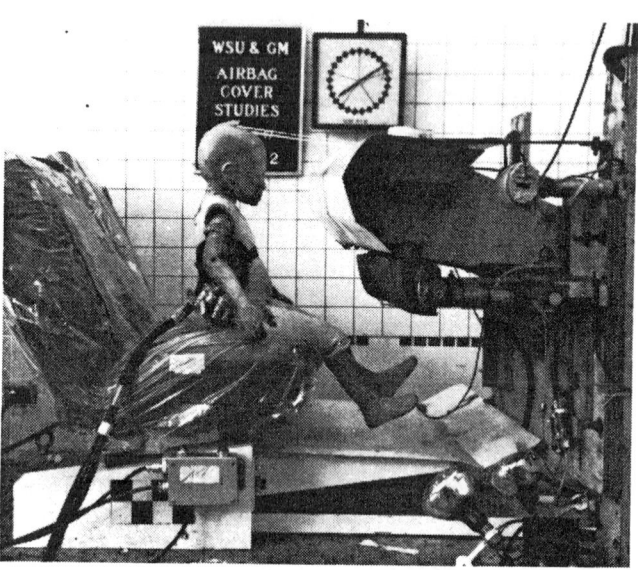

Fig. 8 - Child dummy test position 5b

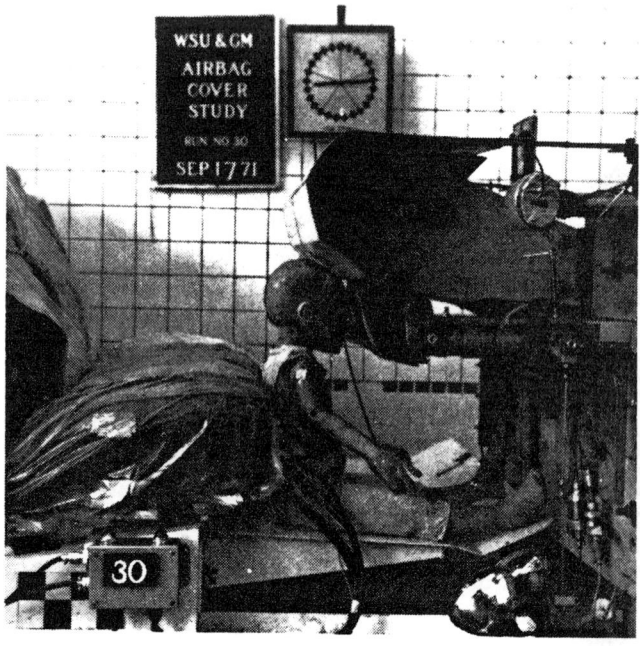

Fig. 6 - Child dummy test position 4

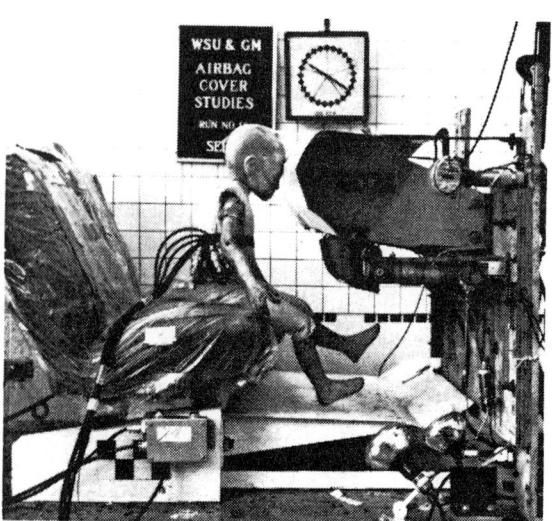

Fig. 9 - Child dummy test position 5c

with his head against the instrument panel and his chest close to it.

DISCUSSION OF EXPERIMENTAL RESULTS

The baboon is a good simulation of the child since it is similar in shape and size, and the internal organs are approximately the same size and in the same location as those of the child. While the baboon is a good simulation of size, shape, and organ similarity, there are major differences that should be noted. They are:

1. The head and brain of the baboon are smaller than those of a child of the same size.

2. The head shape is considerably different with a larger protruding muzzle and considerably heavier neck and head musculature.

3. The temporal muscles are very large compared to those of the child.

4. The thorax of the baboon is not as broad and flat as that of the human.

The dynamics should be similar between the baboon and the child except that the animal is anesthetized and, consequently, is limp. This could correspond to a sleeping child. Also, investigators have observed that much higher accelerations and angles of hyperextension are required before injury results in the baboon when it is subjected to hyperextension accelerating forces. Therefore, one would expect the injuries to be comparable with the baboon having the same organ vulnerability to injury, except that greater energies are required for the same injuries for the animals than for children under otherwise identical conditions. Thus, it appears that noninjury to the baboon is a necessary, but not sufficient, requirement for noninjury to the child. In other words, if the baboon is not injured, there is no way to be sure that a child will not be injured under the same condition. If the baboon is injured, it is fairly certain that the child will be injured to a greater extent. This is particularly true for the head and neck region where the disparity between the baboon and human child is greater than in the abdominal and thoracic areas. It is essential, therefore, that the system be designed to prevent injury to the baboon since any injury would be magnified in the child.

The results from exposure to the statically deployed airbag in each position will be discussed.

POSITION 1 - Four exposures were made in position 1 (Fig. 3) as indicated in Table 1. The injuries consisted of a dislocated clavicle (collarbone) at the sternum, and abrasions on the elbows. The clavicle dislocation occurred in run 1 in which the emergency tether was used. It is hypothesized that the tether produced the forces on the clavicle to cause dislocation. Run 14 made at a later date with the same animal without the emergency tether and a smaller orifice area resulted in only abrasions on the elbow. The difference in orifice area and the difference in tether conditions in the two runs makes it impossible to ascertain the exact cause of the difference between the two. However, observation of the high-speed movies of the experiment lead the investigators to the conclusion that the clavicle dislocation was caused by the tether and, consequently, should not be considered as an injury attributable to the airbag inflation.

POSITION 2 - In position 2 (Fig. 4) with the animal crouching on the seat and its muzzle against the cover, an indication of concussion based on loss of lid reflex was noted for all runs in which the reflex was checked. Loss of reflex ranged from 40 s to 8 min for these three exposures. Abrasions and lacerations were observed in three of the five exposures. Run 15 (Table 1) with the smaller orifice (0.285 in^2) appeared to be the most severe from a concussive standpoint, with loss of lid reflex for 8 min after the exposure. In addition, on this run a broken tooth was observed and blood was noted behind the cornea of the right eye. The tongue was also lacerated.

Position 2 was chosen as being the most vulnerable for head and neck injury. The position is difficult for a child to assume and would probably occur only with a sleeping child during a panic stop in which the child would slide forward on the seat. In either case, the conditions for the child would probably be considerably different than those encountered in the crouched position 2 which is fairly normal for an animal. If the child's head is extended over the seat next to the deploying bag, it appears that injury potential is great since a larger head mass, smaller neck, and lighter musculature of the child makes him more prone to injury from this exposure.

All of the position 2 runs in which the animal was checked for lid reflexes resulted in an indication of concussion through loss of reflex. It should be pointed out that the loss of reflex is probably affected by the amount of anesthetic (Sernylan) used. Since the dose varies with the length of time the animal is maintained in the anesthetized condition, the depth of anesthesia varies and can effect the reflex measurement.

POSITION 3 - Run 5, position 3 (Fig. 5) resulted in the only fatal injury, and was the last run made with the emergency tether. The autopsy showed the fatality to be the result of a badly lacerated, or ruptured, liver. Three other runs were made under identical conditions with two different animals in an effort to repeat the injury or to determine whether the fatal injury was due to the artifact introduced by the emergency tether. No apparent injury resulted from any of the other runs in this series, so it appears that the injury was, in fact, due to the tether rather than the exposure to the inflating airbag. This conclusion was further strengthened by observation of the high-speed movies which show the animal being propelled over the seat back and sustaining substantial concentrated force in the spine and liver area when the emergency tether jerked tight at the end of the fall.

Four more runs in position 3 were made with the smaller orifice as a further measure of the injury potential from the position. There was no serious injury in any of the four runs with the smaller orifice with the only injury noted being an abrasion of the left elbow and a broken tail.

POSITION 4 - Position 4 (Fig. 6) with the animal simulating a child seated on the floor with his back against the front seat, and his head slightly extended and against the instrument panel, resulted in no apparent injury to baboon A when subjected to inflation with the 0.285 in^2 orifice. Autopsy immediately after this run revealed no trauma that would have resulted in long-term injury to the animal.

Baboon C was subjected to the same condition in run 19, and had a loss of lid reflex for about 6 min indicating a concussion. This was the only run other than those in position 2 in which concussion was indicated. An autopsy performed after the run showed no gross damage to the brain or brain stem area.

In position 4, the child would be particularly vulnerable to neck injury since the head would be forced rearward while the torso is stopped by the seat. The combination of hyperflexion and the direct acceleration of the head from the deploying airbag presents a severe potential for head injury. Fortunately, this is probably a rare position for a child so the exposure is expected to be minimal.

POSITION 5 - Positions 5a-c (Figs. 7-9) are normal upright seated positions with different fore-and-aft locations on the seat. The effect of bag slap and different distances from the panel is of particular interest. Both the pressure and membrane forces change with position and, apparently, have a major effect on the potential injury. Three runs were made on the same animal at 6, 12, and 18 in forward of the rearmost position of the bag. Exposure is primarily to the thorax rather than the head, as observed from the high-speed movies.

Extensive lacerations and abrasions resulted from the three impacts to the same animal, including trauma of the chest, chin, tongue, penis, arms, and legs. The vital signs after run 21 were abnormal with erratic heart rate and blood pressure still present the following day. Autopsy after the third run showed a lacerated or ruptured liver which, while not fatal, was close to a fatality. A clot had formed on the lesion (injury) and the animal would probably have survived. However, the injury was near fatal as evidenced by the ease with which the laceration could be extended by means of light finger pressure.

All of the runs in position 5 were made with the large orifice. Only one animal was used in the three runs so there is no way to establish the cumulative effect of multiple runs with the same animal. Further, the smaller orifice should be investigated to determine whether the reduced flow would reduce the severity of the exposure. Also, it will be necessary to study the three different locations in position 5 with different animals to determine whether one of the three locations is more dangerous than the others, or whether all three have the same potential for injury. Additional runs in positions 5a-c with the smaller orifice and individual animals are necessary to complete the investigation of this particular position which is the most common position to be expected in the vehicle.

GENERAL DISCUSSION

In an effort to modify the head and thorax response to the static deployment of the airbag in the five positions studied, similar exposures are being made with the child dummy. In ...tions 2, 4, and 5a-b the head accelerations were up to 450 g, which is far beyond the tolerable limit. Peak thorax accelerations of 180 g were observed in position 4 with positions 2 and 5 having thorax accelerations in excess of 100 g. These are only preliminary results, but the high readings are consistent and indicate that the system under evaluation does present a serious hazard to children in several exposure positions.

Simple calculations of the velocity of the deploying airbag lead to some startling results. Measuring the distance from the stored airbag to the face and chest of the normally seated occupant results in a distance of approximately 30 in, or 2-1/2 ft for this installation. The time required to inflate the bag is in the order of 25-30 ms. A simple calculation shows that the average velocity of the bag is in the order of 100 ft/s by the time it gets to the fully inflated position. With an average of 100 ft/s, the peak velocities are in the order of 150 ft/s, or approximately 100 mph or more. Even though the mass of the portion of the bag which strikes the occupant is comparatively low, the impact from the high velocities can present problems with, at least, superficial injuries. This is the well-known bag slap phenomenon.

While the bag slap may cause superficial injuries due to the high velocity/low mass impact, the membrane action as the bag reaches the maximum pressure produces larger forces on the occupant. The forces are greater than the bag inertia forces plus the internal bag pressure on the occupant over the area in contact. The bag tends to envelope the occupant, and as the pressure increases the membrane action of the bag surrounding the occupant tends to cause the bag to take the shape of a sphere with much larger forces applied than the pressure times area force. Although the bag pressure is only in the order of 2-3 psi, the large area involved and the angles in the membrane mode result in large forces that can cause injury to the occupants.

The experimental setup used in this program included a canvas safety net to catch the animal if it was catapulted over the seat back or to one side. The setup had no B-post, header, roof rail, or roof to add to the injury from impact to these other rigid members. Consequently, the injuries studied were only due to the direct airbag deployment and did not include secondary injuries from impact to vehicle interior components.

CONCLUSIONS

The following conclusions are reached based on the results of the experimental program reported herein:

1. The deploying airbag in the system studied has sufficient force to propel a 29-34 lb baboon (or a child of similar weight) over the front seat back. The animal was propelled over the seat back in positions 1, 3, and 5c. These positions are not considered dangerous to life insofar as the animal is concerned for the inflation exposure only. However, there is no car top or internal components in the experimental setup used to provide secondary injuries so, consequently, the total injury potential was not included in this study.

2. In most positions where the head is in the path of the

airbag, the incidence of concussion as indicated by a loss of lid reflex was large. The head was in the path of the deploying airbag in positions 2 and 4, and concussion indications were present in four out of the five runs checked. The concussions were not severe enough to cause brain damage observable at autopsy. It should be noted that baboons are extremely difficult to concuss from a head impact due to the heavy musculature on the head and the small brain size.

3. Injuries to the thoracic and abdominal organs are likely when the airbag strikes the torso as observed from lesions during autopsy.

4. Superficial soft tissue injuries such as abrasions, contusions, and lacerations result from direct contact with the airbag; especially when the airbag fabric slides over the skin.

5. Fracture of bones is not a major problem with the animals used in these experiments. However, difference in head and neck geometry of the baboon and child could result in child injuries including neck fractures. Preliminary dummy experiments indicated that when the head is exposed to the deploying airbag, the accelerations are above the tolerable level.

6. With the present configuration of the airbag as studied in this program, there is danger of head and internal organ injuries to a child during static inflation.

7. The greatest danger of injury to the child appears to be the torso impact observed in positions 1, 3, and 5c. When standing on the floor, kneeling on the seat, or in a normal seated position, the airbag impacts the torso. The combined pressure and membrane forces are high enough to cause internal injuries. A pressure and/or rate of inflation control should be investigated as a means of minimizing injuries.

8. If the head is in the path of the deploying airbag, it is concluded that injury is likely to occur in the form of brain or neck injury to a child. Fortunately, the number of exposures to positions 2 and 4 is probably low.

760815

Comparison Between Child Cadavers and Child Dummy by Using Child Restraint Systems in Simulated Collisions

D. Kallieris, J. Barz, G. Schmidt, G. Heess, and R. Mattern
University of Heidelberg

Abstract

At present, numerous restraint systems for children applied in vehicles are in general considered for the use on the back seats. Up to now, only impact tests with dummies and animals have been carried through by these systems. Out of the great number of children seats and belts we used a system (deformable safety impact table combined with a lap-belt) which has been investigated by us during frontal impacts utilizing two dummies and four cadavers of children in the age of 2,5 up to 11 years having body weights of 16 up to 31 kg. The tests have been conducted on the deceleration-sled track at the Institute of Legal Medicine of the University Heidelberg. Impact velocities of 30 km/h and 40 km/h at a medium deceleration of 20g have been chosen. None of the test subjects showed injuries to the inner organs; however, numerous muscular hemorrhages as well as hemorrhages of discs and ligaments were noticed. The HIC values lay between 100 and 500; accelerations in x-direction up to 44g and in z-direction up to 85g occurred at the head. Lap-belt forces of 160 up to 400daN were measured. A weak point of the investigated system is that the child's movements are considerably limited, a factor also noticed in other child restraint systems; however, the protective function proved to be an advantage. The movements during the impact, pictured by high-speed cameras, essentially differ from those of adults wearing 3-point belts. The maximum flexion of the vertebral column is, due to the system, located in the transition of the thoracic to the lumbar vertebral column and the flexion angles amounted about 90°. As expected were the maximum head displacements in relation to a sled-fixed axis dependent on the impact velocity and the body height, and ranged between 50 cm (crash velocity 30 km/h, body height 97 cm) and 90 cm (crash velocity 40 km/h, body height 139 cm). The movements will be analysed; the anatomical and mechanical causes are going to be investigated. Finally will the results be compared with similar dummy tests investigated by us. Due to these differences in the dummy and cadaver behavior the necessity is pointed out to examine all restraint systems by cadaver tests.

INVESTIGATIONS REGARDING EFFECTIVE CHILD PROTECTION have been underway since the 1950s. (Roberts V.L. and McElhaney J.H.-(1)*, Stalnaker R.L. and Melvin J.W. (2)). Dye E.R. (3) reported on his experiences when evaluating a comprehensive series of then available child restraint devices and documented a number of criteria which should be applied in the evaluation of potential child seats or restraint devices. Aldman (4) reported on the development of a rearward-facing child seat for use in Swedish cars. Appoldt (5) discussed dynamic tests of child restraint systems manufactured by Rose Manufactures & Co. Siegel et al (6) related the devices of the various types of child seats to the type and frequency of the injury patterns as found in accident investigations. They recommended the use of lap-belts for children over four years of age.

In order to reduce or elminate the number and **severity of injuries** to child occupants in car accidents numerous restraint systems were developed in the following years. A suitable restraint system has to be designed to properly match the child's size. This means, according to the size or weight of the child, appropriate systems have to be used from the period of infancy to the time that the child is large enough to be properly restrained by an adult lap-belt.

For young infants, who are not able to support themselves in a seated position, carry cot type devices are available held to the vehicle's seat by straps and are designed to prevent the child falling out of the cot during an impact. In the age group of the 8 months to 4 years old, when the child can sit up, usually a moulded

---

*Numbers in parentheses designate References at end of paper

bucket seat strapped to the car's seat is used. Loads occurring during an accident are spread to both shoulders and the pelvis when using a diagonal-belt combined with a lap-belt or are spread to one shoulder and the pelvis if a shoulder- and lap-belt combination if used. In systems without shoulder-belts padded torso impact surfaces are mostly available and the loads of the lap-belt are transferred by padded large-sized layers to the abdominal region.

For children of four to 12 years the moulded bucket seat is replaced by a child safety harness. Here too, a similar restraint combination, as it is used for the 8 months to 4 years old is designed in such a manner to ensure that the load is applied to the strong parts of the body.

Use was made of child dummies in corresponding age to test the now available child restraint devices which are technically developed to such an extent in order not to fail during an impact. National and international regulations respectively standards (7,8,9,10) are in existence regarding the investigation of child restraint systems in cars. Contrary to the German standard which indicates no biomechanical values in children limits US Standard No. 213, among other things, the head acceleration to not more than 67g in the test dummy.

In technical literature only little data is found on injuries to children protected by an restraint device in an accident. Herbert et al (11) reported on serious impact accidents including 16 children restrained by devices approved by the Standards Association of Australia. No injury was recorded for fifteen of these children; the sixteenth suffered fatal injuries because of an ejection as the child was too loosely restrained with a restraint device not matching his body weight.

Stalnaker and Melvin (2) reported on 224 children (5 years and younger) who were passengers in car accidents. Thirty-one of these children were restrained by an adult lap-belt or by children restraint devices. No deaths or serious injuries occurred among the restrained children. Five of the 12 children restrained by a child seat and nine of the 19 children restrained by an adult lap-belt showed no injuries. Among the 193 children who were not restrained, three were killed and seven others suffered serious injuries.

Lowne (12) compared accident injuries of unrestrained and restrained children in the same car. In an accident evaluation involving over 100 children he arrived at the conclusion that more than half of the serious injuries might have been prevented if correctly fitted child devices had been worn.

Schreck and Patrick (13) simulated frontal impacts with a five-point harness child restraint system at impact velocities of 20, 25 and 30 mph, juvenile chimpanzees were used as test subjects. In the tests no bone fractures or essential soft tissue injuries were observed.

No biomechanical data of restrained and unrestrained child cadavers is available that has been investigated in simulated accidents through defined crash conditions and exact load measurements. A reason might be that most children killed in accidents are injured and thus are unsuited for crash tests.

In the paper submitted the results of four frontal impacts conducted with four restrained child cadavers will be discussed. Two further tests with child dummies serve for the comparison between child cadaver and child dummy behavior.

METHOD AND MATERIAL

The tests were conducted with impact velocities of 30 km/h (1 test) and 40 km/h (5 tests) utilizing the deceleration-sled at the Institute of Legal Medicine of the University Heidelberg (Kallieris (14); the deceleration pulse shape corresponded to a trapezium (Schmidt et al (15), the medium sled deceleration amounted between 18 and 23g.

The child restraint system consisting of a 50 mm broad standard belt (18% elongation at a load of 1000 kp) was used as a lap-belt and put around a safety table made of expanded polystyrene (Fig. 1). The semi-cylindrically formed safety-table with its large-sized bearing supports the abdominal region during the impact. Thereby, the upper part of the body and the neck--head region remain free; this restraint system is recommended for children of three to 12 years.

VW-standard front seats were at our disposal during the tests. The lap-belt anchorage points were the same as in the 3-point belt adult tests (Schmidt et al (16) and lie within the variation

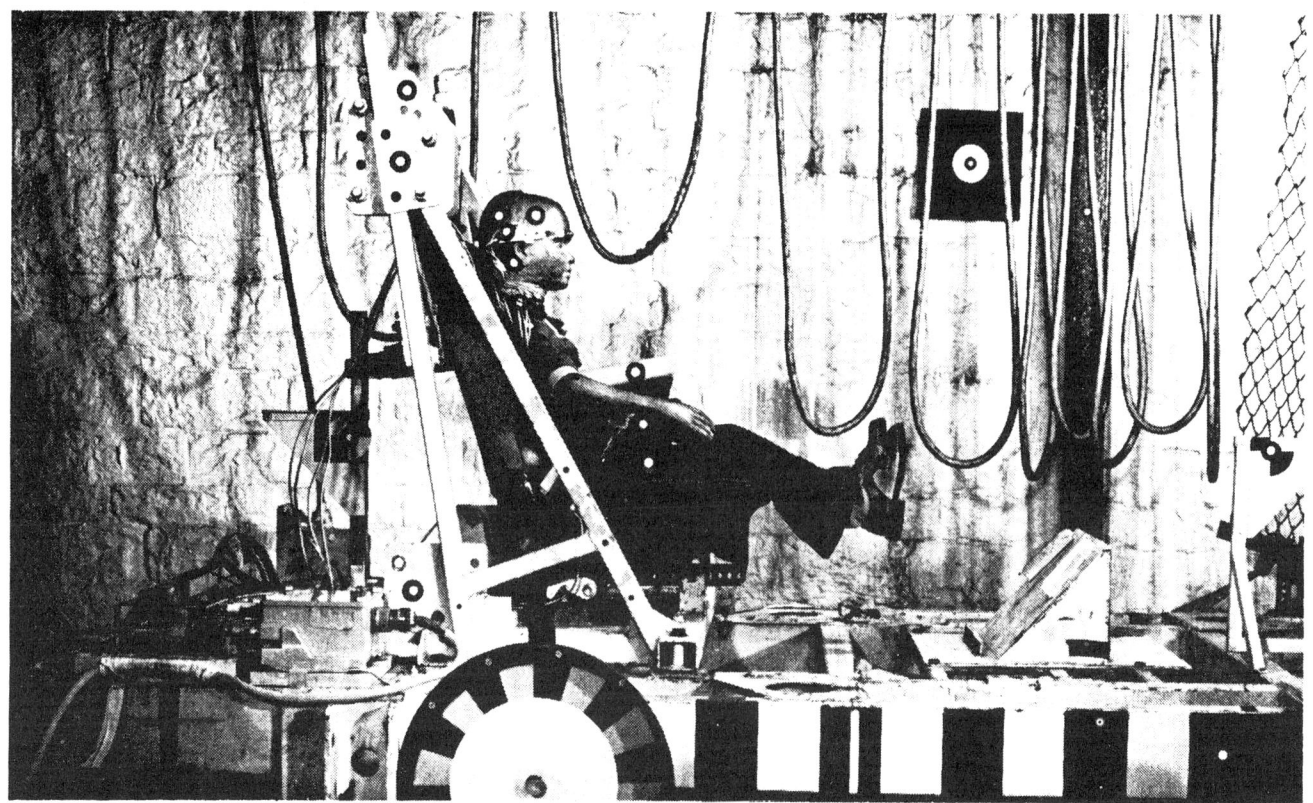

Fig. 1 - Deceleration sled with test subject and child restraint system

range of European vehicles.

Four unembalmed child cadavers (Table 1) in the age of 2,5 up to 11 years had been utilized; the time between death and test amounted 16 up to 120 hours.

The rigor mortis at hip and knee was treated in such a manner to obtain a sitting position. Prior to the test the rigor mortis of the various body parts had been judged and classified into four degrees. In order to better compare the child tests two further experiments with a 6-year old Alderson VIP-6C child dummy were conducted.

INSTRUMENTATION

The test-sled was instrumented to measure acceleration and velocity during each test. In two tests with child cadavers and two tests with child dummies we measured the acceleration of the right and left side at the head in x- and z-direction. The transducers were applied to an especially fabricated mounting which again was fastened to a metal ribbon (Fig. 2); the ribbon was adjustable according to the size of the head and was fastened to the skull bone by means of screws. The head measurement locations as well as the x- and z-axis of the accelerometers are defined in the intersection of the Frankfort plane perpendicular through the external auditory channel (Walker et al (17).

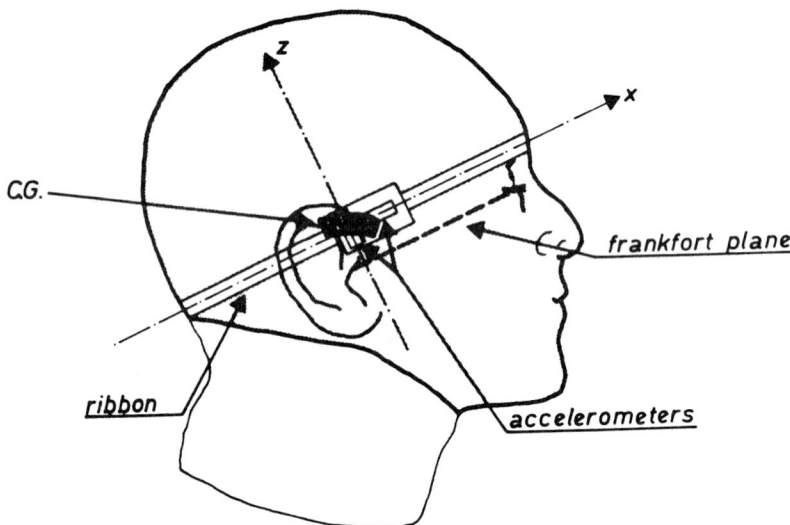

Fig. 2 - Location of the accelerometers at the head

This configuration enables the calculation of the resultant acceleration in the gravity center of the head as well as the head injury criterion. In the right and left lap-belt measurements of the belt loads were accomplished with strain-gauge transducers. The photographic coverage included one Hitachi 16 mm high-speed camera, located laterally (90°) to the sled, having a speed of 1000 frames per second; a Photosonics 16 mm high-speed camera which was adjusted in front of the sled having a speed of 500 frames per second; an occasionally used Hycam high-speed camera and an Arriflex 16 mm camera were located in the right and left front (30°) with a frame rate corresponding to 500 resp. 80 pictures per second. For quick-look information one Graphcheck sequence camera was used laterally to the sled, set at intervals of about 25 milliseconds.

A FM Telemetry System with a constant bandwidth, according to IRIG-standard, was used to record the measuring data and it comprised 10 measuring channels in one multiplex system. A trailing cable transmits the multiplex signal which is directly recorded by a channel on an analog magnet tape. Immediately after the test the measuring channels of the multiplex system can be demodulated and, in order to enable a first review of the results an UV-recorder was used. For the final evaluation the measuring data will be reworked by means of a process-computer.

RESULTS AND DISCUSSION

Evaluation of the Measuring Techniques -
A total of 6 tests was conducted using four child cadavers and two child dummies (Alderson VIP-6C) (Table 1). In one cadaver test (V 36/75) the impact velocity amounted 30 km/h, in all other test runs crash speeds of 40 km/h were utilized. In all experiments the sled was decelerated at about 70 ms with corresponding stopping distances of 21 cm (v=30 km/h) and 29-32 cm (v=40 km/h). All tests showed maximum lap-belt forces at 70 ms after the impact (this corresponds to the end of the sled deceleration phase) (Fig. 3-8). The peaks of the belt forces correspond to the weight of the test subjects i.e., the forces increase by increasing body weight.

Table 1 - Test Results

CADAVER

No. / Sex	Age Years	Length cm	Weight kg	Sled veloc. km/h	decel. g	Beltforce KN right	left	Res. Head decel. g	HIC	Head displ. cm	degree of injury	Bending angle in the transit.thor.-lumb.vertebr.Col. deg.
36/75 ♂	2.5	97	16	30.7	18	1.6	-	-	-	50	I	85
38/75 ♀	6	125	27	40.0	20	2.5	3.2	-	-	90	0 - I	90
39/75 ♂	6	124	30	40.4	21	2.8	3.8	33.5	102	65	I - II	88
41/75 ♂	11	139	31	40.0	21	2.9	3.7	94	523	90	II	93

Dummy (Alderson VIP - 6C)

No.		Length cm	Weight kg	Sled veloc. km/h	decel. g	Beltforce KN right	left	Res. Head decel. g	HIC	Head displ. cm	degree of injury	Bending angle deg.
1/76		121	21.5	40	23	2.7	4.0	40	229	71	-	27
2/76		121	21.5	40	22	3.1	4.3	45	260	70	-	25

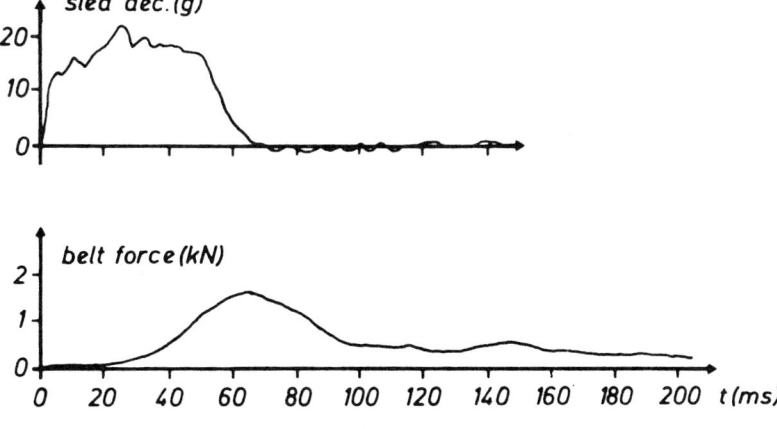

Fig. 3 - Sled deceleration and belt force time histories of test run V 36/75

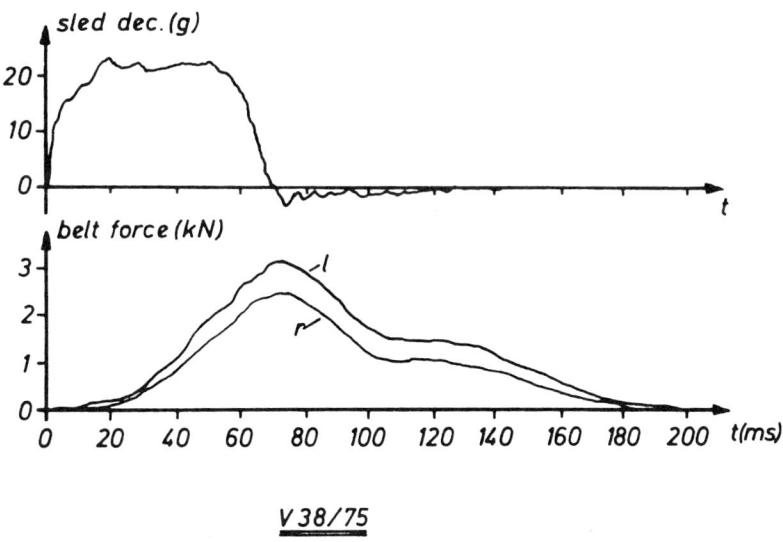

Fig. 4 - Sled deceleration and belt force time histories of test run V 38/75

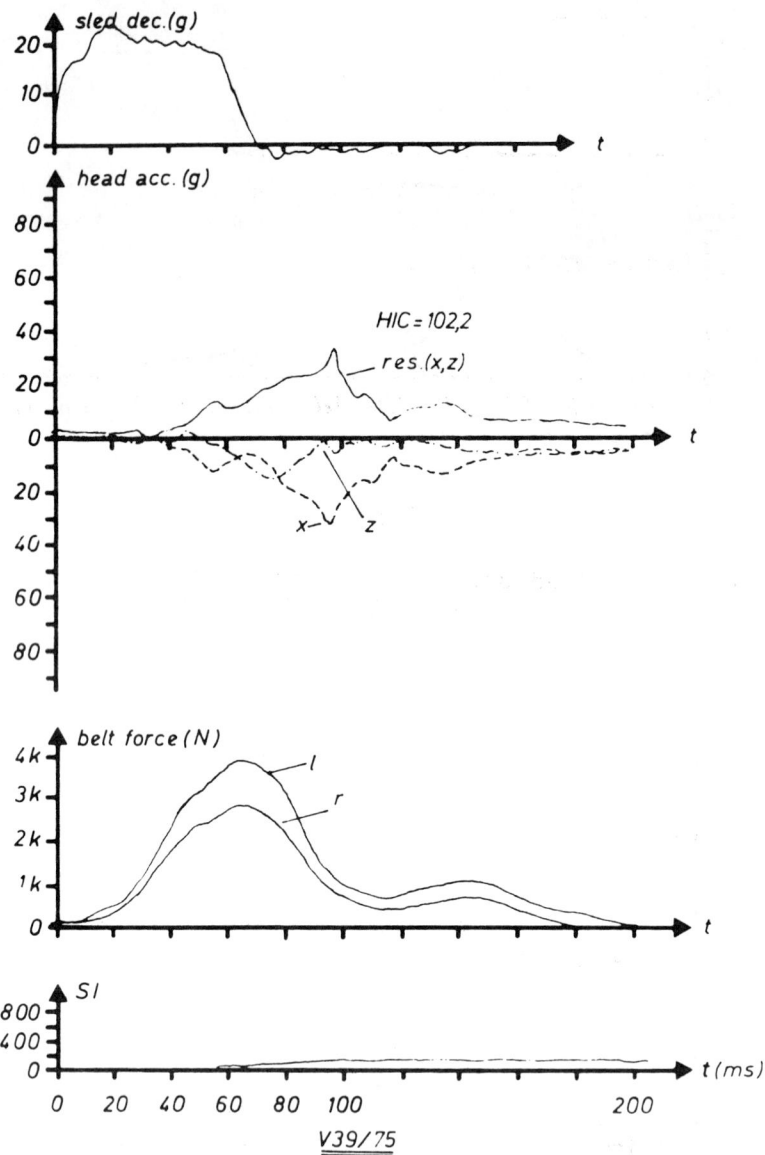

Fig. 5 - Sled deceleration, head acceleration, belt force and SI time histories of test run V 39/75

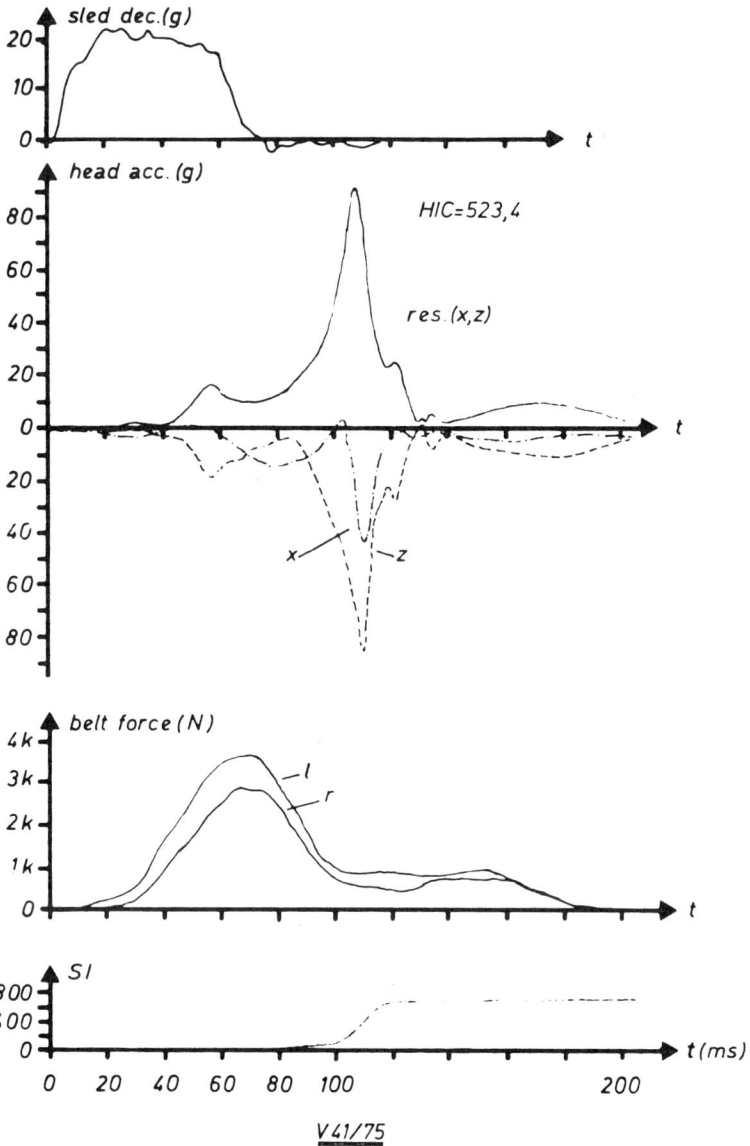

Fig. 6 - Sled deceleration, head acceleration, belt force and SI time histories of test run V 41/75

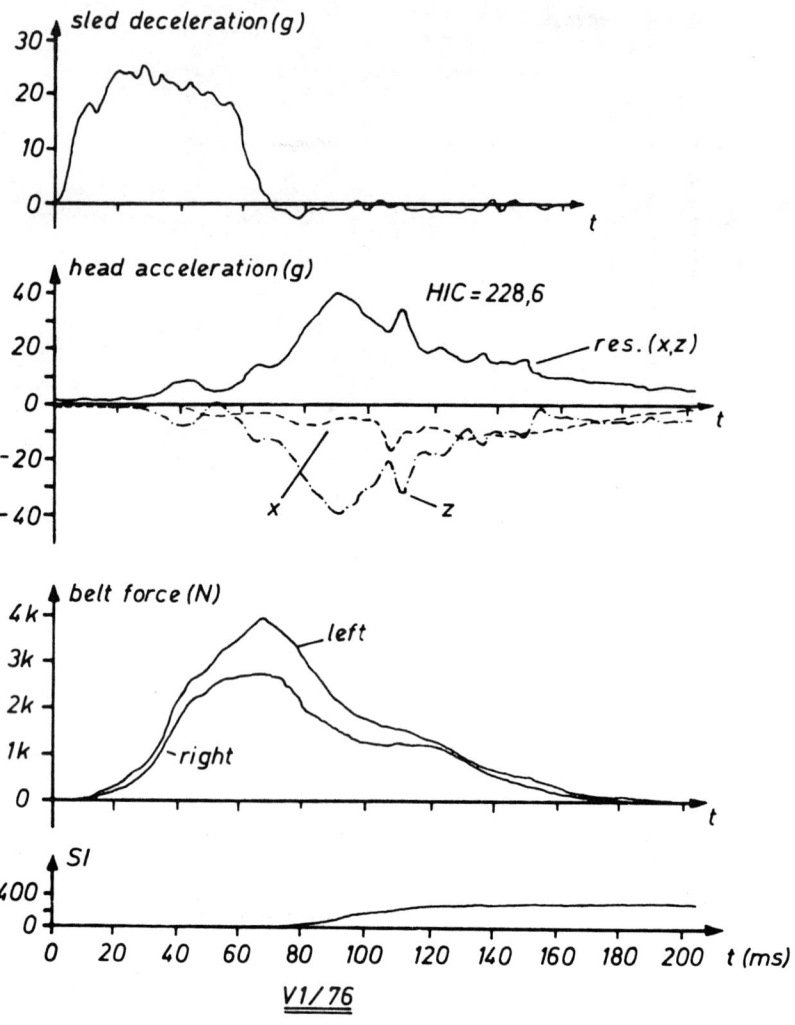

Fig. 7 - Sled deceleration, head acceleration, belt force and SI time histories of test run V 1/76

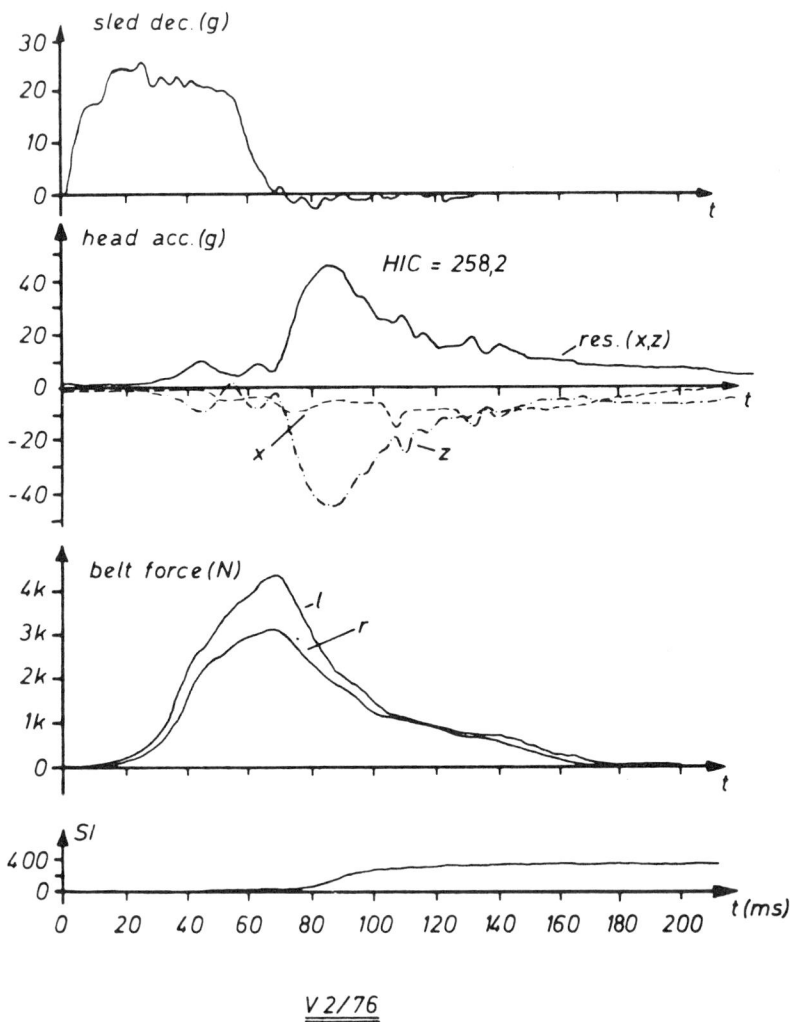

Fig. 8 - Sled deceleration, head acceleration, belt force and SI time histories of test run V 2/76

In test runs V 39/75 and V 41/75 we observed the maximum loads to be in accordance with the tested child cadavers of nearly the same body weight (30 kg and 31 kg) (Fig. 5-6). However, despite a lesser body weight of the dummy we observed higher maximum belt forces. Corresponding damages could be noted on the safety-table (Fig. 9a, 9b). A reason, on one hand, might be the stiffness of the dummy as against the elasticities of a child cadaver; on the other hand, a great part of the forces can be absorbed by propping the feet against the footrest (Fig. 13 - Cadaver). In the dummy test no use was made of the footrest.

Except for test V 36/75 we measured belt forces on the right and left side of the lap-belt; thereby, the belt force measured on the right side was always lower than the one on the left side. As it could be seen in the frontal frame of the high-speed camera the safety table and the corresponding lap-belt were more stronger loaded on the left side than on the right side.

The resultant deceleration at the center of gravity of the head is reached in about 70 to 110 ms after the beginning of impact and amounts 33,5 g and 94 g in cadavers of about the same weight but of different heights (124 cm and 139 cm) (V 39/75, V 41/75). As gathered from the optical evaluation the high value of 94 g was only reached because both upper arms touched the accelerometers. In the two dummy tests the resultant decelerations at the center of gravity in the head amount 40 g and 45,5 g. The computerized HIC and SI values varied like the resultant head decelerations.

Optical Evaluation - The kinematics of the body motion during the impact phase in a child cadaver test and a dummy test are described in a series of typical frames selected of lateral shots of a high-speed camera. Fig. 10 shows the body bearing of both the cadaver and the dummy at 2 ms prior to the impact. The head of the cadaver was strapped to keep it in an erect position; the strap was provided with a predetermined breaking point in order to influence the kinematics of the body motion as less as possible. Because of the dummy's stiffness was a seated position easily obtained. Twenty-eight ms after the impact both subjects were at first translatory moving forward whereas in the child cadaver a small rotating of the head around the lower cervical vertebral

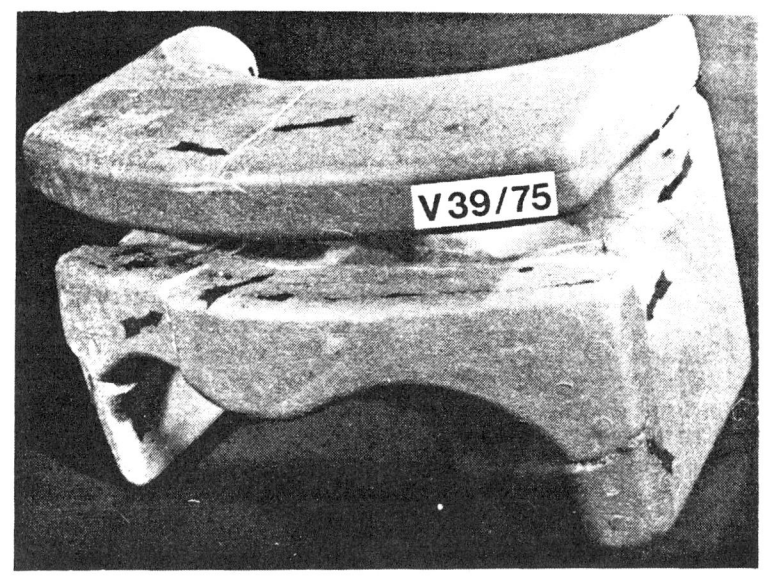

a. Test run V39/75

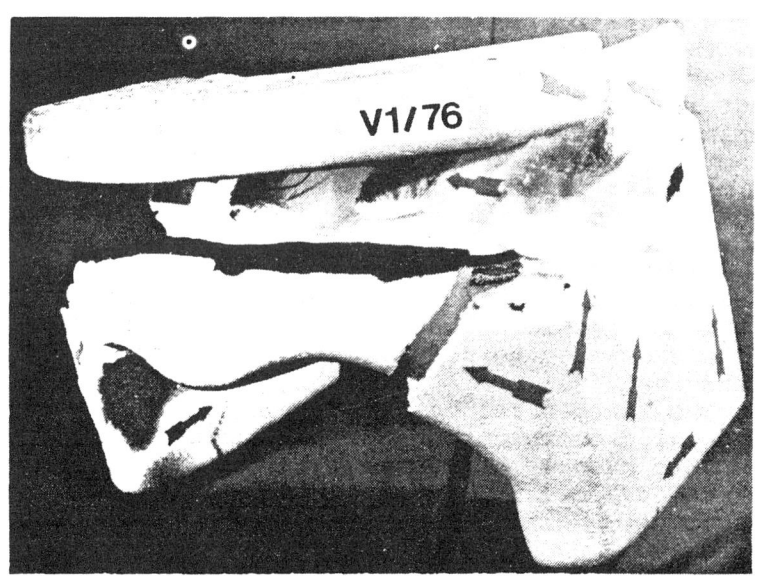

b. Test run V1/76

Fig. 9 - Damages to the safety table

column was seen. At this time the rotation of the tables and the increase of the belt load had already commenced in both tests (Fig. 11). A beginning of the rotation of the dummy's head and a rotation of the safety table in clockwise direction of about 40° was observed 56 ms after impact (Fig. 12). The rotation of the table at about 20° occurred in the cadaver test at the same time; the rotation of the cadaver's head was decelerated for about 5 ms as against the dummy.

The torso rotating around the safety table was clearly seen at 84 ms after the impact. The region of the thoracic and lumbar vertebral column remained extended in the dummy while in the cadaver a flexion at the transition of thoracic and lumbar vertebral column of about 50° was observed (Fig. 13). While the rotation of the safety table amounts about 45° in the cadaver test, it is about 75° in the dummy test. At this time, the course of the belt load in both tests is in the descending branch, the values of the resultant head deceleration approaching maximum. The following Fig. 14 shows the increasing flexion of the subjects around the safety table by reaching the maximum decelerations in the center of gravity of the head.

The maximum displacements of 62 cm in the cadaver and 67 cm in the dummy were reached in about 110 ms (Fig. 15). In the following Fig. 16 the largest displacement of the dummy's head in z-direction (about 32,5 cm) was observed at about 138 ms after impact. At this time, also the largest rotation of the safety tables of about 90° was reached in both tests.

Fig. 17 shows the secondary phase, the rebounding of the subjects 227 ms after the beginning of deceleration. A much stronger flexion of the cadaver's torso as against the dummy could be observed.

The kinematical behavior of a child cadaver and a child dummy during the impact phase has been more closely evaluated by a laterally mounted high-speed camera. The principle is the optical pursuit of single targets which are in dependence on the time. These targets are installed on the body surface and the safety table. The relative stability of the optical targets is here too an essential prerequisite. The moment of the crash is marked by flash-light, the time is recorded by a speed-constant time indicator installed in the field of view of the camera.

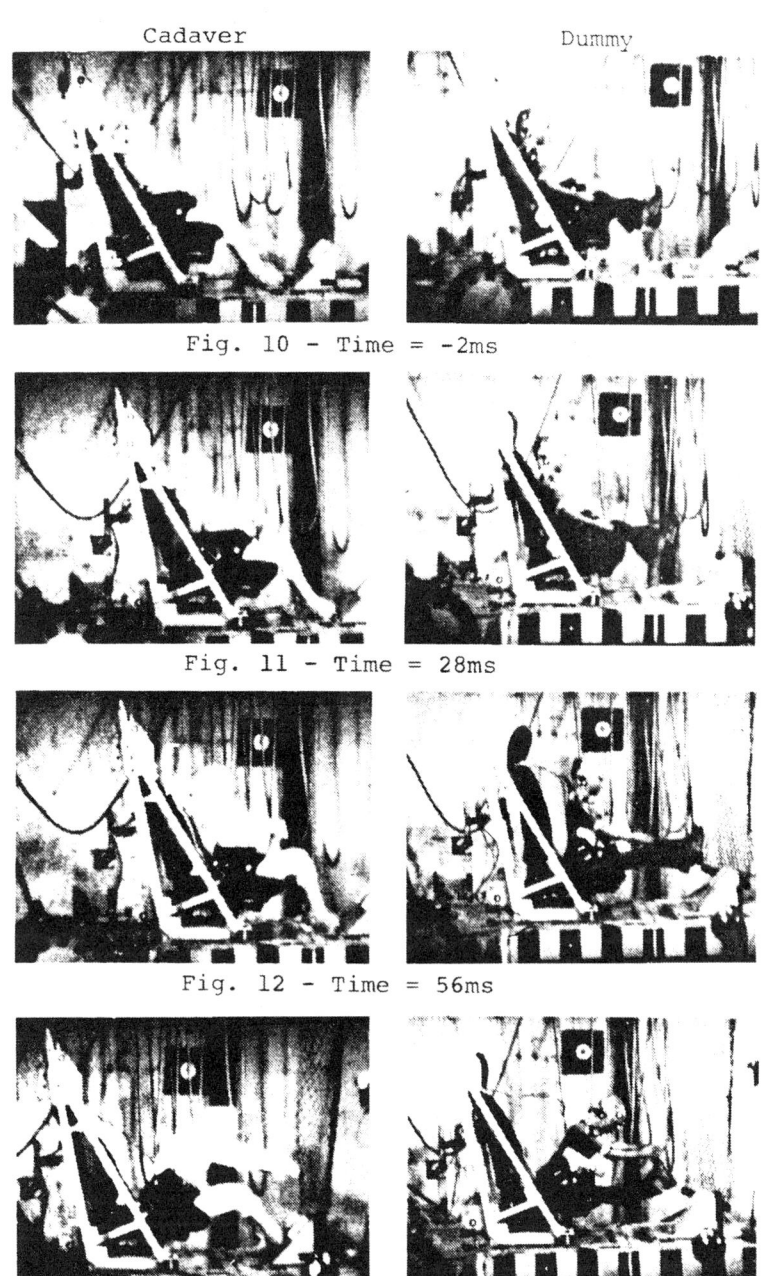

Fig. 10 - Time = -2ms

Fig. 11 - Time = 28ms

Fig. 12 - Time = 56ms

Fig. 13 - Time = 84ms

High speed cine frames

Cadaver　　　　　Dummy

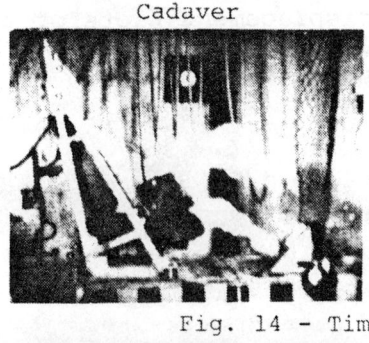

Fig. 14 - Time = 96ms

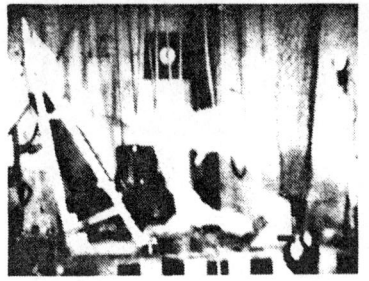 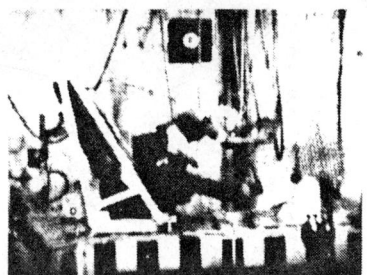

Fig. 15 - Time = 110ms

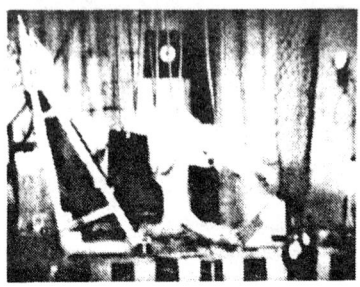 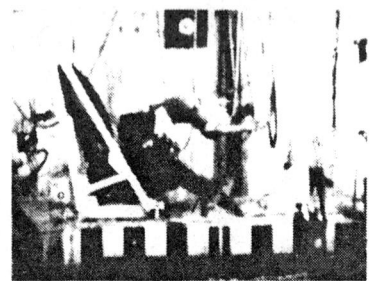

Fig. 16 - Time = 138ms

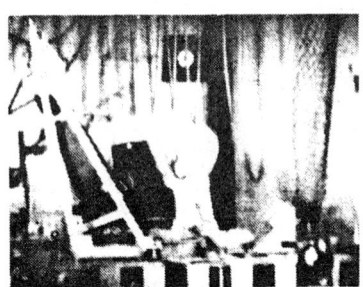 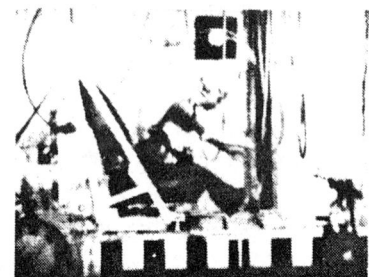

Fig. 17 - Time = 227ms

High speed cine frames

Fig. 18 shows the displacement plots of the targets which are installed on the cadaver and on the dummy to be observed in relation to each other and in relation to the sled-fixed axis S1/S2. Comparisons of the cadaver's respectively the safety table's targets among one another serve for the angle determination. Of interest is thereby the angle between head and upper cervical spine, the angle between head and entire cervical spine, the flexion at the transition of the cervical spine and the thorax; and, dependent on the system, the observed maximum flexion at the transition of the thoracic-lumbar vertebral column. No targets were installed on the pelvis and at the transition of the thoracic and lumbar vertebral column as this region was covered by the safety table.

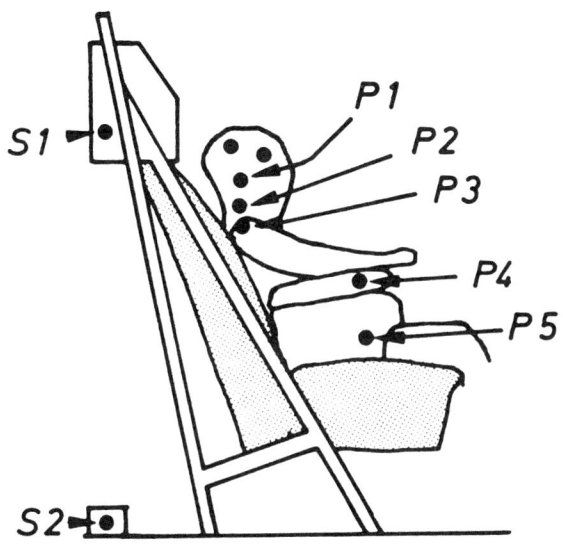

Fig. 18 - Locations of the optical targets

The high-speed films were evaluated by means of a motion analyzer combined with a Hewlett packard calculator and plotter by using a suitable computer program which contained corresponding mathematical filter functions. Thus, displacement plots, angle and angle velocities of the provided points on the subject have been calculated.

Fig. 19a and 19b show the displacement plots of both tests. The movement pattern of the marked body parts is on principle the same. It was noticed in the cadaver test (especially head-center, neck and safety table) that the transitional phase of the primary forward movement to the secondary backward movement was of longer duration than in the dummy test which showed a rather short-time turn. Although the sitting height of the dummy (64,5 cm) as against the sitting height of the cadaver (70 cm) was 5,5 cm smaller we observed larger head displacements in x- and z-direction in the dummy contrary to our experiences in adults (Kallieris et al (18). The forward movement of the cadaver was impeded with the feet standing on the footrest while this was not the case in the child dummy test because of its smaller body height. The deviation of the displacement plot of the shoulder target in z-direction in the cadaver as against the corresponding target in the dummy may be given as a reason for the movability of the targets on the clothing. The larger displacement of the shoulder target in the cadaver as against the dummy results from the own shoulder movement while the hands are tossed forward.

The following figures 20, 21 and 22 show the angles of the axes P1/P3, P2/P3, P1/P2 and P4/P5 as against the sled-fixed axis S1/S2 in dependence on the time; thereby, at the time of impact the angles were equal to zero. After a translatory displacement of the optical targets we noticed the flexion angle always commencing earlier in the dummy test than in the cadaver test, also showing a more gradient increase; therefore, angle maxima are sooner reached in the dummy than in the cadaver. Beside the time difference we observed about the same maxima flexion angles of the axes P1/P3 and P4/P5 corresponding to 136° and 90° in the dummy and cadaver. While in the dummy the axis P2/P3 reached the maximum of 134° in 130 ms, we still noticed a further increase of the corresponding angle at 190 ms in the cadaver. The maximum flexion angle of the axis P1/P2 amounted 138° in the dummy and was reached 140 ms after impact, while it amounted 153° in the cadaver and was reached 160ms after impact.

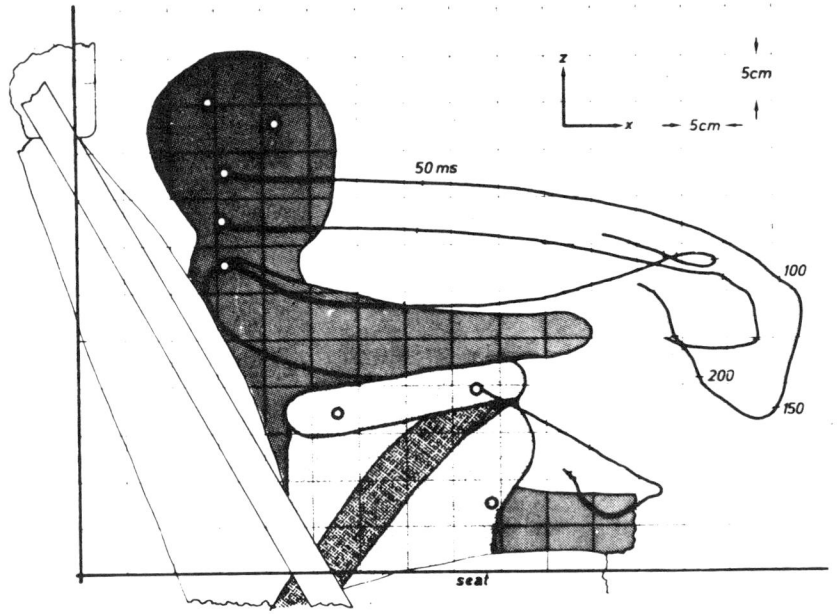

a. Cadaver

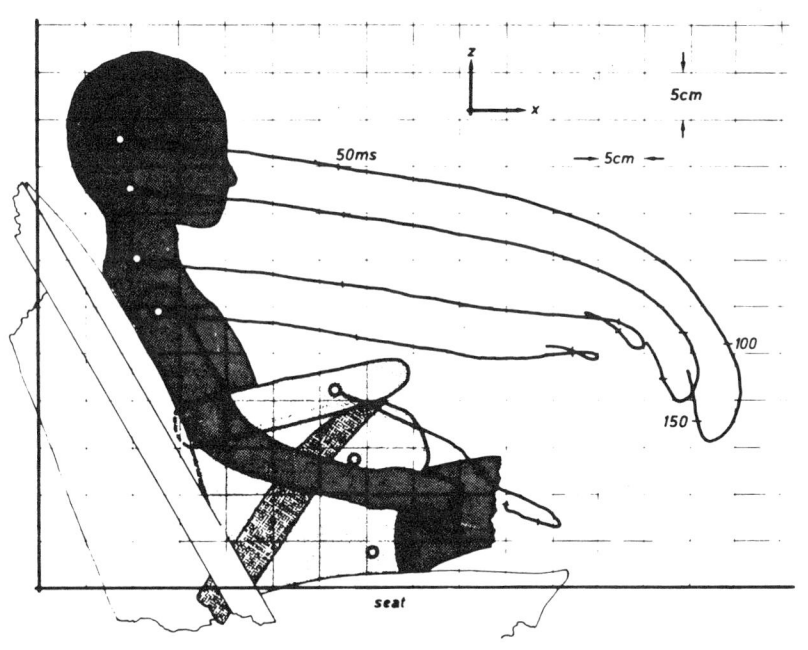

b. Dummy

Fig. 19 - Displacement plots of the photographic targets, mounted on the head, neck, shoulder and safety-table

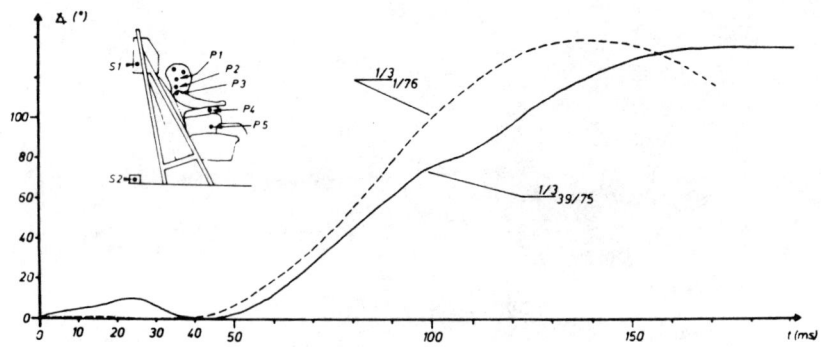

Fig. 20 - Angle time history of the axis P1/P3 against the sled-fixed axis S1/S2 (V39/75 cadaver, V1/76 dummy)

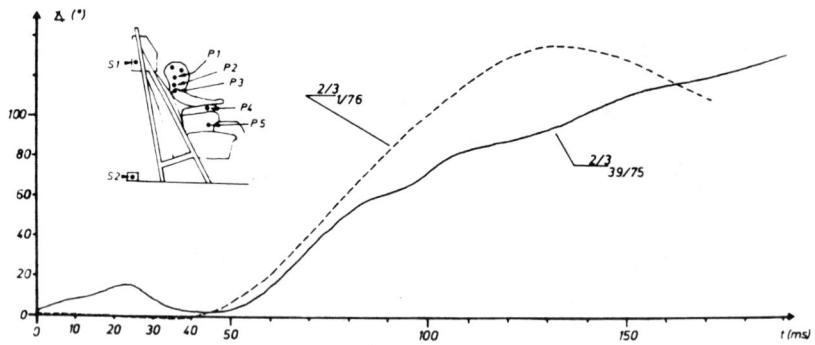

Fig. 21 - Angle time history of the axis P2/P3 against the sled-fixed axis S1/S2 (V39/75 cadaver, V1/76 dummy)

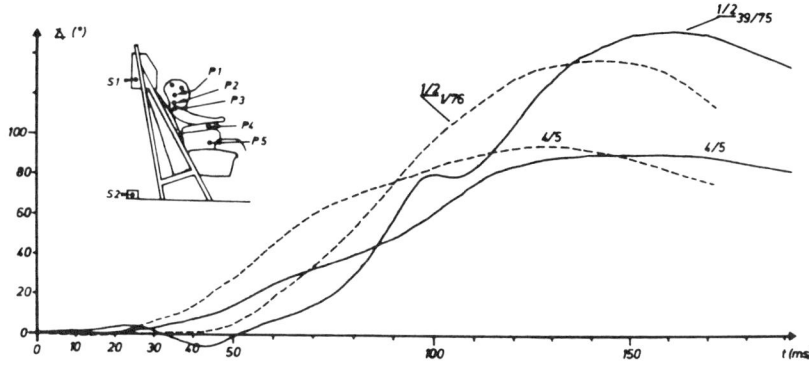

Fig. 22 - Angle time history of the axes P1/P2, P4/P5 against the sled-fixed axis S1/S2 (V39/75 cadaver, V1/76 dummy)

Fig. 23, 24 and 25 show the angular velocity time history of the axes P1/P3, P2/P3, P1/P2 and P4/P5 as against the sled-fixed axis S1/S2 of both impact tests. In the dummy test we obtained maxima of 39 to 43rad/s in the time between 73 ms and 88 ms showing a symmetrical course in all axes. The angular velocity time history in the cadaver test always showed two maxima in the axes P1/P3 and P2/P3 lying before and after as well as below the dummy maxima. Two maxima of the axis P1/P2 in the cadaver test are above the dummy test maxima whereas the first maximum in test V 39/75 (cadaver) was reached about 3 ms later than in the test V 1/76 (dummy).

Injuries - In the medical examination we found no visible injuries on the body surface of the four child cadavers. The brain as well as thoracic and abdominal organs were also uninjured. Fractures of ribs and pelvis as well as fractures of the spinal column and the extremities did not occur. Only the muscular and the ligamentous system of the spinal column showed minor injuries in three of the four examined cadavers. In test run V 38/75 the diagnosis was aggravated because of an advanced sepsis; therefore, the lacking of visible injuries does not allow the conclusion that no injuries at all occurred. The certainly

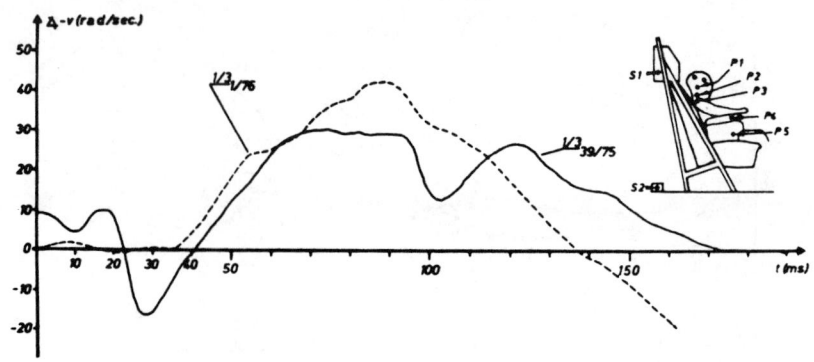

Fig. 23 - Angular velocity time history of the axis P1/P3 against the sled-fixed axis S1/S2 (V 39/75 cadaver, V 1/76 dummy)

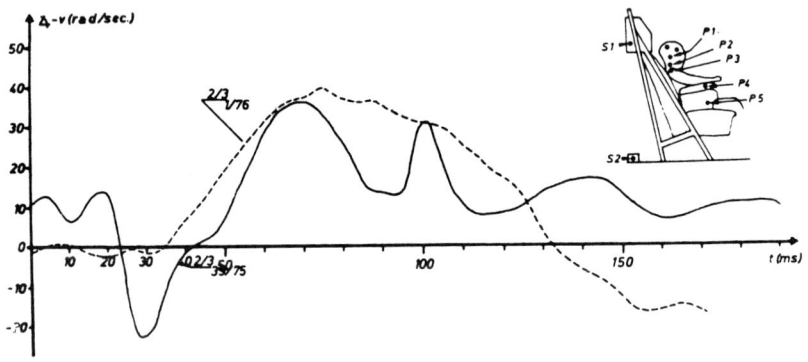

Fig. 24 - Angular velocity time history of the axis P2/P3 against the sled-fixed axis S1/S2 (V 39/75 cadaver, V 1/76 dummy)

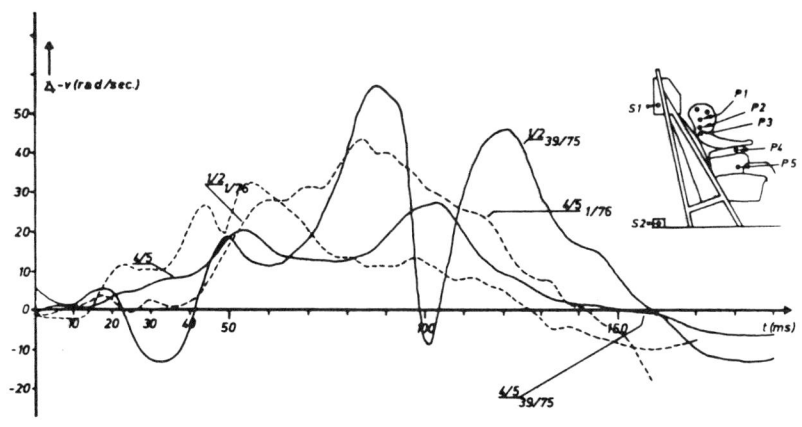

Fig. 25 - Angular velocity time history of the axes P1/P2 and P4/P5 against the sled-fixed axis S1/S2 (V 39/75 cadaver, V 1/76 dummy)

usable injury findings of test runs V 36/75, V 39/75, V 41/75 can be classified in the severity degrees I and II (Kallieris et al (18).

Following injuries were found:

Test run V 36/75:
Preparation findings:

Right side:	Membrana atlanto-axialis covered with blood; interspinal hemorrhage of Th 4/5
Left side:	Hemorrhage of 0,5 cm in the beginning of musculus obliquus capitis superior
At both sides:	Two hemorrhages of 0,5 cm each in the medium muscular layer in the height of L4 (2 cm of the processus spinosus' center)
Saw findings:	No pathological findings in one of the three sectional planes

Test run V 38/75:

Preparation findings:	Muscular system to a great extent autolytically changed; no findings
Saw findings:	No pathological findings

Test run V 39/75:

Preparation findings:

Right side:	Between C7/Th1 on the musculus serratus posterior superior a hemorrhage of 1 x 1 cm
At both sides:	On the level of Th11 to L4 striped hemorrhages in the medium muscular layer, size 4 x 2 cm (2 cm of the processus spinosus center)

Saw findings:

Median cut:	Epidural hemorrhage (thickness 0,3 cm) of C7 to L4
Left side cut:	Hemorrhages in the foramina intervertebralia of C6/7, C7/Th1
Right side cut:	Hemorrhages on the foramina intervertebralia of C1/2, C2/3, Th9/10, Th10/11, Th11/12, Th12/L1

Test run V 41/75:

Preparation findings:

Right side:	Interspinal hemorrhages of C7/Th1, Th1/2, Th2/3, Th3/4. Between Th8 to L4: Eight hemorrhages of 0,2 cm to 0,5 cm in the medium muscular layer
Left side:	In the beginning of musculus rectus capitis posterior minor and obliquus capitis superior was a hemorrhage of about 0,5cm. Hemorrhages of the multifidi (medium muscular layer) of C7 to Th8. Three 0,5 cm hemorrhages in the

Saw findings:

Median cut: Laceration of intervertebral disc No. 4 at the lower neck edge (0,4cm). Epidural hemorrhage of Cl to Thl and of Th9 to L5 (0,3-0,5 cm) range L2 to L4 directly above the processus mamillaria

Left side cut: Increased hemorrhages continuing in the foramina intervertebralia of the entire cervical spine as well as in the Th12, L1/2, L2/3, L3/4

Right side cut: Also continued hemorrhages around the spinal cord into the foramina intervertebralia of Th3/4, Th4/5, Th5/6, Th10/11, Th11/12, Th12/L1 and into all foramina intervertebralia of the cervical spine

In the cadaver and dummy tests induced the applied system (semi-cylindrically shaped safety-table combined with a lap-belt) after a translatory initial phase a rotation around the body axis also involving the safety table. The displacement plots of head, neck and shoulder were on principle similar in dummy and cadaver. However, the differences are significant where injuries could be determined in the medically examined cadavers, especially to the vertebral column. Contrary to the infantile vertebral column which shows a relatively great movability in all segments remains the thoracic and lumbar vertebral column rigid in the dummy. Flexions are therefore displaced to the hip or the cervical spine. Corresponding to it did we observe flexions not worth mentioning during the evaluation of the motional behavior of the vertebral column. In the child cadavers flexion angles up to 90° were noticed in the thoracic-lumbar transition.

Injuries to the cervical spine caused by a strong flexion of the head as well as injuries of the thoracic-lumbar transition could be expected and were confirmed in our tests.

In utilizing the same impact velocity (Schmidt et al (15) a significantly smaller injury degree follows from the comparison with vertebral column injuries in adult cadaver tests (3-point automatic belts). This can be attributed to the greater elastical deformability of the infantile body. A further factor might be the plastic qualities of the safety table. Both prerequisites lead to an extension of the stopping distance. The plastic qualities of the safety table proved to be a desirable factor in the course of the deceleration kinematic. Moreover, the belt load was decisively diminished because of the large table surface; we observed in our tests no injuries to inner organs of the lower thorax and the upper abdominal region. The threshold of injuries is an impact velocity of 40 km/h; therefore it can be assumed that this restraint system offers a sufficient protection up to this velocity.

CONCLUSIONS

The four child cadaver and two dummy tests lead to following conclusions:
The child cadaver and child dummy kinematic is similar during the frontal impact. Also the belt load time history as well as the course of the resultant head decelerations correspond to a great extent. Depsite of a lower dummy weight we measured higher force maxima than in the cadaver. Significant differences could be observed in the flexion behavior of the vertebral column. The dummy is therefore suited for preliminary examinations of child safety devices, however, child cadaver tests are indispensable for the investigation of the tolerance limit. In the investigated system the tolerance limit was reached using an impact velocity of 40 km/h. Emphasis is given to a satisfactory attribute of the system, namely the large-sized influence of the semi-cylindrically shaped safety table which causes a lower compressive load on the abdominal region and thus protects the inner organs.

ACKNOWLEDGMENT

We want to thank the Volkswagenwerk AG for the technical assistance and the Daimler Benz AG supporting the film evaluations.

REFERENCES

1. V.L.Roberts and J.H.McElhaney, "Dynamic Performance of Child Seating Systems." Paper 720971 Proceedings of the 16th Stapp Car Crash Conference, Detroit, Michigan, 1972.

2. R.L.Stalnaker and J.W.Melvin, "Evaluation of Current Production and Prototype Child Restraint Systems in the USA." Proceedings of the International Meeting on Biomechanics of Trauma in Children, Lyon, France, 1974. Publ. by IRCOBI.

3. E.R.Dye, "Automobile Crash Protection for Children." Passenger Car Design and Highway Safety, 1962.

4. B. Aldman, "A Protective Seat for Children" Proceedings of the 8th Stapp Car Crash Conference, Detroit, Wayne State University Press, 1966.

5. F.A.Appoldt, "Dynamic Tests of Restraints for Children." Proceedings of the 8th Stapp Car Crash Conference, Detroit, Wayne State University Press, 1966.

6. A.W.Siegel, A.M.Nahum and M.R.Appleby, "Injuries to Children in Automobile Collisions." SAE Transactions Vol. 77, 1968.

7. DIN 4849, "Kindersicherungseinrichtungen in Kraftfahrzeugen."

8. British Standard BS AU 157, "Children's restraining devices, April 1973.

9. Revised Version of MVss 213, "Child restraint standard." Draft, 1 March 1974.

10. ECE Draft, June 73, Draft Regulation, "Restraining devices for child occupants."

11. D.C.Herbert, B.A.Vazey, J.M.Wyllie, R.G.Vaughan and V.Leitis, "Evaluation of Australian Child Restraints." Proceedings of the 17th Stapp Car Crash Conference, Oklahoma City, Oklahoma, 1973.

12. R.L.Lowne, "Injuries to Children involved in Road Accidents." Proceedings of the International Meeting on Biomechanics of Trauma in Children. Lyon, France, 1974. Publ. by IRCOBI.

13. R.M.Schreck and L.M.Patrick, "Frontal Crash Evaluation Tests of a Five-Point Harness Child Restraint." Proceedings of the 19th Stapp Car Crash Conference, San Diego, Cal., 1975.

14. D.Kallieris,"Eine Fallgewichtsbeschleunigungsanlage zur Simulation von Aufprallunfällen." Prinzip und Arbeitsweise. Z. Rechtsmedizin 74, 25 (1974).

15. G.Schmidt, D.Kallieris, J.Barz, R.Mattern and J.Klaiber, "Neck and Thorax Tolerance Levels of Belt-Protected Occupants in Head-On Collisions" Proceedings of the 19th Stapp Car Crash Conference San Diego, California, 1975.

16. G.Schmidt, D.Kallieris,J.Barz and R.Mattern, "Results of 49 Cadaver Tests Simulating frontal Collisions of Front Seat Passengers." Proceedings of the 18th Stapp Car Crash Conference, Warrendale, Penns., 1974.

17. L.B.Walker, E.H.Harris and U.R.Pontius, "Mass, Volume, Center of Mass and Mass Moment of Inertia of Head and Head and Neck of Human Body." Proceedings of the 17th Stapp Car Crash Conference Oklahoma, Oklahoma City, 1973.

18. D.Kallieris, B.Meister and G.Schmidt, "Reactions observed of the cervical spine during frontal crashes of belt protected cadavers." Proceedings of the 2nd International Conference on Biomechanics of Serious Trauma, Birmingham, 1975, Publ. by IRCOBI.

801313

Biomechanical Data of Children

G. Stürtz
Daimler-Benz AG

IN THE PAST YEARS the main point of research in the field of passive safety was to reduce accident consequences for adult occupants of passenger cars. The increasing efficiency of adult passenger restraint systems favoured by a rising belt-wearing quota have been supplemented by numerous measures for the interior safety of motor cars. This makes it necessary in the framework of solutions with high use/cost-value, to include those for exterior safety to a greater extent. Due to its rising share in traffic accidents, the group of "children" is becoming more and more important.

Since there seem to be important differences when comparing children with adults, we need specific knowledge of the relevant anthropometry and biomechanical loading capacity of children, not only for the protection of children as car occupants, but also for an efficient layout of vehicle exteriors to protect children and persons from 15 years of age on, for instance as pedestrians.

The main objective of this study is therefore the investigation, collection, and discussion of biomechanical-relevant anthropometric and development characteristics as well as biomechanical load limits by using different methods. Additional tendencies of the biomechanical loading capacity of children's bodies are shown also. This is supplemented by the definition of injury and protection criteria against irreversible injuries.

When talking about "critical load values" in the following, the load on the body is that under which an initial considerable damage of the organism takes place - destruction of a cell; irreversible injury - for instance, when bone fractures occur or primary organs rupture.

When talking about "protection criteria", the load - up to strain or compression damage of a cell; reversible injury - is meant which statistically lies well beneath the level of critical load values, i.e. which will cause no irreversible injuries at all or only to a very

---
ABSTRACT

Up till now, biomechanical data have been determined mostly for older adults. Only few results are known for middle-aged persons and almost nothing is known about biomechanical levels of the injury tolerance of children. The limited knowledge of biomechanical data of children is contrary to the increasing need for an efficient layout of exterior vehicle elements as well as restraint systems. Therefore, the following methods were used to find out biomechanical load limits as well as tendencies of the loading capacity of children:
- extensive research of medical/technical literature has given results concerning the overall organism, body tissue, head, thorax, abdomen, pelvis, and lower extremities.
- mechanics of similitude have given results for the head region. (Data Scaling)
- analysis of real pedestrian accidents has given results for the head region and lower extremities.
- repetition tests of real traffic accidents using modified anthropometric dummies have given results for the head, neck, thorax, abdomen, pelvis, and lower extremities.

Based on these results, biomechanical critical load values as well as protection criteria will be given with regard to frontal/dorsal as well as lateral/medial body load directions.

This paper was worked out at the Technical University Berlin.

small percentage. The level of the "protection criteria" is dependent on whether they refer to living human beings (injury criteria) or to loadings measured on a dummy (protection criteria).

EVALUATION OF LITERATURE

According to Faerber (1)* only a limited amount of knowledge of the biomechanical loadability of the human body has been found, and this knowledge is almost exclusively limited to the age group adults. For children such data are either nearly non-existent or can only be found in form of tendencies of the biomechanical loadability (2).

For several years a literary research was carried out concerning this topic (3). Out of the literature sections found, 21 have been selected which contain data with regard to load characteristic values and which are also of relevance in the field of passive safety. These biomechanical data were exclusively obtained through post mortem tests and accident simulation (scaling from adult data). In one publication, data are estimated with the aid of animal tests. The biomechanical data are supplemented by qualitative statements which refer for instance to age-dependent tendencies of the biomechanical loadability of the human body and also to typical anthropometric development characteristics of the child.

The results of the literature study with their characteristic values are shown in Fig. 1 to 4 containing information for the following body regions:
- overall organism
- body tissue/skin, arteries
- head region/skull, brain
- thorax/ribs
- abdomen/general, intestines, liver, spleen
- pelvis, urogenital region
- lower extremities/femur, tibia

Wherever the study was similarily carried out for different age groups, the load characteristic values of the other age groups are also stated as a supplement.

In general, it should be mentioned that the number of test objects ranged from n = 1 to 48 with 10 as an average, but for half of the cases it was only 5, i.e. a number of statements must be considered as not proven based upon their total number of cases. The abbreviations used for test objects employed in the figures have the following meaning:

lav living, accident victim
pwb postmortem, whole body
pbp postmortem, body parts
lwa living, whole body of animals

The abbreviations used e.g. for load characteristic values in the figures have the following meaning:

+x, +y, +z loading direction related to the overall body in standing upright position:
frontal - dorsal (x)
lateral - medial (y)
caudal - cranial (z)

a_{max} maximum acceleration

a_e effective or average acceleration

t   acceleration time

HIC   Head Injury Criterion

F_B ultimate load

M_B ultimate moment

$\sigma_{B,R}$ ultimate stress, breaking strength

τ_B ultimate shear strength

δ_R strain limit

p   unit pressure (also above normal pressure (*))

E_B fracture energy

A   cross-sectional area

z,d,b,t   indices for tension, thrust, bending, torsion

OVERALL ORGANISM - The only statement made with regard to the loadability of the overall organism of children (4), Fig. 1, cannot be used because of the estimation of the real load value contained therein when reconstructing accidents. According to Yamada (5), the tendency is a decreasing loadability of the whole organism the younger the children are, or when considering adults, the older they are. Persons around the age of 20 show the highest loadability.

BODY TISSUE SKIN, ARTERIES

Skin - The average breaking strength of the skin (6) with children up to the age of 10 is $\sigma_R = 10.8$ Nmm^{-2} and is thus lower than that of adults. The test area with the lowest breaking strength is the scalp of children ($\sigma_R = 38$ Nmm^{-2}). In contrast to the breaking strength, the strain limit of children's skin is with $\delta_R = 47\%$ essentially higher than that of adults.

From birth to the age of 35 the thickness of the skin doubles, but starts decreasing with further age (7).

Arteries - The average breaking strength of artery tissue of children

---

* Numbers in parentheses designate References at end of paper.

body-region part	Lit. No:	object	type of loading, remarks	n (/)	load direction	a_{max} (g)	a_e (g)	t (ms)	HIC	σ_R (Nmm^{-2})	δ_R (%)
overall organism	(4)	lav	reconstructed falls of children without death	5		36-160		20-6			
body-tissue /skin	(6)	pbp	quasistatic tensile test with stripes of skin of 10 cm lenght, 1 cm width and same thickness								
			children until 10 y, pilose head skin	6	±y					3.8	
			" neck	6	±z					6.3	
			" chest	6	±z					12.1	
			" abdomen	6	±z					11.8	
			" back	6	±z					15.1	
			" bottom	6	±z					13.4	
			" upper arm	6	±z					13.7	
			" lower arm	6	±z					11.5	
			" thight	6	±z					9.0	
			" shank	6	±z					11.1	
			children until 3 y, general	6	approx. ±z					7.4±1.6	47
			children until 10 y, general	6	approx. ±z					10.8	
			(pers.15 until 50 y, general)	44	approx. ±z					15.8±0.8	34.3
			(pers. over 50 y, general)	71	approx. ±z					20.1±1.1	30.5
/artery tissue general (neck arteries)	(5)	pbp	quasistatic tensile test								
			children 0-9 years	8	longit. and					1.3(1.5)	88(129)
			children and adulescens (10-19 years)	8	transvers.					1.2(1.5)	114(129)
			(average adult)	8	average					0.9(1.1)	81(86)
head region /skull	(9)	lav	estimated tolerable values for children of 3-6 years by mechanics of similitude at the child's skull		±x	44-74		8.2-7.7			
					±y	37-58		6.0-5.6			
/skull + brain	(11)	lav	reconstructed falls of children under 8 years, brain injuries AIS 2	5	-z	350-400		3	1700-2800		
			" " " AIS 5	1	-z	600	350	2.5-3.0	11000		

Fig. 1 - Biomechanical load limits of the whole body, body tissue as well as head region

up to 9 years is $\sigma_R = 1.3$ Nmm^{-2} and thus higher than the corresponding values for adults. However the strain limit with $\delta_R = 88$ % is only slightly higher (5). On the whole the neck artery has the highest breaking strength with $\sigma_R = 1.5$ Nmm^{-2} and a strain limit of $\delta_R = 129$ % and is thus significantly above the corresponding values for adults.

General - The considerably higher neck/trunk mass relationship of children, which for example is 3.9 times higher with a three-year-old child than with an adult, causes a far higher specific load of the neck region (danger of hyperflexion). The ossification of children's neck is only completed at the age of 6 to 7 (8), (9).

HEAD REGION / SKULL, BRAIN

Skull - The limits of direct loading of the skulls of children were established through estimations by mechanics of similitude (9) and are therefore too uncertain to be used as absolute values. Nevertheless, they show the tendency of a slighter loadability as compared to adults. Moreover, the fontanelles of the skull have closed only by the age of 2 to 3 years and the ossification of the skull is only finished by the age of 6 to 7 years.

The higher elasticity of children's skulls up to the point of fracture is especially detrimental. The consequence can be brain contusions sometimes in connection with impression fractures (8).

In comparison to adults the child has a relatively smaller face and a proportionately larger skull (10).

Skull, Brain - The load values of the skull/brain-region of children, found when reconstructing accidents (11), must still be considered uncertain because of the estimations contained therein.

The hypophysis with children lies in a zone neutral to vibrations and is therefore - contrary to adults - especially protected against impact traumas. When a child's skull suffers a blow, we have a summation of effects; on one hand osseous vibration mechanisms propagate to the dura and subdural region and thus to the brain. On the other hand, mass shifts of the child's brain occur which result in an intracranial drop in pressure and are decisive for the effect of the respective impact force. The spatial extension of the "Contre-Coup" center is an expression of the seriousness of the damage (12).

THORAX / RIBS - The breaking load for dynamic bending of the 6th as well as the 7th rib of children under the age of 14, see Fig. 2, is on the average 234 N with a rib compact unit area of 15.5 mm^2 and an absorption of work up to the point of fracture of 7.5 Nm (13). However, the value of 7.5 Nm was calculated too high, as this value was equated with the kinetic energy of the

body-region part	Lit. No.	object	type of loading, remarks	n (/)	load direct.	F_B (N)	t (ms)	p (Nmm^{-2})	σ_R (Nmm^{-2})	ϵ_R, δ_R (Nm; %)
ribs	(13)	pbp	quasistatic bending load of the 6th and 7th rib, children ≤ 14 years	3	±x	F_B=240 196-294				
			dynamic bending load of the 6th and 7th rib with 40-45 kg children ≤ 14 years, v=2.9 m/s	17	±x	196-471 F_B=234	approx.2			(7.5)
			(persons 15 - 64 years, v=2.0 m/s)	65	±x	F_B=372	approx.2			(3.7)
			(persons ≥ 65 years, v=1.7 m/s)	31	±x	F_B=173	approx.2			(2.8)
small intesti. (large intest.)	(5)	pbp	quasistatic tensile load children 0 - 9 years	7	longit. and trans- versal average				0.96 (1.08)	δ_R 74 (126)
			children and adolescens 10 - 19 years	7					0.86 (0.94)	149 (175)
			(average adult)	7					0.57 (0.56)	66 (126)
liver	(14)	pbp	quasistatic compression load child 10 years, first ruptures	1	appr.±x	2649		0.24		
		"	" , multiple ruptures	1	appr.±x	3414		0.15		
			(persons ≥ 15 years, first ruptures)	10	appr.±x	1554		0.15		
			(" , multiple ruptures)	10	appr.±x	3110		0.16		
spleen	(15)	pbp	quasistatic compression load child 10 years, first ruptures	1	appr.±x	785		0.16		
		"	" , multiple ruptures	1	appr.±x	981		0.17		
			(persons ≥ 15 years, first ruptures)	8	appr.±x	388		0.07		
			(" , multiple ruptures)	8	appr.±	844		0.15		
abdomen overall	(17)	pwb	dynamic loading of the abdominal region by mass diversion over great surface deformable table, children 2 - 11 years injuries of the muscles and ligaments of the vertebrea (AIS 2)	4	-x	F_{Bmax} 5700- 6600	70			
	(16)	lwa	dynamic loading of the abdominal region of "mini pigs" by a unelastic rear spoiler (AIS 3), transferred to children of 8 - 12 years	12	-x	981	20			
pelvis/ uro-genital region	(19)	lav	dynamic frontal accidental loading by a lap belt, children of 7 - 12 years, no contact injuries occured ($\bar{a}_{Hip}$ = 15 - 40 g)	3	-x	F_B=6013 -8907	0.52-0.90			

Fig. 2 - Biomechanical load limits of the thorax as well as abdomen

test body prior to the load phase without e.g. subtracting the remaining energy of the test body after the end of the fracture in every individual case. If it is assumed a mean yielding of 15 to 20 mm up to the point when the fracture begins, as it was stated in a few cases for the age group up to 14 years, then the average absorption of work up to the point of fracture is approx. 3.5 to 4.7 Nm.

In the case of a blunt frontal load to a child's thorax the overall break load of the 1st to 7th rib, with assumed equal clamp conditions can be reckoned to be 1.6 kN. Proceeding from the always constant distance of the two rib supports of 80 mm, the mean ultimate bending moment of every single rib can be calculated to be $\bar{M}_{bB}$ = 4.7 Nm.

A large part of the child's skeleton (especially in infancy) still consists of cartilage which has less strength but higher flexibility when compared with bones (8). This means that although fractures are rarer and increased compression loads to inner organs occur. When compared with adults, the child's thorax has a proportionately larger heart (10). Likewise, the child's trunk is proportionately larger than that of adults. The result is that the center of gravity of a child's body is situated relatively higher than in adults. That means that on one hand, a larger part of the body lies above the lap belt for instance, and on the other hand, a rotation - also a shift to the front - of the upper trunk around a possible diagonal shoulder belt is favoured.

ABDOMEN / INTESTINES, LIVER, SPLEEN, GENERAL

Small and Large Intestine - With children up to the age of 9, the breaking strength of the small and large intestine under quasistatic load is on the average σ_R = 0.96 to 1.08 Nmm^{-2}. The strain limit is δ_R = 74 to 126 % (5). Thus the breaking strength is 50 to 55 % above the corresponding values for adults but the strain limit is almost on the same level.

Liver, Spleen, General - The loadability limit of liver and spleen is higher with a ten-year-old child than with persons from 15 years of age on (14), (16), (17).

In postmortem tests, a frontal dynamic load applied to a large contact area of the abdominal region of four children aged 2 to 11 which resulted in no injuries of the abdominal region (17) with maximum resulting forces of

5700 to 6600 N in a retaining belt of an abdominal cushion. If the dynamical belt angle is assumed to be 35 to 45 degrees from the horizontal line, the horizontal maximum load results in 4000 to 5400 N. For a period of time exceeding 20 ms, the resulting horizontal reaction force was not higher than 2800 to 3800 N. The resulting injuries (of AIS 1 - 2) were distributed over the entire vertebrae with regard to muscles and ligaments, whereby vertebrae bending angles of 85 to 95 degrees (!) were determined between thorax and lumber region.

The abdominal region with children is proportionately larger and protrudes considerably (18). This is due to the relatively small costal arch and pelvis in connection with the less-developed abdominal muscles, the lordosis of the lumbar vertebrae, as well as the thick subcutaneous tissue. Abdominal organs, such as the liver for instance, which in infants takes up two fifths of the abdomen, is not protected by the costal arch as is the case with adults. The same applied to the urinary bladder which with children does not lie in the area of the pelvic bones.

PELVIS / UROGENITAL REGION - In reconstructions of dynamic-frontal loads of three children in the age group of 7 to 12 years, no contact injuries were found (19). These children were protected by lap belts. However a mean belt strength of 6012 to 8907 N was estimated through the acceleration of vehicle passenger compartment, and a "mean unit pressure" of 0.52 to 0.90 Nmm^{-2} was present. However, in the real cases, the lap belt will certainly load to a great extent the pelvic bones, thereby causing an unit pressure of the urogenital region beneath 0.52 Nmm^{-2} above normal pressure.

With children the pelvis is relatively soft and small and up to the age of 10 no ilias-spies have yet developed (18). The rounded pelvis palms, together with the thick subcutaneous tissue, cause a negative submarining effect of the child's pelvis under a lap belt. This is only partly compensated by the lordosis of the lumbar vertebrae of children.

LOWER EXTREMITIES / FEMUR, TIBIA

The source of the investigated specimens with regard to the lower extremities was defined as taken from (fresh) autopsy (22, 23, 25, 31) for example from normal healthy subjects (21). They were mostly killed in accidents (20, 28, 30) without being bedridden for a long time, that is to say, without having pathological bone alterations (30).

Femur - The ultimate stress measured under a quasistatic load to children's femurs is, when bending, between 150 and 207 Nmm^{-2} or, when tension is being applied, between 55 and 102 Nmm^{-2} for children up to the age of 13 (20), (21), Fig. 3. The ultimate bending moment was found to be 52 Nm for a 2,5-year-old child in (22) and 210 Nm for a 13-year-old child by calculations using the respective resistance moment of the bone compact area.

Proceeding from the method mentioned with Martin (21) and the data of other publications (20), (22), the quasistatic ultimate bending moment of children's femurs is calculated as follows.
Children:
7,0 years (approx. 50 % child pedestrian)
M_{bB} = 97 - 109 Nm
3,6 years (approx. 5 % pedestrians)
M_{bB} = 52 - 61 Nm

According to Asang (24), the dynamic bending load limit of the tibia with a pulse time duration of 10 ms is approx. 20 % higher than the quasistatic load limit. Transferring this to the femur, the dynamic ultimate bending moment
- <u>dynamic femur fracture criteria</u> -
is calculated to be 116 - 131 Nm (7-year-old child, femur outer diameter d_{Fa} = 19 mm) or 62 - 73 Nm (3,6-year-old child, d_{Fa} = 16.5 mm). Correspondingly the dynamic femur fracture criterion with adults is calculated to be 1100 - 1320 Nm (95 % pedestrians, body height 175 cm, d_{Fa} = 40 mm).

When dynamic axial load is applied to the infant femur, the epiphysical plane of the growing femoral head and neck constitute a considerable weak point. For loads applied above the knee region in the direction of the hip joint and almost axial to the femur, the quasistatic fracture limit is calculated based upon the quasistatic ultimate stresses of the femur head-epiphysical plane found with Stanley (25), as well as from statements also found in it.
Children:
6,0 years (approx. 50 % child passenger)
F_{dB} = 1550 N
3,0 years (infant as passenger)
F_{dB} = 870 N

If the relation of dynamical to quasistatic ultimate stress is assumed also to be approx. 1.2, then we can assume the dynamic fracture forces
- <u>dynamic "axial" femur fracture criteria</u> - to be 1800 N respectively 1000 N.

When a bending load is applied, the

body-region	Lit. No:	object	type of loading, remarks	n (/)	load direct.	F_B (N)	M_{bB} (Nm)	σ, τ (Nmm^{-2})	E_B/A (Nm/mm^{-3})	E-Modul (kNmm^{-2})
femur	(20)	pbp	quasistatic bending of femur segments of the medial third, average values by several regions of the bone diameter calculated		±$\overline{xy}$			σ_{bB}		
			children < 5 years	5				150-177	1.6-2.2	8.2-9.9
			children ≧ 5 years	4				184-207	1.5-2.2	11.4-13.8
			(persons ≧15 years)	9				188-225	1.0-1.8	12.1-16.2
femur	(21)	pbp	quasistatic bending loading of femur segments		±$\overline{xy}$			σ_{bB}		
			child 2,5 years	1			52	212		
			child 13,0 years	1			210	232		
femur	(22)	pbp	quasistatic tensile loading of femur segments, mean value of several probations	48	± z			$\sigma_{zB} \pm s$		E-Modul±s
			children 0 - 2 weeks					55± 7.1		10.5± 2.1
			" 3 - 5 month					59± 2.8		11.4± 2.9
			" 7 -11 month					77± 7.5		18.3± 5.2
			" 1,5 - 2,2 years					89± 8.8		22.5± 7.0
			" 4,0 -13,0 years					102±13.3		33.3± 6.7
			(persons 18 - 40 years)					104±12.3		35.3± 8.0
			(persons 70 - 85 years)					83±13.3		22.5± 5.7
femur	(23)	pbp	quasistatic tensile loading of femur segments		± z			σ_{zB}		
			children ≧ 6 month	8				57-132		7.0-17.1
			child 14 years	1				176		22.4
femur	(25)	pbp	quasistatic compression loading of the femur head epiphysis		± y			τ_{dB}		
			children < 6 years	17				0.3-1.4		
			children ≧ 6 years	6				0.6-1.4		

Fig. 3 - Biomechanical load limits of the femur

elasticity module of the infant femur compacta is 8.2 - 13.8 kN/mm^2. Therefore, children under the age of 5 are clearly below the corresponding values of adults (20). Children aged 5 and older are only slightly below. When compared with the bony tissue of adults, the infant bone has a smaller elasticity module, less ultimate bending stresses and fewer ash residues (20). The infant bone shows a higher fracture bending and absorbs more energy and this occurs as a tendency also after begin of fracture.

The middle third of the femur shaft as well as of the tibia and fibula has the highest tissue strength (26) with epiphysical lines at the end of the hollow bones (27). Fractures in the later area are of special importance as they can cause growth arrest. The special fracture mechanism and the typical fracture forms of the children's age result from the strength and strain properties of the infant bony tissue. The so-called brittle fracture of the adult is therefore in contrast to the deformation fracture of the child (21).

Tibia - On the average the quasistatic torsion ultimate moment of the tibia is 33.0 ± 11.4 Nm for children aged 5 to 14. The elastic torsion limit, however, is 23.0 ± 8.0 Nm (28). Both values are thus smaller than those for adults, see Fig. 4. This is explained simply by the smaller bone "compacta" area. There are no statements to be found in the literature concerning ultimate stresses of the infant tibia, but several data are to be found concerning ultimate moments. The bending ultimate moment was approx. 93 to 179 (299) Nm with a total number of six children aged 4 to 14. These, however, were mathematical estimations apart from one value of 162 Nm (12-year-old child) (29, 30, 31, 32). According to Asang (30), the bending ultimate moment of the tibia is three times as high as the torsion ultimate moment. The most endangered cross section of the tibia is at the "lower-third-point" (transition from the distal to the medial third). This is based upon its "compacta" area (28).

Proceeding from the values mentioned with Lange (28) for the mean outer diameter of the "compacta" area at the "lower-third-point", and assuming the same bending ultimate stress for tibia and femur, the quasistatic bending ultimate moment of the child's tibia can be calculated as follows:
7,0 years (approx. 50 % child pedestrian)
M_{bB} = 44 - 49 Nm
3,6 years (approx. 5 % pedestrian)
M_{bB} = 15 - 18 Nm

If we assume the dynamic bending limit load of the tibia to be approx. 20 % higher than the quasistatic one, as was found by Asang (24), then the dynamic bending ultimate moment at the "lower-third-point" - <u>dynamic tibia fracture criteria</u> - is calculated to be 53 - 59 Nm (7-year-old child, outer diameter of tibia d_{Ta} = 14.6 mm) and 18 - 22 Nm (3,6-year-old child, d_{Ta} = 10.9 mm). The corresponding dynamic tibia fracture criterion with adults is calculated to be 500 - 600 Nm (95 % pedestrian, d_{Ta} = 30.7 mm).

The energy absorption up to the point of fracture is in the elastic field with the child's tibia 29 %, and with adults, however, only 19 % of

body-region	Lit. No:	object	type of loading, remarks	n (/)	load direct.	F_B (N)	M_B (Nm)	σ (Nmm^{-2})	E_B (Nm)	E-Mod. (kNmm^{-2})
tibia	(28)	pbp	quasistatic tension loading of the complete tibia children 5 - 14 years, elastic limit ($\bar{\varphi}_{elastic}$ 14.9°) " , fracture limit (persons 16 - 20 years, elastic limit ($\bar{\varphi}_{elastic}$ 12.4°) " , fracture limit	30 30 16 16	app.±z		$M_B \pm s$ 21.8±8.0 33.0±11.4 59.4±13.6 100.1±28.8		$E_B \pm s$ 3.0±1.1 10.3±4.0 6.5±1.7 34.8±1.4	
tibia	(29)	pbp	quasistatic bending loading of the complete tibia child 12 years calcul. with (28) by tibia head diameter child 12 years, elastic limit " , fracture limit extrapolated fracture bending moment dependent on tibia head diameter child 7 years calcul. with (28) by tibia head diameter child 7 years, elastic limit " , fracture limit	1	± x		M_{bB} approx. 93 approx. 123 approx. 69 approx. 88			
tibia	(30)	pbp	quasistatic bending loading of the complete tibia child 12 years, masculin, fracture limit	1	assumption x		M_{bB} 162			
tibia	(31)	pbp	ascertain of a fracture criterium for dynamic bending load of a child with a body mass of 32 kg		/ unknown		M_{bB} 93			
tibia	(32)	pbp	quasistatic bending load of the complete tibia in her middle, the arm of lever for the half fracture load is a sixth of the tibia lenght child 4 years, arm of lever by (28) approx. 30 mm children 14 y, " " 65 mm	1 4		902 5494-7652	M_{bB}^* 14 179-299			

* own mathematical calculation of the quasistatic bending load

Fig. 4 - Biomechanical load limits of the tibia

energy absorbed after begin of fracture. Likewise the elastic "bending limit moment" of the infant tibia is 70 % of the bending ultimate moment and with adults it is only 59 %.

CONCLUSIONS - The publications evaluated here show how great the uncertainty of the known biomechanical critical load values still is. Their mostly slight statistic significance is caused especially by the small number of cases which, moreover, refer only partly to the dynamic kind of load which is relevant for accidents. Corresponding critical load values are especially missing for the highly-endangered head region and for the abdominal and pelvis region. They are totally missing for the neck-vertebrae region. Acceptable values have been derived for the body surface (skin), the thorax region and especially for the lower extremities.

MECHANICS OF SIMILITUDE (Data Scales)

TRANSLATIONAL ACCELERATION - Translational head acceleration limits for the children's group can be estimated from the critical load values of adults by using the mechanics of similitude. When the force is either applied to a large contact area or indirectly with a translational acceleration of the head, the brain is pressed against the inner skull wall due to its inertia. This brings about a pressure gradient within the skull with a subpressure and sometimes cavitation opposite to the impact occur. An other consequence is the unit pressure at the point of impact.

Haynes, for instance, states that with adults in case of a frontal unit pressure on the brain below 2.1 bar for periods of time shorter than 6 ms, brain injuries are not yet to be expected (33). When arbitrarily assuming the same unit pressures between the brain and the skull exists, without effect for either adult or the child, then the permissible translational head acceleration for children can be estimated by mechanics of similitude as follows:

$$a_C = a_A \left(\frac{m_A}{m_C}\right)^{1/3} \qquad [1]$$

a = translatoric brain acceleration
m = brain mass
C, A = indices for child resp. adult

Proceeding from the protection criterion of ECE R 21, which stipulates for the head impact area on the dashboard that the resulting head acceleration does not exceed a value of 80 g for longer than 3 ms, a value which can be deduced from the Wayne-State-University-Curve (34), is used here as a reference value for adults. Data of the brain mass are to be found in the Geigy Tables (35). For example m = 1.36 kg (1.29 - 1.43 kg) for the brain of adults and 1.09 respectively 1.26 kg for the brain of 3- and 6-year-old children. Putting these values in the equation No. 1, the calculations for children are as follows:

3 years $a_3 = 80 \left(\frac{1.36}{1.09}\right)^{1/3} [g]$ $a_3 = 86.1$ g

6 years $a_6 = 80 \left(\frac{1.36}{1.26}\right)^{1/3} [g]$ $a_6 = 82.1$ g

The translational protection criteria found for indirect loads or loads applied to large contact areas do not differ essentially from those for adults. In contrast to this according to Fayon (9), the tolerability of translational accelerations of the skull-brain region in case of direct load - influence of skull rigidity - was estimated to be in general below the values for adults.

ROTATORIC ACCELERATION - A similar relation can be deduced according to Ommaya (36) for the estimation of rotational accelerations of the head region:

$$\alpha = \alpha_o \left(\frac{m_o}{m}\right)^{2/3} \quad [2]$$

α = rotational acceleration
o = index for rhesus monkey

Based upon i n d i r e c t l y - applied rotational head accelerations during tests with live rhesus monkeys (m_o = 0.1 kg), 50 % of all cases with skull brain traumas were diagnosed as below α_{oi} = 40000 rad/s^2 for periods of time of 10 ms. If we put the values of the brain mass of 3- or 6-year-old children in the equation No. 2, then the calculations for children are as follows:

3 years α_{3i} = 40000 $\left(\frac{0.1}{1.09}\right)^{2/3}$ [rad/s^2]

α_{3i} = 8140 rad/s^2

6 years α_{6i} = 40000 $\left(\frac{0.1}{1.26}\right)^{2/3}$ [rad/s^2]

α_{6i} = 7390 rad/s^2

Thus the values found are above those for adults which are calculated to be α_{Ai} = 7020 rad/s^2. The corresponding values for periods of time of 3 ms are α_{3i} = 81400 rad/s^2, α_{6i} = 73900 rad/s^2, and α_{Ai} = 70200 rad/s^2. Shear loads to the blood-vessel system with ruptures of bridge veins can be considered to be the cause of injuries in the case of indirectly-applied rotational head accelerations. As according to Yamada (5), the breaking strength of arterial tissue with children is approx. 40 % higher than the corresponding value for adults; therefore even higher values can be expected with children.

A supplementary study of the tolerability of rotation accelerations of the head region of rhesus monkeys - whereby the load was applied d i r e c t l y to the head and outside the center of gravity (37) - showed, with α_{od} approx. 11000 rad/s^2 (m_{od} = 0.085 kg) for time durations of 10 ms, an essentially inferior loadability. When putting the brain mass of the 3- and 6-year-old child into equation No. 2, then our calculations for children are as follows:

3 years α_{3d} = 11000 $\left(\frac{0.085}{1.09}\right)^{2/3}$ rad/s^2

α_{3d} = 2008 rad/s^2

6 years α_{6d} = 11000 $\left(\frac{0.085}{1.26}\right)^{2/3}$ rad/s^2

α_{6d} = 1823 rad/s^2

The values found are also above those values found for adults with α_{Ad} = 1732 rad/s^2 for time durations of 10 ms. With a probability of 50 %, they will cause skull brain traumas. The corresponding values for periods of time of 3 ms are α_{3d} = 9100 rad/s^2, α_{6d} = 8300 rad/s^2, and α_{Ad} = 7900 rad/s^2. Because a child's skull is less rigid, the direct application of the force means a generally higher endangering of the child. Therefore, the derived values for children could still be considerably reduced.

When deducing injury criteria to protect against irreversible skull brain injuries from the found load limits, those which reach approx. 75 % of the critical load value would result in the following loadings for time durations of 10 ms. Indirectly applied force:
child 3 years, α_{3Pi} = 6000 rad/s^2
child 6 years, α_{6Pi} = 5500 "
adult   , α_{APi} = 5300 "
Directly applied force:
child 3 years, α_{3Pd} = 1500 "
child 6 years, α_{6Pd} = 1400 "
adult   , α_{APd} = 1300 "

Without considering possible but partly unknown differences of acceptable unit pressures of the brain between children and adults as well as concerning the higher breaking strength values of the blood-vessel system of children (5), a tendency analysis of the loadability of the infant head region, by means of mechanics of similitude (scaling) under frontal translational head acceleration, shows on the whole, nearly the same loadability as when compared with adults. However, this is inversely proportional to the age with rotational loads. The tendencies found only refer to the head region, in particular to the skull/brain region and permit no statements as to the overall region of head plus neck.

ANALYSIS OF REAL PEDESTRIAN ACCIDENTS OF CHILDREN

Proceeding from in-depth single-case-analyses of real traffic accidents involving children (38), the point is to investigate the most important parameter of the seriousness of the accident, in other words: the vehicle impact speed and its traumatic influence. Therefore, groups of the same vehicle/body region combination must be studied. For similar vehicle front geometries, i.e. based upon single front contour types, two body regions of children can be found which are hit with sufficient frequency by the same vehicle elements such as front hood and bumper, for instance. Based upon the possible seriousness of the suffered trauma, the lowest irreversible injury severity degree, i.e. AIS 2 (39), (e.g. Skull Brain Trauma of first degree, SBT 1), is especially appropriate also with regard to its frequency. As an example for pedestrians a frequency of 31 % results for the body regions with an injury level of AIS 2, and only one of 25 % from AIS 3 upward (40). This means also that if this load limit isn't exceeded up to a vehicle impact speed of 11 m/s - under which about 60 % of all injured pedestrians are found (41) -, a reduction of 49 % of AIS 2 and only one of 19 % from AIS 3 upward would then be possible.

HEAD REGION - From the curve of accumulative frequency of vehicle impact speeds (v_{KF}) for head injuries of AIS 2 shown in Fig. 5 - all of them are SBT 1 - and which are caused by the impact to the front hood of pontoon/trapezoid (P/T) vehicle front contours, it can be seen that 50 % (of all injuries) with children are located under v_{KF} = 9.7 m/s. None of these children suffered any fracture of the head region. In one case, only a tooth was lost.

The curve of accumulative frequency for persons from 15 years on, which is given here as a supplementary comparison, shows that 50 % of all head injuries of AIS 2 are under v_{KF}=9.4 m/s. Here, too, all head injuries from AIS 2 were of SHT 1. In one case, however, it was accompanied by a simple skull fracture of AIS 2.

According to Appel (42) the vertical impact speed (relative to the vehicle) of the head (v_{KT}) of adults onto the front hood is, with the same v_{KF}, 15 to 20 % higher than that of children. From that we can deduce a difference of the mean values of v_{KT} of approx. 1.6m/s and thus can conclude, as a tendency, that the direct loadability of child-

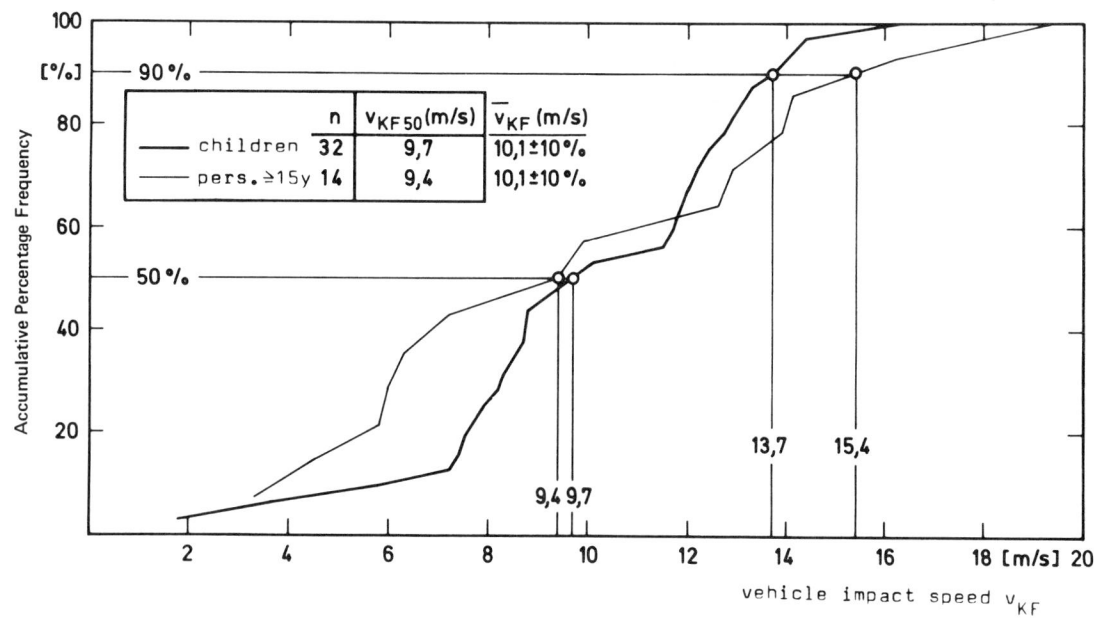

Fig. 5 - Accumulative percentage frequency of vehicle impact speeds with P/T - front contours for cases with pedestrians (children, persons ≥ 15 years) which suffered a first degree skull brain trauma by a head/front hood impact

ren's head region is smaller than that of persons aged 15 and on. The actual v_{KT} of children with this front contour type is, however, according to Appel (42) approx. 25 % beneath v_{KF}. Therefore, with present vehicle fronts we can deduce a mean value of v_{KT} of approx. 7 m/s which cause SHT 1.

Taking into consideration a maximum elastic skull deformation of approx. 15 mm with children as well as considering an elastic/plastic depth of deformation of 2 x 5 mm for the front hood in the average, then a mean head deceleration of children of 109 g for a time duration of 7 ms can be calculated from the impact speed of 7.3 m/s.

LOWER EXTREMITIES - In order to find the median value of vehicle collision speeds in cases with fractures of the lower extremities, single-case-analyses were selected where the cause of the injury was found to be the bumper of P/T front contours. With children these fractures were mostly located in the medial third of femur and tibia/fibula, and with persons aged 15 and older in the medial third of tibia/fibula. The fractures were examined on the basis of the injury severity degree AIS 2 and 3, Fig. 6.

For children the median value of vehicle collision speeds for cases with fractures of degree AIS 2 is 9.4 m/s and is thus higher than the one for persons aged 15 and older (8.4 m/s). As a tendency, this means that the lower extremities of children are less inclined to break with similar absolute vehicle front geometry, i.e. by an impact to the average actual vehicle front structure. The median values of v_{KF} for fractures of the severity degree AIS 3 supplement this by showing that with children this injury severity degree is already reached with considerably lower impact speeds than with persons aged 15 years and older. However, it must be pointed out here that AIS 3 with children always means a dislocated fracture and with persons aged 15 and over this normally means an open fracture.

Proceeding from the analysis of real traffic accidents, the tendency is found that when a, for the most part, direct translatoric load is applied, the head region of children has a smaller load capacity than with adults. For children, with regard to the lower extremities, there is a tendency for a higher specific pedestrian accident loadability based upon similar front geome-

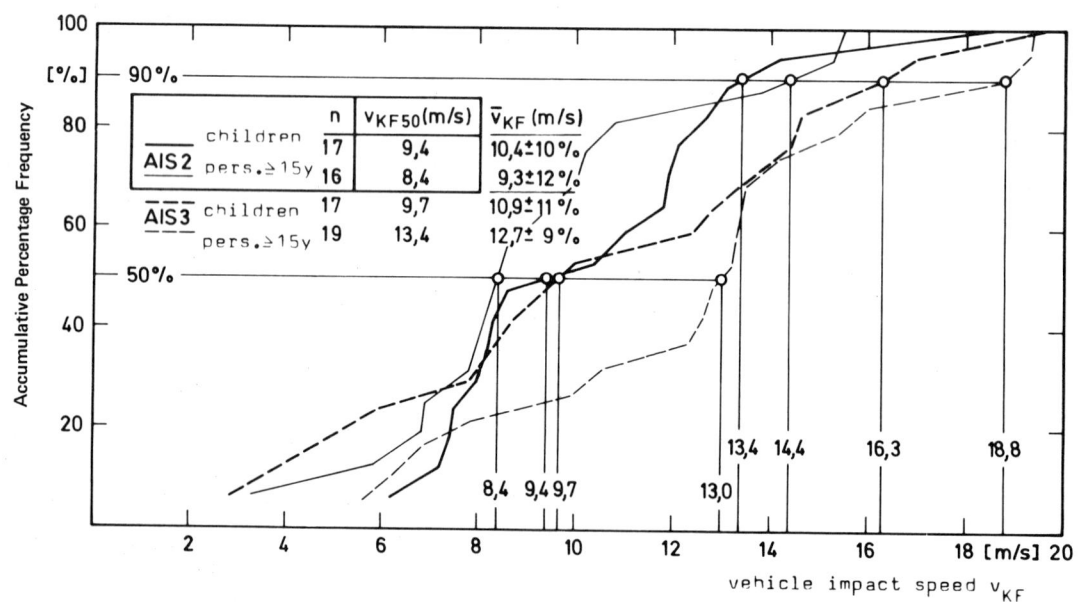

Fig. 6 - Accumulative percentage frequency of vehicle impact speeds with P/T - front contours for cases with pedestrians (children, persons ≥ 15 years) which suffered a fracture of AIS 2 or 3 in the lower extremities by a bumper/lower extremities impact

tries and on the lower limit of irreversible injuries (AIS 2).

REPETITION OF REAL TRAFFIC ACCIDENTS USING ANTHROPOMETRIC DUMMIES

Even in the future it will not be possible to carry out postmortem tests with infant bodies apart from a few single-cases, i.e. a very small number of cases. Therefore, the only efficient way to find biomechanical critical load values or to define injury or protection criteria is to re-enact real case child traffic accidents using appropriate anthropometric dummies, i.e. with similar kinematic behaviour to that of living human being, see also (40), (43). The latter is done under consideration of all vehicle, traffic participant and accident parameters influencing the trauma, but also with regard to a high reproducibility of the test results.

The bases for this are also in-depth single-case-analyses of traffic accidents involving children. They have been representatively selected for this type of accident. The aim is the correlation of dummy measured/calculated values, i.e. mechanical load values with real injuries or medically defined injury severity degrees in contrast to the most often used method to transfer load values found by means of postmortem tests to anthropometric dummies.

On one hand, load values, which can be found and correlated by repetition tests, have the level of estimated biomechanical data, and on the other hand, they serve to define protection criteria against irreversible injuries. When these dummies are used to evaluate the aggressiveness of external vehicle elements of the efficiency of safety measures, for instance, with the help of the correlations found, the significance of the measured loading for the organism can be estimated directly.

This method has several advantages especially for the children's group, when considering on repetition tests of real accidents with child pedestrians as well as restrained child car occupants:
- during the primary collision, children up to middle-sized ones are not thrown onto pontoon-shaped vehicles, but remain positioned on the primary contact areas, with the contributing effect of a high test reproducibility.
- child restraint systems for small-sized children, which reduce the mass-forces of the child by energy absorbtion of a frontal deformable table with area contact have the advantage that in frontal collision modes, these deformations in the repetition tests

can be compared to those found in real cases.

This research is based on a sample of 200 medical and technical in-depth single-case-analyses of child pedestrian accidents as well as one of 93 cases with child car occupants using a special type of child restraint system, both groups mainly from traffic accident research programms (38). The real cases, 25 in all, are taken therefore from a large enough number of traffic accidents, mostly with injured children. Therefore, it is advisable that a selection mode could be used for finding out appropriate cases for repetition. This means that the selected cases are close to the average real accident, as well as close to the anthropometric data of the selected dummies.

CHILD PEDESTRIAN ACCIDENTS

<u>Test Apparatus</u> - In order to allow as much evidence as possible concerning body segments, an Alderson VIP 6 c anthropometric dummy (Fig. 7) was modified by substitute additional measuring gauges which are also of importance, especially for the pedestrian collision (Fig. 8 giving details). With the aim of high test reproducibility, the main influencing accident parameters on kinematics as well as loading of the dummy were found to be repeatable by the impact test facility (Fig. 9). Some of these are for instance: impact speed of the car, breaking deceleration at time of impact, primary impact point on the vehicle and dummy, position of the upper and lower limbs. Because of the low influence of walking speed to the position of the child's head/bonnet impact, due to its low body height, the latter was not simulated in order to achieve better reproducibility of the test results. Post-crash vehicle and dummy are positioned in the initial phase of collision to find out the correlated contact areas.

<u>Real Accidents</u> - Based on the in-depth single-case-analyses of real child pedestrian accidents (38), 10 cases were selected which correspond to a requirement list. As the head is the most traumatised body region of child pedestrians, two-wheel riders, as well as car occupants, of the cases selected, eight show a primary first degree skull brain trauma (SBT 1) for the child and two cases show one of a third degree.

<u>Comparison Real Accident/Dummy Test</u> - A survey of the selected real cases, as well as of the worked-out impact tests, is given by Fig. 10. The vehicle impact speed is varied mostly within the ranges of the real accident. The aim is to have the test in the lower, as well

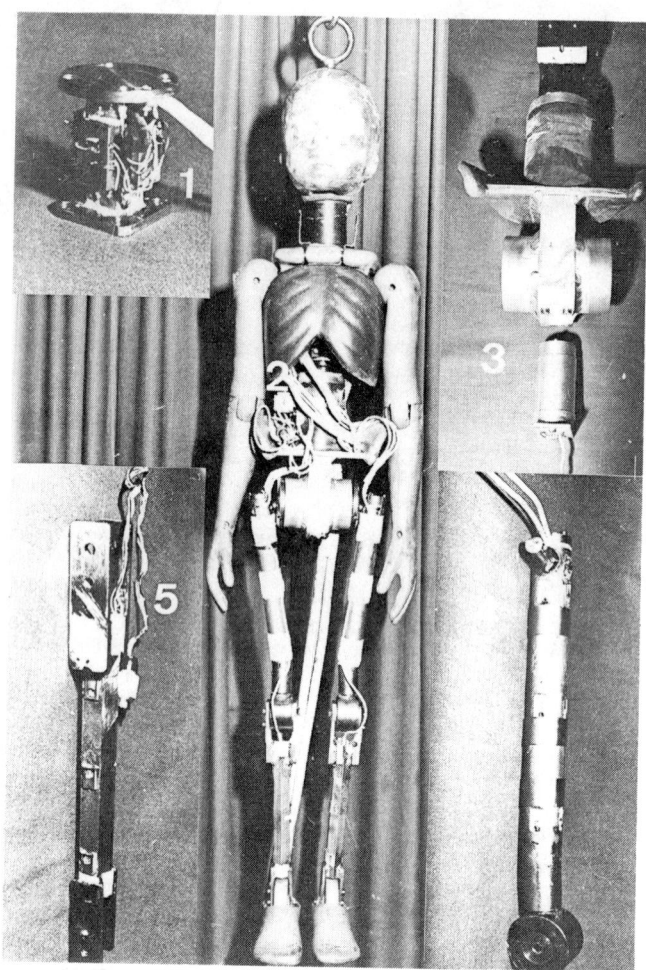

Fig. 7 - Modified Alderson VIP 6c:
1 measuring neck, 2 abdominal accelerometers, 3 tube for pelvis accelerometers, 4 femur, 5 tibia/fibula

as the upper limit, possibly even in the middle of the real impact speed range. Each test set consists of more than two repetition tests designed to provide information on the consistency of results.

A detailed comparison of the real accident data as well as those of the repetition tests regarding the head region is shown by Fig. 11. The peak value of resultant head acceleration (a_{Hrmax}), the maximum resultant value for time durations greater or equal to 3 ms ($a_{Hrg}(\geq 3ms)$), and the Head Injury Criterion (HIC) were taken from the measuring signals.

The impact directions of the head show a good correlation. For the evaluation of the correlation of the vehicle damage due to the head impact as the main parameter, the plastic depth of penetration is shown in the right column. The real depth values must be taken as approximated values. Because the local stiffness of the bonnet is influenced by the position of bracings, additional information is given regarding its position to the vicinity of bracings.

Reproducibility of Test Results - The distribution of test results also contains the distribution resulting from the desired change of the impact speed. For the HIC the average spread in the test series is found with ± 23 %, for the a_{Hrmax} as well as $a_{Hrg}(\geq 3ms)$ with ± 15 %. Together with other body regions, the average spread in the test series for measured/calculated values of the dummy loading is as follows:

head	15 - 23 %
neck	6 - 15 %
thorax	10 - 19 %
abdomen	12 - 23 %
pelvis	10 - 23 %
lower extremities	10 - 12 %

Correlations - Because the test impact speed was mostly in the range

<u>Head (Cranium)</u>

Triaxial acceleration ± 750 g

<u>Neck (C7 area)</u>

Transverse force ± 10000 N
Anterior - posterior force ± 10000 N
Cranial force ± 5500 N
Transverse bending ± 500 Nm
Anterior - Posterior bending ± 500 Nm

<u>Chest (Thorax)</u>

Triaxial acceleration ± 750 g

<u>Abdomen</u>

Anterior - posterior acceleration ± 750 g
Vertical acceleration ± 750 g

<u>Pelvis</u>

Triaxial acceleration ± 750 g

<u>Upper Leg (Femur)</u>

Transverse bending ± 350 Nm
Anterior - posterior bending ± 350 Nm

<u>lower Leg (Tibia/Fibula)</u>

Transverse bending ± 300 Nm

Fig. 8 - Measuring ranges of the modified VIP 6c

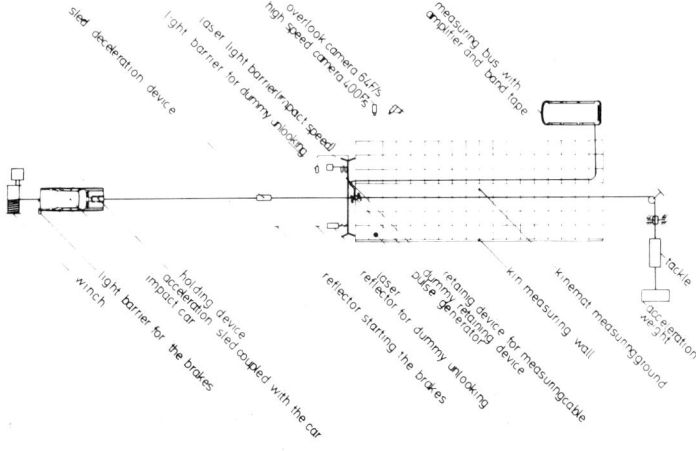

Fig. 9 - Pedestrian impact test facility

Case Test	Passenger Car	Vehicle Impact Speed [m/s]	Braking Deceler. at Imp. [m/s²]	Body Stat [m]	Ped Imp Dir [Clock]	Pedestr Impact Speed [m/s]	Position of lower Extrem.
1 1.1 1.2 1.3	Opel Kadett B	8.4-10.0 9.2 8.4 8.5	7.3-8.9 7.8 7.3 7.2	1.29 1.21 1.21 1.21	8 8 8 8	slow run standing " "	RL f LL " " "
2 2.1 2.2	Opel Kadett B	8.2-10.9 10.1 10.2	5.0-6.0 6.6 6.6	1.25 1.21 1.21	9 9 9	running standing "	unknown LL f RL "
3 3.1 3.2 3.3	Renault R 4	11.3-12.5 11.8 11.8 12.4	7.1-8.0 6.3 5.9 5.8	1.10 1.21 1.21 1.21	3 3 3 3	running standing " "	RL f LL " " "
4 4.1 4.2	Renault R 4	7.8-9.6 9.1 9.0	7.1-8.7 6.6 6.9	1.33 1.21 1.21	9 9 9	running standing "	RL f LL " "
5 5.1 5.2	Opel Rekord C	7.5-10.0 9.3 7.7	5.0-6.5 7.6 6.6	1.21 1.21 1.21	9 9 9	running standing "	RL f LL " "
6 6.1 6.2 6.3	Opel Rekord C	10.1-11.0 10.7 11.0 11.3	7.1-8.0 7.4 7.1 7.1	1.20 1.21 1.21 1.21	3 3 3 3	slow run standing " "	LL f RL " " "
7 7.1 7.2	Renault R 16	7.6-8.7 9.4 8.7	7.1-8.7 8.1 8.1	1.18 1.21 1.21	3 3 3	running standing "	LL f RL " "
8 8.1 8.2 8.3	VW K 70	11.8-13.0 12.2 11.8 12.7	7.3-8.9 7.4 7.5 7.4	1.12 1.21 1.21 1.21	10 10 10 10	slow run standing " "	RL f LL " " "
9 9.1 9.2 9.3	VW K 70	13.4-15.4 12.7 13.0 13.1	7.3-8.9 7.7 7.5 7.3	1.12 1.21 1.21 1.21	3 3 3 3	running standing " "	RL r LL " " "
10 10.1 10.2	Opel Kadett A	11.2-12.4 11.9 11.8	7.1-8.0 8.3 7.9	1.28 1.21 1.21	9 9 9	running standing "	RL f LL " "

Fig. 10 - Accidental data from real accidents as well as repetition tests

of the real accident, all of the recorded maximum load characteristic values of a body region within a test series could be the studied correlated value with the exception that the area and type of impact wouldn't be comparable to the real accident. Should there be only two instead of three acceptable cases in a test series, then their arithmetic mean value is taken as an additional third value for an equal consideration of each series.

The correlations found for the head region are shown here in greater detail. The accumulative percentage frequency of HIC and resultant head accelerations correlated to real injuries of SBT 1 is shown by Fig. 12.

The results of test 4.1 and 4.2 are not included because a shoulder impact occured in every test which is contrary to the real accident. For the HIC, 50 % of the values are located unter 840 and for a_{Hrg} ($\cong$ 3ms) they are under 83 g, as well as for a_{Hrmax} under 143 g. The arithmetical mean values of the test series show a biomechanical distribution with a standard deviation of $\pm$ 50 % for $\overline{HIC}$ = 1031, $\pm$ 23 % for $\overline{a}_{Hrg}$ ($\cong$ 3ms) = 95 g and $\pm$ 32 % for $\overline{a}_{Hrmax}$ = 161 g. Fig. 13 can be used to find a correlated range of reversible child head injuries from which level - effective (average) acceleration - and time duration of loading can be taken. Also shown is the Wayne-State-University-Curve for cerebral concussion (34), (44). Because the direct head/frontend impact can be accepted as the cause of the injury; and the indirect head acceleration can also be a factor of the trauma, the effective resultant head accelerations are shown for both groups.

The consequence of calculated loading values restricted to a limited time duration shows that the borderline of irreversible head injuries with children is reached by a lower direct loading in contrast to adults. The limited time duration is, nevertheless, of special

Case Test	Primary Head Injury	Head Imp. Dir. [Clock]	a_{Hr} Peak [g]	$a_{Hr} \geq 3ms$ [g]	a_{Hei} [g]	t_i [ms]	a_{Hev} [g]	t_v [ms]	SI	HIC	Vehicle Damage b Head Imp Depht [cm]
1	Scull Brain Trauma1	7/8									1.0 med.
1.1	laceration left	7	147	67	50	13	17	75	530	345	0.3 med.
1.2	paretal, Scull Cal.	7	136	73	48	15	24	77	640	339	0.3 med.
1.3	Fract. left paret.	7	104	78	58	12	28	64	610	365	1.0 med.
av	AIS 3		129	73					593	350	
2	Scull Brain Trauma3	9									2.5 soft
2.1	Subdural Haematoma	9	66	57	52	17	38	67	840	683	2.0 soft
2.2	Scull Frac.le pare.	9/10	233	102	70	18	52	56	2260	1283	2.5 soft
av	AIS 5		150	80					1530	974	
3	Scull Brain Trauma1	6									3.0 soft
3.1	Bruise on Scull	5	112	68	58	17	41	55	1020	764	3.3 soft
3.2	occipital	5	69	59	46	19	38	55	720	613	2.6 soft
3.3		5	105	73	41	24	39	62	1050	747	3.5 soft
av	AIS 2		95	67					930	708	
4	Scull Brain Trauma1	12									0.5 soft
4.1	Bruise with lacerat	1	50	41	27	18	20	73	220	164	1.0 soft
4.2	on Forehead	12/1	45	33	22	21	19	70	180	147	0.9 soft
av	AIS 2		48	37					200	156	
5	Scull Brain Trauma1	9/10									0.2 med.
5.1	Bruise left lateral	9	223	121	73	17	36	70	2330	1881	0.3 med.
5.2		9	182	126	59	18	31	72	1470	1134	0.3 med.
av	AIS 2		203	124					1900	1508	
6	Scull Brain Trau2/3	1									0.5 soft
6.1	Subdural Haematoma	1	141	98	65	13	40	57	1170	650	0.4 soft
6.2	Bruise with lacerat	1	156	121	77	13	49	54	1710	1023	0.5 soft
6.3	on Forehead	1	154	102	77	16	57	51	2050	1528	0.5 soft
av	AIS 5		150	107					1643	1067	
7	Scull Brain Trauma1	11									0.8 soft
7.1	Abraison on Fore-	11/12	194	140	56	18	31	76	1770	1380	0.5 soft
7.2	head	12	138	84	45	18	24	86	780	449	0.2 soft
av	AIS 2		166	112					1275	914	
8	Scull Brain Trauma1	11									1.0 med.
8.1	Bruise on Forehead	11	108	76	73	15	46	70	1590	1131	0.3 med.
8.2	Lost of one Incisor	11	141	120	64	15	51	51	1660	1023	0.3 med
8.3		11	204	137	87	14	65	52	3140	2191	0.7 hard
av	AIS 2		151	111					2130	1448	
9	Scull Brain Trauma1	5/6									0.5 soft
9.1	Bruise on Scull	5/6	218	98	94	12	55	56	2780	1552	0.9 soft
9.2	occipital	5/6	283	103	96	12	60	55	3690	1826	0.8 soft
9.3		5	330	186	133	11	67	58	6330	4103	1.1 med.
av	AIS 2		277	129					4267	2493	
10	Scull Brain Trauma1	12/1									0.7 soft
10.1	Laceration on For-	10	124	77	54	18	39	57	1120	622	1.3 soft
10.2	head	10/11	146	84	51	15	33	52	970	572	1.0 soft
av	AIS 2		135	81					1045	597	

a_{Hei} effective resultant head acceleration by direct contact

a_{Hev} effective resultant head acceleration by the whole veh.impact

t_i, t_v puls time durations

Fig. 11 - Comparison of test-measured values with real injuries for the head region

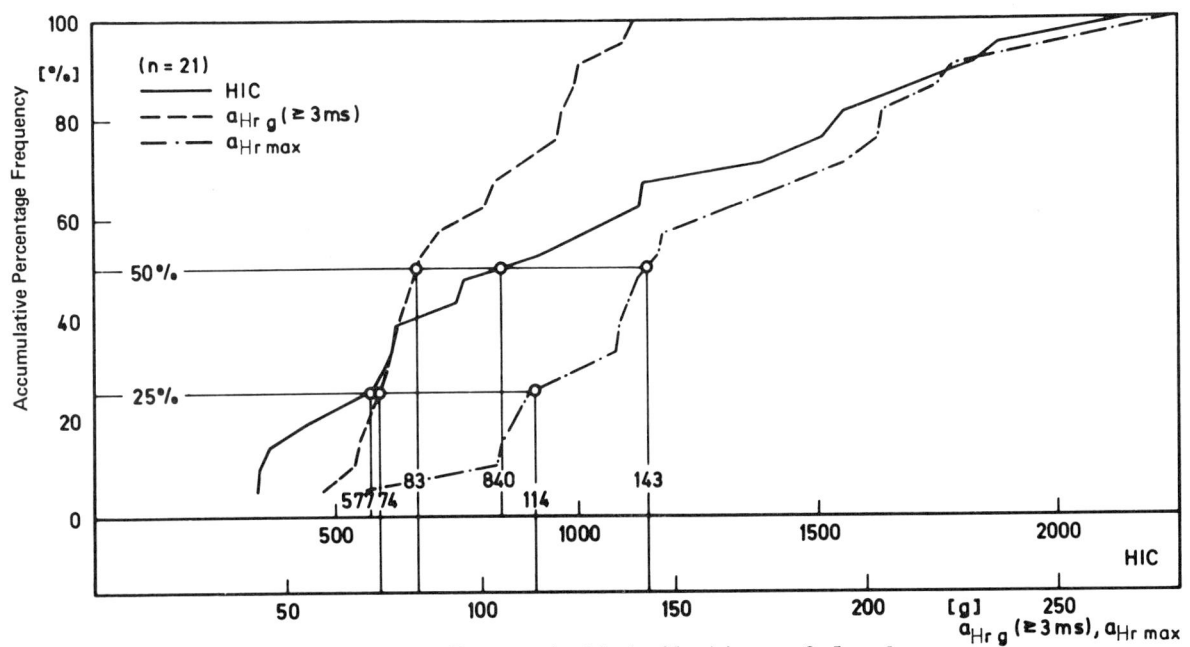

Fig. 12 - Percent distribution of load values from the head region of the VIP 6c which are correlated to real injuries of first degree skull brain trauma (SBT1)

importance for the layout of safety devices in pedestrian collisions.

Loading Ranges, Protection Criteria - A summary of the correlated dummy-measured/calculated loading values (Fig. 14) shows that for the head region there are only results regarding irreversible injuries and for the neck area there are only reversible ones. The other body regions, however, show results for both groups of injury severity.

For the definition of biomechanical protection criteria to prevent irreversible injuries, the upper range of reversible loadings has to be looked for, but as a result it can be seen that both distributions are overlapping. Therefore, two types of protection criteria can be defined:

- SKO gives complete protection against irreversible injuries, only reversible injuries (AIS 1) are tolerated.
- SK1 with an accepted portion of, for instance, 25 % irreversible injuries.

Of the irreversible injuries to the body regions of the children there, in the selected cases, are either no or only a small number of low level irreversible injuries to the body regions of children. Therefore, the frequency of irreversible injuries must be deduced from the load distribution of reversible correlated injuries - or loadings - on the level of defined load levels. The body regions best suited for this are for instance the thorax and the lower extremities. The irreversible injuries from AIS 2 and 3 which are located at the lower limit of irreversible injury degrees show that for the thorax 84 % of the AIS 1 values are located under an SI of 754 as well as 25 % of the irreversible injuries, and their correlated dummy load values are also under this level. For the lower extremities there are 64 % of reversible injuries - or loadings - and 25 % of irreversible ones ranging under $F_{Esä}$ (equivalent quasistatic force causing the same maximum bending moment) 1550 N.

Therefore, protection criteria for body regions seem to be meaningful when covering 75 % of the correlated reversible injuries - or loadings - and thereby tolerating about 25 % of the irreversible injuries (SK1). On the other hand, those criteria which cover about 50 % of reversible injuries - or loadings - and where no irreversible injuries are expected (SKO) are also shown in Fig. 14. To find SKO, part of the lower range of irreversible injuries is taken for the neck, thorax, and abdominal region including also 50 % of the correlated reversible injury severity degrees (AIS<2).

CHILD OCCUPANT ACCIDENTS

Test Apparatus - Repetition tests for vehicle occupants in identical accident situations are very extensive, but on the other hand the child restraint system, described before, can give by itself information with regard to the maximum reaction force in similar dynamic loadings. There exists the possibility to use a crash simulator with idealized deceleration pulses. The accident parameters are chosen in such a way that the same deformations are recorded by the dummy in the restraint system just like they are found in real cases. The system used in a Römer-Peggy I and II which include a plastic deformable frontal shield. The tests were carried out on a Hydro-Pneumatic-Crash Simulator with the use of a sled seat with the structure of a soft back seat and an anthropometric dummy - Alderson VIP 3c - with additional acceleration transducers mounted in the abdominal region at the lumbar vertebra by a clamp (Fig. 15 and 16).

Test Results - As explained above, the analysis needs the mathematic functional connection between load value of the child and deformation of the shield under dynamic crash loading, especially with regard to the way of the integrated belt in the shield. The maximum loading for the abdominal contact region is, first, the maximum horizontal table-belt-force (F_{Admax}) and, second, the resultant abdominal acceleration (a_{Armax}). F_{Admax} is calculated by using the cosine of the dynamic table-belt-angle β (29 to 45°) with $F_{Admax} = F_{rmax} \cdot \cos\beta_{dyn}$. The dependency of F_{Admax} on the maximum static displacement of the shield is shown in Fig. 17 for two different types of the system. Static measurements of the difference between pre- and post-crash values are taken from a reference seat shell considering frontal and lateral deformation of the belt in the shield.

Real Accidents - The real cases are taken from three groups of documentation concerning 93 children using restraints. These groups are composed of the traffic accident research programs in Hannover and Berlin and are supplemented by police reports from the city of Hannover, as well as the traffic accident documentation of Römer-Britax (45).

All 15 cases selected are close to the value VIP 3c even with regard to frontal impact directions and documented deformations in the shield. Among these cases there was only one with an injury of AIS 1 (case 11, Fig. 18) from a type of blunt abdominal trauma "without consequences".

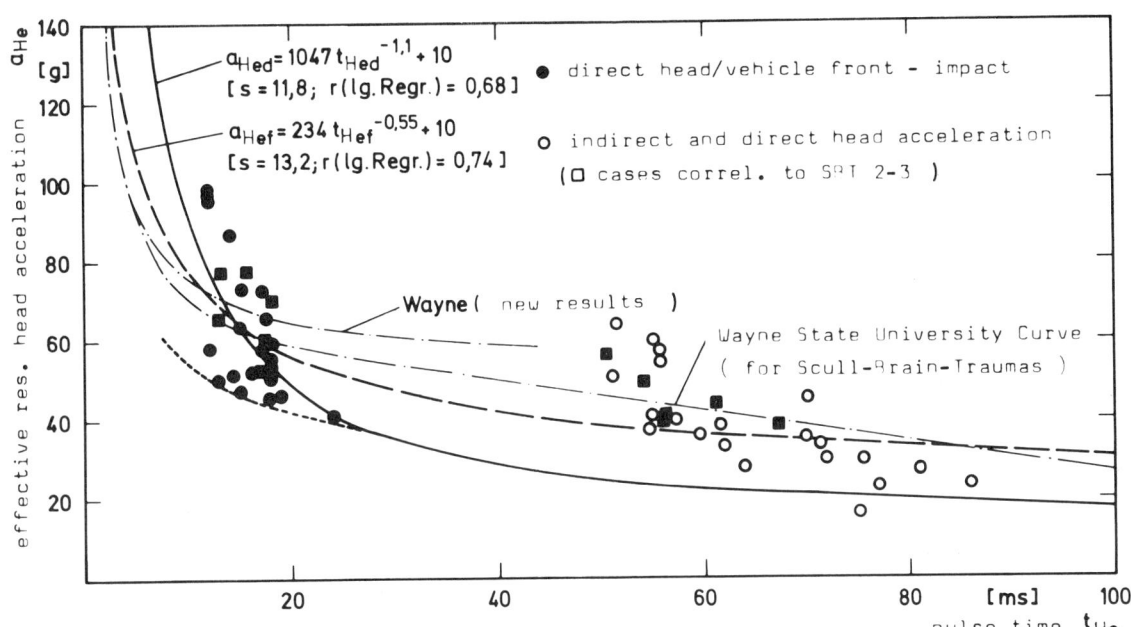

Fig. 13 - Effective resultant head acceleration versus pulse time duration for the direct dummy head/vehicle front end impact as well as for the direct plus indirect phase of the whole vehicle impact (first degree skull brain trauma○●)

body region	load charact. value	reversible injuries (loadings): number n	ΣH 50	ΣH 75	av. value $\bar{x}$	stand. dev. s	irreversible injuries: number n	ΣH 25	ΣH 50	av. value x	stand. dev. s	protection criteria: SKI	SKO
head	type and severity						7	SHT1					
	HIC						21	577	840	1031	517	600	350
	a_{Hrg} (≥3 ms) [g]						"	74	83	95	22	70	60
	$a_{Hr\,max}$ [g]						"	114	143	161	52	110	70
	$a_{He} = f(t_{He})$						$a_{Hed} = 1047\, t_{Hed}^{-1,10} + 10$ [g]				11,8 g		
							$a_{Hef} = 234\, t_{Hef}^{-0,55} + 10$ [g]				13,2 g		
neck	injury severity degree	9	AIS 0										
	$F_{HS\,max}$ [N]	27	825	993	810	312						990	880
	$M_{H\,max}$ [Nm]	"	92	98	90	13						100	90
	$F_{HC\,max}$ [N]	"	1930	2343	1978	541						2300	1900
	$F_{HSe} = f(t_{HSe})$	"											
thorax	injury severity degree	6	AIS 0				3	AIS 2 ÷ 3					
	SI	18	300	433	573	707	9	754	980	1051	226	750	300
	a_{Trg} (≥3 ms) [g]	"	58	70	67	36	"	87	94	103	12	85	55
	$a_{Tr\,max}$ [g]	"	59	78	83	62	"	106	154	146	26	105	55
	$a_{Te} = f(t_{te})$	$a_{Te} = 174\, t_{te}^{-0,62} + 10$ [g]				15,6 g	$a_{Te} = 457\, t_{te}^{-0,78} + 10$ [g]				6,7 g		
abdomen	injury severity degree	6	AIS 0				4	AIS 4 ÷ 5					
	SI_A	18	370	433	371	156	12	1720	2430	2321	693	400	350
	a_{Arg} (≥3 ms) [g]	"	57	66	53	16	"	104	136	130	12	65	55
	$a_{Ar\,max}$ [g]	"	73	90	79	16	"	145	221	208	39	90	70
	$a_{Ae} = f(t_{Ae})$	$a_{Ae} = 724\, t_{Ae}^{-1,07} + 10$ [g]				6,9 g	$a_{Ae} = 2399\, t_{Ae}^{-1,26} + 10$ [g]				7,9 g		
pelvis	injury severity degree	8	AIS 0				2	AIS 2					
	SI_B	24	710	1800	1214	[illegible]	6	-	1285	1184	316	700	500
	a_{Brg} (≥3 ms) [g]	"	87	140	100	52	"	-	93	95	36	85	60
	$a_{Br\,max}$ [g]	"	118	172	143	72	"	-	108	118	38	115	85
	$a_{Be} = f(t_{Be})$	$a_{Be} = 2570\, t_{Be}^{-1,35} + 10$ [g]				7,8 g							
lower extremities	injury severity degree	10	AIS 0 ÷ 1				5	AIS 2 ÷ 3					
	F_{Esa} [N]	30	1385	1760	1613	1039	15	1550	3930	4499	3104	1600	1400
	$M_{E\,max}$ [Nm]	"	211	276	248	129	"	250	533	504	251	250	220
	$M_{Fmr\,max}$ [Nm]	"	139	190	174	109	"	-	-	-	-	190	140
	$M_{T/Fm\,max}$ [Nm]	"	116	157	129	40	"	-	-	-	-	160	115
	$F_{Eqe} = f(t_{Eqe})$	"					$F_{Eae} = 3,24 \cdot 10^3\, t_{Ee}^{-1,85} + 250$ [N]				923 N		

▭ original values for the determination of SKI

Fig. 14 - Summary of correlated dummy-measured/calculated load values as well as derived or recommended protection criteria against irreversible injuries (≙ AIS 2)

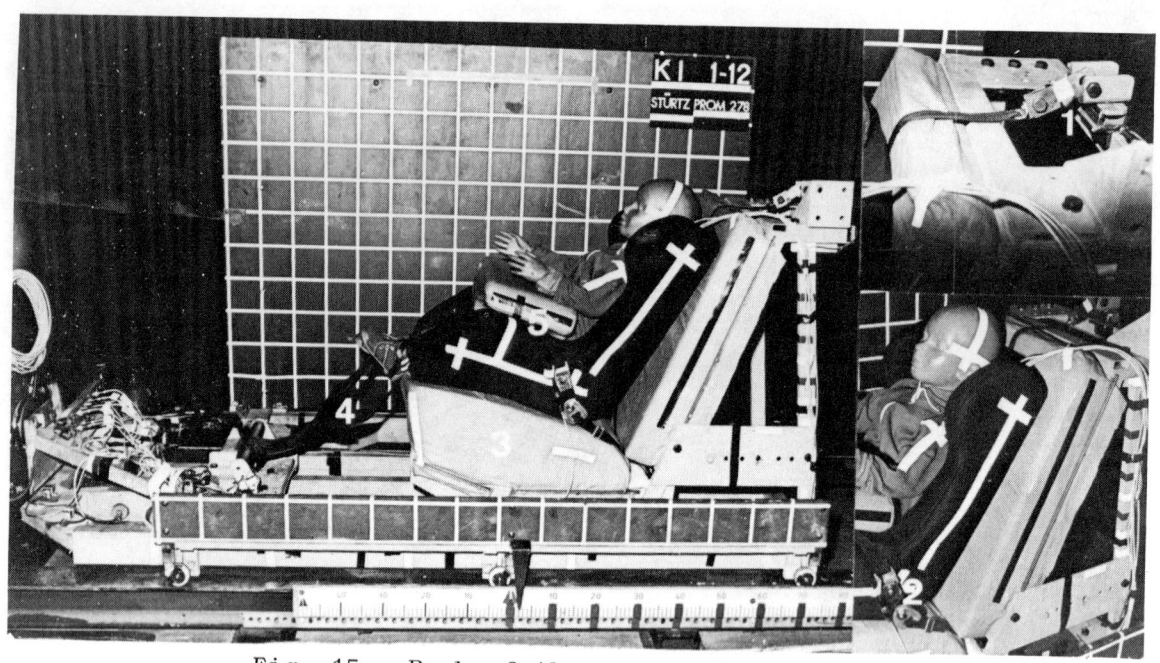

Fig. 15 - Back of the opened VIP 3c with visible abdominal accelerometers opposite to the impact side

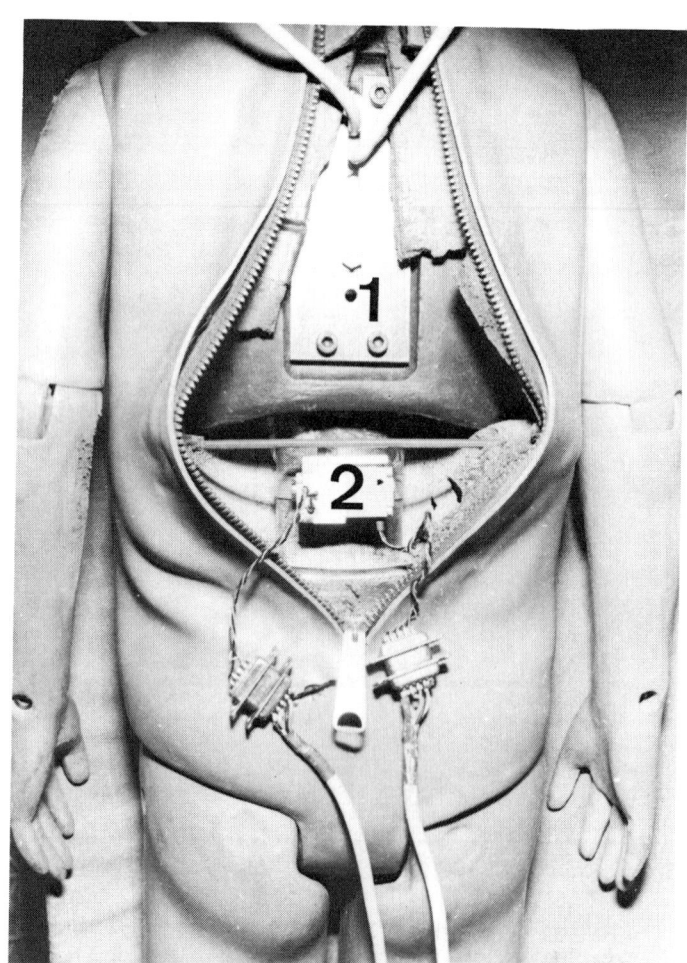

Fig. 16 - Partial view of the hydro-pneumatic catapult with a mounted soft rear seat, the type of child restraint system used as well as the VIP 3c

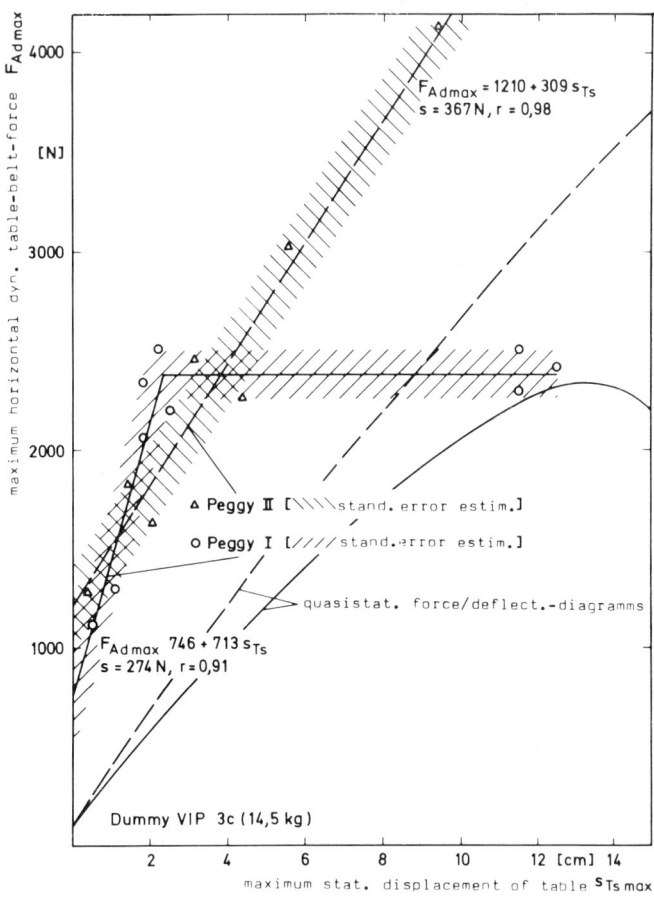

Fig. 17 - Maximum horizontal dynamic table-belt-force versus maximum static forward displacement (post crash measured) of the tables from Peggy I and II

Correlations, Loading Ranges - In Fig. 19, 50 % of the correlated reversible injury severity degrees (AIS<2) are located under SI_{Ard} = 92 - values are related to the mass of the real child ($_{rd}$) -, a maximum abdominal unit pressure P^*_{Admax} of 9.5 N/cm^2, and a maximum resultant abdominal force F_{Admax} of 1385 N, as well as a maximum resultant abdominal acceleration $a_{Arrdmax}$ of 26 g (SK0). 75 % of the values are lower than SI_{Ard} = 176, P^*_{Admax} = 14.2 N/cm^2, F_{Ad} = 2180 N, and $a_{Arrdmax}$ = 31 g (SK1). The observed upper range of reversible injuries - or loadings - resulting from direct frontal abdominal surface loadings can be estimated from case 11 with F_{Admax} = 2380 $\pm$ 5 % (N), P^*_{Admax} = 16.2 $\pm$ 11 % (N/cm^2), a_{Arrd} = 44 $\pm$ 11 % (g), $\overline{a}_{Aerd}$ = 25.0 $\pm$ 16 % (g) (effektive value) as well as SI_{Ard} = 377.

DISCUSSION, REPETITION TESTS - The obtained results are all dependent on the dummy used, a modified Alderson VIP 6c and 3c, which means that these are correlated values. Because these dummies show a similar kinematic behaviour to that of living human beings, the results can also give an estimation of the area of biomechanical tolerance levels of children, but on the other hand, they can be used for the evaluation of safety devices.

As dummy measuring values show on the average shorter and higher signals compared to those of living human beings, the correlated load values are in their overall level somewhat higher than the real biomechanical load values of the single body regions.

BIOMECHANICAL CRITICAL LOADINGS AND PROTECTION CRITERIA OF CHILDREN / CONCLUSIONS

In the previous sections biomechanical load limits - especially biomechanical critical loading - as well as injury (P) and protection criteria were ascertained by different methods. In the following, a selection of suitable and expressive results are shown. Seperated

case No:	abdominal injuries	KSE Peggy Typ	s_{Ts} max. [cm]	s_{St} [cm]	people age sex [y,m]	body height [cm]	body mass [kg]	waist breadth [cm]	R Repre-sentat. [-]	F_{Ad} max. [N]	P_{Ad} max. [N/cm²]	a_{Arrd} max. [g]	SI_{Ard}	a_{Aerd} [g]	t_{Ae} [ms]
1 2311	none	I	not visuable from outside		3,0 m	100	15	15,8 ±1,0	0,48	1050 ±26%	6,5 ±32%	14,3 ±20%	25 ±93%	7,3 ±34%	123 ±10%
2 R 34	none	I	0,5	0,2	2,0 f	70	12	13,7 ±0,9	0,58	1113 ±19%	8,0 ±21%	19,0 ±19%	48 ±83%	8,7 ±35%	105 ±12%
3 R 50	none	I	0,5	0,2	1,5 f	80	12	14,4 ±0,8	0,70	1113 ±16%	7,6 ±24%	19,0 ±19%	48 ±83%	9,1 ±35%	105 ±12%
4 R 31	none	I	0,8	0,5	4,0 m	102	17	16,0 ±1,2	0,80	1310 ±16%	8,0 ±18%	16,8 ±17%	38 ±45%	8,2 ±27%	96 ±13%
5 R 44	none	I	0,8	0,3	1,0 f	74	10	13,7 ±0,7	0,73	1310 ±16%	9,4 ±21%	24,4 ±17%	142 ±45%	13,9 ±27%	96 ±13%
6 R 57	none	I	1,3	0,5	2,5 f	90	13	14,9 ±0,9	0,79	1470 ±15%	9,7 ±21%	21,6 ±15%	122 ±27%	14,8 ±22%	83 ±15%
7 R 40	none	I	2,0	2,0	6,0 f	115	19	16,2 ±1,5	0,85	2160 ±10%	13,7 ±18%	22,9 ±10%	73 ±18%	14,2 ±14%	65 ±11%
8 R 42	none	I	3,5	3,5	2,6 m	89	13,5	15,0 ±0,9	0,64	2380 ±5%	15,6 ±11%	35,9 ±11%	226 ±10%	21,4 ±19%	65 ±11%
9 R 33	none	I	11,0	11,0	1,6 m	82	12,5	14,9 ±0,8	0,56	2380 ±5%	15,7 ±10%	38,7 ±11%	274 ±10%	23,1 ±19%	65 ±11%
10 R 30	none	I	11,5	11,5	2,0 m	88	12	14,7 ±0,9	0,71	2380 ±5%	15,9 ±11%	40,4 ±11%	303 ±10%	24,0 ±19%	65 ±11%
11 2488	AIS1*	I	11,5	11,5	1,5 f	82	11	14,4 ±0,8	0,34	2380 ±5%	16,2 ±11%	44,0 ±11%	377 ±10%	25,0 ±16%	65 ±11%
12 P 1	none	II	not visuable from outside		1,0 m	77	12	14,0 ±0,7	0,42	800 ±34%	5,6 ±38%	14,0 ±33%	48 ±100%	11,0 ±31%	117 ±9%
13 3031	none	II	0,2	0,2	1,7 m	86	12	15,1 ±0,8	0,76	1270 ±21%	8,3 ±15%	22,4 ±21%	58 ±100%	13,3 ±26%	89 ±12%
14 R 54	none	II	1,5	1,5	1,5 f	86	11	14,4 ±0,8	0,65	1680 ±16%	11,4 ±22%	29,3 ±17%	156 ±55%	17,9 ±21%	84 ±13%
15 R 39	none	II	2,0	2,0	3,0 m	96	13,5	15,1 ±1,0	0,80	1870 ±14%	12,1 ±21%	26,3 ±16%	112 ±46%	15,7 ±19%	82 ±13%
av.value $\bar{x}$	-		-	-	2,3 7m 8 f	88	13	14,8 ±0,9	0,65	1644 ±15%	10,9 ±20%	25,9 ±17%	137 ±49%	15,2 ±24%	87 ±12%
stand.dev. s	-		-	-	1,4	12	2,4	0,8	0,15	567	3,7	9,7	110	6,0	20

+ abdominal wall contusion (AIS1) as well as blunt abdom. trauma without conseq. (AIS1)

Fig. 18 - Accidental and occupant parameters from the real cases as well as from the test series, including accident consequences respectively dummy-measured loadings

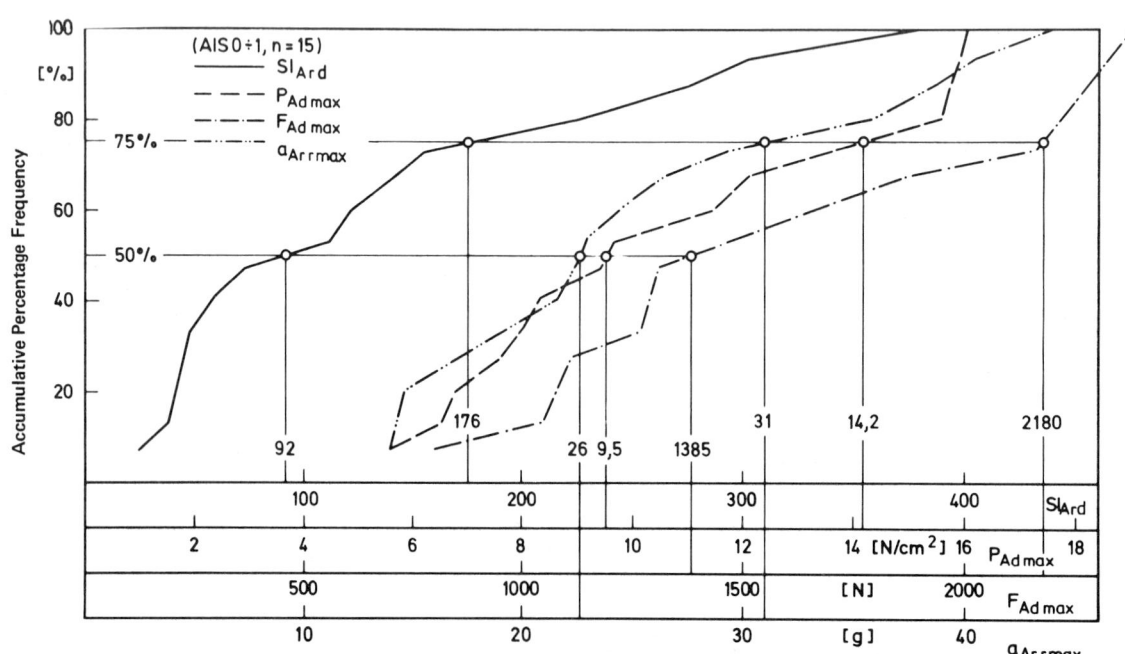

Fig. 19 - Percent distribution of load values from the abdominal region of restrained child car occupants correlated to reversible injury severity degrees as well as loadings without injury consequence

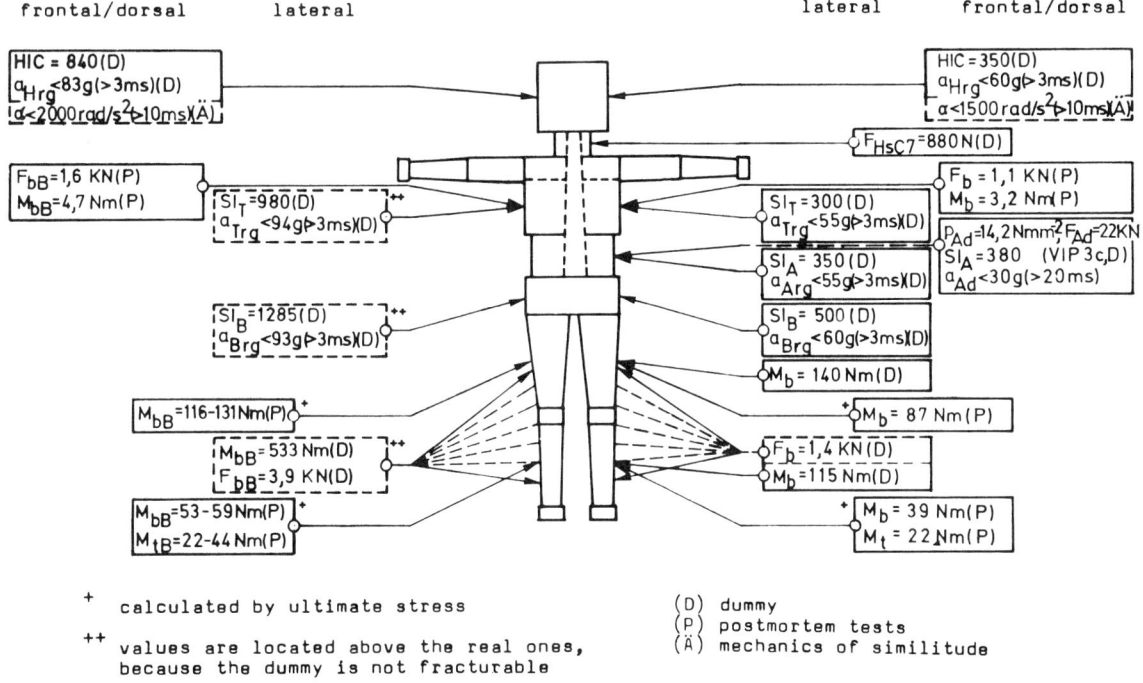

Fig. 20 - Biomechanical load limits and protection criteria of body regions from 6 to 7 (respectively 3) year old children for direct - for the neck indirect - loadings under frontal/dorsal respectively lateral impact directions

into loading directions in Fig. 20, biomechanical critical loadings are listed in detail with regard to the different body regions of children. The protection criteria SKO is also shown in order to consider young children to a far-reaching extent because their fracture moments and forces are far lower, due to their smaller moment of resistance.

The most significant data of load characteristic values are framed in the drawings by a dark line. The data with only limited validity have been framed with a broken line. The values of the head and thorax region as well as those of the lower extremities, also the dynamic axial femur injury criteria with 800 N (3y) resp. 1400 N (6y), can be taken as significant biomechanical critical loadings. Because the derivation of the protection criteria (SKO) necessitates knowing the lower range of load values which cause irreversible injuries, it is possible to determine such limit values by comparing the distributions for reversible and irreversible injuries. Particularly for the "exterior collision", in other words, the pedestrian impact, first protection criteria against irreversible injuries of children have been deduced. For the lower extremities, bending moments in the "lower-third-point" of long hollow bones have priority as opposed to impact forces. This is because the consequences of the latter are strongly dependent on the vertical height of their resulting application of force and therefore are not evident criteria.

REFERENCES

1. E. Faerber, H. A. Gülich, A. Heger, G. Rüter, "Biomechanische Belastungsgrenzen". Bundesanstalt für Straßenwesen, Unfall- und Sicherheitsforschung Straßenverkehr, Köln / West Gernamy, 3, 1976.

2. A. R. Burdi, D. F. Huelke, R. G. Snyder, G. H. Lowrey, "Infants and Children in the Adult World of Automobil Safety Design: Pediatric and Anatomical Considerations for Design of Child Restraints." Biomechanics, Great Britain, Vol. 2, pp. 267 - 80, 1969.

3. DIMDI-Medlars, Köln, "Search Order 02544 No: 004." 1976.

4. R. G. Snyder, "Impact Injury Tolerance of Infants and Children in Free Fall." Proc. 13th AAAM Conf., Illinois, USA, 1969.

5. H. Yamada, "Strength of Biologi-

cal Materials." Williams a. Wilkins Company, Baltimore, USA, 1970.

6. I. G. Fazekas, "Uber die Reißfestigkeit der Haut verschiedener Körperregionen." Deutsche Zeitschrift für gerichtliche Medizin, West Germany, 64, pp. 62 - 92, 1968.

7. H. Holzmann, G. W. Korting, D. Kobelt, H. G. Vogel, "Prüfung der mechanischen Eigenschaften von menschlicher Haut in Abhängigkeit von Alter und Geschlecht." Arch. klin. exp. Derm., West Germany, 239, pp. 355 - 67, 1971.

8. A. Shelness, C. Seymour, "Children as Passengers in Automobiles: The Neglected Minority on the Nations Highways." USA, Pediatrics, Vol. 56, No. 2, pp. 271 - 84, 1975.

9. A. Fayon, C. Tarrière, "Essai de définition de la tolerance de la tête des jeunes enfants." Proc. 1st Int. Meeting on Biomech. of Trauma in Children, Lyon, France, Sept. 1974.

10. G. A. Ryan, "Child Restraint Requirements - A Medical Viewpoint." Seat Belt Seminar, Melbourne, 9 - 11 March 1976.

11. D. R. Foust, B. M. Bowman, R. G. Snyder, "Study of Human Impact Tolerance Using Investigations and Simulations of Free-Falls." Proc. 21st Stapp Car Crash Conf., New Orleans, USA, Oct. 1977.

12. C. Christmann, "Zum Stoßmechanismus am kindlichen Hirnschädel." Verh. Anat. Ges. 71, pp. 1309 - 13, 1977.

13. M. Theis, "Untersuchung der dynamischen und statischen Biegebelastung frischer menschlicher Rippen in Abhängigkeit zu Alter und Geschlecht." Inaugural-Dissertation, Ruprecht-Karl-Universität Heidelberg, West Germany, 1975.

14. I. G. Fazekas, F. Kosa, G. Jobba, E. Meszaros, "Die Druckfestigkeit der menschlichen Leber mit besonderer Hinsicht auf die Verkehrsunfälle." Zeitschrift für Rechtsmedizin, West Germany, 68, pp. 207 - 24, 1971.

15. G. Fazekas, F. Kosa, G. Jobba, "Beiträge zur Druckfestigkeit der menschlichen Milz bei stumpfen Krafteinwirkungen." Archiv Kriminologie, Berlin, West Germany, 149, pp. 158 - 74, 1972.

16. E. Gögler, A. Best, H. H. Braess, H. E. Burst, G. Laschet, "Biomechanical Experiments with Animals on Abdominal Tolerance Levels." 21st Stapp Car Crash Conf., New Orleans, USA, Oct. 1977.

17. D. Kallieris, J. Barz, G. Schmidt, G. Heess, R. Mattern, "Comparison between Child Cadavers and Child Dummy by Using Child Restraint Systems in Simulated Collisions." 20th Stapp Car Crash Conf., Detroit, USA, Oct. 1976.

18. N. O. Hasslev, O. Due, J. Hirsto, R. N. Torgersen, "Children in Cars." Departments Offsetcentral, Stockholm, Nordisk Trafiksikkerheds Rad, Rep. 11A, 1976.

19. A. W. Siegel, "Injuries to Children in Automobil Collisions." 12th Stapp Car Crash Conf., Detroit, USA, 1968.

20. J. D. Curvey, G. Buttler, "The Mechanical Properties of Bone Tissue in Children." The Journal of Bone and Joint Surgery, Vol. 57 - A, No. 6, pp. 810 - 14, 1975.

21. R. B. Martin, P. J. Atkinson, "Age and Sex-related Changes in the Structure and Strength of the Human Femoral Shaft." J. Biomechanics, Great Britain, Vol. 10, pp. 223 - 31, 1977.

22. H. Vinz, "Die festigkeitsmechanischen Grundlagen der typischen Frakturformen des Kindesalters." Zentralblatt für Chirurgie, West Germany, 45, pp. 1509 - 14, 1969.

23. C. Hirsch, F. G. Evans, "Studies on Some Physical Properties of Infant Compact Bone." Acta Orthopaedica Scandinacia, Kobenhaven, 35, pp. 300 - 13, 1965.

24. E. Asang, "Biomechanik des Beines in der Skitraumatologie." Mschr. Unfallheilk., West Germany, 78, pp. 56 - 71, 1975.

25. M. K. Stanley, "Shear Strength of the Human Femoral Capital Epiphyseal Plate." J. Bone Joint Surg. (AM) 58, pp. 94 - 103, 1976.

26. G. Herrmann, H. Liebowitz, A. Arnold, "Mechanics of Bone Fracture, Treatise on Fracture." Academic Press, New York, USA, Vol. 7, pp. 771 - 840, 1971.

27. W. Swoboda, "Das Skelett des Kindes." Georg Thieme Verlag, West Germany, 78, 1969.

28. J. Lange, "Verhalten der Tibia von Kindern und Jugendlichen unter Drehbelastung." Inaugural-Dissertation, TU München, West Germany, June 1976.

29. E. Asang, G. Wittmann, "Experimentelle und praktische Biomechanik des menschlichen Beines." Med. u. Sport XIII, West Germany, 8, 1973.

30. E. Asang, P. Posch, R. Engelbrecht, "Experimentelle Untersuchungen über die Bruchfestigkeit des menschlichen Schienbeines." Monatsschrift Unfallheilkunde, West Germany, 72, pp. 336 - 44, 1969.

31. R. P. Mack, "The Biomechanics of Childrens Skibindings." Journal of Sport Medicine, Vol. 2, No. 3, pp. 154 - 62, 1974.

32. M. Jäger, C. Dietschi, M. Ungethüm, "Über das Verhalten der unversehrten und durchbohrten Tibia bei Biegebeanspruchung." Arch. Orthop. Unfall-Chir., West Germany, 76, pp. 188 - 94, 1973.

33. A. L. Haynes, H. R. Lissner, "Experimental Head Impact Studies." Proc. 5th Stapp Car Crash Conf., Springfield, USA, 1961.

34. V. R. Hodgson, L. M. Thomas, P. Prasad, "Testing the Validity and Limitations of the Severity Index." Proc. 14th Stapp Car Crash Conf., Ann Arbor, Michigan, USA, Nov. 1970.

35. Documenta Geigy, "Wissenschaftliche Tabellen." I. R. Geigy A. G. Pharma, Basel, Schweiz, 7. Edition.

36. A. K. Ommaya, P. Yarnell, A. E. Hirsch, E. H. Harris, "Scaling of Experimental Data on Cerebral Concussion in Subhuman Primates to Concussion Threshold for Man." Proc. 11th Stapp Car Crash Conf., USA, 1967.

37. A. K. Ommaya, A. E. Hirsch, "Tolerance for Cerebal Concussion from Head Impact and Whiplash in Primates." J. Biomechanics, Great Britain, Vol. 4, pp. 13 - 21, 1971.

38. G. Stürtz, "Mainpoints of the Endangering by Different Vehicle Front Contours, their Element / Body Region Combination, as well as the Type of Injuries Produced." Proc. 4th Int. Conf. on the Biomechanics of Trauma, Goeteborg, Sweden, Sept. 1979.

39. Joint Committee of AMA, SAE & AAAM, "The Abbreviated Injury Scale (AIS), 1976 Revision." AAAM, Morton Grove, Illinois, USA, 1976.

40. G. Stürtz, "Repetition of Real-Child Pedestrian Accidents Using a High Instrumented Dummy." Proc. 3rd Int. Meeting on The Simulation and Reconstruction of Impacts in Collisions, IRCOBI, Lyon, France, Sept. 1978.

41. "Beitrag zur Biomechanik des Kindes, Anforderungen an die Äußere und Innere Sicherheit von Kraftwagen." Technical University Berlin, Institute of Automotive Engineering, Rep. No. 265, 1979.

42. H. Appel, G. Stürtz, A. Kühnel, "Pedestrian Safety Vehicle - Design Elements - Results of in-Depth Accident Analyses and Simulations." International Symposium on Automotive Technology & Automation, Wolfsburg, West Germany, 1978.

43. G. Stürtz, "Correlation of Dummy-Loadings with Real Injuries of Children by Repetition Tests." Proc. 5th Int. Conf. on Biomechanics of Impacts, IRCOBI, Birmingham, England, Sept. 1980.

44. L. M. Patrick, "Human Tolerance Impact-Basis for Safety Design." SAE Paper 65 0171.

45. "Accident Reports of Römer-Britax." Inc., Ulm, West Germany, 1977.

826047

Responses of Animals Exposed to Deployment of Various Passenger Inflatable Restraint System Concepts for a Variety of Collision Severities and Animal Positions

H. J. Mertz, G. W. Nyquist, and D. A. Weber
General Motors Corporation

G. D. Driscoll and J. B. Lenox
Southwest Research Institute

ABSTRACT

This paper summarizes the results of tests conducted with anesthetized animals that were exposed to a wide range of passenger inflatable restraint cushion forces for a variety of impact sled—simulated accident conditions. The test configurations and inflatable restraint system concepts were selected to produce a broad spectrum of injury types and severities to the major organs of the head, neck and torso of the animals. These data were needed to interpret the significance of the responses of an instrumented child dummy that was being used to evaluate child injury potential of the passenger inflatable restraint system being developed by General Motors Corporation. Injuries ranging from no injury to fatal were observed for the head, neck and abdomen regions. Thoracic injuries ranged from no injury to critical, survival uncertain. Graphs are presented that show associations between the severity of the animal injuries by body region and selected measured animal responses and restraint system-accident characteristics. Caution must be used in interpreting the significance of these injuries relative to the expected performance of passenger inflatable restraint systems since aggressive restraint system concepts and accident conditions were selected for some tests in order to produce severe injuries.

INTRODUCTION

An important consideration in the development of a passenger inflatable restraint system is to assess the significance of the interactions that may occur between deploying cushions and children who may be close to the instrument panel at the time of deployment (1-8). Analyses by Takeda and Kobayashi (8), Stalnaker et al. (9) and Montalvo et al. (10) have demonstrated that children may be close to the instrument panel in a variety of positions and postures at the instant of a collision either due to their precrash "seated" position or due to the effects of preimpact braking. Tests sponsored by General Motors at Wayne State University (1) and by Volvo at Chalmers University (7) have shown that it is possible to produce significant brain, heart, liver and spleen injuries in anesthetized animals exposed to the impacts of deploying cushions of several concepts of passenger inflatable restraint systems. In the GM program, anesthetized baboons and chimpanzees were used as child surrogates. The Volvo program used anesthetized pigs. Unfortunately, no attempt was made in either program to develop a test device (instrumented child dummy) to aid in understanding the relationships between the observed animal injuries and the cushion-collision interaction forces. However, these programs did demonstrate the need to consider such interactions in the development of passenger inflatable restraint systems (2,3).

When General Motors started its development of a second-generation passenger inflatable restraint system, the interaction between the deploying cushion and the "out-of-position" child was again identified as a topic requiring further study. Concurrent with their inflatable restraint development program, GM initiated a program to develop a test device (an instrumented, 3-year-old child dummy) that could provide measures of the various cushion interaction forces thought to be associated with the type of injuries observed in the previous animal test programs. Such an instrumented child dummy was developed by GM (11) and was used extensively in their second-generation, passenger inflatable restraint development program. While the child dummy provided measurements to make relative comparisons between different passenger inflatable restraint concepts, no biomechanical data existed that would allow intepretations of the dummy responses relative to the severities of injuries that a child might experience in similar exposure environments. An animal test program was needed to provide such a basis. This paper presents the results of the test program that was conducted to obtain the animal injury data. Correlations between the observed animal injuries and corresponding child dummy response measurements are not discussed in this paper. That analysis is the subject of a separate paper by Mertz and Weber (12).

PROGRAM SCOPE

The program conceived was to subject anesthetized animals to a broad range of passenger cushion deployment-simulated collision exposure environments. The specific animal exposure environments were to be selected from child dummy tests that produced a wide range of dummy responses. It was anticipated that test conditions selected by this process would produce a wide range of animal injury types and severities that could be associated with the measured dummy responses.

Southwest Research Institute (SwRI) was contracted by GM to carry out the animal testing portion of the animal injury-child dummy response correlation study. The specific test conditions, test hardware, and animal positions were prescribed by GM based on their child dummy test results. SwRI was responsible for conducting the animal tests and documenting the types and severities of the injuries experienced by the animals.

Physiological measurements such as electrocardiogram (ECG), aortic blood pressure, evoked response, pinch withdrawal and palpebral reflex were made. Blood samples were drawn for gas analysis to aid in assessing the significance of pulmonary injuries. Since past experience had shown that serious internal organ trauma in animals may not be clinically diagnosed (1), all surviving animals were sacrificed usually 24 hours posttest, and gross necropsies were performed. Histopathology was done on the brain, spinal cord, heart and lungs.

A team of medical specialists was formed by SwRI to assess the significance of the observed animal injuries. The team consisted of a neurophysiologist, a neuropathologist, a cardiac pathologist, a cardiologist, a pulmonary specialist and a SwRI Senior Research Physician who served as the medical team leader. The medical specialists were directed to assess the severity of the animal injuries as if the injuries had occurred to a three-year-old child. In addition, each specialist was asked to develop a "dictionary" for his specialty that would describe the types of lesions observed and the injury severity ratings ascribed to the injuries. These dictionaries were to be "living" documents; that is, the specialists were encouraged to revise them based on the results of control tests that were conducted during the program. The medical team leader was responsible for the final injury severity ratings assigned to each test animal.

Each animal injury was assigned two injury severity values. One described the short-term consequences of the injury in terms of threat-to-life (TL value) and the other described the long-term consequences in terms of the potential for permanent impairment (PI value). General descriptions of the TL and PI severity classifications are given in Table 1. The TL descriptors were taken from "The Abbreviated Injury Scale—1980 Revision" (13). However, the injury descriptions contained in the dictionaries developed by the medical specialists are more detailed than those given by The Abbreviated Injury Scale, since each animal was necropsied and much more detailed injury information was available than would be available for a similar human injury. On the other hand, very little data were available on the long-term consequences of the animal injuries, since the animals were usually sacrificed 24 hours postimpact. For the most part, the PI ratings were based on the medical specialist's judgment of the most probable long-term consequences of the various injuries. While the PI ratings are quite subjective, they do serve an important need to rank the severities of brain, cervical spine and heart injuries relative to the potential for permanent impairment of major body functions.

To provide mechanical indicators of the severity of the various exposure environments, accelerometers were attached to the heads and torsos of the animals. The placement and procedure used to mount the accelerometers were chosen so as to not induce injury during the impact

Table 1. General descriptions of threat-to-life (TL) and permanent impairment (PI) injury severity classifications.

TL VALUE	DESCRIPTION OF THREAT-TO-LIFE CATEGORIES
0	NO INJURY
1	MINOR (NOT LIFE-THREATENING)
2	MODERATE (NOT LIFE-THREATENING)
3	SERIOUS (NOT LIFE-THREATENING)
4	SEVERE (LIFE-THREATENING, SURVIVAL PROBABLE)
5	CRITICAL (LIFE-THREATENING, SURVIVAL UNCERTAIN)
6	MAXIMUM (NOT SURVIVABLE)

PI VALUE	DESCRIPTION OF PERMANENT IMPAIRMENT CATEGORIES
0	NO INJURY
1	MINOR (POTENTIAL FOR SOME IMPAIRMENT OF MINOR BODY FUNCTION)
2	MODERATE (SOME IMPAIRMENT OF MINOR BODY FUNCTION)
3	MAJOR (POTENTIAL FOR IMPAIRMENT OF MAJOR BODY FUNCTION, IF UNTREATED)
4	SUBSTANTIAL (PARAPLEGIA)
5	EXTENSIVE (QUADRIPLEGIA)
6	TOTAL (IRREVERSIBLE COMA/DEATH)

or compromise the animal's ability to withstand the impact.

CARE AND USE OF ANIMALS

Southwest Research Institute (SwRI) Animal Medicine Program and Facilities are approved by the American Association for Accreditation of Laboratory Animal Care and the United States Department of Agriculture. Approval by these organizations is based on guidelines of the Animal Welfare Act of 1970 and the Guide for Care and Use of Laboratory Animals. In addition, all protocols involving animal care and testing are subjected to a review by the SwRI Animal Care Committee. This program was reviewed and approved by the SwRI committee as well as the General Motors Corporation Animal Use Committee.

TEST PROTOCOL

Preimpact

Two to three days prior to a test, two pigs whose weights were within the desired range of 15 ± 1 kg were selected as test candidates from the pig herd maintained at SwRI for the test program. These animals were sedated, weighed, depilated and given a physical examination by the veterinarian. Radiographs were taken of each animal and were examined for possible skeletal fractures and abnormal bone growth. On the day of the test, one of the pigs was selected as the test pig, the other serving as the backup. The test pig was sedated and an extensive set of anthropometric measurements was made. Then the animal was anesthetized and incisions were made to expose both femoral arteries. A blood pressure catheter was inserted into one femoral artery and was advanced towards the heart to the level of the xiphoid process. A 16-gauge catheter was placed in the other femoral artery for the purpose of drawing blood samples for gas analyses.

Just prior to transporting the animal to the sled facility, an accelerometer mounting bracket was applied to the animal's nose using two screws located in the midsagittal plane and a wire wrapped around the plate through the animal's mouth. A polyurethane foam solution was injected between the plate and the snout, and when cured, provided a stable accelerometer mounting bracket.

At the test facility the animal was connected to the physiological monitoring equipment and monitored at 15-minute intervals for one hour prior to the placement of the animal on the impact sled. At each interval the following parameters were recorded: blood pressure, 6-lead ECG, heart rate, respiration, rectal temperature, reflex responses to toe and ear pinch, palpebral reflex, pupil size and reactivity to light, and muscle tonus. Drugs were administered in sufficient dosages to produce an animal that was immobile and had adequate pain suppression while retaining good neurological response levels for the physiological testing.

During this hour monitoring period, the accelerometers and the tethering harness were attached to the animal. Four uniaxial accelerometers were mounted to the nose bracket. Three of these accelerometers were positioned with their sensitive axes orthogonal with two of the axes lying in the midsagittal plane of the animal's head. The fourth accelerometer was mounted with its sensitive axis lying in the midsagittal plane, oriented parallel to the sensitive axis of the ventro-dorsal accelerometer and positioned 38 mm closer to the tip of the animal's snout. Two configurations of accelerometers were used for the torso. For the first configuration, a triaxial accelerometer package was attached to the animal's spine at the level of the sixth thoracic spinous process using a nylon strap that encircled the animal's chest. After several tests, it became apparent that this configuration had the potential to injure the thoracic spinous process during rebound into the seat for some of the animal positions. To alleviate this condition, a second configuration consisting of four uniaxial accelerometers was developed. Three of the accelerometers were mounted to the sternum, one each at the presternal protuberance, mid sternum, and xiphoid process. Their sensitive axes were oriented ventral-dorsally, normal to the sternum. The fourth accelerometer was mounted to the thoracic spine at the level of the sixth spinous process. Its axis was oriented ventral-dorsally, normal to the spine. All four accelerometers were encased in individual, thin rubber disks that were held in place by tape that encircled the animal's thorax. This configuration produced no indications of inducing any injury to the animal.

After the one-hour monitoring period was completed, blood was drawn for gas analysis and a complete set of visual and somatosensory evoked responses were taken. The animal was then taken to the sled and placed in the desired position. The animal was held vertically by a tether that was released just prior to cushion deployment. Its buttocks were supported by the seat, floor or foam blocks depending on the choice of animal position. Longitudinal and lateral position of the animal was maintained by paper tape that prevented the animal from translating rearward during the time the sled was being accelerated to the desired velocity, yet let the animal translate forward freely during the collision simulation. The tape was easily torn by the deploying cushion or by the rebound of the animal and had no effect on the animal's kinematics in response to the deploying cushion.

Once the animal was positioned it usually took ten minutes to balance and calibrate the instrumentation and go through the sled firing procedure. During this time the animal's position and physiological responses were continually monitored. Drugs were administered as required to assure a motionless animal with acceptable physiological response levels.

Postimpact

After the impact, the sled was moved under an exhaust fan to change and filter the interior air of the body buck, a safety procedure used when a number of tests are contemplated using sodium azide inflators. When visible emissions had abated, the body buck was opened and a preliminary examination of the animal was done by the attending medical doctor or veterinarian, who wore a respirator. Photographs were taken of the animal's position. The animal was then removed from the buck, sponged off and carried to the medical observation table where the physiological monitoring equipment was reconnected. The one-hour monitoring procedure described under preimpact was repeated. Two full sets of evoked responses were obtained during this period for comparison with the pretest data.

At the end of the one-hour postimpact monitoring period, blood was drawn for gas analysis. The blood pressure catheter was removed and the incision closed. The animal was transported to the SwRI X-ray facility where a full set of postimpact radiographs were taken. From the X-ray facility, the animal was returned to its holding cage for observation. At the end of the observation period (usually 24 hours), the animal was sedated and blood was drawn for gas analysis. Then, the animal was transported to the Necropsy laboratory where it was sacrificed and the gross necropsy was performed by the veterinary pathologist.

TEST CONDITIONS

The test conditions were selected by GM based on their analysis of child dummy tests that they had conducted at GM. For each animal test conducted at SwRI, a similar child dummy test was conducted at GM. This procedure was used to allow associations to be drawn between the observed animal injuries and corresponding measured child dummy responses. A summary of the test conditions is given in Table 2.

Simulated Crash Pulses—Three different sled deceleration pulse shapes were used during the test program. The severity of these simulated collisions can be described by their mean sled decelerations and velocity changes. Two constant-deceleration pulse shapes were used. The most severe pulse had a 14.5 g deceleration level with a change in velocity of 56 km/h. The other had a constant deceleration level of 8.4 g with a velocity change of 33.6 km/h. The third pulse shape was more trapezoidal and represented a car-to-car impact of longer duration. It had a mean deceleration level of 4.3 g and a velocity change of 28.5 km/h, and this was the mildest collision pulse used. The sled pulse used for each animal test is listed in Table 2.

Animal Positions—Seven basic animal positions, each representing a possible child position (9, 10), were used in the deployment tests. Examples of each position are shown in Figures 1 through 7. Table 3 provides descriptions of each position, distances between landmarks on the animal and the interior that were used in positioning the animals, and rationales for selecting each position for testing. Figure 8 shows the locations of the animal positioning landmarks relative to car interior landmarks. Deviations from these nominal dimensions were made during the course of the program in an effort to maximize the severity of the cushion/animal interaction. The nominal position and deviation for each animal test are given in Table 2.

Positions 1, 6 and 7 were used in preliminary tests that were conducted to select the animal species to be used as the principal surrogate for the test program. In the actual test program only Positions 1-5 were used. Position 6 was not used because the preliminary tests showed that the interaction between the animal and cushion was unpredictable for this position. In one test, the cushion deployed over the top of the animal's head. In a second test of the same position, the cushion deployed under the animal's chin. Position 5 was used instead of Position 6 in the test program in order to eliminate this inconsistency of cushion-animal interaction. Position 7, a side-facing position of the animal, was not used in the test program because the preliminary tests showed that the injury types and severities for this position were comparable to those of Position 1, the front-facing equivalent of Position 7.

Inflatable Restraint Systems—A summary of the inflatable restraint system concepts used for the various

Table 2. Summary of test conditions.

ANIMAL NUMBER	SLED KINEMATICS VEL. (km/h)	SLED KINEMATICS ACC. (G)	INFLATOR TYPE	INFLATOR ACTUATE (ms)	CUSHION TYPE	FOLD TYPE	COVER TYPE	ANIMAL POSITION NOMINAL	DEVIATIONS FORE-AFT (mm)	DEVIATIONS UP-DOWN (mm)	SEAT TYPE	SEAT POSITION
PIG 8	50.8	13.2	2	22	2	3	NONE	1	0	0	MODIFIED	FORWARD
PIG 9	54.9	14.3	2	20	2	1	NONE	1	0	6U	MODIFIED	FORWARD
PIG 10	56.8	14.8	2	20	2	2	NONE	1	0	0	MODIFIED	FORWARD
PIG 12	56.5	14.8	2	20	2	3	NONE	1	0	0	MODIFIED	FORWARD
PIG 13	56.8	14.8	2	20	2	1	NONE	2	19A	13U	MODIFIED	REAR
PIG 14	57.0	14.9	2	21	2	1	NONE	2	0	0	MODIFIED	REAR
PIG 15	57.0	14.8	2	20	2	3	NONE	1	16F	25U	MODIFIED	FORWARD
PIG 16	56.6	14.7	2	21	2	3	2	3	0	0	STD.	REAR
PIG 17	55.9	14.6	2	21	2	1	2	3	0	0	STD.	REAR
PIG 18	54.5	14.0	3	20	1	1	1	2	0	0	MODIFIED	REAR
PIG 19	33.3	8.4	4	28	1	1	1	2	44F	25D	MODIFIED	REAR
PIG 21	33.6	8.5	3	28	1	1	1	3	44F	13D	STD.	REAR
PIG 22	33.8	8.5	3	28	1	1	1	2	44F	25D	MODIFIED	REAR
PIG 23	33.8	8.4	3	18	1	1	1	2	0	0	MODIFIED	REAR
PIG 24	55.7	14.2	5	20	3	3	3	1	0	0	MODIFIED	FORWARD
PIG 25	34.0	8.6	5	28	3	3	3	1	0	0	MODIFIED	FORWARD
PIG 26	33.6	8.5	5	28	3	3	3	3	13F	0	STD.	REAR
PIG 29	33.6	8.5	6	29	4	1	3	2	0	0	MODIFIED	REAR
PIG 35	34.2	8.6	5	26	4	1	3	2	0	0	MODIFIED	REAR
PIG 38	33.7	8.6	5	28	4	1	3	2	0	0	MODIFIED	REAR
PIG 41	32.9	8.3	5	36	4	1	3	2*	13A	25U	MODIFIED	FORWARD
PIG 44	33.5	8.5	5	28	4	1	3	2*	0	25U	NONE	PADDING
PIG 46	32.9	8.3	3	0	1	1	1	3	44F	13D	STD.	REAR
PIG 47	33.4	8.3	3	29	1	1	1	3	44F	13D	STD.	REAR
PIG 51	33.6	8.3	7	27	5	4	3	1	6F	0	MODIFIED	FORWARD
PIG 52	33.8	8.3	7	28	5	4	3	3	6F	0	STD.	REAR
PIG 67	34.6	8.8	9	28	5	4	3	3	3F	3U	STD.	REAR
PIG 68	32.6	8.2	8	28	6	4	3	4	0	0	STD.	MID
PIG 69	34.2	8.6	8	27	6	4	3	3	6F	0	STD.	REAR
PIG 70	33.2	8.4	9	29	5	4	3	2	0	0	MODIFIED	REAR
PIG 72	33.4	8.5	9	28	5	4	3	2	3F	25U	MODIFIED	REAR
PIG 80	28.3	4.2	10	25	7	5	3	3	30F	0	STD.	REAR
PIG 81	28.5	4.3	10	25	7	5	3	1	51F	3U	MODIFIED	REAR
PIG 83	28.8	4.3	10	25	7	5	3	*3	41F	51D	STD.	REAR
PIG 84	28.8	4.3	10	25	7	5	3	2	51F	0	MODIFIED	REAR
PIG 85	28.9	4.3	10	25	7	5	3	4	0	0	STD.	MID
PIG 87	28.4	4.2	10	25	7	5	3	3	57F	51D	STD.	REAR
PIG 88	28.6	4.4	10	25	8	5	3	3	60F	51D	STD.	MID
PIG 89	28.4	4.2	10	25	8	5	3	2	51F	0	STD.	REAR
PIG 91	28.7	4.3	10	25	8	5	3	1	32F	38U	STD.	REAR
PIG 93	28.4	4.2	10	25	8	5	3	4**	-	-	STD.	MID
PIG 94	28.1	4.3	10	25	8	5	3	4	0	0	STD.	MID
PIG 151	28.6	4.2	10	25	8	5	3	5	0	0	STD.	MID
BAB 6	55.9	14.3	2	20	2	1	2	3	13F	6U	STD.	REAR
BAB 7	28.3	4.2	10	25	8	5	3	4	0	0	STD.	MID
BAB 8	28.6	4.2	10	25	8	5	3	5	0	0	STD.	MID

NOTES: * LOWER TORSO RESTRAINED BY STRAP
** TETHER SUPPORT RELEASED PRIOR TO SLED DECELERATION. PIG NOT IN POSITION 4 AT TIME OF CUSHION DEPLOYMENT.

animal tests is given in Table 2. Ten different types of inflators were used in combinations with eight types of cushions, four types of cushion folds, and three types of covers. Inflators 1, 3 and 4 were compressed gas inflators. The other inflators used sodium azide to generate the cushion inflation gases. All ten inflators had different gas flow characteristics. Cushions 1 through 4 were "circular cylinder designs" of diferent volumes and incorporated an internal knee restraint cushion (2). Cushions 5-8 were different concepts of "L-shaped" cushions (14). Fold 1 was an "accordion" fold that was symmetrically folded on top and bottom. This fold allowed the cushion to be deployed horizontally rearward. Folds 2-5 were different versions of a "top pleated" fold. These were asymmetrically folded with the bottom most part of the cushion being the layer nearest the cushion door. This type of fold restricted the initial rearward movement of the cushion and resulted in a more upward cushion trajectory. Cover 1 was a foam-filled construction. Covers 2 and 3 were injection moldings of different lengths and cross-sectional shapes.

Front Seat Description—Production type seats were used for the tests. In some instances, the seat cushion and frame had to be modified in order to place the animal in the desired position. For these tests, the front of the seat frame was removed and the thickness of the cushion padding was adjusted to give the desired seat height. Table 2 gives a summary of the seat positions and indicates whether or not the seat was modified for the various tests conducted.

ANIMAL SPECIES SELECTION

The primary consideration for the selection of an animal species to be used as the child surrogate for the test program was that its weight and size be comparable to a 3-year-old child, since that size child dummy was being used by GM in their passenger inflatable restraint system development program (11). Three animal species, the chimpanzee, the baboon and the pig, were considered as candidates for the animal model. Based on comparable

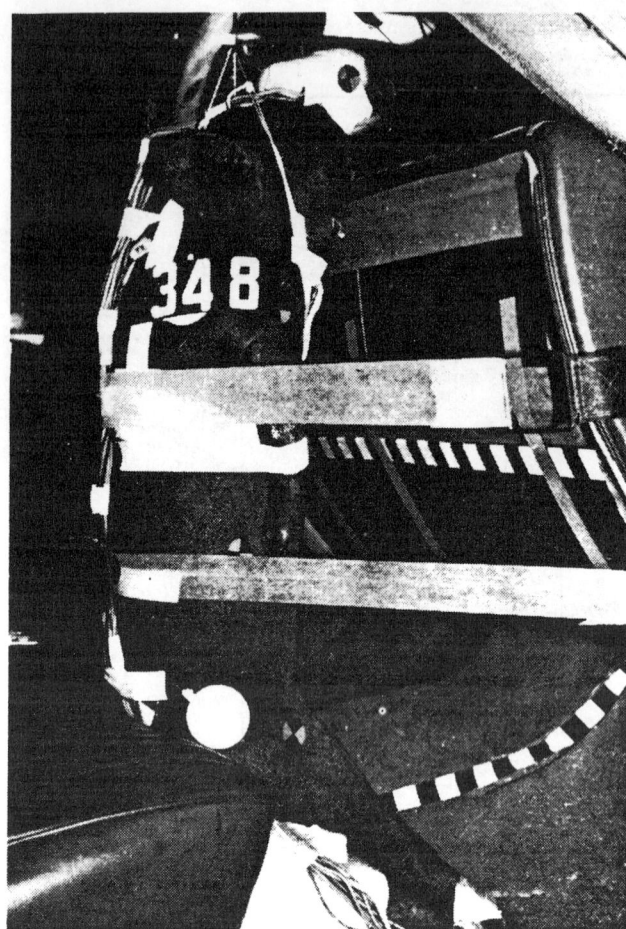

Figure 1. Animal position 1.

size and shape, the chimpanzee was the most logical choice. However, the test protocol required that each animal be impacted only once and necropsied for injury identification. This procedure required that a large quantity of animals be available for testing in order to meet the program objective of producing a broad spectrum of injury types and severities. A sufficient quantity of chimpanzees was not available to meet this program requirement. Consequently, only the baboon and pig were considered as possible animal models for this program.

The pig was selected as the animal model for the 3-year-old child for the following reasons:

i) it was available in large enough quantities to support the test program,
ii) it had more favorable anthropometric characteristics for its chest and abdomen than the baboon,
iii) its physical stage of development was similar to a 3-year-old child's, and
iv) it appeared to be more susceptible to injury than the baboon based on the results of a preliminary test program.

Limited testing was to be done with baboons for comparison purposes. The following is a detailed discussion of the reasons the pig was selected as the primary animal model for the test program.

Size and Shape Considerations—Table 4 gives typical size and shape measurements for the baboon, pig and a 3-year-old child of comparable weights. The pig was considered the preferred animal model over the baboon for investigating the potential for child thoracic and abdominal injuries since the breadths and circumferences of its chest and abdomen compare more favorably to the child's. Both the pig and the baboon have a major anthropometric deficiency as a child thoracic injury model in that their chest depth-to-width ratios are the inverse of the child's. Because of this geometric difference, both animals' fore-aft chest stiffnesses are much greater than the child's resulting in greater force levels required to produce compression type injuries to the thoracic organs.

For assessing the potential for child neck injuries, the pig has an advantage over the baboon since its head-neck length compares more favorably to the child's. However, both species have a number of major deficiencies as neck injury models. The pig has no chin protuberance for interacting with the deploying cushion since its neck attaches to the rear of its skull, resulting in its snout being somewhat aligned with its cervical spine. In contrast, the

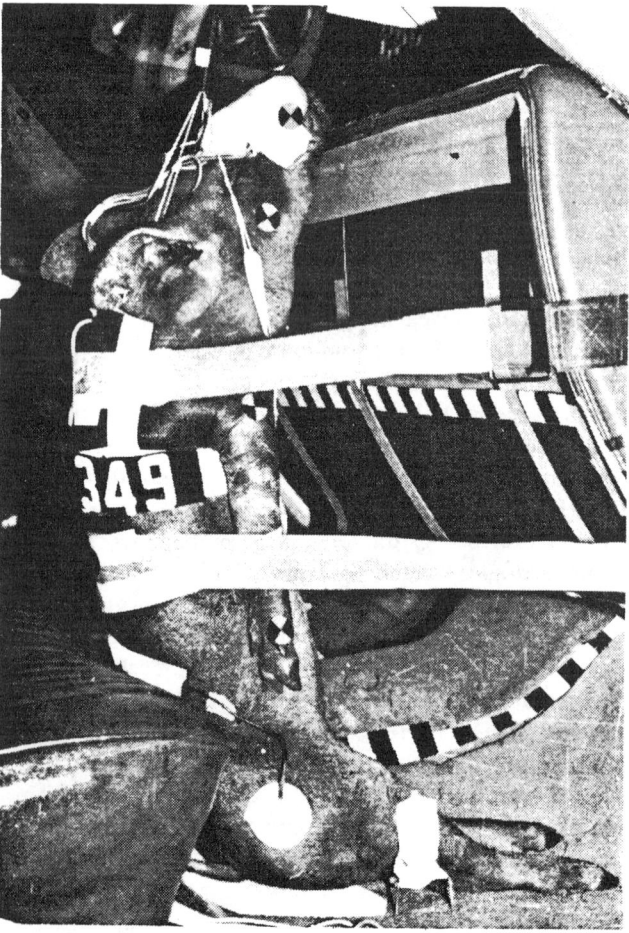

Figure 2. Animal position 2.

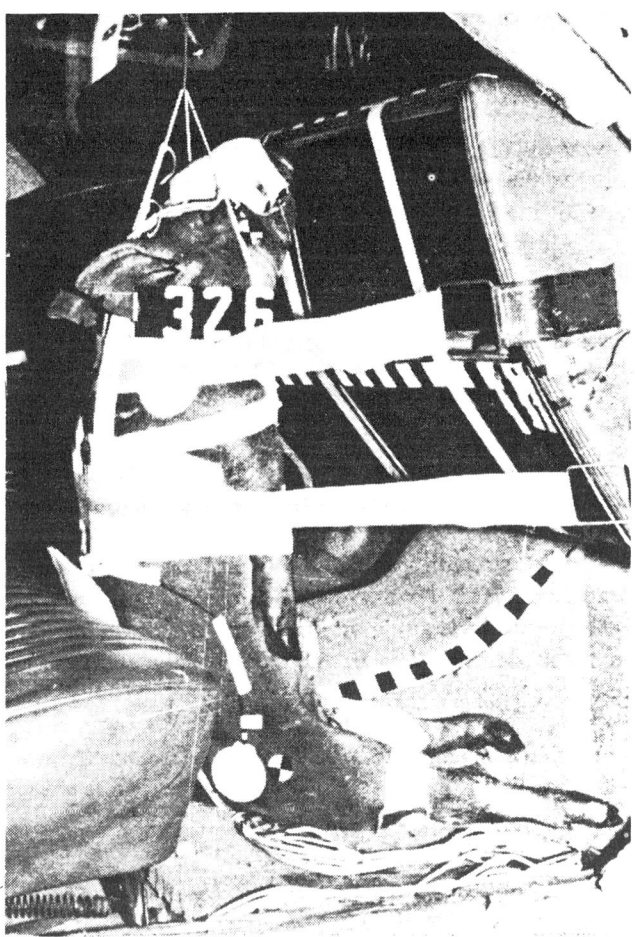

Figure 3. Animal position 3.

baboon's neck attaches to the base of the skull similar to the human. However, its long muzzle provides an accentuated, simulated chin protuberance. The fore-aft range of motion of the pig's head-neck structure is much less than the child's, resulting in a smaller degree of rearward motion required to produce a hyperextension neck injury. The baboon can undergo a greater degree of hyperextension than the child. The pig's neck circumference is twice as large as the child's due to its large dorsal neck muscles. However, these muscles have little influence on its head-neck kinematics since the animal is anesthetized. The cervical vertebrae of the pig and child are of similar size.

Neither animal species is considered a good model for assessing the potential for child brain injuries since their brains are much smaller in size than a child's.

Physical Development Consideration—The ages of a baboon and pig of comparable weight of a 3-year-old child are 4.3 years and 10 weeks (0.19 years), respectively (Table 4). To estimate an age of equivalent physical development for these animals, the animal's age was multiplied by the ratio of the ages that humans (15.5 years) and the animals (baboon—4.0 years and pig—0.7 years) begin to produce mature sperm. These calculations gave equivalent physical development ages of 16.6 and 4.2 years for the baboon and pig, respectively. Based on this analysis, the state of physical development of a pig and a 3-year-old child of similar weight are quite comparable. The baboon's physical development is much more advanced.

Injury Susceptibility Consideration—To determine if either species was more susceptible to injury than the other, a preliminary test series was conducted using 5 pigs and 5 baboons. Four pigs and four baboons were tested in Positions 1 and 7 with two of each species exposed in each of the two positions. A single test of each species was conducted in Position 6. Examples of these animal positions are shown in Figures 1, 6 and 7. The inflatable restraint system used for these preliminary tests consisted of Inflator 1, Cushion 1, Fold 1 and Cover 1. The sled pulses were characterized by a 13.6 g plateau and a 50 km/h velocity change. The cushion was actuated 21 ms after the beginning of the simulated collision event. A standard bench seat was used in the full forward position for these tests. The injury types and severities produced by these exposures are given in Table 5.

For Positions 1 and 7, the cushion-animal involvements were quite similar and produced similar types of injuries.

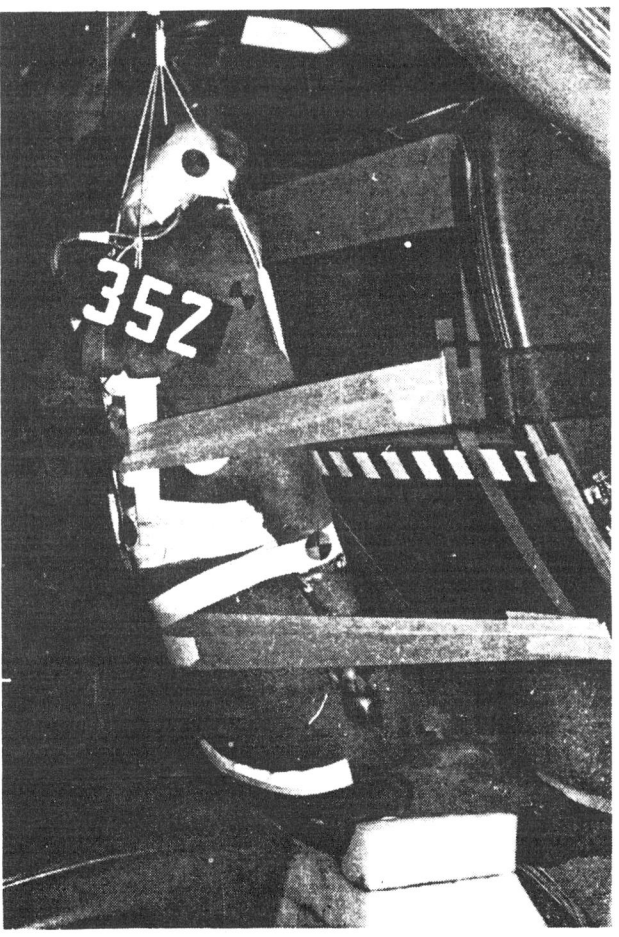

Figure 4. Animal position 4.

Table 3. Description of Animal Positions.

ANIMAL POSITION			ANIMAL TO INSTRUMENT PANEL REFERENCE		SELECTION RATIONALE
POS. NO.	FIG. NO.	DESCRIPTION	REFERENCE POINTS	DISTANCE (mm)	
1	1	SPINE VERTICAL, HEAD ABOVE I.P. BROW, XIPHOID 50 MM ABOVE CENTERLINE OF INFLATOR.	XIPHOID TO INFLATOR CENTERLINE	325 REAR 50 ABOVE	• EXPOSE ABDOMEN TO DEPLOYING CUSHION/COVER. • EXPOSE HEAD AND NECK TO UPWARD DEPLOYING L-CUSHION DESIGN.
2	2	SPINE VERTICAL, SNOUT ON I.P. BROW, XIPHIOD AT SAME LEVEL OF INFLATOR CENTERLINE.	XIPHIOD TO INFLATOR CENTERLINE	300 REAR 0 ABOVE	• EXPOSE THORAX TO DEPLOYING CUSHION/COVER.
3	3	SPINE VERTICAL, SNOUT AT I.P. BROW, PRESTERNAL PROTUBERANCE AT LEVEL OF TOP OF COVER.	PRESTERNAL PROTUBERANCE TO INFLATOR CENTERLINE	290 REAR 115 ABOVE	• EXPOSE HEAD/NECK TO DEPLOYING CUSHION/COVER.
4	4	SIMILAR SNOUT & PRESTERNAL PROTUBERANCE LOCATIONS AS POSITION 3, LOWER TORSO ROTATED FORWARD PARALLEL TO COVER.	PRESTERNAL PROTUBERANCE TO INFLATOR CENTERLINE	240 REAR 115 ABOVE	• EXPOSE HEAD/NECK AND TORSO TO DEPLOYING CUSHION/COVER.
5	5	SPINE 30° TO HORIZONTAL, SNOUT MIDWAY BETWEEN TOP OF COVER AND I.P. BROW.	TIP OF SNOUT AND I.P. PANEL	AGAINST I.P. PANEL	• EXPOSE HEAD/NECK TO UPWARD DEPLOYING L-CUSHION DESIGN.
6	6	SPINE HORIZONTAL, SNOUT JUST ABOVE TOP OF COVER.	TIP OF SNOUT & I.P. PANEL	AGAINST I.P. PANEL	• EXPOSE HEAD/NECK TO COMPRESSION LOADING OF DEPLOYING CUSHION/COVER.
7	7	SAME AS POSITION 1 EXCEPT ANIMAL IS FACING LEFT INSTEAD OF FORWARD, SHOULDER AGAINST I.P. BROW.	XIPHIOD TO INFLATOR CENTERLINE	325 REAR 100 ABOVE	• EXPOSE SIDE OF ABDOMEN TO DEPLOYING CUSHION/COVER • DETERMINE EFFECT OF ORIENTATION OF INJURY TYPE AND SEVERITY.

Table 4. Typical size, shape and mass measurements for 15 kg pigs, baboons, and children.

MEASUREMENT	AVERAGE OF 5 PIGS	AVERAGE OF 4 BABOONS	3-YEAR-OLD MALE CHILD	
			VALUE	REF.*
AGE (YEARS)	0.19	4.3	3	-
EQUIVALENT CHILD AGE (YEARS)**	4.2	16.3	3	-
MASS (kg)	14.9	15.2	14.9	15
SEATED HEIGHT (mm)	746	641	592	15
HEAD-NECK LENGTH (mm)	241	147	226	15
HEAD WIDTH (mm)	111	110	136	15
FORE-AFT HEAD MOTION (DEG)	45	110	105	12
NECK CIRCUMFERENCE (mm)	421	271	243	15
CHEST CIRCUMFERENCE (mm)	529	509	516	15
CHEST BREADTH (mm)	138	110	165	15
CHEST DEPTH TO BREADTH RATIO	1.33	1.44	0.67	15
ABDOMINAL CIRCUMFERENCE AT UMBILICUS (mm)	580	392	486	15
ABDOMINAL BREADTH AT UMBILICUS (mm)	147	125	165	15

NOTES:

* NUMBERS REFER TO PAPERS IN LIST OF REFERENCES

** EQUIVALENT CHILD AGE = $\frac{\text{HUMAN PUBERTY AGE}}{\text{ANIMAL PUBERTY AGE}} \times (\text{ANIMAL TEST AGE})$

The pig, however, appeared to experience more severe injuries. For Position 6, the animal-cushion interactions were quite different. The cushion deployed under the pig's snout driving the animal upwards and rearwards, hyperextending its neck. For the baboon, the cushion deployed

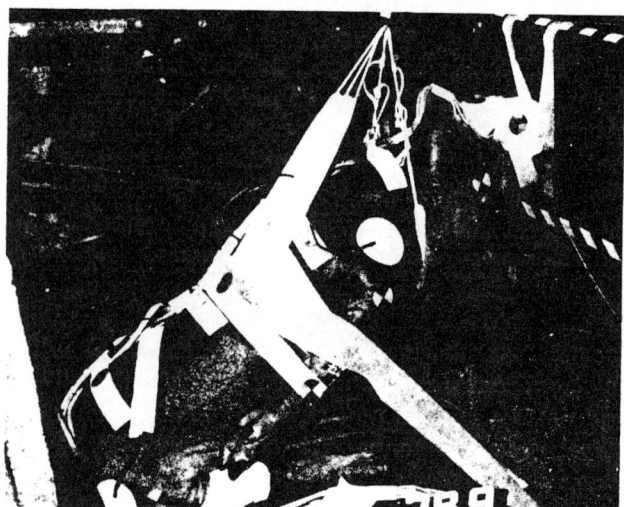

Figure 5. Animal position 5.

Table 5. Summary of animal injuries and severities for the preliminary test series.

BODY REGION INJURED ORGANS	ANIMAL POSITION 1				ANIMAL POSITION 7				ANIMAL POS. 6	
	PIG 1 (TL)	PIG 3 (TL)	BAB 1 (TL)	BAB 3 (TL)	PIG 2 (TL)	PIG 4 (TL)	BAB 2 (TL)	BAB 4 (TL)	PIG 5 (TL)	BAB 5 (TL)
HEAD										
BRAIN	6	2	3	3	2	3	3	2	6	3
NECK										
CERVICAL SPINE/CORD	4	0	0	3	0	3	0	0	4	2
TRACHEA	3	0	0	3	0	2	2	3	0	2
THORAX										
THORACIC SPINE	0	0	0	3	0	3	3	0	0	3
RIBS	0	2	0	0	0	0	0	0	2	0
HEART	3	0	0	0	0	3	0	0	0	0
LUNGS	3	2	1	0	1	1	3	1	3	0
ABDOMEN										
DIAPHRAGM	2	2	0	0	0	2	0	0	0	0
LIVER	4	2	2	3	3	3	3	1	2	0
GALL BLADDER	0	0	0	3	0	0	0	0	0	0
SPLEEN	0	3	3	3	0	4	0	0	1	0
INTESTINES	0	0	2	2	0	0	2	2	1	0
MESENTERY	1	2	1	1	0	1	0	0	1	0
KIDNEY	0	0	0	1	0	0	0	0	0	0
BLADDER	0	0	1	0	0	0	0	0	0	0

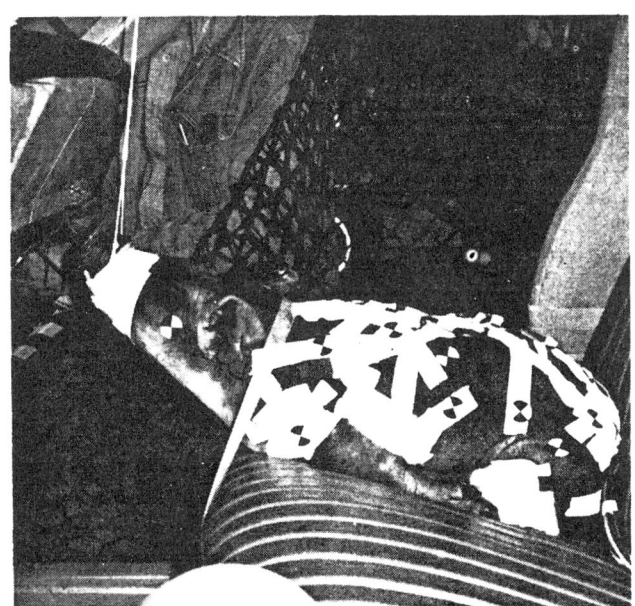

Figure 6. Animal position 6.

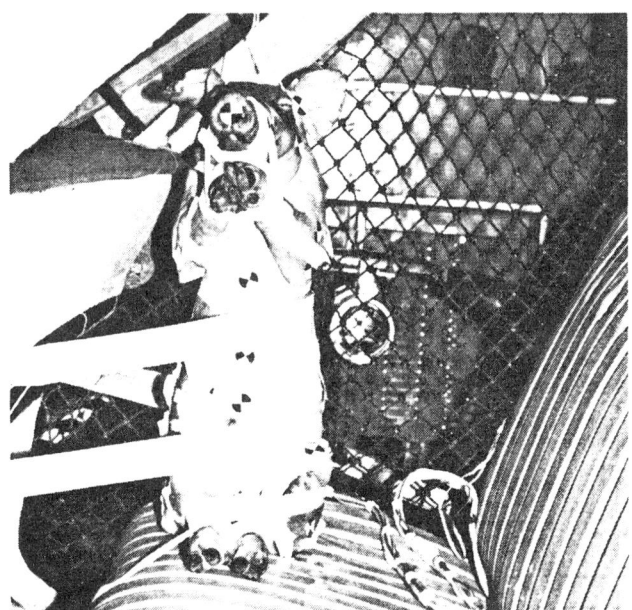

Figure 7. Animal position 7.

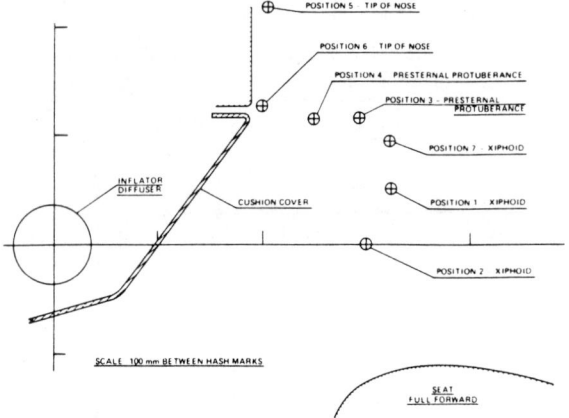

Figure 8. Locations of animal positioning landmarks relative to car interior landmarks.

over its head and there was minimum cushion-animal interaction. Based on these limited tests, the pig appeared more susceptible to injury than the baboon.

TEST RESULTS

Forty-three pigs and three baboons were subjected to the deploying cushion-collision interaction forces. The means and standard deviations of pertinent size, shape and mass measurements of these animals are given in Table 6. A summary of test results is given in Table 7 for each animal exposed to the deployment-collision forces for the test conditions given in Table 2. The peak internal inflator pressure is given in Table 7 for all the gas generating inflators. No pressures are listed for Inflators 3 and 4 which used compressed gas. Care should be exercised in interpreting the HIC and peak resultant head acceleration values since head acceleration was not measured at the center of gravity of the animal's head. Overall injury severity ratings in terms of threat-to-life (TL) and threat-of-permanent impairment (PI) are given for the body regions of the head, neck, thorax and abdomen.

For the pig tests, threat-to-life injuries ranging from 0 to 6 were observed for the head, neck and abdominal regions. Thoracic injuries ranged from TL equal to 0 to 5. The most significant pig injuries were subdural brain hemorrhages, partial transection of the cervical cord, rupture of the apical odontoid ligament, excessive straining of the membranes and ligaments surrounding the atlas-occipital region, cervical spine fractures, lung and heart contusions, persistent abnormal ECG readings, extensive rib fractures, liver tears, and lumbar spine fractures. Five of the animals (Pigs 8, 14, 15, 16 and 17) died as a result of their injuries. These test results indicate that the primary program objective of obtaining a wide spectrum of injury types and severities to the head, neck and torso regions was achieved.

The three baboon tests provided results similar to those observed in the preliminary test series. The baboon injury types were similar to the pigs, but the severities were somewhat less.

Caution must be used in interpreting the significance of these animal injuries relative to the expected performance of passenger inflatable restraint systems in general. It must be remembered that the objective of the study required using very aggressive passenger inflatable restraint system concepts for some of the tests in order to produce severe injuries to the animals. Because severe injuries were produced does not imply that all passenger inflatable restraint system concepts are aggressive. The fact is animals were exposed to several passenger inflatable restraint system concepts that were much less aggressive than the systems used to produce many of the severe animal injuries.

DISCUSSION OF RESULTS

Significant Animal Injuries

Head Injuries—Seven of the forty-six animals had significant (TL or PI ratings equal or greater than 3) head injuries. A summary of these injuries is given in Table 8. Four of these animals (Pigs 8, 15, 16 and 17) suffered fatal brain injuries. A photograph of the brain of Pig 8 is shown in Figure 9. Note the extensive subdural hemorrhage.

Table 6. Means and standard deviations of pertinent size, shape and mass measurements for the tested animals.

MEASUREMENT	PIGS MEAN	PIGS STD. DEV.	PIGS COEFF. VAR.	BABOONS MEAN	BABOONS STD. DEV.	BABOONS COEFF. VAR.
AGE (YEARS)	0.20	0.02	10%	5.2	0.8	15%
BODY MASS	15.7	1.0	6%	16.0	1.5	9%
BRAIN & SPINAL CORD	0.096	0.006	6%	0.183	0.005	3%
HEART	0.091	0.015	16%	0.068	0.007	10%
LIVER	0.490	0.078	16%	0.305	0.035	11%
SPLEEN	0.039	0.011	28%	0.028	0.019	68%
LEFT KIDNEY	0.044	0.006	14%	0.029	0.005	17%
RIGHT KIDNEY	0.042	0.006	14%	0.028	0.004	14%
SEATED HEIGHT	723	34	5%	661	13	2%
HEAD - NECK LENGTH	219	19	9%	125	6	5%
HEAD BREADTH	108	5	5%	110	6	5%
NECK CIRCUMFERENCE	448	28	6%	247	60	24%
STERNUM LENGTH	161	12	7%	159	12	8%
CHEST BREADTH	144	17	12%	112	17	15%
CHEST DEPTH	186	17	9%	146	7	5%
CHEST CIRCUMFERENCE	542	17	3%	499	54	11%
ABDOMINAL CIRCUM.	600	27	5%	463	11	2%
ABDOMINAL BREADTH	143	24	17%	143	16	11%

NOTES: BODY AND ORGAN MASSES GIVEN IN kg.
DIMENSIONS GIVEN IN mm.

Table 7. Summary of test results.

ANIMAL NUMBER	PEAK INFLATOR PRESSURE (Mpa)	HIC*	PK. HEAD RESULT. ACC.* (G)	PEAK V-D SPINE ACC. (G)	PEAK V-D STERNUM ACC.** (G)	PEAK BLOOD PRESSURE (mm Hg)	HEAD (TL/PI)	NECK (TL/PI)	THORAX (TL/PI)	ABDOMEN (TL/PI)
PIG 8	19.0	--	--	--	--	375	6/6	6/6	5/3	0/0
PIG 9	14.4	--	--	114	--	570	2/1	0/0	3/1	3/2
PIG 10	17.0	19300	675	101	--	500	4/3	0/0	2/1	2/1
PIG 12	16.7	8570	350	120	--	310	2/0	4/4	3/2	2/1
PIG 13	18.4	1080	164	147	--	530	0/0	3/3	4/3	5/4
PIG 14	15.2	2470	143	152	--	600+	3/2	4/4	5/4	6/6
PIG 15	17.4	10300	494	132	--	490	6/6	6/6	4/2	4/4
PIG 16	16.1	22800	798	--	--	370	6/5	5/4	3/2	2/1
PIG 17	15.7	6270	264	--	--	600	5/4	5/4	4/3	4/2
PIG 18	--	7410	321	259	--	325	4/2	3/3	4/3	4/2
PIG 19	--	1760	146	--	--	390	0/0	2/1	1/0	1/0
PIG 21	--	5060	309	--	--	530	1/1	3/3	3/1	0/0
PIG 22	--	3790	240	--	--	610	2/1	4/4	2/1	3/1
PIG 23	--	--	--	--	--	280	0/0	3/1	3/1	2/1
PIG 24	6.0	--	--	93	--	190	2/2	3/4	2/1	2/1
PIG 25	6.8	1350	180	55	--	210	0/0	5/5	2/1	2/1
PIG 26	5.6	1120	133	48	--	210	2/1	4/4	2/1	0/0
PIG 29	7.1	1760	193	69	--	380	2/1	3/4	2/1	4/2
PIG 35	5.5	--	--	121	--	240	2/2	0/0	4/3	4/2
PIG 38	5.9	1980	136	104	--	390	2/2	0/0	3/2	0/0
PIG 41	4.7	433	94	79	--	230	2/1	0/0	1/0	0/0
PIG 44	4.6	102	53	--	--	210	0/0	0/0	1/0	0/0
PIG 46	--	897	194	--	--	360	2/2	0/0	1/0	2/1
PIG 47	--	1770	151	--	--	260	0/0	3/3	2/1	1/1
PIG 51	9.8	866	103	46	--	195	0/0	0/0	(3/2)	2/1
PIG 52	10.3	2140	175	61	--	235	1/0	3/4	2/1	2/1
PIG 67	11.0	1220	121	84	--	220	2/1	0/0	1/1	2/1
PIG 68	6.1	--	--	57	--	400	2/1	3/2	3/2	3/2
PIG 69	5.5	1270	137	60	--	200	0/0	0/0	1/0	0/0
PIG 70	11.1	1020	170	52	--	260	2/1	4/4	2/1	0/0
PIG 72	11.6	765	164	63	--	330	0/0	0/0	2/0	2/2
PIG 80	10.8	455	132	38	1040U	145	2/1	0/0	0/0	0/0
PIG 81	10.6	325	100	35	1260U	160	0/0	1/1	1/0	0/0
PIG 83	10.9	450	93	43	685U	178	1/0	0/0	1/0	0/0
PIG 84	11.3	765	190	97	1110U	110	0/0	3/3	1/0	0/0
PIG 85	9.7	2440	184	166	1400L	420	0/0	3/4	2/0	0/0
PIG 87	9.7	1400	252	78	1740M	205	0/0	2/1	1/0	0/0
PIG 88	8.9	620	168	62	1340L	255	1/0	0/0	1/0	1/1
PIG 89	9.4	345	107	63	1300L	220	0/0	0/0	2/1	0/0
PIG 91	9.2	335	76	27	1520M	220	1/0	0/0	1/0	0/0
PIG 93	9.7	1850	221	97	570U	480	0/0	3/4	2/1	1/1
PIG 94	9.3	3000	332	86	2220L	625	2/1	4/4	2/1	4/3
PIG 151	9.5	1015	128	23	103U	250	1/1	0/0	2/1	0/0
BAB 6	13.0	3480	167	--	--	400	1/1	0/0	2/1	2/1
BAB 7	9.7	4810	243	297	2340U	490	1/0	3/3	3/1	4/3
BAB 8	9.5	2650	215	30	1190L	270	0/0	2/1	2/0	3/2

NOTES:
* NOT MEASURED AT CENTER OF GRAVITY OF THE HEAD
** ACCELEROMETER GIVING PEAK RESPONSE: U-UPPER, M-MID, L-LOWER.
( ) - THORACIC INJURY MAY HAVE OCCURRED PRETEST

Neck Injuries—Twenty-four of the forty-six animals experienced significant neck injuries. Table 9 gives a summary of these injuries. Two of the animals (Pigs 8 and 15) suffered fatal neck injuries. Pig 8 had a subluxation of the atlanto-occipital joint with torn joint ligaments and extensive subdural and subarachnoid hemorrhages of the cervical cord. Pig 15 had a fracture of the dorsal arch of C5 including the articular process and a partial transection of the cervical cord at the level of C5.

The most frequent neck injury observed was hemorrhage within the atlas-occipital joint capsules and/or hemorrhage dorsal of the membrane covering the midsagittal-ventral aspect of the atlas-occipital junction. Such hemorrhages were observed in twenty of the twenty-four animals with significant neck injury and appeared to be a good indicator of the onset of damage to the apical odontoid ligament, the ligament extending from the tip of the odontoid process to the occiput. In a number of instances, hemorrhage of the apical odontoid ligament was observed and was rated as TL/PI = 3/4.

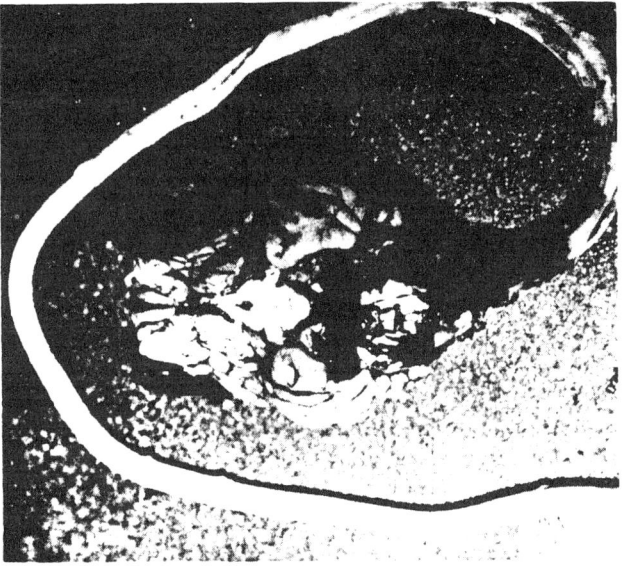

Figure 9. Brain of pig 8 showing extension subdural hemorrhage.

Table 8. Summary of animals with significant brain injuries.

ANIMAL NUMBER	HEAD INJURY SEVERITY (TL/PI)	INJURY DESCRIPTION	COMMENTS
8	6/6	DURAL SINUS LACERATION, EXTENSIVE SUBDURAL AND SUBARACHNOID HEMORRHAGE. NO PALPEBRAL REFLEX RESPONSE.	PIG DIED 12 MINUTES POSTIMPACT OF HEAD/NECK INJURIES.
15	6/6	SEVERE CONTUSION OF BRAIN STEM & CERVICAL CORD. NO PALPEBRAL REFLEX RESPONSE.	PIG DIED 2 1/4 MINUTES POSTIMPACT OF HEAD/NECK INJURIES.
16	6/5	SEVERE SUBDURAL & SUBARACHNOID HEMORRHAGE OF BRAIN STEM. ABSENT, DIMISHED, THEN ABSENT PALPEBRAL REFLEXES.	PIG DIED 39 MINUTES POSTIMPACT OF HEAD/NECK INJURIES.
17	5/4	DIFFUSE SUBARACHNOID HEMORRHAGE. ASYMMETRIC, THEN ABSENT PALPEBRAL REFLEXES. MARKED DEPRESSED RESPIRATION AND BLOOD PRESSURE.	PIG DIED 55 MINUTES POSTIMPACT OF APPARENT BRAIN STEM INJURY.
10	4/3	ACUTE BRAIN CONTUSION, ISCHEMIC, LEFT DORSAL TEMPORAL LOBE. ABSENT, THEN DEPRESSED PALPEBRAL REFLEXES.	
18	4/2	DIFFUSE BRAIN CONTUSION. PALPEBRAL REFLEXES DIMINISHED FOR 30 MINUTES POSTIMPACT.	RESPIRATION AND BLOOD PRESSURE DEPRESSED FOR 10 MINUTES POSTIMPACT.
14	3/2	PARENCHYMAL HEMORRHAGE. ASYMMETRIC, THEN ABSENT PALPEBRAL REFLEXES.	PIG DIED 24 MINUTES POSTIMPACT DUE TO BLOOD LOSS FROM SEVERELY LACERATED LIVER.

Fractures of the cervical spine were observed in three animals (Pigs 15, 17 and 68). Pig 15 had a fracture of the lateral arch of C5 including the articular process which resulted in partial transection of the cervical cord. This fracture was rated TL/PI = 5/4 because of the consequences of the fracture relative to severe damage to the cord. Pig 17 experienced a similar type fracture of C6 without involvement of the articular process or cord and was rated as TL/PI = 4/3. Both of these fractures were rated more severe than the rating given in the AIS-80 code (13) because of the potential for severe cord damage. Pig 68 experienced a simple fracture of the spinous process of C7 which was rated as TL/PI = 3/2.

Significant pathological changes in the cervical cord were found in only four of the twenty-four animals (Pigs 15, 25, 12 and 47) that had significant neck injuries. Pig 15 had the most severe cord trauma, a partial transection which was rated as TL/PI = 5/3. Pig 47 had cord damage rated as TL/PI = 3/3 without any evidence of cervical spine damage. It is difficult to understand how the cord could be damaged without attendant cervical spine damage. Perhaps the pathological observations of petechial hemorrhages is an artifact of the histology or necropsy protocol.

Thoracic Injuries—Sixteen of the forty-six animals had significant thoracic injuries. These injuries are summarized in Table 10. None of the animals experienced fatal thoracic lesions; however, Pigs 14 and 8 did suffer critical (TL/PI = 5/4 and 5/3, respectively) thoracic injuries. Pig 14 had extensive rib fractures, a first and second degree AV block followed by an incomplete right bundle branch block, and pathological damage to the heart and lungs. This animal died 24 minutes postimpact of blood loss from a severely lacerated liver. Pig 8 had a fracture of the body of T8, profound bradycardia and pathological damage to the heart and lungs. This animal died two minutes postimpact of fatal head and neck injuries.

Twelve of the sixteen animals had significant pathological damage to the heart. Six had significant lung damage. Significant changes in ECG occurred in five animals, including one baboon. Five animals had rib fractures with Pig 14 having the most extensive fractures. Three animals (Pigs 8, 18 and 68) had thoracic vertebral fractures. The heart lesion noted for Pig 51 may not have been related to the impact since histology indicated that it may have been an old injury.

In a number of cases, the overall thoracic injury rating is more severe than any of the individual ratings. These

Table 9. Summary of animals with significant neck injuries.

ANIMAL NUMBER	NECK INJURY SEVERITY (TL/PI)	CERVICAL SPINE SPINAL CORD (TL/PI)	CERVICAL SPINE ATLAS-OCCIPUT JOINT DAMAGE (TL/PI)	CERVICAL SPINE FRACTURE (TL/PI)	OTHER (TL/PI)
PIG 8	6/6	2/2	6/6	0/0	
PIG 15	6/6	5/3	4/4	5/4	PARTIALLY SEVERED CERVICAL MUSCLE (3/3).
PIG 25	5/5	3/2	5/5	0/0	
PIG 16	5/4	2/1	4/4	0/0	
PIG 17	5/4	1/0	3/3	4/3	
PIG 26	4/4	2/1	4/4	0/0	
PIG 94	4/4	2/1	4/4	0/0	
PIG 70	4/4	0/0	3/4	0/0	HEMORRHAGE, ATLAS-AXIS JOINT (3/3).
PIG 22	4/4	0/0	4/4	0/0	
PIG 14	4/4	2/2	4/4	0/0	
PIG 12	4/4	3/2	4/4	0/0	HEMORRHAGEIC CERVICAL MUSCLE (3/2).
PIG 85	3/4	0/0	3/4	0/0	
PIG 52	3/4	0/0	3/4	0/0	
PIG 29	3/4	0/0	3/4	0/0	
PIG 24	3/4	0/0	3/4	0/0	
PIG 93	3/4	1/0	3/4	0/0	
BAB 7	3/3	0/0	3/3	0/0	
PIG 18	3/3	2/1	3/3	0/0	
PIG 13	3/3	0/0	3/3	0/0	
PIG 84	3/3	0/0	3/3	0/0	
PIG 21	3/3	0/0	0/0	0/0	HEMORRHAGE, ATLAS-AXIS JOINT (3/3).
PIG 47	3/3	3/3	0/0	0/0	
PIG 68	3/2	0/0	0/0	3/2	
PIG 23	3/1	0/0	0/0	0/0	CONTUSED MUCOSAL SURFACE, LARYNX (3/1).

Table 10. Summary of animals with significant thoracic injuries.

ANIMAL NUMBER	THORACIC INJURY SEVERITY (TL/PI)	LUNG DAMAGE (TL/PI)	HEART DAMAGE (TL/PI)	ECG (TL/PI)	RIB FRACTURE (TL/PI)	OTHER (TL/PI)
PIG 14	5/4	3/1	3/2	4/4	3/2	
PIG 8	5/3	4/2	4/2	4/2	0/0	FRACTURE OF BODY OF T8 (3/3).
PIG 35	4/3	2/0	4/3	2/1	0/0	
PIG 18	4/3	2/1	3/2	3/2	2/1	FRACTURE OF SPINOUS PROCESSES OF T4-T7 (2/1).
PIG 17	4/3	3/1	3/2	3/3	2/1	
PIG 13	4/3	2/1	3/2	0/0	0/0	HEMORRHAGE, VENA CAVA (3/2).
PIG 15	4/2	4/2	3/1	0/0	0/0	
PIG 68	3/2	2/1	3/2	0/0	0/0	FRACTURE OF SPINOUS PROCESS OF T1 (2/1).
PIG 51	3/2	1/0	3/2	0/0	0/0	HEART LESION MAY NOT BE IMPACT RELATED.
PIG 38	3/2	2/1	3/2	0/0	0/0	
PIG 16	3/2	2/1	3/2	2/1	0/0	
PIG 12	3/2	0/0	3/2	0/0	1/0	
BAB 7	3/1	2/1	1/0	3/0	0/0	
PIG 23	3/1	2/1	2/1	0/0	0/0	BLOOD STAINED FORTH IN BRONCHI (3/1).
PIG 21	3/1	3/1	2/1	0/0	0/0	
PIG 9	3/1	3/1	1/0	0/0	0/0	

Table 11. Summary of animals with significant abdominal injuries.

ANIMAL NUMBER	ABDOMINAL INJURY SEVERITY (TL/PI)	LIVER (TL/PI)	DIAPHRAGM (TL/PI)	SPLEEN (TL/PI)	KIDNEY (TL/PI)	GALL BLADDER (TL/PI)	INTESTINE (TL/PI)	OTHER (TL/PI)
PIG 14	6/6	6/6	3/1	0/0	0/0	0/0	0/0	
PIG 13	5/4	5/4	0/0	0/0	2/1	0/0	0/0	MESENTERY HEMORRHAGE (3/1).
PIG 15	4/4	4/4	3/1	0/0	0/0	0/0	0/0	
BAB 7	4/3	4/3	0/0	2/1	3/2	0/0	3/2	SEVERE HEMORRHAGE OF OMENTUM (3/2) & PORTAL VEIN (4/3).
PIG 94	4/3	4/3	2/1	0/0	0/0	0/0	0/0	
PIG 35	4/2	4/2	0/0	0/0	0/0	0/0	0/0	
PIG 29	4/2	4/2	0/0	0/0	0/0	2/1	0/0	
PIG 18	4/2	4/2	0/0	0/0	0/0	0/0	0/0	
PIG 17	4/2	4/2	0/0	0/0	0/0	0/0	0/0	
BAB 8	3/2	1/1	0/0	0/0	0/0	3/2	2/1	
PIG 68	3/2	3/2	0/0	0/0	2/1	0/0	0/0	
PIG 9	3/2	3/2	0/0	0/0	0/0	0/0	3/2	
PIG 22	3/1	3/1	0/0	0/0	0/0	0/0	0/0	

higher severity ratings reflect the possible synergistic effect of multiple significant thoracic injuries.

The most frequent gross cardiac pathology observations were subendocardial petechiae and/or ecchymoses of the interventricular septum and/or papillary muscle of the left ventricle. Such hemorrhages were observed in both impacted animals and in non-impacted, control animals. Since it was not possible to separate the artifactually jinduced hemorrhages from impact-induced hemorrhages, all such hemorrhages were rated as impact induced. Changes in the animal handling and euthanasia techniques were instituted in an attempt to reduce the occurrence of artifactually induced hemorrhages.

Abdominal Injuries—Thirteen of the forty-six animals, including two of the three baboons, had significant abdominal injuries (Table 11). The liver was the most frequently injured abdominal organ. Nine of the fourteen animals had lacerated lobes and/or junctional tears of the liver which were rated as TL equal to four or greater. Pig 14 died 24 minutes postimpact of blood loss from the severely lacerated liver shown in Figure 10. Pig 13 had a deep rent on the right lobe of the liver that resulted in ischemic necrosis of the parenchyma, peripheral to the tear, Figure 11.

Distribution of Various Mechanical Response Measurements Within Discrete Injury Classifications

For each animal, the mechanical response measurements listed in Table 7 were paired with threat-to-life (TL) injury severity ratings for selected body regions. HIC's were paired with the TL ratings for the head, peak

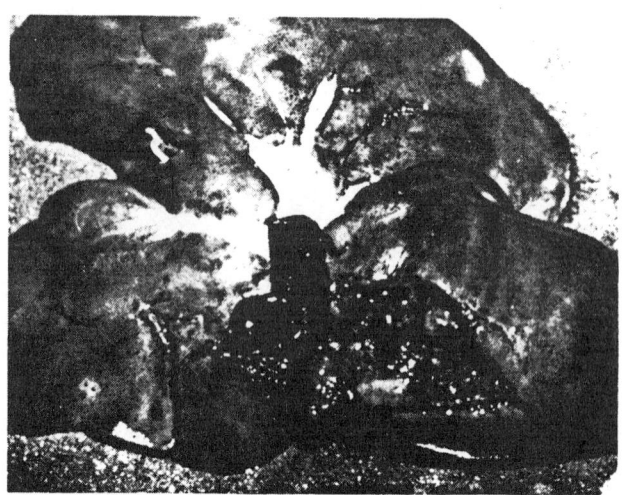

Figure 10. Severely lacerated liver of pig 14.

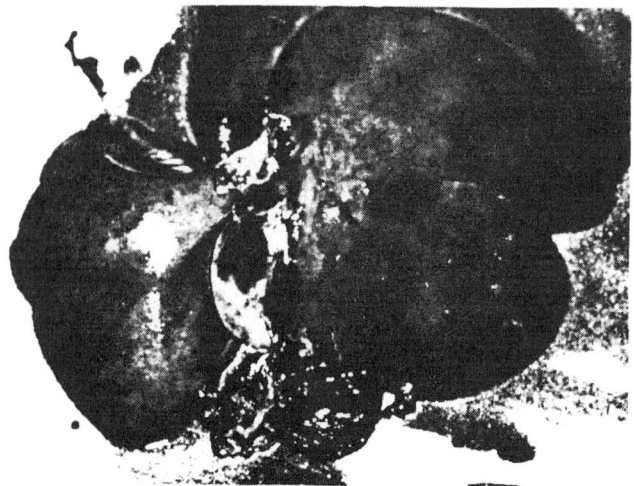

Figure 11. Ischemic necrosis of the liver of pig 13 peripheral to the laceration.

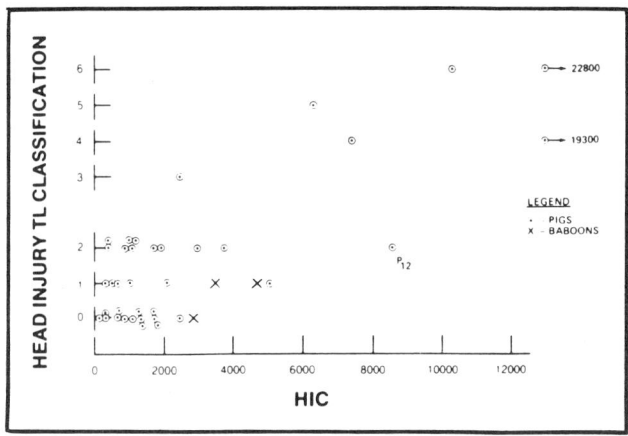

Figure 12. Distributions of head HIC values within the various head TL classifications.

resultant head accelerations with neck injury TL ratings, and peak ventro-dorsal thoracic spine accelerations with the thorax and the abdomen TL ratings. These pairings are displayed in Figures 12 through 15 for the body regions of the head, neck, thorax and abdomen, respectively. The thoracic injury rating for Pig 51 was not plotted since the injury could have occurred pretest. The thoracic and abdominal injury ratings for Baboon 8 were not plotted because the sensivity axis of the thoracic spine accelerometer was not aligned with the direction of the cushion-animal interaction force for the animal position that was used (see Figure 5). The TL ratings are shown as discrete classifications, ranked in terms of increasing injury severity. Linearity of severity should not be assumed between the integers assigned to the various classifications.

Note that for a given body region, many of the mechanical response ranges for the various discrete TL classifications overlap. Two possible reasons for these overlaps are: i) the animals have different levels of injury susceptibility, and ii) the measured response values chosen may not be the most appropriate indicators of the injury severity rating of the body region. It may be that a given injury type can be produced by a variety of mechanisms,

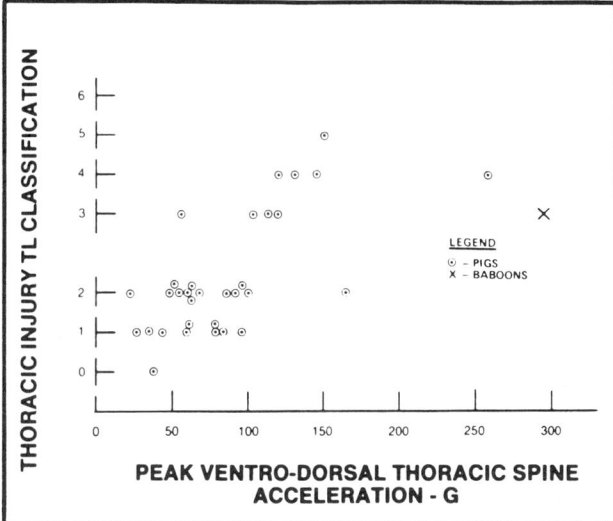

Figure 14. Distributions of peak ventro-dorsal thoracic spine acceleration values within the various thoracic TL classifications.

each related to a different physical parameter or combinations of parameters. The implication of these overlaps is that given a value of one of the measured responses, the injury severity classification for the corresponding body region is not uniquely defined. In such cases, one must speak of the probability for various levels of injury severity.

In several cases, an extreme of a mechanical response range for a given body region and injury severity classification appears to be an outlier. Such outliers could be due to a number of causes such as mechanical response measurement artifacts, undiagnosed injuries, or injuries that occur as the result of procedural techniques and not the test environment. For example, Pig 12 had a HIC of 8570, but only a moderate head injury (see Figure 12,

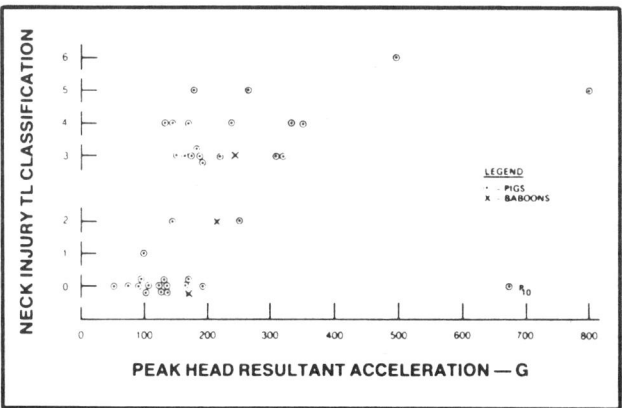

Figure 13. Distributions of head resultant acceleration values within the various neck TL classifications.

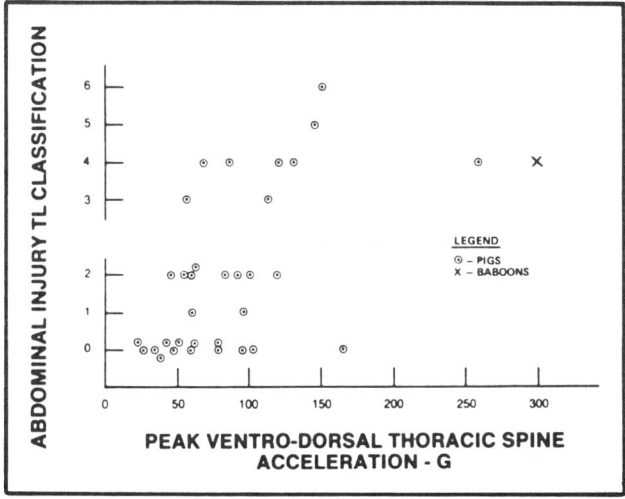

Figure 15. Distributions of peak ventro-dorsal thoracic spine acceleration values within the various abdominal TL classifications.

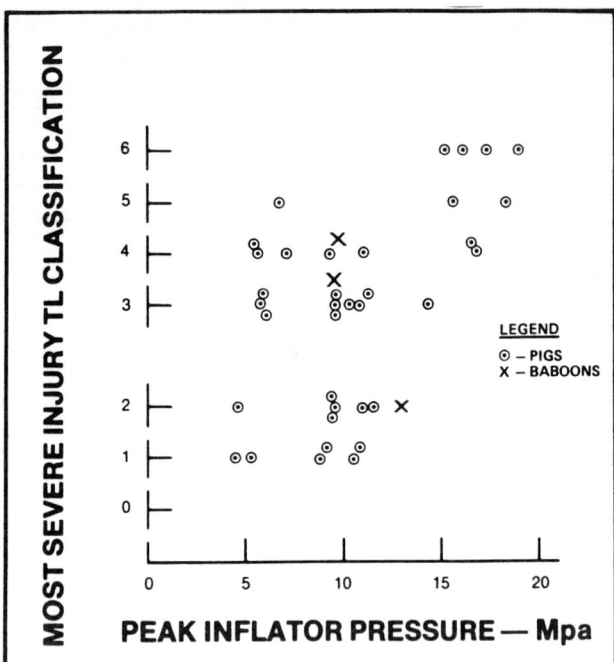

Figure 16. Association between peak inflator pressure and most severe injury.

TL = 2 Classification). The resultant head acceleration of Pig 12 had two distinct peaks and the HIC time interval contained both peaks. The HIC value for either peak, individually, would be lower and probably would be more representative of the severity of the head impact environment. As a second example of an outlier, Pig 10 had peak resultant head acceleration of 675 g's without any apparent neck injury (Figure 13, TL = 0 Classification). In this case, it is quite possible that Pig 10 had an undiagnosed neck injury since the dissection technique used to detect neck injuries was not developed until later in the program.

Peak inflator pressure was paired with the highest TL rating experienced by the animal. A plot of these pairings is given in Figure 16. Note the strong association between the more aggressive inflators (peak pressures of 15 Mpa or greater) and the more severe injuries (TL's of 5 and 6).

SUMMARY

Forty-six anesthetized animals (forty-three pigs and three baboons) were subjected to a variety of deploying cushion-collision interaction forces which produced a broad spectrum of injury types and severities to the major organs of the head, neck and torso of the animals. The severity of the animal injuries were rated as if the injuries were sustained by a 3-year-old child. For the pig tests, threat-to-life (TL) injuries ranging from no injuries (TL = 0) to non-survivable injuries (TL = 6) were identified for organs of the head, neck and abdomen. Thoracic organ injuries ranged from no injuries (TL = 0) to critical injuries (TL = 5). The more significant injuries were subdural brain hemorrhages, partial transection of the cervical cord, rupture of the apical odontoid ligament, excessive straining of the membranes and ligaments surrounding the atlas-occipital region with attendant hemorrhaging, cervical spine fractures, lung and heart contusions, persistent abnormal ECG readings, extensive rib fractures, liver tears and lumbar spine fractures. Five of the pigs died as a result of their injuries. Three baboons were used in the program and experienced similar, but less severe injuries than pigs that were exposed to similar test environments. The animal injury data were needed to interpret the significance of the responses of a specially instrumented child dummy (11) that was being used in GM's passenger inflatable restraint development program. That interpretation is the topic of a separate paper by Mertz and Weber (12).

ACKNOWLEDGEMENTS

The program described in this paper was a multi-disciplinary project requiring the efforts of many people. The authors would like to express their appreciation to the instrumentation, sled and animal care staffs of Southwest Research Institute for handling the many details of conducting the tests; to the medical specialists for their interpretation of the animal injuries and to the management and staffs of Passenger Inflatable Restraint group of Fisher Body and the Inflatable Restraint Project Center of Current Product Engineering of General Motors Corporation for their support of this project. A special note of thanks is given to Vernon Lancaster who handled the logistics of the test hardware and to Dr. K. D. Carey and Ned Zamora his assistant who conducted the animal necropsies.

LIST OF REFERENCES

1. Patrick, L. M. and Nyquist, G. W., "Airbag Effects on the Out-of-Position Child", 2nd International Conference on Passive Restraints, SAE 720442, 1972.
2. Campbell, D. D., "Air Cushion Restraint Systems Development and Vehicle Application", 2nd International Conference on Passive Restraints, SAE 720407, 1972.
3. Klove, E. H. and Olgesby, R. N., "Special Problems and Considerations in the Development of Air Cushion Restraint Systems", 2nd International Conference on Passive Restraints, SAE 720411, 1972.
4. Smith, G. R., Hurite, S. S., Yanik, A. J., and Greer, C. R., "Human Volunteer Testing of GM Air Cushions", 2nd International Conference on Passive Restraints, SAE 720443, 1972.
5. Wu, H., Tank, S. C., and Petrof, R. C., "Interaction Dynamics of an Inflating Air Bag and a Standing Child", SAE 730604, 1973.

6. Lundstrom, L. C., "Rating Air Cushion Performance to Human Factors and Tolerance Levels", Fifth International Technical Conference on Experimental Safety Vehicles, 1974.
7. Aldman, B., Anderson, A., and Saxmark, O., "Possible Effects of Airbag Inflation on a Standing Child", Proceedings of the International Meeting on Biomechanics of Trauma in Children, Lyon, France, 1974.
8. Takeda, H. and Kobayashi, S., "Injuries to Children From Airbag Deployment", 8th International Technical Conference on Experimental Safety Vehicles, 1980.
9. Stalnaker, R. L., Klusmeyer, L. F., Peel, H. H., White, C. D., Smith, G. R., and Mertz, H. J., "Unrestrained, Front Seat, Child Surrogate Trajectories Produced by Hard Braking", Proceedings of the Twenty-Sixth Stapp Car Crash Conference, October 20-22, 1982.
10. Montalvo, F., Bryant, R. W., Mertz, H. J., "Possible Positions and Postures of Unrestrained Front-Seat Children at the Instant of Collision", Proceedings of the Ninth International Technical Conference on Experimental Safety Vehicles, Nov. 1-4, 1982.
11. Wolanin, M. J., Mertz, H. J., Nyznyk, R. S., and Vincent, J. H., "Description and Basis of a Three-Year-Old Child Dummy for Evaluating Passenger Inflatable Restraint Concepts", Proceedings of the Ninth International Technical Conference on Experimental Safety Vehicles, Nov. 1-4, 1982.
12. Mertz, H. J., and Weber, D. A., "Interpretations of the Impact Responses of a 3-Year-Old Child Dummy Relative to Child Injury Potential", To Be Published.
13. The Abbreviated Injury Scale—1980 Revision, AAAM, Morton Grove, IL, 1980.
14. United States Patent 4290627, "L-Shaped Inflatable Restraint Cushion", Sept. 22, 1981.
15. Snyder, R. G., Schneider, L. W., Owings, C. L., Reynolds, H. M., Golomb, D. H., Schork, M. A., *Anthropometry of Infants, Children, and Youths to Age 18 For Product Safety Design*, SP450, SAE, Warrendale, PA, 1977.
16. Diffrient, N., Tilley, A. R., Bradagjy, J. C., "Design Requirements for Infants and Children", *Human Scale (TM) 1/2/3*, MIT Press, Cambridge, 1974.

826048

Interpretations of the Impact Responses of a Three-Year-Old Child Dummy Relative to Child Injury Potential

H. J. Mertz and D. A. Weber
General Motors Corporation

ABSTRACT

An analysis is presented that was used to interpret the significance of response measurements made with a specially instrumented, 3-year-old child dummy that was used to evaluate child injury potential of the second-generation, passenger inflatable restraint system that was being developed by General Motors Corporation. Anesthetized animals and a specially instrumented child dummy, both 3-year-old child surrogates, were exposed to similar inflating-cushion, simulated collision environments. The exposure environments were chosen to produce a wide spectrum of animal injury types and severities, and a corresponding broad range of child dummy responses. For a given exposure environment, the animal injury severity ratings for the head, neck, thorax and abdomen are paired with dummy response values corresponding to these body regions. These data are used to develop relationships that can be used to predict the probability of an animal experiencing significant injuries to these body regions based on the child dummy response measurements. A rationale is developed for interpreting the predicted animal injury severities relative to child injury severities.

INTRODUCTION

A specially instrumented, 3-year-old child dummy (1) was used to evaluate the performance of the second-generation, passenger inflatable restraint system being developed by General Motors Corporation. While it was possible to assess the performances of various inflatable restraint concepts based on the relative magnitudes of the child dummy response measurements, no basis existed to interpret these measurements relative to child injury potential. In previous studies by General Motors Corporation (2) and Volvo (3), anesthetized baboons, chimpanzees and pigs were used as child surrogates to estimate the child injury potential of various passenger inflatable restraint concepts. Unfortunately, no attempt was made in either program to develop a test device (instrumented child dummy) to aid in understanding the relationships between the observed animal injuries and the cushion-collision interaction forces.

To develop a basis for interpreting the responses of the child dummy relative to child injury potential, an animal test program was again needed. The program proposed was to expose anesthetized animals and the specially instrumented child dummy to similar deploying cushion-collision interaction environments. Exposure environments were chosen to produce a wide range of animal injury types and severities, and a corresponding broad spectrum of child dummy responses. This scheme would allow association to be made between the animal injury severity ratings for the head, neck, thorax, and abdomen and the dummy response measurements for the corresponding body regions. A detailed description of the animal test program and observed animal injuries is given by Mertz et al. (4). The following describes the analyses that were done of that animal injury data and the corresponding child dummy response data to estimate child injury potential due to inflating cushion-collision interactions.

PAIRED ANIMAL INJURY AND CHILD DUMMY RESPONSE DATA

Animal Tests

Forty-three pigs and three baboons were subjected to a spectrum of deploying cushion-collision interaction forces, with each animal being subjected to a single exposure (4). Physiological measurements made pre- and postimpact were: blood pressure, 6-lead ECG, heart rate, respiration, rectal temperature, visual and somatosensory evoked responses, reflex responses to toe and ear pinch, palpebral reflex, pupil size and reactivity to light, muscle tonus, and blood gases. Drugs were administered in sufficient dosages to assure that the animal was immobile and had adequate pain suppression while retaining good neurological response levels for the physiological testing. If the animal survived the exposure, it was sacrificed usually 24 hours posttest. A detailed gross necropsy was performed on all animals. Selected sections of the brain, spinal cord, heart and lungs were examined microscopically.

The resulting physiological and pathological data were evaluated by a team of medical specialists that consisted of a neurophysiologist, a neuropathologist, a cardiac pathologist, a cardiologist, a pulmonary specialist and a biomechanics specialist/physician who was the team leader. The medical specialists were directed to assess the severity of the animal injuries as if the injuries had occurred to a 3-year-old child. When all the injuries for a given animal had been rated, injury severity ratings in terms of threat-to-life (TL) and permanent impairment (PI) were assigned to the body regions of the head, neck, thorax and abdomen. For the head, neck and abdomen, the overall body region TL ratings ranged from no injuries (TL = 0) to nonsurvivable injuries (TL = 6). Thoracic injury severity ratings ranged from no injuries (TL = 0) to critical injuries (TL = 5). In the following analysis, these TL ratings for the four body regions of each animal will be paired with corresponding child dummy response measurements. The PI ratings will not be used in this paper.

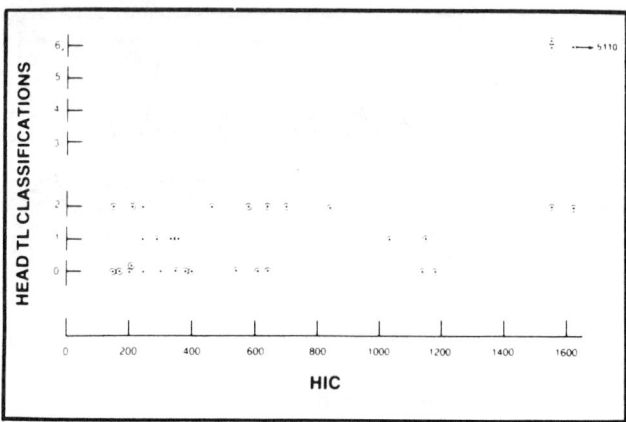

Figure 1. Paired child dummy HIC values and animal head TL values.

SELECTION OF CHILD DUMMY AND ANIMAL TEST DATA

For each animal exposed, a similar test was conducted using the instrumented child dummy. High-speed films of paired animal and dummy tests were reviewed to determine if the kinematics of the animal and dummy were similar. In a number of cases, gross differences in kinematics were noted. Data from those tests were excluded from the correlation analysis. A comparison of inflator characteristics was made between paired dummy and animal tests. In several cases, gross differences were noted in the performance of the inflators and the results of those tests were excluded from further analysis. The remaining paired animal and child dummy data were subjected to the following analysis.

ANALYSIS OF CHILD DUMMY AND ANIMAL TEST DATA

The head injury severity TL rating for each animal was paired with the child dummy HIC value that was measured in a similar exposure environment. These pairings are depicted in Figure 1. Similar pairings were done for the head TL ratings and peak child dummy neck tensions (Figure 2), the neck TL ratings and peak child dummy neck tensions (Figure 3), the thoracic TL ratings and peak child dummy upper-spine resultant accelerations (Figure 4) and maximum rate of chest compressions (Figure 5), and the abdominal TL ratings and peak child dummy lower-spine resultant accelerations (Figure 6) and maximum rate of abdominal compressions (Figure 7). Child dummy neck tensions were paired with head TL ratings (Figure 2) because the significant head injuries that were produced in the test program were subdural hemorrhages that appeared to be related to rapid rearward displacement of the animal's head relative to its torso. Neck tension along with HIC were thought to be good indicators of severity of this kinematic behavior. Conse-

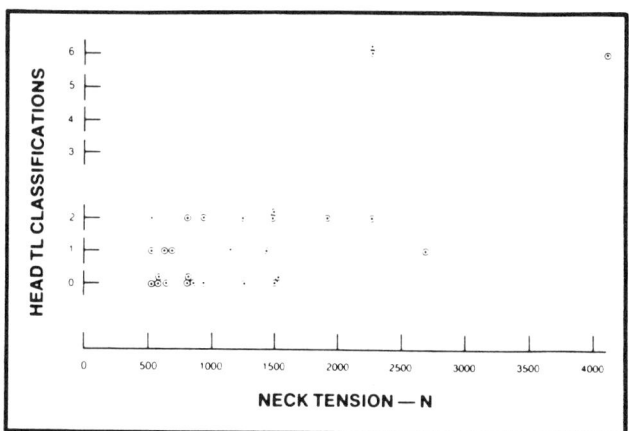

Figure 2. Paired child dummy neck tension values and animal head TL values.

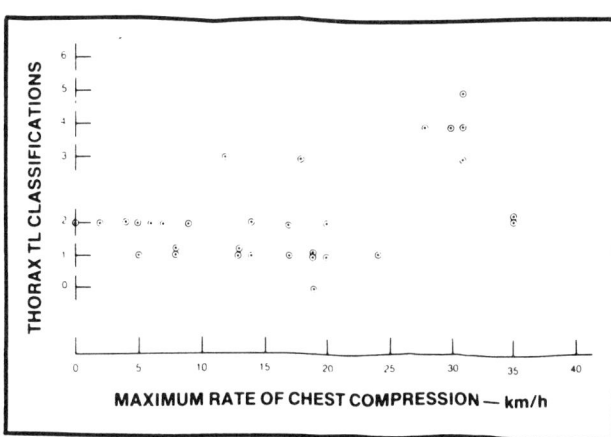

Figure 5. Paired child dummy maximum rate of chest compression values and thoracic TL values.

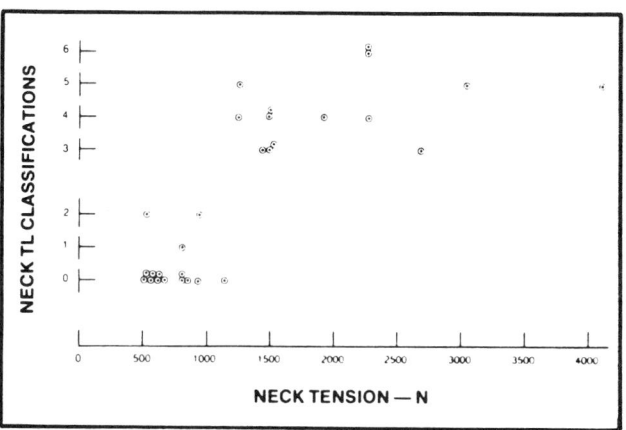

Figure 3. Paired child dummy neck tension values and animal neck TL values.

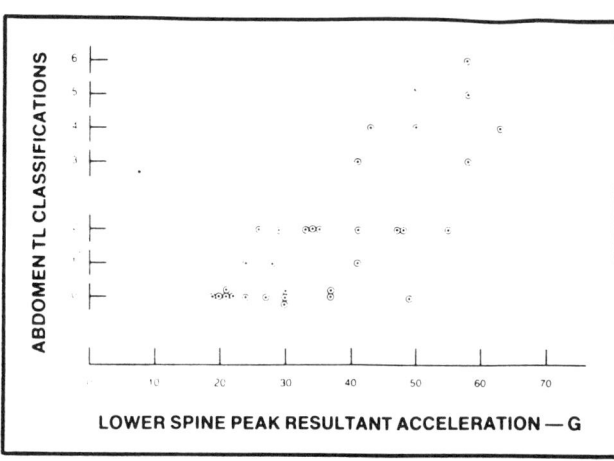

Figure 6. Paired child dummy peak lower-spine resultant acceleration values and animal abdominal TL values.

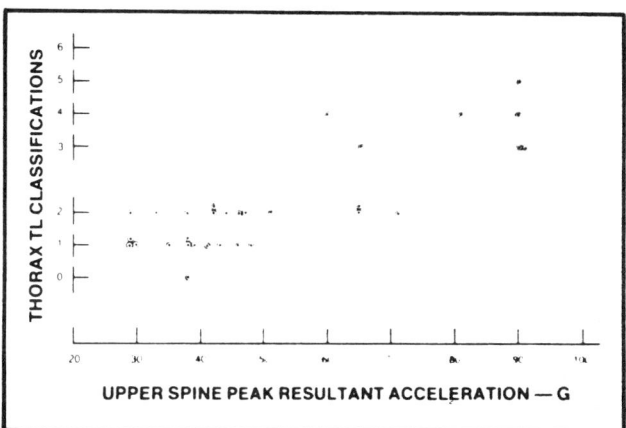

Figure 4. Paired child dummy peak upper-spine resultant acceleration values and animal thoracic TL values.

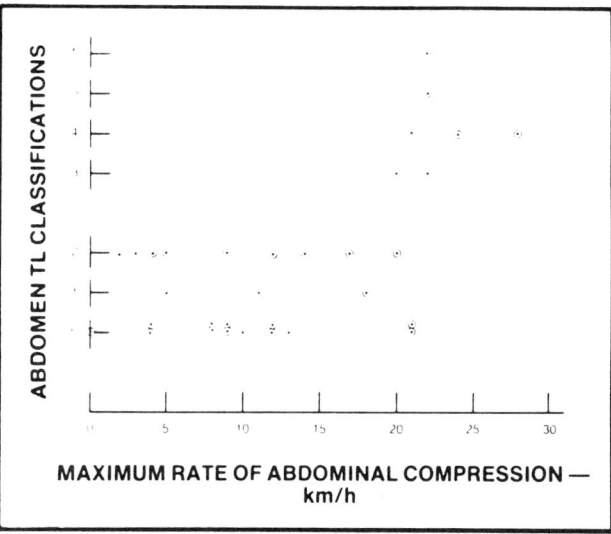

Figure 7. Paired child dummy maximum rate of abdominal compression and animal abdominal TL values.

quently, both child dummy responses were paired with the animal's head TL ratings.

To emphasize that linear relationships do not exist between the integer values assigned to the various injury severity classifications, adjacent TL classifications shown on Figures 1-7 are separated by a space. A larger space is used between the TL = 2 and TL = 3 classifications to distinguish between significant injuries (TL = 3, 4, 5 and 6) and nonsignificant injuries (TL = 0, 1 and 2).

DISCUSSION OF ANIMAL INJURY—CHILD DUMMY RESPONSE ASSOCIATIONS

Extremes of Injury Severity Classifications

The extremes of the range of the child dummy response data for a given body region and TL classification are bounds for the child dummy response value that is associated with 50 percent of the animals experiencing that level of injury severity for the prescribed body region. The lowest child dummy response value of the range is a conservative estimate of the 50 percent value, while the largest value is a nonconservative estimate. The actual 50 percent value will lie somewhere between the extremes and will not be, in general, the mean value of the child dummy response data associated with the given TL classification.

Distribution of Dummy Response Data for a Prescribed TL Classification and Body Region

There are two important features of the distribution of dummy response data for a prescribed TL classification and body region that need to be considered. First, the mean value of the child dummy response data for a given injury severity classification and body region is always greater than the child dummy, 50 percent response value. To understand why the mean value is a nonconservative estimate, the procedure used to select the test conditions must be examined. Test conditions were selected to obtain a broad range of child dummy response data for the body regions of the head, neck, thorax and abdomen. It was conjectured that the selection process would result in exposure environments that would produce a wide spectrum of animal injury types and severities, which it did. The test conditions were not selected to determine what levels of the child dummy response would correspond to the thresholds of the various injury severity classifications for the four body regions of the animal population that was tested. Such an approach would have required conducting multiple tests (6 or greater) for many, many levels of child dummy responses. Hundreds of animals and a similar number of inflatable restraint systems would be needed, both of which were clearly inconsistent with the program time frame and resources. With the approach that was used, it is unlikely that any animal was exposed to the exact test condition needed to produce the levels of injury severities that resulted. For this reason, the measured child dummy response values that were paired with the resulting injury severity ratings are greater than (very seldom equal to) the threshold values for the animal. Consequently, the mean value of the child dummy response data for a given injury severity classification and body region is greater than the 50 percent value.

A second important feature is that the distribution of the child response data within a given injury severity classification for a given body region can be highly dependent on the investigator's choice of test conditions. This feature can be illustrated by the following example.

Assume that all the animals have the same well-defined thresholds (child dummy HIC values of 600, 1000, 1500) for TL = 2, 3 and 4 head injuries. With this assumption, all child dummy HIC values between 600 and 999 will be paired with animal TL's of 2 and all HIC values between 1000 and 1499 would be paired with TL = 3 head injuries. The investigator selects his test matrix so that the child dummy HIC values range from 500 to 2000. If he chooses to conduct most of his tests for the TL = 3 range (1000 to 1499) close to the threshold of 1000, then the average for the TL = 3 classification will be close to 1000. However, if he chooses instead to conduct most of his test for this range close to 1499, then the average will be close to 1499. An even distribution of tests over the range will give an average close to 1250. All three of these mean HIC values are dependent on the investigator's choice of exposure environments and are nonconservative estimates of the child dummy 50 percent value for the threshold of TL = 3 injuries, which in this example is 1000.

Overlap of Ranges of Child Response Data of Adjacent Injury Severity Classifications

If in the preceding example the assumption was made that the animals had different thresholds of dummy HIC values for TL = 3 head injuries, then an overlap in HIC values would exist between the ranges of the TL = 2 and TL = 3 injury severity classifications. Let's assume further that the actual ranges of HIC values for the TL = 2 and 3 classifications are 600 to 1000 and 800 to 1500, respectively. Then, for HIC values within the overlap (800 to 1000), an uncertainty exists as to the injury severity level that a given animal might experience. For HIC values within the overlap, estimates of the percent of animals experiencing TL = 2 and TL = 3 head injuries are needed.

One approach to estimating these percentages is to assume that the thresholds of HIC values for TL = 3 injuries are normally distributed within the overlap. Implicit in this assumption is the requirement that the HIC value corresponding to the mid-point of the overlap is the child dummy 50 percent value. To estimate how the percent of animals experiencing TL = 3 head injuries varies, all the HIC values within the overlap (both those associated with TL = 2 injuries and TL = 3 injuries) are ranked ordered. These HIC values are assigned median ranking values based on their order numbers (5). The lowest and highest median ranking values and their corresponding HIC values are plotted on normal probability paper. A line drawn through these two points provides estimates of the percent of animals expected to experience TL = 3 head injuries for various child dummy HIC values. The median ranking values of the other HIC values within the overlap are not plotted since their distribution can be biased by the investigator's choice of test conditions.

It is possible that the test conditions and/or animals are chosen so that there is no overlap of the HIC values paired with TL = 2 and TL = 3 head injuries. If such is the case, then the 50 percent HIC value is taken as the average of the highest HIC value corresponding to a TL = 2 head injury and the lowest HIC value corresponding to a TL = 3 head injury. The highest TL = 2 HIC value is assigned the median ranking value of 0.2063 and the lowest TL = 3 HIC value is assigned a value of 0.7937. These are the median ranking values for the first and third order numbers for a sample size of three (5).

Both of these approaches have two shortcomings. The lowest HIC value within the overlap will usually be greater than the threshold HIC value for that animal and the highest HIC value will be less than the threshold HIC value for its corresponding animal. Thus, the median ranking value assigned to the lowest HIC value will be somewhat less than the true median ranking value for that HIC value. The reverse is true for the median ranking value assigned to the highest HIC value. The implications of these shortcomings are that the percent of the animals experiencing TL = 3 head injuries is underestimated for HIC values below the 50 percent value and overestimated for HIC values greater than the 50 percent HIC value. For the case where there is no overlap, the reverse of this implication is true, since the roles of the lowest TL = 3 HIC value and the highest TL = 2 HIC value are interchanged in defining the median ranking values. In both cases, the error in estimating the child dummy 50 percent value depends on how close the median rankings assigned to the extreme HIC values are to their true values.

APPLICATION OF MEDIAN RANKING TECHNIQUE TO ANIMAL INJURY—CHILD DUMMY RESPONSE ASSOCIATIONS

A review of the data shown on Figures 1-7 indicates that in most cases there is considerable overlap between the ranges of child dummy responses for the various injury severity classifications for a given body region. Within these overlaps, one must speak of the percent of animals expected to experience various levels of injury severity for a given value of child dummy response. The median ranking technique discussed previously can be applied to these data if the seven classifications of injury severity can be reduced to two. This can be accomplished by defining two groups: significant injuries (TL = 3, 4, 5 and 6) and nonsignificant injuries (TL = 0, 1 and 2). The results of applying the median ranking technique to the data shown on Figures 1-7 grouped in this manner are given in Figures 8-14, respectively. The percent of animals expected to have nonsignificant injuries for a given body region is 100 percent minus the percent estimated to have significant injuries. The curves of Figures 8-14 should not be construed as showing causative relationships, since the analysis is based on associations made of measured child dummy responses and observed animal injuries. These curves can be used to define a set of child dummy response values corresponding to any prescribed percent of significant animal injuries for the body regions of the head, neck, thorax and abdomen.

RELATIONSHIP BETWEEN OBSERVED ANIMAL INJURIES AND POSSIBLE CHILD INJURIES

The curves shown in Figures 8-14 provide estimates of the probable occurrence of significant animal injuries for various levels of measured child dummy responses. What

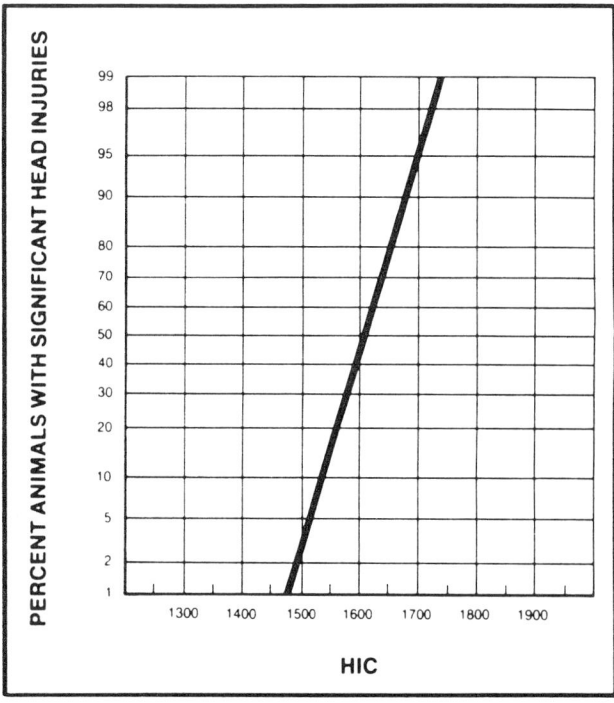

Figure 8. Percent of animals experiencing a significant head injury (TL greater than 2) as a function of child dummy HIC.

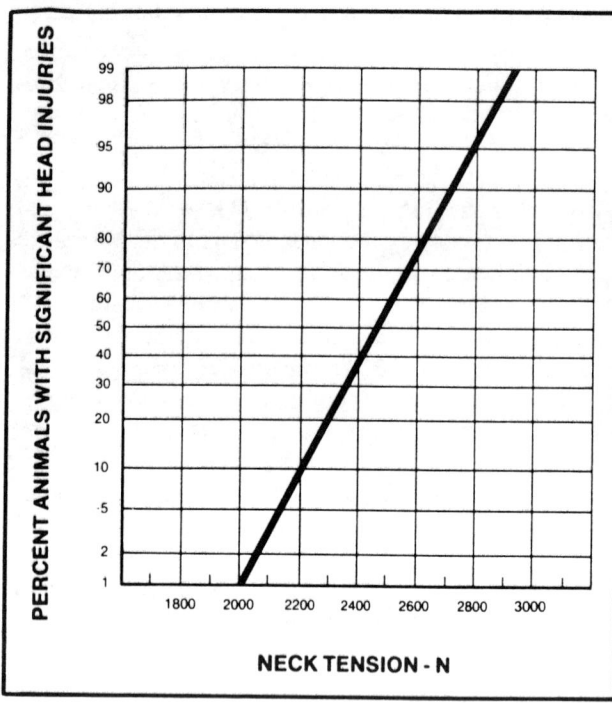

Figure 9. Percent of animals experiencing a significant head injury (TL greater than 2) as a function of child dummy neck tension.

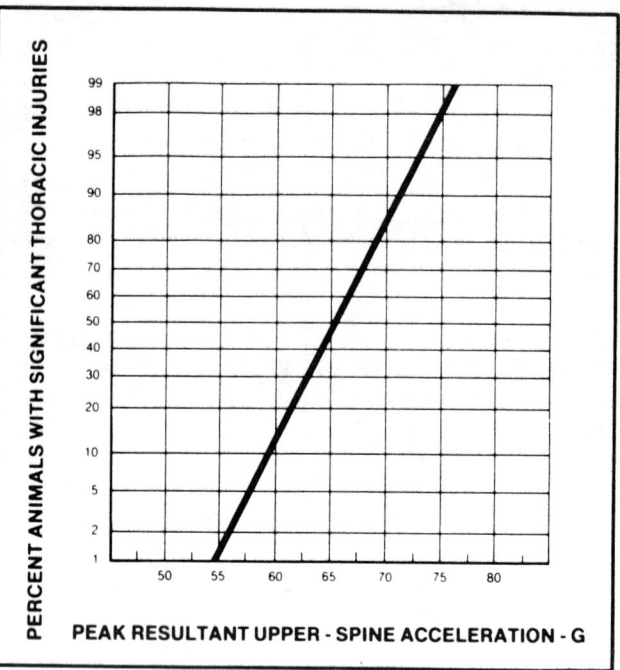

Figure 11. Percent of animals experiencing a significant thoracic injury (TL greater than 2) as a function of child dummy peak upper-spine resultant acceleration.

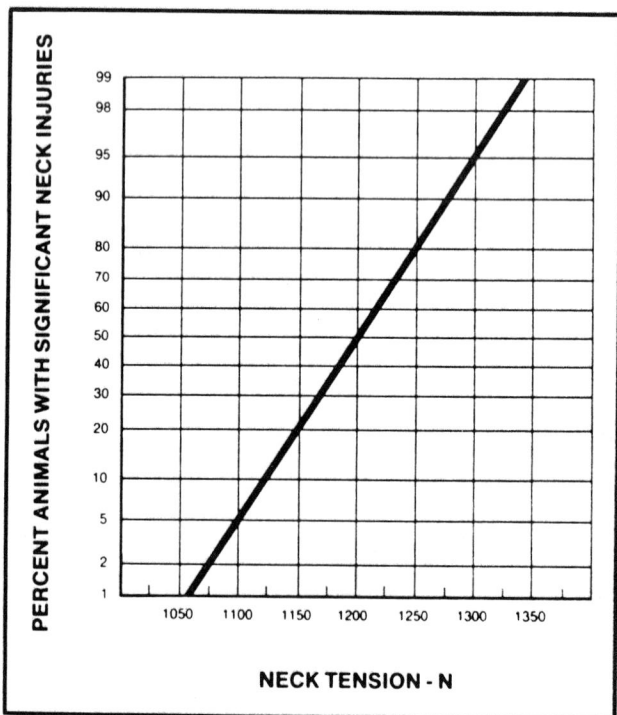

Figure 10. Percent of animals experiencing a significant neck injury (TL greater than 2) as a function of child dummy neck tension.

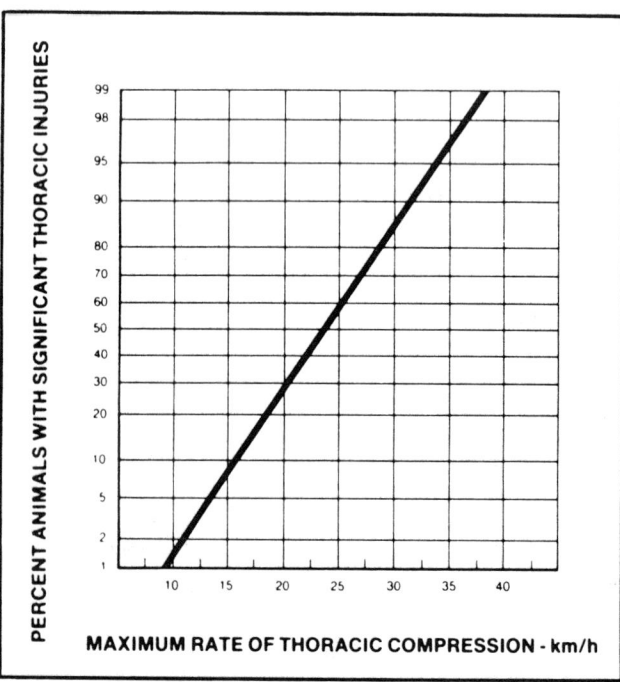

Figure 12. Percent of animals experiencing a significant thoracic injury (TL greater than 2) as a function of child dummy maximum rate of chest compression.

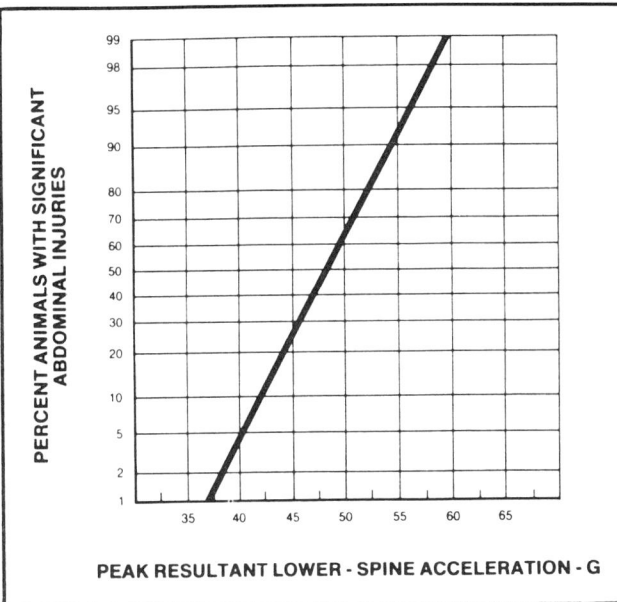

Figure 13. Percent of animals experiencing a significant abdominal injury (TL greater than 2) as a function of child dummy peak lower-spine resultant acceleration.

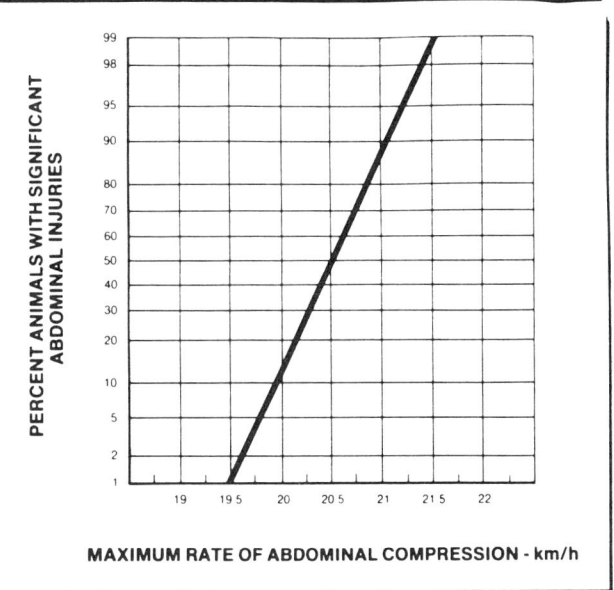

Figure 14. Percent of animals experiencing a significant abdominal injury (TL greater than 2) as a function of child dummy maximum rate of abdominal compression.

is desired are curves giving estimates of the probable occurrence of significant child injuries for various levels of measured child dummy responses. One approach to developing such relationships is to infer the probabilities of significant child injuries from the probable occurrence of animal injuries given by the curves of Figures 8-14. To develop such inferences, a comparison of the geometric, inertial and strength characteristics of the child and the animal must be made.

Animal Species Selection Rationale

The primary considerations used in selecting an animal species for the test program (4) were that its weight and size be comparable to a 3-year-old child, which was the size of the child dummy being used by GM to evaluate various passenger inflatable restraint system concepts. It was reasoned that animal surrogates that had overall geometric and inertial characteristics that were similar to the child would experience similar cushion-collision interaction forces as the child. Three animal species, the chimpanzee, the baboon and the pig, were considered as animal models. Based on comparable size and shape, the chimpanzee was the logical choice. However, chimpanzees could not to be obtained in sufficient quantities to carry out the proposed number of tests. Consequently, only the baboon and the pig were considered as possible child surrogates. While testing was done with both animal species, the majority of the tests were conducted using anesthetized pigs for the following reasons:

1. The pig's thoracic and abdominal breadths compared more favorable to the child's (Table 1). The implication of this consideration is that the thoracic-abdominal cushion interaction would be more comparable to those of the child.

2. The state of physical development of a 15 kg pig was estimated to be quite comparable to a 3-year-old child based on a comparison of human versus pig puberty ages (Table 1). The equivalent child age of the 15 kg pig was estimated to be 4.2 years while that of the baboon was 16.3 years. The implication is that the strength of the anesthetized pig would be similar to that of a child.

3. Based on a limited test program (4) where pigs and baboons were subjected to similar deploying cushion-collision environments, the pig experienced similar, but in some tests, more severe injuries than the baboon. This result is consistent with the previous implication that the physical development of the 15 kg pig is not as advanced as the 15 kg baboon. Using the apparently more injury prone pig would provide a more conservative estimate of the expectation of significant injuries.

Animal Model Deficiencies

There are a number of geometric and response differences between the pig and the baboon, and more importantly between either animal and the child. These differences can influence the interactions between the deploying cushion and the subject, and consequently, affect the resulting injury pattern.

Table 1. Typical size, shape and mass measurements for 15 kg pigs, baboons and children (4).

MEASUREMENT	AVERAGE OF 5 PIGS	AVERAGE OF 4 BABOONS	3-YEAR-OLD MALE CHILD VALUE	REF.*
AGE (YEARS)	0.19	4.3	3	-
EQUIVALENT CHILD AGE (YEARS)**	4.2	16.3	3	-
MASS (kg)	14.9	15.2	14.9	6
SEATED HEIGHT (mm)	746	641	592	6
HEAD-NECK LENGTH (mm)	241	147	226	6
HEAD WIDTH (mm)	111	110	136	6
FORE-AFT HEAD MOTION (DEG)	45	110	105	7
NECK CIRCUMFERENCE (mm)	421	271	243	6
CHEST CIRCUMFERENCE (mm)	529	509	516	6
CHEST BREADTH (mm)	138	110	165	6
CHEST DEPTH TO BREADTH RATIO	1.33	1.44	0.67	6
ABDOMINAL CIRCUMFERENCE AT UMBILICUS (mm)	580	392	486	6
ABDOMINAL BREADTH AT UMBILICUS (mm)	147	125	165	6

NOTES:
* NUMBERS REFER TO PAPERS IN LIST OF REFERENCES.

** EQUIVALENT CHILD AGE = $\frac{\text{HUMAN PUBERTY AGE}}{\text{ANIMAL PUBERTY AGE}}$ × (ANIMAL TEST AGE)

Neither animal's head is geometrically similar to the child's. The pig's head size is comparable to a child's; however, its shape is not due to its snout. The baboon's head is much smaller than a child's, and is characterized by a pronounced muzzle, similar to a dog's head. These characteristics will influence how their heads interact with deploying cushions.

The brain sizes of both animals are much smaller than the child's. Consequently, neither animal is considered a good model for predicting the potential for child brain injury due to direct head impact. However, such impacts were rare events in the test program. The significant head injuries that were produced in the program were massive subdural hemorrhages that appeared to be related to rapid rearward displacement of the animal's head relative to its torso and not to direct head impacts.

For assessing the potential for child neck injuries, the pig has an advantage over the baboon since its head-neck length compares more favorably to the child's. However, both species have a number of major deficiencies as neck injury models. The pig has no chin protuberance for interacting with the deploying cushion since its neck attaches to the rear of its skull resulting in its snout being somewhat aligned with its cervical spine. In contrast, the baboon's neck attaches to the base of the skull similar to the human. However, its long muzzle provides an accentuated, simulated chin protuberance. The fore-aft range of motion of the pig's head-neck structure is much less than the child's, resulting in a smaller degree of rearward motion required to produce a hyperextension neck injury.

The baboon can undergo a greater degree of hyperextension than the child. The pig's neck circumference is twice as large as the child's due to its large dorsal neck muscles. However, these muscles had little influence on its head-neck kinematics since the animal was anesthetized. The cervical vertebrae of the pig and child are of similar size.

The pig has a major anthropometric deficiency as a child thoracic injury model in that its chest depth to width ratio is the inverse of the child's (Table 1). Because of this geometric difference, the pig's fore-aft chest stiffness is greater than the child's resulting in greater force levels required to produce compression type injuries to the thoracic organs. This geometric difference could result in the pig underestimating the possibility of the child experiencing thoracic organ injuries due to chest compression. The baboon also has this geometric deficiency.

An in-depth study of the influences of all these various deficiencies is beyond the scope of this paper. A study was undertaken to investigate the influences of the neck deficiencies since significant neck injuries were the most frequent animal injury (Figure 3). The results of that study, when completed, will be the subject of a separate paper.

Interpretations of Measured Child Dummy Responses Relative to Child Injury Potential

The approach used to estimate the possibility of child injuries for GM second-generation, passenger inflatable restraint development program was to assume that a 3-year-old child would experience similar injury types and severities as the anesthetized animals. The curves shown in Figures 8-14 were used to provide a preliminary estimate of the probability of significant child injury based on measured child dummy responses. The final estimates were based on these preliminary estimates, tempered by the knowledge of the various animal model deficiencies discussed previously.

SUMMARY

A technique is given for estimating the potential for significant child injury due to deploying cushion-collision interactions forces based on measurements made with a specially instrumented, child dummy. These estimates should be tempered by the various geometric and response deficiencies noted for the animals that were used as child injury models. This approach proved quite useful in evaluating various concepts of a second-generation, passenger inflatable restraint system that were being developed by GM. The use of this approach should reduce the need for animal testing in any future inflatable restraint development program.

Section 6:
Modeling, Simulation, and Instrumentation

760771

A Biodynamic Model of the Human Spinal Column

S. A. Tennyson and A. I. King
Wayne State University

EXTENSIVE EXPERIMENTATION HAS BEEN conducted to determine the response of the spinal column to +G_z impact acceleration. Studies employing anesthetized animals were carried out by Beeding and Cook (1) with swine and bears and by Stapp (2,3) with swine and chimpanzees to establish injury patterns above tolerance limits. Kazarian et al. (4) employed the rhesus monkey to study spinal fracture patterns sustained during high amplitude, short duration impacts.

Human cadaveric subjects have been used to determine vertebral strain patterns and spinal injury mechanisms. Vulcan et al. (5) reported on the significance of bending on the spinal column. Prasad et al. (6) presented evidence of the load-bearing role of articular facets. This role was subsequently firmly established by Hakim (7). Load transimssibility via the abdominal-thoracic cavities was investigated by Tennyson and King (8).

The effect of spinal musculature remains to be investigated. Experimentation employing cadavers or anesthetized animals as test subjects cannot measure its possible effect on the biodynamic response of the torso.

Electromyographic (EMG) activity in the postero-lateral spinal musculature was recorded by Tennyson and King (9) during whole-body acceleration of unanesthetized dogs which were subjected to low level impacts of 3 to 5 g. Evidence of involuntary muscle response leads naturally to such questions as
1. What are the magnitudes of muscle forces developed?
2. Do they affect loading patterns along the spinal column?
3. Can they affect the overall kinematic response of the spinal column?

A useful tool in obtaining an insight into these questions would be a mathematical model of the spine. The use of one which has been validated against experimental data would render the results more credible.

A MATHEMATICAL MODEL OF THE SPINE

Any valid model for the spine should include both the salient features of the vertebral column and the associated musculature. The vertebral column model should be formulated such that the effects of natural spinal curvatures, eccentric inertia loading and felxion due to bending become apparent. The muscle model should describe the physiological mechanisms which bring about an active component of tension as well as the passive response. Anatomical distribution of predominant muscle groups along the vertebral column should be represented. Any external constraints to the system such as seat and shoulder belts and seat back support should be present.

SPINE MODELS - A number of spinal models have been formulated. A comprehensive two-dimensional discrete parameter model was proposed by Prasad and King (10) and was successfully validated against experimentally measured intervertebral loads during whole-body +G_z acceleration of human cadaveric subjects. It has also successfully modelled the 'ramping' phenomenon of the torso in rear-end (+G_x) automobile impacts in a study by Prasad et al. (11). A natural extension of this model would then be a reformulation to include the effects of muscular response in the impact situations to which it can be applied.

MUSCLE MODELS - Bahler (12) and Wilkie (13) have shown that skeletal muscle can be described as a force generator within a viscoelastic system. Constitutive equations represented the force generator as a function of muscle stretch and stretch rate and neural delay time.

---ABSTRACT---

A biodynamic model of the spine simulated the action of spinal musculature on the head, vertebral bodies and pelvis in the midsagittal plane. Muscle was treated as a force generator whose contractile force was dependant on muscle stretch, stretch rate and neural delay time. Eight model runs were conducted with and without muscle, simulating +G_z and -G_x impact acceleration. The model predicted that spinal musculature was incapable of affecting overall spinal column kinematics. However, as a result of muscle contraction, significantly higher local axial forces were predicted in the discs and facets than were predicted when muscle was absent.

Experimentally validated three component models of skeletal muscle have appeared in the literature. Bahler (12) described muscle as a non-linear force generator bridged by a non-linear viscous element in series with a non-linear elastic element, and presented model validation data for tension, displacement and velocity histories of an isolated rat gracilis anticus muscle which was electrically stimulated. Soechting et al. (14) validated a similar linear model against rotational motion of the human forearm which had been subjected to an abrupt change in load.

PROPRIOCEPTIVE RESPONSE IN MUSCLE - Physiologically, muscle spindles are in parallel with the main motor fibers and sense stretch and stretch rate. In the simplest proprioceptive response, termed a stretch reflex, nerve impulses generated at a spindle receptor travel along an afferent nerve fiber to synapse in the spinal cord with α-motor neurons. These motor neurons in turn carry efferent nerve impulses to the main motor fibers (extra fusal fibers) initiating muscle contraction. The finite time required for this proprioceptive response to occur is the neural delay time.

The frequency of afferent discharge by the spindle receptors is proportional to the magnitude of stretch and stretch rate. Spindle receptor sensitivity can be modified by γ-efferent motor neurons which are under higher neuronal control. The γ-efferents innervate the muscle spindles and have been divided into two classes by Crowe and Matthews (15); those which affect sensitivity to stretch and those which affect sensitivity to stretch rate.

Poppele and Terzuolo (16) established that a linear relationship exists between afferent and efferent signals in the stretch reflex circuit. An increase in α-motor neuron discharge increases firing rate of individual extra-fusal fibers and additionally brings about recruitment of more extra-fusal fibers within the muscle. The maximum developable tension which muscle can exhibit in response to a strong efferent imput is termed muscular tetany.

As muscle is only capable of exerting tension, movements about a joint, such as flexion and extension, require that musculature be composed of paired sets in order to provide synergistic action.

THE POSTERO-LATERAL SPINAL MUSCULATURE - Deep musculature of the spinal column is divided in three longitudinal muscle masses, each comprising many overlapping fascicles (Gray, 17). These muscles act as extensors of the vertebral column and, in the cervical region, they extend the head.

The transversospinalis system is the deepest and most medial muscle group consisting of a number of different muscle tracts which join one vertebra with another or span one or more vertebra. Included in this grouping are the interspinalis, rotatores, multifidus, spinalis, semispinalis and semispinalis capitis.

The longissimus system is lateral to the transversospinalis system and consists of overlapping fasicles extending from all the vertebrae to the head. The longissimus thoracis and lumborum are the strongest muscles of the trunk having their origin at the iliac crest of the pelvis and insertions in all the lumbar and thoracic vertebrae. The longissimus cervicis and capitas are continuations of the longissimus thoracis, having their insertions in the cervical vertebrae and on the mastoid part of the temporal bone.

The iliocostalis system is lateral most with its caudal fasicles originating on the ilium and cranial fasicles extending to the seventh cervical vertebra.

ASSUMPTIONS FOR THE MODEL - Basically, the biodynamic model of the spine simulates the action of the spinal musculature on a discrete parameter vertebral column model conceptually similar to the one developed by Prasad and King (10). It is, thus, a two-dimensional model which can simulate motion of the head, the pelvis and the 24 vertebrae in the midsagittal plane. Each segment was treated as a rigid body and was assigned to carry a portion of the torso weight which was eccentric with respect to the centerline of the spine. The rigid bodies assumed a trapezoidal shape and were arranged to simulate the spinal curvatures as closely as possible. The dual load path through the spinal column was modelled by treating the intervertebral discs and posterior vertebral structure as massless deformable elements. The disc is an elastic element capable of simultaneously resisting axial and shear loads and bending moments. The posterior vertebral structure (facets) was taken to be a spring element which could transmit axial and shear forces. Auxiliary forces were added to the appropriate vertebrae to simulate external contact forces, such as loads due to the shoulder harness, the lap belt and the seat back. It was also possible to simulate chin-chest contact.

The following assumptions were made in the development of the muscle model:

1. All load transmitting (passive) elements in the posterior structure of the spine including the passive component of muscle were included in the facet model. That is, in compression the 'facet' represented facet joint and spinous process interaction. In tension, the facet model simulated the action of the facet joints, spinous ligaments and passive muscle components.

2. The active mode elements or force generators linked vertebra to vertebra posteriorly and were essentially in parallel with the facets.

3. The muscle contractile force was taken to be a linear function of stretch and stretch rate.

4. The transversospinalis system was represented by the active elements which linked adjacent vertebra.

5. The longissimus and iliocostalis systems were represented by a 'linked' muscle system with an insertion at every vertebral level and the head. The contractile force was based

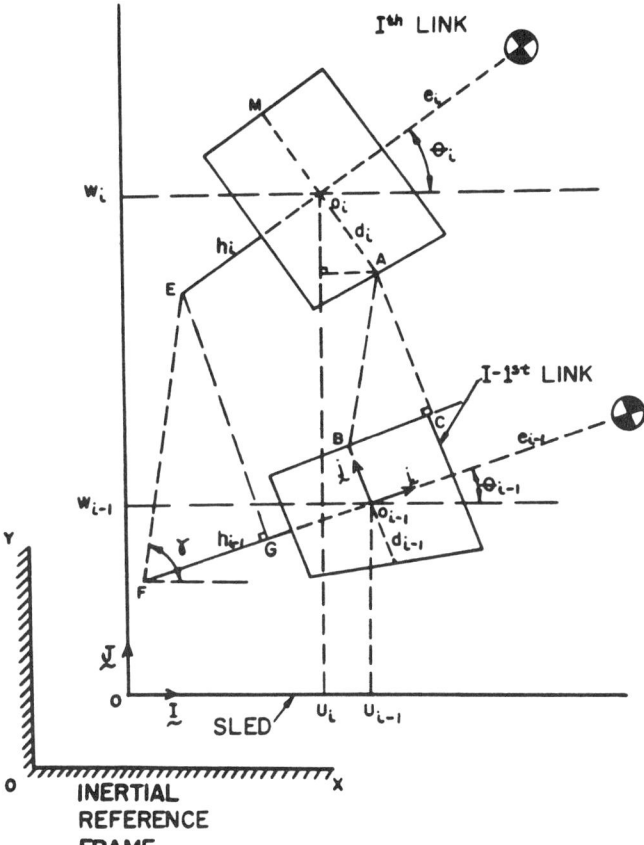

Fig. 1 - Configuration of two adjacent vertebrae

on a summation of the activity in the individual active elements. This muscle system was anchored inferiorly in the pelvis.

6. A numerical scheme was developed to store the activity of each contractile element for subsequent recall so that a variable neural time delay of up to 100 ms could be simulated.

7. As the predominant passive response of the spinal column was one of flexion during the 200 ms of $+G_z$ acceleration, only the extensor half of the spinal musculature was modelled.

8. Muscular tetany was represented by setting a maximum allowable force developable by any particular muscle.

9. Neural activity was confined to the 'stretch reflex' phenomenon and the γ-efferent effect remained constant.

MUSCLE KINEMATICS - The position vector for any muscle connecting two adjacent links at points E and F in Figure 1 is given by:

$$\underline{M}_i = (U_i - U_{i-1} - h_i \cdot \cos\theta_i + h_{i-1} \cdot \cos\theta_{i-1})\underline{I} \\ + (W_i - W_{i-1} - h_i \cdot \sin\theta_i + h_{i-1} \cdot \sin\theta_{i-1})\underline{J} \quad (1)$$

where U_i = x- coordinate of vertebra i
W_i = y- coordinate of vertebra i
Θ_i = angular position of vertebra i
h_i = displacement from origin, O_i

i = 1 to 26, 1 for the pelvis and 26 for the head

The velocity vector for this muscle is:

$$\underline{\dot{M}}_i = (\dot{U}_i - \dot{U}_{i-1} + h_i \cdot \dot{\Theta}_i \cdot \sin\theta_i - h_{i-1} \cdot \dot{\Theta}_{i-1} \cdot \sin\theta_{i-1})\underline{I} + (\dot{W}_i - \dot{W}_{i-1} - h_i \cdot \dot{\Theta}_i \cdot \cos\theta_i + h_{i-1} \cdot \dot{\Theta}_{i-1} \cdot \cos\theta_{i-1})\underline{J} \quad (2)$$

Muscle stretch is then the difference between the value of current muscle length and its original length $|\underline{MO}_i|$.

$$DML_i = |\underline{M}_i| - |\underline{MO}_i| \quad (3)$$

The time derivative of Eq. 3 becomes the muscle stretch rate and is given by

$$\dot{DML}_i = \dot{Mu}_i \cdot \cos\gamma_i + \dot{Mw}_i \cdot \sin\gamma_i \quad (4)$$

where $\dot{Mu}_i$ = component of $\underline{\dot{M}}_i$ in $\underline{I}$ direction,
$\dot{Mw}_i$ = component of $\underline{\dot{M}}_i$ in $\underline{J}$ direction,
and γ_i = arctan (Mw_i/Mu_i)
where Mu_i = component of $\underline{M}_i$ in $\underline{I}$ direction
and Mw_i = component of $\underline{M}_i$ in $\underline{J}$ direction.

The value of the afferent nerve impulse generated, α_i, is then the weighted sum of Equations 3 and 4:

$$\alpha_i = D1_i \cdot DML_i + D2_i \cdot \dot{DML}_i \quad (5)$$

where $D1_i$ and $D2_i$ are the sensitivity factors determined by the dynamic and static γ-efferents respectively.

MUSCLE FORCES - A numerical scheme was devised to model neural delay time. At 1 ms intervals during model simulation a pair of data points, α_i (nerve impulse) and t (time), were stored for each muscle. At discrete time intervals, an algorithm developed by Akima (18) was used to determine the slopes at each of the data points. The coefficients of a third order polynomial could then be computed and stored for the segment between each pair of points. These polynomial coefficients could be recalled at any later time to calculate an α_i which would reflect the exact neural delay. Thus, at any new integration time step during the simulation the appropriate values of α_i were provided to the muscle force equations.

These values of α_i in a physiological sense became the efferent portion of the nerve impulse acting on the muscle to generate muscle contractile force, MF_i. It was taken to be directly proportional to α_i,

$$MF_i = FO_i \cdot \alpha_i \quad (6)$$

where FO_i is the proportionality constant Equation 6 is thus the constitutive equation for the muscles. The program ensured that each MF_i was greater than or equal to zero.

The muscle forces acting on each particular vertebral link are then summed with the facet forces, disc forces and disc moments, as shown in Figure 2, in the equations of motion to determine the overall dynamics of the spine.

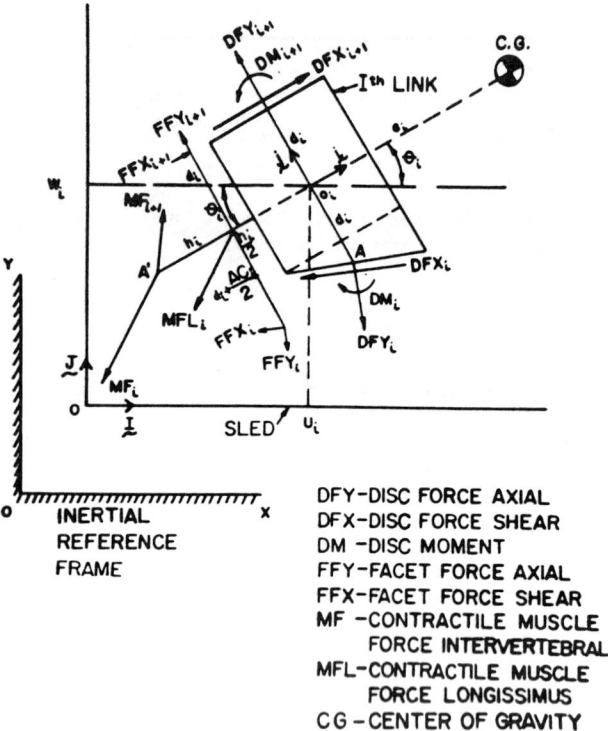

Fig. 2 - Free body diagram of the ith vertebra

DFY-DISC FORCE AXIAL
DFX-DISC FORCE SHEAR
DM -DISC MOMENT
FFY-FACET FORCE AXIAL
FFX-FACET FORCE SHEAR
MF -CONTRACTILE MUSCLE FORCE INTERVERTEBRAL
MFL-CONTRACTILE MUSCLE FORCE LONGISSIMUS
CG -CENTER OF GRAVITY

CHOICE OF PARAMETERS - Model constants for the spinal column were taken from those used by Prasad and King (10) for the validation of human cadaver runs with the exceptions of the facet constants. In order that the effects of the active muscle component on spinal column dynamics could be accentuated, elastic constants of the facets were reduced by a factor of 2 to 4. However, the facet loading pattern still remained consistent with that reported by Hakim (7). Each intervertebral (transversospinalis) muscle attachment was at a distance of h_i from the vertebral body origin along the $\underline{i}$-axis, as shown in Figure 2, to represent an attachment to the spinous process. The 'linked' muscle was assumed to act at a distance of $\frac{1}{2}h_i$ along the $\underline{i}$-axis in order to represent an attachment to the accessory process.

The qualitative effects of the γ-efferent sensitivity factors $D1_i$ and $D2_i$ have been represented mathematically by Houk (19), Crowe (20), Poppele and Bowman (21) and McRuer et al. (22) but not quantified. In his non-linear model of frog muscle Bahler (12) found the contractile force to be directly proportional to stretch and to the square root of stretch velocity. In their evaluation of neuromuscular parameters in human arm Soechting et al. (14) derived values of $D1_i/D2_i$ which ranged from 0.005 to 0.027 with a large standard deviation in $D2_i$. For this study a value for $D1_i/D2_i$ was set at 0.005 and D2 was assumed to be equal to unity when the unit of length in Equation 5 was in inches. As the stretch rate values normally were on the order of 10^2 to 10^3 times larger than those of the stretch values, the use of 0.005 gave approximately equal weight to the effects of stretch and stretch rate. If the ratio $D1_i/D2_i$ was set at 0.05, the slope of contractile muscle force-time curve approached that of a step function, implying that too much weight was given $D1_i$.

There is a lack of data in the literature for the muscle force proportionality constants $F0_i$. Its values were chosen based on muscle contractile forces reaching maximum allowable values (muscular tetany) during a high g-level impact. Morris et al. (23) estimated that the deep back muscle tension at the level of the 5th lumbar disc could be as high as 6672 N (1500 lb) when lifting weights of 890 N in a flexed position. Based on this data a limit of 6672 N was set for the 'linked' muscle system. For the intervertebral muscles a limiting value of 556 N was assumed. The proportionality constant $F0_i$ was assigned a value of 4448 N for the 'linked' muscle system, 1334 N for the lumbar-thoracic muscles and 1112 N for the cervical intervertebral muscles. These values assured that maximal allowable muscle forces could be developed during a higher $+G_z$ model run, since it was found that α_i normally varied between zero and unity.

In distributing the 'linked' muscle force among the vertebrae and head, 80% of the force was assumed to be equally distributed among the lumbar-thoracic vertebrae and the remaining 20% among the cervical vertebrae and head.

Proprioceptive response of muscles has been studied by many investigators. Muscle response delay time in the human arm was found to be 60-80 ms by Hammond (24) and 90-140 ms by Soechting et al. (14). Foust et al. (25) found response delay for human neck extensors to be 54-87 ms and Tennyson and King (9) found response delay for spinal musculature in dogs to be 24-44 ms. This delay includes the time required to stretch muscle and to complete the reflex arc (neural delay time). It is measured from the time of onset of acceleration to the first increase in EMG activity. The peak EMG derived force occurs some time after the neural delay. Hannan et al. (26) and Inman et al. (27) observed that actual muscle tension reached a peak about 80 ms after the occurrence of the peak of the EMG derived force.

Based on the above information, delays of 20 and 35 ms were chosen to represent strictly a neural delay. Delays of 95 ms were used to include the mechanical delay in developing peak force as observed by Hannan et al. (26) and Inman et al. (27).

ANALYSIS OF MODEL RESULTS - Eight model runs were conducted to simulate three different impact situations. Runs 10A, 11A and 12A were of short duration, 100 ms $+G_z$ pulse, and relatively low peak acceleration to simulate 'pancaking' type crashes of aircraft or helicopter or a recreational vehicle running over a large bump. The occupants were restrained with a lap belt only. Runs 13A, 14A, 15A and 16A were of longer duration, 240 ms $+G_z$ pulse, which can

TABLE 1

SUMMARY OF MODEL RUNS CONDUCTED

Model Run No.	Acceleration Level	Restraints	Active Muscle
10A	$+G_z$, 200 g/s onset for 30 ms, const. 6 g for 70 ms	Lap belt	Not included
11A	$+G_z$, 200 g/s onset for 30 ms, const. 6 g for 70 ms	Lap belt	Included, 95 ms neural delay
12A	$+G_z$, 200 g/s onset for 30 ms, const. 6 g for 70 ms	Lap belt	Included, 35 ms neural delay
13A	$+G_z$, 213 g/s onset for 30 ms to 6.4 g peak, -40 g/s for 10 ms to 6 g, const. 6 g to 240 ms	Shoulder belt and lap belt	Included, 20 ms neural delay
14A	$+G_z$, 213 g/s onset for 30 ms to 6.4 g peak, -40 g/s for 10 ms to 6 g, const. 6 g to 240 ms	Shoulder belt and lap belt	Not included
15A	$+G_z$, 213 g/s onset for 30 ms to 6.4 g peak, -40 g/s for 10 ms to 6 g, const. 6 g to 240 ms	Shoulder belt and lap belt	Included, 35 ms neural delay
16A	$+G_z$, 213 g/s onset for 30 ms to 6.4 g peak, -40 g/s for 10 ms to 6 g, const. 6 g to 240 ms	Shoulder belt and lap belt	Included, 95 ms neural delay
17A	$-G_x$, const. 0 g for 14 ms, 370 g/s onset for 22 ms to 8.1 g peak, -30.7 g/s for 264 ms to 0 g	Shoulder belt and lap belt	Included, 95 ms neural delay

simulate pulses experienced by jet pilots on an ejection training tower restrained with lap and shoulder belts. Run 17A was conducted to compare model response with experimental data collected by Ewing and Thomas (28) in which human volunteers were subjected to $-G_x$ impact acceleration. The conditions for all runs are given in Table 1. Muscular contraction was simulated in all runs except 10A and 14A.

RUNS WITH SHORT DURATION PULSE - A common passive kinematic response for all $+G_z$ model runs was increasing spinal flexure with time. Flexure is first caused by the initial curvature which brings about a 'collapsing' effect and then by bending which is developed due to the anterior eccentricity of the torso center of gravity.

In Runs 10A through 12A, the pelvis lifted off the impact seat within 20 ms after the end of the acceleration pulse. However, spinal flexure continued to develop as shown in Figures 3 and 4. The pelvis lift-off can be seen from Figure 5 by noting the rapid decrease of seatpan load to zero and by the development of a lap belt load.

From Figures 5 and 6 it is evident that for Run 10A the discs and facets tended to unload into tension after pelvic lift off. For Runs 11A and 12A, the muscles were then stretched due to the combined effects of unloading of the spine and increased flexion. With a 95 ms neural delay (Run 11A), maximal muscle tension developed at about 220 ms, as shown in Figure 7. Concurrent with the peak muscle tension, it is seen from Figure 8 that there was a second compression peak in the discs in which the loads sustained were more than double those for the first peak. As shown in Figure 3, muscle response for Run 11A did not affect the spinal column kinematics significantly.

In Run 12A, with a 35 ms delay, two muscle tension peaks occurred, the first from 120 ms to 160 ms and the second at about 220 ms, as shown in Figure 9. Again Figure 10 shows compression peaks occurring in the discs, concurrent with the muscle tension peaks. The facets were also forced into compression, as shown in Figure 11. Note that the magnitude of muscle tension in the first peak of Run 12A was less than that in Run 11A due to the fast neural response. However, as indicated in Figure 4, muscle contraction in Run 12A limited forward excursion of the spinal column and head after 180 ms.

RUNS WITH LONG DURATION PULSE - Figure 12 shows the increased kyphosis developed in the cervical spine when a shoulder belt is added as a restraint. In addition to the natural flexural reaction of the spine, the cervical vertebrae and head are the only segments not restrained if shoulder belts are used. The cervical discs and facets tend to unload and go into tension due to spinal kyphosis, as shown in Figures 13 and 14. In these figures, the abscissa indicates vertebral level starting with the pelvis at 1.00 and ending with the head at 26.00.

In Run 16A, with a 95 ms neural delay, maximal muscle contraction occurred at about 220 ms as shown in Figure 15 and concurrently the discs and facets were forced into compression as shown in Figures 16 and 17. Figure 12 shows that this muscle contraction did not significantly affect the spinal column kinematics.

Run 15A was made with a 35 ms neural delay. Maximal muscle tension peak was attained at 150 ms and a second muscle contraction was in

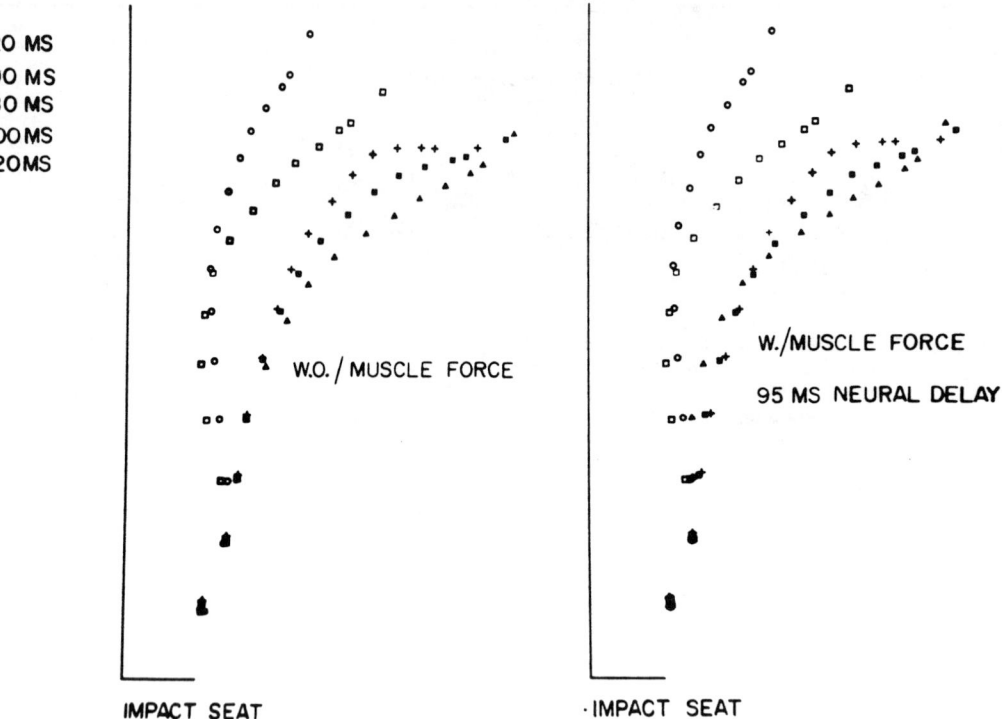

Fig. 3 - Comparison of spinal flexion without and with muscle (95 ms neural delay). 6g, 100 ms pulse run without shoulder belt. (Lowest link is pelvis; uppermost link is head)

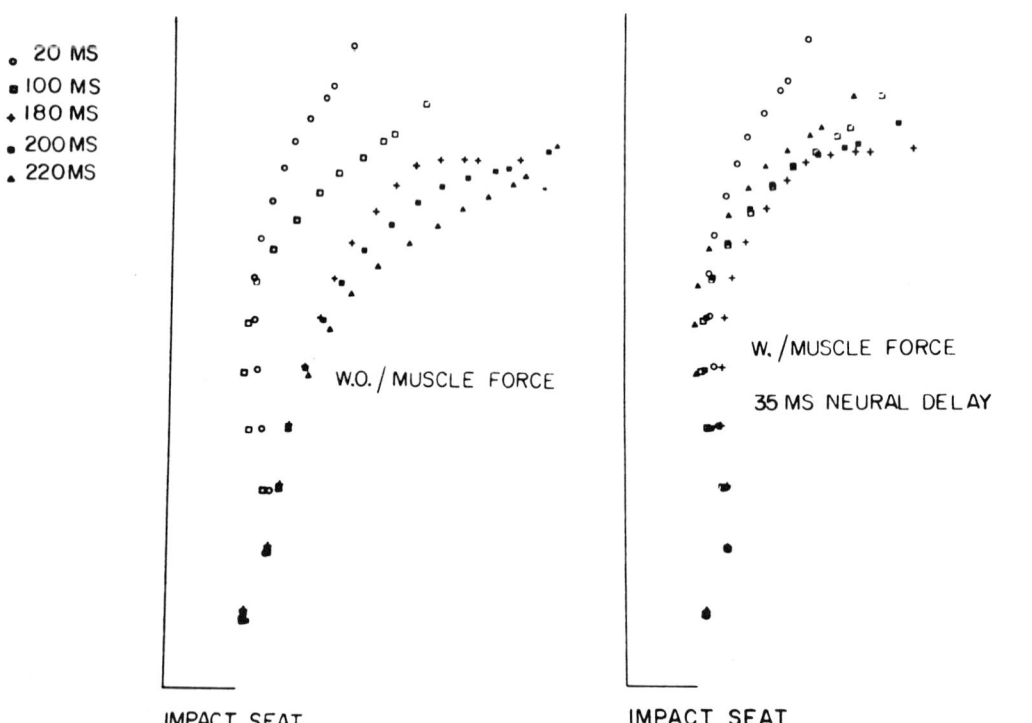

Fig. 4 - Comparison of spinal flexion without and with muscle (35 ms neural delay). 6g, 100 ms pulse run without shoulder belt

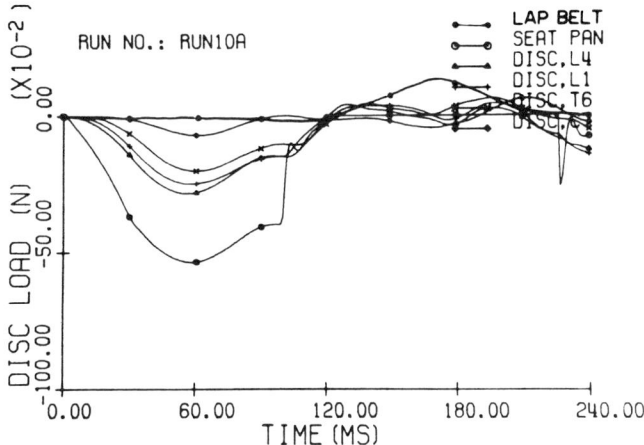

Fig. 5 - Disc axial and lap belt loads for a 6 g, 100 ms pulse run with no muscle

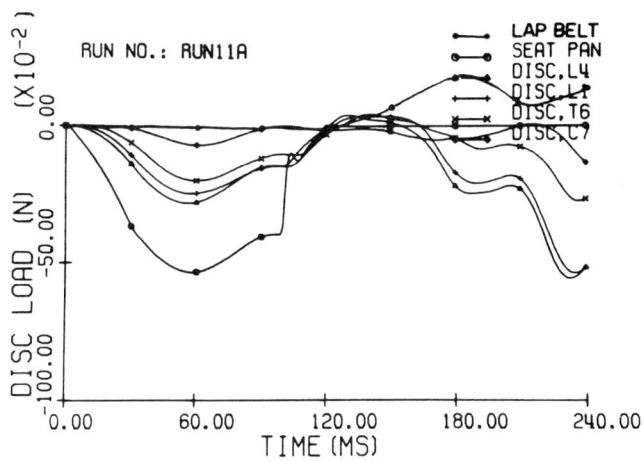

Fig. 8 - Disc axial and lap belt loads for a 6 g, 100 ms pulse run with muscle (95 ms neural delay)

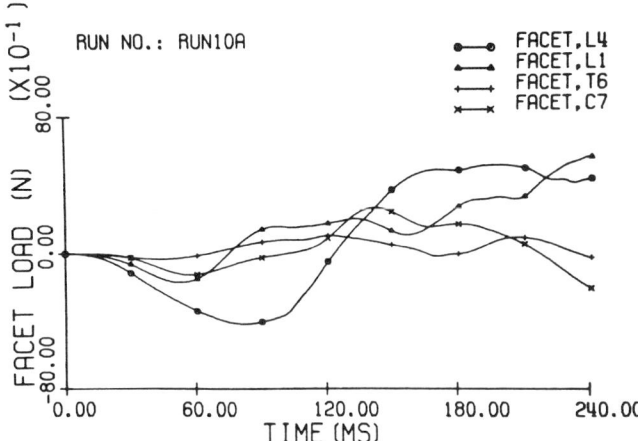

Fig. 6 - Facet loads for a 6 g, 100 ms pulse run with no muscle

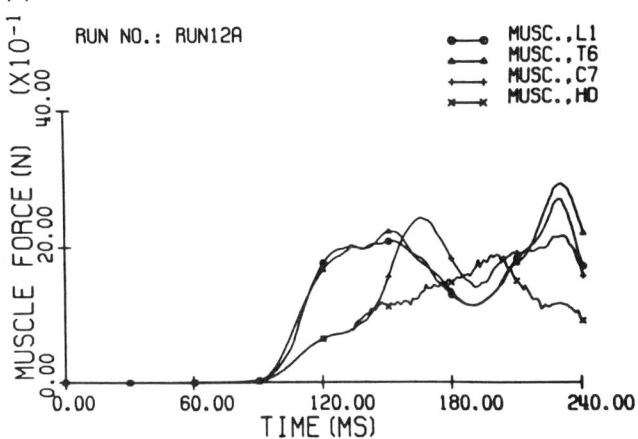

Fig. 9 - Muscle forces for a 6 g, 100 ms pulse run (35 ms neural delay)

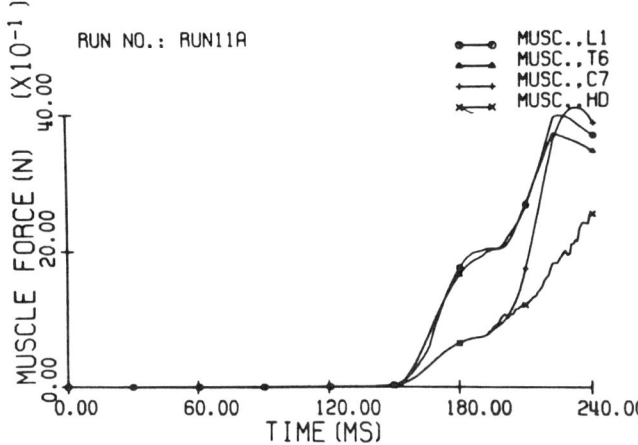

Fig. 7 - Muscle forces for a 6 g, 100 ms pulse run (95 ms neural delay)

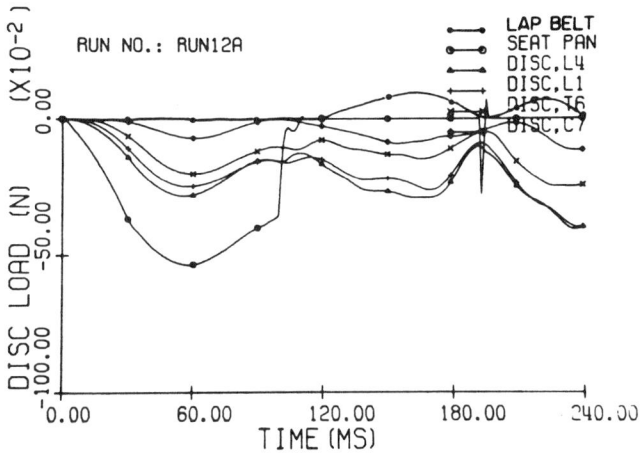

Fig. 10 - Disc axial and lap belt loads for a 6 g, 100 ms pulse run with muscle (35 ms neural delay)

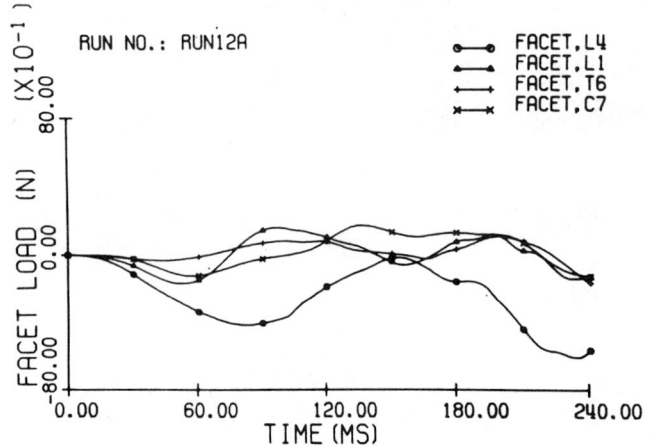

Fig. 11 - Facet loads for a 6 g, 100 ms pulse run (35 ms neural delay)

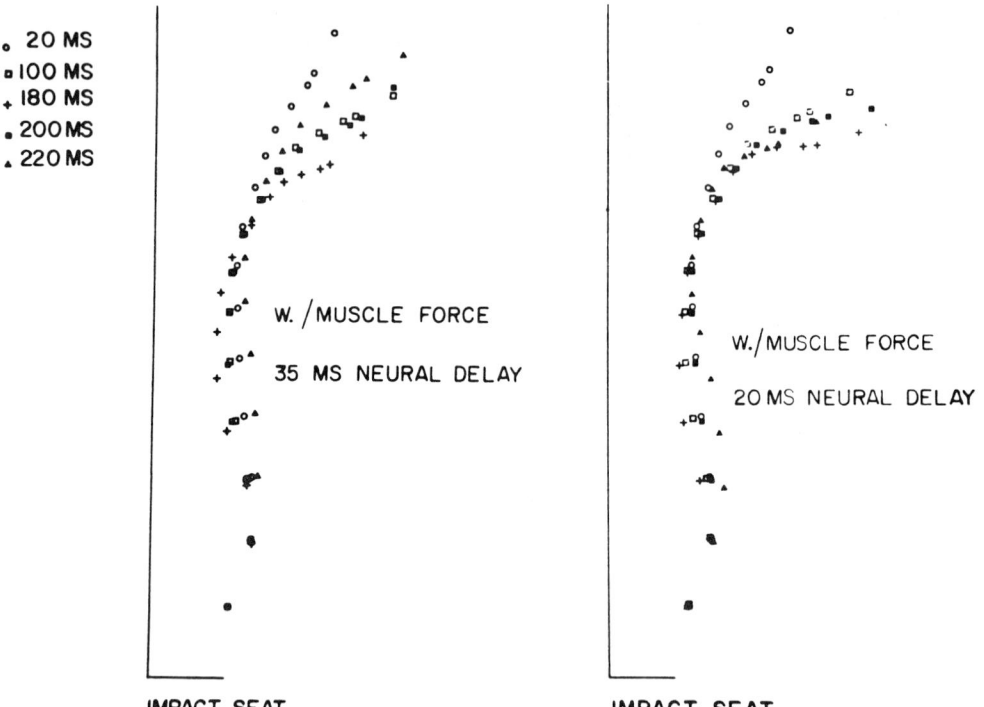

Fig. 12 - Comparison of spinal flexion without and with muscle (95 ms neural delay) 6 g, 240 ms pulse run with shoulder belt

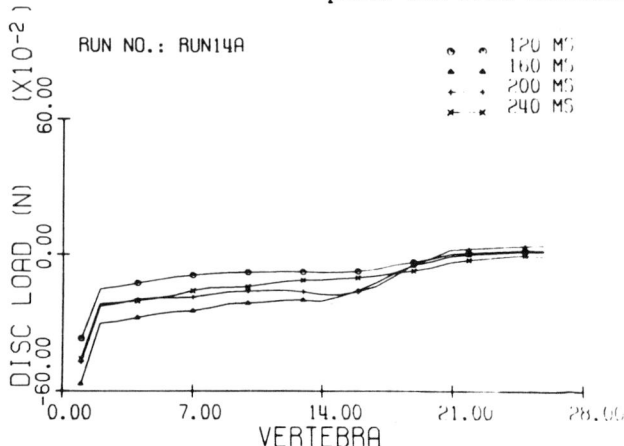

Fig. 13 - Distribution of disc axial loads along the spinal column for a 6 g, 240 ms pulse run without muscle

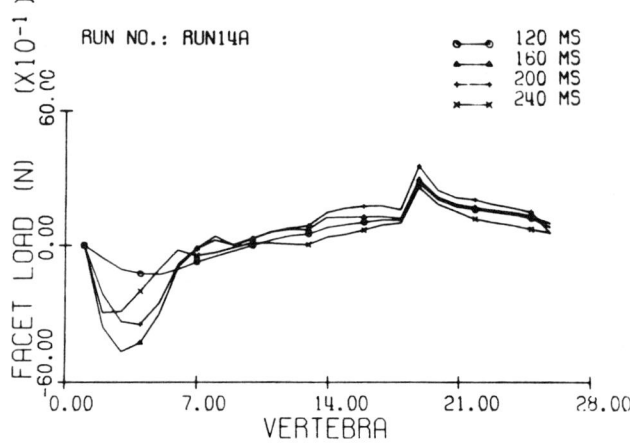

Fig. 14 - Distribution of facet loads along the spinal column for a 6 g, 240 ms pulse run without muscle

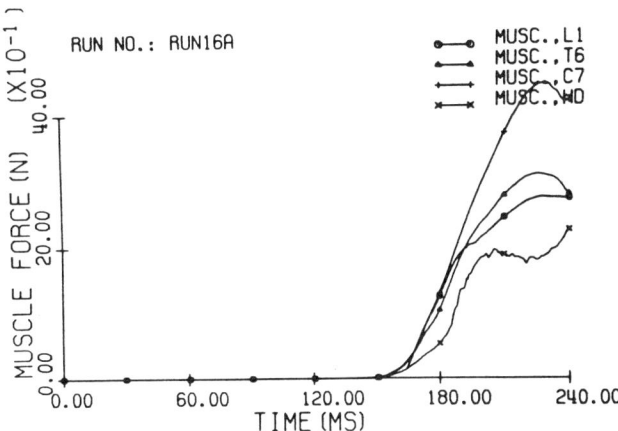

Fig. 15 - Muscle forces for a 6 g, 240 ms pulse run (95 ms neural delay)

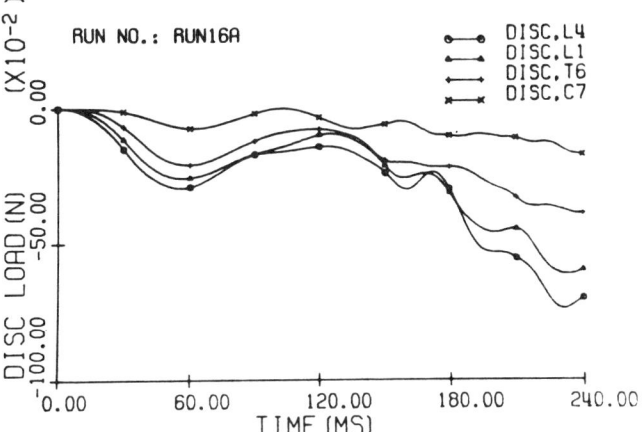

Fig. 16 - Disc axial loads for a 6g, 240 ms pulse run (95 ms neural delay)

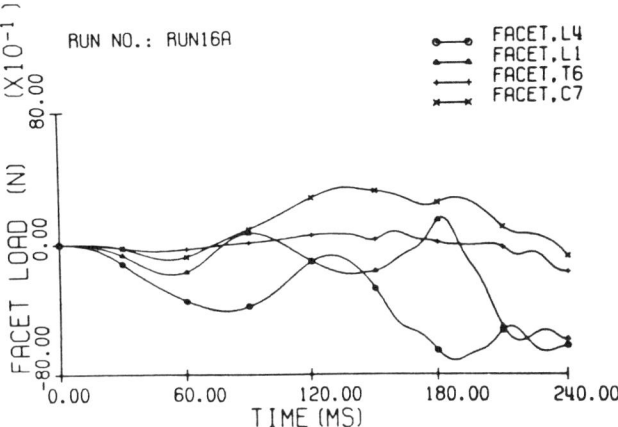

Fig. 17 - Facet loads for a 6 g, 240 ms pulse run (95 ms neural delay)

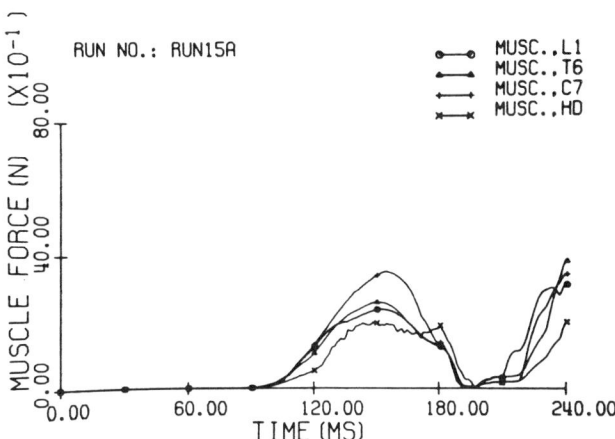

Fig. 18 - Muscle forces for a 6 g, 240 ms pulse run (35 ms neural delay)

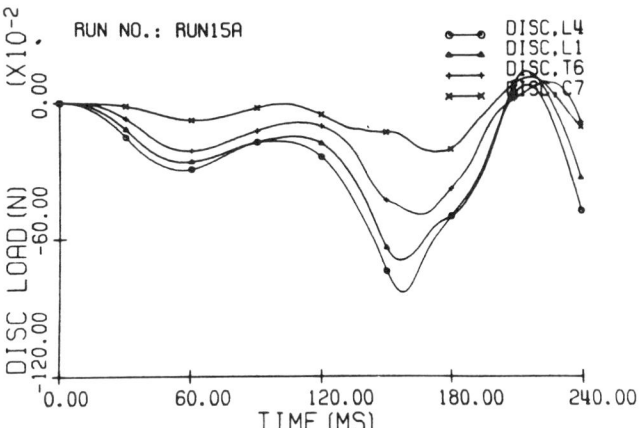

Fig. 19 - Disc axial loads for a 6 g, 240 ms pulse run (35 ms neural delay)

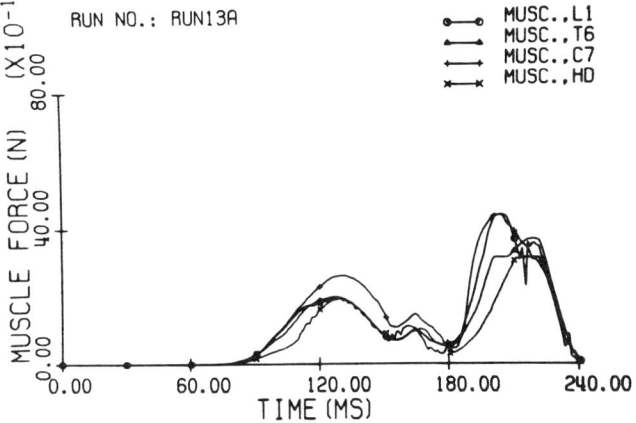

Fig. 20 - Muscle forces for a 6 g, 240 ms pulse run (20 ms neural delay)

progress at 240 ms, as shown in Figure 18. A second compression peak in the discs is shown in Figure 19. This is associated with the muscle tension peak at 150 ms and its magnitude is 2½ times that of the initial disc compression peak. Run 13A, with a 20 ms neural delay, had maximal muscle tension peaks at 130 ms and 200 ms as shown in Figure 20. A second compression peak in the discs, shown in Figure 21, is associated with the muscle tension peak at 130 ms.

It had a magnitude two times that of the initial disc compression peak. A third compression peak three times larger than the first peak can be attributed to the muscle tension peak occurring at 200 ms. In Run 14A, there was no active muscle component and the second and subsequent peak loads in the disc were less than the first peak shown in Figure 22.

Figure 23 shows spinal column kinematics for Runs 15A and 13A. For both runs, the initial muscle contraction arrested forward flexion by 200 ms and spinal column extension took place. In Run 15A, at 220 ms, spinal column extension was continuing but in Run 13A, the entire spinal column was forced in compression due to the second muscle contraction which took place at 200 ms.

GENERAL EFFECTS OF MUSCLE ACTION - Figure 24 shows spinal column shapes for Runs 10A, 11A, 12A, 14A, 15A and 16A at 200 ms. In runs with a 95 ms neural delay, the degree of spinal flexion is almost the same as that in runs without active muscle. In fact the only effect of muscular contraction is to shorten the column. With a 35 ms neural delay, forward flexion was restricted by a faster muscular response. It must be taken into consideration, however, that these simulations were designed to accentuate muscle action by excluding the effects of mechanical delay and by setting a high allowable muscle tension limit. This limit is probably not achievable for a relatively low level impact. Indeed, the 'linked' muscle system developed tensions which approached and reached the maximum allowable tension limit during these runs. This would indicate that at higher g-levels and with the same maximum tension limits, increased inertial loading would overcome any stabilizing effects by the muscles, even if the actual muscle response time were within the 20 to 30 ms times employed here.

Run 13A indicated that shortening neural delay time from 35 to 20 ms was not an advantage in extending the spinal column but caused

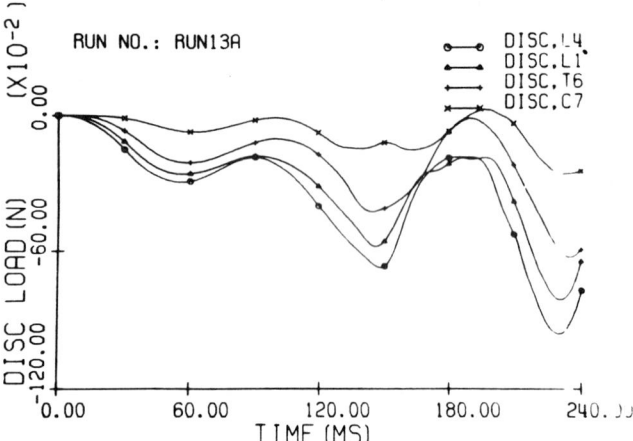

Fig. 21 - Disc axial loads for a 6 g, 240 ms pulse run (20 ms neural delay)

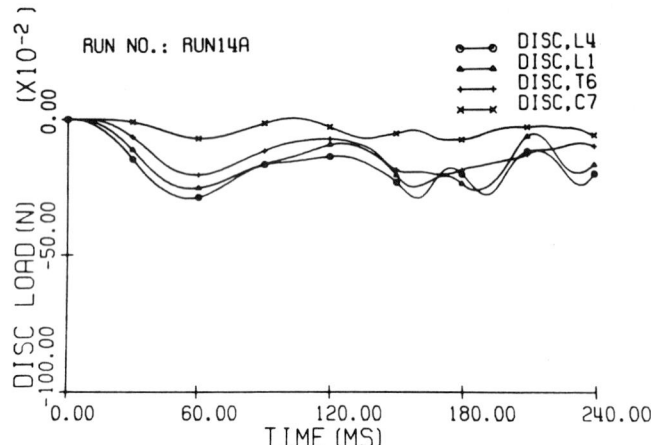

Fig. 22 - Disc axial loads for a 6 g, 240 ms pulse run without muscle

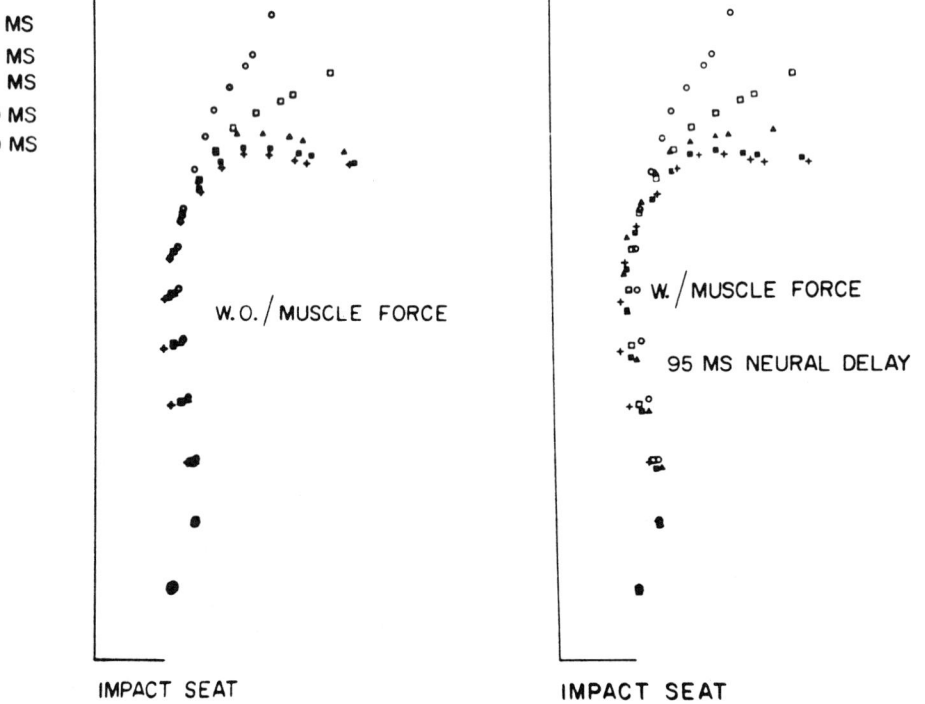

Fig. 23 - Comparison of spinal flexion with muscle for 35 ms and 20 ms neural delays. 6 g, 240 ms pulse run with shoulder belt

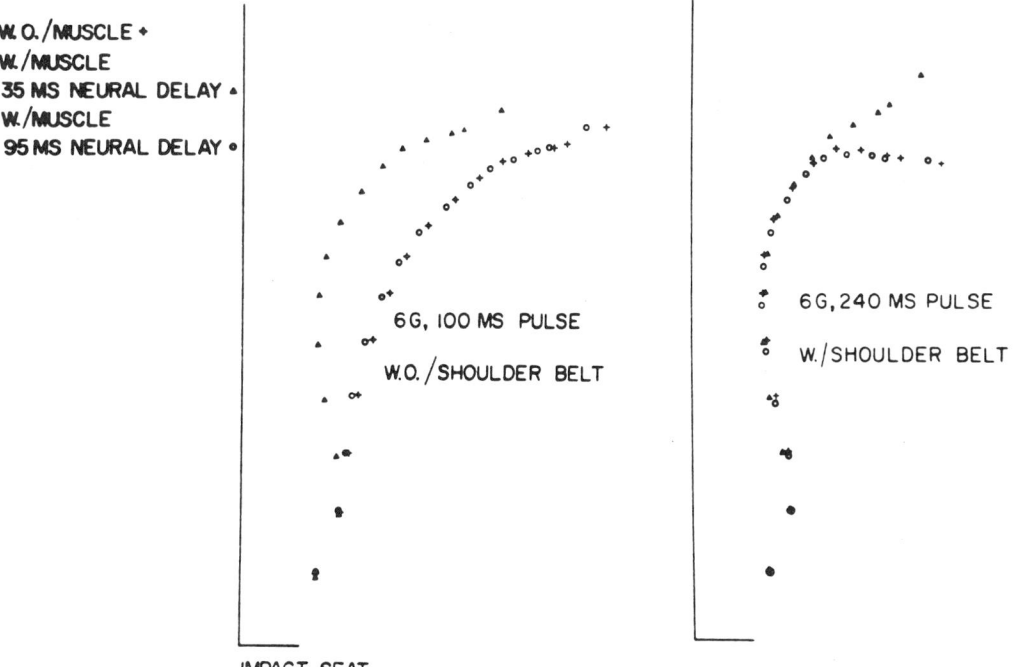

Fig. 24 - Comparison of spinal shapes at 200 ms for six different runs

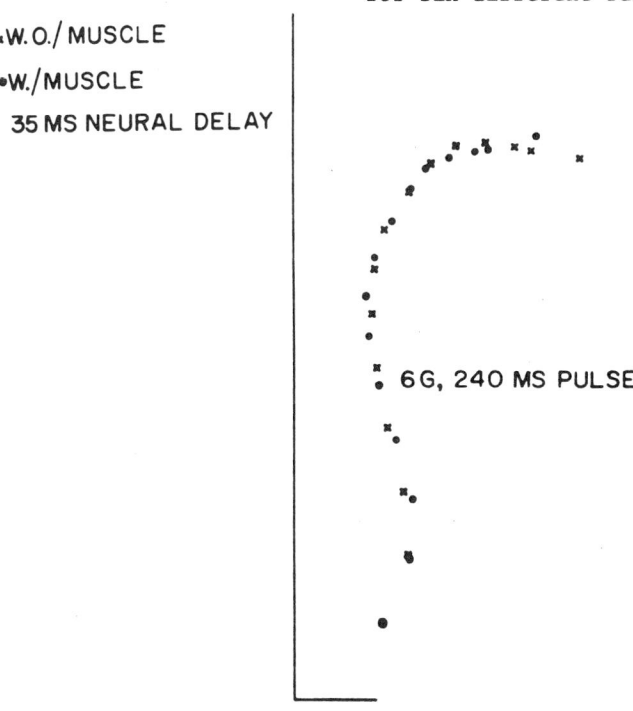

Fig. 25 - Comparison of spinal flexion at 160 ms with and without muscle

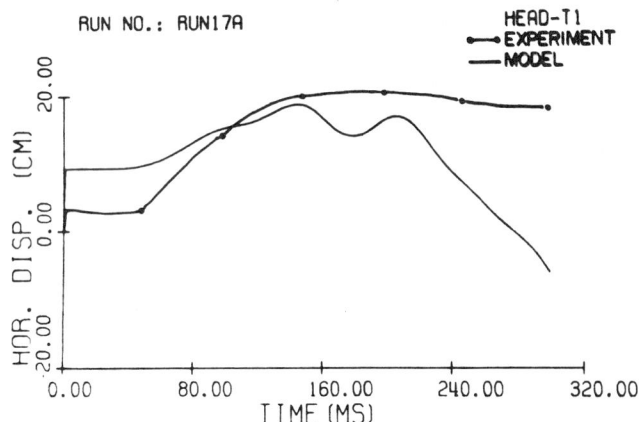

Fig. 26 - Horizontal displacement of head center of gravity with respect to T1 during $-G_x$ acceleration

a pronounced compressive effect. In fact, as pointed out previously, increased compressive loads were supported by the discs and facets during all muscle contractions. The overall effect was a shortening of the spinal column as the muscle system attempted to limit flexion. This is borne out in Figure 25 which compares spinal column shapes for Runs 14A and 15A at 160 ms.

This model indicates that the musculoskeletal structure of the spinal column is inadequate to provide stability during $+G_z$ acceleration when large inertial moments are present. The muscle attachments to bone are in close proximity to the joints upon which they act, that is, the facet joints and the discs. This kind of a leverage system is good for providing large, fast displacements but has poor mechanical advantage. Thus, in the situation modelled, as large inertial moments are generated about the disc and facet joints due to spinal flexure, the muscles respond by generating large contractile forces. However, due to their poor mechanical advantage, they are ineffective in stopping the forward flexion of the spinal column.

$-G_x$ SIMULATION - Ewing and Thomas (28) have reported on the kinematic response of the human head and neck to $-G_x$ acceleration. Model output was compared to head acceleration and dis-

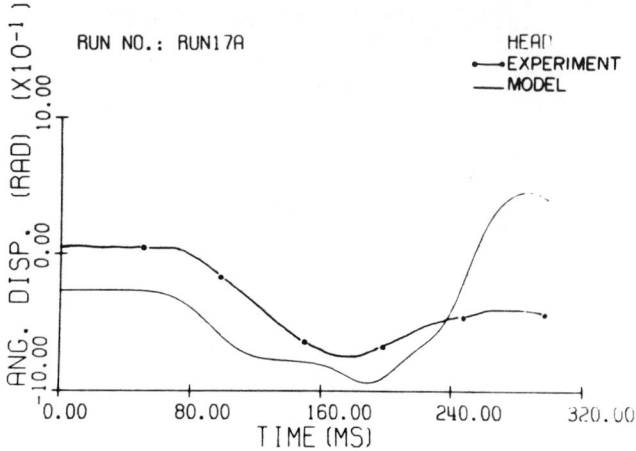

Fig. 27 - Angular displacement of head during $-G_x$ acceleration

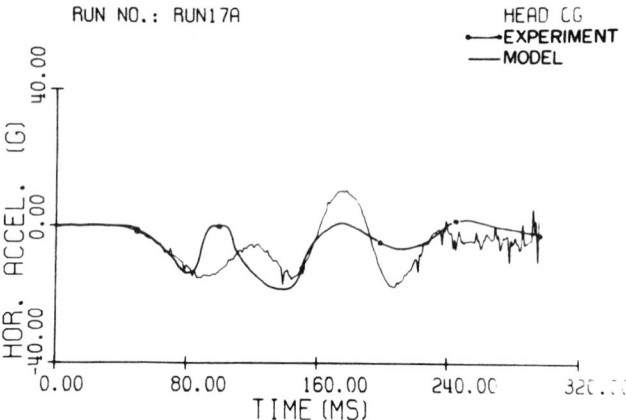

Fig. 28 - Horizontal acceleration of head center of gravity during $-G_x$ acceleration

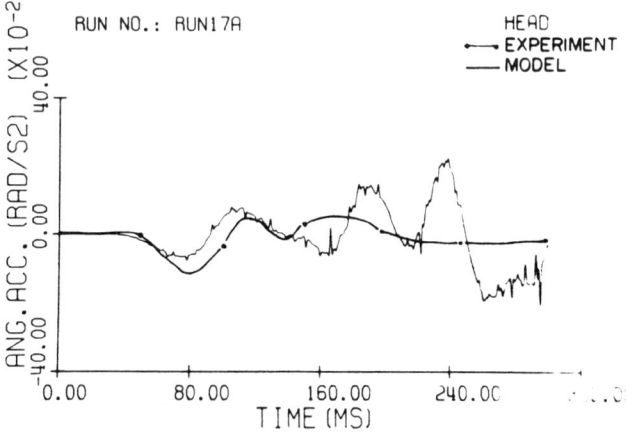

Fig. 29 - Angular acceleration of head during $-G_x$ acceleration

placement of a human volunteer (Subject #12), of approximately the same weight and sitting height as that used in the model. The acceleration pulse in the model closely matched that of the test run made by Ewing and Thomas (28).*
Allowable peak muscle forces were set at 3336 N (750 lb) for the 'linked' muscle and 334 N for

---

* The run is for Subject # 12, 370 g/sec onset, 8.3 g peak as shown in plot #6 on page 1-2.

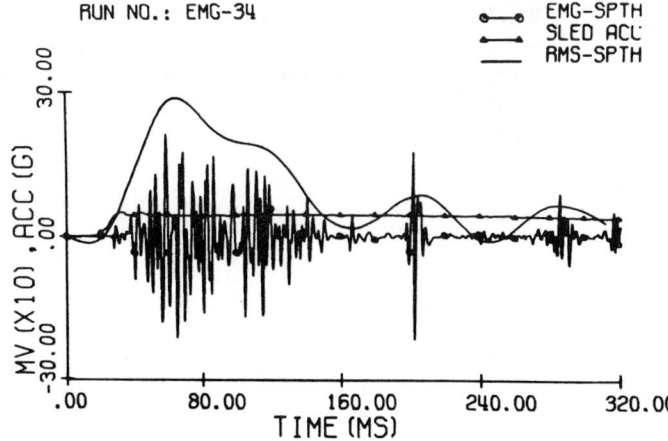

Fig. 30 - EMG activity and EMG derived force for the spinalis thoracis muscle during a 5 g $+G_z$ impact

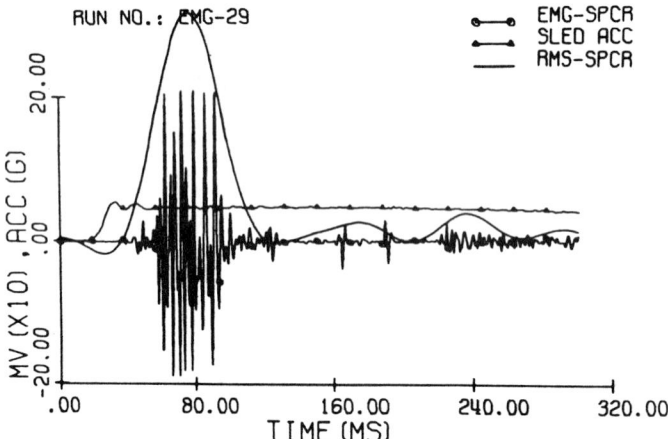

Fig. 31 - EMG activity and EMG derived force for the Spinalis cervicis muscle during a 5 g $+G_z$ impact

the intervertebral muscles. Muscle force proportionality constants were assumed to be 2224 N for the 'linked' muscle and 667-890 N for the intervertebral muscles. Figures 26 through 29 show a comparison of head horizontal and angular displacement and head horizontal and angular acceleration. In general, for at least the first 200 ms, the model output correlated well with experimental data, except for larger experimental displacement peaks and some phase difference in the accelerations. This run was a preliminary validation attempt and as such, its output indicated that with proper adjustment of input parameters, better correlation could be achieved. Furthermore, in the experiment, after 200 ms the volunteer was able to voluntarily stabilize his head position whereas in the model, dynamic rebound brought about further involuntary displacements.

MUSCLE MODEL FORCES COMPARED TO EMG FORCE - Figures 30 through 32 are typical of strong EMG bursts measured in the thoracic, cervical and lumbar regions, respectively, of canine spinal musculature during $+G_z$ acceleration. Derived muscle force proportional to the EMG signals are shown superimposed on the EMG. These muscle forces were obtained from a root mean square

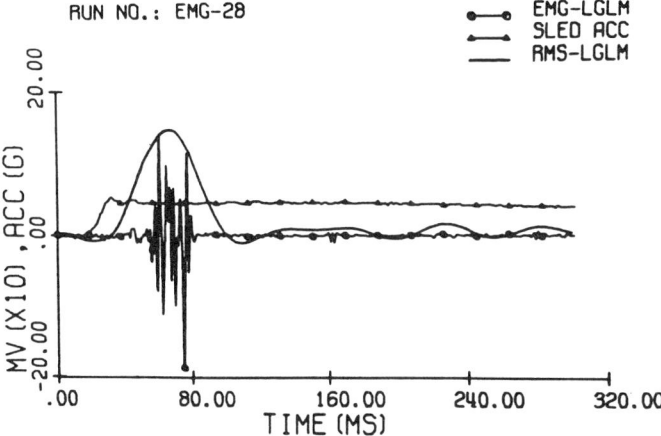

Fig. 32 - EMG activity and EMG derived force for the longissimus lumborum muscle during a 5 g $+G_z$ impact

analysis of the EMG signals and were filtered digitally by a fast Fourier Transform described by Tennyson and King (9). The EMG activity normally occurred in a series of bursts with short quiescent periods in between as opposed to a continous signal. Thus, the cyclical forces predicted by the model correspond in form to those derived from actual muscle activity.

As shown in Figure 33, the average time to reach the EMG derived peak force was 90 ms. Adding to this an 80 ms muscle mechanical delay yields a predicted muscle force peak at 170 ms. The model predicted peak forces at about 150 ms for a 20 ms neural delay and peak forces at about 220 ms for a 95 ms neural delay (which also included the mechanical delay). Thus, input parameters chosen for the model resulted in peak force times which were correlatable to those deduced from experimental data.

CONCLUSIONS

1. A spinal muscle model was formulated which generated forces correlatable in form and time to muscle forces derivable from actual experimentation.

2. Spinal muscles are ineffective in affecting overall spinal column kinematics during high level $+G_z$ acceleration.

3. Contractile forces of the muscles added significant compression loads throughout the spinal column to the discs and facets.

4. The magnitudes of muscle forces generated in these relatively low g-levels (3 to 6 g) are more likely encountered at a much higher g level such as during a 20 g pulse for pilot ejection. However, added to the inertial loads at higher g-levels, the effects of maximal muscle contraction could add significantly to the problem of spinal fractures.

5. The effects of muscles were not evident until about 150-200 ms into the run.

6. With further refinement of parametric inputs, the model should be able to closely correlate kinematic response to $-G_x$ acceleration.

The predictions of this model could have important implications in cervical injuries re-

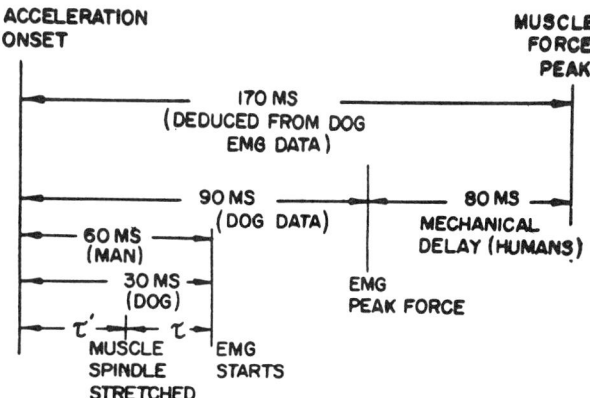

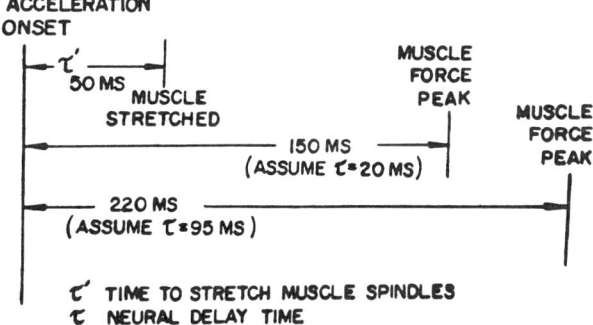

Fig. 33 - Comparison of muscle response predicted by model against experimental data

sulting from such events as parachute opening shock, aircraft 'ditching' into the ocean and 'head-spearing' type tackling in football. In future modelling, careful consideration should be given to the cervical recion, particularly the unique configuration of the first and second cervical vertebrae. As hyperextension could be involved, inclusion of the anterior musculature would be necessary. Analysis of relative motions between the cervical vertebrae and the determination of maximum shearing and bending moments would be useful criteria in predicting injuries.

REFERENCES

1. Beeding, E.L., Jr. and Cook, J.E., "Correlation Tests of Animals and Humans," Proceedings 5th Stapp Automotive Car Crash Conference, Univ. of Minn., Minneapolis, 1962, pp. 125-32.

2. Stapp, J.P., "Tolerance to Abrupt Deceleration," Collected Papers on Aviation Medicine, AGARDograph No. 6, Butterworth Scientific Publication, 1955, pp. 122-69.

3. Stapp, J.P., "Human and Chimpanzee Tolerance to Linear Decelerative Force," Paper presented at Conference on Problems of Emergency Escape in High-Speed Flight at Wright-Patterson Air Force Base, Ohio, 1952.

4. Kazarian, L.E., Hahn, J.W. and von-Gierke, H.E., "Biomechanics of the Vertebral Column and Internal Organ Response to Seated Spinal Impact in the Rhesus Monkey (Macaca Mulatta)," Proceedings 14th Stapp Car Crash Conference, SAE, New York, 1970, pp. 121-43.

5. Vulcan, A.P., King, A.I., and Nakamura, G.S., "Effects of Bending on the Vertebral Column During $+G_z$ Acceleration," Aerospace Medicine, Vol. 4, 1970, pp. 294-300.

6. Prasad, P., King A.I., and Ewing, C.L., "The Role of Articular Facets During $+G_z$ Acceleration," Journal of Applied Mechanics, Vol. 41, 1974, pp. 321-26.

7. Hakim, N.S., "An Experimental Study and Finite Element Analysis of the Mechanical Response of a Vertebra," Ph.D. Dissertation, Wayne State University, 1976.

8. Tennyson, S.A., and King, A.I., "Effect of Intra-Abdominal Pressure on the Spinal Column During $+G_z$ Acceleration," Advances in Bioengineering, ASME, New York, 1974, pp. 95-97.

9. Tennyson, S.A., and King, A.I., "Electromyographic Signals of the Spinal Musculature During $+G_z$ Impact Acceleration," Presented at the 1976 Meeting of the International Society for the Study of the Lumbar Spine, Bermuda, 1976.

10. Prasad, P., and King, A.I., "An Experimentally Validated Dynamic Model of the Spine," Journal of Applied Mechanics, Vol. 41, 1974, pp. 546-50.

11. Prasad, P., Mital, N., King, A.I., and Patrick, L.M., "Dynamic Response of the Spine During $+G_z$ Acceleration," Proceedings of 19th Stapp Car Crash Conference, SAE, Inc., Warrendale, Pa, 1975, pp. 869-97.

12. Bahler, A.S., "Modeling of Mammalian Skeletal Muscle," IEEE Transactions on Biomedical Engineering, Vol. BME-15, 1968, p. 249.

13. Wilkie, D.R., "Mechanical Properties of Muscle," British Medical Bulletin, Vol. 12, 1956, pp. 177-82.

14 Soechting, J.F., Stewart, P.A., Duffy, J., Hawley, R.H., and Paslay, P.R., "Evaluation of Human Neuromuscular Parameters," Journal of Dynamic Systems, Measurement, and Control, Transactions ASME, Series G, Vol. 93, 1971, pp. 221-26.

15. Crowe, A. and Mathews, P.B.C., "The Effects of Stimulation of Static and Dynamic Fusimotor Fibers on the Response to Stretching of the Primary Endings of Muscle Spindles," Journal of Physiology, Vol. 174, 1964, pp. 109-31.

16. Poppele, R.E., and Terzuolo, C.A., "Myotatic Reflex: Its Input-Output Relation," Science, Vol. 159, 1968, p. 743.

17. Gray, H., "Anatomy of the Human Body," Goss, C.M., ed., 29th American Edition, Lea and Febiger, Philadelphia, 1973.

18. Akima, H., "A New Method of Interpolation and Smooth Curve Fitting Based on Local Procedures," Journal of Association of Computing Machinery, Vol. 17, 4, 1970, pp. 589-602.

19. Houk, J.C., Cornew, R.W., and Stark, L., "A Model of Adaption in Amphibian Spindle Receptors," Journal of Theoretical Biology, Vol. 12, 1966, p. 196.

20. Crowe, A., "A Mechanical Model of the Mammalian Muscle Spindle," Journal of Theoretical Biology, Vol. 21, 1968, p. 21.

21. Poppele, R.E., and Bowman, R.J., "Quantitative Description of Linear Behavior of Mammalian Muscle Spindles," Journal of Neurophysiology, Vol. 33, 1970, p. 59.

22. McRuer, D.T., Magdaleno, R.E., and Moore, G.P., "A Neuromuscular Activation System Model," IEEE Transactions on Man-Machine Systems, Vol. MMS-9, 1968, pp. 61-71.

23. Morris, J.M., Lucas, D.B., and Bresler, B., "The Role of the Trunk in Stability of the Spine," Biomechanics Laboratory, Univ. of California, Berkeley, 1961, Report No. 42.

24. Hammond, P.H., "An Experimental Study of Servo Action in Human Muscular Control," Third International Conference on Medical Electronics, p. 190, 1960.

25. Foust, D.R., Chaffin, D.B., Snyder, R.G., and Baum, J.K., "Cervical Range of Motion and Dynamic Response and Strength of Cervical Muscles," Proceedings 17th Stapp Car Crash Conference, SAE, New York, pp. 285-308, 1973.

26. Hannan, A.G., Inkster, W.C., and Scott, J.D., "Peak EMG Activity and Jaw Closing Force in Man," Journal of Dental Research, Vol. 54, 1975, p. 694.

27. Inman, V.T., Ralston, H.J., Saunders, J.B. de C.M., Feinstein, B., and Wright, E.N., Jr., "Relation of Human EMG to Muscle Tension," Electroencephalography and Clinical Neurophysiology, Vol. 4, 1952, pp. 187-94.

28. Ewing, C.L., and Thomas, D.J., "Human Head and Neck Response to Impact Acceleration," Naval Aerospace Medical Laboratory, NAMRL Monograph 21, August, 1972.

Finite Element Simulation of the Occupant/Belt Interaction: Chest and Pelvis Deformation, Belt Sliding and Submarining

D. Song, F. Brun-Cassan, and J. Y. Le Coz
Peugeot/Renault

P. Mack and C. Tarrière
Renault DSE

F. Lavaste
ENSAM Paris

ABSTRACT

In frontal impact, the occupant/belt interaction is essential to obtain a good simulation of the occupant dynamic behaviour. Nevertheless, current mathematical models do not allow a realistic representation of this interaction to be obtained. Especially they are not adapted to simulate two important phenomena : the chest and pelvis deformation under the belt loading, and the belt sliding on the occupant.

This paper deals with a tridimensional finite element model which allows an improved simulation of this interaction. The Hybrid III dummy, restrained by a 3-point retractor belt, was aimed, with a finite element program (RADIOSS). The model consisted of two parts : a deformable part representing, by means of springs and shell elements, the belt system, the thorax and the- pelvis ; a rigid part representing, with rigid shell elements, the other components of the system. The belt was simulated by shell elements with a elasto-plastic material law. For the pelvis/lap belt modelling, special attention was given to the iliac spine function and the abdomen deformation effect as well as the belt sliding over the pelvis, essential for the submarining investigation. For the chest/shoulder belt interaction, the whole chest surface was considered as being deformable, in order to take account of its influence on belt sliding. A series of subsystem tests was firstly used to validate the chest and pelvis model : a belt loaded by an impactor, the pelvis loaded by a lap belt, the thorax loaded by an impactor and by a shoulder belt. Then the complete model was evaluated by comparing with sled tests, special attention being paid to the submarining. The correlation of analytical predictions with test data is presented.

1. INTRODUCTION

In frontal impact, the dynamic response of a belted occupant is essentially conditioned by the interaction of his torso with the belt system. Conditions of occupant impacts with others protection devices, such as air bag for example, are also closely linked with this interaction. For frontal impact analysis with mathematical models, the quality of the occupant/belt interaction approach is therefore primordial.

The principal method used in the past for simulating this interaction is based on a spring and rigid body approach. The belt is divided into different segments and each segment is modelled by a spring, while the occupant torso is represented by a system composed of rigid bodies. Springs simulating the segments which restrain directly the occupant are fixed to these rigid bodies in order to simulate the occupant/belt interaction. This is the technique used by most of the rigid body CVS softwares, such as MVMA2D, CAL-3D and MADYMO [1,2,3].

Compared to the reality of the occupant/belt interaction, this method has several shortcomings, in particular :

1) It only allows simulation of the belt slip along its own length. Slip in others directions is impossible to account for, such as for example the upward slip of the lap belt over the iliac spines, which can sometimes lead to the submarining. Recourses to artificial astuteness, such as attaching the lap belt to small ellipsoids [4], seem too far from the physical reality.

2) It does not allow a realistic repartition of belt loads over the occupant torso. In fact, with this method, belt loads on the occupant are simplified as point forces and the application points are fixed during impact. So effects of belt bearing point change over occupant can not be accounted for.

3) With this method, it is delicate to define characteristics of the springs simulating belt segments. They can not be deduced directly from the webbing characteristics, because the torso compliance has to be integrated in their definition. In order to do that, subsystem tests are necessary and these have to be repeated when webbing characteristics or belt path over the torso are modified.

In order to reduce these inconveniences, some rigid body CVS software packages were enhanced by introducing more advanced features. In CAL-3D a "harness belt system" option allows a description of belt slip by using a collection of reference points and by introducing slip conditions which control the movement of these points on ellipsoids representing the occupant torso [5,6]. In MADYMO a finite element feature was added which allows belt description with linear triangular membrane elements [7]. Nevertheless applications of these features for belt slip modelling are limited by the fact that the occupant torso has to be modelled by ellipsoid rigid bodies.

The finite element modelling of both occupant torso part and belt part appears to be the most promising option for improving the simulation of the occupant/belt interaction. Nevertheless, until now, investigations into this subject remain insufficient. The few approaches presented in the literature seem still too simplified to allow a satisfactory simulation of this interaction [8,9].

This paper describes the development of an FEM approach which allows simulation of the principal aspects of the occupant/belt interaction in a realistic way. The emphasis was in particular to simulate the belt slip over the chest and pelvis and the deformation of these under belt loading. Special attention was also directed towards the simplicity of approach in order to make it a frontal impact analysis tool, more powerful and realistic than the spring/rigid body approach, and less CPU-time consuming than a detailed finite element representation.

This study was carried out with an available finite element package RADIOSS [10]. The target occupant was the 50th percentile frontal impact dummy HYBRID-III [11].

2. SUBSYSTEM MODELLING

Three key elements of the occupant/belt interaction - belt, thorax and pelvis - were firstly modelled and validated with respect to a series of subsystem tests.

2.1 BELT MODELLING

The quality of the occupant/belt interaction simulation is conditioned by that of the belt representation.

It was decided to investigate firstly the belt modelling in the following configuration as it represented the simplest problem with a minimum of variables. It involved the simulation of the impact of a cylindrical mass upon a belt strap which was fixed at its two extremities to a rigid support. Figure 1 shows the experimental set up for the test configuration. The choice of such an impact loading of the belt was to observe its behaviour under dynamic contact. The impactor mass is 8.25 kg ; two impact velocities used were 2.5 m/s and 3.7m/s. The displacement and acceleration of impactor were measured, and from this the belt tension is deduced.

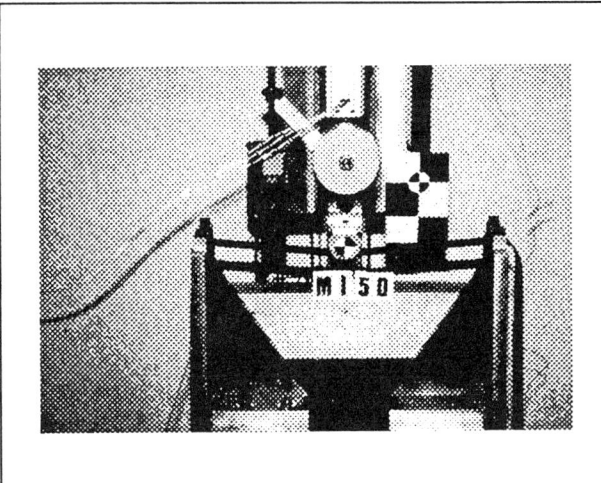

Figure 1. Belt test set up

Figure 2 shows the model simulating these tests. Shell elements were used to model the belt. The "One point integration in thickness" option was used to obtain the membrane behaviour of shell elements. The size of each element is identical and corresponds to a third of belt breadth. The impactor was treated as a rigid body. Its contact surface is represented by rigid shell elements.

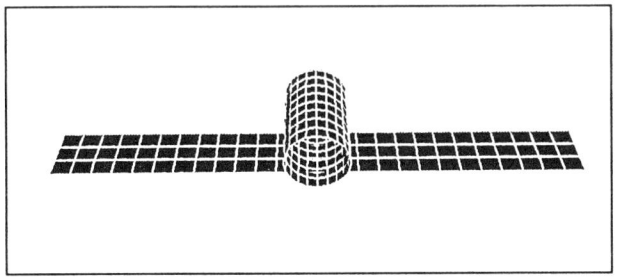

Figure 2. Belt and impactor model set up

The elasto-plastic law is used to characterize these elements.

$$\sigma = \begin{cases} E\varepsilon & (\varepsilon \leq \varepsilon_0) \\ (A + B\varepsilon_p^n) & (\varepsilon \geq \varepsilon_0) \end{cases}$$

Where E is Young's modulus, A elastic limit, B hardening coefficient and ε_p plastic deformation

Figure 3 shows the definition of the law according to experimental data from belt static tests. Poisson's ratio was assumed 0.2 and the thickness of elements is that of the belt.

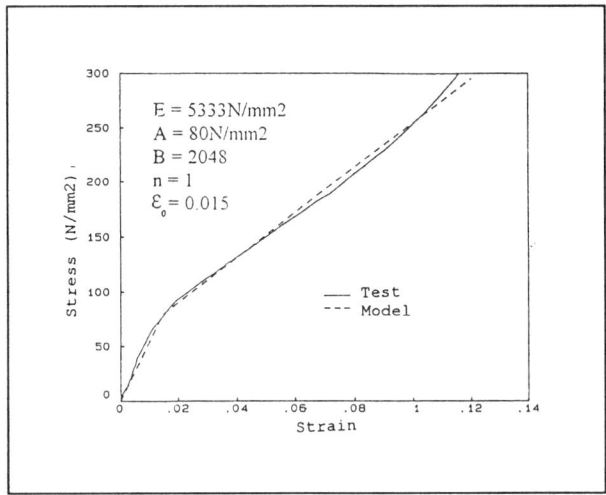

Figure 3. Approach of quasi-static belt elongation test data by a elesto-plastic law

Figure 4 compares the time histories of the displacement and acceleration of the impactor, and the belt tension for model and experiments. The belt model prediction matches well with experimental results.

Based on this model, a parametric study was carried out for belt thickness and Poisson's ratio. The thickness does not influence the model behaviour if the force-deflection relationship is conserved. By varying the Poisson's ratio between 0.1 and 0.4, model responses are almost identical.

2.2 THORAX MODELLING

Figure 5 shows the thorax model developed. It is composed of a rigid body carrying its inertia and an envelope in shell elements representing the real thorax contact surface. This envelope is attached to the "thorax" rigid body by general springs (springs which allow control of the 6-DOF movement between two nodes by defining the force-deflection and damping velocity relationships for both translation and rotation). Such a spring is created behind each node of the frontal surface of the thorax.

The thorax surface is divided into two parts : the frontal surface discretized in deformable shell elements and the thorax back in rigid shell

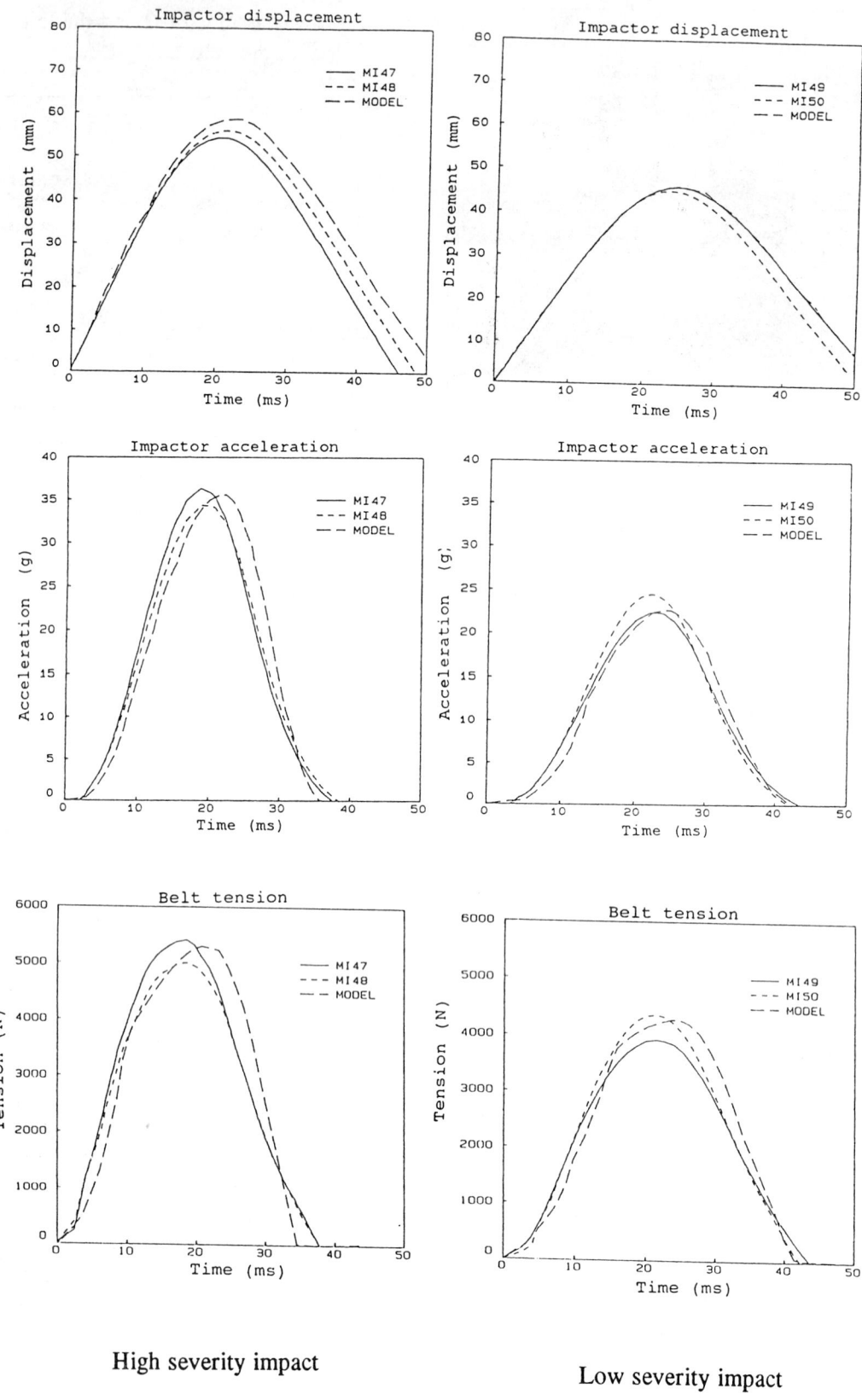

Figure 4. Belt model response compared to experimental results

elements. These latter ones were inserted into the "thorax" rigid body. General springs were classed into three groups according to their stiffness :

Group 1 : "Sternum" springs
Group 2 : "lower thorax" springs.
Group 3 : "shoulder" springs

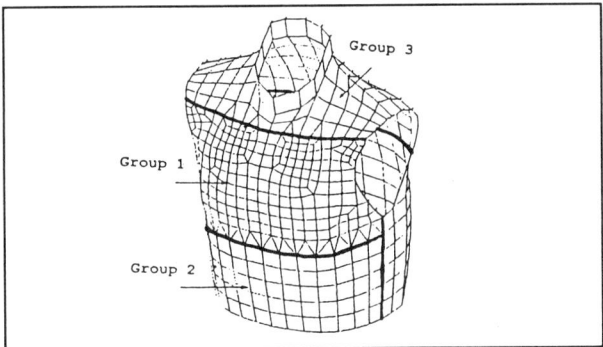

Figure 5. Thorax model

Characteristics of shell elements and general springs used are :

Shell elements

Young's Modulus = 1.5 N/mm2

Poisson's Ratio = 0.2

Thickness = 3 mm

Springs

Group 1 : K = 0.155 N/mm, C = 0.55 N.s/m
Group 2 : K = 0.6 N/mm, C = 0.55 N.s/m
Group 3 : K = 15.5 N/mm, C = 0.55 N.s/m

In all, 997 nodes, 558 shell elements (156 rigid elements) and 419 springs were used to model the thoracic portion. The number of nodes and elements were significantly reduced compared to a full finite element thorax description, such as the model developed by Yang et al [12] where, for the description of the ribs and spine box alone, 1996 nodes and 1582 elements had been used.

Two types of test were used to evaluate this model.

Evaluation with impactor tests : This was based on the HYBRID-III thorax calibration test results. Two standard impact velocities - 4.3 m/s and 6.7 m/s respectively - were simulated.

Taking into account the decoupling movement between the thorax assembly and the others segments of the occupant in the first 20 milliseconds, i.e. the loading phase of impact, an effective mass of 24.9 kg was used in the model. This mass corresponds to the sum of the thorax and uppers extremities masses. The impactor was treated as a rigid body with its contact surface discretized in shell elements.

Figure 6 illustrates the thorax shape at 0 and 20 ms for the 6.7 m/s test. A comparison of the impact force and chest deflection between the model and the test is presented in figure 8. The agreement is satisfactory for the loading phase. Similar results can be obtained for the 4.3 m/s test.

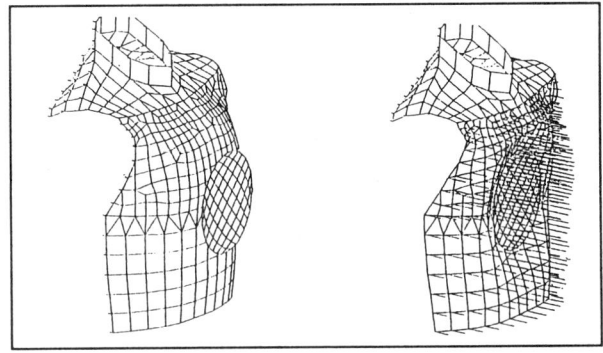

Figure 6. Impacted thorax at 0 and 20 ms

Evaluation with belt tests : A series of tests was conducted by INRETS to study the HYBRID-III thorax behaviour under belt loading [13]. As shown in figure 7, the dummy is laying on a rigid flat surface. A seat belt strap is placed across the thorax and compresses this one when the belt is loaded by an impactor.

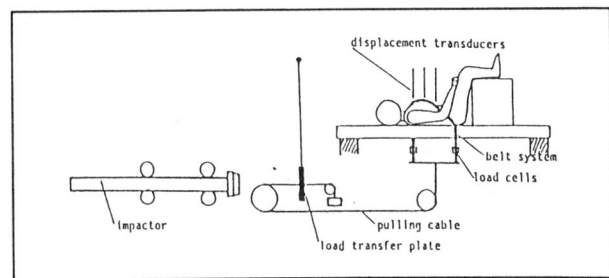

Figure 7. Thorax belt test set up

Two tests were chosen to evaluate the thorax model behaviour for its interaction with a belt :

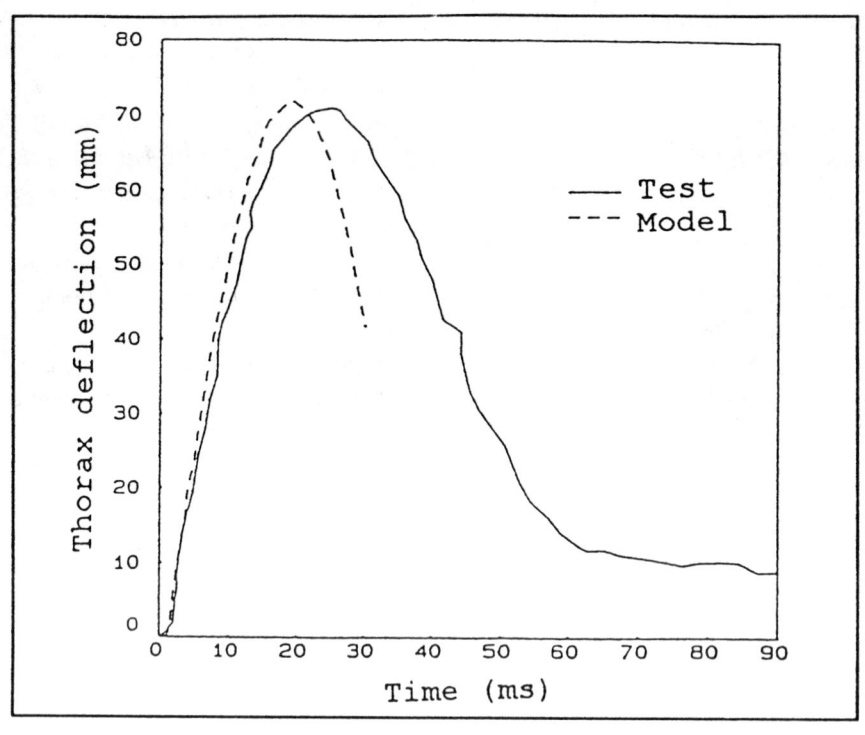

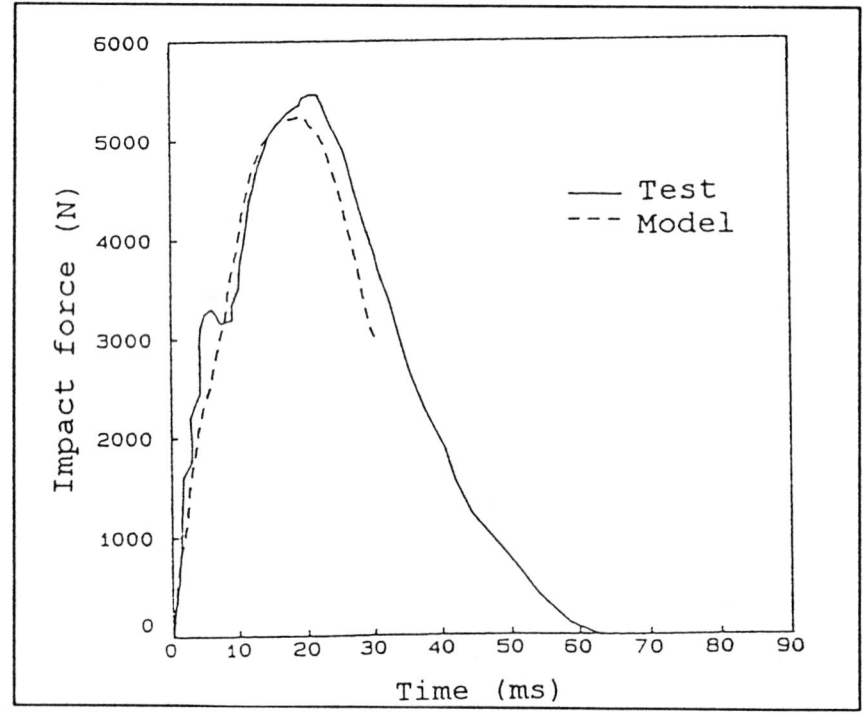

Figure 8. Comparison of contact force and thorax deflection between model and experiment for 6.7 m/s pendulum impact

THC89 :
Impactor mass = 22.4 kg
Impact velocity = 7.3 m/s
THC83 :
Impactor mass = 76.1 kg
Impact velocity = 3.4 m/s

Figure 9 shows the model simulating these tests. The cylindrical surfaces in shell elements in the model were to simulate pulleys used in the tests which guide the belt during impact. The chest/belt interaction is modelled by using a master surface/slave surface contact algorithm. The interfaces were defined between belt and shoulder, sternum and lower thorax surface.

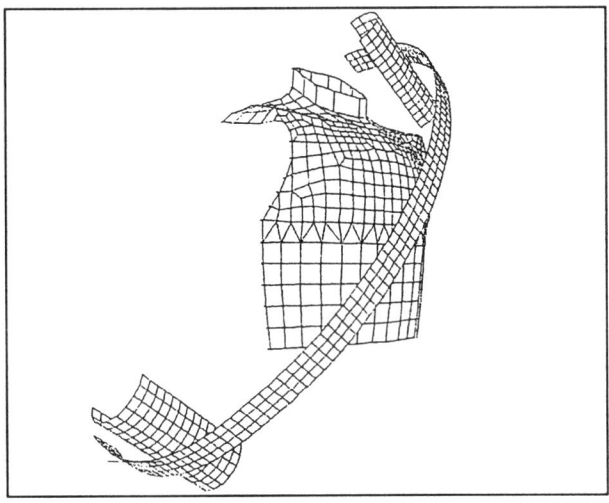

Figure 9. Model for thorax belt test

The belt was loaded in two ways. The first one consists in distributing the impactor mass to the boundary belt nodes and assigning the initial impactor velocity to the nodes.

A comparison of calculated and measured values of thorax deflection and belt tension is presented in figure 10 for test THC 83. The principal difference lies in the time for reaching peak values. This can be explained partly by existing plays in the experimental set up and the energy loss in the cable path.

Another way for loading the belt is to assign directly the measured belt tension to the boundary belt nodes. In this case the model behaviour is evaluated by comparing the chest deflection. Figure 11 shows the agreement between model and experiment for test THC83. Figure 12 shows the model configuration at 35 ms for test THC89. Figure 13 illustrates the calculated thorax deformation form and the experimentally reconstructed one, for test THC83, at the instant where the maximum thoracic deformation was reached. The thorax compliance under belt loading is quite satisfactory.

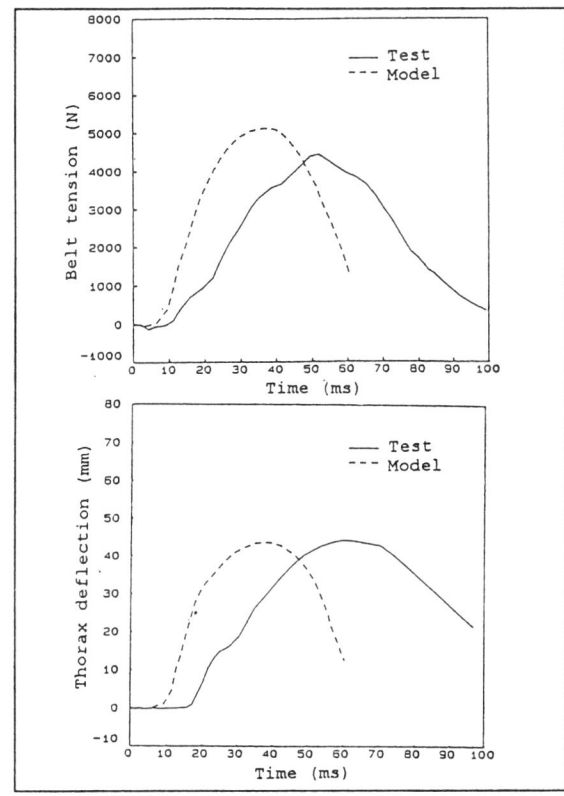

Figure 10. Comparison of belt tension and thorax deflection between model and experiment for test THC 83.

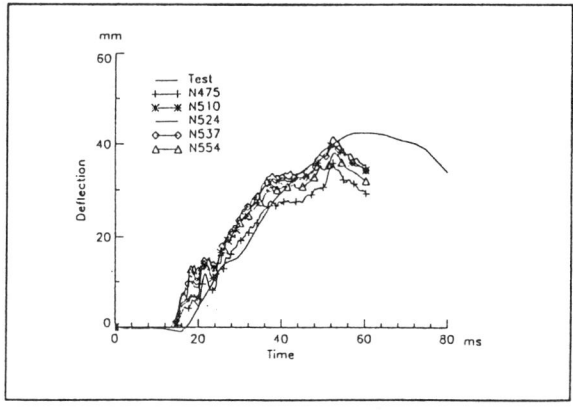

Figure 11. Comparison of thorax deflection for test THC 83

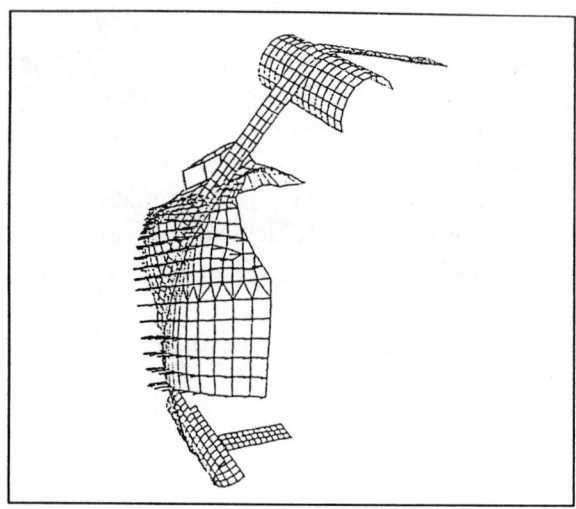

Figure 12 Model configuration at 35 ms

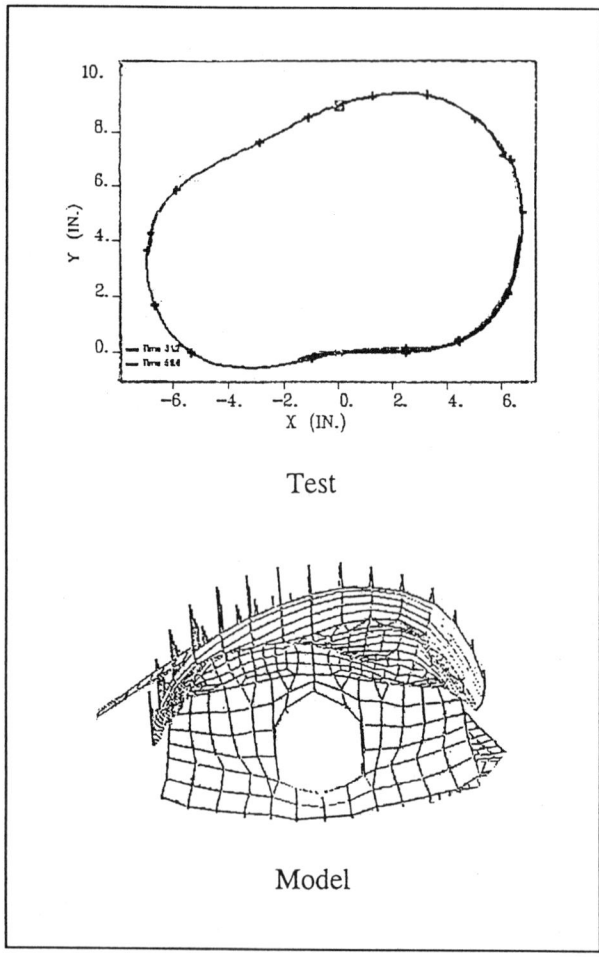

Figure 13. Calculated deformed thorax shape viewed from toe to head and experimentally reconstructed thorax deformation contour at the moment where the maximum thoracic deformation was reached

2.3 PELVIS MODELLING

A pelvis model should account for the essential role of the iliac spine for the pelvis/lap belt interaction, in particular for the submarining risk. To do this, it is necessary to model the iliac foam and skin compression under belt loading, and also the iliac spine shape effects.

Figure 14 shows the pelvis model developed. Four shell element groups were used to model the exterior pelvis surface as well as the front iliac spine shape. Groups 1 and 2 represent the pelvis surface part which can enter into contact with the lap belt. The group 3, representing the rest of the surface, was used for the pelvis/seat cushion modelling. The group 4 describes the iliac spine front shape which influences directly the belt slip over the pelvis surface. In all, 995 nodes and 919 elements (639 rigid elements) were used.

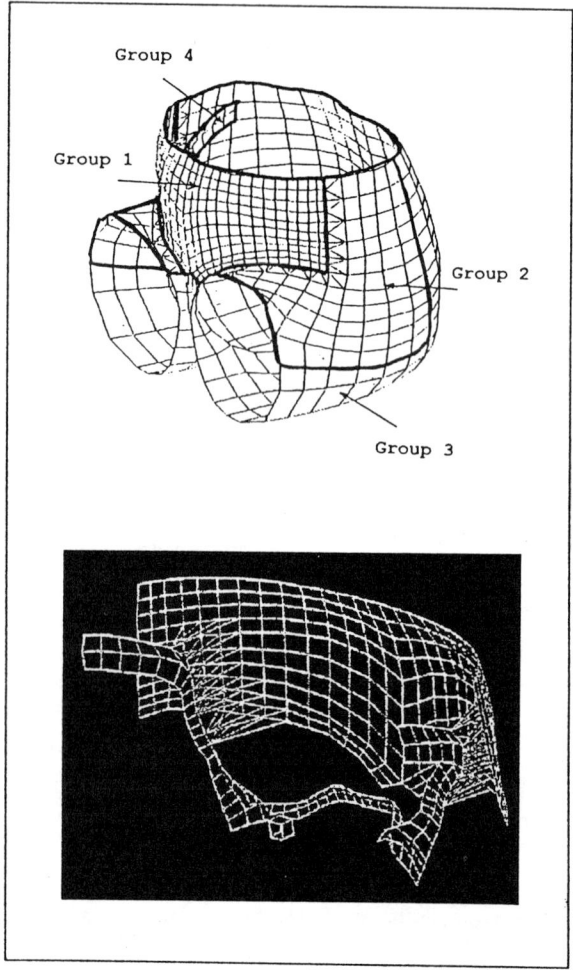

Figure 14. Pelvis model

The pelvis inertia is carried by a "pelvis" rigid body. Shell elements of groups 3 and 4 were inserted in this rigid body and consequently are rigid. Elements of group 1 are deformable and those of group 2 rigid. These elements were disconnected from group 3 and were attached to iliac spine elements with 64 general springs. These springs, with the aim of simulating the foam in front of the iliac spine, were guided along the A-P direction of the pelvis. Their characteristics were calculated according to the foam strain/stress relationship and their length. In total, four stiffness were distinguished (Figure 15).

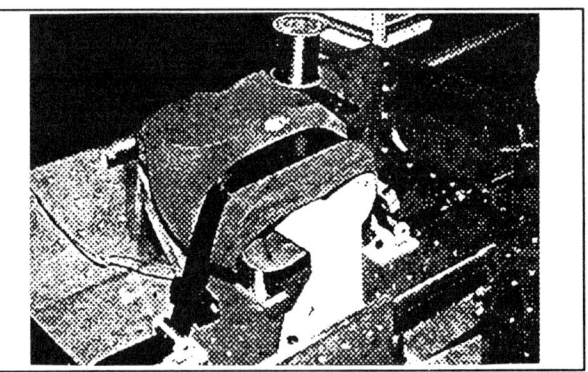

Figure 16. Pelvis belt test set up

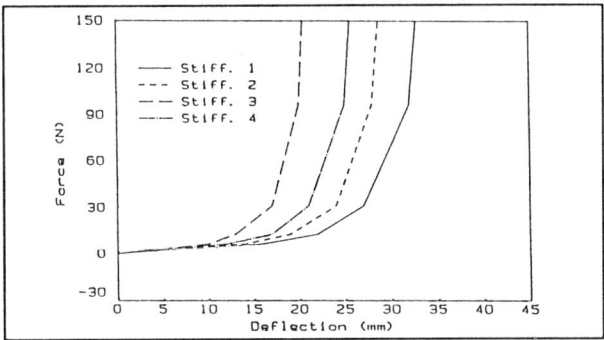

Figure 15. Iliac springs stiffness

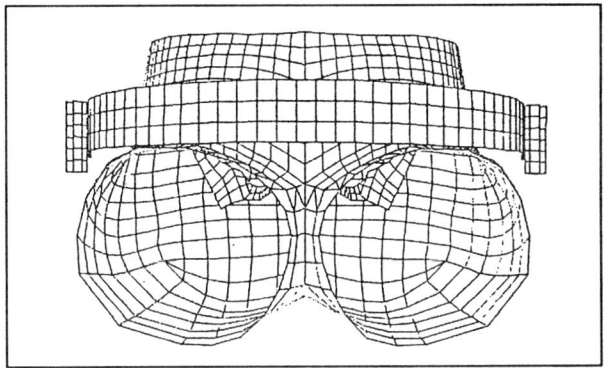

Figure 17. Model for pelvis belt test

Quasi-static tests were carried out to evaluate this model in a relatively simple configuration. Figure 16 shows the experimental set up. The pelvis is fixed rigidly and was compressed by loading the belt with two cranks. The belt path over the pelvis can be adjusted by moving two pulleys guiding the belt during test. A piece of tissue was placed between belt and pelvis to account for the clothing influence on friction. Two configurations were tested, one leading to submarining and the other not.

Figure 17 shows the model simulating the tests. A constant velocity of 0.5 m/s was assigned to the boundary belt nodes for loading the belt.

<u>Simulation of configuration without submarining</u> : In this case, as illustrated in figure 19 (a), shell elements and general springs were compressed under belt loading and the belt was hooked to the iliac spine. Figure 18 shows a comparison of the belt tension between model and experiment.

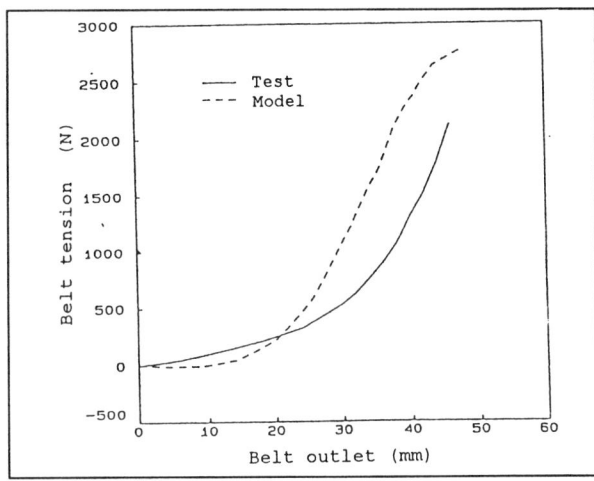

Figure 18 Comparison of predicted belt tension with quasi-static test results

<u>Simulation of configuration with submarining</u> : We can observe in this case an upward belt slip which ends up passing over the iliac crest ; such movement corresponding to the occurence of submarining. Figure 19 (b) shows the model shape at the moment where the belt reached its slip limit.

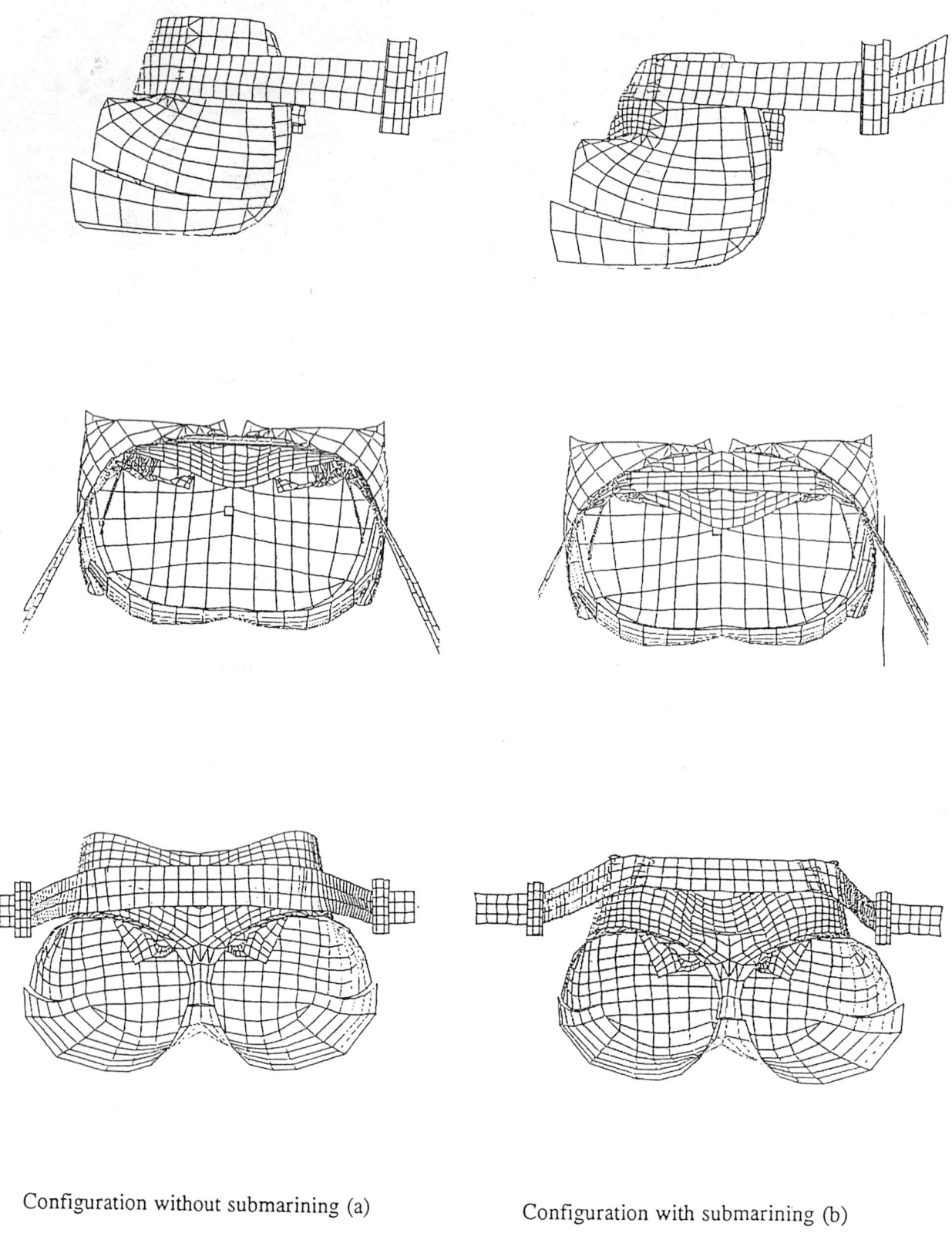

Configuration without submarining (a)　　　Configuration with submarining (b)

Figure 19. Comparison of belt position and deformed pelvis for configurations with and without submarining

3. OCCUPANT/BELT INTERACTION MODELLING IN SLED TESTS

Based on the subsystem models of the belt, thorax and pelvis outlined above, the occupant/belt interaction in a vehicle crash environment will be examined in this section. The target system was composed of the HYBRID-III dummy restrained by a 3-point retractor belt, a seat and a toeboard.

3.1 MODEL DESCRIPTION

Occupant

As shown in figure 20, the full dummy model is a combination of preceding thorax and pelvis models with a RADIOSS rigid body H-III model. The latter was constructed using data in the literature [14,15] and consisted of 15 rigid bodies representing respectively the head, neck, thorax, lumbar spine, pelvis, upper legs, lower legs, feet, upper arms and lower arms/hands assemblies. Connections between these segments were modelled with general springs. The relative rotation between adjacent segments was governed by a torque-angle relation, a dry friction constant and a damping constant for each rotation axis. The surface of each segment was approached by ellipsoid dicretized in shell elements.

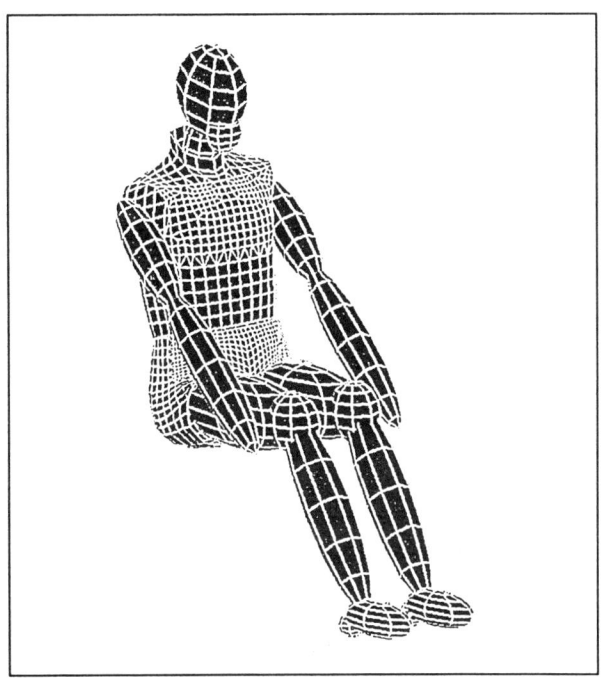

Figure 20. Full dummy model

Restraint System

The idea of modelling the total belt by shell elements was thrown out. On the one hand, the surface shape of the belt material as a whole is very complex, in particular for the D-ring part and stalk buckle part where belt surface warping is difficult to represent ; on the other, it is not more advantageous to model with shell elements the belt segments which can not enter into contact with the occupant surface than with springs.

A combination of springs, rigid bodies and shell elements was used to model the belt system (Figure 21).

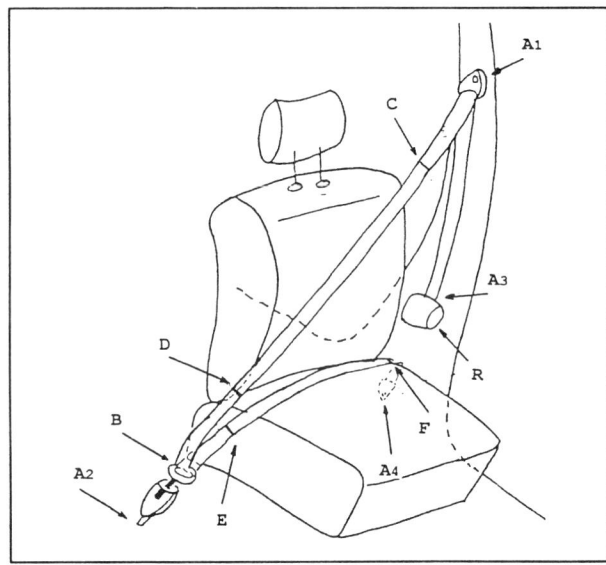

Figure 21. Belt system layout

1) Belt parts in contact with occupant : Segments **CD** and **EF**, in contact with the occupant surface, were modelled with shell elements. At the ends of two segments triangular rigid shell elements were used in order to obtain a good link between belt shell elements and springs modelling the others parts of the belt.

2) Belt parts without contact with occupant : Segments A_3A_1C, **DBE** and FA_4 can not enter into contact with occupant and were modelled by spring elements -a simple spring for segment FA_4 and two 3-node springs respectively for segments A_3A_1C and **DBE** in order to account for the belt material transfer at the D-ring and the stalk buckle.

3) <u>Friction</u> : Tension in the upper shoulder belt is greater than that in the retractor part owing to the friction between D-ring and belt material. It is the same for the lower shoulder belt and inboard lap belt. The friction effect was accounted for by installing two simple springs (between point A_1 and point **C** for D-ring friction and between point **B** and point **E** for stalk buckle friction).

4) <u>Film spooling effect</u> : This was simulated by a 1D spring which links the extremity point A_3 of the spring A_3A_1C to the anchorage **R**.

5) <u>Stalk</u> : A rigid body was used to represent the stalk. It is attached to the sled by a general spring with which the stalk rotation about anchorage A_2 and the deformation of the latter can be accounted for.

The whole sled system was treated as a rigid body to which 4 rigid shell elements were attached simulating contact planes of the seat back, seat cushion, floor and toeboard. In all 3439 nodes, 2655 shell elemnts (1751 rigid elements) and 577 springs were used for the model. The crash pulse is applied as a velocity input.

Interfaces

The contact of the occupant with the belt was modelled using a master surface/slave surface contact interface algorithm. Two interfaces were defined between shoulder belt and thorax (shoulder, sternum and lower thorax) and between lap belt and pelvis . The master surfaces are those of the thorax and the pelvis.

Contacts between occupant and sled interior surface are between rigid surfaces. A rigid surface contact interface algorithm was used for modelling these contacts. Each contact is defined by a force-penetration function and a dry friction constant. The following interfaces were defined :

Pelvis/seat cushion
Right foot/toeboard
Left foot/toeboard

3.2 MODEL EVALUATION WITH RESPECT TO SLED TESTS

The model evaluation proceeded in two steps. In the first step, the system model was evaluated for configurations without submarining. In the second, several important parameters that affect significantly the submarining were varied in order to evaluate the model behaviour for the submarining simulation.

Simulations without submarining

To serve as experimental references for model evaluation, two sled tests were conducted with a change in velocity of 35-65 km/h, and a peak acceleration of 15-35 g (Figure 22). The HYBRID-III dummy was restrained by a 3-point retractor belt, a rigid seat and a toeboard.

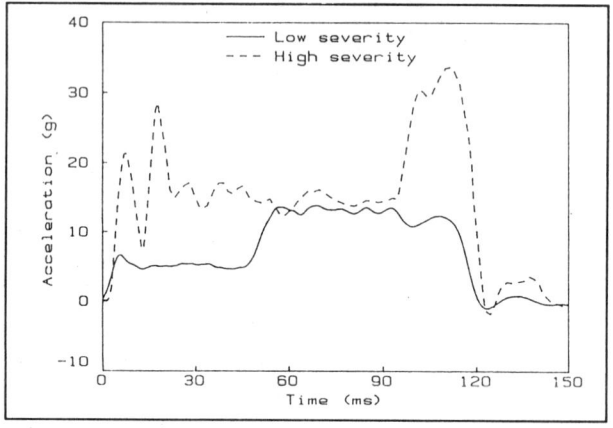

Figure 22. Impact pulses

The occupant and belt kinematics, thorax and pelvis accelerations as well as belt tensions are the most interesting criteria for evaluating the occupant/belt interaction simulation.

Figures 23 and 24 illustrate the model configurations at 0, 70, 110 and 150 ms, compared to the kinematics obtained from experimental film analysis for the low severity test. The sequence of events given by the model matches well with experimental tests. For both tests, we can observe a tendency of right-upwards shoulder belt slip over the chest, as can be seen in the corresponding tests. But a friction constant superior to 0.5 was needed for the belt/thorax interface so that the belt does not slip off the chest surface across the neck. For the lap belt, the skin and foam in front of the iliac spine were collapsed under belt loading; the belt was hooked to the iliac spine with a friction constant of 0.3 between pelvis skin and belt material. Figure 25

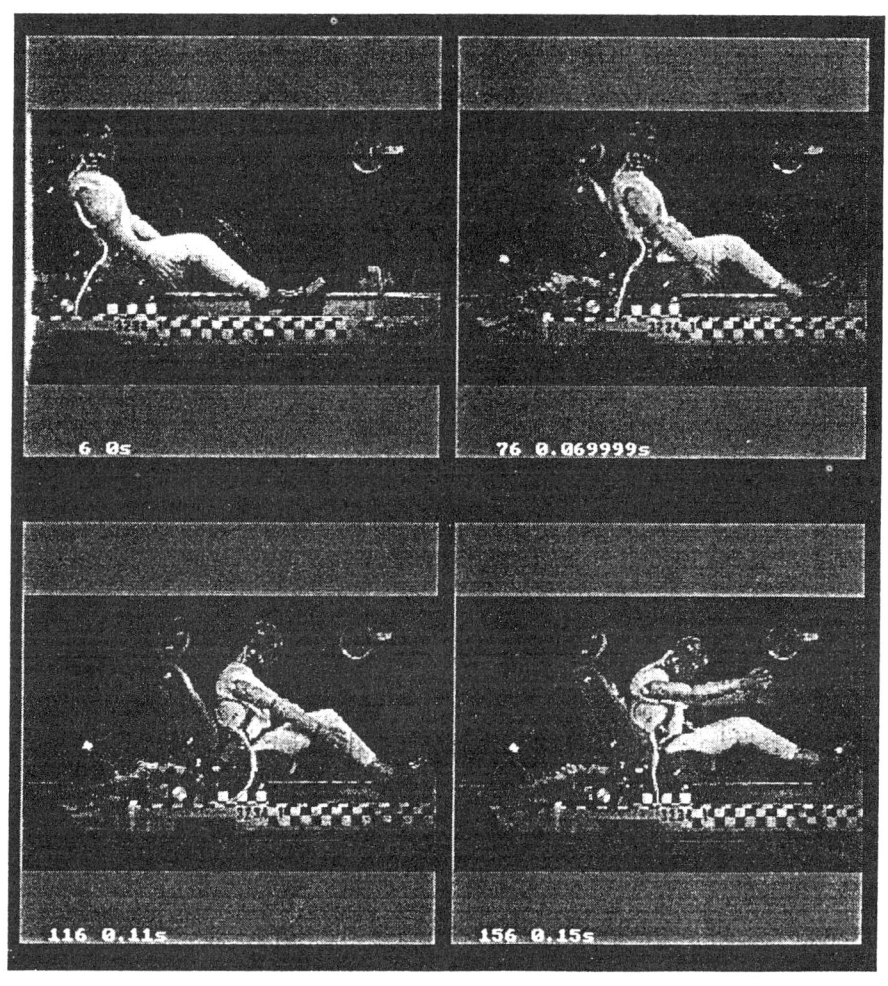
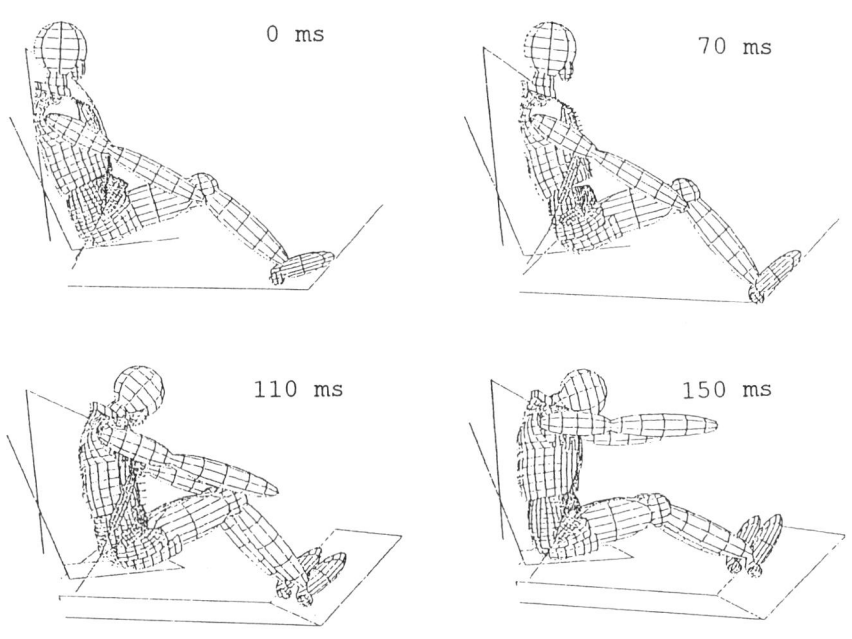

Figure 23. Model kinematics compared to experiment

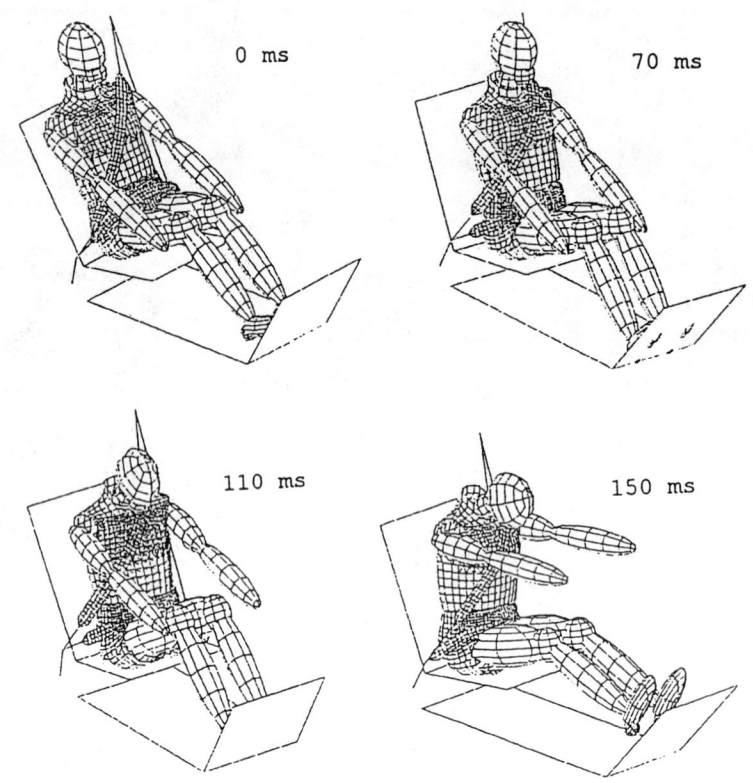

Figure 24. Model kinematics in perspective view

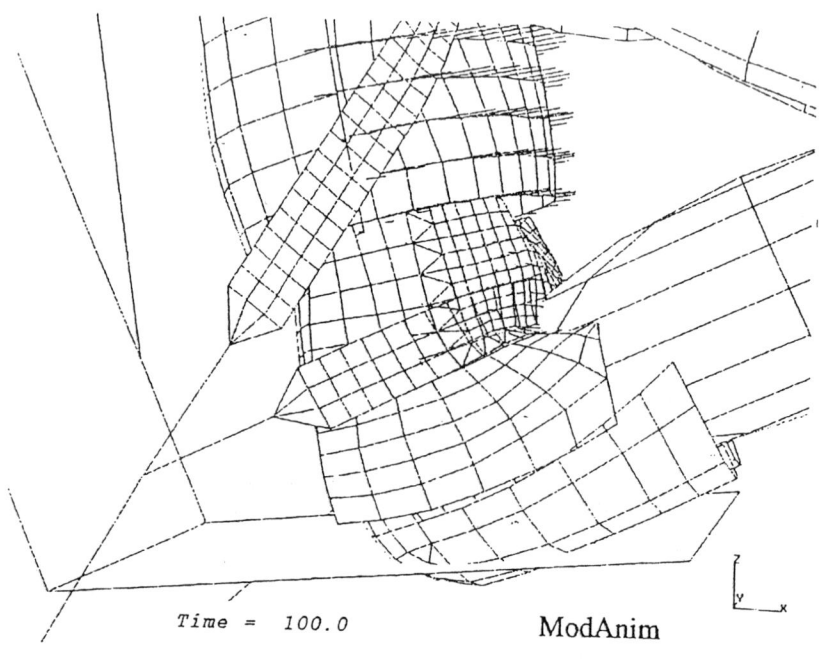

Figure 25. Lap belt position relative to the deformed pelvis for configuration without submarining

shows the deformed shape of the pelvis at 100 ms for the low severity test.

The calculated time histories with the model are presented together with experimental results. Belt loads are presented in figure 26. The resultant acceleration for the thorax and pelvis are presented in figure 27. As can be seen in the figures, there is in general a reasonable agreement between models responses and experimental results. A more accurate definition of some parameters of the system model should reduce the level of deviation between model and experiment. It is noted that, for belt loading, the model/test correlation is better than that of the test THC83 simulation for thorax model evaluation (Figure 10). In fact, in the THC83 simulation the experimental belt tension, as for the thoracic deflection, reached his peak value less quickly than the model prediction because of existing plays in the experimental set up and the energy loss in the cable path. These are difficult to simulate in the model representation of the experimental set up.

Simulations with submarining

The lap belt - to - pelvis angle, seat cushion characteristic and friction level between belt material and pelvis clothing are the most significant parameters on the submarining occurrence.

Three simulations were performed by varying these parameters. The baseline dataset used corresponds to the above model with the low severity impact pulse.

Run 1 :
Reducing the friction constant from 0.3 to 0.1
Run 2 :
Replacing the rigid cushion stiffness by a softer one (Figure 28)
Run 3 :
Moving lap belt anchorages back 100 mm.

For run 1, the model kinematics show that the lap belt was always maintained in front of the iliac spine during impact and there was not submarining. For run 3, similar belt kinematics can be observed.

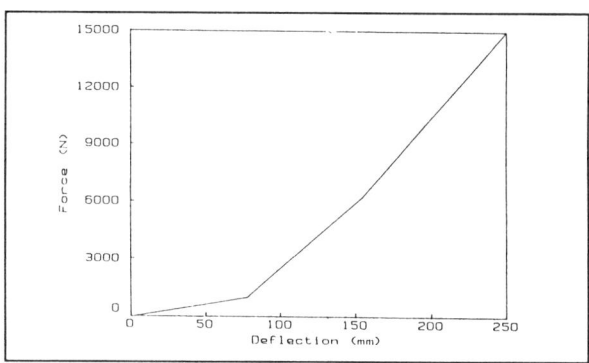

Figure 28. Stiffness of soft seat cushion

For run 2, the seat cushion stiffness was insufficient to resist the downwards motion and rear rotation of the pelvis. These motions changed progressively the lap belt - to -pelvis angle. When this angle reached a critical angle, the lap belt slipped over the iliac crest, that corresponding to the occurrence of submarining. Figure 29 shows the deformed pelvis and the belt position relative to the pelvis about this moment. After its passage over iliac crests, the lap belt was totally unhooked from the pelvis, as illustrated in figure 30

Figure 31 presents calculated lap belt loads for run 2 along with the baseline results. One can observe a sudden drop of lap belt load for run 2, a typical indication of submarining occurrence. Nevertheless, this model can not yet calculate the force transmitted by lap belt to the abdomen after its passage above the iliac spine. As a consequence, the calculated belt load does not present a second peak, as in experiments with submarining, which results from the belt interaction with the lumbar spine.

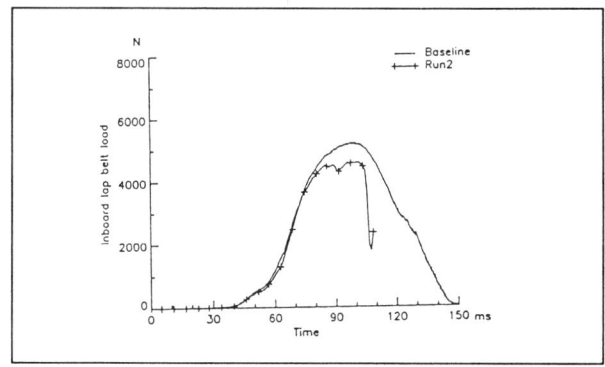

Figure 31. Comparison of lap belt load for run 2 (submarining) and baseline run (no submarining)

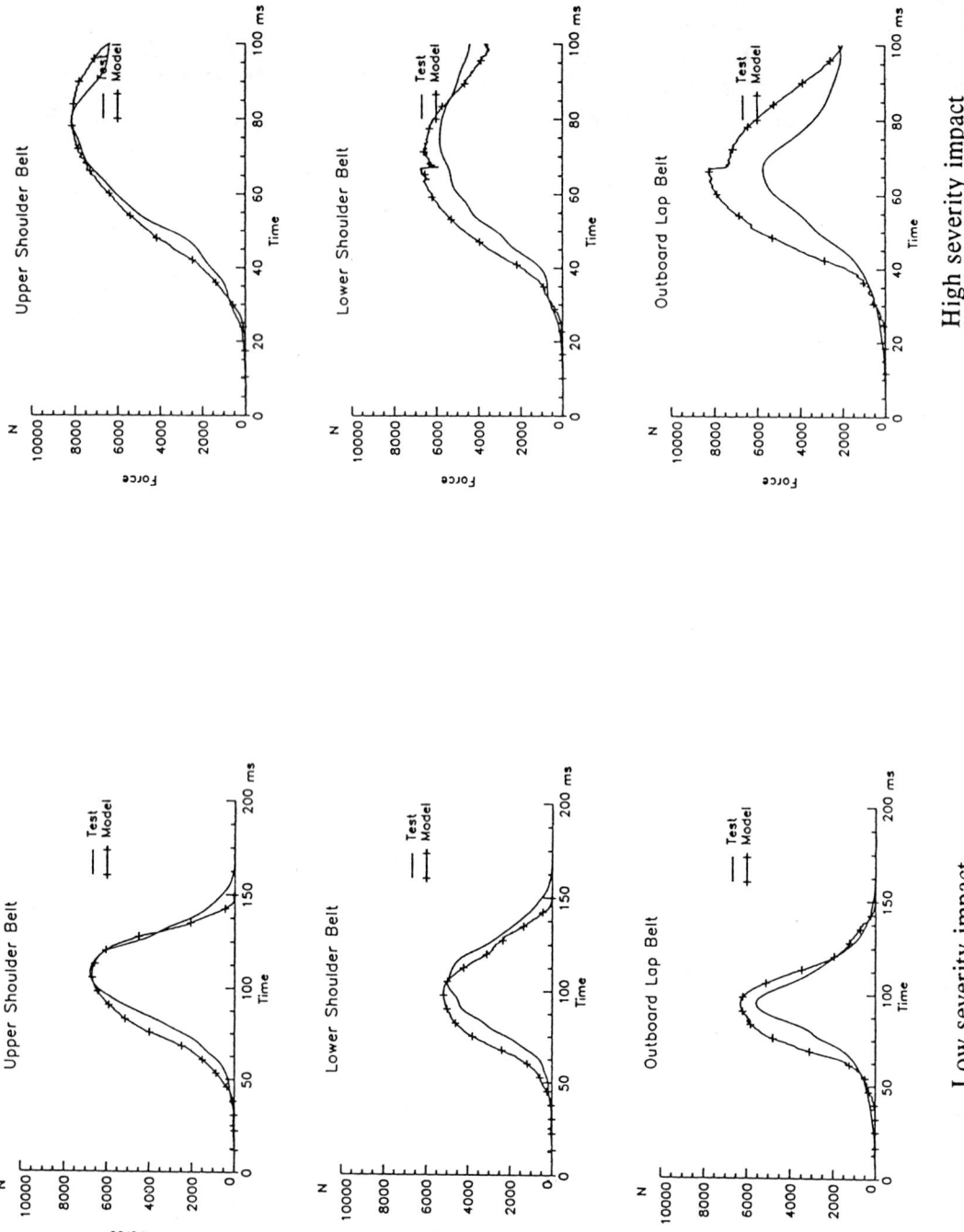

Figure 26. Comparison of belt loads

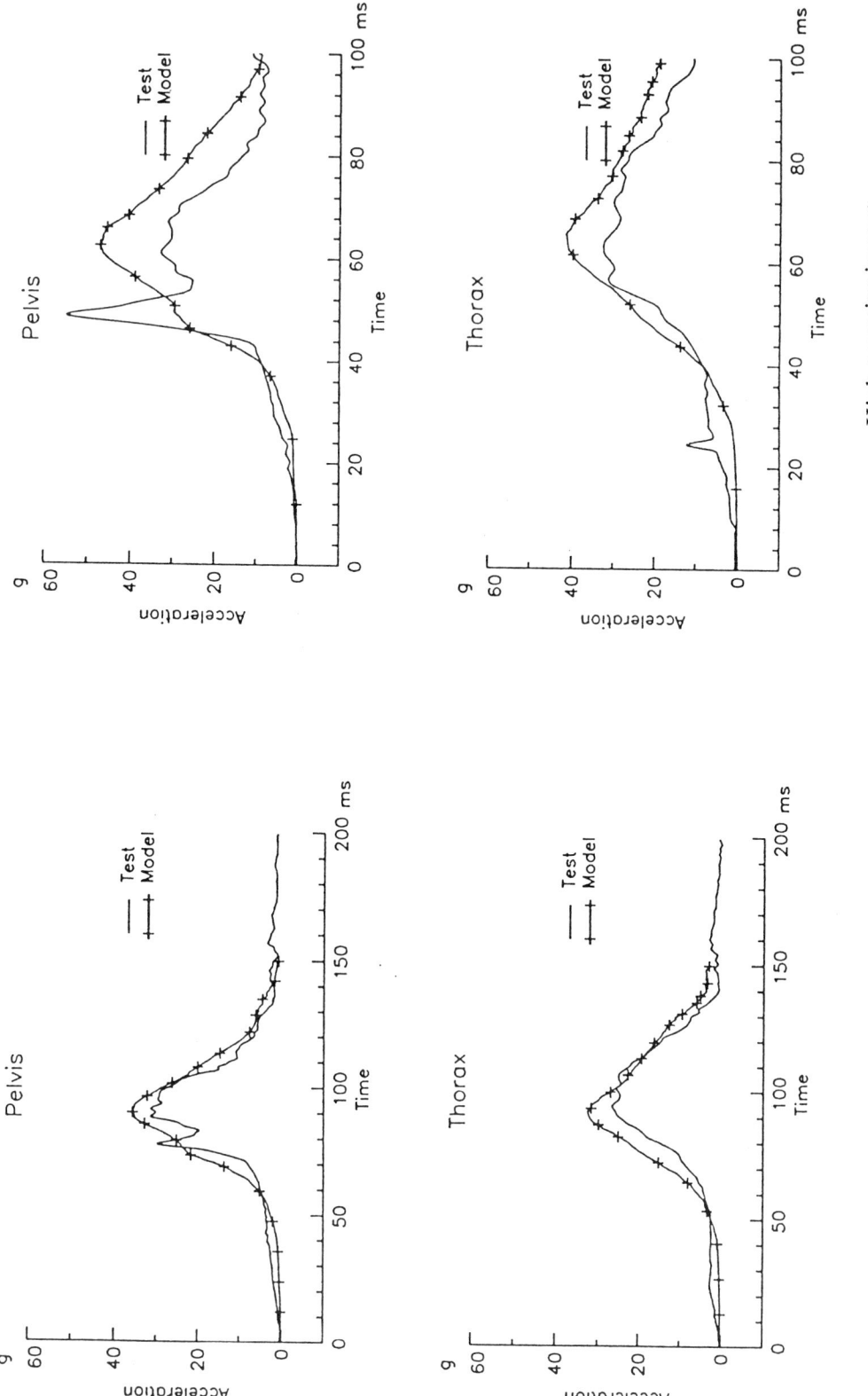

Figure 27. Comparison of accelerations

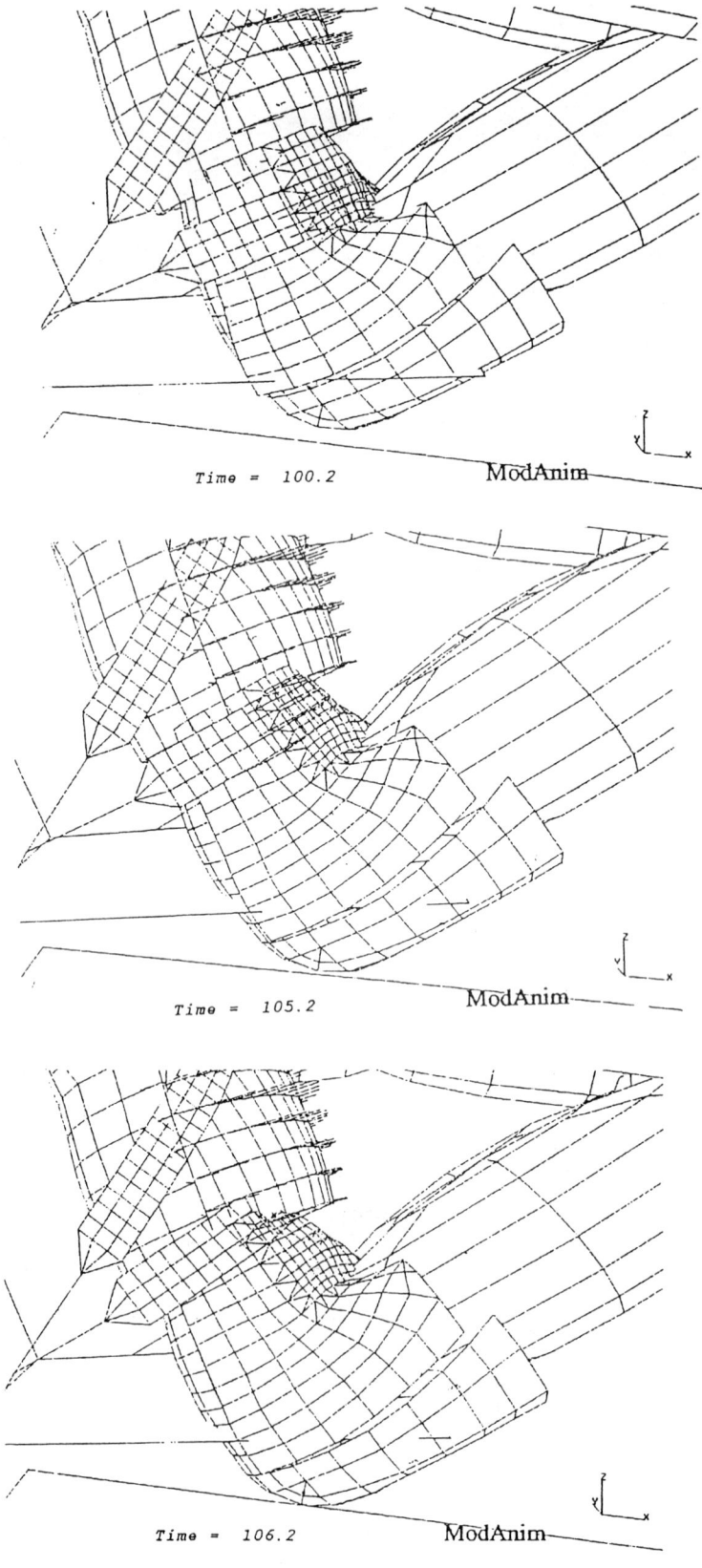

Figure 29. Passage of lap belt over iliac crests - beginning of submarining

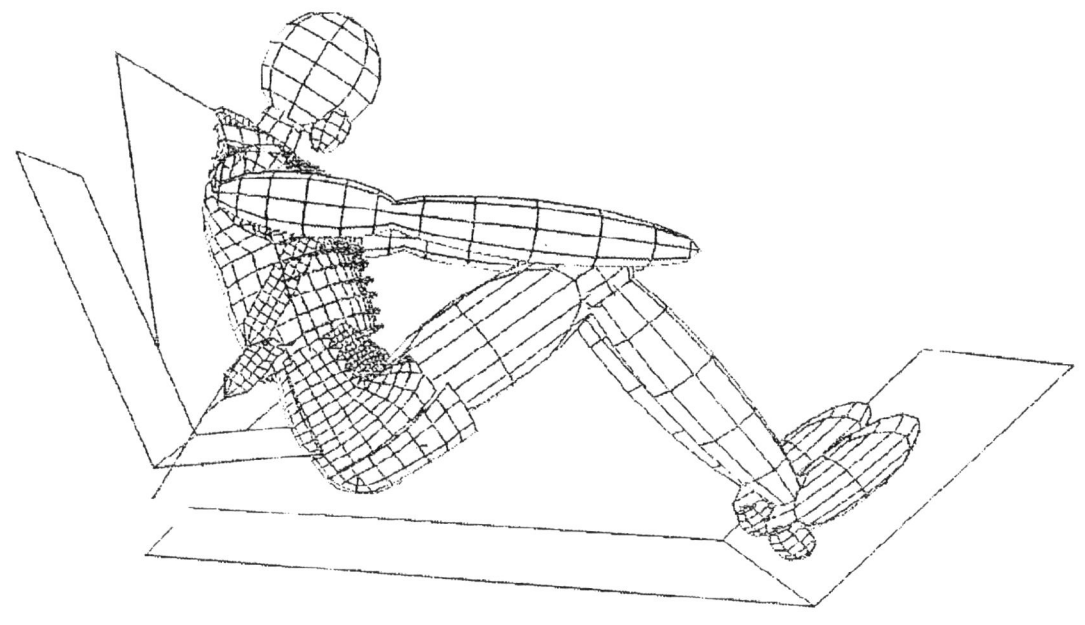

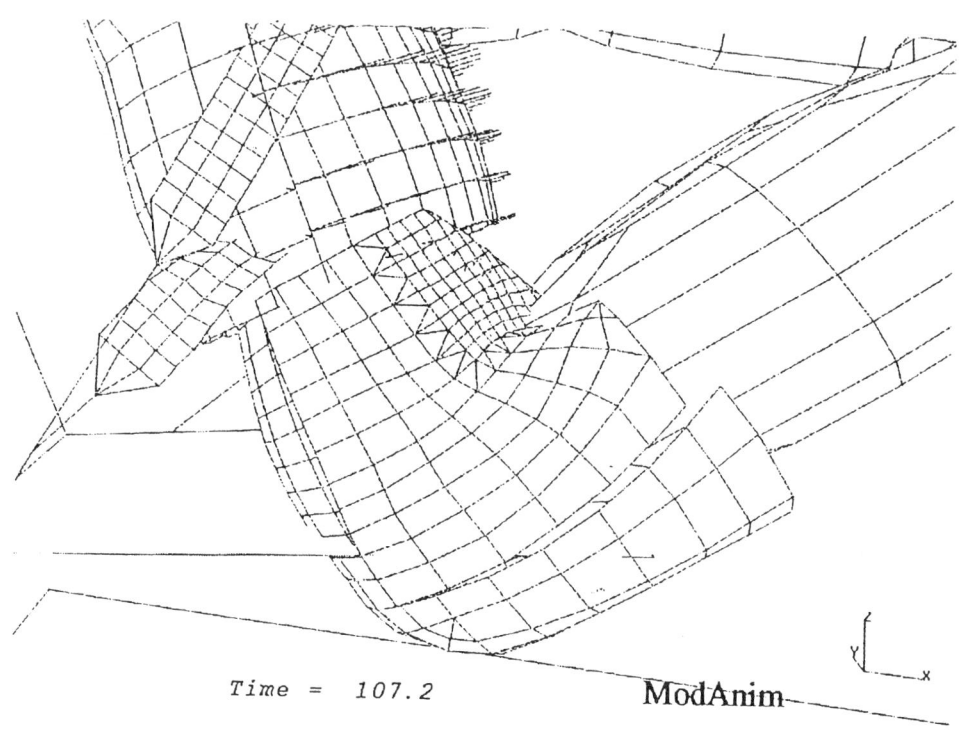

Figure 30. Model kinematics after the passage of lap belt over iliac crests

4. SUMMARY AND CONCLUSION

A finite element approach to the occupant/belt interaction in frontal impact was developed. The target system was the 50th percentile HYBRID III dummy restrained by a 3-point retractor belt. Three key elements of the occupant/belt interaction - belt, thorax and pelvis - were firstly modelled and validated with respect to four subsystem configurations : a belt loaded by a cylindrical surface impactor, the dummy pelvis compressed by a lap belt, the dummy thorax loaded by an impactor and by a shoulder belt. Based on these subsystem models, the occupant/belt interaction in a vehicle crash environment was modelled. The model was evaluated with respect to two sled tests of different severities for configurations without submarining. The model behaviour for submarining simulation was examined by varying some parameters that affect significantly such type of occupant kinematics.

This approach allows simulation, in a realistic way, of the principal aspects of the occupant/belt interaction, and in particular the belt slip over the thorax and pelvis and the deformation of these under belt loading. In general, a good agreement between model and experiment can be observed. For submarining simulation, the model allows the detection of submarining occurrence through lap belt kinematics and its tension time history.

This model is an approach more powerful and realistic than spring/rigid body approach and less CPU-consuming than a detailed finite element representation. With enhancements of some aspects of the model, such as a more realistic description of the seat structure and a direct simulation of friction in the D-ring and stalk buckle, this approach should allow a satisfactory simulation of a belted occupant response. The modelling methodology could be also extended easily for simulating the interaction of others human surrogates with a belt system.

ACKNOWLEDGEMENTS

The authors wish to thank J. Uriot, M. Moutreuil, S. Mairesse and F. Bendjellal for their assistance in many aspects of this project.

REFERENCES

1. Bowman, B.M., Bennett, R.O., and Robbins, D.H., "MVMA Two-Dimensional Crash Victim Simulation", Version 4, Final Report UM-HSRI-79-5-1, Hight Traffic Safety Research Institute, June 1979.

2. Fleck, J.T., Butler, F. and Deleys N., "Validation of the Crash Victim Simulator", Final Report DOT-HS-806280, Volume I-IV, August 1982

3. MADYMO Users Manuals, Version 4.3, April 90, TNO Road-Vehicles Research Institute, Delft, the Netherlands

4. Bosio, A.C., "Simulation of Submarining with MADYMO", Proceedings of the Second International MADYMO Users Meeting, 1990.

5. Butler, F.E., Fleck, J.T., "Advanced Restraint System Modeling", Air Force Report AFAMRL-TR-80-14, May, 1980.

6. Deng, Y.C., "Developement of a Submarining Model in the CAL3D Program", SAE Paper No. 922530, 36th Stapp Car Crash Conference, 1992.

7. Fraterman, E. and Lupker, H.A., "Evaluation of Belt Modelling Techniques", SAE Paper No. 930635, SAE International Congress & Exposition, Detroit, Michigan, 1993.

8. Sturt, R., Walker, B.D, MILES, J.C. and Giles, A. "Modelling the Occupant in a Vehicle Context-an Intergrated Approch", 13th International Conference on Experimental Safety Vehicles, 1991.

9. Midoun, D.E., Rao, M.K., and Kalidindi, B., "Dummy Models for Crash Simulation in Finite Element Programs", SAE Paper No. 912912, 35th Stapp Car Crash Conference, 1991.

10. RADIOSS Users Manuals, Version 2.1, July 1992, MECALOG, les Ulis, France

11. Faster, J.K., Kortge J.O., and Wolanin M.J., "Hybrid III - A Biomechanically-Based Crash Test Dummy", SAE Paper No. 770938, 21th Stapp Car Crash Conference, 1977.

12. Yang, K.H., Pan, H., Lasry, D. and Hoffmann, R., "Mathematical Modelling of the Hybid III Dummy Chest with Chest Foam", SAE Paper No. 912892, 35th Stapp Car Crash Conference, 1991.

13. Cesari, D., and Bouquet, R; "Behaviour of Human Surrogates Thorax under Belt Loading", SAE Paper No. 902310, 34th Stapp Car Crash Conference, 1990.

14. Wismans, J., and Hermans, J.H.H, "MADYMO 3D Simulation of HYBRID III Dummy Sled Tests", SAE Paper No. 880645, SAE International Congress & Exposition, Detroit, Michigan, 1988.

15. Kaleps, I., and Whitestone J., "HYBRID III Geometrical and Inertial Properties", SAE Paper No. 880638, SAE International Congress & Exposition, Detroit, Michigan, 1988.

942207

Finite Element Modeling of Gross Motion of Human Cadavers in Side Impact

Yue Huang, Albert I. King, and John M. Cavanaugh
Wayne State University

ABSTRACT

Seventeen Heidelberg type cadaveric side impact sled tests, two sled-to-sled tests, and forty-four pendulum tests have been conducted at Wayne State University, to determine human responses and tolerances in lateral collisions. This paper describes the development of a simplified finite element model of a human occupant in a side impact configuration to simulate those cadaveric experiments. The twelve ribs were modeled by shell elements. The visceral contents were modeled as an elastic solid accompanied by an array of discrete dampers. Bone condition factors were obtained after autopsy to provide material properties for the model. The major parameters used for comparison are contact forces at the level of shoulder, thorax, abdomen and pelvis, lateral accelerations of ribs 4 and 8 and of T12, thoracic compression and injury functions V*C, TTI and ASA. A total of four runs to simulate Heidelberg type sled tests, eight runs to simulate pendulum tests and two runs to simulate sled-to-sled tests were performed. Chest band data from the latest sled-to-sled tests were compared with the calculated deformable chest contours. It is found that there is a fair agreement between model results and experimental data. The model can be used to estimate the current chest injury parameters of an elderly occupant involved in a side impact. However, an accurate anatomical representation of the head, neck, shoulder and pelvis was not attempted, and the calculated stresses and strains have not been compared with human data.

INTRODUCTION

The National Highway Traffic Safety Administration (NHTSA) requires that all passenger cars sold in the U.S., after 1996, should pass a side impact test specified by the new Federal Motor Vehicle Standard (FMVSS) 214. In this test, the side impact dummy or SID in a normal sitting position is impacted by a moving barrier with a crabbed angle of 27 degrees. The injury is evaluated by the Thoracic Trauma Index (TTI) developed by Eppinger et al (1984) and Morgan et al (1986). Per FMVSS 214, the TTI limit is 85 g for four-door cars and 90 g for two-door cars. Cavanaugh et al (1993) studied a total of sixty-one cadaveric side impact sled tests from the combined database of NHTSA and Wayne State University (WSU). They developed an injury criterion called Average Spine Acceleration (ASA), which is obtained by integrating the T12-Y spinal acceleration to obtain spinal velocity, and by taking the slope of the spinal velocity pulse between a specified range of minimum and maximum spinal velocity. ASA was found to be as effective as TTI in predicting cadaveric injuries of AIS 4 or greater, even though ASA uses only one data channel. In the SID dummy, ASA worked much better than TTI in predicting the benefits of soft padding over stiff padding. Currently, there are four possible injury parameters to predict chest injuries, including two acceleration-based injury criteria, TTI and ASA, and two deflection-based injury criteria, C (compression) and V*C (Viscous Criterion) developed by Viano and Lau (1985) and Lau and Viano (1986).

Huang et al (1994) developed a side impact MADYMO human model to predict injury parameters TTI, C and V*C. The model was validated against 17 cadaveric sled tests and 44 pendulum tests. A total of 10 parameters for each run was used for validation. The average difference between model output and average experimental results was 12 %. ASA was not included in that paper since ASA had not been developed at that time. Recently, the model was modified to compute ASA. Model results and experimental data were in satisfactory agreement. The MADYMO model was used to study the effect of air space, padding, reduction in door velocity and of shoulder engagement as a sequel to a preliminary model by King el al (1991). However, the MADYMO model suffers from a basic limitation in that it is based on rigid body dynamics. In order to specify a meaningful interaction between the occupant and door trim, the MADYMO model requires a combined stiffness of both parts involved in the interaction. It will be costly to obtain this contact stiffness if experiments are required. Therefore, a more detailed model is needed to study those issues in detail.

Finite element analysis has been used to study human response. Plank and Eppinger (1989) generated a finite element model of the thorax in a frontal impact configuration, and ran it utilizing a finite element code called DYNA3D. It was shown that this simplified model could predict thoracic force-deflection characteristics with reasonable accuracy.

Under the sponsorship of the Centers for Disease Control (CDC) and Wayne State University, finite element modeling of human occupants in side impact was initiated in 1992. This paper presents the development of a simplified finite element model of a human occupant interacting with the side structure of a vehicle, to predict the current chest injury parameters - C, VC, TTI and ASA.

THE EXPERIMENTAL DATA BASE

The experimental data base used for side impact modeling has been reported by Huang et al (1994) in their MADYMO paper. For the sake of completeness, the same data base is provided in this paper.

Sled Impacts

A total of 17 cadaveric side impact tests have been conducted so far. The data from these tests constitute the experimental base for the validation of the model. A brief description of the test set-up and an up-dated summary of the test results is provided in this paper, while details of these tests can be found in Cavanaugh et al (1993) and Zhu et al (1993).

All of 17 the side impact tests were conducted on the Wayne Horizontal Accelerator Mechanism III (WHAM III) which is a pneumatically powered deceleration sled. The deceleration distance was set to a very low value (about 200 mm) to ensure that the sled was completely stopped before the side impact occurred. The test subject was placed in a seated position, at one end of a 1.2-m long bench seat, the long-axis of which was parallel to the direction of motion of the sled. At the other end of the bench seat, an instrumented barrier was erected to stop the test subject and to measure the forces of impact at the level of the shoulder, thorax, abdomen, pelvis and knee. The cadaver impacted this barrier at approximately 0.45 m/s less than the pre-impact speed of the sled, based on film analysis data. To minimize the loss of speed of the cadaver, the surface of the bench seat was made of Teflon™ and the cadaver sat on a piece of plastic sheet so that friction was minimized. Although the basic set-up was very similar to that described by Marcus et al (1983), it should be noted that separate forces were measured at each of the four levels of the torso for the first time, in side impact cadaveric tests. These are, therefore, the most desirable data that can be used to validate a model which seeks to simulate the response of the four regions of the torso individually. The deformation of the thorax was measured optically using photo targets and high speed cinematography.

In addition to the 9 load cells on the barrier, there was additional instrumentation on the cadaver; namely, head, chest and spinal accelerometers and photo targets on the shoulder and thorax to measure regional deformation, for both padded and unpadded impact with the barrier. Strategically placed high speed cameras were used to record the impact and to provide optical data for analysis.

Summary of Sled Test Data

A summary of the experimental data from the 17 sled tests done so far can be found in Table 1. The first eight tests were impacts against a rigid wall and three of those were done with a 150 mm rigid pelvic offset. That is, the pelvis was stopped 150 mm before the rest of the torso by an offset rigid barrier. The remaining nine tests were padded impacts in which the principal padding used was a cardboard or paper honeycomb material, identified in the table as PH. The crush strength of the honeycomb was given in terms of its pressure rating in pounds per square inch (psi). For a nominal strength of 15 psi, its actual strength after precrush is 8-11 psi (55-76 kPa). There was also a change in the arm position in Tests 14 through 17 in which the arm was raised so that the thorax was completely exposed to the padded wall. Partial interaction of the arm occurred in Tests 1 through 13 since the arm was flexed anteriorly about 15 deg relative to the mid-axillary line. Table 1 also provides relevant data on the cadavers, the scaling factors to be used to scale the force and acceleration data and the maximum value on the Abbreviated Injury Scale (AIS) seen in the neck (NE), shoulder (SH), thorax (TH), abdomen (AB) and pelvis (PE). The AIS range of 0 to 6 indicates gradations of injury from none to maximum (currently untreatable).

It can be seen from the injury data that, for the thorax, the AIS was between 4 and 5 for rigid wall impacts. When 15-psi paper honeycomb was used AIS was reduced to 0 to 2 in four cadavers, with two older cadavers sustaining an AIS of 4 in Tests 13 and 14. It should also be noted that the 15 psi paper honeycomb used in Test 14 was a single piece from the shoulder to the abdomen. In the other tests, the padding was cut up into rectangular pieces 100 mm high and approximately 400 mm long. The thickness of the padding ranged from 75 to 150 mm.

Pendulum Impacts

Viano et al (1989) performed a series of 44 lateral pendulum impacts to the thorax, abdomen and pelvis of 14 unembalmed cadavers at nominal velocities of 4.5, 6.7 and 9.4 m/s. The pendulum had a mass of 23.4 kg and a diameter of 150 mm. Impacts to the thorax and abdomen were carried out at an angle of 30 degrees to the transverse

Table 1 WSU/CDC Cadaveric Sled Tests: Test Conditions and Injury Summary

RUN NO.	RUN DATE	PELVIC OFFSET (IN.)	PAD WALL PAD	PAD THICK. (IN.)	SLED VEL. (M/S)	CAD. NO.	MASS (KG)	HT. (M)	AGE	SEX	LAMDA	NE	SH	TH	AB	PE
SIC01	1-20-89	6	NO	0	8.9	UM6	70.5	1.76	61	M	1.021	0	2	5	2	2
SIC02	1-30-89	6	NO	0	9.1	187	49.5	1.63	64	F	1.148	3	2	5	2	3
SIC03	2-03-89	6	NO	0	10.5	188	70.0	1.75	37	M	1.023	0	0	5	0	2
SIC04	4-03-89	0	NO	0	9.1	215	57.6	1.63	69	M	1.092	3	2	4	2	2
SIC05	4-10-89	0	NO	0	6.7	216	44.0	1.72	67	M	1.194	0	0	4	0	0
SIC06	4-27-89	0	NO	0	9.0	217	61.2	1.82	60	M	1.070	0	2	4	0	2
SIC07	5-16-89	0	NO	0	6.7	206	74.8	1.70	66	M	1.001	0	2	4	0	0
SIC08	8-10-89	0	NO	0	6.6	UM12	73.9	1.62	64	F	1.005	3	2	5	3	0
SIC09	0-26-89	0	ARSAN	3	9.2	280	54.9	1.65	61	F	1.110	3	2	5	0	3
SIC10	1-17-90	0	15 PH*	6	8.7	317	62.1	1.71	60	M	1.065	0	0	2	0	0
SIC11	2-22-90	0	15,23 PH*	4	8.9	330	55.3	1.65	54	F	1.107	0	0	2	0	0
SIC12	3-01-90	0	23,31 PH*	4	8.9	335	54.4	1.43	68	F	1.113	0	0	5	0	0
SIC13	4-12-90	0	15,23 PH*	4	8.3	338	66.7	1.61	62	M	1.040	0	0	4	0	0
SIC14	7-17-90	0	15,23 PH*	4	9.4	360	55.3	1.74	72	M	1.107	3	2	4	2	0
SIC15	8-09-90	0	15,23 PH*	4	8.9	386	68.9	1.54	43	F	1.028	0	2	0	0	0
SIC16	2-21-91	0	16,23 PH*	3	8.9	462	56.7	1.70	58	F	1.098	0	2	4	4	2
SIC17	6-11-91	0	15,23 PH*	6	8.9	503	93.0	1.80	65	M	0.931	0	2	2	0	0

* SIDEWALL PAD: PH SIGNIFIES PAPER HONEYCOMB,
 15, 16, 23, 31 ARE MANUFACTURER'S RATED COMPRESSIVE STRENGTHS IN PSI.

NE = NECK, SH = SHOULDER, TH = THORAX, AB = ABDOMEN, PE = PELVIS

SIC 09: PADDING 3" THICK 0.9 PCF CLOSED CELL FOAM ENTIRE HEIGHT OF SIDEWALL.

SIC 10: 6" THICK 15 PSI PADDING USED ENTIRE HEIGHT OF SIDEWALL.

SIC 11: 4" THICK 15 PSI PADDING USED AT THORAX & ABDOMEN BEAMS, 23 PSI AT SHOULDER & PELVIC BEAMS.

SIC 12: 4" THICK 23 PSI PADDING USED AT THORAX & ABDOMEN BEAMS, 31 PSI AT SHOULDER & PELVIC BEAMS.

SIC 13: 4" THICK 15 PSI PADDING USED AT THORAX & ABDOMEN BEAMS, 23 PSI AT SHOULDER & PELVIC BEAMS.

SIC 14: ONE PIECE OF 4" THICK 15 PSI PADDING USED AT SHOULDER, THORAX, ABDOMEN BEAMS; 23 PSI AT PELVIC BEAM.

SIC 15: 4" THICK 15 PSI PADDING USED AT THORAX & ABDOMEN BEAMS, 23 PSI AT SHOULDER & PELVIC BEAMS.

SIC 16: 3" THICK 16 PSI VERTICEL USED AT THORAX & ABDOMEN BEAMS, 23 PSI HONEYCOMB AT SHOULDER & PELVIC BEAMS.

SIC 17: 6" THICK 15 PSI PADDING USED AT THORAX & ABDOMEN BEAMS, 23 PSI AT SHOULDER & PELVIC BEAMS.

SIC01-13: ARMS DOWN (ANGLE APPROXIMATELY 15 DEGREES ANTERIOR TO MID-AXILLARY LINE).

SIC14-17: ARMS UP TO EXPOSE LEFT SIDE OF THORAX TO DIRECT IMPACT.

(side-to-side) axis of the torso, directed at the center of gravity of the torso and approaching it from an anterolateral direction. Such impacts resulted in an absence of ribcage rotation and a pure compression of the torso. The impact force was measured by means of an accelerometer on the pendulum and chest deflection was obtained by an analysis of high speed film data. Response data in the form of force-deflection curves were obtained for each body region at each of the three velocities and a Logist analysis was performed to determine the tolerance limits of these body regions in terms of the injury functions V*C and C. The criteria for a 50% probability of an AIS 4 thoracic injury were found to be 1.65 m/s and 39.8 % respectively for V*C and C. The Thoracic Trauma Index (TTI) was not measured. Torso compression was computed based on the full undeformed body width. However, this does not mean that it is half as large as the C computed using the half torso width because the non-impacted side is also deformed during impact. In one of our latest tests using the EPIDM chest band developed by Eppinger (1989), the non-impacted side deflection was about 35% of the total chest deflection.

THE FINITE ELEMENT MODEL

General Requirements of the Model

When this project was initiated, some requirements were set forth for the development of the model:

1. The model should predict the current injury

parameters for the chest in side impact, including C, VC, TTI and ASA. The model should also provide chest deformation contours which cannot be obtained from the MADYMO model. However, this first generation side impact FEM model at WSU was not required: (a) to predict head, neck, shoulder and pelvic responses and (b) to generate new injury criteria based on stresses or strains since relevant experimental data were not available.

2. The model can be used to interact with automotive side structures. It is not sufficient to model the chest only, since the whole torso is struck by the door in a car-to-car side impact, and the shoulder and pelvis provide additional load paths as shown by King et al (1991), Huang et al (1994) and Deng (1988).

3. Assessment of the model will be based on a comparison of injury functions C, V*C and TTI with experimental data. However, the difference of the force and acceleration responses between model results and experimental data are also estimated for both sled and pendulum tests.

4. Computing time should be reasonable when the model is run with a commercial finite element code.

Geometry

The geometry of the human body is very complex, varies from person to person and is affected by posture. However, a single geometrical shape had to be selected for the model. Since most of the cadaveric data were scaled to those of a 50th percentile male with a body weight of 75 kg, it is reasonable to select the 50th percentile male at this initial stage of the study. The geometry of the rib cage was based on drawings provided by the Transportation Research Institute of the University of Michigan (1983). These drawings provided the coordinates of key anatomical landmarks. The half chest width (including skin) was chosen to be 175 mm, which is slightly smaller than that measured from the drawings. It should be mentioned that the drawings were not designed for quantitative measurements. The contour of the head, neck, shoulder, pelvis and limbs were also estimated based upon the drawings, but greatly simplified.

Rib Cage

The twelve ribs and the sternum were modeled with shell elements (Figure 1a). Since the thickness of a shell element does not affect the size of the integration time step, a larger time step than that of a corresponding brick element was used to reduce computing time. Twenty elements were used to model a single rib, and the minimum length of the elements was 7.4 mm. The time step of the model was controlled by the smallest rib element and was 0.003 ms.

The vertebral column serves as a support for the rib cage and undergoes much less strain than the ribs and internal organs. Thus, it has an insignificant effect on thoracic deformation. Therefore, each vertebra and intervertebral disc were modeled with only eight elements, as shown in Figure 1b. Nevertheless, connectivity among the ribs, spinal column and the viscera were maintained to provide a stable numerical solution.

Visceral Contents

Visceral contents have a viscous response, which should be included in the model. Again, a detailed description of each organ, such as the heart and kidney, will create too many elements, if connectivity among organs, the rib cage and spinal column are required. Visceral injuries were not modeled because in our cadaveric side impact tests, most of the observed injuries were rib fractures (Cavanaugh et al 1993). They were represented by 8-node elements composed of a soft viscous isotropic and homogeneous material and were made to fill the rib cage, accompanied by an array of discrete dampers, as shown in Figure 1c. It should be noted that the calculated stresses and strains of the visceral contents are not be taken literally because specific organs were not identified in the model. Although PAM-CRASH can simulate a viscoelastic material with shear relaxation behavior, it cannot be used in this model because its shear modulus is a function of simulation time and not nodal velocity. In order to model both the elastic and viscous response of the visceral contents, they were modeled as elastic solid elements accompanied by damping (dashpot) elements which were strategically placed within the rib cage and shown as lines between nodes in Figure 1d, which is a typical cross-section of the rib cage. The same arrangement of dampers was used at each level from T1 to T12. Dashpot elements were not placed between the nodes of the visceral contents, because either a huge number of damping elements was required or numerical difficulties would be encountered when an extremely soft material was subjected to a concentrated load. The current damping matrix did not optimally simulate the viscous effect. Ideally, an non-linear material model, with a high Poisson's ratio and a damping matrix between its nodes, should be developed to simulate the internal viscera.

Muscles and Ligaments

The muscles and ligaments between ribs were simply modeled by a single layer of membrane elements. The integumentary system (skin) and part of the outer muscles were modeled as solid elements with a stiffening property which allowed the skin to contact vehicular surfaces without bottoming out. A foam model (Type 21 in PAM-CRASH) was used to model the skin.

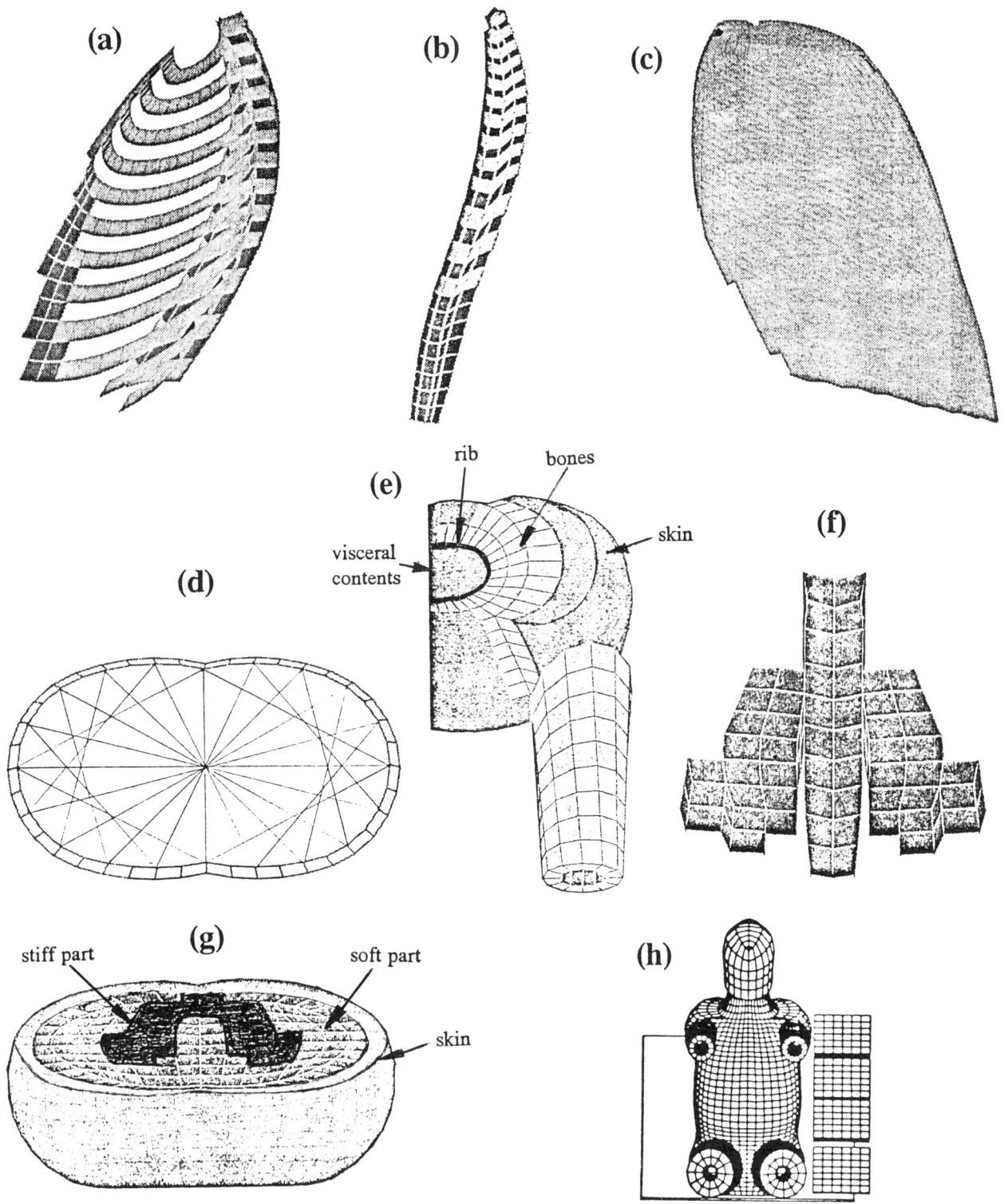

Figure 1. The finite element model. (a) Rib cage. (b) Spinal column. (c) Visceral contents. (d) Damping matrix. (e) Shoulder and arm. (f) Lumbar spine and pelvic ring. (g) Pelvis. (h) A frontal view of the whole model.

Shoulder and Upper Arm

Modeling of the shoulder and pelvis was also important to obtain the appropriate inertial properties. Without these parts, TTI (Thoracic Trauma Index) could not be obtained, and C (compression) and V*C could not be correctly estimated since interaction of the shoulder and pelvis with the side door is a key factor for the thoracic injury parameters as mentioned above in Requirement No. 2. The shoulder consists of the clavicle, scapula and several muscles. In the interest of a simple model, the shoulder complex was represented by a group of isotropic elastic elements. Part of the upper arm was also included in the "shoulder", otherwise, too much force would be transmitted through the shoulder joint. A transverse section of the shoulder model is shown in Figure 1e. It includes skin, bones and within the shoulder, ribs and visceral contents. Anatomically, it is not a replica of the human shoulder. The foam model (Type 21 in PAM-CRASH) was used to simulate the skin and bones by a judicious choice of material properties, to enable the shoulder to withstand a 10-m/s impact without numerical difficulties such as negative volumes.

Several other meshes for the shoulder were also tested, but the results were not good. An hourglass mode or an unstable total energy state was encountered. These tested meshes included: (a) a beam between the shoulder joint and sternum to represent the clavicle; (b) a separate model of the scapula and muscles which was coupled to the original rib cage by a contact surface and (c) a shoulder model which was connected to the rib cage by nodal connectivity (partly) and a contact surface. The shoulder mesh used in the current model was not totally satisfactory, although it yielded the best result among the meshes considered. A finer mesh for the shoulder can solve these problems if increased model size and decreased time steps are acceptable.

The skin and muscles of the arm were modeled by a layer of solid elements, and the long bone was simulated by shell elements which were assumed to be rigid (Figure 1e). The shoulder joint was defined as a spherical joint, and a contact surface was used between the arm and torso, to prevent the arm from penetrating the torso.

Pelvis and Thigh

A transverse section of the pelvis is shown in Figure 1g. The model was simplified and represented by a stiff part to represent the lumbar spine and pelvic ring (Figure 1f), and a soft part to represent muscles.

The mass of both lower extremities comprises 20 % of the total body weight. Neglecting this part greatly affected the distribution of the inertial properties, and thus a coarse mesh for the thighs was necessary. The thigh was treated the same as the arm. The skin and muscles were represented by two layers of soft solid elements, and the long bone was represented by rigid shell elements. A spherical joint was specified between the thigh and the pelvis to simulate the hip joint. A contact surface was specified between the thigh and pelvis.

Head and Neck

The head and neck responses were not considered in the current model. However, in order to preserve a proper global motion, the neck and head were also modeled using a coarse mesh. The head was modeled as shell elements and defined as a rigid body. The cervical spine was not modeled. The neck was modeled as solid elements and had nodal connectivity with the shoulder. The head and neck were connected by a rigid link.

Whole Model

The whole model is shown in Figure 1h. The barrier, including shoulder, thoracic, abdominal and pelvic beams, was modeled as solid elements. This configuration was similar to that used in the WSU sled test, as described in the Test Setup and Procedures. These four beams were specified either as rigid bodies to simulate a rigid wall impact, or as deformable elements to simulate a padded wall impact. For the Heidelberg type test, the contact wall was fixed and the subject had a lateral initial velocity. For the sled-to-sled test, the contact wall was given a velocity pulse, for it moved towards and impacted an initially stationary subject.

The overall model contained 9308 eight-node solid elements (including padding), 2384 four-node shell and membrane elements and 514 two-node dashpot elements.

Material Properties

Material properties are important in determining the appropriate response of the human model. The bone condition factor (BCF) of ribs 6 and 7 was measured, using a bending test method, for each of the 17 cadavers used by Cavanaugh et al (1993) after an autopsy was performed. The average Young's modulus was found to be 9.0 Gpa, and was used in the current model. This value is smaller than 12.0 Gpa used by Plank and Eppinger (1989). The sternum and vertebrae were assumed to have the same properties as the rib. The compressive and tensile response of intervertebral discs are very different (Yamada, 1970), and the estimated Young's modulus ranges from 3.82 MPa (tension) to 24.5 Mpa (compression). The value assumed by Plank and Eppinger (1989) for Young's modulus of the intervertebral discs was 10.3 MPa. This value was incorporated in the current model. The stress - strain curve of muscle is highly non-linear (Yamada, 1970), and the average Young's modulus of the muscle was found to be 0.02 Gpa for the initial 20 % of elongation. The visceral contents in the current model were not representative of any specific organ, and their stiffness was adjusted to provide the best thoracic

Table 2 Material Properties for the FEM Human Model

Name	E GPa	v	Density kg/m^3
Ribs, sternum, vertebrae	9.000E+00 (Test data)	0.30 (Viano, 1986) (Plank, 1989)	4790 (Nahum, 1985) (Plank, 1989)
Costal cartilage	3.000E+00	0.42 (Viano, 1986)	2768 (Plank, 1989)
Intervertebral disc	1.030E-02 (Plank, 1989)	0.20 (Plank, 1989)	2768 (Plank, 1989)
Visceral contents	8.420E-06	0.47	1000
muscle	2.000E-02 (Yamada, 1970)	0.30	1000
Pelvis stiff part	7.100E-03	0.30	1200
Pelvis soft part	4.740E-04	0.30	1000
Dashpot	damping coefficient: 10 Ns/m		
Skin	stiffness: 30 kpa @ 40 % compression		
Shoulder bones	stiffness: 120 kpa @ 40 % compression		

compression. The damping coefficient of the dashpot elements was chosen to be 10 Ns/m. This damping coefficient did not provide adequate damping to the visceral contents as can be seen from the thoracic contact force results. However, if this coefficient was made too large, the calculated force - deflection curve would become unrealistic for a pendulum impact to the thorax. Yamada (1970) found that the average Young's modulus of the costal cartilage was 26 MPa, for the initial 10 % of elongation. However, if this value was input to the model, the model did not provide a chest contour similar to the chest band data. A much larger value (3 Gpa) for the costal cartilages was used in the current model. The thickness of costal cartilage was assumed to be 3.5 mm, which can be less than that of the real one. The material properties of the pelvic elements were fitted to provide an overall response similar to that from the cadaveric sled and pendulum tests.

In the selection of parametric values, major consideration was given to the thorax by providing the closest possible match between model results and experimental data related to thoracic compression and deformable chest contours. For the abdomen, not too many options were available because the properties of visceral contents were fixed when matching the thoracic response. For the pelvis, the aim was to obtain a balanced response between the sled and pendulum tests. The difficulty encountered in simulating the shoulder is further explained in the Section on Model - Experimental Comparisons. The properties of the major materials used in the model are listed in Table 2. The references are in parentheses.

Padding

The padding was modeled with a foam material available in PAM-CRASH called Urethane Foam (Type 21) or Crushable Foam (Type 2). A stiffening effect could be specified. A series of 54 dynamic impacts to the padding was conducted to determine padding properties, a part of which has been reported by Cavanaugh et al (1992). The dynamic tests were performed at 4.5-5.0 m/s with a pneumatically driven linear impactor of 16.3 kg mass and a 0.15 m (6 inch) diameter impact face. A 25 mm thick piece of Ensolite was attached to the face of the impactor to reduce spikes at initial contact. Deflection was measured with a linear potentiometer centered in the pad and attached to a 152 mm x 152 mm (6 by 6 inch) thin aluminum plate at the front of the pad. Contact force was measured by means of a load cell mounted on the impactor. The inertial effect of the mass in front of the load cell was mass-corrected to yield the true contact force which is equal to the measured contact force minus the product of the mass and impactor acceleration.

Analysis

The finite element model was run on PAM-CRASH, an explicit finite element code provided by the ESI of the France. It took about eight hours to complete one model run on a SPARC 10 SUN station. Figure 2 shows the total

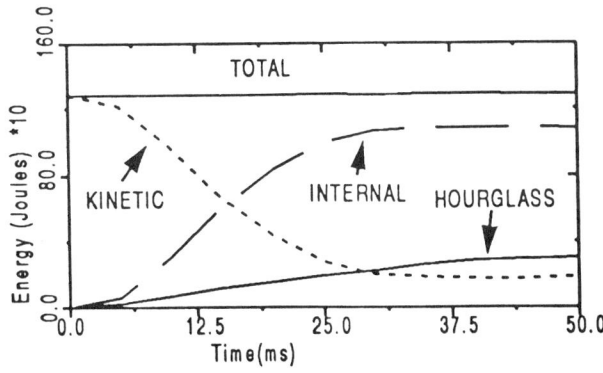

Figure 2. The calculated total, internal, kinetic and hourglass energies.

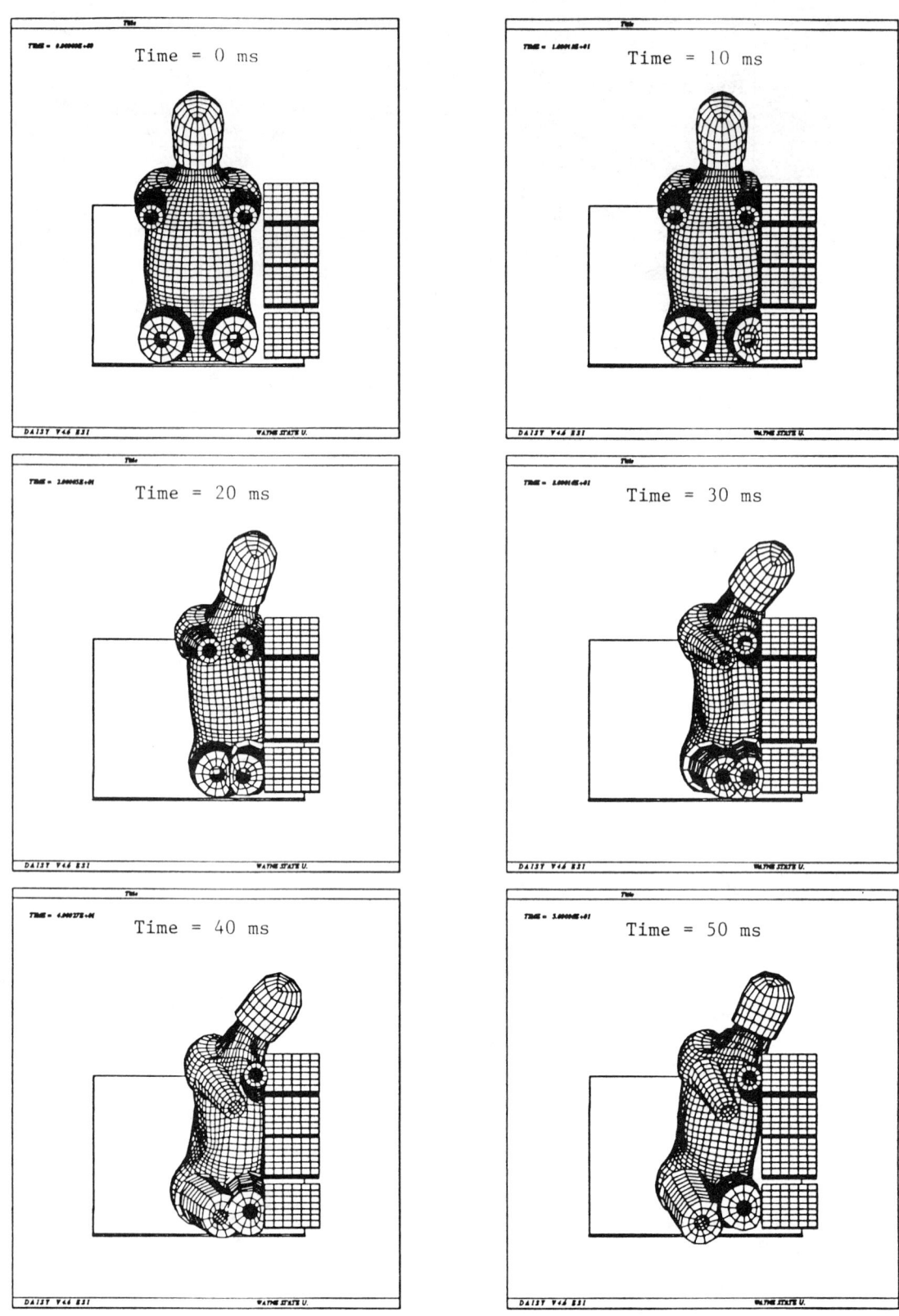

Figure 3. The kinematics of a rigid wall impact at 8.6 m/s.

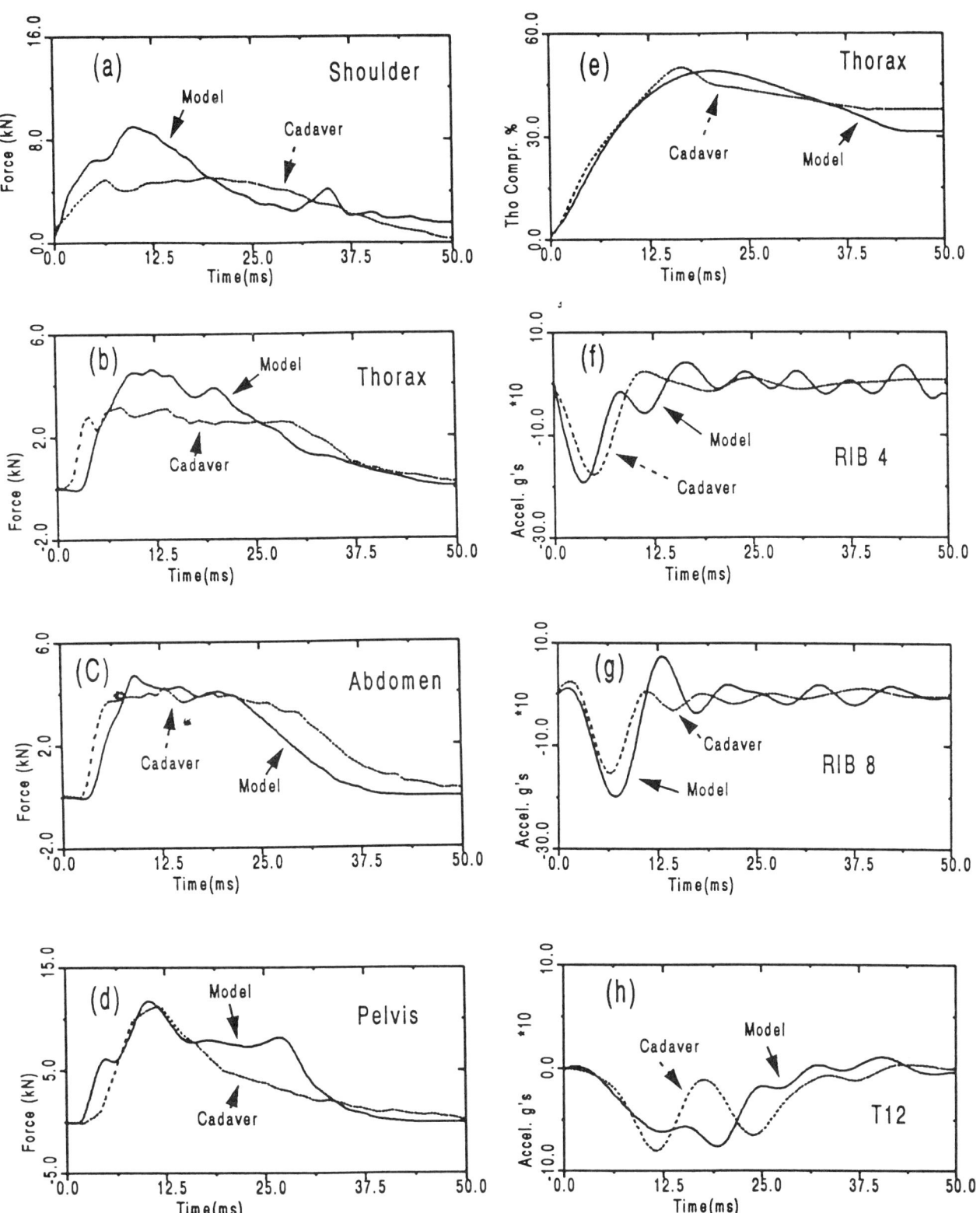

Figure 4. Comparison of model and experimental time histories for a rigid wall impact at 8.6 m/s.
(a) Shoulder force. (b) Thorax force. (c) Abdomen force. (d) Pelvis force. (e) Rib 4 acceleration.
(f) Rib 8 acceleration. (g) T12-Y acceleration.

energy, internal energy, kinetic energy and hourglass energy, for a rigid wall sled impact with an initial velocity of 6.2 m/s. As can be seen in the figure, the total energy was stable.

MODEL - EXPERIMENTAL COMPARISONS

The principal parameters used for comparison were the four contact forces, thoracic compression (C), lateral accelerations of Ribs 4 and 8 and of T12, and the three injury parameters - V*C, TTI and ASA. It should be noted that C and V*C were based on the impacted-side half torso width in the sled tests since full chest compression was not available experimentally, but in the pendulum tests, the half chest compression was not available and the full chest compression was used for comparison.

Rigid Wall Sled Impacts

To avoid confusion, simulations using the finite element model will be denoted as Model as opposed to cadaveric experiments which are referred to as Side Impact Cadaveric (SIC) Tests. The "SIC" designation was used in previous publications and refers to the same series of tests. Two model runs were made to simulate rigid wall impacts at nominal sled velocities of 6.7 m/s and 9 m/s without pelvic offset (Runs 1 and 2 respectively). The rigid wall impact with a 150-mm pelvic offset was not included due to a numerical difficulty (negative volume). It should be noted that in these comparison runs, the velocity of the test subject was assumed to be 0.45 m/s less than the average sled velocity for each test condition. The kinematics for Run 2 are shown in Figure 3, which is similar to that of the cadaver test observed from the high speed film except for the shoulder. Model and experimental time histories for this run are compared in Figure 4. It is seen that there is a reasonably good fit for the contact forces of thorax, abdomen and pelvis, the lateral accelerations of Ribs 4 and 8 and of T12, and thoracic compression. As for the injury parameters which were summarized in Table 3, there is also a relatively good fit. The shoulder did not behave very well, and the model predicted a higher contact force from 3 ms to 20 ms. If the stiffness of shoulder elements was reduced, the shoulder contact force would decrease and the shoulder compression would be too large. The major problem is that the shoulder was simply compressed and there was no inward rotation as observed in the experiment. When using a beam to represent the clavicle, the shoulder rotated but the calculated total energy was not stable. This may be due to the coarse mesh for the shoulder. Similar results for Run 1 were obtained and their peak values are compared in Table 3. The average errors refer to differences in peak values between model predictions and experimental results of all parameters in the table. Some may appear to be rather large but if the overall time-history is examined, the fit is reasonable.

Padded Wall Sled impacts

The same comparisons are made for Run 3, a padded run made at 8.3 m/s (cadaveric velocity), with averaged data from SIC 11, 13, 15 and 17. The other two tests (Tests 10 and 14) in which the 15-psi pad was used for the thorax and abdomen were not included in the validation because the 23-psi pad was not used for the shoulder and pelvis. The pad had a rated initial crush strength of 159 kPa (23 psi) for the shoulder and pelvis and 103 kPa (15 psi) for the thorax and abdomen. In order to chose an appropriate material model and parameters for the padding, a separated finite element model of the padding was developed to simulate the linear impactor tests referred to the last section. The force-deflection curves of a 15-psi pad are compared in Figure 5. Although the model result does not follow test data precisely, the model is still acceptable considering the difficulty of modeling a very soft paper honeycomb. In actual tests, the honeycomb had an initial force spike and a loss in strength as it crushes, while the model does not. The comparison of force-deflection curves for ARSAN padding is shown in Figure 6.

The kinematics of the whole model is shown in Figure 7. The time histories for the contact forces, lateral

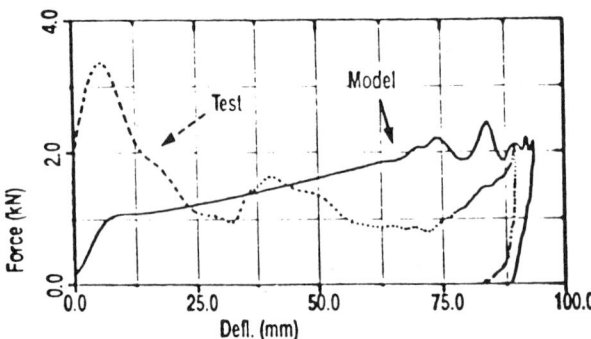

Figure 5. Comparison of model and experimental force-deflection curves of the 15-psi paper honeycomb for a linear impactor test at 4.7 m/s.

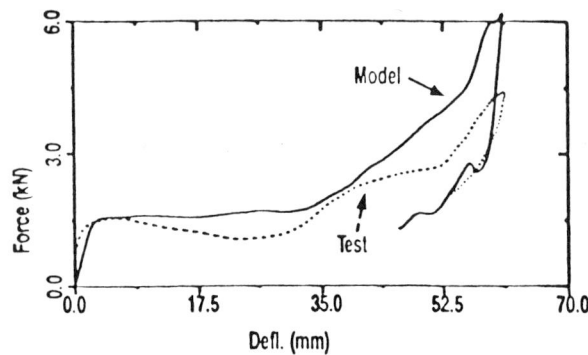

Figure 6. Comparison of model and experimental force-deflection curves of ARSAN 601 for a linear impactor test at 4.7 m/s.

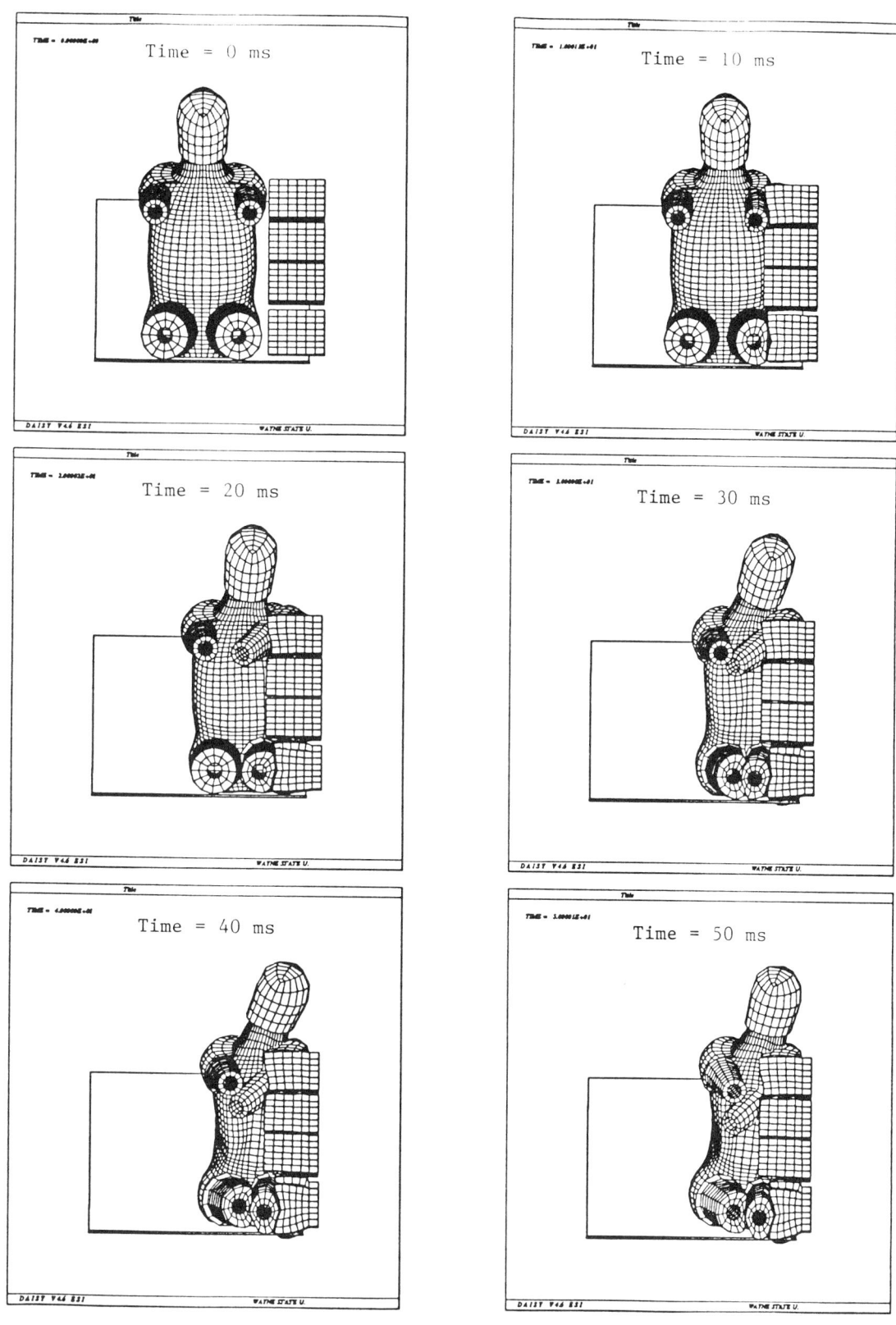

Figure 7. The kinematics of a padded wall impact at 8.3 m/s, using 15/23 psi paper honeycomb.

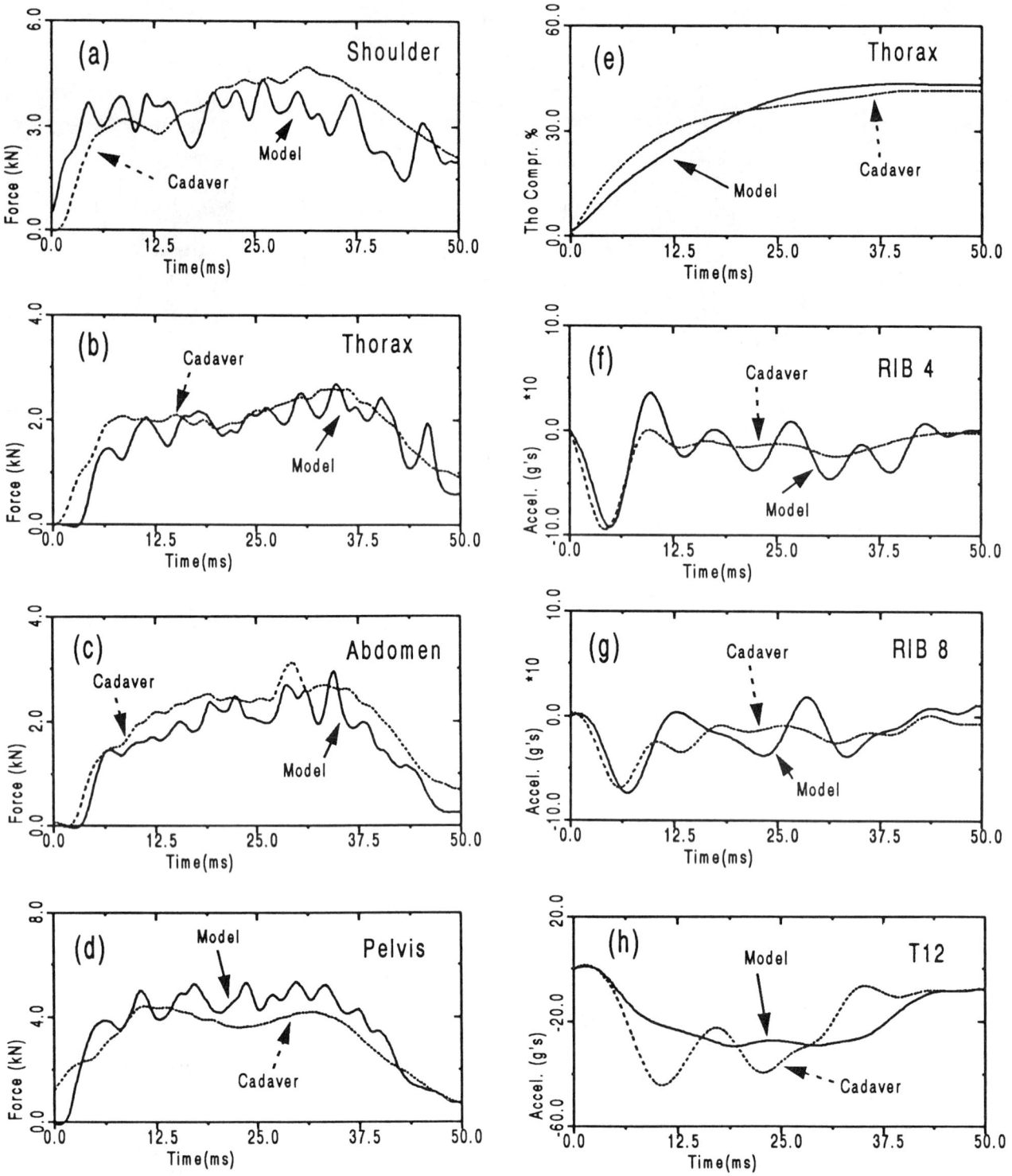

Figure 8. Comparison of model and experimental time histories for a padded wall impact at 8.3 m/s, using 15/23 psi paper honeycomb. (a) Shoulder force. (b) Thorax force. (c) Abdomen force. (d) Pelvis force. (e) Rib 4 acceleration. (f) Rib 8 acceleration. (g) T12-Y acceleration.

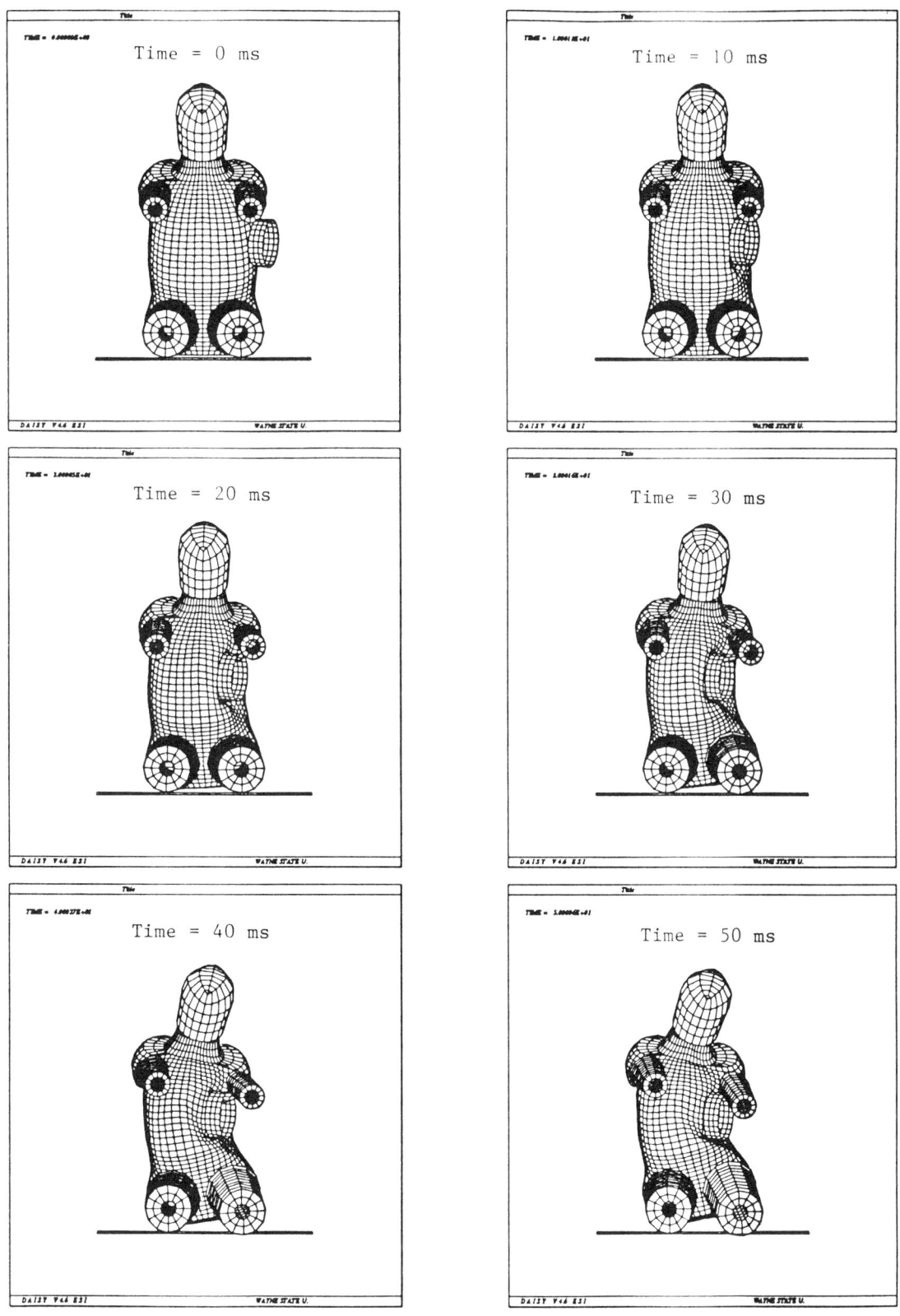

Figure 9. The kinematics of a pendulum impact to the thorax at 6.5 m/s.

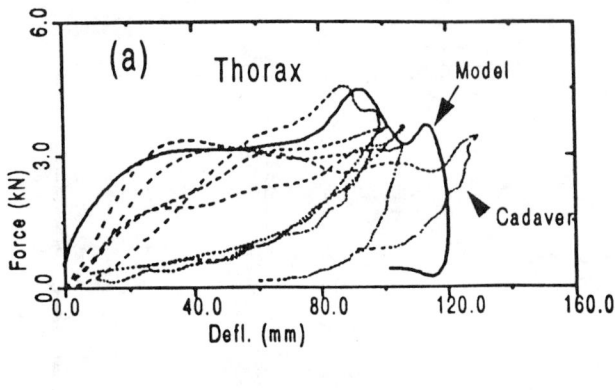
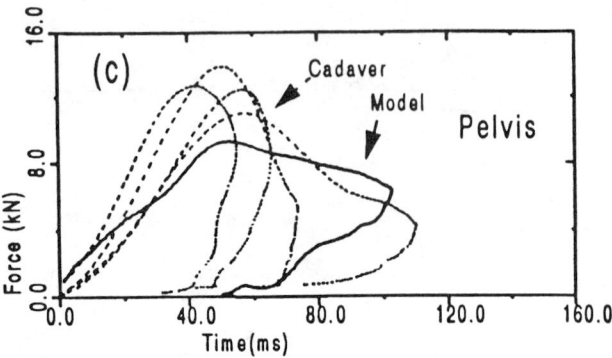
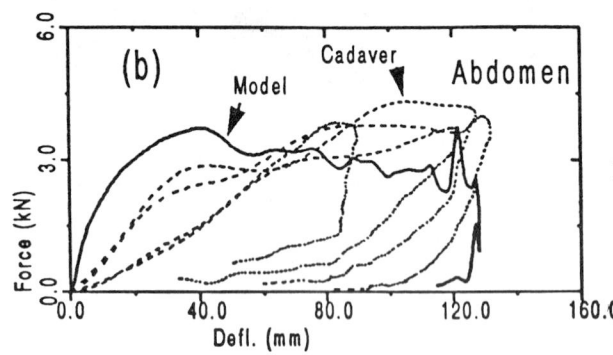

Figure 10. Comparison of model and experimental force-deflection curves for pendulum impacts.
(a) Pendulum impact to the thorax at 6.5 m/s.
(b) Pendulum impact to the abdomen at 6.5 m/s.
(c) Pendulum impact to the pelvis at 9.5 m/s.

accelerations and thoracic compression are shown in Figure 8. Again there is fairly good agreement between the analytical and experimental results. SIC Test 9 used a pad made of ARSAN 601. It was modeled in Run 4. The peak values for Runs 3 and 4 are compared with peak experimental data in Table 3. The values of C and V*C in Table 3 are based on half chest width.

Pendulum Impacts

The comparison against pendulum impacts was carried out by plotting the force-deflection curve predicted by the model on the same graph as those obtained experimentally. The predicted response for the chest, abdomen and pelvis all fell well within the scatter of the experimentally derived curves for all three speeds of impact. The kinematics for a thoracic impact at 6.5 m/s are shown in Figure 9. Figure 10 shows representative curves of thoracic and abdominal response for a 6.5-m/s impact, and pelvic response for a 9.5-m/s impact. The peak values of force, deflection and V*C for all three body regions, for both model and the experimental data are shown in Table 4. The values of C and V*C in Table 4 are based on full chest width.

CHEST CONTOURS

Recently, two additional cadaveric side impact tests, using a sled-to-sled test setup, have been conducted at Wayne State University. This setup involved a bullet sled, a target sled and a simulated door. The bullet sled struck the initially stationary target sled and the simulated door at a velocity of 13 m/s. The door then impacted the cadaver seated on the target sled. The door velocity pulse was

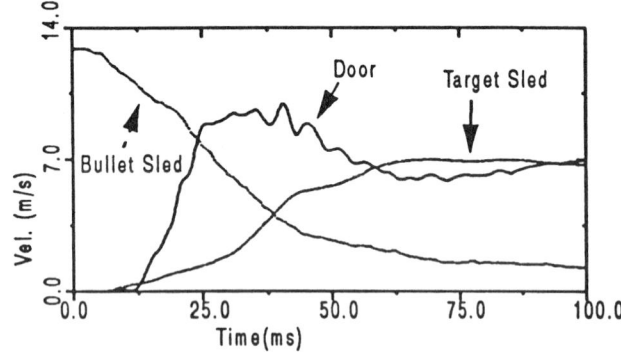

Figure 11. The velocity profiles used in the sled-to-sled cadaveric tests.

programmed to simulate a real car-to-car side impact. The velocity profiles of the door, target sled and bullet sled, used in the cadaver tests, are shown in Figure 11. The first and second velocity peaks of the door are 10 m/s and 7 m/s, respectively. The simulated door has four contact beams instrumented with load cells which are similar to those of the Heidelberg type sled tests referred to previously. The cadavers were instrumented with multiple accelerometers and an EPIDM chest band with 40 strain gages. Unfortunately, 48 data channels for both of the tests, including those of the barrier forces and accelerations of the cadavers, were lost due to the failure of an on-board data acquisition system. However, the chest band data were acquired by another data acquisition system and are available for model and experimental comparisons.

In one cadaver test, there was 102 mm (4 inch)

Table 3 Comparison of the model against sled test data

Model or Cadaver Run No.	Impact Conditions	Shd Force (N)	Thorax Force (N)	Abd Force (N)	Pelvis Force (N)	Thorax C (%)	Thorax V*C (m/s)	TTI* (g's)	ASA (g's)	Avg Error (%)
Model 1	Unpad	6450	2500	2652	7270	40.0	1.0	91	33.8	
SIC5,7,8	6.2 m/s	3051	2194	2748	6450	46.0	1.3	89	24.0	21.9
Model 2	Unpad	9002	4024	4708	11734	49.1	1.7	137	53.4	
SIC4,6	8.6 m/s	5072	3148	4227	11131	53.2	1.6	128	47.9	16.2
Model 3	Padded	4342	2645	2945	5332	43.5	0.7	61	25.3	
SIC11,13,15,17	15,23 PH	4699	2589	3109	4417	40.4	0.9	69	22.8	11.3
Model 4	Padded	6590	4727	4500	7159	64.1	2.3	103	30.5	
SIC9	ARSAN 601	4121	4025	3585	7891	66.1	2.0	92	37.4	18.2

* TTI = { Max(R4, R8) + T12 } / 2

Table 4 Comparison of the model against pendulum impact data

Run No.	Impact Conditions	Impact Vel (m/s)	Model or Cadaver	Forces (N)	Deflection (mm)	V*C (m/s)	Avg. Error (%)
6	Thorax	4.3	Model	3040	95	0.5	
			Cadaver	2240	75	0.6	24.4
7		6.7	Model	4478	120	1.0	
			Cadaver	3660	108	1.1	13.4
8		9.5	Model	6769	134	1.8	
			Cadaver	6670	148	2.1	7.4
9	Abdomen	4.3	Model	2044	98	0.5	
			Cadaver	1990	93	0.8	16.8
10		6.7	Model	3745	128	1.0	
			Cadaver	3940	108	1.3	15.0
11		9.5	Model	6631	144	1.9	
			Cadaver	6910	138	2.2	7.9
12	Pelvis	4.3	Model	3671	60	---	
			Cadaver	5360	44	---	34.0
13		9.5	Model	9319	102	---	
			Cadaver	12440	73	---	30.9

space, but there was no padding, between the rigid door and the test subject. The cadaver was a 66 year-old male and had a body weight of 122 lbs. The autopsy data showed that there were: (1) 11 rib fractures on the impacted side; (2) 3 rib fractures on the non-impacted side; (3) multiple fractures and avulsion in the superior ramus of pubis and (4) separated disc between C4 and C5.

In the other cadaver test, there was a pad of 102-mm thick (23 psi paper honeycomb for the shoulder and pelvis beams, 15 psi for the thorax and abdomen beams), but there was no space between the simulated door and the test subject. The cadaver was a 59 year-old male and had a body weight of 126 lbs. The injuries included: (1) 10 rib fractures on the impacted side; (2) 4 rib fractures on the non-impacted side; (3) fracture and separation on the impacted side clavicle. There was no injury in the neck and pelvis.

The door and the seat (target sled) velocity pulses (Figure 11) were used as input to the computer model. Two model runs were conducted to simulate the sled-to-sled tests. A comparison of the deformed chest shapes is shown in Figure 12 and 13, for both cases. To obtain the modeled chest contour, the closest nodes on outer body surface to the boundary of a mid-sternum section, perpendicular to the spinal column, were projected to the mid-sternum plane as points on the contour, as shown in the figures. These points were simply connected by lines and were not interpolated, which could cause the discontinuity in the contour at the left mid-axillary line. As shown in the figures, the model response was quite human-like, and confirmed that non-impacted side deflected about 35% of the total chest deflection, as observed experimentally. The experimental and model results shows that the impacted side chest deformation is less but the duration is longer in the padded wall impact than in the rigid wall impact. However, both cadavers had the similar chest injuries. Due to the limited number of the tests, no conclusion can be drawn from this study regarding the effect of padding and the effect of space.

DISCUSSION

This finite element and previous MADYMO models are an effort to predict side impact response of a near side occupant. They are based on cadaveric data obtained at the shoulder, thorax, abdomen and pelvis. The average age of the cadavers used in the experiments was 60. They are representative of elderly occupants, and it is not known if the cadaver is weaker than a live occupant. These can be treated as safety factors in automotive design. However, finite element modeling can provide a new technique to estimate the response of a strong and young occupant based on the response of the weak and old cadavers, if the ratios of their material properties are available and their geometries are assumed to be the same. The finite element model does not do a better job than the MADYMO model, in the comparison of the model and experimental results. However, the finite element model has much better contact surface, which does not rely on the combined stiffness of both parts involved in the contact. Therefore, it would be easier and more accurate to use the finite element model to interact with detailed models of the door trim, armrest and side airbag.

Due to the limitation of the current technology, it is necessary to simplify the complicated human geometry. The model in this study used a very coarse mesh to represent an average human with a body weight of 75 kg. It can be used to estimate the chest injury functions of an elderly occupant involved in a side impact. However, to predict shoulder and pelvic responses, the mesh of the shoulder and pelvis should be improved.

The material properties and the constitutive laws of the human tissues should be studied in greater detail. Development of new material model is necessary to simulate the highly non-linear and rate dependent soft tissues. A viscous fluid-like element can help simulate the fat and water content in the body.

This finite element model has been shown to be able to predict the deformation pattern of the chest. These chest contours provide much more information than the chest compression C based on the film analysis. However, more chest band data are needed, to develop a procedure to calculate C and V*C or other injury functions based on the chest band.

It should be noted that the calculated stresses and strains of the visceral contents are meaningless and cannot be used to predict injury, since all of the organs were lumped together. No attempt was made to compare stresses or strains between the model and experimental results since such experimental data were not available. Therefore, this model does not provide an alternative to predicting injuries based the stresses or strains. It is recommended that strain gages be used to measure the strains of some bones for model development, in the future cadaveric tests.

CONCLUSIONS

1. A three-dimensional finite element human model, using a coarse mesh, has been developed to simulate near-side occupant response to a side impact.

2. The model has been compared with the cadaveric tests of 14 different test conditions. The average difference between the model result and experimental data is 18.1%.

3. The model is useful in the estimation of thoracic injury parameters for padding, armrest, side airbag and door designs.

4. The shoulder and pelvic portion of the model needs

to be improved. The predicted stresses and strains were not compared with experimental data and should not be used to assess injuries.

ACKNOWLEDGEMENTS

This work was supported in part by the Centers for Disease Control (Grant No. CCR 502347). PAM-CRASH was provided by the ESI of the France. The EPIDM chest band was provided by NHTSA. We wish to thank Drs. Paul C. Begeman and King H. Yang for advice and for providing an excellent software environment, Mr. Warren Hardy, Matt Mason, Jr., and the rest of the Bioengineering staff who conducted the experiments.

REFERENCES

Cavanaugh JM, Zhu Y, Huang Y, King AI (1992) Mechanical properties of various padding materials used in cadaveric side impact sled tests. SAE Paper No. 902354. In: Analytical Modeling and Occupant Protection Technologies, pp. 109-124. SAE International Congress and Exposition, Detroit, Michigan, Feb. 24-28, 1992.

Cavanaugh JM, Zhu Y, Huang Y, King AI (1993) Injury and response of the thorax in side impact cadaveric tests. Proc. of the 37th Stapp Car Crash Conf. SAE Paper No. 933127.

Deng YC (1988) The importance of the test method in determining the effects of door padding in side impact. Proc. of the 33rd Stapp Car Crash Conference.

Eppinger RH, Morgan RM (1982) Side impact data analysis, Ninth International Conference on Experimental Safety Vehicles.

Eppinger RH, Marcus JH, Morgan RM (1984) Development of dummy and injury index for NHTSA's thoracic side impact protection research program. SAE Paper No. 840885, Government/Industry Meeting and Exposition, Washington, D.C.

Eppinger RH (1989) On the development of a deformation measurement system and its application toward developing mechanically based injury indices. Proc. of the 33rd Stapp Conf., SAE Paper No. 892426.

Plank GR and Eppinger RH (1989) Computed dynamic response of the human from a finite element model. Proc. of the 12th International Technical Conference on Experimental Safety Vehicles. Goteborg, Sweden.

Huang Y, King AI, Cavanaugh JM (1994) A Madymo model of near-side human occupants in side impact. Journal of Biomechanical Engineering, Vol. 116, May 1994.

FMVSS 214, 49 CFR Part 571 (1990) Federal Motor Vehicle Safety Standard No. 214, Side Impact Protection. Federal Register, Docket No. 88-06, Notice 8, RIN 2127-AB86, Vol. 55(210), Oct. 30, 1990.

King AI, Huang Y, Cavanaugh JM (1991) Protection of occupants against side impact. Proc. of the 13th International Technical conference on Experimental Safety Vehicles, Paper No. 91-S5-0-04.

Lau IV and Viano DC (1986) The viscous criterion - basis and applications of an injury severity index for soft tissues. Proc. 30th Stapp Car Crash Conference, pp. 123-142, SAE Paper No. 861882.

Nahum AM and Melvin J (1985) The biomechanics of trauma. Appleton-Century-Crofts, Norwalk, Connecticut.

National Highway Traffic Safety Administration of University of Michigan (1983) Anthropometry of motor vehicle occupants: specifications and drawings.

Morgan RM, Marcus JH, Eppinger RH (1986) Side Impact - the biofidelity of NHTSA's proposed ATD and efficacy of TTI. SAE Paper No. 861877, 30th Stapp Car Crash Conference.

Marcus JH, Morgan RM, Eppinger RH, Kallieris D, Mattern R, Schmidt G (1983) Human response to injury from lateral impact. Proc. of the 35th Stapp Conf., SAE Paper No. 831634.

Viano and Lau IV (1985) Thoracic impact: a viscous tolerance criterion. Tenth International Conference on Experimental Safety Vehicles, Oxford, England, pp. 104-144.

Viano DC (1986) Biomechanics of bone and tissue: a review of material properties and failure characteristics. SAE paper No. 861923.

Viano DC, Lau IV, Asbury C, King AI, Begeman P (1989) Biomechanics of the human chest, abdomen, and pelvis in lateral impact. 33rd Annual Proc. of AAAM, pp. 367-382.

Yamada H (1970) Strength of Biological Materials. The Williams and Wilkins Company Baltimore, 1970.

Zhu JY, Cavanaugh JM, King AI (1993) Pelvic biomechanical response and padding benefits in side impact based on a cadaveric test series. Proc. of 37th Stapp Conf., pp. 223-233, SAE Paper No. 933128.

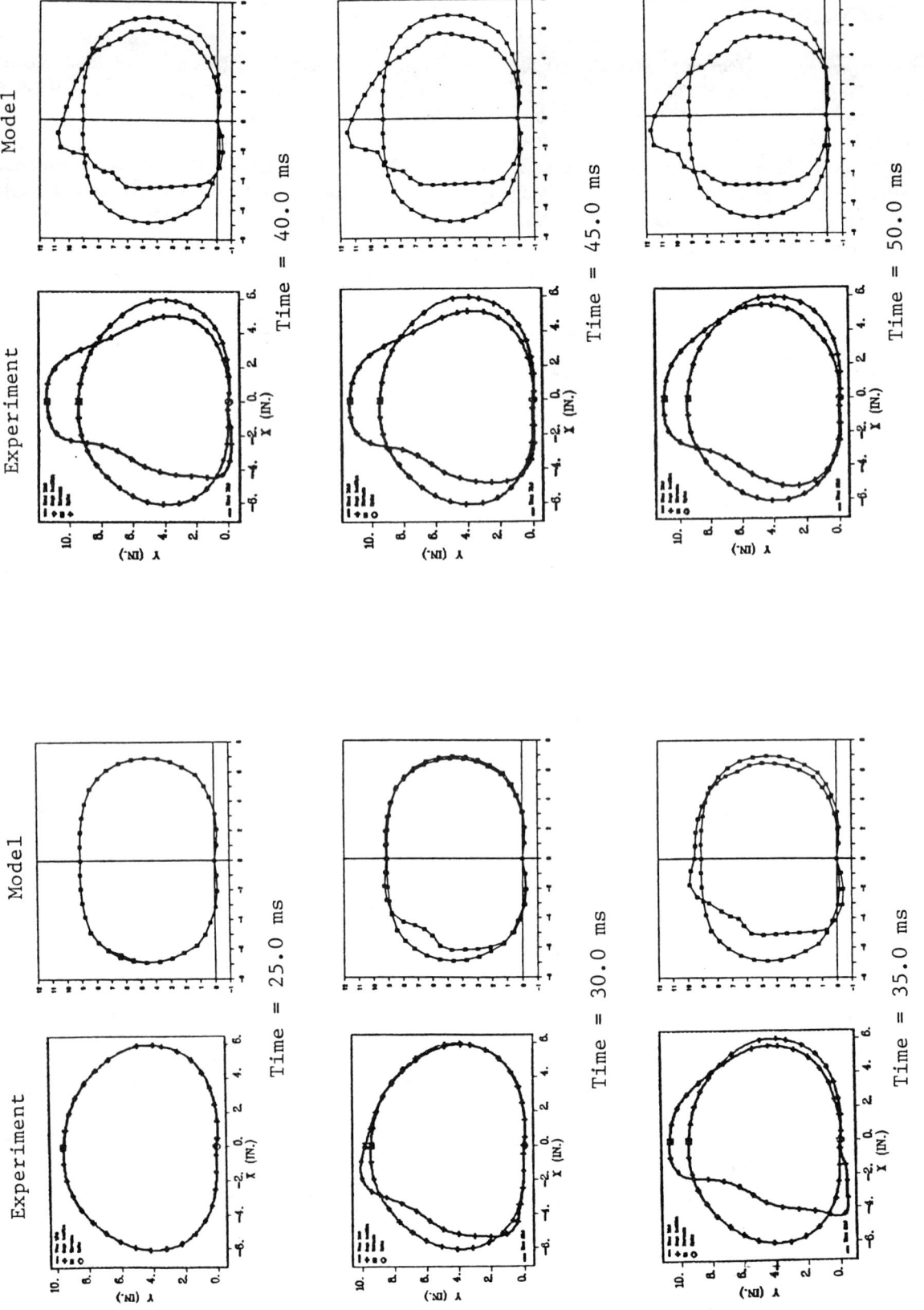

Figure 12. Comparison of the chest contours for a rigid wall sled-to-sled impact with 100 mm space.

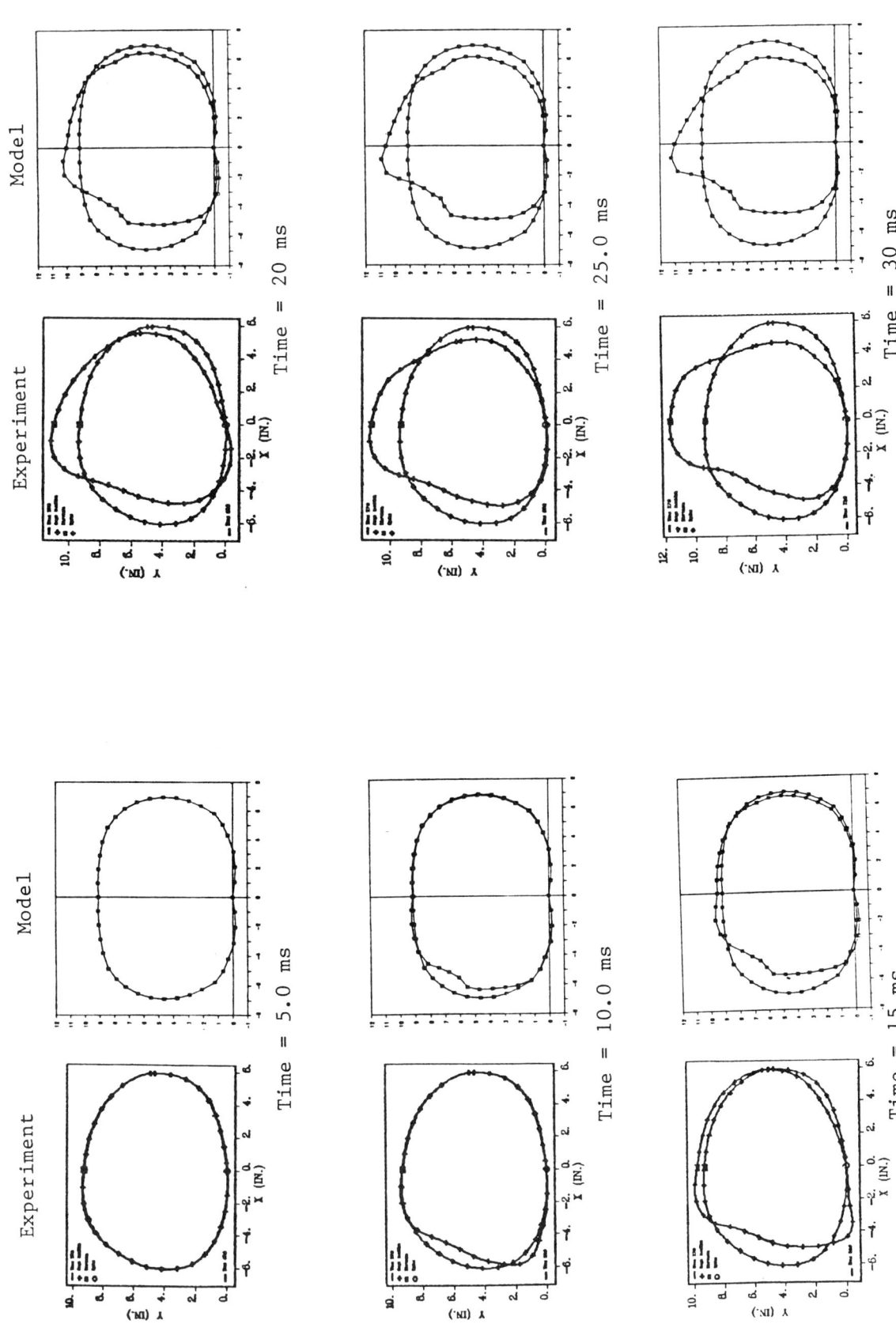

Figure 13. Comparison of the chest contours for a padded wall sled-to-sled impact with no space.

942223

Development of an Abdominal Deformation Measuring System for Hybrid III Dummy

Shin-ichi Ishiyama, Koji Tsukada, Hidekazu Nishigaki, Yasuaki Ikeda, and Shigeru Sakuma
Toyota Central R & D Labs., Inc.

Fumio Matsuoka, Yoshihisa Kanno, and Shigeki Hayashi
Toyota Motor Corporation

ABSTRACT

A new abdominal deformation measuring system for Hybrid III dummy has been developed in order to evaluate the abdominal injury by using the dummy. From the dynamic abdominal deformation of the dummy, the abdominal compression velocity V, the compression ratio C, and the maximum value of the product VC, expressed as $[VC]_{MAX}$, can be calculated.

This abdominal deformation measuring system consists of an abdominal insert having the same compression characteristics as those of the human body, a dynamic deformation sensor, and an analysis program. The abdominal insert is made of elastic foam rubber and has a shape fitted to Hybrid III. The deformation sensor in a band shape is a thin stainless steel band with 25 strain gauges on it. Each strain gauge measures the curvature on its mounted position. Since the deformation sensor is located along the surface of the dummy abdomen, the sensor deforms as the dummy surface deforms. The analysis program calculates the distribution of curvature in the longitudinal direction of the sensor and the deformation of the abdomen during an impact. This system makes it possible to obtain the abdominal deformation in the impact tests using a cylindrical bar or a lap belt within an error of 10 %.

According to the automobile accident statistics from 1984 through 1992 collected by the National Accident Sampling System (NASS), the total injuries of AIS≥3 occurred to occupants wearing seat belts consist mainly of the injuries to thorax (27%), head (19%), thigh (11%), and abdomen (8%). The number of abdominal injury is the 4th largest. The main contact points of the vehicle in abdominal injury are steering wheel (44%) and seat belts (16%).

To reduce abdominal injury in vehicle accidents, the following steps are necessary:
(1) definition of abdominal injury criterion of the human body (relationship between injury level and physical quantity),
(2) development of a dummy abdominal structure having similar characteristics to those of the human body,
(3) development of a system for measuring abdominal injury criterion using dummy.

Recent studies on abdominal injury mechanisms, criteria and tolerances are reviewed by Rouhana [1] in detail. Among these studies, Eppinger et al. [2], in the development of Thoracic Trauma Index (TTI) for side impact, correlated injuries of upper abdominal organs (i.e. liver, kidney, spleen) with the acceleration of ribs and vertebrae. Brun-Cassan [3], Lau and Viano [4] [5], however, reported that abdominal injury has no correlation with the acceleration. Melvin et al. [6], Stalnaker et al. [7], and Miller [8] confirmed the correlation between abdominal compression deformation and abdominal injury by impact tests using animals or unembalmed cadavers. Meanwhile, Rouhana et al. [9] and Viano et al. [5] reported the correlations are relatively poor.

Some studies on abdominal injury report that abdominal injury corresponds well to the product of abdominal deformation velocity V and compression deformation ratio C. Based on these studies, two measures of abdominal injuries are proposed. One is the abdominal injury criterion (AIC) proposed by Rouhana et al. [10,11], which evaluates abdominal injury from the maximum deformation velocity V_{MAX} and maximum compression C_{MAX} obtained by experiments using animals. The other measure is the viscous response criterion, a refined injury

---
* Numbers in square brackets indicate references at end of paper.

criterion of the AIC, proposed by Viano and Lau [12, 5]. They argue that the maximum value of the product of velocity-time history and compression-time history $[V(t) \times C(t)]_{MAX}$ well corresponds to the abdominal injury.

In the second place, we describe the dynamic response of abdomen to the impact loading to the human body. It is generally considered that abdomen has different responses in different abdominal regions and loading directions. In the studies on the accidental safety, abdomen is commonly divided into three regions: upper abdomen covered with ribs, middle abdomen and lower abdomen. Loading directions often refer to frontal collision and side impact. The response of lower abdomen in frontal collision was studied by Cavanaugh et al. [13]. They examined abdomen response of unembalmed cadavers in the collision with a 25 mm diameter cylindrical bar at impact velocities of 6.1 and 10.4 m/s. Nusholtz et al. [14] applied impact load to the 12th thoracic vertebra with steering wheel, and examined response characteristics in the impact velocity range of 3.9-10.8 m/s. Miller [8] obtained response characteristics from the impact load applied to the mid abdomen of swines in the impact velocity range of 1.6-6.6 m/s. Characteristics of upper abdomen of various kinds of primates were obtained by Stalnaker and Ulman [15]. Since the response characteristics of upper abdomen and middle abdomen have not yet been clarified, the response characteristics of lower abdomen obtained by Cavanaugh et al. [13] are recommended as those of the human abdomen [1].

As for the abdominal response characteristics to side impact, Walfisch et al. [16] obtained armrest load to unembalmed cadavers at impact velocities of 4.5 and 6.3 m/s. Viano et al. [5] obtained force-deflection responses for lateral abdominal impact at velocities of 4.8, 6.8 and 9.4 m/s.

Thus, various criteria of abdominal injury have been proposed, and studies on abdominal impact response have advanced so far. However, the method of measuring abdominal injury to evaluate vehicle safety has not yet been established.

On the other hand, development of Trauma Assessment Device (TAD), the revised dummy for Hybrid III, is now in progress. Schneider et al. [17] proposed many thorax structural designs for the advanced dummy. However, they made only a little mention of dummy abdomen: abdominal should have the same characteristics as those reported by Rouhana et al. [18] so that the intrusion of vehicle components could be measured. If abdominal viscous criterion is regarded as an appropriate measure for the estimation of injury, the proposal on TAD's abdominal structure and measuring method could be considered insufficient.

There are two main abdominal injury measuring systems for dummy developed so far. The first system is the foam-filled air bladder insert developed by Mooney and Collins [19]. In this system, however, the measurement accuracy of the deflection obtained by pressure-deflection calibration curve is unsatisfactory, and pressure-deflection responses are affected by the shape of impactor and the height of the position impacted. The other system is the crushable styrofoam insert abdomen developed by Rouhana et al. [20]. The F-S characteristics of this insert agree with that of human cadavers in low velocity deformation ($\leq$3 m/s). This insert allows us to perform easy measurement of abdominal deformation. However, since this insert shows only maximum deformation, time-history of the deformation cannot be obtained. Thus, there is no successful method for measuring abdominal injury using a dummy.

Recently, a newly developed injury measuring method for the dummy, External Peripheral Instrument for Deformation Measurement (EPIDM), was reported by Eppinger [21]. In this system, deformation pattern is obtained as a time-history response from the bending strain in a thin steel band called "chest band" during impact. This method has been used for the measurement of chest deformation.

This paper describes an abdominal deformation measuring system developed for Hybrid III dummy. The objectives and special features of this system are as follows:

(1) Since the system is installed in Hybrid III dummy, we determined the shape and dimension of the abdominal structure to fit the abdominal inner dimension of the currently used dummy.

(2) The response characteristics of lower abdomen of human cadavers obtained by Cavanaugh [13] were adopted as those of human abdomen. We selected a foamed rubber material suited for this purpose.

(3) The system have the capability of evaluating abdominal viscous criterion (VC). Therefore, the system should have the performance of measuring the deformation velocity of abdomen V and deformation ratio C in the form of time-history response during impact.

(4) The abdominal deformation measuring system utilizes a thin steel band with one end fixed and the other end free.

CALCULATION METHOD OF ABDOMINAL DEFORMATION

Figure 1 shows the rough sketch of Toyota Abdominal Deformation Analyzing System (TADAS). The calculation algorithm of abdominal deformation is extended from that of the thoracic deformation measuring system (EPIDM) developed by Eppinger [21]. While EPIDM utilizes a sensor shaped a thin steel band having a closed contour, TADAS has the one having an open end. This is the main difference between EPIDM and TADAS. Therefore, the two systems are different in the boundary conditions and the calculation method of deformation pattern. However, both the systems adopt the same principle that the deformation pattern is obtained from the curvature distribution along a steel band. The calculation method in our system takes two steps: the calculation of the curvature distribution from the discrete bending strains on a steel band, and the calculation of the deformation pattern of the steel band from the curvature distribution. The two steps are described in the following sections.

CALCULATION OF THE CURVATURE - Figure 2 illustrates the sensor on which n strain gauges are mounted. A thin steel band is put on x, y plane, where s is the longitudinal coordinate, s=0 is a fixed end, and s=l is a free end. To measure the bending strains, n pieces of uniaxial strain gauges (i=1,n) are bonded on the center line of the thin steel band surface. If the steel band deforms with the abdominal surface change during impact, the bending strain ε_i and curvature k_i at point i have the following relation:

$$\varepsilon_i = \frac{t}{2} k_i \quad (1)$$

where,
t : thickness of the steel band.

From the n discrete measured curvatures k_i (i=1,n), curvature distribution k(s) along the total length of the band ($0 \leq s \leq l$) is approximated by the following steps.

According to the beam theory of the structural analysis, when a uniform load is applied to a band, the curvature distribution k(s) is expressed by a quadratic equation. Therefore, we assume the curvature distribution k(s) between point i and point i+1 to be the following quadratic equation.

$$k(s) = a_{i,i+1} + b_{i,i+1}s + c_{i,i+1}s^2 \quad (2)$$
$$: (i=1, n-1)$$

The unknown coefficients $a_{i,i+1}$, $b_{i,i+1}$, $c_{i,i+1}$ are calculated under the following conditions.
(1) From the curvature (k_1, k_n) at the positions with strain gauge mounted (s_1, s_n), the following expressions can be obtained:

$$k_i = a_{i,i+1} + b_{i,i+1}s_i + c_{i,i+1}s^2_i \quad (3)$$
$$: (i=1, n-1)$$

$$k_{i+1} = a_{i,i+1} + b_{i,i+1}s_{i+1} + c_{i,i+1}s^2_{i+1} \quad (4)$$
$$: (i=1, n-1)$$

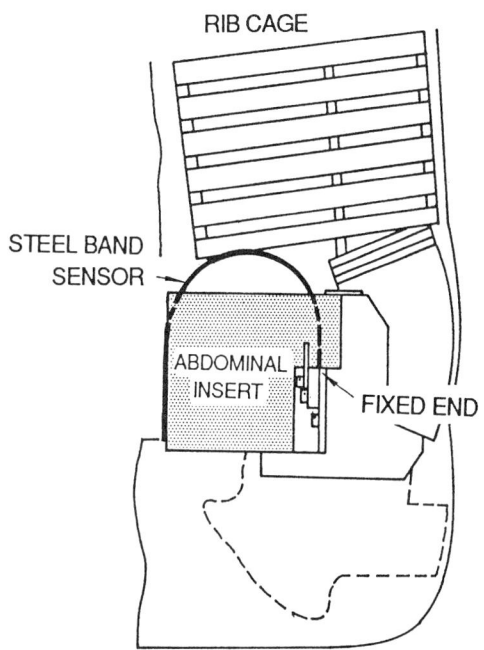

Figure 1 TOYOTA Abdominal Deformation Analyzing System (TADAS)

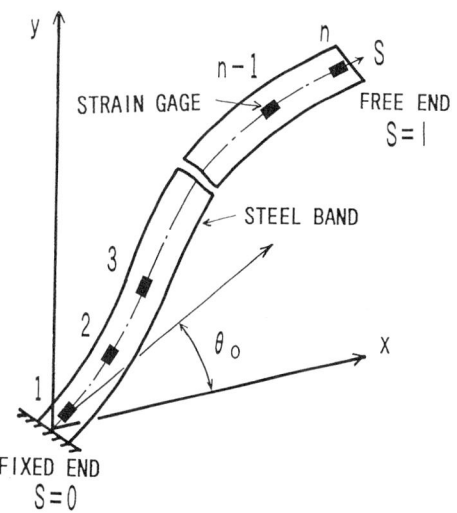

Figure 2 Sensor with n strain gauges

(2) From the continuity of the first derivatives of the curvature at the positions (s_1, s_n), the following expressions can be obtained:

$$b_{i,i+1} + 2c_{i,i+1}s_{i+1} = b_{i+1,i+2} + 2c_{i+1,i+2}s_{i+1} \quad : (i=1, n-2) \quad (5)$$

(3) Equation (2) has $3n-3$ unknown coefficients. Since the number of equations (3)-(5) is $3n-4$, one more equation must be defined to solve the equations. Providing the complete fixing of the band at the origin $s=0$, another equation is introduced:

$$\left(\frac{dk(s)}{ds}\right)_{s=0} = b_{1,2} = 0 \quad (6)$$

where, the section between gauge positions 1 and 2 is extended to the section between the origin and gauge position 2. We chose the gauge position 1 to be as close to the origin as possible in order to minimize the error caused by the extension of the section between 1 and 2.

Equations (3)-(6) give the unknown coefficients $a_{i,i+1}$, $b_{i,i+1}$ and $c_{i,i+1}$ in equation (2), which provide the curvature distribution $k(s)$ in the longitudinal direction of the band. The calculation process is described as follows:

From the equations (3) and (4),

$$c_{i,i+1} = -\frac{1}{s_i + s_{i+1}} b_{i,i+1} + \frac{k_i - k_{i+1}}{s_i^2 - s_{i-1}^2} \quad (7)$$
$$: i=1, n-1$$

Substituting $b_{i,i+1}$ and $b_{i+1,i+2}$ in equation (7) into equation (5),

$$c_{i+1,i+2} = -\frac{s_i - s_{i+1}}{s_{i+1} - s_{i+2}} c_{i,i+1} + \frac{k_i - k_{i+1}}{(s_i - s_{i+1})(s_{i+1} - s_{i+2})} - \frac{k_{i+1} - k_{i+2}}{(s_{i+1} - s_{i+2})^2} \quad (8)$$
$$: i=1, n-2$$

From equation (7),

$$b_{i,i+1} = -(s_i + s_{i+1}) c_{i,i+1} + \frac{k_i - k_{i+1}}{s_i - s_{i+1}} \quad (9)$$
$$: i=2, n-1$$

From equation (3),

$$a_{i,i+1} = k_i - b_{i,i+1} \cdot s_i - c_{i,i+1} \cdot s_i^2 \quad (10)$$
$$: i=1, n-1$$

Consequently, the coefficients $a_{i,i+1}$, $b_{i,i+1}$ and $c_{i,i+1}$ are obtained as follows:

1) $c_{1,2}$ from equation (7)
2) $c_{i+1,i+2}$; $i=1, n-2$ from equation (8)
3) $b_{i,i+1}$; $i=2, n-1$ from equation (9)

and

4) $a_{i,i+1}$; $i=1, n-1$ from equaiton (10)

With the calculation steps described here, all the unknown coefficients can be determined, and the curvature distribution $k(s)$ can be obtained.

CALCULATION OF THE DEFORMATION PATTERN - From the curvature distribution obtained in the previous section, deformation curve of the abdominal surface was calculated in x, y coordinates. The coordinates and notations are illustrated in Figure 3.

The section between two positions with strain gauge i and $i+1$ is divided into small segment ds. The curvature distribution is assumed to be constant (a part of an arc) in each small segment. From the geometrical relations shown in Figure 3, increments Δx and Δy in x and y coordinates are expressed as follows:

$$\Delta x = \cos(\theta_s + \Delta\theta_s/2) \cdot ds \quad (11)$$
$$\Delta y = \sin(\theta_s + \Delta\theta_s/2) \cdot ds \quad (12)$$

where,

$$\theta_s = \theta_{s=0} + \int_0^s k(s)\, ds \quad (13)$$

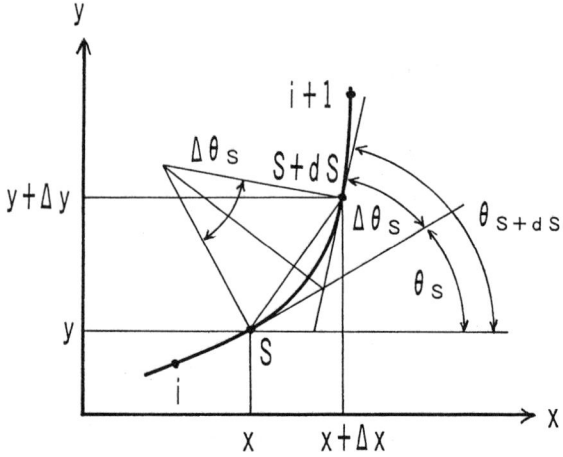

Figure 3 Coordinates and notations

$$\Delta\theta_s = \theta_{s+ds} - \theta_s = -\left|\int_s^{s+ds} k(s)\,ds\right| \cdot (\text{sign of } K(s))$$

θ_0; angle at origin (s=0)   (14)

When the curve is convex in x direction, the sign of k(s) is plus, and vice versa.

The deformation pattern in x, y coordinates can be obtained by the numerical integration of the increments Δx and Δy in equations (11) and (12).

NUMERICAL VERIFICATION - Next, the accuracy of the calculation method described in the previous sections was numerically verified. An example is shown in Figure 4. In this example, a quadratic deformation curve was chosen as an input pattern to simulate the deformation of a 296 mm long steel band.

First, to evaluate the effect of the number of gauges n, nine or fifteen points on the band at equal spaces (n=9,15) were assigned to provide curvatures at each point. Using the curvatures, we calculated deformation patterns by using the method described in the previous sections. Second, to evaluate the effect of the distance between the origin and the first gauge point s_1, the deformation patterns were examined in the two cases for s_1=2 mm and 5 mm.

To calculate the deformation patterns in x, y coordinates, 5000 increments in the numerical integration have been used over the total band length.

The calculation results are shown in Figure 5. When n=9 is given, some difference between the input pattern and the calculated pattern is observed. When n=15 is given, however, there is hardly any difference between the two patterns. As to the first gauge point, the nearer the gauge locates to the origin, the more accurately the calculated pattern is obtained.

TRIAL MANUFACTURE OF DEFORMATION MEASUREMENT SENSOR

Eppinger [21] has developed the "chest band" to measure the thoracic deformation pattern during impact. He used a closed band of 0.38 mm in thickness, 12.7 mm in width and 1168 mm in length. The bending strain at a position on the band is measured with four strain gauges forming a bridge. The band is covered with rubber compound. The spaces between the gauges ranged 7.35-9.8 cm. Since the thorax contains relatively rigid rib cage, deformation distributes throughout thorax and large local deformation does not occur. Abdominal injury, on the other hand, involves large local deformation when it collides against seat belt and steering wheel because abdomen is soft. Therefore, using the calculation method described in the previous section, we investigated the possibility of measuring the large local deformation by a sensor newly developed.

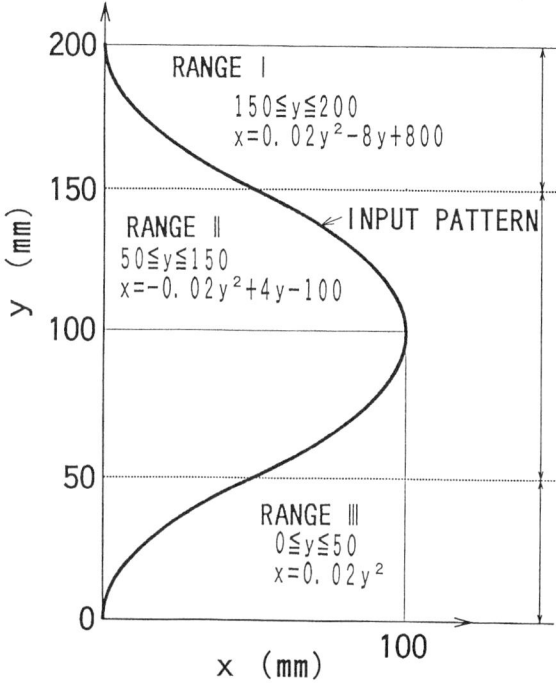

Figure 4 Example of deformation shape used to verify calculation algorithm

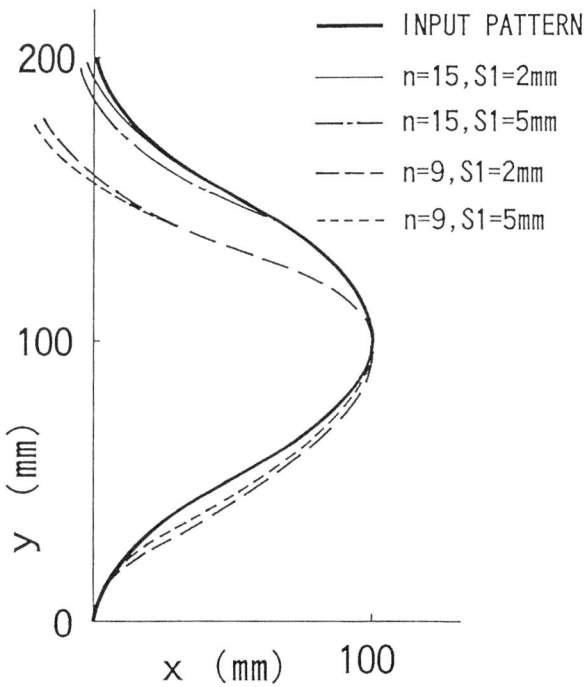

Figure 5 Comparison of input pattern and calculated results (n: number of strain gauges, S1: distance of 1st gauge from fixed end)

SENSOR CONSTRUCTION - The outlook and detailed dimensions of the sensor are shown in Figure 6 and Figure 7, respectively. The sensor consists of a steel band and two lead harnesses. The sensor must have:
(1) low rigidity in bending and easy deformability,
(2) no possibility of occurrence of longitudinal strain.

For this reason, from the stainless steel tapes on the market, we chose a stainless steel tape (sus 301) of 0.1 mm in thickness and 12.7 mm in width to use as the steel band. The length of the steel band was designed to be 350 mm. We used a uni-axis foil type strain gauge of 1 mm in gauge length and 0.03 mm in thickness. Fifteen strain gauges were mounted on the surface of the stainless tape at a space of 2 cm. For making the circuit, one active gauge in Wheatstone bridge method was adopted. To make the rigidity of the harness small compared with that of the steel band, two ribbon-type lead harnesses are located by both the sides of the steel band.

The sensor was designed so that the frictional force between the sensor and the abdominal material will be minimized. To reduce the tensile strain of the steel band in the longitudinal direction, the top and bottom surfaces of the sensor were covered with a sheet of Teflon (polytetrafluoroethylene, t=0.13 mm). On the surface of the abdominal structure, a sheath made of Teflon film (t=0.08 mm) was attached with double pasted tape. The sensor was inserted into this sheath. The frictional force was reduced as much as possible by the low friction between Teflon materials.

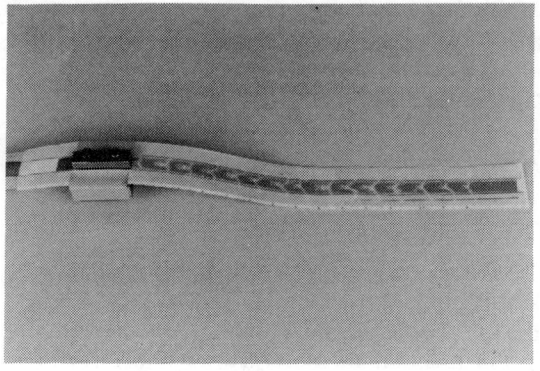

(a) Whole structure

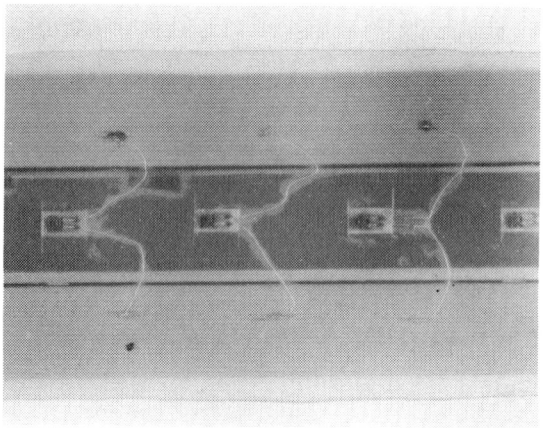

(b) Enlarged picture of sensor

Figure 6 Outlook of sensor (a trial piece)

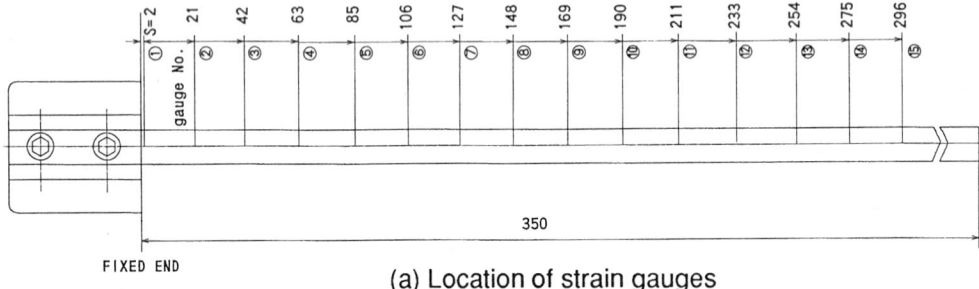

(a) Location of strain gauges

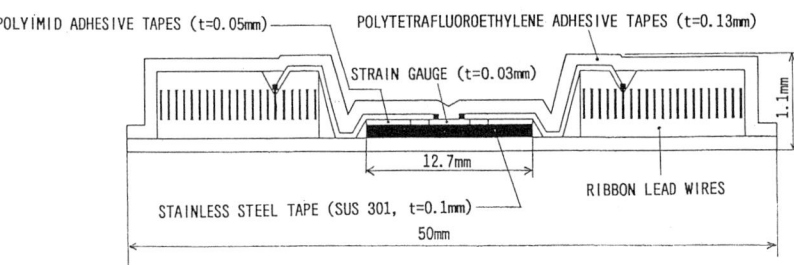

(b) Schematic cross-section of sensor

Figure 7 Detail design of sensor (a trial piece)

VERIFICATION OF THE METHOD BY STATIC TESTS - Static tests were performed to confirm the possibility of measuring large deformation of soft materials. The method of the static tests is shown in Figure 8. In the static tests, the sensor was put on a block of foamed urethane located on the bed of a universal static load tester, Autograph. The sensor and foamed urethane were compressed with a cylindrical bar of 50 mm in diameter. One end of the sensor was fixed, and the other was free. Actual deformation pattern was read by a scale simultaneously with the measurement.

Table 1 shows the results of the measured strains for a deformation of 80 mm. Figure 9 illustrates the curvature distribution obtained by strain gauges. Figure 10 shows the comparison between actual deformation (test no.1) and the calculated deformation pattern obtained by the method previously described. The number of increments in the calculation of the deformation pattern is 5000 to the whole length of the sensor. The measured and calculated deformation patterns from the fixed end to

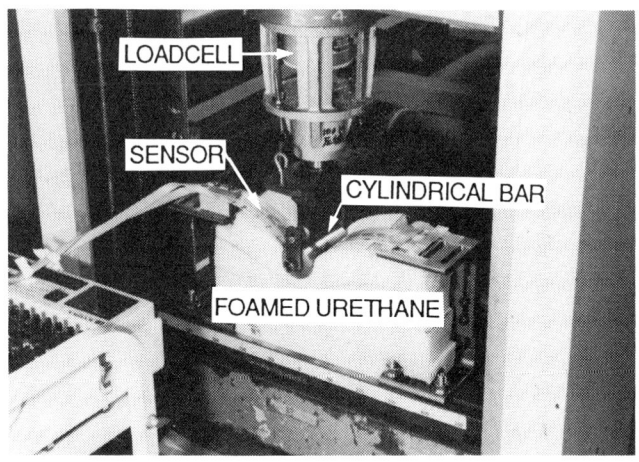

Figure 8 Test setup (static compression test)

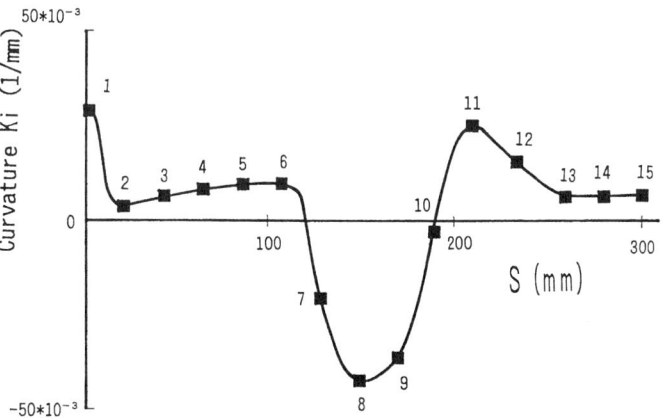

Figure 9 Curvature K_i obtained by strain gauges

Table 1 Measured strains at 80mm deflection ($*10^{-6}$)

GAUGE No	1	2	3	4	5	6	7	8	9	10	11	12	13	14	15
TEST 1	2125	220	455	588	689	728	-1601	-3191	-2766	-154	1850	1157	518	495	497
TEST 2	2037	308	444	560	646	692	-1323	-3070	-2607	-633	1600	1170	557	612	821

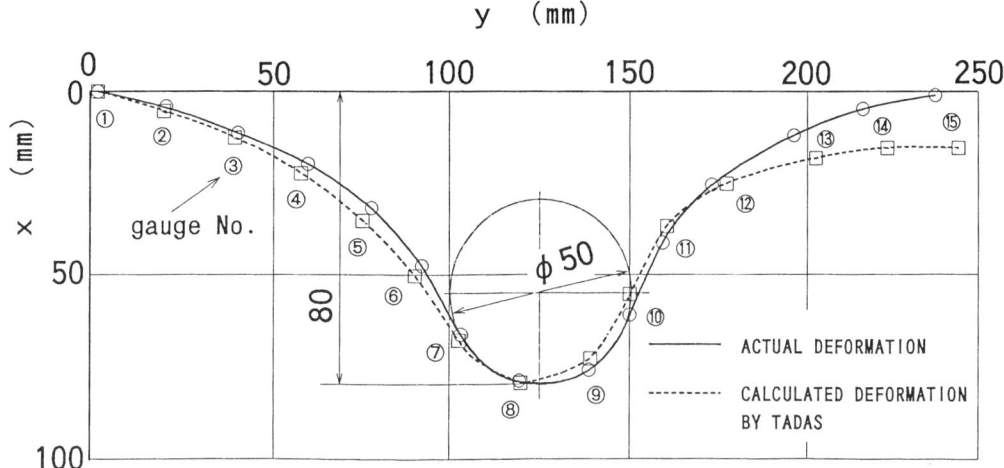

Figure 10 Comparison between actual deformation and calculated deformation patterns under static compression test (y=0: fixed end)

the maximum deformation position agree well with each other. However, the difference in deformation pattern near the free end is relatively large. Nevertheless, this difference is of little importance, because the measurement is aimed for obtaining the maximum deformation with high accuracy.

SELECTION OF DUMMY ABDOMINAL INSERT MATERIAL

The dynamical response characteristics of human abdomen under the impact loading were measured by Cavanaugh et al. [13] using unembalmed cadavers. In their study, a cylindrical bar of 25 mm in diameter was used as the impactor. Impact velocities were 6.1 and 10.4 m/s.

Based on their study, we investigated four materials by dynamic tests to find a dummy abdominal material having the same force-deflection response characteristics. The test method is shown in Figure 11. Abdominal material (175 mm wide, 300 mm long, and 150 mm thick) was fixed on a rigid wall. The tip of the impactor is a cylindrical bar of 25 mm in diameter which is of the same shape as that used in their study. The physical properties of the materials offered by the material production company are shown in Table 2. In the table, rubber hardness was measured with a spring-type hardness tester.

A series of force-deflection curves was obtained at an impact velocity of 6 m/s. The deflection was calculated from the deceleration of the impactor. Figure 12 compares the results of the measurement with their test results.

The results in Figure 12 indicates that the material most fitted for the human characteristics is the material D (EPT15). In the actual dummy abdomen, however, abdominal insert is supported not by a plane, but mainly by a spine. Additional tests showed that the rigidity of the abdomen supported by the dummy spine decreased by 20 % as compared to that supported by a rigid plane. This indicates that the dummy abdominal material most fitted for the human characteristics is the material B (Neoprene 15) in Table 2. Figure 13 shows the characteristics of Neoprene 15 compared to the human characteristics. As a result, the force-deflection characteristics of Neoprene 15 is found to fit with the human characteristics obtained by Cavanaugh et al. We used Neoprene 15 as the dummy abdominal insert as described in the next section.

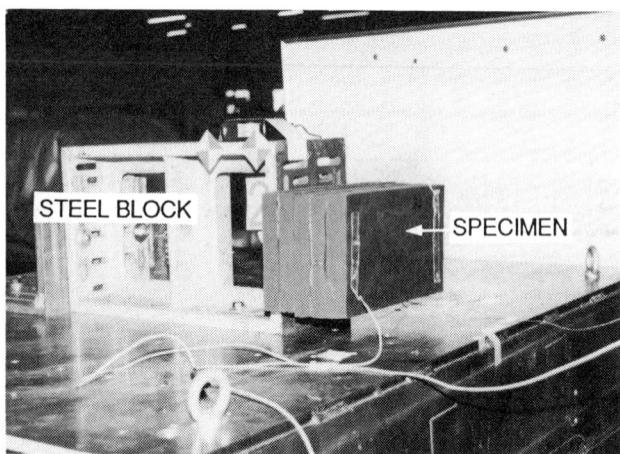

Figure 11 Test setup on abdominal material for dummy

Table 2 Test specimens for abdominal insert

MATERIAL CODE	MATERIAL NAME	CHEMICAL STRUCTURE	RUBBER HARDNESS (DEGREE)
A	NEOPRENE 30	POLYCHLOROPRENE	30
B	NEOPRENE 15		15
C	EPT 25	ETHYLEN PROPYLENE TERPOLYMER	25
D	EPT 15		15

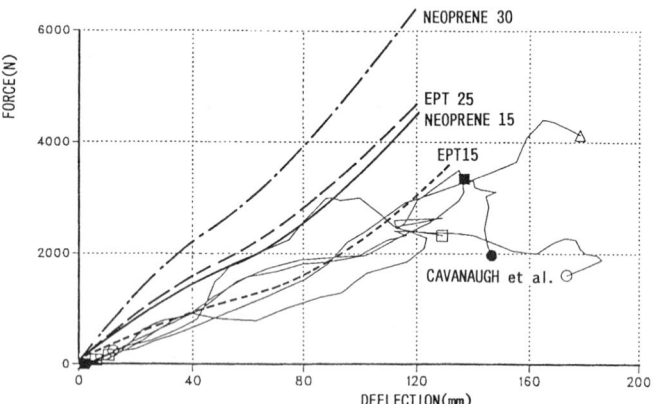

Figure 12 Impact response of abdominal materials for dummy (supported on plane surface)

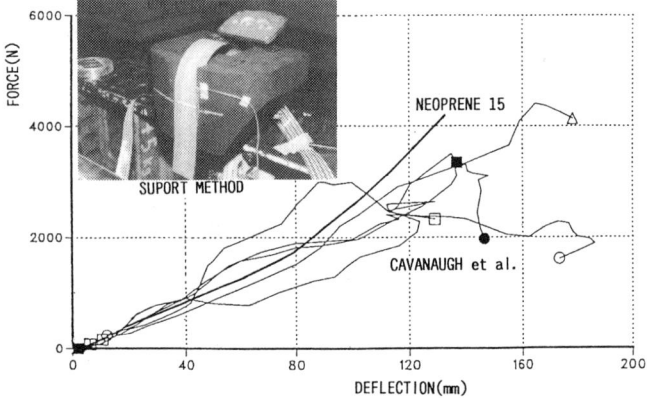

Figure 13 Impact response of Neoprene 15 (supported by spine of dummy and plane surface)

ABDOMINAL DEFORMATION MEASURING SYSTEM

Toyota Abdominal Deformation Analyzing System (TADAS) for Hybrid III dummy was assembled by the sensor and the abdominal material described in the previous sections. The usefulness of the system was evaluated by impact tests using a cylindrical bar and a lap belt. The outlook of the system is shown in Figure 14. The sensor was improved to measure the impact responses as accurately as possible.

MEASURING SYSTEM - We manufactured an abdomen which fits to the abdominal configuration of Hybrid III dummy from the foamed rubber (Neoprene 15) illustrated in Table 2. The drawing of the abdomen for the machining is shown in Figure 15.

Six sheets of 30 mm thick Neoprene 15 were laminated and machined. To prevent the rotation of the abdomenal insert during impact, a sheet of cloth, which is usually used for car seat, was inserted between the second and third layers of the Neoprene 15 with a protrusion from under the bottom surface of the abdomen. The protrusion was held by two pieces of aluminum plates (20 mm wide, 78 mm long and 3 mm thick, each) with three bolts (size M4). Two pieces of aluminum plates were fastened to the frontal end of the lumber spine bracket of the dummy with two bolts (size M8). The fastening method is shown in Figure 16.

To fix the end of the sensor, a set of clamping elements was used together with the sensor band. The clamping elements consist of three parts, a fixing plate, a fixing block, a sensor protector, and two clamping bolts of size M6. The clamping method of the sensor is shown in Figure 17. The fixing plate of the clamping elements of the sensor was fastened on

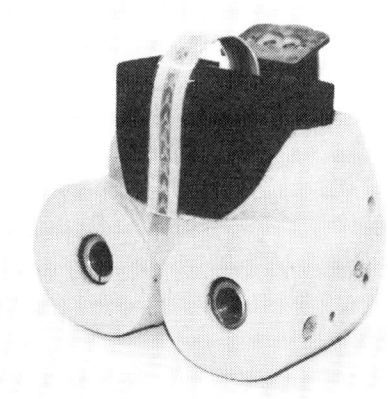

Figure 14 Picture of TADAS

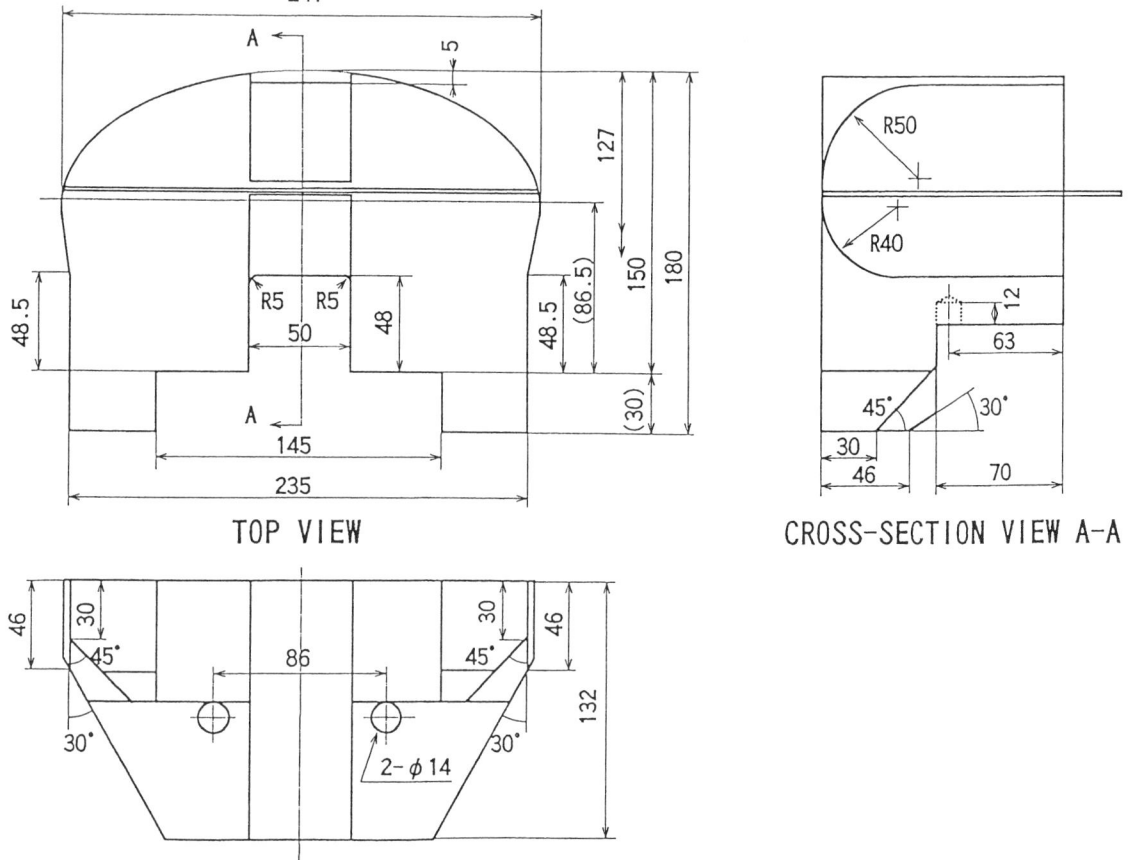

Figure 15 Print of the abdominal insert for Hybrid III dummy

the frontal surface of a newly designed attachment. The attachment is welded to the lumber spine bracket in the lower frontal region of the spine of the dummy. The sensor extends from the fixed end to the upper region along the spine, turns frontward, and reaches the frontal surface of the abdomen forming U curve. This initial curve is made to ensure the mobility of the sensor even when dynamic large local deformation occurs, to avoid the generation of tensile strain in steel band, and to prevent a bending fracture at the fixed end of the sensor. Furthermore, to prevent the bending fracture at the fixed end of the sensor, the corners of the clamping elements of the sensor were machined roundly.

The outlook and the structure of the sensor are shown in Figures 18 and 19, respectively. Although the fundamental performance of the sensor was confirmed by the static tests, the following were further improved for the impact tests:

(1) The length of the steel band was increased to 384 mm. The number of the strain gauges was also increased to 25. The spaces of the gauges were 10-20 mm to give smaller spaces where larger curvature is expected and larger spaces where smaller curvature is expected.

(2) The thickness of the wire harness was equalized to that of the steel band with strain gauges on it in order to prevent the jumping action of the steel band during impact. To decrease the thickness of the wire harness, a flexible print circuit (FPC) was newly developed. Figure 20 shows an enlarged picture of the FPC. In designing the FPC, we adopted a pattern that enables the electric resistance of the leading wire of all the 25 strain gauges to be almost the same, and that enables the bending rigidity of the sensor to be uniform in the longitudinal direction. Furthermore, by the introduction of FPC instead of ribbon-type harness, the bending rigidity of the harness became much smaller than the one used for static tests.

(3) The sensor was inserted in the sheath made of Teflon pasted on the frontal surface of the dummy abdomen, and used for the measurement.

The sensor installed in TADAS has the spring characteristics of a thin and light steel band, which

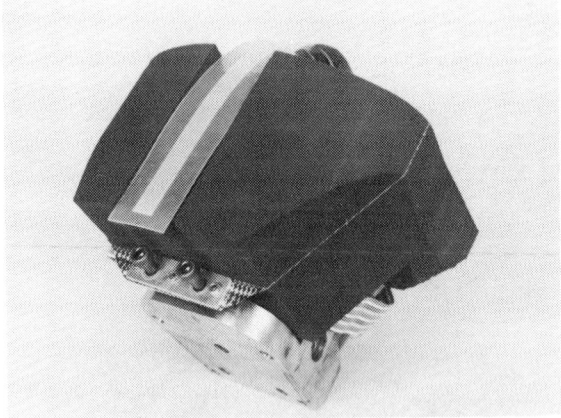

Figure 16 Fastening method of abdominal insert to dummy

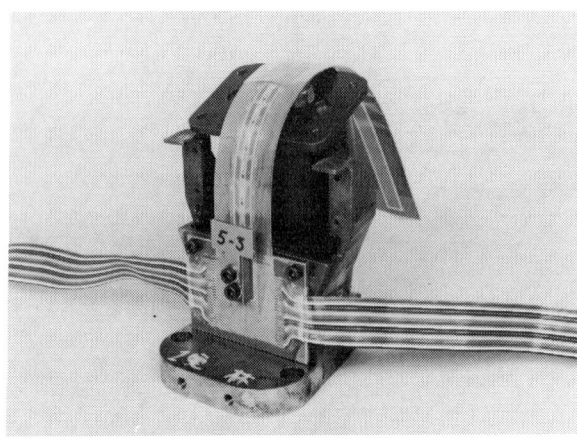

Figure 17 Fixing method of deformation measurement sensor to dummy

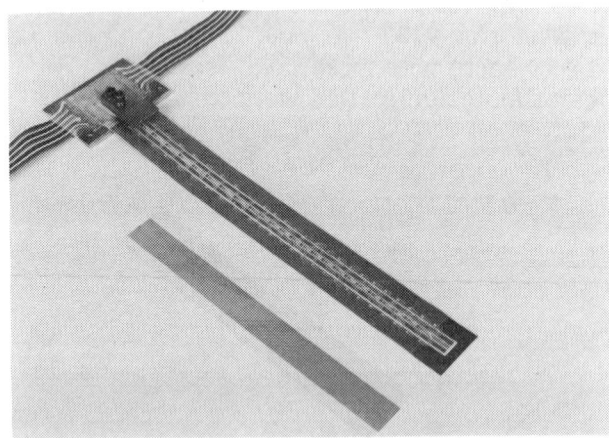

(a) Whole structure and sheath

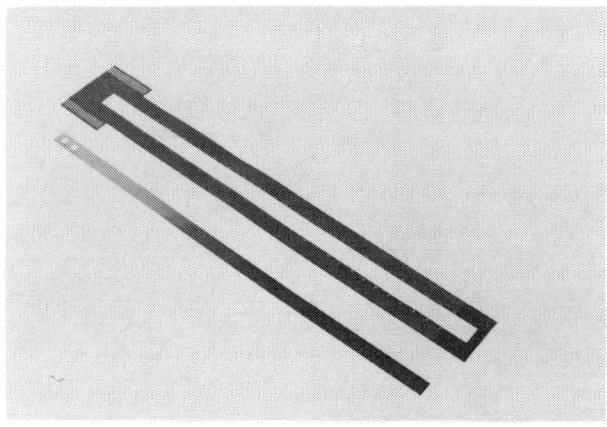

(b) Flexible printed circuit

Figure 18 Outlook of sensor (an improved piece)

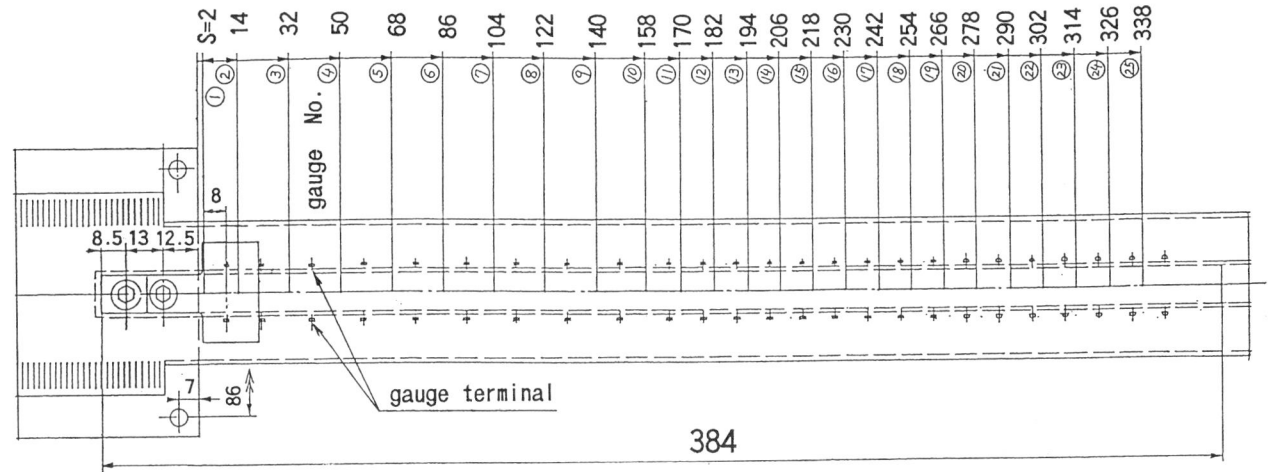

(a) Location of strain gauges

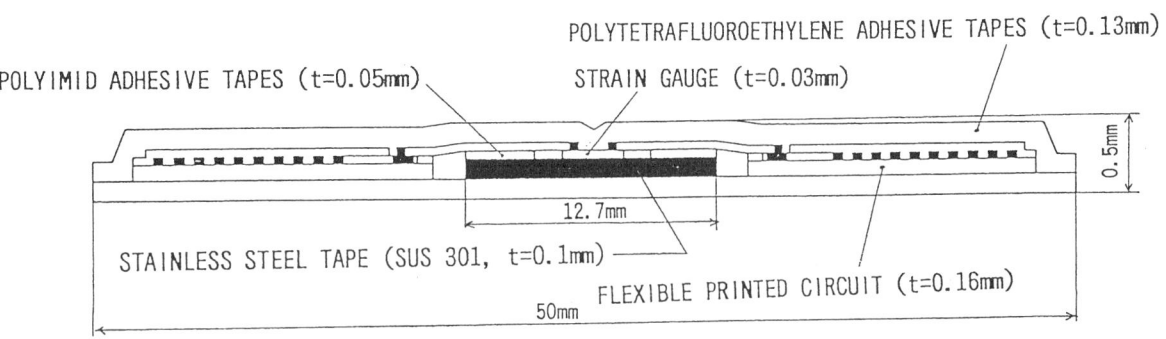

(b) Schematic cross-section of sensor

Figure 19 Detail design of sensor (an improved piece)

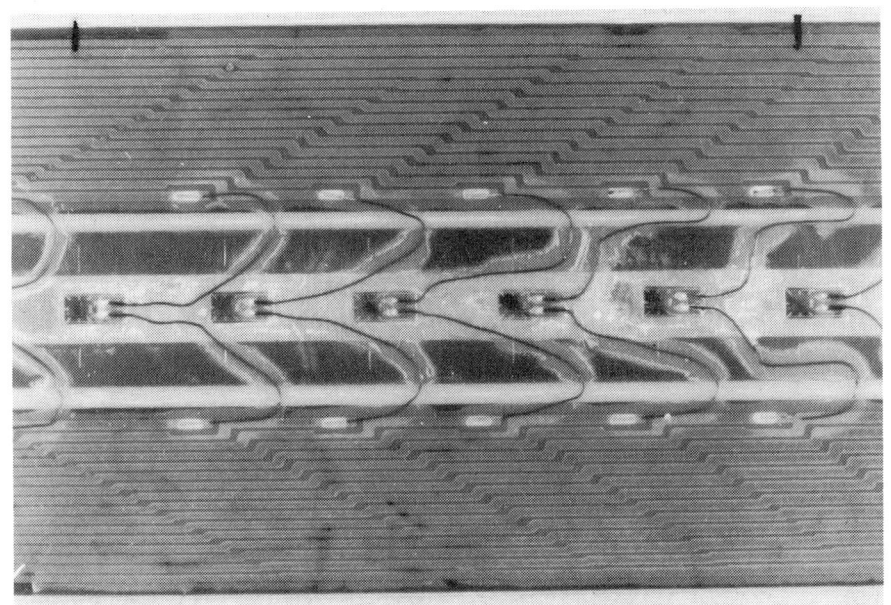

Figure 20 Outlook of flexible printed circuit

results in the advantages of smaller damping and better response.

In measuring the abdominal deformation using TADAS, the initial strains of the sensor were balanced in the Wheatstone bridge by putting the sensor on a flat surface. The sensor was then installed in the dummy abdomen forming U curve. Thus, TADAS makes it possible to measure automatically the deformation pattern just before the collision of impactor (t=0), as well as time-history of the abdominal deformation during impact.

IMPACT TEST USING CYLINDRICAL BAR IMPACTOR - To confirm the usefulness of the TADAS, impact tests were performed using an impactor. A linear stroke type testing device called "Pedestrian Protection Tester" was used for the test. The impactor was a cylindrical bar of 50 mm in diameter and 20 kg in mass. The impact velocity was 3.1 m/s. The deformation was measured by TADAS, and also analyzed with a high speed movie. Figure 21 shows the method of impact test using the cylindrical bar impactor. The center line of flight of the impactor is located at 31 mm from the top surface of the abdomen. This location corresponds to 101 mm upward from the the upper surface of the lumber-spine bracket of the dummy.

Figure 22 illustrates the test results. In the figure, the solid lines show the results for TADAS, and the dotted lines show the results for the high speed movie. There is hardly any difference between the results for TADAS and those for the high speed movie in regard to the abdominal deformation before the impact (t=0 ms). Both the deformation patterns during impact agree well. At 40 ms, the difference in intrusion between TADAS and movie (approximately 96 mm) was about 7 %. The maximum value [VC]$_{MAX}$ of the viscous criterion [VC] was calculated from these results using the abdominal depth (206 mm) of the Hybrid III dummy. The maximum value [VC]$_{MAX}$ was 0.7 m/s when TADAS was applied, and 0.8 m/s when the movie was used.

IMPACT TEST USING LAP BELT - Impact tests using a lap belt were performed. A 48 mm wide lap belt was fixed to the tip of the testing device using a clamping frame.

The maximum penetration chosen was 110 mm. This value corresponds to the amount of compression when the probability of abdominal injury of AIS ≥ 3 is 50 % in low velocity loading range (impact velocity ≤ 3 m/s), which was summarized by Rouhana et al [20] [22] for a mid-sized male Hybrid III dummy.

The impact velocity of the lap belt was 3 m/s referring to the above papers. The mass of the moving part of the impactor chosen was 21.1 kg by equating the kinetic energy at the impact with the deformation energy of the abdominal insert.

The location of impact was 89 mm upward from the upper surface of the lumber-spine bracket of the dummy. The deformation pattern was analyzed by TADAS and the high speed movie. The method of the belt impact test is shown in Figure 23.

Figure 24 shows the result at an impact velocity of 2.91 m/s. In the figure, the solid lines show the results for TADAS, and the dotted lines show the results for the high speed movie. The difference in the abdominal deformation between TADAS and the

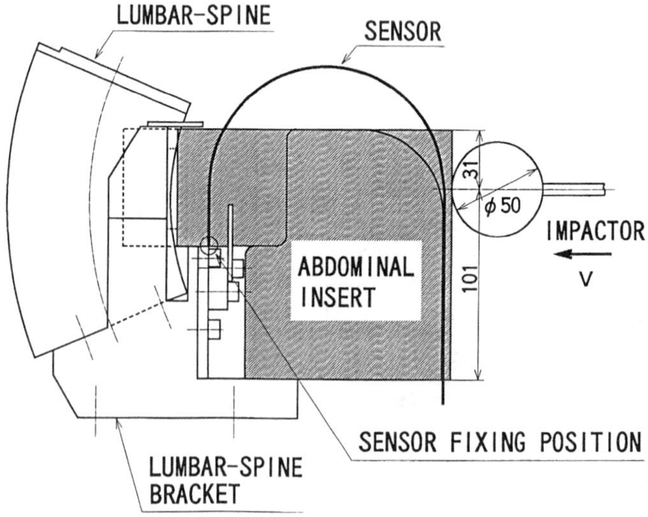

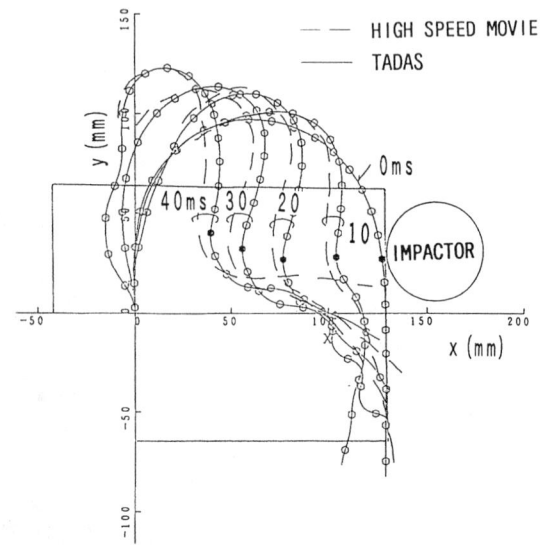

Figure 21 Impact test setup by cylindrical bar impactor

Figure 22 Deformation of abdominal insert during impact by using cylindrical bar impactor (V=3.1 m/s)

high speed movie was 2-5 mm at the collision point with a lap belt before the impact (t=0ms). Both the deformation patterns during impact correspond well to each other, and the moving process of the lap belt towards upper part of the abdomen can be clearly observed.

At an impact velocity of 2.91 m/s and a time of 50 ms, the maximum deformation was 87 mm for the TADAS measurement and 89 mm for the high speed movie: the error was 2 %.

Figure 25 shows the result at an impact velocity of 5.15 m/s. This velocity condition was tried since the maximum penetration at the impact velocity of 2.91 m/s was about 20% smaller than that intended under the impact velocity of 3 m/s. At an impact velocity of 5.15 m/s and a time of 30 ms, the difference was comparatively large. After the impact with a velocity of 5.15 m/s, some plastic deformations of the steel band caused by bending were observed near the fixed end, although no plastic deformations of the steel band were found in the distant region from the fixed end.

From this observation, in the test of the impact velocity of 5.15 m/s, it is considered that the bottoming of the lap belt occurred and the lap belt compressed the abdominal insert which, in turn, plastically bent the steel band largely near the fixed end of the sensor, and, this plastic deformation of the steel band made the measuring error larger than that of the case without the bottoming of the lap belt. For this reason, to perform the tests in which the bottoming of the abdominal insert occurs, further improvement of the present sensor protector is necessary to prevent the bending fracture of the steel band near the fixed end.

DISCUSSION ON THE CALIBRATION PROCEDURE - The usefulness of TADAS has been evaluated, in which the measurement of the initial strain, and the calculation of the deformation were carried out in the following steps:
(1) Since the deformation pattern of the sensor is unknown when the sensor is installed in the abdominal insert, the initial strains of the sensor were balanced in the Wheatstone bridge by putting the sensor on a flat surface.
(2) After that, the sensor was installed in the insert and the shape of the sensor at the set-up was calculated from the strains at that time.
(3) Then, the time-history of the deformation pattern of the abdominal insert during impact was calculated from the dynamic strains.

To reduce the amount of work in the set-up process and save the time for the calculation, the following procedures can be considered:
(1) To eliminate the measurement of the initial strains by putting the sensor on a flat surface, the abdominal

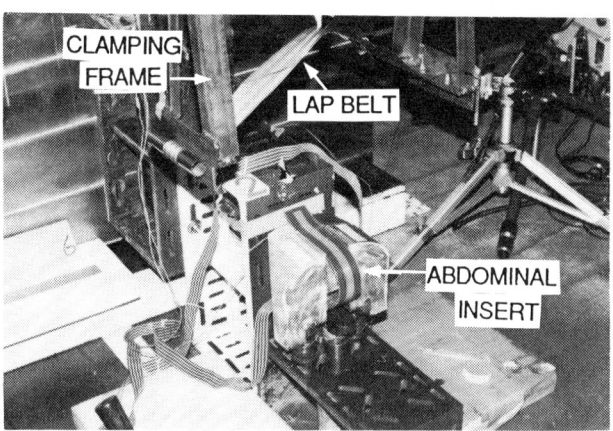

Figure 23 Impact test setup by using lap belt

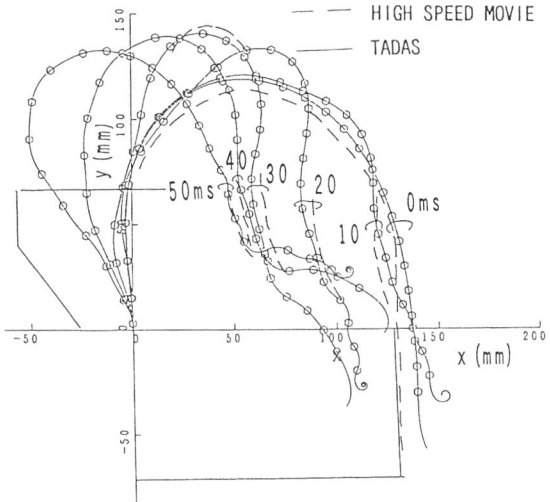

Figure 24 Deformation of abdominal insert during impact by using lap belt (V=2.91m/s)

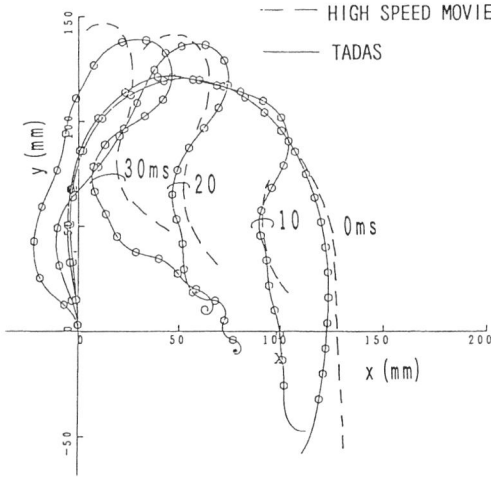

Figure 25 Deformation of abdominal insert during impact by using lap belt (V=5.15m/s)

insert is machined with some prescribed shape like those shown in Figure 14 or Figure 21.
(2) The sensor is fixed along the surface of the abdominal insert which has a prescribed shape.
(3) The initial strains are measured after the sensor is fixed along the surface of the abdominal insert.

If we used the latter method, we could eliminate the measurement of the initial strains by putting the sensor on a flat surface and expected the reduction of the total number of the calculation of the deformation patterns.

Nevertheless, if the latter method were used, there may be some problems about the accuracy of the measuremnt of the deformation patterns of the abdominal insert during impact. These problems would be caused by the increase of the frictional force due to the constrains of the steel band movement during impact or by the estimation error of the positions of strain gauges after the set-up to the insert.

CONCLUSIONS

Toyota Abdominal Deformation Measuring and Analyzing System (TADAS) for Hybrid III dummy has been developed and its usefulness was evaluated. The following conclusions have been obtained:
(1) A steel band sensor to measure the abdominal deformation of the Hybrid III dummy during impact was developed. Using a system consisting of a sensor and a calculation software, abdominal deformation pattern can be determined from the discrete curvatures obtained from the bending strains of 25 strain gauges mounted on a steel band with one end fixed and the other end free. Using this system, the abdominal deformation during impact can be measured in the form of time-history response.
(2) A surrogate abdominal material fitted for Hybrid III dummy has been found which has the same response characteristics as those of human abdomen at an impact speed of 6 m/s.

Nevertheless, the following items are required for improving TADAS:
(1) Our sensor cannot be used again when some plastic deformation of the steel band occurs. For the case when the bottoming of the sensor occurs, further improvement of the present sensor protector is necessary to prevent the bending fracture of the steel band near the fixed end.
(2) Further studies are needed to obtain abdominal materials having the same characteristics as those of human abdomen in a wide range of impact velocity. For this purpose, the characteristics of human abdomen must be further clarified.

In the future, to develop TADAS for practical use, it will be necessary to improve the system to include accurate measurements associated with steering wheels and seat belts.

REFERENCES

[1] Rouhana S.W., "Biomechanics of Abdominal Trauma," Accidental Injury: Biomechanics and Prevention, Springer-Verlag, pp.391-428, 1993.

[2] Eppinger R.H., Morgan R.M. and Marcus J.H., "Side Impact Data Analysis," Ninth International ESV Conference Proceedings, pp.244-250, 1982.

[3] Brun-Cassan F., Pincemaille Y., Mack P. and Tarriere C., "Contribution and Evaluation of Criteria Proposed for Thorax-Abdomen Protection in Lateral Impact," Eleventh International ESV Conference Proceedings, SAE 876040, pp. 289-301, 1987.

[4] Lau I.V., and Viano D.C., "How and When Blunt Injury Occurs - Implications of Frontal and Side Impact Protection," 32nd Stapp Car Crash Conference Proceedings, SAE 881714, 1988.

[5] Viano D.C., Lau I.V., Asbury C, King A.I. and Begeman P., "Biomechanics of the Human Chest Abdomen, and Pelvis in Lateral Impact", Proceedings of the 33rd Association for the Advancement of Automotive Medicine, pp. 367-382, 1989.

[6] Melvin J.W., Stalnaker R.L. and Roberts V.L. and Trollope M.L., "Impact Injury Mechanism in Abdominal Organs," 17th Stapp Car Crash Conference Proceedings, SAE 730968, pp.115-126, 1973.

[7] Stalnaker R.L., Roberts V.L. and McElhaney J.H., "Side Impact Tolerance to Blunt Trauma," 17th Stapp Car Crash Conference Proceedings, SAE 730979, pp.377-408, 1973.

[8] Miller M.A., "The Biomechanical Response of the Lower Abdomen to Belt Restraint Loading," J Trauma 29(11): 1571-1584, 1989.

[9] Rouhana S.W., Ridella S.A. and Viano D.C., "The Effect of Limiting Impact Force on Abdominal Injury: A Preliminary Study," 30th Stapp Car Crash Conference Proceedings, SAE 861879, pp. 65-79, 1986.

[10] Rouhana S.W., Lau I.V. and Ridella S.A., "Influence of Velocity and Forced compression on the Severity of Abdominal Injury in Blunt, Nonpenetrating Lateral Impact," GMR Research Publication No. 4763, 1984.

[11] Rouhana S.W., Lau I.V. and Ridella S.A., "Influence of Velocity and Forced compression on the Severity of Abdominal Injury in Blunt, Nonpenetrating Lateral Impact", J Trauma 25(6): 490-500.

[12] Viano D.C. and Lau I.V., "Thoracic Impact: A Viscous Tolerance Criteria", Tenth international

ESV Conference Proceedings, 1985.

[13] Cavanaugh J.M. Nyquist G.W., Goldberg S.J. and King A.I., "Lower Abdominal Tolerance and Response", 30th Stapp Car Crash Conference Proceedings, SAE 861878, pp.41-63, 1986.

[14] Nusholtz G.S., Kaiker P.S. and Lehman R.J., "Steering System Abdominal Impact Trauma," UMTRI Report No. 88-19, MVMA, 1988.

[15] Stalnaker R.L. and Ulman M.S., "Abdominal Trauma-Review, Response, and Criteria," 29th Stapp Car Crash Conference Proceedings, SAE 851720, pp.1-16, 1985.

[16] Walfisch G., Fayon A., Tarriere C., Rosey J.P., Guillon F., Got C., Patel A. and Stalnaker R.L., "Designing of a Dummy's Abdomen for Detecting Injuries in Side Impact Collision," Fifth International IRCOBI Conference Proceedings, pp.149-164, 1980.

[17] Schneider L.W., Rouhana S.W., Haffner M.P., Eppinger R.H., King A.I., Hardy W.H., Salloum M.J., Beebe M.S. and Neathery R.F., "Development of an Advanced ATD Thorax System for Improved Injury Assessment in Frontal Crash Environments," 36th Stapp Car Crash Conference Proceedings, SAE 922520, pp.129-155, 1992.

[18] Schneider L.W., Ricci M.J., Salloum M.J., Beebe M.S., King A.I., Rouhana S.W. and Neathery R.F. (in press), "Design and Development of an Advanced ATD Thorax system for Frontal Crash Environments, Volume 1: Primary Concept Development. Final report on NHTSA Contract No. DTNH22-83-C-07005. U.S. Department of Transportation, National Highway Traffic Safety Administration, Washington, D.C.

[19] Mooney M.T. and Collins J.A., "Abdominal Penetration Measurement Insert for the Hybrid III Dummy", SAE Technical Paper 860653, 1986.

[20] Rouhana S.W., Viano D.C., Jedrzejczak E.A., McCleary J.D., "Assessing Submarining and Abdominal Injury Risk in the Hybrid III Family of dummies," 33rd Stapp Car Crash Conference Proceedings, SAE 892440, pp.257-279, 1989.

[21] Eppinger R.H., "On the Development of a Deformation Measurement System and Its Application Toward Developing Mechanically Based Indices," 33rd Stapp Car Crash Conference Proceedings, SAE 892426, pp.21-28, 1989.

942226

Mathematical Modelling of the BioSID Dummy

Mark Fountain, Paul Altamore, and John Skarakis
Royal Melbourne Institute of Technology

Oliver Spiess
Technical University of Berlin

ABSTRACT

The objective of this work was to create mathematical models of the BioSID side impact test dummy, for use in side impact simulation studies. Two dummy models were created - a multibody model, and a finite element model. The models have been validated according to the procedures described in the BioSID User's Manual[1]. The responses of both models were within the required corridors for most of the specified calibration tests, and during these test conditions the behaviour of the models correlated well with physical dummies.

The models are now being tested in numerical side impact models of the vehicle. Each dummy model is particularly suited to different tasks: The multibody model is used in a lumped-mass model of the vehicle side structure, for studying the door padding and door intrusion characteristics. The finite element dummy model is implemented into finite element models of vehicles, allowing the vehicle-dummy interaction to be studied in much greater detail than is possible with physical testing or with lumped-mass models.

Both types of modelling technique have inherent advantages and disadvantages. Examples from the models are used to highlight these traits, and recommendations are made regarding techniques which will improve the ability of mathematical models to represent vehicle occupants.

INTRODUCTION

Passenger cars in Australia will soon be required to pass safety standards for both frontal and side collisions that they have previously not been required to satisfy. General Motors-Holden's Australia (GMH) and the Royal Melbourne Institute of Technology (RMIT) have therefore engaged in a three-year joint research project to improve the level of occupant protection in the GMH range of cars.

To achieve the highest possible levels of occupant protection during side impacts, GMH chose to develop their cars using the most realistic test conditions. Studies[2] have indicated that the BioSID is a more biofidelic dummy than the SID. For this reason it was selected for use in the development of the side impact protection systems at GMH.

The new safety standards create many new challenges for engineers and designers. Experimental testing alone will not be a practical way to achieve these goals. RMIT is utilising computer simulations to support the physical test programs conducted at GMH's Safety Test Laboratory. It is necessary to be able to accurately predict the response of the dummy during collisions if such simulations are to provide useful results. Representative mathematical models of the dummy are therefore required. However, such models of the BioSID dummy were not available. Therefore, GMH and RMIT developed a multibody model and a finite element model of the BioSID dummy.

RMIT had previously used separate programs for occupant modelling and for finite element structural modelling. The latest release of Madymo enables both finite element and multibody features to be combined in the same model, and this method was used to develop the dummy models. The ability to combine different types of models gives the user tremendous flexibility in the way models are constructed. For example, a multibody occupant model can now be combined with a finite element vehicle model, and vice-versa, within the same program. Also, structural models or occupant models can be constructed using a combination of the two techniques.

BioSID (Biofidelic Side Impact Dummy) was developed in 1989 because the International Standards Organisation judged that neither the SID nor the EUROSID were sufficiently biofidelic for the assessment of side impact safety[3]. The BioSID represents a fiftieth-percentile adult male during lateral impact conditions, and shows excellent biofidelity for responses of the head, neck, shoulder, thorax, and abdomen responses, and fair biofidelity for the arm and pelvis responses[4]. Currently, the BioSID is not specified for use in any side impact standards, and it is not certain if this situation will change[5]. Many organisations are using the BioSID for development purposes, and using the SID mainly for compliance testing. Perhaps it is for these reasons that there have been few mathematical models of the BioSID developed.

DESCRIPTION OF MODELS

MULTIBODY MODEL - The BioSID has several features that other side impact dummies do not have. For example, the BioSID has five ribs compared to three in the EuroSID. The multibody model was constructed to capture in the simplest possible way all of the features of the physical dummy. This meant that (usually) one rigid body was used to represent each distinct part of the dummy. This approach is consistent with most multibody dummy models, although a recent version of the EuroSID model released by TNO uses a more sophisticated method[6]. The BioSID model was made up of 25 rigid bodies, joined by a combination of Cardan Joints, Flexion-Torsion Joints, Revolute Joints, Bracket Joints, and Translational Joints. 33 ellipsoids were used to describe the shape and contact surfaces of the dummy. The model was created using MADYMO V5.0[7], and is shown in Figure 1.

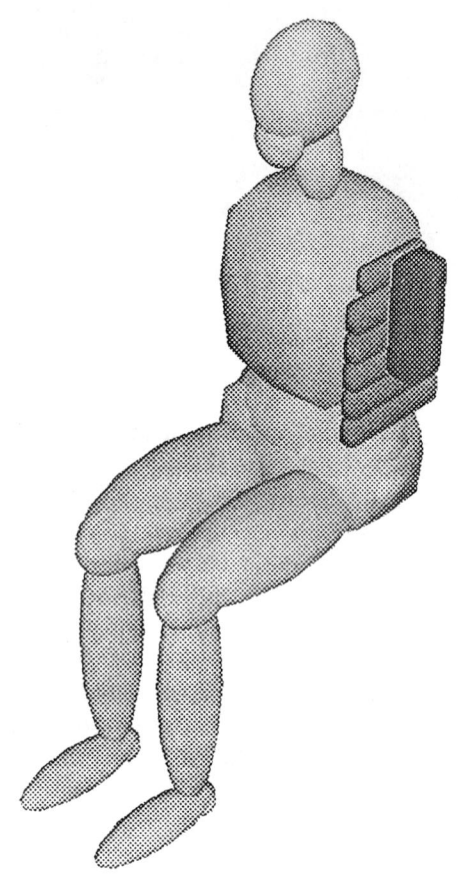

Figure 1. Multibody Model of BioSID Dummy

The spine box was represented by one rigid body. At the lower end, it was connected to the lumbar spine with a Flexion-Torsion Joint. At the top, the neck was connected using another Flexion-Torsion Joint. The shoulder, thoracic, and abdominal ribs were modelled as single rigid bodies, which were connected to the spine box using Translational Joints. The masses of each of these bodies were set equal to the total individual rib mass. Corrections were made during the data analysis to account for the inertial effects of mass distribution in the ribs of the physical dummy. Kelvin Elements were used to represent the non-linear stiffness and damping characteristics of the ribs. The non-linear response of the ribs was caused by the large rib deflections that are possible with the BioSID, and the addition of a damping material on the inside of the ribs. Figure 2 shows the BioSID ribset and a schematic representation of the multibody ribset model.

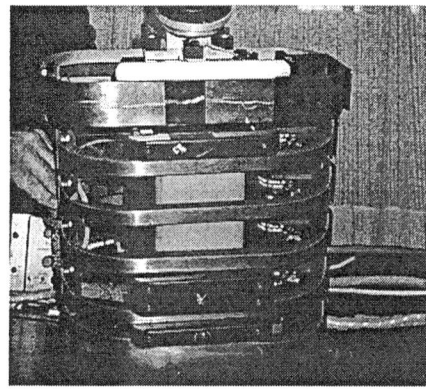

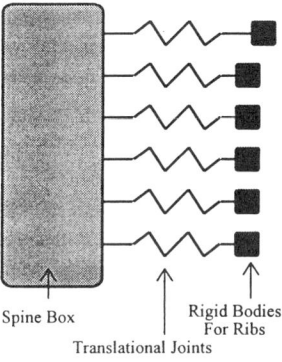

Figure 2. BioSID Ribset and Multibody Ribset Model.

The thoracic and abdominal ribs are covered with an Ensolite™ foam. This foam was represented by ellipsoids for which non-linear stiffness and damping functions were prescribed. The rib wrap foam is supported by a polyurethane backing sheet which, along with the foam, acts as a coupling between the ribs. Thus, even when there is an impact which does not cover the entire foam area, more than one rib can deflect. Kelvin Elements were used to represent the stiffness of this coupling.

The method of representing the ribs as single lumped masses was chosen because of its simplicity, and because the method has been proven to be suitable for modelling dummy rib structures[6]. The main limitation of this approach is that it will give accurate results only when the direction of impact is close to perpendicular to the dummy. During most test conditions this should not cause any serious problems. The ribs of the physical BioSID are guided so that they can only deflect by a significant amount in the lateral direction. However, it is possible that under certain impact conditions this modelling method will lead to inaccuracies.

The arm was represented by a single body, connected to the shoulder rib with a Revolute Joint. The shoulder plug was represented with one ellipsoid. Six ellipsoids were used to represent the arm. One ellipsoid represented the steel backing plate in the arm. There was one large ellipsoid which was used only for visualisation, and which had no effect on the model response. Four smaller ellipsoids represented the arm foam. The BioSID shoulder-arm assembly is shown in Figure 3, along with the multibody representation.

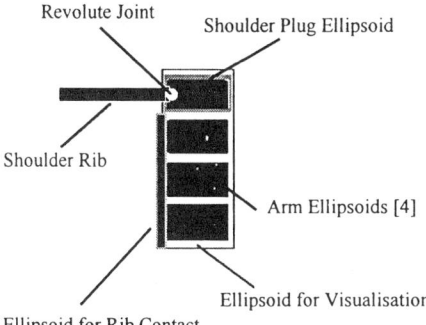

Figure 3. BioSID Shoulder-Arm Assembly and Multibody Model.

Initially only one ellipsoid was used to describe the arm foam, but this did not transfer the loads correctly when small impactors were used. The arm was tested using two, three and four ellipsoids to represent the foam, with four being required to correctly transfer the loads to the thoracic ribs and shoulder. This problem demonstrates one of the limitations of the rigid body method. The force-deflection characteristic that is specified is reliant upon the geometry of the impacting surface. If the impact conditions during a simulation are different to those used to develop the model, inaccuracies can occur.

The BioSID pelvis is constructed of a steel structure shaped to represent a human pelvis, with iliac wings, etc. This is covered with a vinyl skin. Located in line with the h-point are pelvis plugs, which are made of a crushable foam material, which must be replaced after each test. The pelvis assembly is shown in Figure 4. There are two possible load paths - through the pelvis plug, and through the iliac wings. The pelvis was modelled as a single rigid body, with one ellipsoid used to represent the pelvis "skin" (with the iliac wings beneath it), and one to represent the pelvis plug. In the current version of the model, all side loads are transferred through the pelvis plug ellipsoid. There is currently no capability to measure the pubic symphysis load or ilium load.

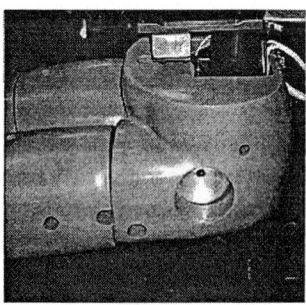

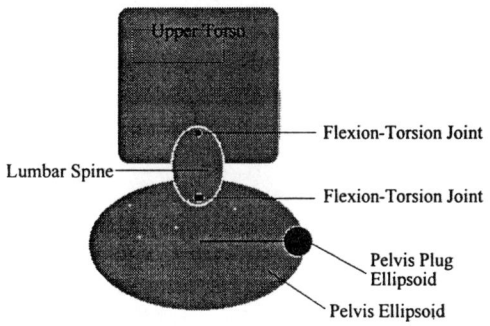

Figure 4. BioSID Pelvis and Multibody Model.

The head, neck, lower legs and feet of the BioSID are taken directly from the Hybrid III. This model used the head, neck, lower legs and feet from the MADYMO Advanced 50th percentile Hybrid III Dummy Database[6]. The upper legs were modelled as Hybrid III legs with different inertial properties.

Experimental Testing - The inertial properties of the components were obtained from a physical test program. Masses, moments of inertia, and principal axes of inertia were measured. The stiffness, damping, and hysteresis of the ribs, arm, pelvis, and rib foam were calculated from quasi-static and dynamic force-deflection data, obtained by testing with an MTS testing machine and with pendulum impacts. The response data for most parts was found by compressing the various parts with an impactor with controlled motion, at various speeds. The forces and displacements were recorded as functions of time. For the pendulum impacts, accelerations were also recorded. These tests were performed on individual dummy parts (such as individual ribs) and sub-systems (such as ribs covered with the foam). Velocity and acceleration time histories were found by differentiation and double-differentiation. The damping and inertial forces were then calculated by subtracting the quasi-static forces from the dynamic forces. The data were then de-coupled, i.e. the stiffness contribution of individual parts during coupled tests was identified, and extracted in a suitable form to be incorporated into the model. The data that were used in the model are included in the Appendix.

This procedure for obtaining the data for the model demonstrates one advantage of the lumped-mass modelling approach over finite element modelling. That is, because many of the deformable parts can be represented by specifying a force-deflection characteristic for a joint or contact surface, the experimental data can often be easily obtained, and without the need for destructive tests. This can be a distinct advantage when parts are expensive or difficult to obtain. However, it has also been shown that sometimes this approach is unsuitable, and experience is needed to select the appropriate method.

The test data are too extensive to be fully included in this paper, but Figure 5 shows an example of tests on the arm. A flat-faced impactor was used to compress the arm with a controlled motion at three different mean velocities. The peak deflection was identical in all tests. Figure 5 shows clearly the influence of the rate of deformation on the response.

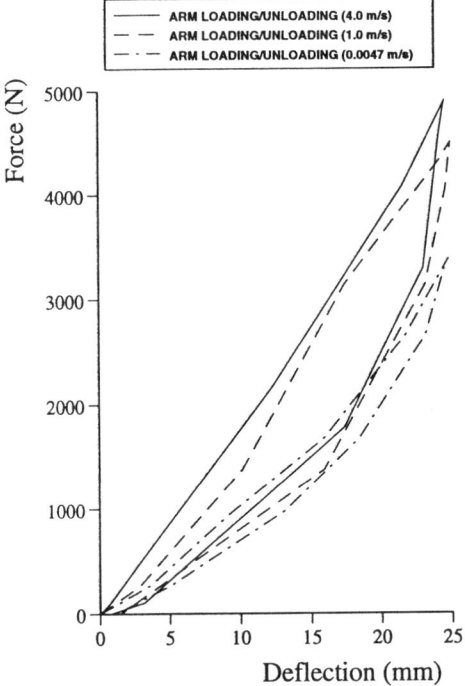

Figure 5: Results of Arm Compression Tests at Different Velocities.

The final step in the development procedure was to validate the model. Most of the validation process followed the requirements of the BioSID User's Manual, although various other impact tests were also performed. Results from the validation tests are presented in a later section.

FINITE ELEMENT MODEL - The explicit finite element code MSC/DYNA[8] was used for the initial development work of the finite element model. With the addition of full finite element capability to Madymo V5.1, the development proceeded in Madymo, and DYNA was no longer used. The reasons for this are discussed in detail in a later section, however the main reasons were the ease of modelling, and the flexibility of being able to combine multibody methods and finite element methods in the same program. Unless otherwise stated, the following discussion describes the modelling process used to create the model in Madymo.

The multibody model (described above) was simplified by the removal of the bodies which represented the ribs, shoulder, and arm foam. This left the pelvis, lumbar spine, spine box, arm backing-plate, neck, head, legs and feet as the remaining rigid bodies. Finite element meshes of the arm, shoulder plug, shoulder rib, rib foam, and abdominal and thoracic ribs were created, and joined with the rest of the model. Four-node shell elements were used to represent the rib steel. The rib damping material, the arm foam, the rib foam, and the shoulder plug were modelled with 8-node solid elements. There were 736 shell elements and 944 solid elements used in the model, in addition to the rigid bodies. The finite element model is shown in Figure 6.

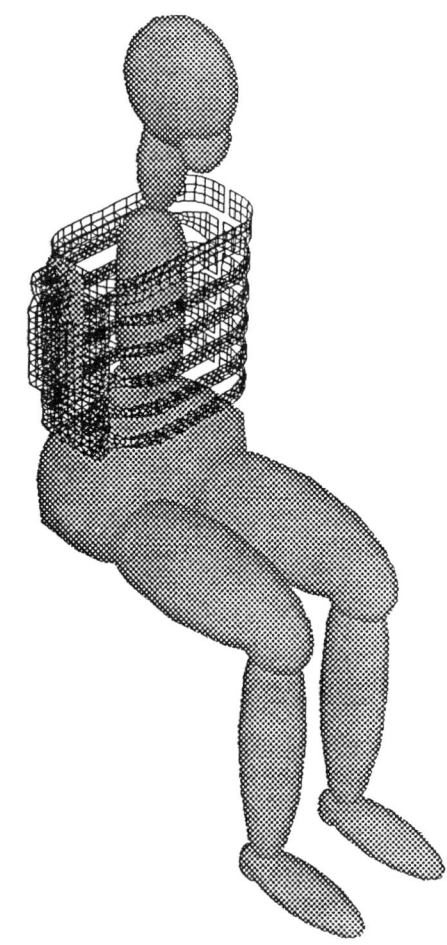

Figure 6. Finite Element BioSID Model
<u>Experimental Tests and Component Modelling</u>
- Only the behaviour of the components were required for the multibody model, but for the finite element model materials properties had to

be obtained. Therefore, in addition to the component tests which were completed as part of the multibody model development, experimental tests were performed to determine the material properties of the rib foam, rib damping material, arm foam, and shoulder plug. Table 1 lists these tests.

TABLE 1. Experimental Tests for F. E. Model

Component/ Material	Test Performed
Shoulder Plug	Quasi-Static Compression
	Dynamic Compression
Rib Foam	Quasi-Static Compression
	Pendulum Impact - 3 m/s and 5 m/s
	Hydrostatic Compression
Shoulder Rib	Pendulum Impact - 3 m/s and 5 m/s
Rib Damping Material	Quasi-Static Tensile Stress-Strain
	Dynamic Tensile Stress-Strain
Arm	Quasi-Static Compression
	Pendulum Impact - 3 m/s and 5 m/s

In some cases the material properties had to be determined from component testing, because of the destructive nature of the tests. Information from the literature[9,10,11] shows large discrepancies in the properties of many materials. It is thought that two main reasons contribute to this. Firstly, it is difficult to select the most suitable material model for items such as foams, etc., until some material tests have been completed and the behaviour is understood. Secondly, the transient nature of the events being simulated usually requires that the material properties include dynamic effects. This can make experiments extremely difficult to perform, so the behaviour is often approximated using quasi-static test data.

Each of the individual component models were validated separately, before performing the calibration tests on the complete dummy. Separate finite element models were created for each of the individual parts, which were then used to validate the material properties, and to assess the suitability of the selected material models, the mesh discretisation, etc. Two examples are presented which demonstrate some aspects of material model selection and validation of the model.

Figure 7 compares the results of a rib foam impact test with the finite element model, using two different material models. In this test the foam was placed on a flat surface, and impacted with a flat-faced pendulum, which covered the entire foam area. DYNA was used for these simulations. Both a viscoelastic model and an elastic-plastic material model compared well with experimental results, although the viscoelastic model overestimated the penetration of the impactor. Although the foam does not actually behave as an elastic-plastic material (i.e. it does not permanently deform during the test) several dummy models[9] use elastic-plastic materials to represent the foam, and with good effect.

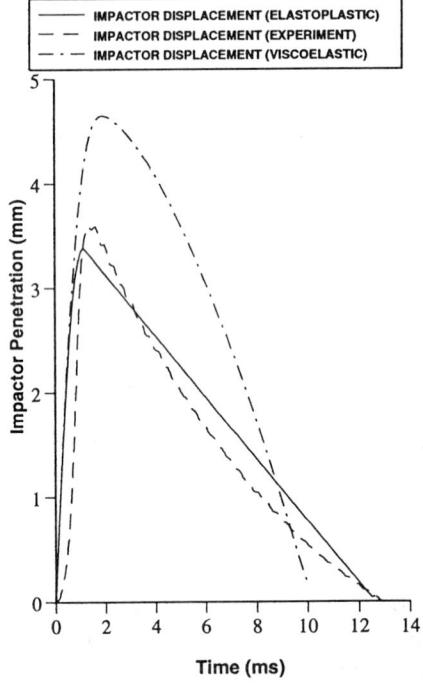

Figure 7. Foam Impact Test Experimental and Simulation Results

A "hysteresis" material model is available in Madymo which allows the user to specify non-linear stress-strain relationships for a material. Different curves can be specified for loading and unloading, thus taking account of hysteresis and energy loss. This material model was used in the final version of the dummy model. It appears to be well suited for modelling elastomeric foams, although strain rate effects are not included.

Figure 8 compares the influence of the rib damping material on the response of the shoulder rib and the thoracic/abdominal rib. The model simulated pendulum impacts to the end of the shoulder rib and abdominal/thoracic rib, where the foam is normally attached. A viscoelastic material was used to describe the rib damping material. In both simulations, the shear moduli of the damping material was varied by an order of magnitude. The response of the shoulder rib was controlled almost totally by the rib steel, and the damping material has very little influence. The abdominal rib response was highly sensitive to the rib damping material. It is therefore inappropriate to use only the shoulder rib for validation of the ribset model.

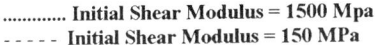
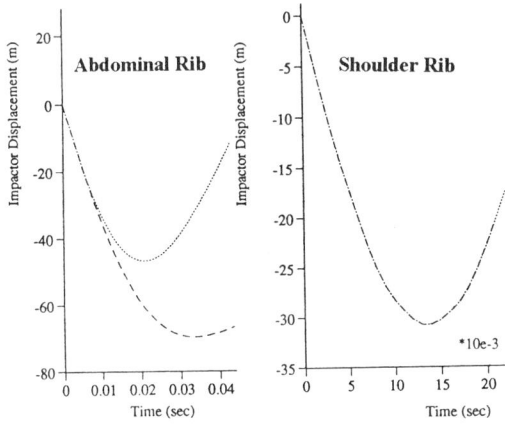

Figure 8. Influence of Rib Damping Material on Response of Shoulder and Abdominal Ribs

A linear elastic material model could also be used for the rib damping material, with reasonable results, but the response was more realistic when a viscoelastic material model was used. A viscoelastic material was not available in Madymo V5.1, so an Eulerian/Maxwell viscoelastic material model for solid elements was implemented by the authors. This model assumes that the volumetric behaviour is linear and the deviatoric behaviour is viscoelastic. The bulk modulus is therefore defined by a constant value, and the shear modulus is defined by an exponential curve that decays as a function of time. The implementation and validation of this material model are discussed in detail in reference [12].

After the material models were finalised, and each component had been validated, the material properties were incorporated into the complete dummy model. Final validation tests were performed on the complete dummy model, according to the requirements of the BioSID User's Manual. The material models and material properties used in the final model are listed in the Appendix.

CALIBRATION TEST RESULTS

MULTIBODY MODEL - The BioSID User's Manual specifies pendulum impacts to the shoulder, pelvis, arm, abdomen, and thorax of the assembled dummy, and defines corridors for the dummy responses. The responses of the models were compared to the specified corridors, and to the responses of physical dummies. The complete test results are too numerous to be included here. Time histories comparing the responses from the model, the specified corridors, and a physical dummy are shown for the pelvis, shoulder, and abdomen impact tests. All responses fell within International Standards Organisation corridors for biomechanical response, and most were also within the BioSID calibration corridors. The results for the pelvis, shoulder, and abdomen tests are shown in Figures 9, 10, and 11, respectively. The level of correlation between the model and the physical dummy shown in these figures is also typical of the responses during the other impact tests. Figure 12 shows the kinematics of the multibody model during the abdomen impact test.

FINITE ELEMENT MODEL - The calibration test results for the finite element model are shown in Figures 13 and 14. As for the multibody model, time histories comparing the responses from the model, the specified corridors, and a physical dummy are shown for the shoulder and abdomen impact tests. The pelvis was the same in both models.

RIGID-BODY BioSID CALIBRATION TEST

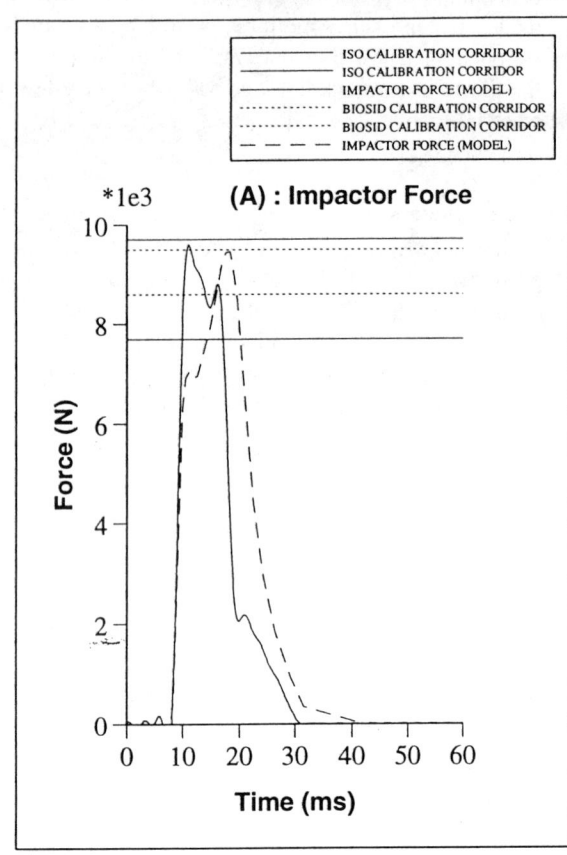
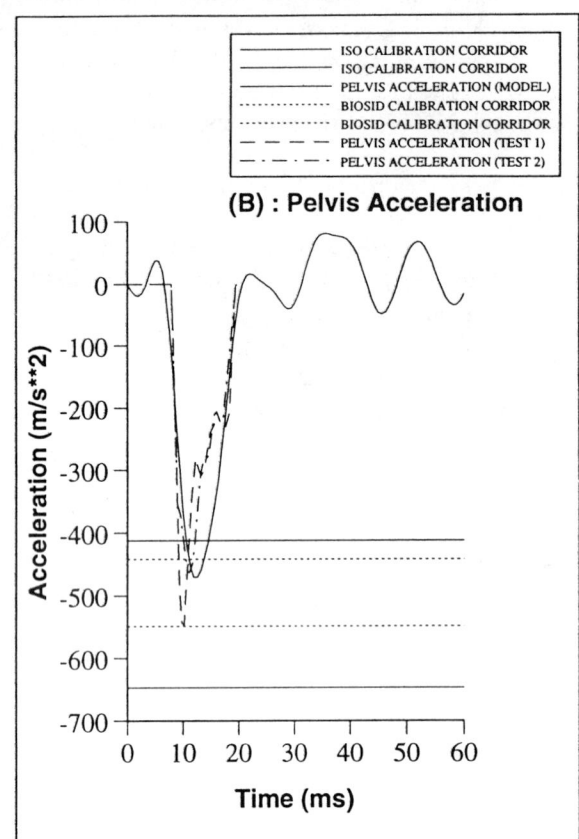

FIGURE 9 : PELVIC IMPACT

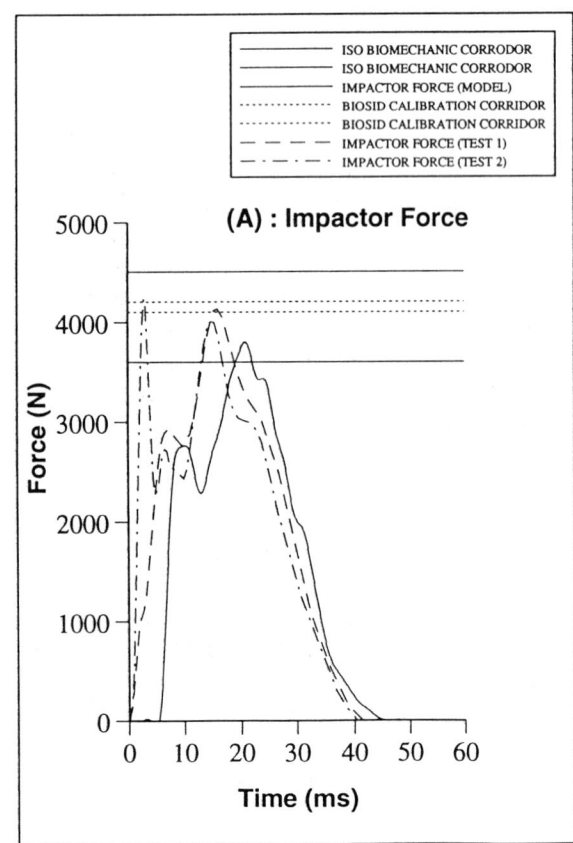
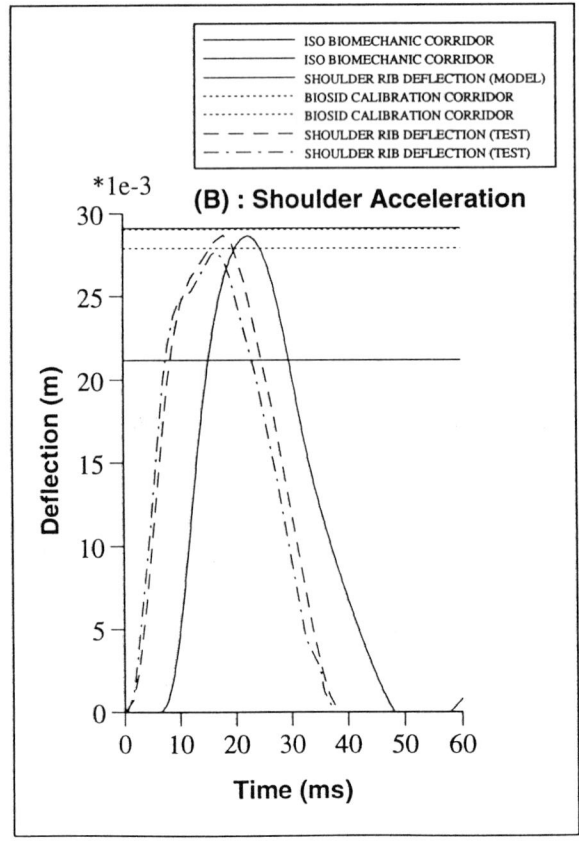

FIGURE 10 : SHOULDER IMPACT

RIGID-BODY BioSID VALIDATION TEST

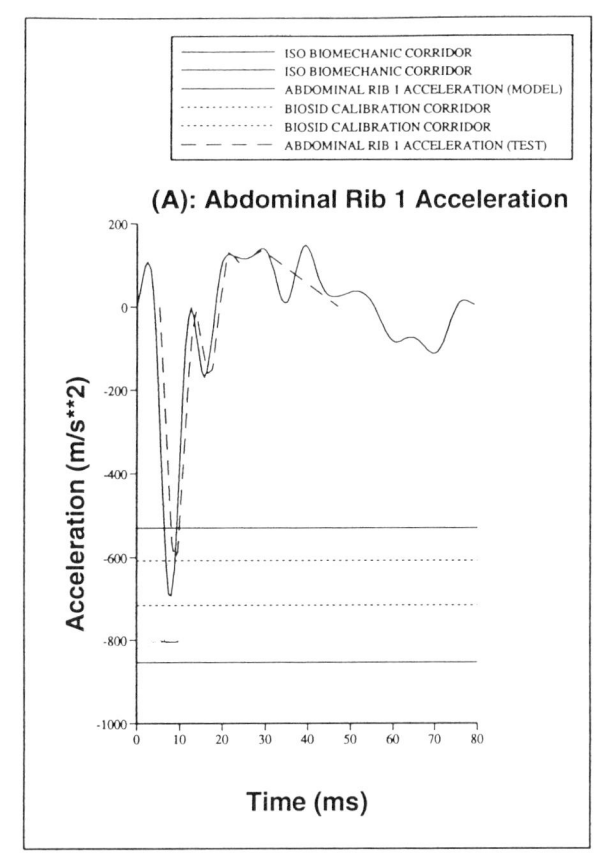
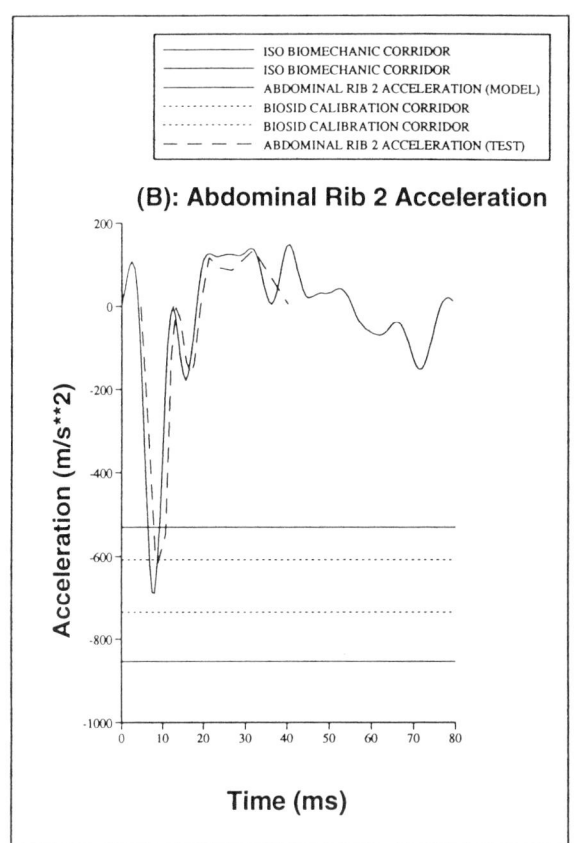
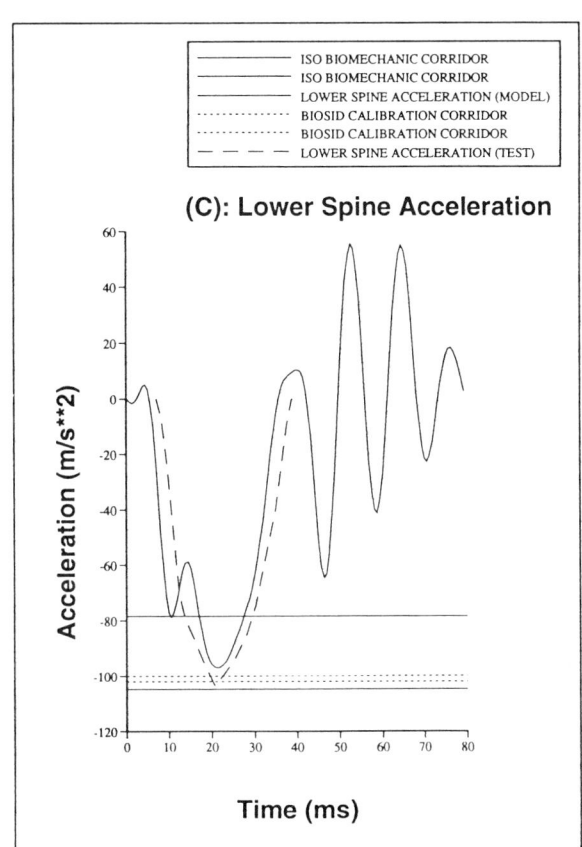
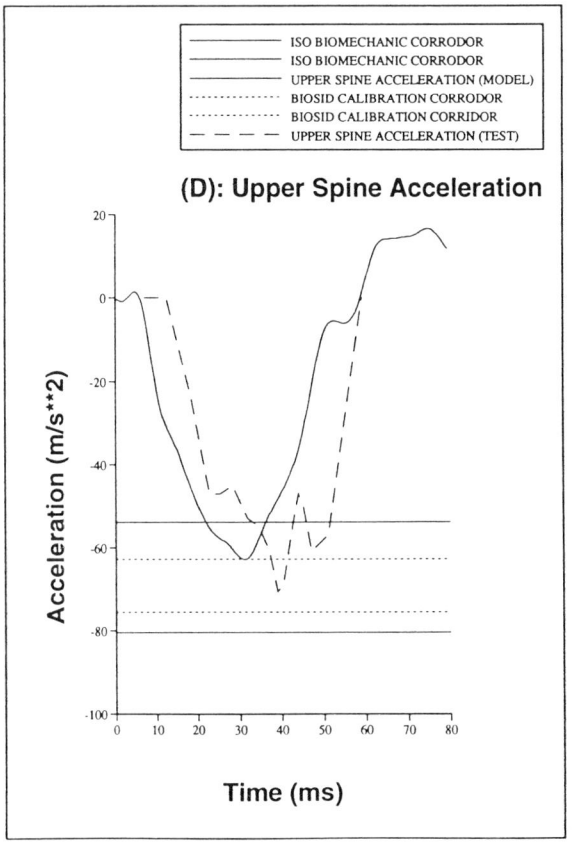

FIGURE 11 - ABDOMINAL IMPACT

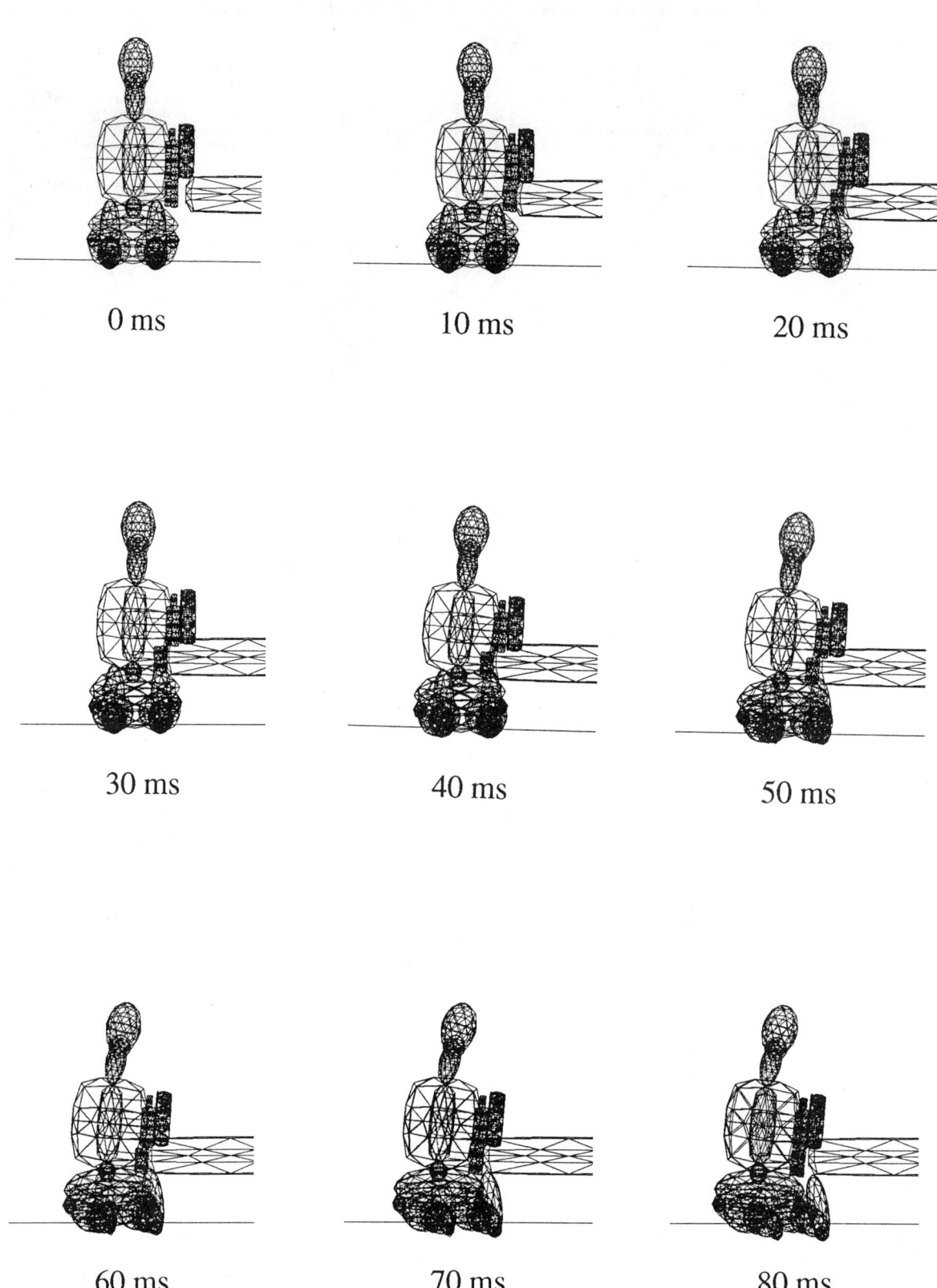

Figure 12. Kinematics of Multibody Model During Abdominal Impact Test.

FEM BioSID CALIBRATION TEST

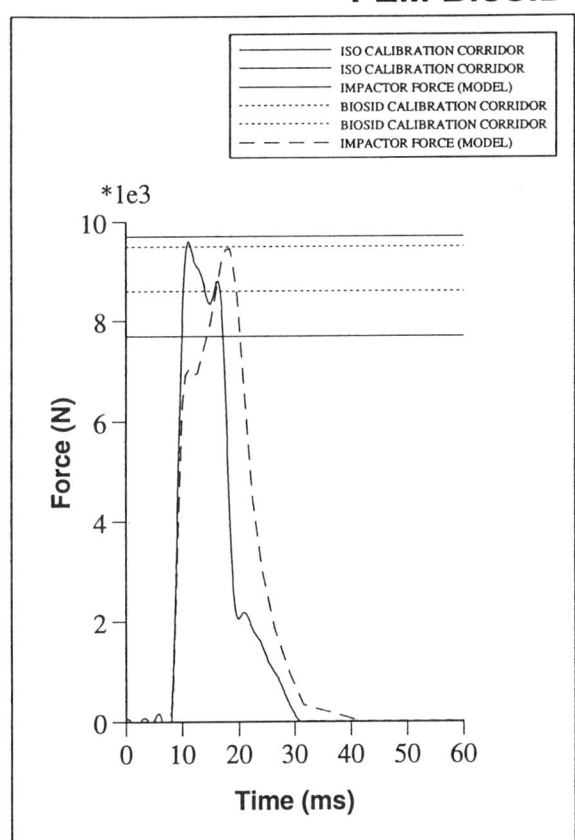
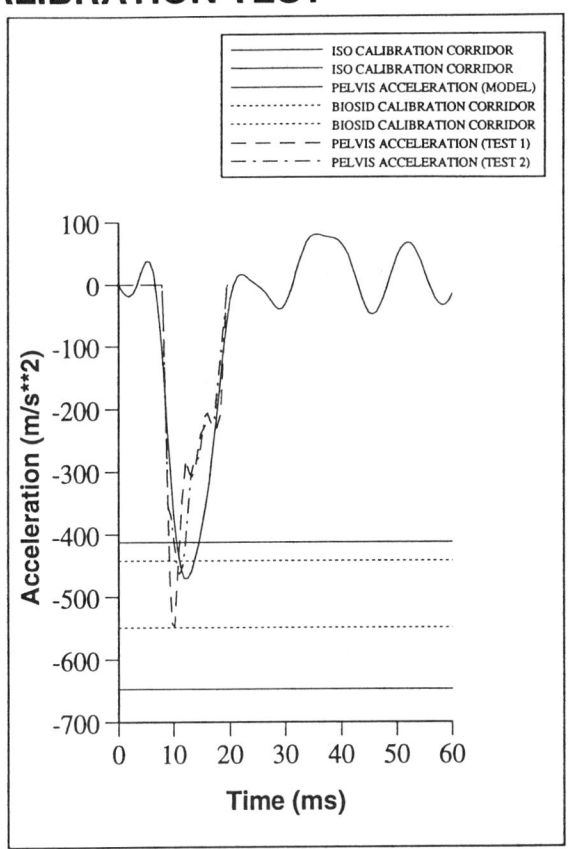

FIGURE 13 : ABDOMINAL RIB IMPACT

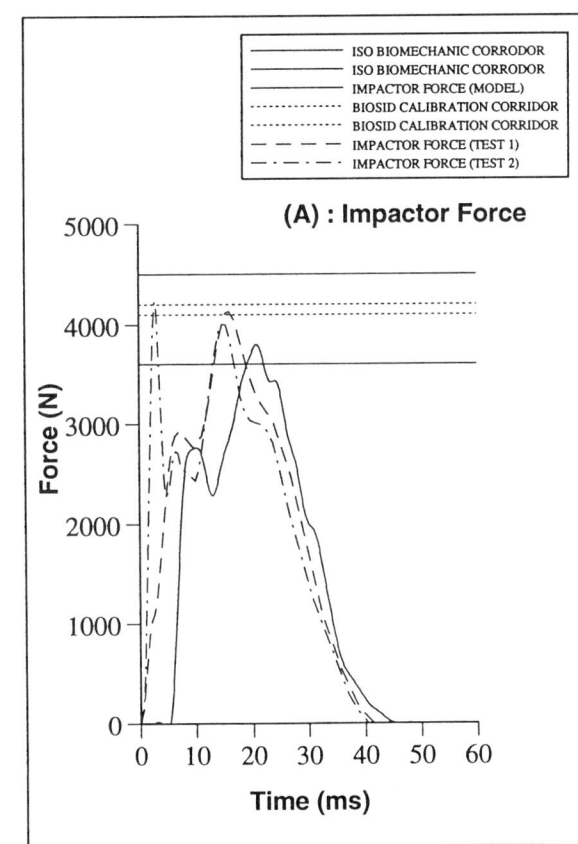
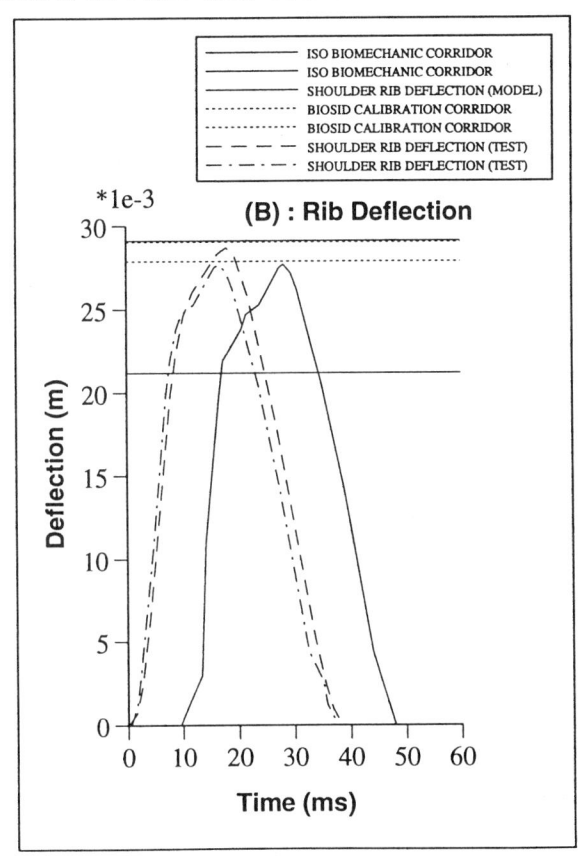

FIGURE 14 : SHOULDER IMPACT

DISCUSSION

Both the multibody model and the finite element model are representative of physical dummies in the specified test conditions. They are now being used to simulate full-scale collisions, to provide more feedback about the performance in different impact conditions. This is a necessary step, because the test conditions that have been used thus far in the validation process are not broad enough to allow total confidence in the models in all impact situations.

Modelling the finite element dummy in DYNA required considerably more effort than in Madymo, particularly with respect to specifying the rigid bodies, kinematic connections, and contact surfaces. For example, to define a rigid body in DYNA the body must first be meshed using finite-elements, and then assigned a rigid material property. Further, these rigid bodies are in general not suitable where contact occurs because nonlinear stiffness or damping cannot be specified for the contact surface. When modelling in DYNA, the pelvis response could not be captured using rigid bodies only, and a finite element "skin" with non-linear material properties had to be placed over the rigid body. This was simply extra modelling effort, and did not return better results or extra information.

The finite element models required much more modelling effort and far greater computing power than did the multibody model. There were many difficulties in obtaining adequate experimental data for the material properties for the rib foam and arm foam. The advantages of the finite element model were not demonstrated during the test conditions that were used to develop the model. These advantages include, potentially, more accurate responses in a wider range of impact conditions, and more information about the interaction with the impacting structures. The multibody model was simpler to develop, with very little processing time needed. However, using rigid multibodies to represent highly deformable contact surfaces did not give accurate results over a wide range of impact conditions. This may be improved by using flexible multibody methods[13], or multiple rigid bodies connected with joints. However, flexible multibody methods can not yet include large strain effects and using multiple rigid bodies may not satisfactorily solve the problems with the contact surfaces.

CONCLUSION

A three dimensional multibody model and a finite element model of the BioSID side impact dummy have been developed. The models have been validated according to the procedures set out in the BioSID User's Manual, and the behaviour of the models correlated well with physical dummies during these test conditions.

For meaningful assessments of vehicle crashworthiness to be made, numerical crash simulations must be able to accurately predict the response of occupants during collisions. The development of improved occupant models should therefore be seen as a priority. Perhaps the most important consideration when developing occupant models is the choice of modelling technique.

In this paper, a rigid multibody and a finite element model of the BioSID dummy have been presented and compared. Both models have advantages and disadvantages which cannot be ignored. The experience of the authors in developing these models has made it clear that it is a tremendous advantage to be able to combine multibody and finite element methods in the same program, because the respective advantages of the techniques can be utilised to maximum effect.

ACKNOWLEDGMENTS

This work was funded by the Australian Research Council and General Motor's-Holdens Australia, as a part of the Collaborative Research Grant "Reduction of Injuries in Automobile Accidents". The inertial properties and some of the component test data was supplied by Mr. Galen Ressler, General Motors Side Impact Safety Centre. Thanks go to Mr. Henk Lupker and Mr. Erwin Poeze, both from TNO Road-Vehicles Research Institute, for supplying the subroutines which allowed the user-defined materials to be implemented.

REFERENCES

1 Society of Automotive Engineers, Warrendale, PA. "User's Manual for the BioSID Side Impact Test Dummy." SAE Engineering AID 24.

2 Beebe, M. "What is BioSID". SAE 900377, Society of Automotive Engineers, Warrendale, PA

3 Irwin, A. et.al. "Comparison of the EUROSID and SID Impact Responses to the Response Corridors of the International Standards Organisation". SAE 890604.

4 Beebe, M. "BioSID Update and Calibration Requirements". SAE 901319, Society of Automotive Engineers, Warrendale, PA

5 Eppinger, R. Personal Communication. 1993.

6 TNO Road-Vehicles Research Institute, "Madymo Database Manual, Version 5.0". 1990.

7 TNO Road-Vehicles Research Institute, "Madymo Users Manual, Version 5.0". 1990.

8 MSC Corporation, "MSC/DYNA User's Manual, Version 3." 1992.

9 Lasry, et.al. "Mathematical Modelling of the Hybrid III Dummy Chest with Chest Foam." SAE 912892 Society of Automotive Engineers, Warrendale, PA

10 Khalil, T. " Hybrid III thoracic Impact on Self-Aligning Steering Wheel by Finite Element Analysis and Mini-Sled Experiment." SAE 912894, Society of Automotive Engineers, Warrendale, PA

11 Khalil, T. Personal Communication, 1993.

12 Altamore, P., Fountain, M. "The Modelling of Viscoelastic Solid Continua using Madymo V5.1". Proceedings of the Fifth International Madymo User's Conference. November, 1994. To Appear.

13 Koppens, W. et.al. "Comparison of modeling Techniques for Flexible Dummy Parts". Proceedings of the 37th STAPP Car Crash Conference, 1993.

14 Pipkorn, B. "A 2D MADYMO BIOSID Dummy." Proceedings of the 3rd International MADYMO Users' Meeting, 1992.

15 MSC Corporation, "MSC/NASTRAN User's Manual, Version 67." 1991.

16 Mecalog SARL "RADIOSS CRASH User's Manual, Version 2.1.6". Les Ulis, France, 1992.

17 Fountain, M., Spiess, O. "The Development of a BioSID Dummy Model Using MADYMO". Research Report for General Motors-Holden's Australia. October 1993

18 Livermore Software. "LS-DYNA 3D User's Manual." 1992.

19 PDA Engineering "P3/PATRAN User's Manual, Version 1.2" 1993.

20 Brujis, W. "Coupled MADYMO-FEM Simulations for the BIOSID Dummy." Proceedings of the 3rd International MADYMO Users' Meeting, 1992.

APPENDIX

MULTIBODY MODEL INPUT DATA - Complete test results are too numerous to be included in this paper. The properties used as input for the models are included here. Table A1 lists the inertial properties of the parts which are unique to the BioSID. Figures A1-A4 show the force-penetration characteristics used for the contact surfaces.

TABLE A1. Inertial Properties Used For Multibody Model

Part	Mass (kg)	Ixx (kg-m^2)*	Iyy (kg-m^2)*	Izz (kg-m^2)*
Pelvis	20.98	0.228	0.203	0.181
Spine Box	19.50	0.216	0.193	0.140
Thoracic Rib	0.645	0.0051	0.0088	0.014
Shoulder Rib	1.485	0.0072	0.0218	0.286
Arm	1.19	0.0035	0.0038	0.0003
Femur	5.59	0.013	0.074	0.074

*Note: All moments of inertia are defined about the centre of gravity of the segment. The x-x axis is defined as the axes which runs from the rear to the front of the dummy (as shown in Figure 1). The y-y axes runs laterally, from left to right. The z-z axis is the vertical axis.

MATERIAL PROPERTIES FOR FINITE ELEMENT MODEL - The material models and material properties used for the finite element dummy are shown in Table A2.

Table A2. Material Properties used in Finite Element Model

Part	Material	Properties
Rib Steel	Linear Elastic	E = 210 GPa ν = 0.3
Rib Damping Material	Viscoelastic	K = 1.01 GPa G_0 = 105 MPa G_∞ = 5.0 MPa β = 1.5s
Rib Foam	Hysteresis	Strain vs. Stress (MPa) Loading Unloading 0.000 0.000 0.000 0.000 0.129 0.108 0.246 0.108 0.350 0.323 0.350 0.155 0.388 0.431 0.391 0.323 0.413 0.539 0.418 0.431 0.429 0.646 0.425 0.539
Arm Foam	Hysteresis	Strain vs. Stress (Mpa) Loading Unloading 0.000 0.000 0.000 0.000 0.095 0.047 0.128 0.000 0.209 0.069 0.268 0.035 0.326 0.099 0.338 0.088 0.350 0.362 0.350 0.200
Shoulder Plug	Linear Elastic	E = 1 MPa ν = 0.495

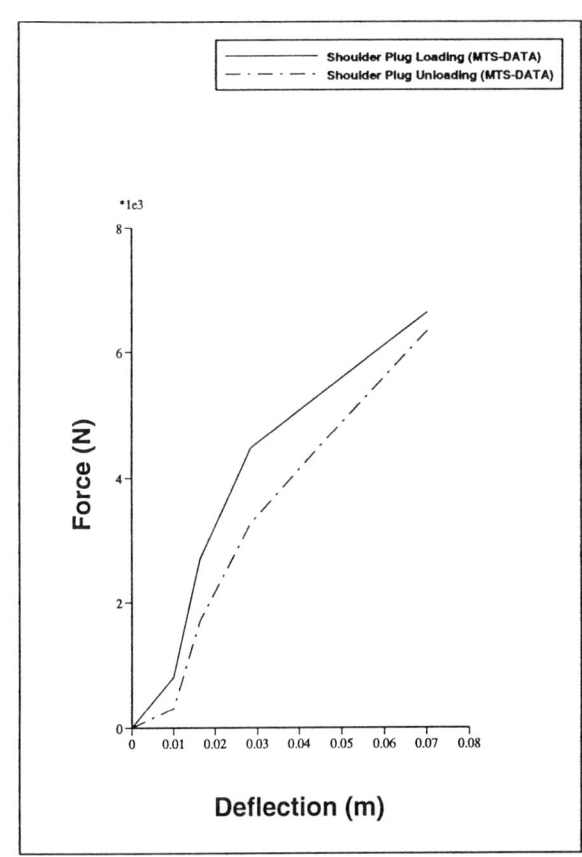

Figure A1 : Shoulder Plug Test Data

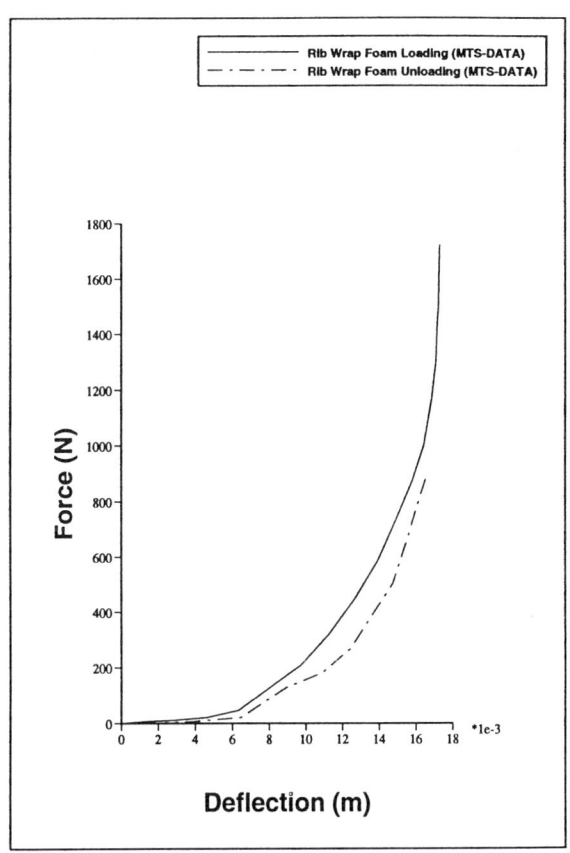

Figure A2 : Rib Wrap Foam Test Data

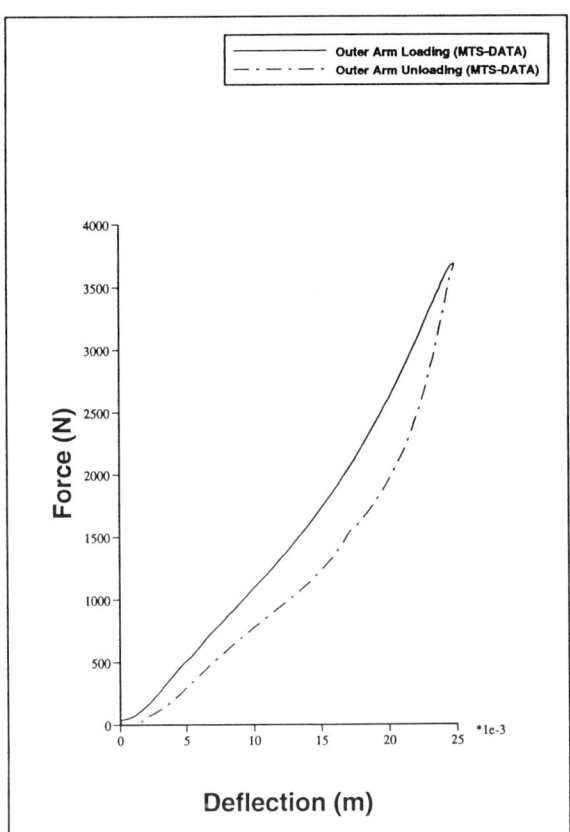

Figure A3 : Arm Test Data

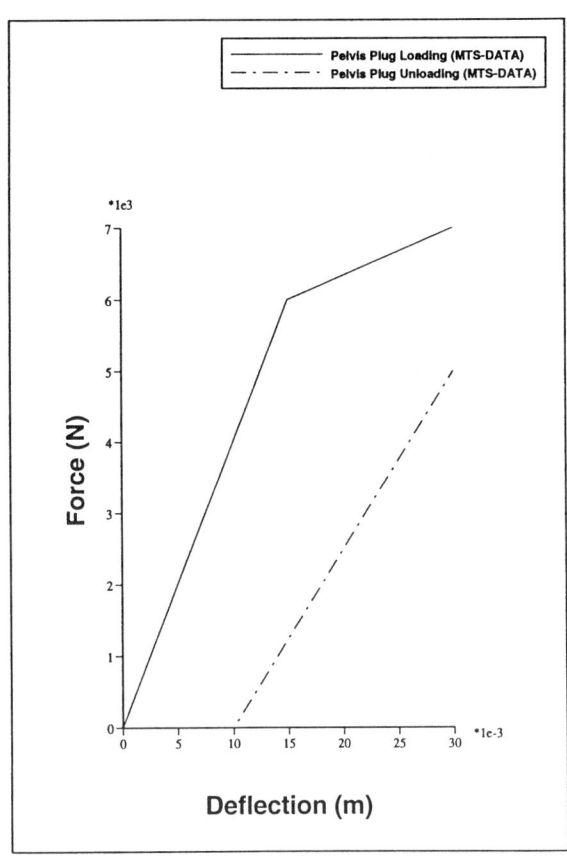

Figure A4 : Pelvis Plug Test Data

942227

Simulation of the Hybrid III Dummy Response to Impact by Nonlinear Finite Element Analysis

T. B. Khalil and T. C. Lin
General Motors Corporation

ABSTRACT

The Hybrid III dummy is an anthropomorphic (humanlike) test device, generally used in crashworthiness testing to assess the extent of occupant protection provided by the vehicle structure and its restraint systems in the event of vehicle crash. Lumped-parameter analytical models are commonly used to simulate the dummy response. These models, by virtue of their limited number of degrees of freedom, can neither represent accurate three-dimensional dummy geometry nor detailed structural deformations. In an effort to improve the state-of-the-art in analytical dummy simulations, a set of finite element models of the Hybrid III dummy segments - head, neck, thorax, spine, pelvis, knee, upper extremities and lower extremities - were developed. The component models replicated the hardware geometry as closely as possible. Appropriate elastic material models were selected for the dummy "skeleton", with the exterior "soft tissues" represented by viscoelastic materials. The impact response of each individual component was determined by explicit integration finite element analysis.

Subsequently, a whole dummy model was assembled from the various segments with appropriate joint characteristics prescribed to allow for dummy articulation. Finally, the thoracic impact force-deformation response was calculated from a ballistic impactor with a mass of 23.4 kg, launched from 2 initial velocities of 6.71 m/s and 4.3 m/s, respectively. The predicted response was compared with standard dummy and human cadavers experimental data. In all calculations, the model response compared favorably with experimental data, and provided a reasonable level of confidence of the model biofidelity.

Introduction

The Hybrid III dummy is an assemblage of mechanical components designed and manufactured to replicate the human body structural response when subjected to mechanical impact, primarily in the midsagittal plane. It is commonly used in the design of restraint systems, ejection seats and in crashworthiness of automobile structures to assess the potential for human harm, should a vehicle crash occur. Also, the dummy is used to certify the vehicle performance in frontal impact with a rigid barrier. Currently there are three dummy sizes developed to represent the midsagittal impact response of the adult population: 5th-percentile female (small), 50th-percentile male (average) and 95th-percentile male (large). The 50th-percentile dummy was developed first with its physical characteristics - height, weight, size, mass distribution, joint locations, etc. - selected to closely match the median of the U.S. adult male population. The other two dummies were derived from the 50th-percentile by geometric scaling [1].

The 50th-percentile dummy was developed at General Motors in the early 1970's [2]. Steel and aluminum components were used to represent human bones, so that the dummy can be used in repetitive testing without damage. The metallic "skeleton" is covered with pliable vinyl skin to give the dummy a reasonable human look and feel. The material properties of the exterior "soft tissues" encapsulating the various dummy "organs", head, neck, thorax, lumbar spine, knees and articulating joints were selected and tuned, so that their responses match human cadaver response when subjected to midsagittal impact loads. Several transducers are strategically located within the dummy, providing 34 channels of data [3] to monitor the dummy kinematics and associated loads and moments

Although the dummy was developed in the early 1970's, it was not accepted by the National Highway Traffic Safety Administration (NHTSA) for use in compliance testing with FMVSS 208 [4] for passive restraints until 1986. Currently, the Hybrid III dummy is widely used in automotive crash testing when the vehicle is subjected to frontal or oblique impact. The most common test is the vehicle compliance impact test with FMVSS 208, where the vehicle is launched from 30 m.p.h. into a rigid barrier. In the test, the dummy kinematics and exerted loads are monitored and compared with established biomechanical human tolerance data. The vehicle crashworthiness is measured by its structural integrity together with its ability to manage the crash energy so that a properly restrained occupant can achieve a high level of protection.

Vehicle crashworthiness is typically achieved by a combination of crash experiments and analytical models. Crashworthiness experiments, particularly when prototype vehicles are used, are extremely expensive. In today's competitive environment, mathematical modeling has been steadily gaining momentum, and it has been quite effective in shortening the design cycle, improving product quality and reducing cost.

This paper is concerned with the development and validation of a detailed FE model of the Hybrid III dummy. The model development initially focused on geometric model building and comparing the impact response of the primary dummy segments - head, neck, thorax, lumbar spine and knee - with corresponding experimental data. Then, all of the dummy segments were assembled with appropriate descriptions of joint characteristics to simulate articulation and relative motion among the various segments. Finally, the assembled dummy, while in a seated position, was subjected

to a ballistic pendulum impact on the thorax and the whole dummy response was compared with a standard test used in dummy calibration. The developed model can enhance our capabilities in:
1. further understanding of the dummy biofidelity and its sensitivity to impact loads of various severities and directions beyond the midsagittal plane;
2. simulations of interactions and calculation of contact loads between restraint systems (air bag, three point belts and knee bolster) and an occupant in typical crash environments;
3. integration with a vehicle structure to develop a vehicle-occupant system model that can be used in crashworthiness studies to assess how variations in vehicle structure can influence the occupant response;
4. advancing the state-of-the-art in dummy development, particularly for nonstandard anthropometry.

Dummy Description

The 50th-percentile Hybrid III dummy (Figure 1), commonly known as an Anthropomorphic (humanlike) Test Device (ATD), represents state-of-the-art in biofidelic impact response in the midsagittal plane. Although the dummy geometry is based on human anthropometric measurements, and its component or subassembly responses closely match human cadaver responses, it does not necessarily behave like a human. In fact its "skeleton" is nonfrangible, constructed from metallic components (steel and aluminum) which provide sufficient durability and maintainability necessary for repetitive use of the device. But the device response can provide sufficient information to enable the prediction of actual human kinematics and joint loads (and/or moments) in dynamic load environments.

The dummy segmentation closely resembles an anatomically based segmentation scheme, so that the subassembly weight and center of gravity location can be easily checked and compared with corresponding human data. The main segments comprising the dummy are described below:

<u>**Head**</u> - The head consists of a hollow cast aluminum, thick shell with uniform thickness which approximates the exterior skull geometry. The occipital portion of the shell is removable to allow for mounting and servicing an accelerometer package located within the shell interior. The aluminum shell is covered with a vinyl skin that closely adheres to the skull to prevent the skin from slipping relative to the skull. The skin's physical properties and thickness were "tuned" to assure similar impact response on a rigid surface, with corresponding cadaver head experiments [5]. The head assembly is instrumented with a triaxial accelerometer, located at the head center of gravity, to monitor its three-dimensional translational acceleration response.

<u>**Neck**</u> - The neck consists of four polymeric, nonsymmetric discs, which are geometrically shaped, including a horizontal slit in the anterior part to provide appropriate flexion-extension kinematics, similar to human cadaver response. The polymeric neck segments are sandwiched between aluminum discs to provide the neck with the necessary structural stiffness. A flexible steel cord is inserted along the neck axis to provide tensile strength. The neck top plate is connected to the head by a pin joint to simulate head rotation about a lateral axis through the occipital condyles. The neck lower part is a serrated bracket that attaches to the thoracic spine box via an adjustable joint to maintain the base plane of the head horizontal, or as demanded by the seating configuration.

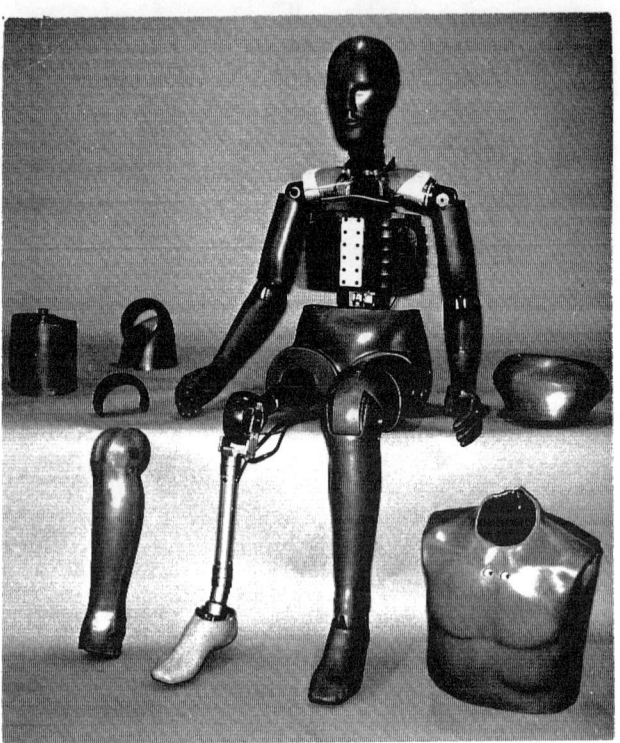

Figure 1. Hybrid III Dummy Interior and Exterior Components

<u>**Shoulders**</u> - The shoulders assembly, consists of cast aluminum articulated linkages between the spine and the upper arms. Rubber blocks, pivots and bushings are inserted among the various parts to allow for flexibility and prevent metal-to-metal contact. The structure is designed to allow for weight control and durability. The whole assembly is contoured to provide a good shoulder-to-belt fit and to provide a realistic setting for 3-point harness evaluation.

<u>**Thorax**</u> - The thorax assembly, consists of six spring steel ribs lined with a damping material along the lateral sides of its interior surface to provide a viscoelastic/damped response. The ribs are connected at the back to a "thoracic spine", manufactured from welded steel plates which resembles a hollow box beam structure. An adjustable bracket is mounted at the top of the steel box to provide support for the neck. An inclined steel plate is mounted at the bottom of the thoracic spine which attaches to the "lumbar spine". The ribs are attached at the front to a plexiglass plate to simulate a "sternum". The thorax assembly is covered with a removable vinyl jacket, with a soft foam pad inserted at the sternum plate. A triaxial accelerometer transducer resides within the thoracic spine, approximately at the assembly's center of gravity, to monitor its three-dimensional acceleration. In addition a displacement transducer is mounted between the sternum and the thoracic spine to measure the chest compression in the midsagittal plane.

<u>**Lumbar Spine**</u> - The lumbar spine is a thick curved cylindrical member, manufactured from stiff "polyacrylate

elastomer" rubber, to provide for a realistic human posture in a car seated position. Two flexible steel cords run through the middle of the cylinder to provide lateral stability while allowing fore and aft mobility. The lumbar spine is secured to the thoracic spine plate and to the "pelvis" by four screws.

Pelvis - The pelvis consists of a cast aluminum structure with a geometry that somewhat resembles a human's pelvic bone structure. It is encased by soft rubber material to approximate the shape of human buttocks, which also houses a triaxial accelerometer.

Lower Extremities - The lower extremities consist of the upper legs, lower legs, knee joints and feet. The upper and lower legs have steel inserts surrounded with soft rubbery material to simulate the look and, to some extent, the feel of human flesh. The knee joints consist of a cast aluminum cap with a steel clevis. The knee joint is constructed in such a way as to allow for applying a pre-specified torque to the pin joint.

Upper Extremities - The upper extremities consist of the upper arms, lower arms and hands. They are constructed from steel shafts with appropriate joints at the shoulders, elbows and wrists to simulate the various degrees of freedom for arm motion. Similar to the lower extremities, all steel components are covered with soft rubbery material.

The segments anthropometry, weights and center of gravity locations can be found in Reference [6]. Table 1 lists a summary of the 50th-percentile Hybrid III dummy inertial properties which were developed for the purpose of lumped parameter modeling.

Table 1. Masses and Moments of Inertia of the 50th-Percentile Hybrid III Dummy.

Segment	Mass (kg)	Principal Moment of Inertia kg cm**2		
		11	12	13
Head	4.5	238.0	180.0	137.0
Neck	1.02	19.0	18.7	9.4
Thorax	`17.5	2801.5	2472.1	1157.9
Abdomen	18.5	1682.4	1449.9	1112.6
Upper Leg*	7.4	1032.7	1031.4	126.2
Lower Leg*	4.16	937.7	929.3	41.8
Foot*	1.78	111.4	109.4	20.6
Upper Arm*	2.76	225.7	218.9	26.2
Lower Arm*	1.67	131.8	129.3	11.5
Hand *	0.6	15.0	12.1	7.2

*Values for one side.

The dummy mass is approximately 78.3 kg. The moments of inertia shown are principal values computed at the C.G. of the component.

Dummy Modeling

During the development process of the dummy, experimental techniques were primarily used to design the various hardware components, so that their mechanical impact responses mimic as closely as possible human cadaver data. To our knowledge, only the thorax development was accompanied by a discrete spring-mass-damper model, developed by Lobdell [7], to simulate its transient response to impact.

Several lumped-parameter models, however, were developed as early as 1963 [8] to simulate occupant response to a vehicle crash pulse. Later, two-dimensional [9] and three-dimensional [10] codes were introduced and became known as Crash Victim Simulation (CVS) codes. In the early 1980's a multi-body code (MADYMO) was developed by TNO [11] to simulate multi-body systems using rigid-body mechanics formulation. The three-dimensional CAL3D code was used to simulate occupant interactions with the steering system, [12] and the MADYMO code [13] was applied to simulate dummy interactions with an inflated air bag. The primary concern in developing these models is accurate representation of occupant kinematics and associated acceleration and forces at each dummy segment center of gravity and of moments at the joints. It must be emphasized, however, that the analyst is required to make some judgments on how the dummy is divided into a group of lumped masses. Also, experimental data to describe the force-deformation response between the dummy and interior components that are likely to be contacted must be provided.

In spite of their limitations, the lumped-parameter models have provided, and still provide, an effective analytical tool, particularly useful for non-intensive calculations. In the hands of an experienced user, they provide an effective design tool. Perhaps the main limitation of the lumped-parameter dummy models lie in their inability to represent the three-dimensional geometry of the dummy and to predict contact forces and deformations associated with dummy impact and interactions with other structures. In fact, in spite of the three-dimensional analytical techniques used to analyze the dummy response, it must rely on unidirectional force-deformation data, measured experimentally, to calculate impact/contact forces.

There is an obvious need to develop detailed dummy models based on deformable structural mechanics and appropriate material description. Such a model can be used in :
1. improving the dummy response, and providing further understanding on how this relatively simple mechanical structure can replicate human response to mechanical impact;
2. design of seats and restraint systems, including belts, air bags and knee bolster;
3. integration with vehicle structures to develop system models to enable the analyst to assess in real time the influence of structural variations and restraint characteristics on occupant protection;
4. shifting from primary reliance on testing environments in vehicle design for crashworthiness to a balanced experimental/analytical method, which can save both time and cost. However, the developments of such detailed models is associated with considerable effort in model building and validation. In addition, the calculation time increases by about an order of magnitude.

Status of FE Dummy Models - The FE technique represents our best mechanics-based knowledge for analyzing the transient response of geometrically complex structures with nonlinear material behavior, subject to large deformations. Dummy modeling is characterized by the following attributes: complex three-dimensional geometry consisting of solids, beams and shells, several materials with elastic, elastic-plastic and viscoelastic behavior, dynamic response persisting for about 100 ms, time-varying boundary conditions from contact impact and interactions with other structures and nonlinear joints that are used in assembling the dummy segments.

The first FE Hybrid III dummy model was presented in 1991 [14]. It simulated the dummy structure by a combination of solid, shell and beam elements. This dummy was represented by approximately 5,000 nodes and 3,000 elements and used explicit-integration, nonlinear FE analysis. Another Hybrid III dummy model was presented in 1991 [15], which simulated the dummy with 5,000 shell elements. However, details of interior dummy component models were not provided. Comprehensive models of the Hybrid III thorax and comparisons with experimental data were developed in 1991 [16, 17]. The current dummy model extends our previous thorax model work [16] to include all dummy segments. Accurate geometric representation of the dummy hardware and component validation against experimental data are the main ingredients which distinguish this dummy model from others, which appeared in the literature thus far.

Analysis - The nonlinear FE code DYNA3D was used for calculating the impact response of the dummy models. A complete description of the code can be found in references [18, 19]. The code utilizes updated Lagrangian mechanics to formulate the semi-discrete equations of motion. The equations of motion are derived by applying the principle of virtual work to a weak form of the momentum equation. The spatially discretized second-order equations in time are solved by a central difference (explicit) technique. This integration technique requires no formulation of the global-stiffness matrix, and thus reduces computer storage and cost. The calculation cost is further reduced by using reduced integration and "hourglass" control to rid the response of the spurious zero energy modes.

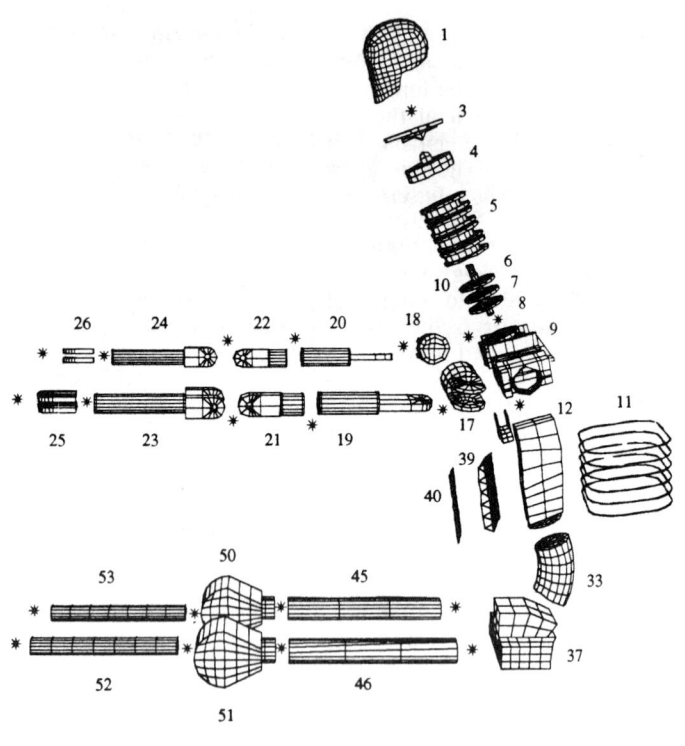

Figure 3. FE Models of the Interior Components of the Hybrid III Dummy and Joint Locations.

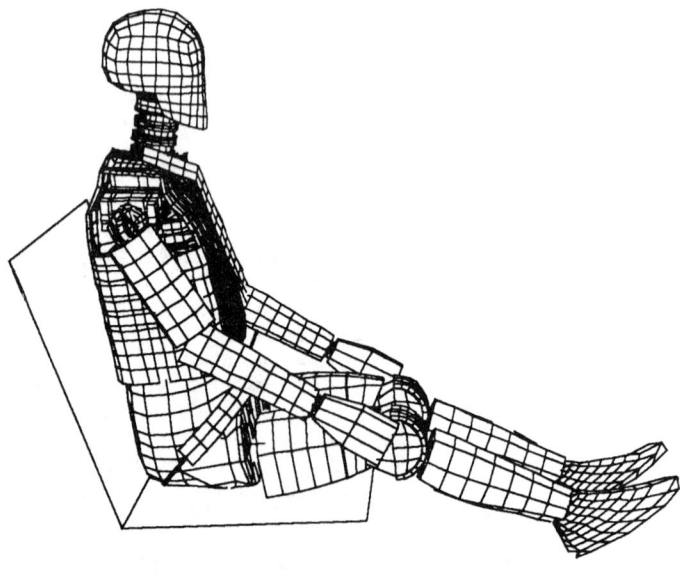

Figure 2. FE Model of the Hybrid III Dummy.

The FE Model - The Hybrid III dummy model, shown in Figure 2, was developed by using the mesh generator INGRID [20] to replicate all dummy components, both interior and exterior. The model at this time, consists of 53 parts, built from a combination of solid elements (6,782), thin shell elements (530) and beam elements (264). The

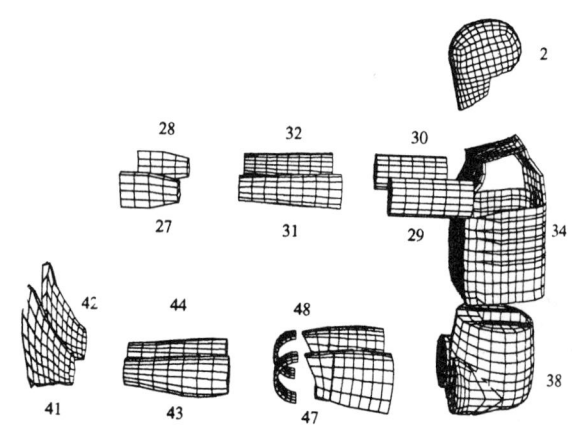

Figure 4. FE Models of the Polyvinyl Exterior Components of the Hybrid III Dummy.

total number of nodes is 13,975. Figure 3 shows the interior parts of the dummy, which are represented by rigid parts with the exception of the lumbar spine, sternum and sternum pad. The exterior skin of the dummy model is shown in Figure 4. Table 2 lists the joints, their stiffness, connecting parts, and motion types. The stiffnesses used here are preliminary values based on lumped-parameter models. They have yet to be verified by comparing the dummy response with sled tests. Table 3 provides a summary of the model parts including their material constitutive types, number of elements and type of element. It can be observed that the majority of the parts constituting the dummy "skeleton" are defined as rigid materials. The deformable materials are: the rib cage, "soft tissues" covering the "skeleton", lumbar spine and neck rubber discs. However, it should be realized that any rigid part can be easily changed to a deformable component once its material properties are specified. The rigid parts characteristics are specified by defining their material mass densities. The deformable material properties are generally considered viscoelastic in shear and elastic in compression. Specific values have been determined experimentally [16] for the thorax segment, and were used for the whole dummy. Some adjustments were necessary to insure that the component's impact response match experimental data. The specific material constants are listed in the Appendix.

Table 2. Description of Joints.

Joint Number	Stiffness kNm/rad	Stiffness kN/m x 10^7	Type
1	0.31		Revolute
6	104.000		Revolute
7	104.000		Revolute
8	10.000		Revolute
9	10.000		Revolute
10	0.1		Revolute
11	0.1		Revolute
12	0.1		Revolute
13	0.1		Revolute
14	0.5		Revolute
15	0.5		Revolute
16	0.1		Revolute
17	0.1		Revolute
18	10, 0.2, 0.1		Spherical Joint
19	10, 0.2, 0.1		Spherical Joint
20	0.005		Revolute
21	0.005		Revolute
22	0.002		Revolute
23	0.002		Revolute
24		1.0	Planar
25		1.0	Planar
26		1.0	Translational
27		1.0	Translational

The dummy parts are grouped into segments somewhat similar to the Hybrid III segmentation as presented in Table 2. These segments and their corresponding part numbers, masses and principal moments of inertia are listed in Table 4. The dummy assembly's mass (without any instrumentation) is 78.8 kg which is almost identical to the actual Hybrid III hardware mass of 78.3 kg. Adjustment of the dummy model mass to account for instrumentation can be trivially achieved by adding lumped nodal masses at the location of the transducers. Also, although not shown, the CG. locations of the various segments were within few millimeters of the hardware segments.

In comparing the model parts' moments of inertia with those from the hardware (Tables 1 and 4), some differences can be observed. The influence of these differences on overall dummy kinematics has not yet been evaluated. Further evaluation of the dummy assembly response in crash environments involving vehicle collision with a barrier and sled tests will be addressed in a future study. Geometric modifications of the component models will be addressed and reconciled to insure that the principal moments of inertia and their orientations agree with data from hardware measurements.

Table 3. Model Part Descriptions and Materials.

Parts	Material	Description	Elements Type	Elements No.
1	Rigid Body	Skull	Brick	768
2	Vioscoelastic	Head Skin	Brick	320
3	Rigid Body	Bracket	Brick	96
4	Rigid Body	Bracket	Brick	44
5	Viscoelastic	Neck	Brick	464
6	Rigid Body	Neck	Brick	48
7	Rigid Body	Neck	Brick	48
8	Rigid Body	Neck	Brick	48
9	Rigid Body	Shoulder	Brick	560
10	Elastic	Neck	Brick	56
11	Elastic	Ribs	Beam	282
12	Rigid Body	Thoracic Spine	Shell	148
17	Rigid Body	Shoulder	Brick	96
18	Rigid Body	Shoulder	Brick	66
19	Rigid Body	Upper Arm	Brick	92
20	Rigid Body	Upper Arm	Brick	90
21	Rigid Body	Upper Arm	Brick	94
22	Rigid Body	Upper Arm	Brick	92
23	Rigid Body	Lower Arm	Brick	108
24	Rigid Body	Lower Arm	Brick	108
25	Rigid Body	Lower Arm	Brick	40
26	Rigid Body	Lower Arm	Brick	40
27	Rigid Body	Hand	Brick	16
28	Rigid Body	Hand	Brick	16
29	Viscoelastic	Upper Arm Skin	Brick	96
30	Viscoelastic	Upper Arm Skin	Brick	96
31	Viscoelastic	Lower Arm Skin	Brick	128
32	Viscoelastic	Lower Arm Skin	Brick	128
33	Elastic	Lumbar Spine	Brick	192
34	Viscoelastic	Chest Skin	Brick	758
37	Rigid Body	Pelvis	Brick	106
38	Viscoelastic	Pelvis Skin	Brick	716
39	Elastic	Sternum	Shell	66
40	Viscoelastic	Sternum Pad	Brick	88
41	Rigid Body	Feet	Shell	126
42	Rigid Body	Feet	Shell	126
43	Viscoelastic	Lower Leg Skin	Brick	112
44	Viscoelastic	Lower Leg Skin	Brick	112
45	Rigid Body	Upper Leg	Brick	48
46	Rigid Body	Upper Leg	Brick	48
47	Viscoelastic	Upper Leg Skin	Brick	48
48	Viscoelastic	Upper Leg Skin	Brick	164
50	Rigid Body	Knee	Brick	68
51	Rigid Body	Knee	Brick	68
52	Rigid Body	Lower Leg	Brick	112
53	Rigid Body	Lower Leg	Brick	112

Component Validation

Head - The FE head model was constructed from three-dimensional solid elements, which represented the interior aluminum shell and the exterior vinyl layer. The occipital removable cap in the hardware was not modeled separately, rather it was considered as an integral part of the whole shell. Also, the interior compartment which accommodates the accelerometer package was not modeled. The exterior head geometry, however, was accurately modeled to represent the engineering design drawings. The dummy inertial properties, based on geometry and mass density (Table 4) closely represent the corresponding values of the hardware. The original head hardware development, including head anthropometry, landmark locations, inertial characteristics and comparisons with human cadaver data can be found in a comprehensive study by Hubbard and McLeod [5].

Table 4. FE Segments Masses and Moments of Inertia.

Parts	Segment	Mass (kg)	Principal Moment of Inertia kg cm**2		
			11	12	13
1, 2	Head	4.52	216.4	206.7	148.2
3, 4, 5, 6, 7, 8, 10	Neck	1.06	20.1	20.09	8.03
9, 11, 12, 17, 18, 34, 39, 40	Thorax	17.3	3091.5	2525.6	1921.5
37, 38, 33	Abdomen	19.4	2379.0	1785.9	1721.2
46, 48, 50	Upper Leg*	6.5	1119.2	1110.6	97.0
43, 52	Lower Leg*	4.57	341.3	333.8	69.6
41	Foot*	1.7	84.8	81.8	21.2
19, 21, 29	Upper Arm*	2.71	161.4	157.6	24.4
23, 25, 31	Lower Arm*	2.3	173.5	173.2	15.8
27	Hand*	0.5	13.1	11.5	3.7

*Values provided for one side.

In a typical crash test, the head is subject to a combination of: inertial load, transmitted through the neck, and direct impact from interacting with the vehicle interior and/or the restraint system. In an indirect impact the head behaves almost like a rigid body. In a direct impact, the exterior vinyl layer plays an important role in the magnitude and duration of the contact force and the associated kinematics. The impact severity is assessed by the Head Injury Criterion (HIC) [21], which is based on a weighted-time integral of the three-dimensional head acceleration measured at the CG. HIC is the acceptable measure for compliance with FMVSS 208. The complete three-dimensional head kinematics describing both head rotation and translation can be calculated from a 12- one-dimensional accelerometer cluster located within the head interior [22].

The dummy head compliance test requires a free drop of the head onto a rigid surface from a height of 376 mm. In the test the head is suspended such that the initial contact with the rigid plate occurs at the forehead as shown in Figure 5. The biomechanical performance requires a peak head acceleration in the range 225 - 275 g measured at the CG. The head acceleration is filtered at SAE filter class 1000.

Two impact simulations of the FE dummy head model, shown in Figure 5, were conducted where the head was allowed to drop freely and impact a rigid surface from initial velocities corresponding to drop heights: 376 and 889 mm, respectively. In the calculations, the aluminum shell was considered rigid and the exterior polyvinyl layer was considered viscoelastic in shear and elastic in compression. This type of simulation resembles a classic Hertzian contact problem [23]. The model acceleration-time response, shown in Figure 6, captured the peak and duration quite well. However it can be observed that the predicted pulse shape is symmetric, unlike what is obtained from the test, where the rebound phase is longer. This asymmetric contact pulse is believed to be due to a difference in energy loss in the rubber material during the approach and rebound phases of contact. This behavior can not be included in the material model with its current formulation, which provides only for symmetric treatment of material response. The HIC values obtained from these pulses were within 7% of the experimental results, and therefore the skewness of the pulse does not seem to significantly influence the results of the FE model. Interestingly, the total energy calculated was not constant during the contact event. It showed a dip almost reflecting the contact pulse. This dip was verified to be due to the

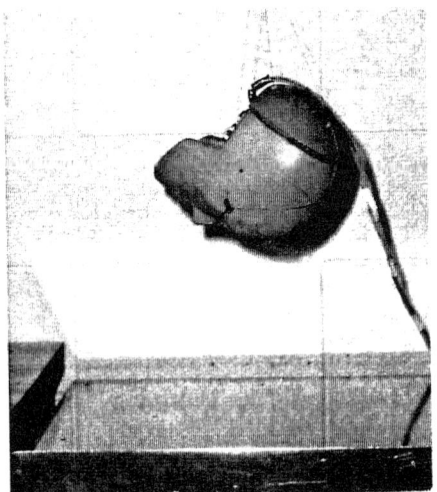

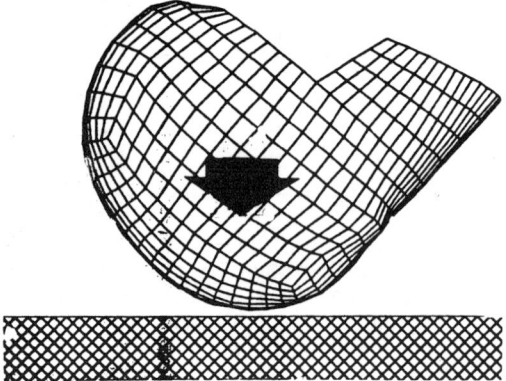

Figure 5. Head Impact Test Setup and Corresponding FE Model.

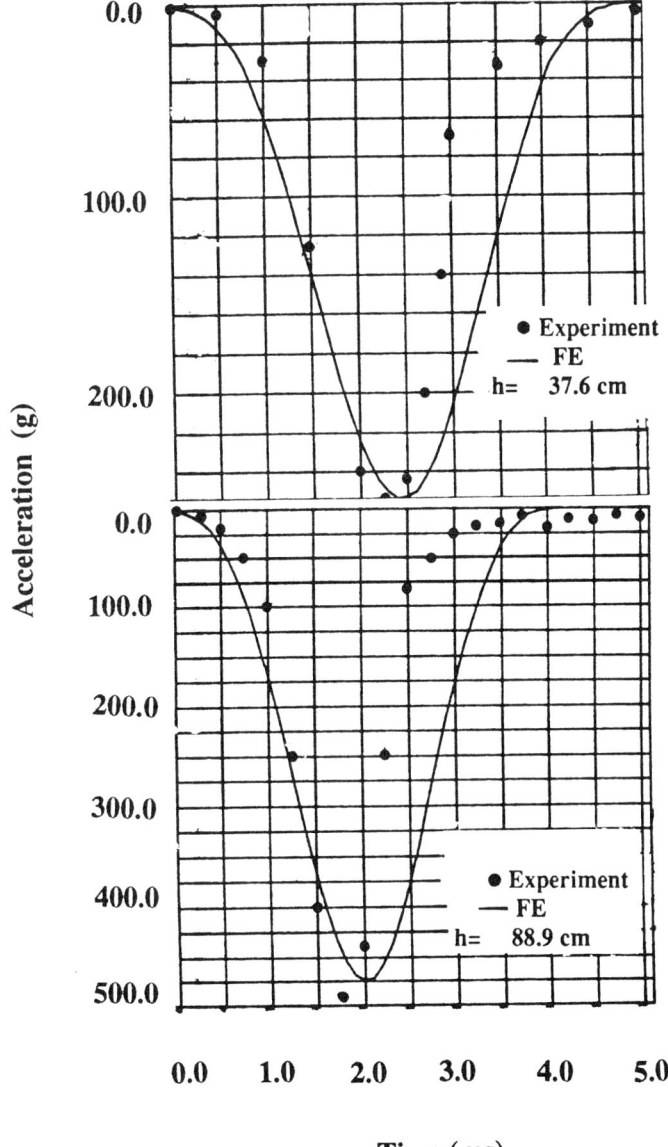

Figure 6. Measured and Calculated Head Acceleration-Time Response

coupling between the deformable outer layer and the rigid shell. When the shell material was treated as deformable this dip disappeared. The model rebound velocity was nearly equal to the initial velocity, indicating little energy loss. The peak accelerations obtained: 255 and 475 g, respectively match closely the experimental data [5].

Neck - The FE neck model (Figure 7d) was developed to simulate the neck hardware described earlier in Section 2.2 using primarily three-dimensional brick elements. The elastomeric viscoelastic disc models contain thin horizontal cuts, about 20 mm deep, in the anterior part of the discs, so together with the disc asymmetry it can simulate the difference in neck stiffness for extension and flexion motions. A contact constraint was defined for each of the disc's slits. The material properties were identified by requiring the model response to match corresponding experimental data. This parameter identification technique or "reverse engineering" can be used in analysis where accurate material properties are difficult to obtain. Specific material constants are included in the Appendix. Figure 7 shows the head-neck assembly, neck hardware and corresponding FE models.

To validate the neck model, the standard procedure described in the Code of Federal Regulations [24] was followed. The test consists of a pendulum drop with pre-specified length, mass and moment of inertia in the vertical plane. For the extension test, the regulation specifies an impact velocity in the range of 5.95 to 6.19 m/s whereas in the flexion test the range can vary from 6.89 to 7.13 m/s. The head-neck assembly attaches to the lower extremity of the pendulum bar in two configurations, as shown in Figure 8, to simulate extension and flexion motions, respectively. The pendulum impact energy is absorbed by an aluminum Honeycomb block. In a drop silo test of a block of Honeycomb material (100 x 100 x 100 mm), at an impact velocity of 7.5 m/s, the pulse had nearly a square shape with a duration of 5.5 ms and a peak force of about 3.9 kN. The pendulum bar is instrumented with a one-dimensional accelerometer mounted on the surface opposite from the contact location with the Honeycomb block. The pendulum deceleration response for extension (flexion) must be in the range of 17.2 - 21.2 g (22.5 - 27.5 g) at 10 ms, 14.0 - 19.0 g (17.6 - 22.6 g) at 20 ms and 11 - 16 g (12.5 - 18.5 g) at 30 ms, and can not exceed 22.0 g (29 g). A load transducer is mounted at the head-neck joint to measure the moment-time response about a lateral axis through the occipital condyles. The measured moment in extension (flexion) should be in the range 52.9 - 80.2 Nm (88.4 - 108.8 Nm) and should occur between 65 - and 79 ms (47 and 58 ms). Also, the moment should decay to 0 Nm between 120 and 148 ms (97 and 107 ms). The head rotation is measured by the rotation of D-plane as shown in Figure 8. The regulation specifies for extension (flexion) a rotation in the range 81 - 106 degrees (64 - 78 degrees) and should occur in the time interval 72 ms - 82 ms (57-64 ms) and should drop to 0 degrees between 147 and 174 ms (113 and 128 ms).

Two FE calculations were obtained to simulate extension and flexion motions, as shown in Figure 8. The models simulated two tests conducted at impact speeds of 6 m/s for extension and 7 m/s for flexion. The simulation kinematics for a time duration of 90 ms, at 20 ms intervals, are shown in Figure 9 for extension and in Figure 10 for flexion, respectively. The overall kinematics appears quite realistic and seems to capture the essential features of the anterior-posterior head-neck motion in the midsagittal plane as observed from actual tests. The calculated response histories from extension and flexion simulations are shown in Figures 11 and 12 for pendulum acceleration, moment at the occipital condyles joint and D-plane rotation, along with corresponding experimental data and compliance ranges. The predicted response matched the experimental data quite well for flexion and extension motions; and they also seem to satisfy the regulation requirements for pendulum acceleration and D-plane rotation. However, it may be noticed that the calculated moments for both extension and flexion are higher than the experimental data by 28% and 23%, respectively. This discrepancy is believed to be due to lack of exact material data. Future improvement of the dummy model should include accurate identification of the deformable components materials response.

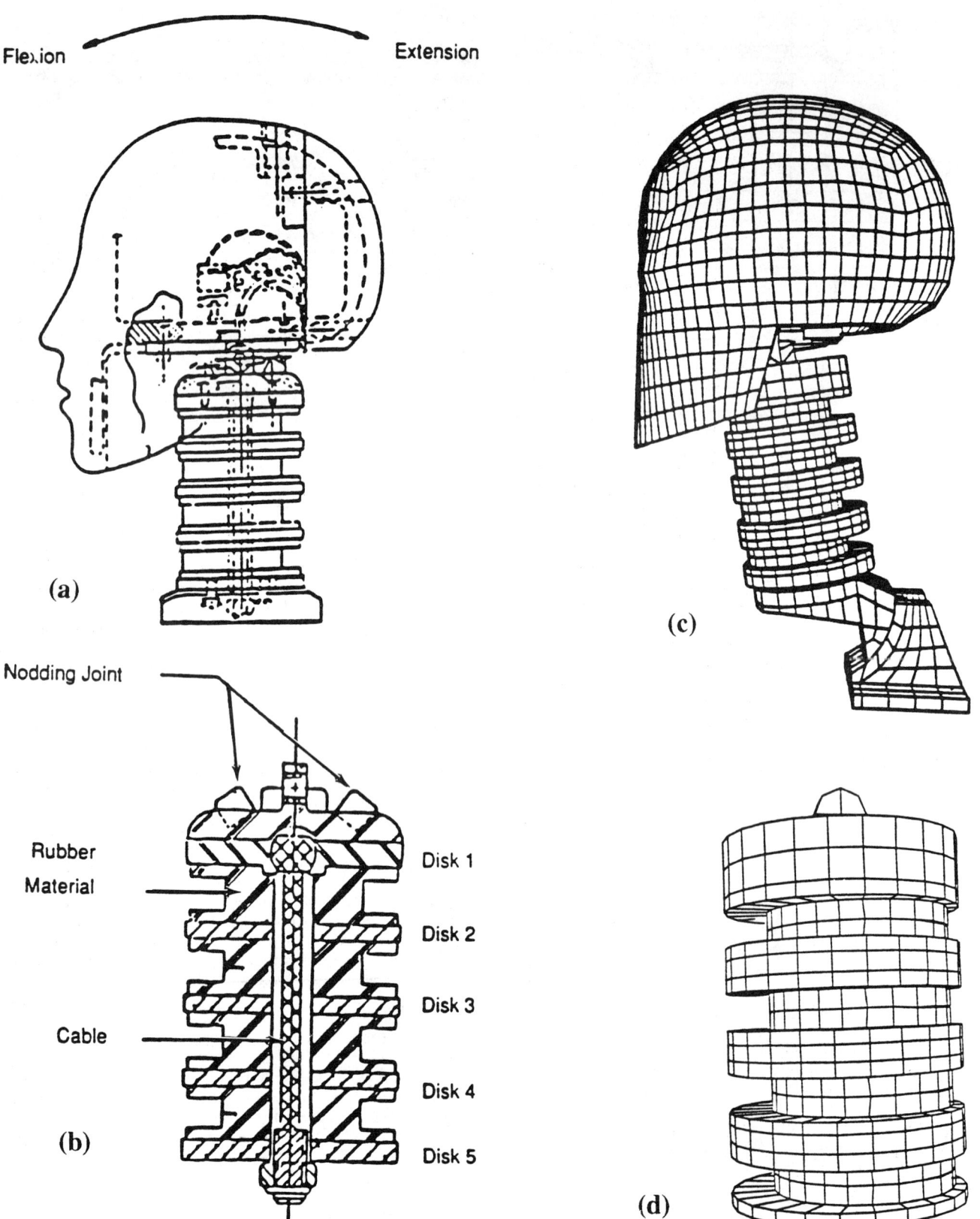

Figure 7. Head-Neck Hardware and Corresponding FE Models

1134

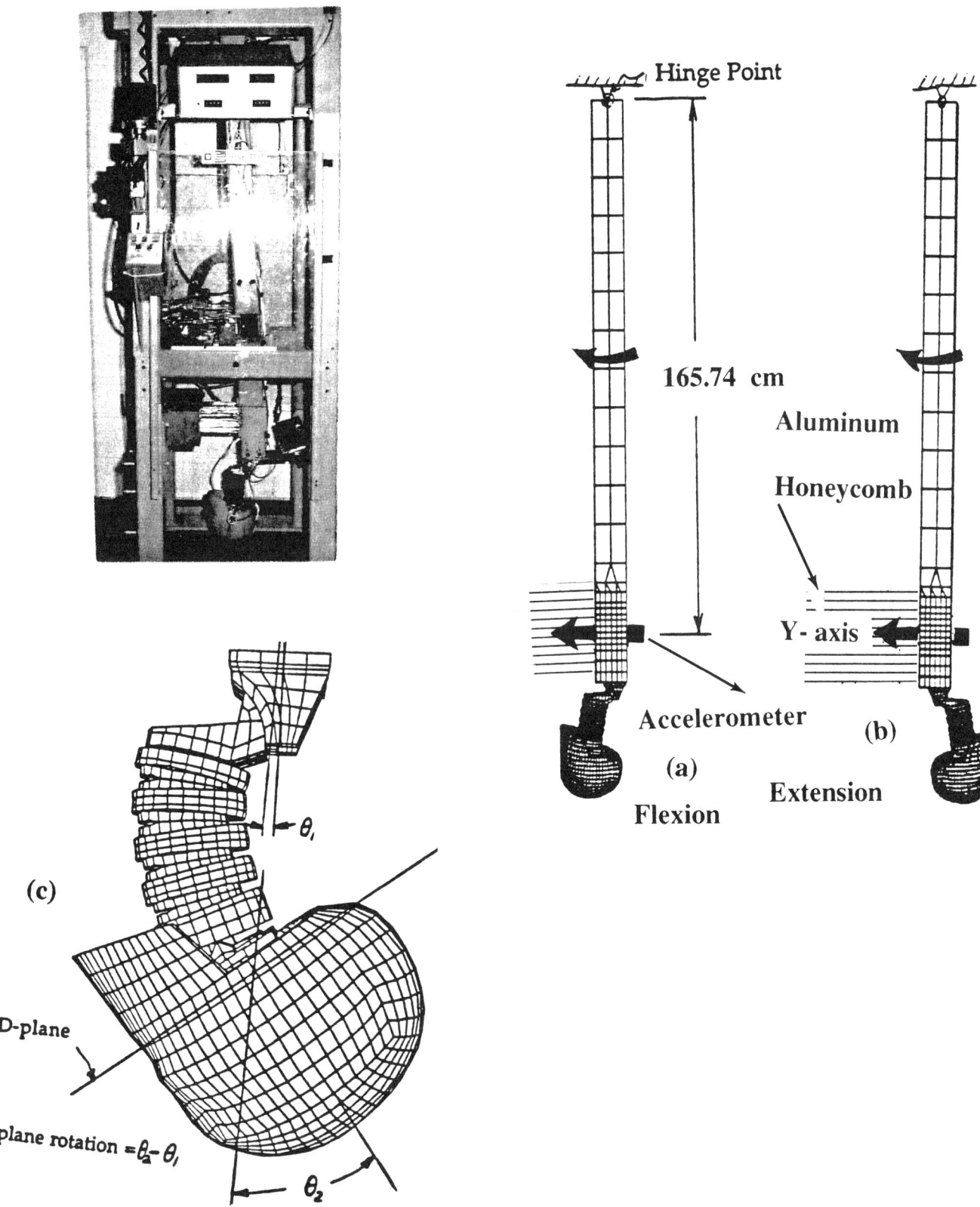

Figure 8. Head-Neck Pendulum Test for: (a) Flexion and Corresponding FE Model; (b) Extension FE Model and (c) D-Plane Rotation Definition.

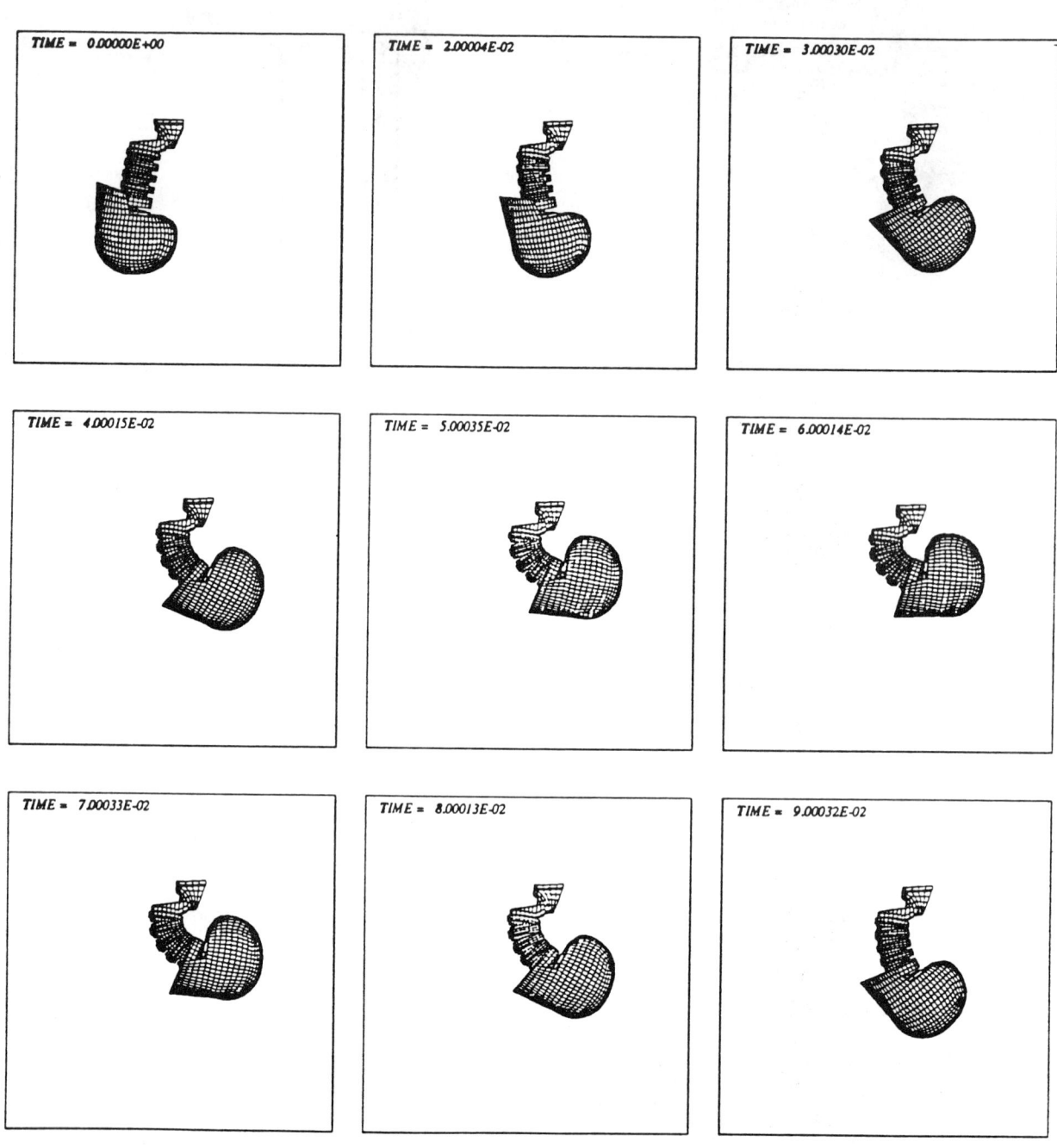

Figure 9. Calculated Head-Neck Kinematics in Extension Motion.

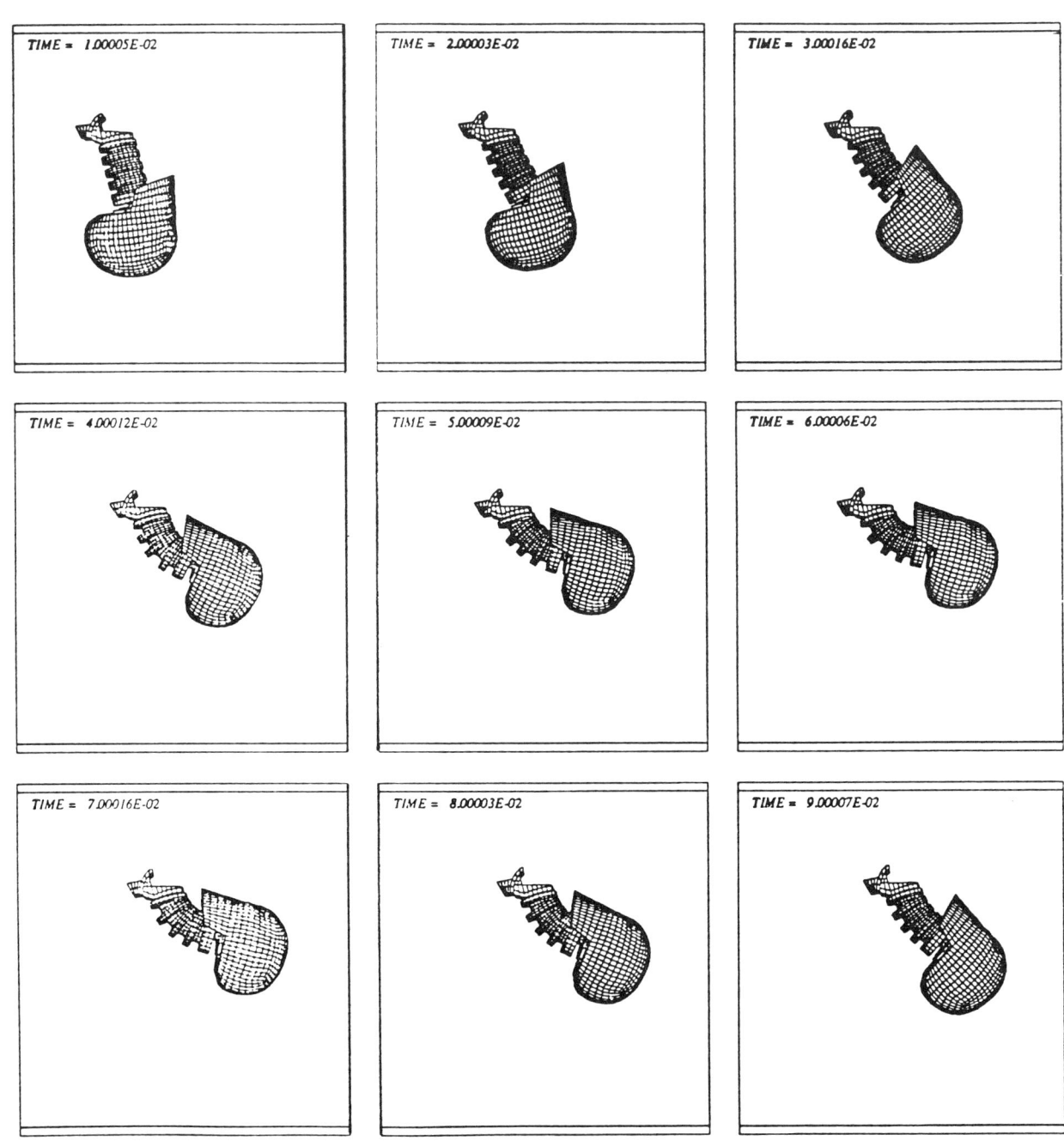

Figure 10. Calculated Head-Neck Kinematics in Flexion Motion.

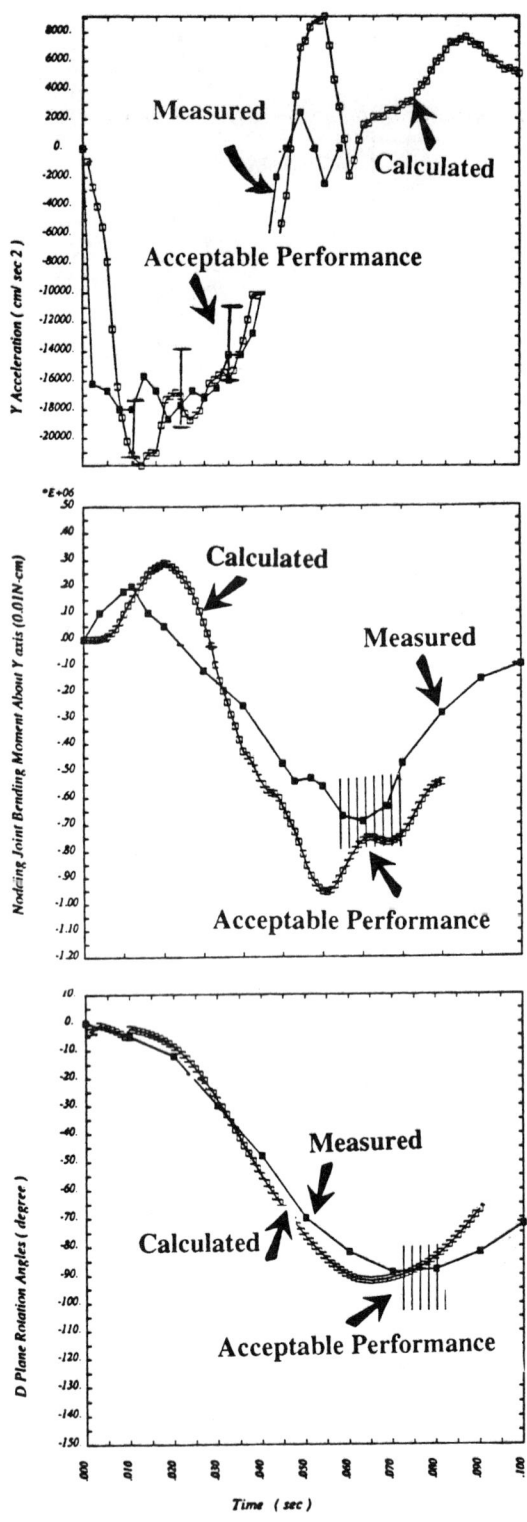

Figure 11. Comparison Between Calculated and Measured Pendulum Acceleration, Nodding Joint Bending Moment and D-Plane Rotation, along with Acceptable Performance Corridors for Extension Motion.

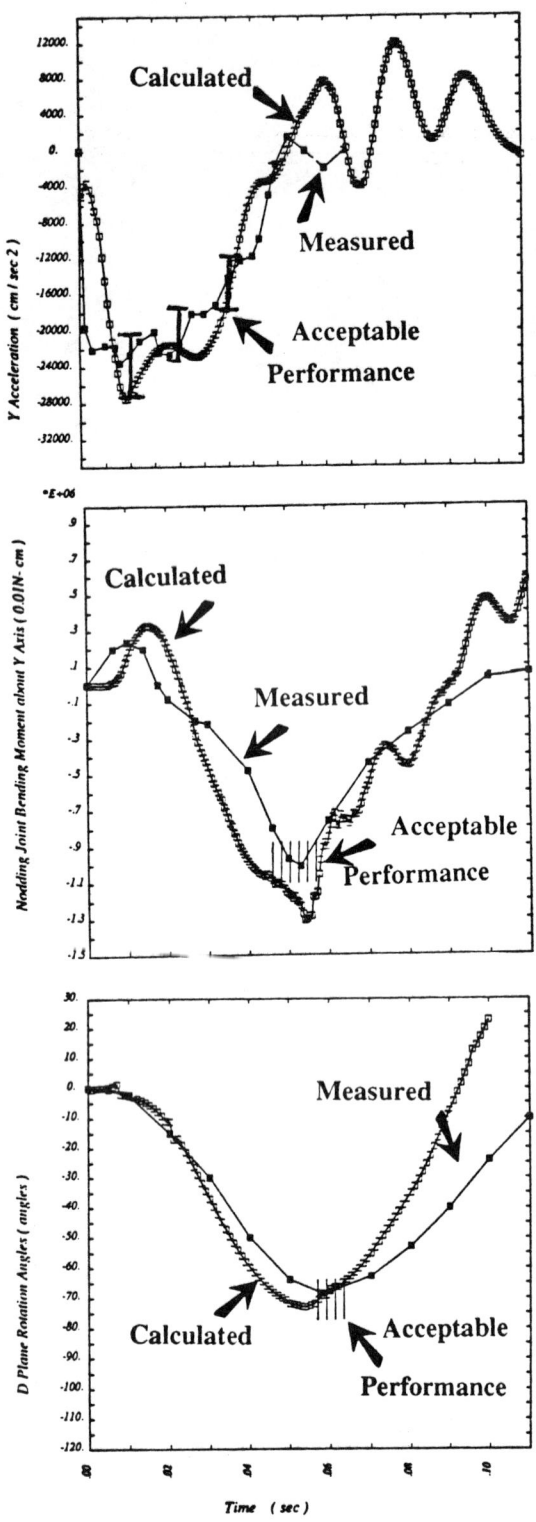

Figure 12. Comparison Between Calculated and Measured Pendulum Acceleration, Nodding Joint Bending Moment and D-Plane Rotation, along with Acceptable Performance Corridors for Flexion Motion.

Thorax - The thorax FE model was developed from several components with their geometry and material properties representing the actual hardware as closely as possible. In a previous publication [16], the development and validation of an isolated thorax model was discussed in detail. In this study, the thorax model response was validated in situ. In addition, an impactor with a mass of 23.4 kg and diameter equal to 150 mm was launched to impact the thoracic mid-region from an initial velocity of 6.71 m/s, similar to the thoracic validation test, as shown in Figure 13, instead of applying a direct force-time pulse, as used previously in thorax validation [16]. Figures 14a and 14b show a midsagittal cross section of the calculated dummy deformations in the time span 0 - 55 ms, at 5 ms intervals. The maximum deformation (65 mm) was reached at 25 ms, which is consistent with experimental data [16]. The calculated force deformation response agreed quite well with measured data from human cadavers, as shown in Figure 15. The comparison with dummy experiments was shown in Reference [16]. A second calculation of the thoracic impact force-deformation response was obtained for an impact velocity of 4.3 m/s, as shown in Figure 16. From the two simulations, it appears that the thorax model captured the essential features of the hardware and accurately represented the thoracic response to impact in the midsagittal plane.

Lumbar Spine - The short curved cylinder representing the lumbar spine was modeled by eight-node brick elements which accurately represented the exterior shape of the component. At this time no attempt was made to include the two flexible cables. Instead, it was assumed that the elastomeric rubber material would dominate the flexural response in the midsagittal plane. It should also be pointed out that the lumbar spine represents the only deformable component of the Hybrid III spine, i.e, no significant deformation is expected, under normal usage of the dummy between the neck and the lumbar spine.

The elastomeric rubber material was represented by a Blatz-Ko rubber model [18]. The large deformation material response is assumed elastic with a Poisson's ratio of 0.463. To identify the shear modulus of the material, an experiment described in reference [25] was simulated, which provided the moment-rotation response of the lumbar spine in the midsagittal plane. In the model a moment-time ramp function was applied at one end of the model while keeping the other end constrained. The calculated deformed shape was then compared with the experimental response to insure that accurate kinematics of the component are captured. By iteratively varying the material shear modulus, it was noted that when G was 460 MPa and the material density was 1.3 gm/cm**3, the model response agreed quite well with experimental data as shown in Figure 17. Accordingly, this model was considered adequate, at this time, to represent the basic behavior of the lumbar spine despite exclusion of the flexible cables.

Knee Joint - The geometry of the knee model is an approximate representation of the hardware as shown in Figure 18. It consists of a cylindrical surface, rigidly attached to the distal end of the femur shaft. A layer of viscoelastic material to simulate the knee padding surrounds the exterior surface of the knee joint. The knee joint articulates with respect to the tibia shaft by a pin joint, and, at this time, does not exactly replicate the femur-knee-tibia complex of the Hybrid III dummy.

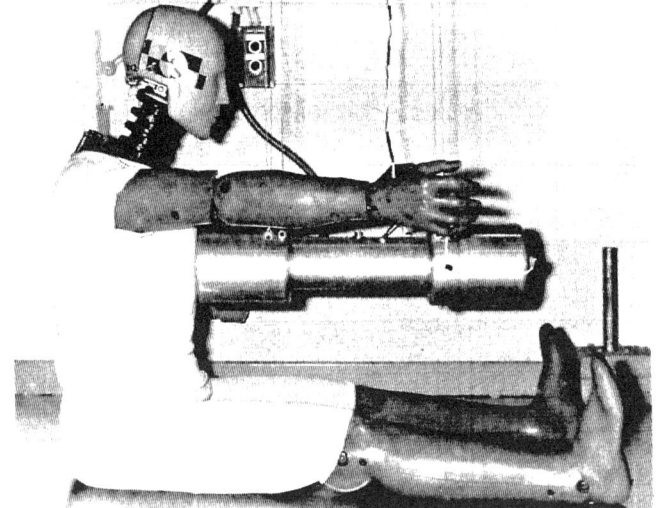

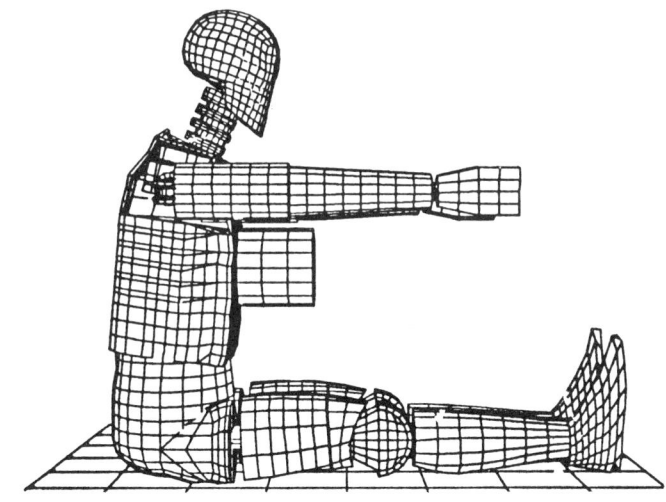

Figure 13. Thoracic Impact Test Setup and Corresponding FE Model

To evaluate the knee padding, an FE model of the knee joint, distal femur, and lower leg was isolated from the dummy model and subjected to pendulum impact along the femoral axis, similar to the test set up, as shown in Figure 18 [2]. The femoral shaft was fixed to simulate the very large mass used in the test. Three cylindrical impactors were used with diameters of 51, 51 and 76 mm and masses: 0.5, 1.5 and 5 kg, respectively [2]. The impactor velocity for all 3 simulations was 2.1 m/s. The knee padding material of the Hybrid III dummy was selected to provide a peak force similar to measurements from human cadaver. In the test, the knee force was calculated from the mass of the impactor and its one-dimensional rigid-body acceleration. A similar procedure was followed in the FE simulations.

The first simulation modeled the 0.5 kg impactor. In this test the material property was assumed viscoelastic in shear and elastic in compression with material constants selected so

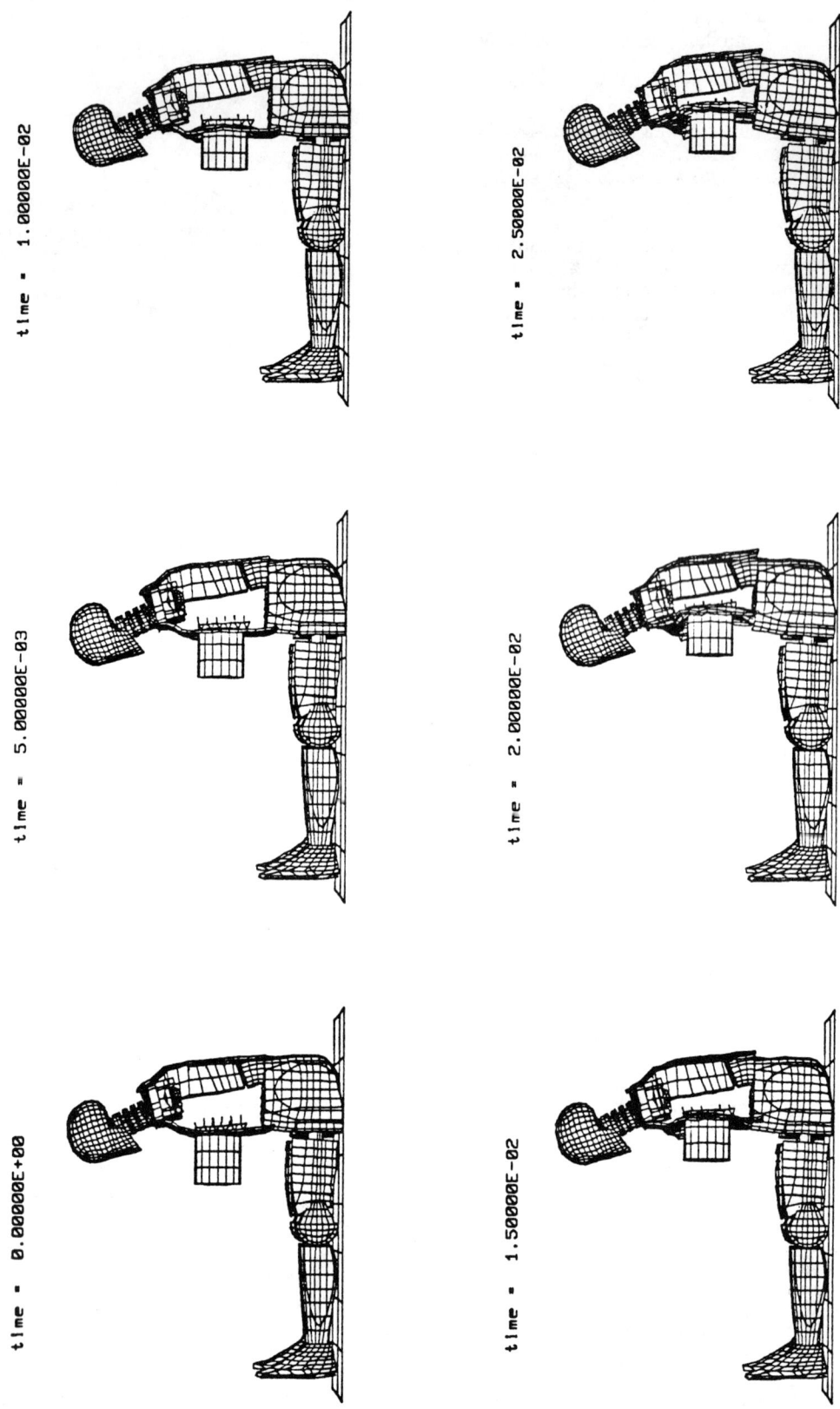

Figure 14a. Dummy Deformations in Time (0-25 ms) from Impact on the Midthorax, Pendulum Mass = 23.4 kg and Initial Velocity = 6.71 m/s.

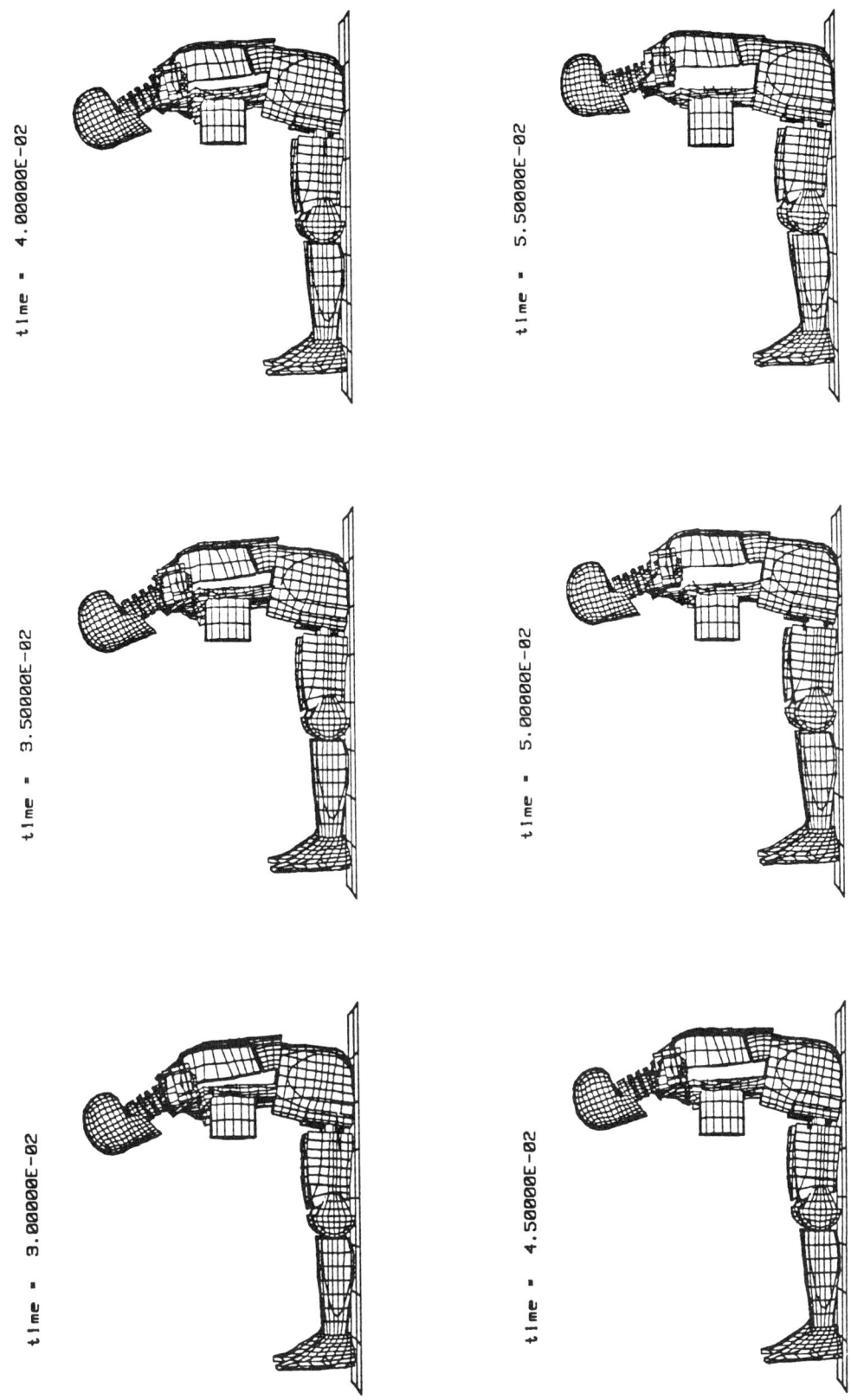

Figure 14b. Dummy Deformations in Time (30-55 ms) from Impact on the Midthorax, Pendulum Mass = 23.4 kg and Initial Velocity = 6.71 m/s.

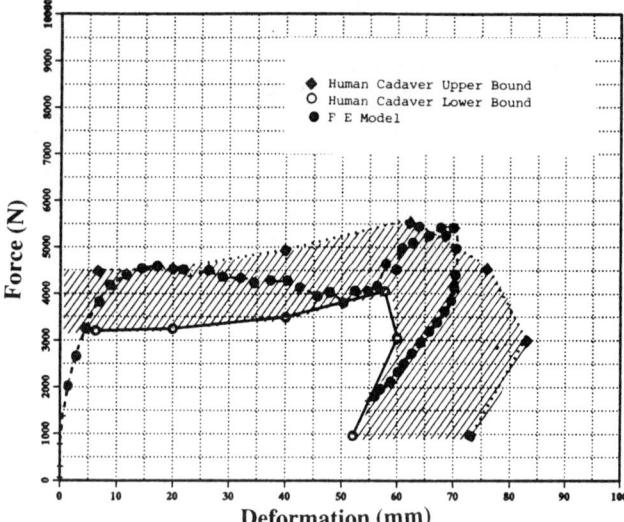

Figure 15. Thoracic Force-Deformation Response from FE Calculation and Human Cadavers Corridors.

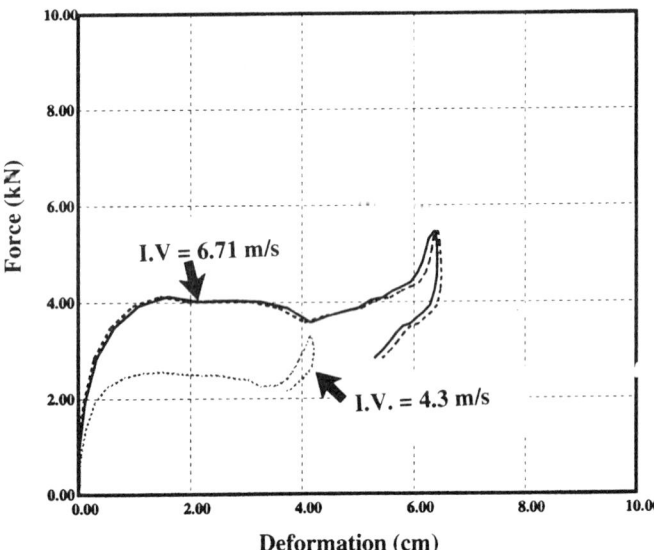

Figure 16. Thoracic Force-Deformation Response from 2 FE Calculations with Pendulum Velocities: 6.71 m/s and 4.3 m/s.

the peak force (1.1 kN) matches closely the measured value from the Hybrid III dummy and human cadavers [2]. The force-time response shown in Figure 19 represented nearly a Hertzian contact force persisting for about 3.5 ms, and the simulation was considered adequate in representing the padding material response. The impact durations are not provided in reference [2]. In the second simulation the impactor mass was increased to 1.5 kg and in the third simulation the mass of the impactor was increased to 5 kg with a diameter of 76 mm, while maintaining the same material properties used in the first simulation. The force time pulses (Figure 19) showed an increase in contact duration to 5.5 and 8.5 ms with peak forces of 2.2 and 5.3 kN. The peak forces agreed quite well with reported experimental data (2.05 and 5.7 kN) [2].

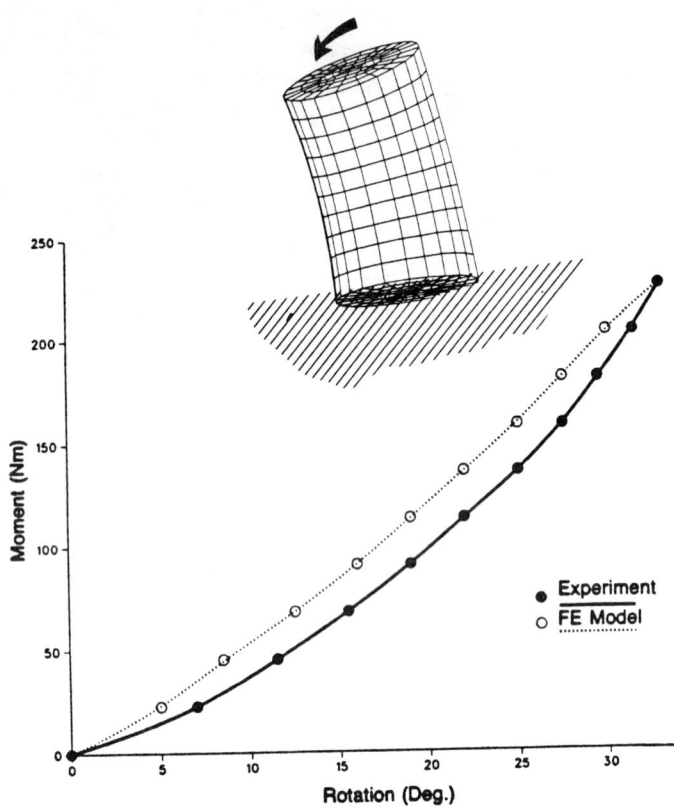

Figure 17. Moment-Rotation Response of Lumbar-Spine from Experiment and FE Calculation.

Conclusions

FE models of the Hybrid III dummy components - head, neck, shoulders, thorax complex, pelvis, upper extremities and lower extremities - were developed to simulate as closely as possible corresponding hardware of the dummy. The dummy "skeleton" consisted of metallic materials (aluminum and steel) covered with polyvinyl soft "skin" to simulate the exterior soft tissues. All metallic parts were assumed rigid, with the exception of the thorax rib cage which was treated as elastic with appropriate discrete dampers to simulate the ribs damping material. Viscoelastic material properties were assigned to all deformable components.

Component validation tests were conducted for the head, neck, thorax, lumbar spine, and knees. The impact responses of all these components agreed quite well with experimental data and provided an acceptable level of confidence in the models. Subsequently, all components were assembled using appropriate joint kinematics and characteristics similar to those used in lumped parameter models of the dummy. The impact response of the whole dummy when subjected to thoracic impact from two initial velocities (6.71 and 4.3 m/s) were calculated. For the 6.71 m/s impact condition the calculated force-deflection response was in good agreement with corresponding experimental data from human cadavers.

Also, the deformed configurations of the assembled dummy assured that all dummy parts are properly connected.

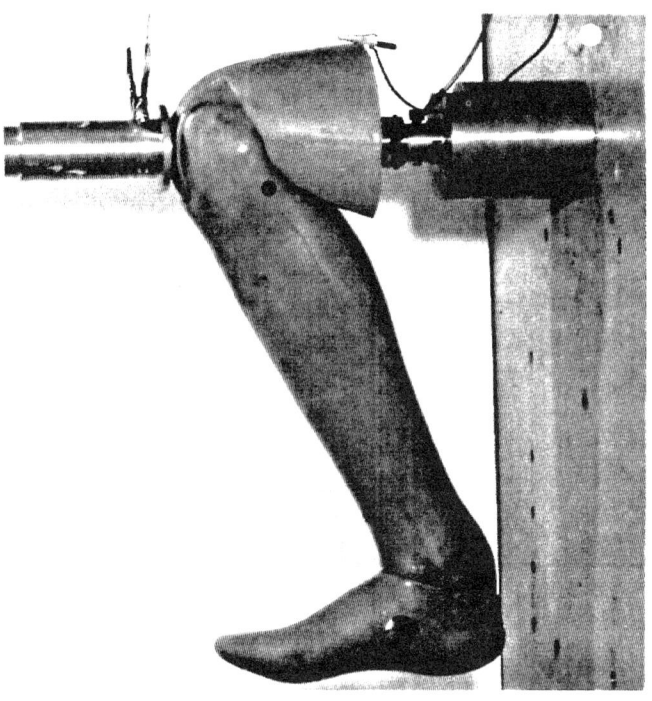

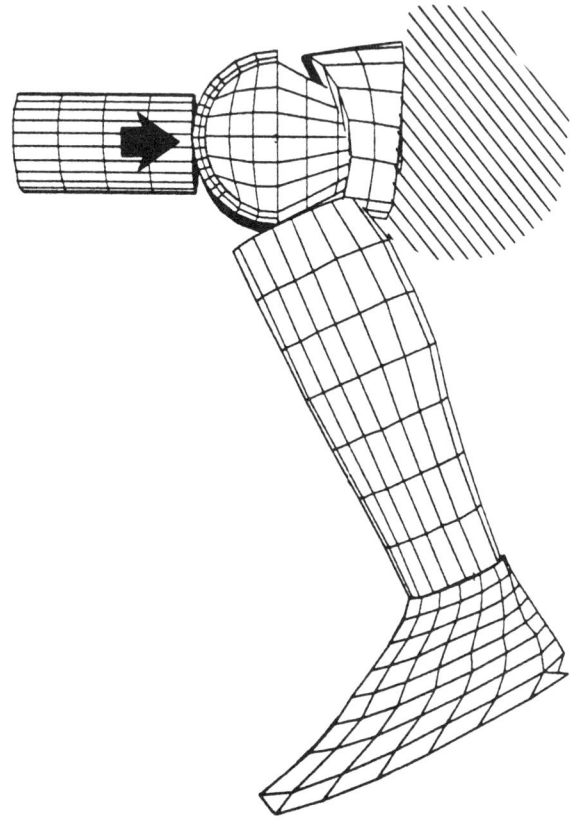

Figure 18. Knee Joint Impact Test Set Up and Corresponding FE Model.

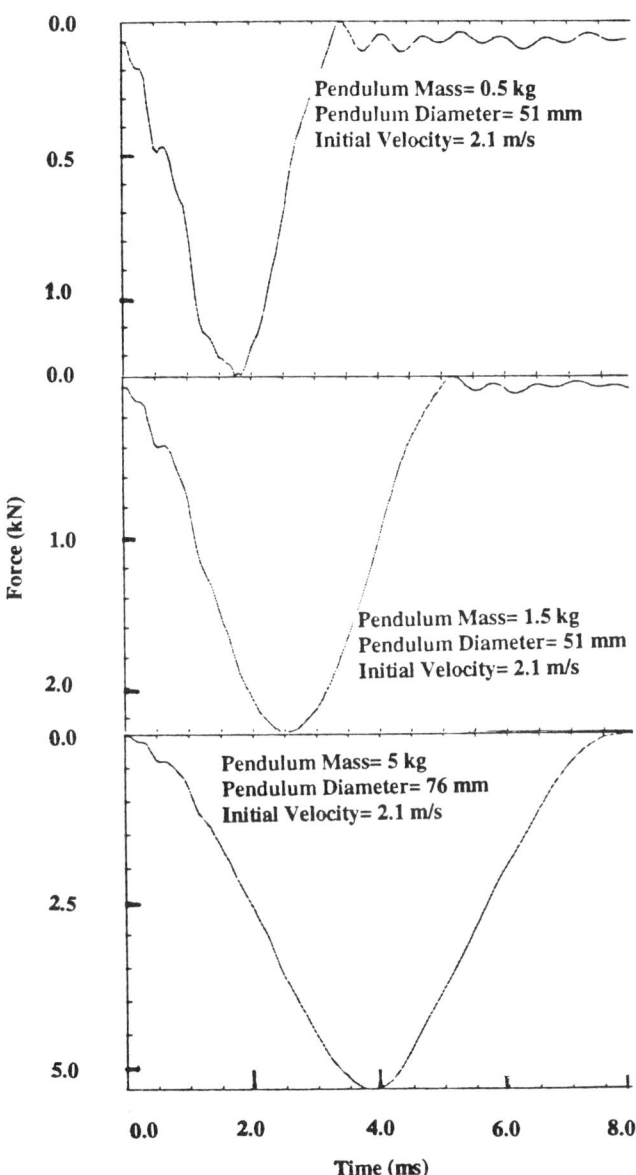

Figure 19. Calculated Force-Time Response from Three Knee Impact Calculations.

Final validation of the assembled dummy with sled tests is yet to be conducted to evaluate the influence of segment inertial properties and joint definitions. Also, the material properties used in this simulation relied primarily on ad-hoc parameter identification. There is an obvious need to identify accurate viscoelastic materials response and incorporate them in the next release of the dummy model, particularly for the neck and the lumbar spine.

ACKNOWLEDGMENTS

The authors appreciate Doug Stillman's efforts in developing the FE models. Thanks are also due to Myong Hwang for conducting FE simulations.

REFERENCES

1. Mertz, H. J., Irwin, A. L., Melvin, J. W., Stalnaker, R. L. and M. S. Beebe, "Size, Weight and Biomechanical Impact Response Requirements for Adult Size Small Female and Large Male Dummies," SAE 890756, International Congress and Exposition, Detroit, Michigan, 1989.
2. Foster, J. K., Kortge, J. O. and Wolanin, M. J., "Hybrid III - A Biomechanically Based Crash Test Dummy," SAE 770938, 21st Stapp Car Crash Conference, 1977.
3. Mertz, H. J., "Anthropomorphic Test Devices", to appear in Accidental Injury: Biomechanics and Prevention, Springer-Verlag, NY, 1993.
4. Federal Motor Vehicle Safety Standards No. 208: Docket 74-14, Notice 11: Federal Register, Volume 42, No. 128, July 1987.
5. Hubbard, R. P. and McLeod, D. G., "Definition and Development of A Crash Dummy Head," 18th Stapp Car Crash Conference, 1974.
6. Harry, G., "Measurement of Hybrid III Dummy Properties and Analytical Simulation Data Base Development," AAMRL-TR-88-005, 1988.
7. Lobdell, T. E., "Impact Response of the Human Thorax," In Proceedings of the Symposium on Human Impact Response, GM Research Laboratories, Warren, Michigan, 1972.
8. McHenry, R. R., "Analysis of The Dynamics of Automobile Passenger-Restraint Systems," 7th Stapp Car Crash Conference, 1963.
9. Robinson, D. H., Bowman, B. M. and Bennett, R. O., "The MVMA Two-Dimensional Crash Victim Simulation," SAE 741195, 18th Stapp Car Crash Conference, 1974.
10. Fleck, J. T., Butler, F. E. and Vogel, S. L., "Three Dimensional Computer Simulation of Motor Vehicles Crash Victims," Vol I-IV, Report Nos. DOT-HS-801507, 508, 509 and 510, 1974.
11. Wismans, J. and Hermans, J. H. A., "MADYMO 3D Simulations of Hybrid III Dummy Sled Tests," SAE International Congress and Exposition, Paper No. 880645, Detroit, Michigan, 1988.
12. Wang, J. T. and Lin, K. H., "A CAL3D Steering System Impact Model", SAE 880654, 1988.
13. Neiboer, J. J., Wismans, J. and Fraterman, E., "Status of the MADYMO 2D Airbag Model," SAE 881729, 1988.
14. Schelkle, E. and Remensperger, R., "Integrated Occupant-Car Crash Simulation with the Finite Element Method: The Porsche Hybrid III-Dummy and Airbag Model," SAE 910654, in Frontal Crash Safety Technologies for the 90's, SP-852, 1991.
15. Midoun, D. E. Midoun, Rao, M. K. and Kalidindi, B., "Dummy Models for Crash Simulation in Finite Element Programs," 35th Stapp Car Crash Conference Proceedings, San Diego, California, 1991.
16. Khalil, T. B. and Lin, K. H., "Hybrid III Thoracic Impact on Self-Aligning Steering Wheel by Finite Element Analysis and Mini-Sled Experiments," 35th Stapp Car Crash Conference Proceedings, San Diego, California, 1991.
17. Yang, K. H., "Mathematical Modeling of the Hybrid III Dummy Chest with Chest Foam," 35th Stapp Car Crash Conference Proceedings, San Diego, California, 1991.
18. Hallquist, J. O., "LS-DYNA3D User's Manual," Livermore Software Technology Corp., Livermore, California, 1991.
19. Hallquist, J. O., "Theoretical Manual for DYNA3D," University of California, Lawrence Livermore National Laboratory, Report No. UCID-19401.
20. Stillman, D. W. and Hallquist, J. O., "LS-INGRID: A Pre-Processor and Three Dimensional Mesh Generator for the Programs LS-DYNA3D, LS-NIKE3D and TOPAZ," Livermore Software Technology Corp., Livermore, California, 1991.
21. Versace, J., "A Review of the Severity Index," Proceedings of 15th Stapp Car Crash Conference, 1971.
22. Hardy, W. N. et. al., "Investigation of the Least Squares Approach to the Calculation of Angular Acceleration for Linear Accelerometry," Proceedings of 15th Annual International Workshop on Human Subjects for Biomechanical Research, 1987.
23. Goldsmith, W., "The Theory of Physical Behavior of Colliding Solids," Edward Arnold Publisher, London, 1960.
24. Code of Federal Regulations, Title 49, Part 572 and Amended Part 572.
25. Deng, Y. C., "Analytical Study of the Interaction between the Seat Belt and a Hybrid III Dummy in Sled Tests," SAE 880648, 1988.

APPENDIX A

Material Properties

The Hybrid III dummy is manufactured from several metallic and nonmetallic parts. The material properties of the metallic parts (Table A.1) were assumed elastic. Their constants were obtained from the open literature, with the exception of the lumbar spine properties, which were identified by matching the model response with test data, using a Blatz-Ko [19] rubber model.

Table A.1

Component	Material Type	E (GPa) x $10^{**}5$	ν	ρ (kg/m**3) x $10^{**}3$
Neck Cable	Steel	40	0.3	7.9
Neck Discs	Aluminum	67	0.3	2.8
Ribs	Steel	200	0.3	7.9
Sternum	Plexiglass	58	0.4	1.2
Lumbar Spine	Rubber	0.1	0.46	1.3

The material properties of the thorax skin, sternum pad and rib damping material were assumed elastic in bulk (hydrostatic compression) and viscoelastic in shear deformations, respectively. The Viscoelastic model used can be written as:

$$G(t) = G_\infty + (G_o - G_\infty)xe^{-\beta t},$$

Where G_o and G_∞ are the short-term and long-term shear modulii and β is the relaxation parameter. We have conducted uniaxial relaxation tests in both tension and compression, respectively, for the thoracic skin material, compression tests for the sternum pad and rib damping material to identify the material constants, according to the previous equation. the tests were conducted at strain rates of 2.5 - 5.0 mm/mm/s. The bulk modulii were identified from standard one-dimensional tests. A summary of the material properties is listed in Table A.2. It should be emphasized that these values describe quasistatic material behavior, and dynamic tests at higher strain rates need to be conducted for accurate representation of the material response in impact environments, typical of vehicle crash. Also, only few samples were tested, and therefore, the data in Table A.2 may not represent all the inhomogeneity that exist in the soft materials of the dummy.

Table A.2

Hybrid III Viscoelastic Material Properties

Component/ Test	Material	Material Coefficients				
		K (MPa)	G_o (kPa)	G_∞ (kPa)	β(s)	ρ (kg/m^3)
Outer Skin/ Tension	Layered Vinyl Rubber	1.53	270	225	0.5	68.8
Outer Skin/Compression	Layered Vinyl Rubber	0.15	30	22	0.6	68.8
Sternum Pad Compression	Urethane Rubber	0.32	45	33	0.6	10.8
Ribs Damping Material/ Tension	Polyviscous	1010	105	5	1.5	183.3

For the purpose of developing the FE component models, the material coefficients in Tables A.1 and A.2 were used as initial values to predict the component responses, which were subsequently compared with corresponding experimental data. In this comparison, discrepancies were noted between calculated component responses and experimental results. To reconcile these differences, it was necessary to modify the soft material properties so that an agreement can be obtained. the final material properties used for the head, neck, thorax, upper extremities, lower extremities, pelvis are listed in Table A.3. Although these properties provided calculated response in reasonable agreement with experimental data, there remains a need to verify their accuracy by further testing of the dummy materials in deformation ranges and strain rates consistent with dummy exposure to impact loads.

Table A.3

Viscoelastic Material Properties of Component Models

Component	Material Coefficients				
	K (MPa)	G_o (kPa)	G_∞ (kPa)	β(s)	ρ (kg/m^3)
Head Skin	22.6	3.3	2.7	0.5	330
Neck Rubber	112.8	16.9	13.8	0.5	2100
Thorax Skin	9.0	1.3	1.1	0.5	700
Sternum Pad	0.3	0.05	0.03	0.7	10
Knee Skin	75.2	10.2	8.1	0.5	330
Upper Extremities	9.0	1.3	1.1	0.5	700
Lower Extremities	9.0	1.3	1.1	0.5	700
Pelvis	9.0	1.3	1.1	0.5	700

RECOMMENDED READING

Most of these papers have been published by SAE and are available in original or photocopy form. For ordering information, contact SAE's Customer Sales and Satisfaction Department, SAE International, 400 Commonwealth Drive, Warrendale, PA 15096-0001, USA, Telephone: 412/776-4970, Fax: 412/776-0790. Copies of papers referenced but not published by SAE must be obtained directly from the publisher listed.

Alem, Nabih M.; Bowman, Bruce M.; Melvin, John W.; Benson, Joseph B., "Whole-Body Human Surrogate Response to Three-Point Harness Restraint," SAE Technical Paper 780895.

The general objective of the Whole-Body Response (WBR) research program was to generate data on the kinematics and response of human surrogates in a realistic automobile impact environment. The program used a test configuration consisting of an idealized hard seat representation of a car seat with a three-point harness restraint system. Three different severity levels of crash test conditions were used. The human surrogates tested in this program were fifteen male cadavers, a Hybrid II (Part 572) Anthropomorphic Test Device and a Hybrid III ATD recently developed by General Motors. In addition, mathematical simulations of the response and kinematics of a 50th percentile male occupant were performed at the three levels of crash severity, using the MVMA Two-Dimensional Crash Victim Simulator. The primary utility of the data generated by this program is for comparing the similarities and differences in response and kinematics of the various types of human surrogates and in pointing out areas that need improvement in both anthropomorphic test devices and mathematical models.

Ashton, S. J., "Factors Associated with Pelvic and Knee Injuries in Pedestrians Struck by the Fronts of Cars," SAE Technical Paper 811026.

The incidence of pelvic and lower extremity fractures is examined by reference to data extracted from police and hospital records. It is shown that the incidence and number of fractures to the pelvis and the lower extremities is strongly dependent on the age of the struck pedestrian and the speed of the vehicle. Pelvic injuries are shown to be more common in elderly females than in other age groups and it is suggested that this is due to elderly females being more likely, with current vehicle front end heights, to sustain a direct blow at the level of the pelvis. Pubic rami fractures appear to result when there are distributed impact forces at the level of the pelvis and acetabular fractures occur when there are concentrated forces applied to the greater trochanter. Injuries to the knee joint ligaments are shown to occur when there is an impact in the vicinity of the knee joint and can occur at speeds as low as 20 km/h although for complete rupture an impact speed of at least 35 km/h is required. It is suggested that the use of a simple impactor to control front structure compliance may not be sufficient and that a test procedure which controls hip reaction forces and knee joint angulation may be necessary.

Cesari, Dominique; Bouquet, Robert; Zac, Rene, "A New Pelvis Design for the European Side Impact Dummy," SAE Technical Paper 841650.

During the phase IV of the EEC biomechanical programme, the available side impact dummies were evaluated and this work concluded that none of the dummies were acceptable. The European Experimental Vehicle Committee set up a working group to build a new side impact dummy to be used in a standard side impact test. The ONSER laboratory was in charge of the development of the pelvis. This paper includes the specifications for the pelvis, agreed to by the EEVC working group dealing with this subject, anthropometric analysis to choose sizes and mass distribution, a description of the shape of the pelvic bone, and the location and the type of transducer (force, acceleration). The design of the hip joint and the use of deformable materials to simulate the pelvic bone deformations are discussed. Results of impactor tests using a dummy fitted with this pelvis are analyzed and their results compared to those of cadaver tests conducted previously. The results of these first tests seem promising and have been completed especially to validate repeatability and durability.

Chumlea, W. Cameron, "Growth of the Pelvis in Children," SAE Technical Paper 831663.

Growth and maturation of the pelvis are complex but the process of endochondral ossification in the pelvis is the same as that in the long bones. Primary ossification of the pelvis is completed about 8 years of age, and secondary ossification is completed in the early twenties. Growth of the pelvis follows that of the rest of the body. The most rapid period of growth is in the first year of life. A stable rate of growth is attained after age 3 years until puberty. Basic sex differences in the adult pelvis are established in early childhood. Exterior dimensions of the pelvis are greater in boys, but interior dimensions of the pelvis are greater in girls. Much of the present knowledge about growth and maturation of the pelvis has come from radiographs. More current knowledge of pelvic growth is needed by those involved in automobile restraint design. Pelvic injuries are not uncommon to children in automobile accidents. A child's body is not similar to an adult's, so the results of pelvic injuries may produce life long problems.

DeSantis Klinich, Kathleen; Burton, Ronald W., "Injury Patterns of Older Children in Automotive Accidents," SAE Technical Paper 933082.

A study of injury patterns of older children (aged 6-12 years) indicates that they may deserve more attention from automotive safety researchers. Although older children represent 43.1% of child occupants involved in accidents taken from the National Accident Sampling System (NASS) database, they receive 55.4% of the injuries suffered by children. A lower restraint usage rate (56.2% compared to 63.4% for younger children) partly accounts for this disproportionate amount of injury. However, when restrained, fewer older children remain uninjured compared to younger children (62.8% vs. 70.8%). The number of older children receiving injuries decreases with restraint use (63.6% injured for unrestrained vs. 37.5% injured for restrained). When comparing injuries to restrained and unrestrained older children, the injuries are generally the same severities, but restraints lead to higher proportions of pelvis/abdomen injuries while reducing the occurrence of whole body injuries. Additional analysis of injury patterns for older children when grouped by minor and serious injuries helps to show areas of potential improvement for each class of injury.

Duval-Beaupere, G.; Guezard, B.; Pignolet, F.; Guillon, F.; Tarriere, C., "In VIVO Measurement of Human Weight Supported by the Successive Anatomical Level from C4 to the Femoral Head," SAE Technical Paper 902306.

Biomechanical studies of the spine require data on the weight supported by each body segment studied. The only data available are from post mortem measurements on one old subject. The Barycontremetre, a gamma ray scanner, provides in vivo measurements. Barycentremetre measurements and full spine radiographs with a single reference system, were used to measure the weights of the arms and the remaining body weight supported by each anatomical level of 17 men and 11 women. Their weights are expressed in absolute terms (kg) and as a percentage of the total body weight. The vertebra level of the scapulohumeral joint is also provided. The range of the individual values may justify using of individual values or mean values supplemented by such other anthropometric values as the upper to lower body segment length ratio.

Horsch, John D.; Hering, William E., "A Kinematic Analysis of Lap-Belt Submarining for Test Dummies," SAE Technical Paper 892441.

A kinematic view of the test dummy pelvis "unhooking" from the lap-belt was developed from a series of sled tests. The dynamics of the test resulted in reducing the vertical angle of the lap-belt and rearward rotation of the top of the pelvis. Both of these motions acted to "unhook" the belt from the pelvis. When a "critical" angle between the belt and pelvis was reached, the belt "slipped" from the pelvic spines and directly loaded the abdomen. In these tests, rearward rotation of the pelvis was a predominant mechanism. The study also identified a threshold test severity. At test severities less than the threshold, the dummy did not submarine and at severities greater than the threshold the dummy submarined. The critical pelvis-to-belt slip angle and threshold test severity associated with the pelvis unhooking from the belt are parameters that can enhance assessment of submarining performance beyond a yes/no evaluation.

Hubbard, R. P.; Reynolds, H. M., "Anatomical Geometry and Seating," SAE Technical Paper 840506.

Published and unpublished data on external body configuration and skeletal geometry, were interpreted with an understanding of functional anatomy to provide information on body positions for different size people in automotive seating. Body positions for erect, lumbar-supported postures are presented for small women, average men, and large men, and this posture is compared to the SAE seating design practice. Also, a reclined posture is described. This paper provides some information and insights which are of use in automotive seat design.

Hubbard, Robert P.; Haas, William A.; Boughner, Robert L.; Canole, Richard A.; Bush, Neil J., "New Biomechanical Models for Automobile Seat Design," SAE Technical Paper 930110.

New models are being developed to represent the geometry and movements of people in seated postures. The positions and motions of the torso skeletal structures for different amounts of lumbar curvature have been studied and represented in side view, two dimensional computer models of the average man, small woman, and large man. Some further developments for the average man include: 1) two dimensional, articulated drafting template, 2) three dimensional computer model of the skeletal system with soft tissue thicknesses added to represent the external body contours on the back of the torso, and 3) model of forces and moments between body segments based on seated posture, body segment masses, and seat surface forces. This paper describes these new biomechanical models and their potential uses in designing seats that more comfortably fit and move with people.

Huelke, D. F.; Lawson, T. E., "Lower Torso Injuries and Automobile Seat Belts," SAE Technical Paper 760370.

Injuries to the lower torso (abdomen, pelvis, and lumbar spine) were studied in front seat, lap-belted, outboard occupants involved in frontal crashes. The data indicate that the "no injury" category is increased by 50% in belt users over unbelted occupants. Of injured lap-belted occupants, only one in five was injured in the lower torso area. Of these injuries, 7 out of 10 were rated as minor. Belts reduce the occurrence of serious injuries in all lower torso regions except the lumbar area. The more serious injuries occur at impact speeds of over 30 mph. Only 5% of the injured lap-belted occupants had critical to life-threatening injuries in the lower torso area. The angle of the seat belt does not appear to be related to lower torso injury severity.

Irwin, Annette L.; Pricopio, Linda A.; Mertz, Harold J.; Balser, Joseph S.; Chkoreff, William M., "Comparison of the EUROSID and SID Impact Responses to the Response Corridors of the International Standards Organization," SAE Technical Paper 890604.

Side impact tests were conducted on the EUROSID and SID to assess their biofidelity compared to the response requirements of the International Standards Organization. The body regions evaluated were the head, neck, thorax, shoulder, abdomen and pelvis. Test conditions and data normalization procedures are outlined in the report. Data plots are given which compare the impact response of each dummy to the ISO requirements. The EUROSID gave humanlike responses for most tests involving padded surface impacts, but its responses were not humanlike for rigid surface impacts. Overall, the EUROSID responses were more humanlike than the responses of the SID.

Kallieris, Dimitrios; Mellander, Hugo; Schmidt, George; Barz, Jurgen; Mattern, Rainer, "Comparison Between Frontal Impact Tests with Cadavers and Dummies in a Simulated True Car Restrained Environment," SAE Technical Paper 821170.

A test series of 12 fresh cadavers and 5 Part 572 dummies is reported. The test configuration is frontal impact sled simulation at 30 mph and aims to simulate the restraint environment of a Volvo 240 car. The test occupants are restrained in a 3-point safety belt. The instrumentation of the surrogates involves mainly 12-accelerometers in chest, 9-accelerometers in head and 3-accelerometers in pelvis. Measured values are given and discussed together with the medical findings from the cadaver tests. The occurrence of submarining with cadavers and dummies is reported. A comparison is also made with earlier work where both field accidents and sled simulations of similar violence have been reported. It is concluded that there exist differences in kinematics between the dummy and the cadaver, although peak chest acceleration is similar in both conditions. The lap belt slides over the iliac crest more frequently in the cadaver tests than in the dummy tests. However, no abdominal injuries were found. The pattern of the observed injuries on the cadavers are similar to what has been earlier reported, although the severity is higher than in comparable field accidents.

Kleerekoper, M.; Feldkamp, L. A.; Goldstein, S. A., "The Effect of Aging on the Skeleton -- Implications for Changes in Tolerance," SAE Technical Paper 861926.

The ability of the skeleton to withstand trauma without sustaining a fracture is a function of its inherent strength. Like any other load-bearing structure, this depends on the amount, distribution and quality of the structural elements. Several disease processes can weaken the skeleton but few diseases affect it to the same extent as the normal aging process, which remains the most common cause of diminished skeletal strength, often to the point where spontaneous fractures occur. In this article we will discuss the effects of aging on the amount, distribution and quality of the skeleton in order to examine why trauma is more likely to result in fracture in the elderly.

Lau, Ian V.; Capp, John P.; Obermeyer, James A., "A Comparison of Frontal and Side Impact: Crash Dynamics, Countermeasures and Subsystem Tests," SAE Technical Paper 912896.

Frontal crashes and near-side crashes were compared and found to be significantly different events. In a frontal crash, the energy to be dissipated from the occupant is constant for a given speed. In a side crash, the energy transferred to a struck-side occupant depends highly on his interaction with the door. That difference has important implications on the choice of countermeasures, injury criteria, and subsystem tests. In a front crash, chest and abdominal injuries occur in the "second" impact when the occupant, acting like a free-flight mass, strikes the interior. Padding can absorb some of the free-flight energy, reduce the impact force, and provide earlier and longer contact of the occupant with the interior. The earlier contact decreases the differential velocity of the occupant to the interior, and the longer contact allows more time and greater distance to dissipate the kinetic energy. These improved energy management effects are reflected by lower deflection-based and acceleration-based chest injury criteria in a frontal crash test when padding is added. In a side impact, chest and abdominal injuries occur when the stationary occupant is "punched" by the enroaching door. Padding also provides an earlier and a longer contact of the occupant with the encroaching door, which prolongs the side impact punch. The prolonged punch can actually increase the net energy transferred from the door to the occupant, which may be reflected by higher deflection-based chest injury criteria. Despite the greater energy transfer, padding actually reduces acceleration-based injury critiera, such as TTI(d), in the same side impact crash test. Traditional subsystem tests, such as sled or pendulum tests, can mimic most effects on an occupant of a frontal crash, but they cannot mimic many essential characteristics of a side crash.

Leung, Y. C.; Tarriere, C.; Fayon, A.; Mairesse, P.; Delmas, A.; Banzet, P., "A Comparison Between Part 572 Dummy and Human Subject in the Problem of Submarining," SAE Technical Paper 791026.

Anthropometric data relative to the pelvis have been obtained from X-rays of volunteers and Part 572 dummy, as well as pelvic bones of 28 human skeletons. Consequently, modifications in the pelvic portion of Part 572 dummy are proposed. These are based on the study in the difference of tendency to submarining, the difference of the pelvic shape, and the abdominal flexibility between Part 572 dummy and the human being. Some submarining parameters are discussed using the experimental results. A method for establishing the criteria of abdominal injuries caused by submarining is also described.

Low, Tah Chuan; Prasad, Priya, "Dynamic Response and Mathematical Model of the Side Impact Dummy," SAE Technical Paper 902321.

A series of rigid wall tests have been conducted at three impact velocities to quantify the dynamic response of the side impact dummy (SID) developed by US DOT. This paper reports the chest, pelvis and head responses of the dummy at various filter frequencies and describes the development and verification of the three-dimensional mathematical model of the side impact dummy utilizing the rigid wall test results. The mathematical model uses the mass distribution and the linkage system of the current part 572, hybrid II dummy which forms the basic platform of the SID. The unique chest of the dummy is modeled by two systems of linkages simulating the rib cage and the jacket. Also included in the model is the internal hardware of the chest, e.g. a damper, rib stopper and a clavicle simulator at the upper spin. The material and linkage models are based on static and dynamic tests of the dummy components. Model verification were carried out at component levels by comparing model and dummy certification test results. The final validation of the whole dummy model was conducted by simulating rigid wall and APR padding tests and comparing with test results.

Melvin, John W.; Mohan, Dinesh; Stalnaker, Richard L., "Occupant Injury Assessment Criteria," SAE Technical Paper 750914.

This paper is a brief review of the complex subject of human injury mechanisms and impact tolerance. Automotive accident-related injury patterns are briefly described and the status of knowledge in the biomechanics of trauma of the head, neck, chest, abdomen and extremities is discussed.

Melvin, John W.; Stalnaker, Richard L.; Alem, Nabih M.; Benson, Joseph B.; Mohan, Dinesh, "Impact Response and Tolerance of the Lower Extremities," SAE Technical Paper 751159.

This paper presents the results of direct impact tests and driving point impedance tests on the legs of seated unembalmed human cadavers. Variables studied in the program included impactor energy and impact direction (axial and oblique). Multiple strain gage rosettes were applied to the bone to determine the strain distribution in the bone. The test results indicate that the unembalmed skeletal system of the lower extremities is capable of carrying significantly greater loads than those determined in tests with embalmed subjects (the only similar data reported in the present literature). The strain analysis indicated that significant bending moments are generated in the femur with axial knee impact. The results of the impedance tests are used to characterize the load transmission behavior of the knee-femur-pelvis complex, and the impact test results are combined with this information to produce suggested response characteristics for dummy simulation of knee impact response.

Myklebust, J.; Sances, A.; Maiman, D.; Pintar, F.; Chilbert, M.; Rauschning, W.; Larson, S.; Cusick, J.; Ewing, C.; Thomas, D.; Saltzberg, B., "Experimental Spinal Trauma Studies in the Human and Monkey Cadaver," SAE Technical Paper 831614.

Compression studies were conducted on the ligamentous thoracolumbar spines of fresh human male cadavers. For comparison, forces were applied to the posterior upper thoracic region of intact seated cadavers. Since thoracolumbar flexion injury routinely involves ligament failure and vertebral body wedge compression fractures, studies were conducted on single vertebral bodies and isolated ligaments. Similar studies were conducted in isolated monkey ligaments. The intact and ligamentous thoracolumbar spines failed predominantly in the region of the thoracolumbar junction at forces from 1113-5110 N. For both the human and monkey cadavers, the anterior longitudinal ligament was the strongest. The human ligaments were 2-5 times stronger than those of the monkey.

Pritz, H. B.; Hassler, C. R.; Herridge, J. T.; Weis, E. B., "Experimental Study of Pedestrian Injury Minimization Through Vehicle Design," SAE Technical Paper 751166.

The overall objective of this experimental investigation of pedestrian/vehicle impacts was to conduct representative impacts of unembalmed cadavers in order to (1) pioneer the establishment of impact tolerance levels for the pelvis and legs of a standing pedestrian and (2) explore the ability of a few selected geometry and compliance modifications to the impacting vehicle to increase the impact velocities that can be tolerated. A series of 15 experimental impacts were conducted which covered a speed range from 10 to 30 mph. Dynamic data obtained included high-speed films and time histories of (1) bumper and hood edge forces, (2) horizontal and vertical ground reaction forces, and (3) pelvic acceleration. The resulting injuries were determined from examination of pre- and post-impact X-rays and detailed pathological dissections, and were assessed as to probable temporary total and permanent partial disabilities. Three of the key results are that (1) injuries to the lower body of an adult pedestrian are strongly dependent upon vehicle design, (2) the pedestrian leg injury mechanism is a complex dynamic event influenced significantly by both the bumper force and the ground friction force, and (3) a threshold tolerance value of pelvic acceleration appears to exist below which pelvic injuries do not occur.

Renaudin, F.; Guillemot, H.; Lavaste, F.; Skalli, W.; Lesage, F.; Pecheux, C., "A 3D Finite Element Model of Pelvis in Side Impact," SAE Technical Paper 933130.

A 50th percentile male pelvis finite element model was designed for impact simulation. Shell elements represented the pelvic bone, which geometry was taken into account. Non linear viscous springs accounted for soft tissues connecting skin to bone structure, and body segments inertia around the pelvis were represented using rigid bodies. Geometric and mechanical characteristics were taken either from literature of by identification to in house experimental results. Three dimensional movements were reproduced by the model for static lateral loading and dynamic lateral impact simulation at two different velocities, 3.5 and 6.5 m/s, with a good agreement with experimental results. This model taken into account pelvic bone geometry, allowing an appreciation of its deformation and therefore injury risk.

Robbins, D. H.; Schneider, L. W.; Snyder, R. G.; Pflug, M.; Haffner, Mark, "Seated Posture of Vehicle Occupants," SAE Technical Paper 831617.

This paper describes the methodology and results from a project involving development of anthropometrically based design specifications for a family of advanced adult anthropomorphic dummies. Selection of family members and anthropometric criteria for subject sample selection were based on expected applications of the devices and on an analysis of U.S. population survey data. This resulted in collection of data for dummy sizes including a small female, a mid-sized male, and a large male. The three phases of data collection included: 1. in-vehicle measurements to determine seat track position and seating posture preferred by the subjects for use in development of laboratory seat bucks; 2. measurement of subject/seat interface contours for fabrication of an average hard seat surface for use in the buck; and 3. measurement of standard anthropometry, seated anthropometry (in the buck), and three-dimensional surface landmark coordinates using standard and photogrammetric techniques. Following data collection, activity was concentrated on data analysis and development of specifications. Data for each subject group were averaged for use in development of two reference resources. One is an epoxy/fiberglass standard reference shell positioned in the average hard seat. The other is an anthropometric specification package consisting of full-size drawings detailing estimates of body linkage, mass, and segmentation data. Final results are presented for the mid-sized male population group.

Rouhana, Stephen W.; Jedrzejczak, Edward A.; McCleary, Joseph D., "Assessing Submarining and Abdominal Injury Risk in the Hybrid III Family of Dummies Part II--Development of the Small Female Frangible Abdomen," SAE Technical Paper 902317.

The frangible abdomen is a crushable styrofoam insert for the abdominal region of the hybrid III family of dummies, which has biofidelity, and assesses the occurence of submarining and its risk of injury. It was first developed for the mid-sized male hybrid III dummy. This paper describes the design of the frangible abdomen for the small female hybrid III dummy, and how to use it to assess the occurrence and the risk of injury from submarining. The force-deflection properties of the mid-sized male insert were scaled to the small female dimension using equal stress/equal velocity scaling. Sled tests were run to compare the kinematic and dynamic performance of the baseline small female hybrid III dummy with the same dummy modified to incorporate the frangible abdomen. The kinematic and submarining performance of the small female hybrid III dummy was unchanged by the addition of the frangible abdomen. The frangible abdomen was easy to install and use, and had excellent repeatability. Injury assessment with the frangible abdomen is based on the depth of foam deformation. Tables and graphs are included which relate the risk of injury to the amount of crush. Issues regarding its use, handling, applicability, spinal injury, belt roping, and unilateral submarining are discussed. Appendices containing information on retrofitting existing dummies, calibration testing of styrofoam, and with more detailed tabulations of sled test data are provided.

Rouhana, Stephen W., "Abdominal Injury Prediction in Lateral Impact--An Analysis of the Biofidelity of the Euro-SID Abdomen," SAE Technical Paper 872203.

European safety community has been actively involved in side impact research and has made significant contributions. One of the most recent is the development of the Euro-SID (European Side Impact Dummy) which contains an abdominal injury detection element. This report details an analysis of the dummy abdomen and the cadaver tests upon which it is based.

Schneider, Lawrence W.; Haffner, Mark P.; Eppinger, Rolf H.; Salloum, Michael J.; Beebe, Michael S.; Rouhana, Stephen W.; King, Albert I.; Hardy, Warren H.; Neathery, Raymond F., "Development of an Advanced ATD Thorax System for Improved Injury Assessment in Frontal Crash Environments," SAE Technical Paper 922520.

Injuries to the thorax and abdomen comprise a significant percentage of all occupant injuries in motor vehicle accidents. While the percentage of internal chest injuries is reduced for restrained front-seat occupants in frontal crashes, serious skeletal chest injuries and abdominal injuries can still result from interaction with steering wheels and restraint systems. This paper describes the design and performance of prototype components for the chest, abdomen, spine, and shoulders of the hybrid III dummy that are under development to improve the capability of the hybrid III frontal crash dummy with regard to restraint-system interaction and injury-sensing capability. The new features include a more humanlike ribcage, a flexible thoracic spine, more humanlike shoulders with load-bearing clavicles connected to the sternum and improved front/back range of motion, a biofidelic frangible abdomen, and an enhanced chest-deflection measurement system capable of monitoring three-dimensional displacements of the ribcage at the sternum and at the left and right regions of the lower ribcage.

Shaw, L. M., "Pelvic Response to Lateral Impact--Padded and Unpadded," SAE Technical Paper 890606.

This paper summarizes pelvic side-impact data obtained from a research program conducted for the U.S. National Highway Traffic Safety Administration. The basic objectives of the program were to develop test methodologies for simulating the side-impact environment, to evaluate vehicle side impact injury response and to develop and evaluate the performance of incorporated padding materials. The data presented and evaluated herein represent the results of characterizing the side-impact responses of a modified VW Rabbit vehicle, duplicating those responses on a dual sled test system and conducting parametric test studies varying impact velocity, occupant-to-door spacing (GAP), padding thickness and padding material. Eighteen unpadded and 21 padded tests are presented as well as the full-scale crash characterization test. Comparisons are made between unpadded and padded pelvic peak accelerations under identical conditions to assess the restraint effectiveness for each padding countermeasure.

Stalnaker, Richard L., "Spinal Cord Injuries to Children in Real World Accidents," SAE Technical Paper 933100.

In the last twelve years, the overwhelming effectiveness of restraining children in the United States, Canada and Europe has been proven in reducing death and injury in automobile accidents. Despite the proven benefits of restraining children, one type of injury has not been prevented. This paper is an analysis of stretch injuries to the spinal cord in the upper thoracic or cervical spine. This paper discusses, in general, spinal cord injuries from a biomechanical point of view. The relationship between various loading conditions and the resulting types of spinal cord injuries is discussed. This paper also examines seven real world automobile accidents. Information for each case includes: vehicles involved, type of roadway, crash Delta-V, occupant direction of motion, restraint type, injuries to occupants, and anthropometry of child with spinal cord injury. A description and location of each spinal cord injury that occurred at the time of the accident is discussed. A discussion of a possible injury mechanism for spinal cord stretch injuries to children is also given. The results of this research indicate that infants should ride in rearward-facing child restraint systems as long as possible. It was noted that the crash Delta-V that resulted in serious spinal cord injury is proportional to the child's age. All but one spinal cord injury could have been prevented if the appropriate child restraint system had been used, or if the one that was used had been used properly. Finally, the spinal cord injuries in this study could not have been predicted by shear forces of bending moments at the top of the neck.

Viano, David C., "Biomechanical Responses and Injuries in Blunt Lateral Impact," SAE Technical Paper 892432.

In a recent series of experiments, fourteen unembalmed cadavers were subjected to forty-four blunt lateral impacts at velocities of approximately 4.5, 6.7, or 9.4 m/s with a 15 cm flat 23.4 kg pendulum. Chest and abdominal injuries consisted primarily of rib fractures with a few cases of lung or liver laceration in the highest severity impacts. There were two cases of public ramus fracture in the pelvic impacts. In this study, biomechanical responses from the individual tests were normalized to the 50th percentile adult male by an established procedure. Corridor and average responses were determined for the scaled force-deflection and force-time data at three impact severities. Since serious injury occured primarily in the highest severity tests, the 6.7 and 9.4 m/s normalized response corridors define the key aspects of biofidelity in blunt lateral impact. The EUROSID and SID dummy have responses that are very different from the essential characteristics of the human impact response as determined in this study. The maximum Viscous response had the best correlation with injury risk for chest and abdominal impacts. A tolerance level of VC = 1.5 m/s for the chest and VC = 2.0 m/s for the abdomen was determined for a 25% probability of serious injury. Maximum compression was similarly set at C = 38% for the chest and at C = 44% for the abdomen. Pelvic tolerance to pubic ramus fracture was set at 27% compression, since acceleration of the hip did not correlate with injury.

Viano, David C., "Biomechanical Responses and Injuries in Blunt Lateral Impact," SAE Technical Paper 892432.

In a recent series of experiments, fourteen unembalmed cadavers were subjected to forty-four blunt lateral impacts at velocities of approximately 4.5, 6.7, or 9.4 m/s with a 15 cm flat 23.4 kg pendulum. Chest and abdominal injuries consisted primarily of rib fractures with a few cases of lung or liver laceration in the highest severity impacts. There were two cases of public ramus fracture in the pelvic impacts. In this study, biomechanical responses from the individual tests were normalized to the 50th percentile adult male by an established procedure. Corridor and average responses were determined for the scaled force-deflection and force-time data at three impact severities. Since serious injury occured primarily in the highest severity tests, the 6.7 and 9.4 m/s normalized response corridors define the key aspects of biofidelity in blunt lateral impact. The EUROSID and SID dummy have responses that are very different from the essential characteristics of the human impact response as determined in this study. The maximum Viscous response had the best correlation with injury risk for chest and abdominal impacts. A tolerance level of VC = 1.5 m/s for the chest and VC = 2.0 m/s for the abdomen was determined for a 25% probability of serious injury. Maximum compression was similarly set at C = 38% for the chest and at C = 44% for the abdomen. Pelvic tolerance to pubic ramus fracture was set at 27% compression, since acceleration of the hip did not correlate with injury.

Viano, David C., "Evaluation of the Benefit of Energy-Absorbing Material in Side Impact Protection: Part II," SAE Technical Paper 872213.

This paper refines the methodology presented in the companion paper linking reductions in biomechanical responses due to force-limiting material to projections of injury mitigation in real-world side impact crashes. The revised approach was used to evaluate the potential injury reducing benefit for the chest and abdomen with either constant crush force or constant stiffness, crushable material in the side door and armrest. Using a simulation of the human impact response, a range in crush force or stiffness was determined which reduced the viscous response from that obtained with a rigid impact. NCSS field accident data for car-to-car side impacts provided information on the occupant exposure and injury as a function of the change in velocity (ΔV) of the struck vehicle. Since the velocity of the side door at contact with the occupant's chest is similar to the ΔV of the struck vehicle, the chest impact velocity in the simulation was assumed equal to the observed ΔV in the NCSS data. This related the simulation data to real-world injury data. Reductions in biomechanical response were related to lower injury risk using a sigmoidal injury probability function. This enabled a calculation of a reduction in injured occupants for the velocity range in which the EA material was effective. Reductions of up to 30% in seriously injured occupants may be possible with a low stiffness EA material that is effective in low-speed (ΔV = 4-8 m/s) crashes, whereas either type of padding was ineffective in high-speed crashes (ΔV > 10 m/s). Index Terms: Automobile safety, Energy absorption, Impact tests, Automobile materials, Occupant protection.

Yoganandan, Narayan; Haffner, Mark; Maiman, Dennis J.; Nichols, Hunter; Pintar, Frank A.; Jentzen, Jeffrey; Weinshel, Steven S.; Larson, Sanford J.; Sances, Anthony Jr., "Epidemiology and Injury Biomechanis of Motor Vehicle Related Trauma to the Human Spine," SAE Technical Paper 892438.

Engineering efforts directed at better occupant safety require a thorough understanding of available epidemiologic data. Epidemiologic studies using clinical as well as accident information facilitates the prioritization of biomechanics research so that controlled laboratory experimentation and/or analytical models can be advanced. This information has also value in dictating levels and types of injury that are critical to the development of anthropomorphic test devices used in crash environments. In this paper, motor vehicle accident related (excluding pedestrians, bicyclists, and motorcyclists) epidemiologic data were obtained from clinical and computerized accident (National Accident Sampling System-NASS) files. Clinical data were gathered from patients admitted to the Medical College of Wisconsin Affiliated Hospitals, and fatalities occurring in Milwaukee County, State of Wisconsin. NASS database with specific focus on spinal injuries of motor vehicle occupants was also used.

Rouhana, Stephen W.; Horsch, John D.; Kroell, Charles K., "Assessment of Lap-Shoulder Belt Restraint Performance in Laboratory Testing," SAE Technical Paper 892439.

Hyge sled tests were conducted using a rear-seat sled fixture to evaluate submarining responses (the lap belt of a lap-shoulder belt restraint loads the abdominal region instead of the pelvis). Objectives of these tests included: an evaluation of methods to determine the occurrence of submarining; an investigation into the influence of restraint system parameters, test severity, and type of anthropomorphic test device on submarining response; and an exploration of the mechanics of submarining. This investigation determined that: 1) slippage of the lap belt off the pelvis due to dynamic loading of the dummy and the resulting kinematics can cause abdominal loading to the dummy in laboratory crash testing; 2) the 5th female dummy submarined more easily than did the Hybrid III in the test environment; 3) motion of the pelvis was controlled using a "pelvic stop", which reduced the submarining tendency for both the 5th female and Hybrid III dummies; 4) shortening the buckle strap length (in conjunction with a pelvic stop) increased the submarining "threshold"; 5) modifying the belt restraint by removing the retractor from the lap-belt and adding a retractor to the shoulder belt (with the standard seat) increased the "threshold" severity for submarining; 6) the occurrence of the belt slipping off the pelvis and loading the abdomen was well correlated to rearward rotation of the pelvis; 7) in addition to standard film analysis, detection of the belt slipping off the pelvis is strongly enhanced by use of a submarining indicating pelvis, pelvic in-line accelerometry, and belt force transducers; and 8) the development of a method to unequivocally detect the occurrence of submarining, and to predict the severity of any resulting injury would greatly strengthen the analysis of restraint performance.

Yoganandan, Narayan; Pintar, Frank A.; Skrade, David; Chmiel, Wayne; Reinartz, John M.; Sances, Anthony Jr., "Thoracic Biomechanics with Air Bag Restraint," SAE Technical Paper 933121.

The objective of the present study was to determine the biomechanics of the human thorax in a simulated frontal impact. Fourteen unembalmed human cadavers were subjected to deceleration sled tests at velocities of nine or 13 m/s. Air bag - knee bolster, air bag, - lap belt, and air bag - three-point belt restraint systems were used with the specimen positioned in the driver's seat. Two chest bands were used to derive the deformation patterns at the upper and lower thoracic levels. Lap and shoulder belt forces were recorded with seatbelt transducers. After the test, specimens were evaluated using palpation, radiography, and detailed autopsy. Thoracic trauma was graded according to the Abbreviated Injury Scale based on autopsy findings. Peak thoracic deformations were normalized with respect to the initial chest depth to facilitate comparison between the specimens. Results indicated that under any restraint combination, regional differences exist in the deformation response between the upper and lower thoracic levels. The air bag - knee bolster tests indicated more uniform compressions of the thorax (based on chest band contours), demonstrated greater maximum lower chest deflections, produced fractures in the lower region of the thorax due to steering wheel contact, allowed greater hip and torso excursion and produced significant steering wheel and column loading with permanent deformations. The air bag - lap belt experiments indicated uniform compressions of the thorax (chest band contours), produced minimal fractures, allowed greater torso excursion but less hip excursion, and produced significant steering wheel and column loading with residual deformations. The air bag - three-point belt system tests indicated high localized compressions of the thorax (chest band contours), produced multiple rib fractures consistent with shoulder belt loading, allowed less hip and torso excursion, and produced virtually no steering wheel and column loading. Based on the contours of thoracic deformation, kinematics and injury patterns, the biomechanical response of the human thorax is different between air bag - three point belt loading compared to the air bag - knee bolster/lap belt restraint combination.

RELATED READING

This Appendix is a collection of papers suggested for related reading by the individuals who assisted with the development of PT-47. Due to space constraints, abstracts for these papers were not included.

Barter, James T.; Emanuel, Irvin; Truett, Bruce, "A Statistical Evaluation of Joint Range Data," WADC-TN-57-311, Wright Air Development Center, Wright Patterson AFB, Ohio, 1957.

Bates, T., (1973) "Abdominal Trauma: A Report of 129 Cases," Postgraduate Medical Journal, 49:285-292.

Baxter, C. F.; Williams, R. D., (1961) "Blunt Abdominal Trauma," Journal of Trauma, 1:241-248.

Bondy, N., (1980) "Abdominal Injuries in the National Crash Severity Study," National Center for Statistics and Analysis Collected Technical Studies, Vol. II: Accident data analysis of occupant injuries and crash characteristics, pp. 59-80. National Highway Traffic Safety Administration, Washington, D.C.

Brun-Cassan, F.; Leung, Y. C.; Tarriere, C.; Fayon, A.; Patel, A.; Got, C.; Hureau, J. (1982) "Determination of Knee-Femur-Pelvis Tolerance from the Simulation of Car Frontal Impacts," Proc. 7th International Conference on the Biomechanics of Impacts, pp. 101-115. IRCOBI, Bren, France.

Buchshaum, H. J., (1968) "Accidental Injury Complicating Pregnancy," American Journal of Obstetrics and Gynecology, 102:752-769.

Chance, G. O., (1948) "Note on a Type of Flexion Fracture of the Spine," British Journal of Radiology, 21:452-453.

Crosby, W. M., (1970) "Pathology of Obstetric Injuries in Pregnant Automobile-Accident Victims," Accident Pathology: Proceedings of an International Conference, pp.204-207. U.S. Government Printing Office, Washington, D.C.

Crosby, W. M.; Snyder, R. G.; Snow, C. C.; Hanson, P. G., (1968) "Impact Injuries in Pregnancy I: Experimental Studies," American Journal of Obstetrics and Gynecology, 101:100-110.

Crosby, W. M.; Costiloe, J. P., (1971) "Safety of Lap-Belt Restraint for Pregnant Victims of Automobile Collisions," New England Journal of Medicine, 284(12):632-636.

Eiband, A. M., (1959) "Human Tolerance to Rapidly Applied Accelerations: A Summary of the Literature," NASA Memorandum No. 5-19-59E. NASA Lewis Research Center, Cleveland.

Engin, Ali E.; Shuenn-Muh-Chen, in Technical Report AAMRL-TR-87-O11 under the title: "Human Joint Articulation and Motion-Resistive Properties," July 1987. Department of the Air Force, Armstrong Laboratory, Wright Patterson Air Force Base, 10 February, 1994.

Gallup, B. M.; St-Laurent, A. M.; Newman, J. A., (1982) "Abdominal Injuries to Restrained Front Seat Occupants in Frontal Collisions," Proc. 26th Conference of American Association of Automotive Medicine, pp. 131-148. AAAM, Morton Grove, Illinois.

Glanville, Douglas A.; Kreezer, George, "The Maximum Amplitude and Velocity of Joint Movements in Normal Male Human Adults," Human Biology, Vol. 9, 1937, pp 197-211.

Hakim, N. S.; King, A. I., (1976) "Programmed Replication of In-Situ (Whole-Body) Loading Conditions During In Vitro (Substructure) Testing of a Vertebral Segment," Journal of Biomechanics, 9:629-632.

Kazarian, L. E.; Boyd, D.; von Gierke, H., (1971) "The Dynamic Biomechanical Nature of Spinal Fractures and Articular Facet Derangement," Linear Acceleration of Impact Type, AGARD Conference Proc. No. CP-88-71, pp. 19.1-19.25. Advisory

Group for Aerospace Research and Development, Neuilly Sur Seine, France.

Kazarian, L. E., (1982) "Injuries to the Human Spinal Column: Biomechanical and Injury Classifications," Exercise and Sports Sciences Review, 9:297-352.

King, A. I.; Cheng, R., (1984) "Kinesiology of the Human Shoulder and Spine," Final Report, DOT Contract No. DOT-HS-5-01232. Wayne State University, Detroit, Michigan (in press).

King. A. I., (1984) The Spine: Its Anatomy, Kinematics, Injury Mechanisms and Tolerance to Impact," The Biomechanics of Impact Trauma, pp. 191-226. Edited by A. Chapon and B. Aldman. Elsevier, Amsterdam.

Lau, V. K.; Viano, D. C., (1981) "An Experimental Study of Hepatic Injury from Belt-Restraint Loading," Aviation, Space, and Environmental Medicine, 52:611-617.

Laubach, Lloyd L., "Range of Joint Motion," NASA Reference Publication 1024, Scientific and Technical Information Office, 1978

Mays, E. T., (1966) "Bursting Injuries of the Liver," Archives of Surgery, 93:92-103.

Melvin, J.; Nusholtz, G., (1980) "Tolerance and Response of the Knee-Femur-Pelvis Complex to Axial Impacts," UM-HSRI-80-27. The University of Michigan, Highway Safety Research Institute, Ann Arbor.

Mertz, Harold J., "Hip Flexion Angle with Knee Flexure," SAE Small Female, Large Male, 3- and 6-Year-Old Dummy Task Group. SAE Committee Correspondence, March 25, 1994.

Nyquist, G. W.; and King, A. I., (1984) "Sagittal Plane Static Bending Response of the Torso," Subcontractor Report on DTNH22-83-C-07005. Wayne State University, Detroit, Michigan

Olinde, H. D. H., (1960) "Nonpenetrating Wounds of the Abdomen: A Report of 47 Cases with Review of the Literature," Southern Medical Journal, 53:1270-1282.

Patwardhan, A.; Vanderby, R.; Lorenz, M., (1982) "Load Bearing Characteristics of Lumbar Facets in Axial Compression," 1982 Advances in Bioengineering, pp. 155-160. American Society of Mechanical Engineers, New York.

Pepperell, R. J.; Rubinstein, E.; MacIsacc, I. A., (1977) "Motor-Car Accidents During Pregnancy," Medical Journal of Australia, 1:203-205.

Perry, J. F., Jr., (1965) "A Five-Year Survey of 152 Acute Abdominal Injuries," Journal of Trauma, 5:53-61.

Prasad, P.; King, A. I., (1974) "An Experimentally Validated Dynamic Model of the Spine," Journal of Applied Mechanics, 41:546-550.

Prasad, P.; King, A. I.; and Ewing, C. L., (1974) "The Role of Articular Facets During +Gz Acceleration," Journal of Applied Mechanics, 41:321-326.

Ramet, M.; Cesari, D., (1979) "Experimental Study of Pelvis Tolerance in Lateral Impact," Proc. 4th International Conference on the Biomechanics of Trauma, pp. 243-249. IRCOBI, Bron, France.

SAE J963 Recommended Practice, "Anthropomorphic Test Device for Dynamic Testing," Report of Automotive Safety Committee, 1968.

Snyder, R. G.; Snow, C. C.; Young, J. W.; Price, C. T.; Hanson, P., (1969) "Experimental Comparison of Trauma in Lateral (+Gy), Rearward-Facing (+Gx), and Forward-Facing (-Gx) Body Orientations When Restrained by Lap Belt Only," FAA report no. AM69-13. Federal Aviation Agency, Office of Aviation Medicine, Washington, D.C.

Society of Automotive Engineers, Human Mechanical Response Task Force. (1985) "Human Mechanical Response Characteristics," SAE J1460. Society of Automotive Engineers, Warrendale, Pennsylvania.

Solheim, K., (1963) "Closed Abdominal Injuries," Acta Chirurgica Scandinavica, 126:579-592.

Sonoda, T., (1962) "Studies on the Strength for Compression, Tension, and Torsion of the Human

Vertebral Column," Journal of the Kyoto Prefectural University of Medicine, Medical Society, 71:659-702.

Steindler, Arthur, "Mechanics of the Hip Joint," Kinesiology of the Human Body, Fifth Printing, Charles C. Thomas, Springfield, Illinois, 1977.

Trollope, M. J.; Stalnaker, R. L.; McElhaney, J. H.; Frey, C. F., (1973) "The Mechanism of Injury in Blunt Abdominal Trauma," Journal of Trauma, 13:962-970.

Vulcan, A. P.; King, A. I.; Nakamura, G. S., (1970) "Effects of Bending on the Vertebral Column During +Gzref advance \U 3.0Acceleration," Aerospace Medicine, 41:294-300.

Walfisch, G.; Fayon, A.; Tarriere, C.; Rosey, J. P.; Guillon, F.; Got, C.; Patel, A.; Stalnaker, R. L., (1980) "Designing of a Dummy Abdomen for Detecting Injuries in Side Impact Collisions," Proc. 5th International Conference on the Biomechanics of Impacts, pp. 149-164. IRCOBI, Bron, France.

Walt, A. J.; Grifka, T. J., (1970) "Blunt Abdominal Injury: A Review of 307 Cases," Impact Injury and Crash Protection, pp. 101-124. Edited by E. S. Gurdjian et al. Charles C. Thomas, Springfield, Illinois.

Williams, R. D.; Sargent, F. T., (1963) "The Mechanism of Intestinal Injury in Trauma," Journal of Trauma, 3:288-294.

Williams, J. S.; Kirkpatrick, J. R., (1971) "The Nature of Seat Belt Injuries," Journal of Trauma, 11:207-218.

Willox, G. L., (1965) "Nonpenetrating Injuries of Abdomen Causing Rupture of Spleen: Report of 100 Cases," Archives of Surgery, 90:498-502.

Wilson, D. H., (1963) "Incidence, Aetiology, Diagnosis, and Prognosis of Closed Abdominal Injuries: A Study of 265 Consecutive Cases," British Journal of Surgery, 50:381-389.

Woelfel, G. F.; Moore, E. E.; Cogbill, T. H.; Van Way, C. W., III (1984) "Severe Thoracic and Abdominal Injuries Associated with Lap-Harness Seatbelts," Journal of Trauma, 24:166-167.

Yamada, H., (1970) "Strength of Biological Materials," pp. 75-80. Edited by F.G. Evans. Williams and Wilkins, Baltimore.

Yang, K. H.; King, A. I., (1984) "Mechanism of Facet Load Transmission as a Hypothesis for Low Back Pain," Spine, 9:557-565.